THINK DOCTOR PUBLICATIONS

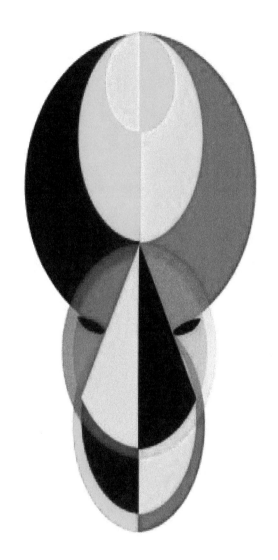

WWW.THINKDOCTORPUBLICATIONS.COM/KEEPBOOKSFREE

THE BRAZILIAN COVID-19 CATASTROPHE

A COLLECTION OF 120 RESEARCH AND OPINION ARTICLES WHICH EXPLORE AND EXPLAIN THE IMPACT OF COVID-19 IN BRAZIL

EDITED BY

DELROY CONSTANTINE-SIMMS

COPYRIGHT PAGE

ABOUT THE EDITOR

Delroy Constantine Simms C.Psychol;. MSc Occupational and Organizational Psychology; BA (Hons) Social Science; BA (Hons) Sociology; BSc (Hons) Psychology; Diploma in Higher Education; PGCert Research Methods, PGCert Coaching PGCert Education; HNC Business Studies & Finance; is a UK registered Counselling Psychologist, and Level A qualified in the use of Ability tests and Level B and B Plus qualified in the use of personality tests and a registered MBTI practitioner. Constantine-Simms has previously taught sociology, psychology, at the Open University; The University of Stirling; Westminster College; and Barnet College. In addition, Constantine-Simms has presented academic papers in Germany, South Africa, The USA, Jamaica, Gambia, and Ethiopia on a variety of psychology related topics. He is also the recipient of the 2001 Lambda Book Award for Best Anthology (The Greatest Taboo: Homosexuality in Black Communities). Constantine-Simms is currently pursuing part-time study at the University of Oxford, while running his book publishing company Think Doctor Publications and other business ventures in the United Arab Emirates.

-
  Rice and Peas For The Soul 1: A collection of 150 Motivational, Inspirational and Moral Stories To make You Think, Reflect and Wonder
- Rice and Peas for the Soul 2
- Rice and Peas For The Soul 3: A Collection of 80 Motivational, Inspirational Stories That Empower, Enthuse and Engage
- Rice and Peas For The Soul 4: A Collection of More Than 45 Motivational, Inspiration and Moving Stories, Which Aim to Stimulate, Stir and Confound.
- Happy To Be Me: A Collection of 50 Poems Reflecting Love Hope and Faith: Volume 1
- Happy To Be Me II: A Collection of 50 Poems Reflecting Love Hope and Faith (Poetry For The Soul Book 2)
- Incidents in the Life of a Slave Girl
- Behind The Scenes
- Fifty Years In Chains: "Includes Interviews With Thirty Former Slaves
- Hearts and Minds: A Resource Book Of 60 Learning Activities To Affirm Diversity and Promote Equality: Volume 1
- Hearts and Minds (Vol. 2): A Resource Book of 30 Learning Activities To Affirm Diversity and Promote Equality.
- Hearts and Minds (Vol. 3): 50 Diversity and Equality Case Studies (Volume 3)
- Changing Hearts and Minds: More Than 90 Training Activities Which Promote Diversity and Equality (Volume 4)
- How To Turn Your I Can't Into I Believe I Can: 30 Excellent Strategies That Will Enable You To Achieve Your True Potential
- Fruit of the Soul 1: A Collection of 30 Stories Which Proves That God's Words Are Not Wasted But Richly Rewarded
- Fruit of the Soul 2: A Collection of 50 Stories of Humility, Compassion and Kindness
-

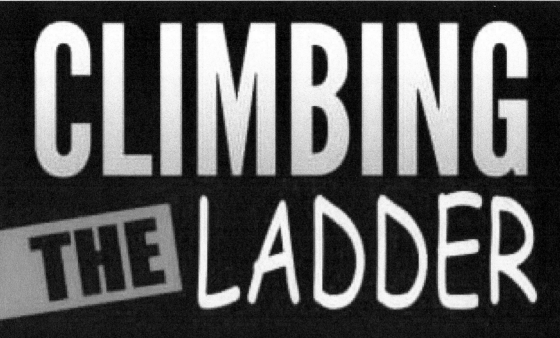

CLIMBING THE LADDER

AN INTRODUCTION TO 15 MENTORING STRATEGIES

DELROY CONSTANTINE-SIMMS

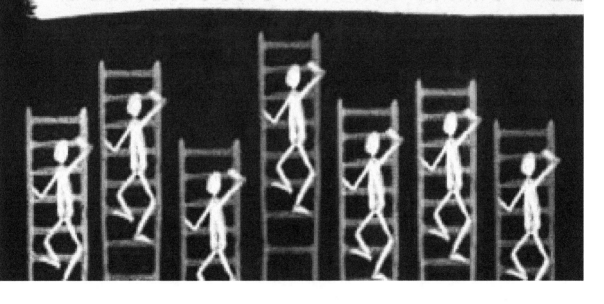

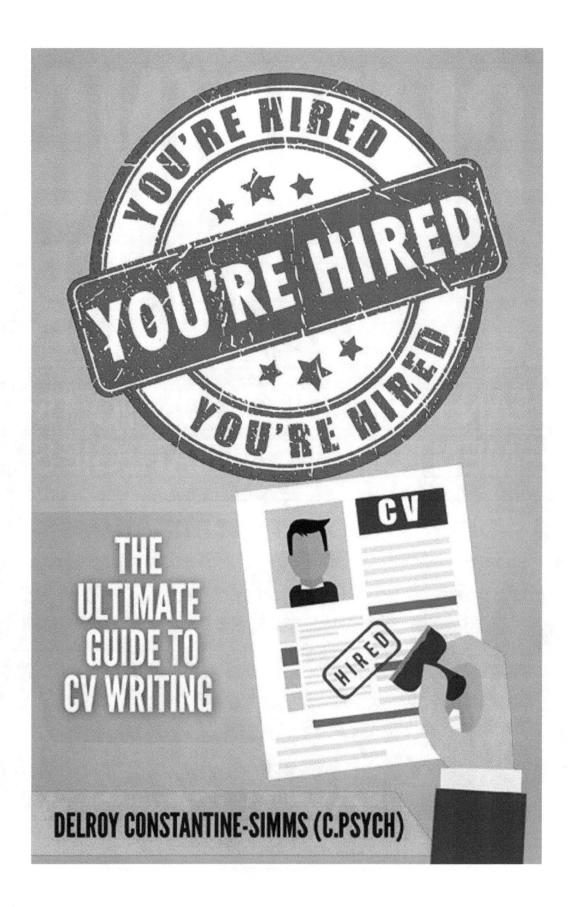

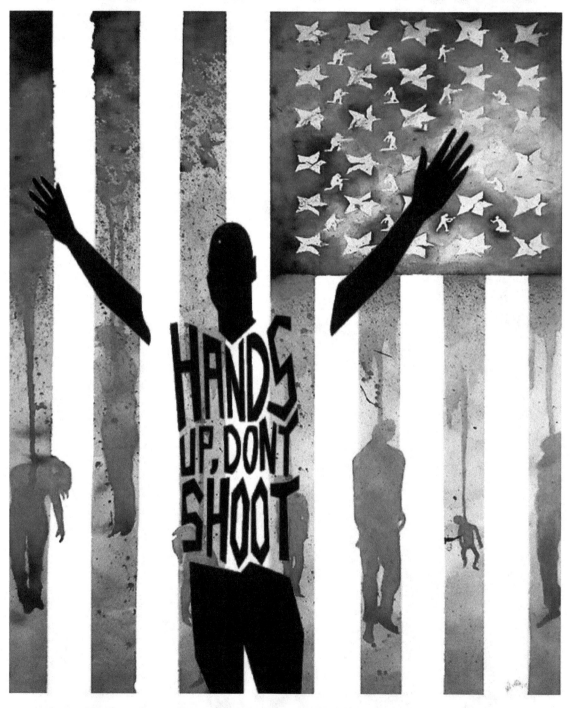

BLACK LIVES MATTER

HANDS UP, DON'T SHOOT

EDITED BY DELROY CONSTANTINE SIMMS

The WILLY LYNCH LETTER

How To Make African-American Slaves For A 1000 Years

(Ed.) Delroy Constantine-Simms

PUBLISHER ACKNOWLEDGMENTS

Cambridge University Press

Oxford University Commons Dream

Elsevier

JAMA Network

Nature Press

PeerJ

PLOS

PubMed Central

Research Gate

REVISTA

Sage Publications

SCIELO

SCILIT

Spring Nature Publishing

SSEN

The British Medical Journal

The Conversation

The Lancet

The Oxford University

Wiley

ACKNOWLEDGMENTS

All HSBCU's

Althea Grant LLB

Angela D. Spence

Angela Davis

Beverley Jones

Christopher Briscoe and extended family

Colin Kaepernick

Collette Empson

Dada Imarogbe

Dale Williams

Dana Belafonte

Dr Colin Sampson

Dr Deborah Gabriel

Dr John Avis

Dr. Gerald Horne

Dr. Helen Deane

Dr. Michael Barnett

Esther Austin

Heath Bailey

Ifeanyichukwu Anthony Ogueji

Heath Town (Wolverhampton)

Ivor Patterson

Rachael and Lemar

Hilda Benette and Family

The Smith Family (Heath Town)

Simms Family (Canada and Jamaica

Reginald Anderson

Rene and Nickell Simpson and Family

Johnson Akintolu

Junia Finn

Karl Finn

Katrina Morris

Marlon Weir

Maud Anderson

Maureen Drackett

Pat Finn

Professor Paul Gilroy

Rashada Balsal-Simms and Family

PREFACE

This comprehensive book is a collection of 120 peer reviewed preprint articles and opinions authored by academics and researchers with a vested interest in the COVID 19 crisis in Brazil. Having read a wide range of material covering the current pandemic, I felt that it was time to contribute to the growing mountain of research information on the COVID-19, in my own right.

I was tempted to join the bandwagon of journalists and academics eager to focus their attentions on the COVID-19 crisis in North America and Europe and Africa. South America was not a consideration. It wasn't until I heard the Brazilian President Jair Bolsonaro, echo Trump like conspiracy theory sentiments, describing the COVID-19 virus as just a little flu. That comment alone, among many others, motivated me to succumb to my journalistic instincts and follow the bandwagon of journalists hoping to explore, explain and offer a wider variety of perspectives regarding the pandemic crisis.

If the truth be said, I really didn't need much motivating to write about the pandemic, my struggle was what to say what had not already been said. After a few weeks of research, I quickly realised that simply writing opinion articles, would not suffice, so I chose the book option instead. I did consider writing a book in my own right, but after assessing the complexity of the issues at hand, I changed direction and opted for the tried and tested book editing route instead.

After reading numerous COVID-19 research abstracts, I soon realised that full research papers were often written in Portuguese or Spanish, I felt this could be an obstacle, but fortunately, I discovered websites with English language versions of COVID-19 Brazilian research material. After screening more than 400 research papers over a five-month period, courtesy of the United Arab Emirates lockdown, I managed to complete this mammoth screening project within twelve weeks.

The selected articles discuss the origin of COVID-19 in Brazil through to the official government response and the economic consequences. As part of the screening process, selected articles were assessed by subject matter specialists, before they were deemed eligible for this book. Academic contributions presented as credible, were excluded for a variety of ethical and methodological reasons. Predictive models while important, were also excluded, the reason being that predictive models are like political polls, they sound good, but rarely present accurate findings.

On the matter of scholarly referencing, numerous contributions were already available as pre-prints or open access documents, hence the diverse use reference and citation conventions within this book. The idea of asking authors to re-edit their work to accommodate a standard referencing style, had crossed my mind, but I decided against making that request, as I knew that most authors would be reluctant to comply. If I was responsible for the initial call for papers, I would have insisted that all contributing authors use the Harvard refencing system, since many haven't, I'm prepared to accept full responsibility for this editing shortcoming. I'm not shunning academic conventions, regarding referencing standards, I'm just being practical, and recognise that editing the references of more than 150 articles, would be an excruciatingly time-consuming process.

I'm confident that book reviewers, will comment on my editorial approach, that's their prerogative, but before they do, I would like to offer them the words of the great South African activist Steve Biko, who said the following, "*I write what I like.* "I would like to state, "*I edit what I like, when I like, however I like*". If this book is adopted by a mainstream publisher, then I'll be more than happy to make the necessary changes, but for now, I'm happy to leave this book as it is while ensuring researchers and academics that the substance and content of this book, reflect the highest academic standards possible.

INTRODUCTION

Brazil is a country of 210 million inhabitants with a third of the country's wealth is in the hands of 1% of the population. Women have an income 41.5% lower than men. There are 12.8 million unemployed, 40 million working as freelancers, or informally, without a regular income.

The tremendous social inequality that marks the country is at the heart of understanding the spread and the destruction produced by COVID 19 in Brazil.

In order to understand parameters of this crisis, readers of this multi-perspective book of more than 160 contributions are initially introduced to the chapter entitled *"The Origin, Transmission And Spread Of COVID-19"* which summarizes how the COVID-19 virus began in China, and eventually Brazil, after the first Brazilian, patient, a 61-year-old businessman tested positive on February 26th, who had recently returned from a trip to Italy. Furthermore, this chapter informs reader, that four days later after he contracted the virus, the press reported an emblematic case of the country's social contrasts, in that a domestic worker who worked in Leblon, a high-class neighbourhood on the south side of Rio de Janeiro, died of COVID-19 after being contaminated by her employer. Consequently, her interaction with friends and family, the disease has expanded from the favelas to the richest areas in many large Brazil.

In order that readers gain a greater appreciation of the varied response to the COVID-19 crisis, the following chapter *"Preparing For The Pandemic Storm"* and *"Failure To Respond And Contain"* enables readers to delineates how the first COVID-19 cases were confirmed in late February 2020, an how President Bolsonaro dismissed COVID-19 interventions that could mitigate the spread of the virus. Unfortunately, Brazil is now paying the price for the lack of integrated coordination in terms of crisis management, such as the slow delivery of test results analysed in public laboratories. Readers are also asked to recognise how and why the absence of central coordination has impacted on Brazil's ability to purchase and distribute respirators and protective equipment, a task that had to be assumed, by local states and counties. Once the Brazilian government managed to organize itself, the procurement process was aggravated by Brazilian diplomatic mistakes which led to delays in the delivery of mechanical respirators.

The chapter *"The Brazilian Health Care Disparities Exposed"* enlightens readers that the first state affected by the lack of hospital beds to treat patients with severe symptoms was Amazona. The situation has been exacerbated by the lack of ventilators, personal protective equipment physicians and health care professionals trained to perform procedures such as intubation. The Amazona situation is an example of the inequity in the distribution of health resources in the current health system consists of public and private assistance, has 7 ICU beds per 100,000 inhabitants for users of the public network and 35 beds per 100,000 inhabitants available to about 25% of the wealthiest population who can afford private plans or insurance, five times more, while explaining that governments solutions to these circumstances vary widely, for example, the state of Maranhão, the governor resorted to an emergency health law to request beds from the private sector, providing financial compensation in the future. In São Paulo, the government rented hospital beds from the private sector.

Perspectives expressed in Chapter *"Brazilian Health Care Disparities Exposed"* and *"Racialized Health in COVID-19 Brazil"* implores readers to recognize health care access reflects long-standing inequalities equality issue in Brazil. Inspired by the British NHS the Brazilian health care system was created to universally treat diseases and promote health, complemented by a network of health care providers. However, 25% of the population with medium and high-income pay for health care plans and insurances which are delivered by an extensive private network of services with excellent hospitals, clinics, and laboratories. The remaining 150 million people who are more likely to be poor black brown or indigenous and favela dwellers who depend on the care provided by a public and universal system, the Sistema Único de Saúde (SUS, Unified Health System), which has long been underfunded. In chapters "**Obesity, Diabetes and Susceptibility to Covid-19**" and "**Converging and Contrasting Age-Related Risks**" begins by informing readers that Brazil has a population that already has high rates of chronic diseases which often affects those with the lowest income. Four out of 10 Brazilian adults have hypertension, diabetes, respiratory diseases, heart disease, and cancer, according to the Instituto Brasileiro de Geografia e Estatística (IBGE, Brazilian Institute of Geography and Statistics). Readers should observe that the long before the current pandemic, chronic diseases were the leading cause of death in Brazil. It's also possible to predict that diseases like COVID-19 would affect the poorest much more severely. The fact that SARS-CoV-2 arrived in Brazil by airplane, through the most privileged class, enabled those in charge of health care, time to tackle the spread of COVID-19 in Brazil, speaks volumes.

Contributions in the chapter "**Preparing For The Pandemic Storm**" and contributions in "**COVID Testing and Diagnostics**" suggests to readers that delays in the preparation and response to the Coronavirus, is because Brazilian health authorities genuinely did not believe that the pandemic would reach Brazil. According to official data, up to May 26th, 2020, the country performed 871,800 tests for the new coronavirus. There were 460,100 reverse transcription polymerase chain reaction (RT-PCR) tests to identify viral RNA performed by public reference laboratories. Another 411.7 thousand tests were performed by the five leading private laboratories in the country (47% of the total). Countries like Italy and Germany have performed millions of tests, and at the time of this publication, China did announce that it had performed 6.6 million tests in the city of Wuhan in 12 days in order to monitor the risk of a second wave of COVID-19, while Brazil's low testing rates have been blamed on a dependence on imports and a lack of national production.

Brazil has been held hostage by the need to import reagents for testing, mechanical ventilators, and personal protective equipment (PPE).At the end of March 2020 for every 1200 tests that arrived daily at the public reference laboratory Instituto Adolfo Lutz, in São Paulo, only 400 results were released. This delay led to a queue of almost 20,000 tests, and a waiting time of 2 weeks or more, thus affecting the entire network of public laboratories in Brazil, forcing different states to seek their own solutions.

Readers are encouraged to dissect the findings expressed in the chapter "**Managing Deaths by Covid-19**" emphasise that Brazil has fast overtaken the countries of Europe to become one of the worst affected globally according to a tally by Johns Hopkins University. In a country of more than 200 million people, many fear the situation could be even worse than the official figures. The underreporting of COVID-19 cases is massive. Researchers have calculated that the actual numbers can be, on average, 7 to 12 times higher than those of the official record. A recent study funded by the federal government and issued on May 25th, brought insightful data in this matter.

Researchers at the Universidade Federal de Pelotas (UPFEI), in Rio Grande do Sul, visited 133 municipalities and collected more than 25,000 blood samples to find out how many people had antibodies against SARS-CoV-2.

The results revealed high rates of infection and underreporting. In the capital city of Recife, in Pernambuco, and the city of Rio de Janeiro, the actual contagion may be 13.4 times greater than the figures reported. In Manaus, up to 20 times. In São Paulo, 11 times. In Breves, on Ilha do Marajó, located in the state of Pará, in northern Brazil, the number of people who had contact with the virus is 87 times higher than the official data reported, platforms such as MonitoraCOVID-19 and the

Observatório COVID-19 Br offer more reliable data, in terms monitoring the true pathway of the COVID-19 disease. The themes discussed in "***Adherence And Resistance To Covid-19 Intervention Strategies***" enables reader to explore and analyse determining factors behind the low adherence of Brazilians and the lack of understanding of the relationship between social isolation and the collapse of the health system and the ambiguous tone of the guidelines. While the then Minister of Health, Dr Luiz Henrique Mandetta, and several governors advocated for measures of protection and social distancing. This chapter concludes by expressing the unfortunate reality, that the number of infected people is growing, while adherence to measures to restrict the spread of COVID-19 appears to be decreasing.

The chapters "***The Efficacy Of Lockdowns***" and "***The Cross Fertilization Of Brazilian***" including "***The Great Coronavirus Denial***" clarifies in varying degrees why President Jair Bolsonaro chose to engage in deadly gamble with COVID-19 by leading anti-lockdown protests by describing COVID-19 as "a little flu". These chapters also describe why Bolsonaro has chosen defies the global consensus on how to tackle the coronavirus pandemic, by leading a movement against science, while defending the immediate use of chloroquine by patients with mild symptoms, despite the lack of evidence. Mental health researchers in "***Evaluating Covid-19 Induced Mental Health Concerns***" argue that pandemics/ epidemics affect physical health and compromises psychosocial integrity, which could result in a high level of psychological suffering and psychosocial maladjustment. This section also asserts that people facing the (COVID-19) outbreak tend to be more susceptible to alterations in physical not necessarily related to clinical symptoms), cognitive, behavioural and emotional aspects.

Worldwide actions against COVID-19 have focused primarily on efforts to contain the acceleration of peak contamination, with questionable success as argued in "***Failure To Respond And Contain***" Perspectives in "***Adherence And Resistance To Covid-19 Intervention Strategies***" explain how people minimises the pandemic by going outdoors without a mask, embraces citizens, while Bolsonaro and his supporter hold public rallies against social distancing, justifies his action lack of adherence COVID-19 intervention and social relationships are discussed in "***Sexual Behaviour in The Midst of The Covid-19***" in Brazilian urban and health policies and their intersections with the sale of sex and the prevention of pandemic disease. This chapter also informs readers as to how the challenges of the COVID-19 pandemic are being met within the context Brazil's organized sex workers in this time of quarantine. Researchers in "***The Cross Fertilization of Brazilian Politics and Covid-19***" continue to debate whether the health crisis has sparked the current political crisis or whether the political crisis has worsened the health problem. This chapter also outlines the growing political polarisation makes it increasingly difficult to control the pandemic, by argues that Bolsonaro harasses governors that have adopted isolation measures, by threatening to restrict the flow of funds to states that do not comply with his anti-isolation and quarantine agenda.

Despite all the pollical games, one thing is clear, Brazil is united in its dismay at the increasing death rates, which certainly guarantee that Brazil is seen as a pariah nation on par with the United States, simply because the leaders of both countries have ignored the science as outlined in the chapter "***The Great Coronavirus Denial***" by engaging in culture wars and most of all placed a higher value on economic over the health of their people. Unfortunately, history will not be kind to either of them or rightly so Furthermore in the chapter ***"How the Pandemic Exacerbates Social Disparities Brazilian"*** contributors outline the invisibility of most vulnerable populations in the eyes of the government. This has translated into the absence of public policies to fight the new coronavirus in the favelas and the outskirts. Thirteen million people are living in high-density populated areas, and in settings that make isolation difficult, often in small spaces shared by numerous people, and without basic sanitation. The lack of assistance and an ever-increasing number of infected people has been the cause of conflicts and demands among slum leaders and public authorities across the Brazil.

In the Palaeopoles favela, in São Paulo, the community hired doctors and ambulances during the pandemic and trained residents as rescuers. In Rio de Janeiro, the network, No's Por Nós Contra o Coronavirus (Us for Us Against Coronavirus), distributed funds, spread information about preventive measures, created brigades to sanitise the favelas, hired doctors, and created its own emergency care network. *The chapter **"Food Supply and Scarcity"*** The impact of the coronavirus crisis on livelihoods and prices has limited access to food in Brazil, particularly for those on lower incomes. Supply chains that fail to cover the "last mile" into poor urban communities are a significant part of the problem, and impressive community initiatives to meet nutritional needs are not enough to bridge that gap.

So far, the issue of food security has been used by the current government mainly for political point-scoring, but there are real steps that it could take to achieve a more resilient, fairer, and healthier food system. Commentators assert in *"**Disaster Looms Large For Indigenous Amazonians**"* that levels of invisibility are such that vulnerable indigenous communities are exposed to the illegal desires of land grabbers and poachers, who are simply taking advantage of a country distracted by the pandemic. As the COVID-19 incidence advances in Brazil the chapter, "***The Economic Future Isn't Bright***", explores how the economic fallout affects different consumer goods and services industries. This comes not long after industries were showing signs of recovery following the country's economic crisis in 2014-2018. Euromonitor International forecasts another year of negative real GDP growth for Brazil in 2020. While we foresee some categories benefiting from spikes in short-term demand, most industries foresee major negative impacts on sales in 2020 and even 2021. This is especially true in services industries, where consumption occasions that did not take place due to the lockdown cannot be made up in future consumption events. Regardless of the industry, however, important common denominators should drive consumer behaviour in Brazil over the next few months

CONTENTS

CHAPTER 1

The Origin, Transmission And Spread of COVID-19..................................1

CHAPTER 2

Preparing For The Pandemic Storm 24

CHAPTER 3

CHAPTER 4

CHAPTER 5

CHAPTER 26

CHAPTER 27

CHAPTER 1

THE ORIGIN, TRANSMISSION AND SPREAD OF COVID-19

1. Routes For COVID-19 Importation in Brazil[1]

Darlan Da S Candido[2], MSc[1], Alexander Watts, PhD [2,3],
Leandro Abade, DPhil [1], Moritz UGKraemer, DPhil [1,4,5], Prof Oliver G Pybus,
DPhil [1,6], Prof Julio Croda, MD, PhD [7,8,9], Wanderson de Oliveira, PhD [7], Kamran
Khan, MD, MPH [2,3], Prof Ester C Sabino, PhD [10], Prof Nuno R Faria, PhD[1,10]

HIGHLIGHT

The global outbreak caused by the severe acute respiratory syndrome coronavirus-2 (SARSCoV-2) has been declared a pandemic by the WHO. As the number of imported SARS-CoV2 cases is on the rise in Brazil, we use incidence and historical air travel data to estimate the most important routes of importation into the country.

INTRODUCTION

Severe acute respiratory syndrome coronavirus-2 (SARS-CoV2) was first detected in Wuhan, Hubei province, China, on December 8th 2019. SARS-CoV-2 infection can cause coronavirus disease (COVID-19) and can lead to acute respiratory syndrome, hospitalization and death. [1]
As of the 12th March 2020, the global SARS-CoV-2 outbreak has been declared a pandemic, with 125,048 cases and 4,613 deaths have been notified by the World Health Organization (WHO)[3] in117countries/territories or areas worldwide The first case in Latin America was confirmed on February 26, 2020, in the São Paulo metropolis, the most populous city in the Southern hemisphere (11 million people Instituto Brasileiro de Geografia e Estatística, www.ibge.gov.br). Self-declared travel history and subsequent genetic analyses confirmed that this infection was acquired via importation of the virus from Northern Italy[2]. Since then Brazil has reported the largest number of cases in Latin America (n=34, as of March 10, 2020). SARS-CoV-2 has been now detected in 7 (26%) of the 27 federal states of Brazil.
So far, transmission of SARS-CoV-2 appears to be primarily sporadic (85.3%, 29/34 are imported cases).Here, we analyse data on airline travellers to Brazil in 2019, who departed from countries that had reported local cases of COVID-19 transmission by March 5th 2020. This information provides insights into which Brazilian cities are most at risk for SARS-CoV-2 importation. We used travel data on all air journeys that had a Brazilian city as their final destination during February and March 2019 as a proxy for flight density during the 2020 COVID-2019 outbreak (see Supplementary Material). We focused on the data for 29 countries that had reported SARS-CoV-2 cases by 5th March 2020. We collated the total number of passengers flying to any Brazilian airport during this period,

---

[1] Epidemiology and Infection, 1-7, doi:10.1017/S0950268818002881 (2018).
[2] Correspondence to Nuno Rodrigues Faria (nuno.faria@zoo.ox.ac.uk)
[3] (who.int/emergencies/diseases/novelcoronavirus-2019/situation-reports).

country population size for 2019 from the United Nations World Population Prospects 2019 database, and the WHO-reported number of COVID-19 cases (as of March 5th, 2020). We used these values to estimate the proportion of infected travellers potentially arriving in Brazilian cities from each country and for each route (additional information can be found in Supplementary Material). No air passenger data from Iran to Brazil was available for our analysis. Between February and March 2019, Brazil received 841,302 international passengers in a total of 84 cities across the country (Figure 1). São Paulo, the largest city in the country, was the final destination of nearly half (46.1%) of the passengers arriving to Brazil, followed by Rio de Janeiro (21%) and Belo Horizonte (4.1%). More than half of the international passengers started they journey in the USA (50.8%) followed by France (7.9%) and Italy (7.5%). The air-travel routes to airports in Brazil with most passengers were USA-São Paulo (23.3%), USA-Rio de Janeiro (9.8%) and Italy-São Paulo (3.4%).

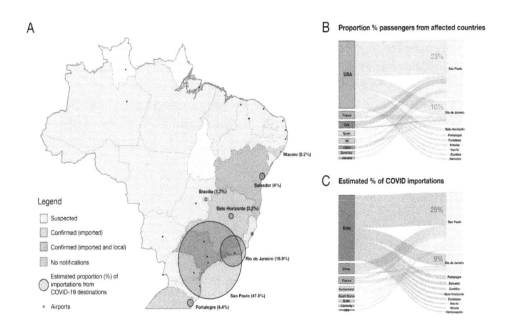

Figure 1. Potential for COVID-19 importation to Brazil. A) Map of Brazilian federal states and Federal District coloured according to COVID-19 notification status (as of March 10, 2020). Circles correspond to the estimated proportion of arrivals from the top 29 destinations (except Iran) that had reported local COVID-19 by 5th March 2020. B) Percentage of passengers for the top-20 routes to Brazilian airports from countries that had reported COVID-19 cases by the 5th March 2020. C) Estimated percentage of importations for the top20 routes from countries that had reported local COVID-19 by the 5th March 2020.To better understand the potential for SARS-CoV-2 introductions to Brazil, we estimate the relative risk of COVID-19 introduction to Brazilian cities by taking into account SARS-CoV2 incidence per international traveller arriving at an airport in Brazil.

We estimate that 54.8% of all imported cases would be expected to come from travellers infected in Italy, 9.3% and 8.3% of the cases would be from travellers infected in China and France, respectively. The route Italy-São Paulo was estimated to comprise 24.9% of total infected travellers travelling to Brazil during this period.

Moreover, we estimate that Italy has been the source location for five of the top 10 most importation routes for infected travellers into Brazil based on the current epidemiological scenario (Supplementary Information). Consistent with this, at least 48% (n=14/29) of the reported imported cases in Brazil have a history of travelling to Italy prior to onset of symptoms, as of 9th March 2020. Six (23.1%) of the confirmed cases that acquired the virus in Italy have been identified in São Paulo (Supplementary Information). We find that the proportion of estimated imported cases by airport of destination is highly correlated with the proportion of detected imported cases. Our study has several limitations. Unfortunately, data from Iran was not available for this analysis. Moreover, our analysis relies on incidence data, and thus the risk of importation will follow changes in epidemic sizes at source locations. In fact, with the reduction in the number of flights leaving from Italy and 51% of flights to Brazil depart from airports in the USA, we should anticipate for an increasing proportion of infected travellers arriving from the USA. Moreover, the estimated risk of importation from China is likely an overestimate as recent measures have extensively decreased the flights to Brazil.

At a time when the number of SARS-CoV-2 cases are steadily growing in Brazil, our findings highlight the high potential for the introduction of new cases in several cities of Brazil, especially in Sao Paulo and Rio de Janeiro metropolises. Rapid identification of locations where clusters of local transmission might first ignite is critical to better coordinate preparedness, readiness and response actions.[3,4] There is critical need for epidemiological, human mobility and genetic data[5] to understand virus transmission dynamics at local, regional and global scales. Continued integration of these data streams should help guide deployment of resources to mitigate COVID-19 transmission.

Authors Affiliation

1. Department of Zoology, University of Oxford, United Kingdom.
2. Li Ka Shing Knowledge Institute, St. Michael's Hospital, Toronto, Canada.
3. Department of Medicine, Division of Infectious Diseases, University of Toronto, Canada.
4. Harvard Medical School, Harvard University, Boston, United States.
5. Computational Epidemiology Group, Boston Children's Hospital, Boston, United States.
6. Department of Pathobiology and Population Sciences, The Royal Veterinary College, London, United Kingdom.
7. Secretaria de Vigilância em Saúde, Coordenação Geral de Laboratórios de Saúde Pública, Ministério da Saúde, Brasília-DF, Brazil.
8. Laboratório de Pesquisa em Ciências da Saúde, Universidade Federal da Grande Dourados, Dourados, Mato Grosso do Sul, Brazil.
9. Fundação Osvaldo Cruz Campo Grande, Mato Grosso do Sul, Brazil.
10. Instituto Medicina Tropical, University of São Paulo, Brazil.

Funding

This work was supported by a Medical Research Council and Fundação de Amparo à

Pesquisa do Estado de São Paulo CADDE partnership award (MR/S0195/1) and a John Fell Research Fund (grant 005166). NRF is supported by a Sir Henry Dale Fellowship (204311/Z/16/Z). DDSC is supported by the Clarendon Fund and by the Oxford University Zoology Department. This work was supported by a Medical Research Council and FAPESP CADDE partnership award (MR/S0195/1) and a John Fell Research Fund (grant 005166). NRF is supported by a Sir Henry Dale Fellowship (204311/Z/16/Z). DDSC is supported by the Clarendon Fund and by the Oxford University Zoology Department.

REFERENCES

1. Zhu, N. *et al.* (2020). A Novel Coronavirus from Patients with Pneumonia in China, 2019. *The New England Journal of Medicine* **382**, 727-733, doi:10.1056/NEJMoa2001017 (2020).
2. de Jesus JG *et al.* (2020). First cases of coronavirus disease (COVID-19) in Brazil, South America (2 genomes, 3rd March 2020) (http://virological.org/t/first-cases-ofcoronavirus-disease-covid-19-in-brazil-south-america-2-genomes-3rd-march2020/409, Virological, 2020).
3. Ministério da Saúde, B(2020).. Brasil amplia monitoramento do coronavírus.(2020). WHO. Critical preparedness, readiness and response actions for COVID-19. (Technical Guidance 2020, https://www.who.int/emergencies/diseases/novelcoronavirus-2019/technical-guidance/critical-preparedness-readiness-and-responseactions-for-covid-19).
4. Kraemer, M. U. G. *et al.* (2020) Reconstruction and prediction of viral disease epidemics.

2. Importation and Early Local Transmission of COVID-19 In Brazil, 2020

Jaqueline Goes de Jesus[1*]Claudio Sacchi[2*]Darlan da Silva Candido[3*]Ingra Morales Claro[1]Flávia Cristina Silva Sales[1] Erika Regina Manuli[1] Daniela Bernardes Borges da Silva[4]Terezinha Maria de Paiva[4] Margarete Aparecida Benega Pinho[4] Katia Correa de Oliveira Santos[4]Sarah Catherine Hill[3] Renato Santana Aguiar[5] Filipe Romero[5] Fabiana Cristina Pereira dos Santos[4] Claudia Regina Gonçalves[2]Maria do Carmo Timenetsky[4]Joshua Quick[6]Julio Henrique Rosa Croda[789]Wanderson de Oliveira[7] Andrew Rambaut[10] Oliver G. Pybus[3] Nicholas J. Loman[6] Ester Cerdeira Sabino[1*]Nuno Rodrigues Faria[1311*]

ABSTRACT

We conducted the genome sequencing and analysis of the first confirmed COVID-19 infections in Brazil. Rapid sequencing coupled with phylogenetic analyses in the context of travel history corroborate multiple independent importations from Italy and local spread during the initial stage of COVID-19 transmission in Brazil.

INTRODUCTION

The severe acute respiratory syndrome 2 (SARS-CoV-2) was first identified in Wuhan, Central China, in early December 2019, and reported to the World Health Organization (WHO) country office in China on December 31, 2019[1]. SARS-CoV-2 infection causes coronavirus-associated acute respiratory disease in humans, a disease named corona virus disease 19 (COVID-19)[2]. COVID-19 is the third documented spill over of a coronavirus from an animal reservoir to humans in the last two decades to have caused a serious public health threat[3]. On January 30, 2020, COVID-19 was declared a Public Health Emergency of International Concern. On March 16, 2020, WHO reported 153,517 confirmed cases across the globe, and 5,735 confirmed deaths in 143 countries, territories or areas. Within Latin America, Brazil is the country with the largest number of confirmed cases. The country has reported 234 cases across 15 federal States; Sao Paulo, Rio de Janeiro and Bahia States have confirmed local transmission[4].

During the early stages of an epidemic disease, molecular surveillance can inform on the tracking and control of the virus spread across the global and at local scales. Moreover, viral genomes can help to design effective molecular diagnostics, improve vaccine design and complement the contact tracking[5,6]. However, the resolution of the transmission networks reconstructed from genetic data will depend on the rate at which genetic changes accumulate across viral genomes. Within outbreaks, short timescales mean that not all the observed changes will become fixed at the population level[7].

To investigate the early transmission dynamics of imported and local cases in Brazil, we set up a genomic observatory in Sao Paulo where we sequenced and analysed two complete SARS-CoV-2 genomes in less than 48 h after the cases confirmation. Here we investigate the transmission patterns from phylogenetic analysis of the earliest six SARS-CoV-2 cases in Brazil.

MATERIALS AND METHODS

Samples from suspected SARS-CoV-2 cases underwent confirmatory diagnostic real-time RT-PCR testing[8] at the Instituto Adolfo Lutz (IAL), the regional reference laboratory for SARS-CoV-2 detection in Sao Paulo State, Southeast Brazil. Samples obtained from the Reference Centre for Arbovirus of Sao Paulo, Adolfo Lutz Institute (IAL) have been processed in agreement with routine surveillance activities from the Brazilian Ministry of Health.

We used the open COVID-19 sequencing available and the bioinformatics protocols developed by the ARTIC network. Sequencing protocols, multiplex PCR primers, and bioinformatic pipelines are described in detail at https://artic.network/ncov-2019. In brief, cDNA synthesis was conducted in duplicate for each sample and the concentration of PCR products was measured using a Qubit dsDNA High Sensitivity kit on a Qubit 3.0 fluorometer. [1] Library preparation was conducted without a barcoding step and libraries were sequenced on an R9.4.1 flow cell using MinKNOW[2] version 19.10.1 for over 12 h. The open-source software RAMPART version 10.5 was used to assign and map reads in real-time. Raw files were base-called with Guppy, demultiplexed and trimmed with Porechop [3]and mapped against reference sequence Wuhan-Hu-1 (GenBank Accession Number MN908947). Variants were called using nanopolish 0.11.3. Low coverage regions were masked with N characters. Coverage for the SPBR1 and SPBR2 was 96.9 and 99.6%, with 552730 and 3461754 mapped reads, respectively (Table S1)[4].

We investigated the transmission dynamics of the early COVID-19 cases in Brazil (SPBR1 to SPBR6) by analysing genetic changes among the early genomes from Brazil belonging to imported and local cases, and by estimating a maximum likelihood phylogenetic tree together with a set of global reference sequences. We added the SBPBR1 and SPBR2 consensus sequences from Sao Paulo to a curated dataset of complete genomes available from GISAID that included four additional sequences from Brazil (available on GISAID of 15th March 2020). A multiple sequence alignment comprising 347 complete genomes from several countries was generated using MAFFT[9] and manually edited. A maximum likelihood (ML) phylogenetic tree was estimated using PhyML version 3.0[10] using a Hasegawa-Kishino-Yano nucleotide substitution model with a gamma-distributed rate variation across sites.

---

[1] (Thermo Fisher Scientific, Waltham, USA).
[2] (Oxford Nanopore Technologies, Oxford, UK)
[3] (https://github.com/rrwick/Porechop)
[4] https://cadde.s3.climb.ac.uk/covid-19/BR1.sorted.bam.

RESULTS

Four of the six patients self-reported travelling from European countries to Sao Paulo city (SPBR1 to SPBR4) (Table S1). Two patients (SPBR5 and SPBR6) reported direct contact with SPBR1 and no travel outside Brazil. Patient SPBR1 (60-65-year-old male) self-reported arriving from Italy on the February 21, 2020he started symptoms on the February 24 and tested positive two days later. Patients SPBR5 and SPBR6 were in direct contact with patient SPBR1 on February 22 and tested positive on February 29, 2020. Figure 1 shows the clade containing Brazilian sequences along with location of infection (squares) and reporting (circles). Our analyses show that the SPBR1 genome is identical to the SPBR5 and SPBR6 contacts (illustrated by zero branch lengths in Figure 1; detailed tree with annotated tips and travel history information for the clade containing Brazilian sequences can be found in the Figure S1).

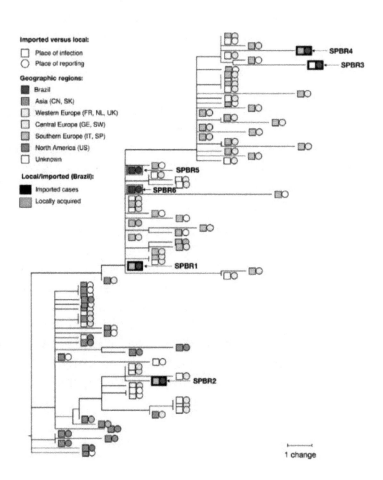

Figure 1 Maximum likelihood phylogeny (n=88) including Brazilian SARS-CoV-2 genomes from the first confirmed cases in Brazil. Squares and circles are coloured according to the place of infection and the place of reporting, respectively. Local cases are highlighted with a grey background, imported cases are highlighted with a black background. A full tree (n=347) can be found in the Supplementary Material (Figure S1).

We found that the SPBR1, SPBR5 and SPBR6 are identical to several other genomes circulating in Italy and elsewhere collected between February 20 and March 2, 2020. The lack of changes among SARS-CoV-2 genomes collected during this period is not surprising given the evolutionary rate of the virus that results in an average of 1 to 2 mutations per month[11]. These data highlight the critical importance of contextualizing phylogenetic information with travel history when investigating early transmission dynamics of SARS-CoV-2. As no epidemiological information was available for SPBR5 and SPBR6, one could not exclude an alternative scenario based on sequencing data alone that would suggest additional independent introductions from Italy or elsewhere. Patients SPBR2, SPBR3 and SPBR4 all reported travelling to Italy, where the of incidence of COVID-19 has been the highest outside Wuhan in China[12]. Consistent with the travel history, sequences from these patients are found interspersed in the tree in agreement with the multiple independent introductions of SARS-CoV-2 to Sao Paulo from Italy. This finding highlights the key role of human mobility in the early stages of the pandemic and is in line with a recent analysis on the risk of importation of COVID-19 based on the history of air traveling data and the incidence data[13]. Given that the air traveling to Brazil from Italy has reduced, it is possible that the proportion of SARS-CoV-2 imported cases from other countries, particularly the USA, may increase[13].

DISCUSSION

Our study provides a snapshot of the early establishment of the COVID-19 pandemic in Brazil, characterized by multiple independent introductions from Italy, followed by local transmission of the virus in Sao Paulo. Phylogenetic analyses are broadly consistent with the patients' self-reported traveling histories. We show that the two genomes associated with local transmission are linked to a patient infected in Italy and are identical to other Italian genomes collected in the same time window. Given the within-outbreak rate of evolutionary change estimated for SARS-CoV-2[11], we caution against inferring directionality of transmission based on genetic data alone. Such inferences can further be overshadowed by incomplete sampling due to delays, reflecting the lack of equitable access to diagnosis and genomic sequencing.

CONCLUSION

Given the findings of the present study, we conclude that phylogenetic data from the pandemic needs to be contextualized with appropriate metadata, including basic demographics, symptoms onset date, the sample collection date, the country of reporting and the self-reported travel history. Joint epidemiological and genomic surveillance of COVID-19 cases will be critical to rapidly identify possible clusters of local transmission in Brazil and in other countries, and to better understand and help mitigating the transmission in the community.

ACKNOWLEDGMENTS

We thank GISAID database for supporting rapid and open access real-time SARS-CoV-2 genomic data sharing. We would like to thank the authors who generated and shared data with the research community and all the patients involved, the staff and research groups who assisted with patient care, sample collection, genome sequencing and data sharing. We thank Josh Quick, Lucy Matkin and Julien Thezé for support.

AFFILIATIONS

[1]Universidade de São Paulo, Instituto de Medicina Tropical de São Paulo, São Paulo, São Paulo, Brazil
[2]Instituto Adolfo Lutz, Laboratório Estratégico, São Paulo, São Paulo, Brazil
[3]University of Oxford, Department of Zoology, Oxford, United Kingdom
[4]Instituto Adolfo Lutz, Centro de Virologia, São Paulo, São Paulo, Brazil
[5]Universidade Federal do Rio de Janeiro, Rio de Janeiro, Rio de Janeiro, Brazil
[6]University of Birmingham, Birmingham, United Kingdom
[7]Ministério da Saúde, Secretaria de Vigilância em Saúde, Coordenação Geral de Laboratórios de Saúde Pública, Brasília, DF, Brazil
[8]Universidade Federal da Grande Dourados, Laboratório de Pesquisa em Ciências da Saúde, Dourados, Mato Grosso do Sul, Brazil
[9]Fundação Osvaldo Cruz Campo Grande, Mato Grosso do Sul, Brazil
[10]University of Edinburgh, Institute of Evolutionary Biology, Edinburgh, United Kingdom
[11]Imperial College, School of Public Health, Department of Infectious Disease Epidemiology, London, United Kingdom

REFERENCES

1. World Health Organization. Critical preparedness, readiness and response actions for COVID-19. [cited 2020 Apr 22]. Available from: https://www.who.int/publications-detail/critical-preparedness-readiness-and-response-actions-for-COVID-19 [Links]

2. Coronaviridae Study Group of the International Committee on Taxonomy of Viruses. The species severe acute respiratory syndrome-related coronavirus: classifying 2019-nCoV and naming it SARS-CoV-2. Nat Microbiol. 2020 In Press. [Links]

3. Andersen KG, Rambaut A, Lipkin WI, Holmes EC, Garry RF. The proximal origin of SARS-CoV-2. Nat Med. 2020;26:450-2. [Links]

4. Brasil. Ministério da Saúde. Notificação de casos de doença pelo coronavírus 2019 (COVID-19). [cited 2020 March 15]; Available from: https://www.saude.go.gov.br/component/content/article/34-page/9895-coronav%C3%ADrus.html? highlight=WyJjb3JvbmF2XHUwMGVkcnVzIl0=&Itemid=101 [Links]

5. Park DJ, Dudas G, Wohl S, Goba A, Whitmer SL, Andersen KG, et al. Ebola virus epidemiology, transmission, and evolution during seven nonths in Sierra Leone. Cell. 2015;161:1516-26. [Links]

6. Gire SK, Goba A, Andersen KG, Sealfon RS, Park DJ, Kanneh L, et al. Genomic surveillance elucidates Ebola virus origin and transmission during the 2014 outbreak. Science. 2014;345:1369-72. [Links]

7. Holmes EC, Dudas G, Rambaut A, Andersen KG. The evolution of Ebola virus: insights from the 2013-2016 epidemic. Nature. 2016;538:193-200. [Links]

8. Corman VM, Landt O, Kaiser M, Molenkamp R, Meijer A, Chu DK, et al. Detection of 2019 novel coronavirus (2019-nCoV) by real-time RT-PCR. Euro Surveill. 2020;25:2000045. [Links]

9. Katoh K, Standley DM. MAFFT: iterative refinement and additional methods. In: Russel DJ, editor. Multiple sequence alignment methods. New York: Humana; 2014. p.131-46. [Links]

10. Guindon S, Dufayard JF, Lefort V, Anisimova M, Hordijk W, Gascuel O. New algorithms and methods to estimate maximum-likelihood phylogenies: assessing the performance of PhyML 3.0. Syst Biol. 2010;59:307-21. [Links]

11. Rambaut A. Phylogenetic analysis of nCoV-2019 genomes. [cited 2020 Apr 22]. Available from: http://virological.org/t/phylogenetic-analysis-of-23-ncov-2019-genomes-2020-01-23/335 [Links]

12. World Health Organization. Coronavirus disease (COVID-2019) situation reports. [cited 2020 Apr 22]. Available from: https://www.who.int/emergencies/diseases/novel-coronavirus-2019/situation-reports [Links]

13. Candido DS, Watts A, Abade L, Kraemer MU, Pybus OG, Croda J, et al. Routes for COVID-19 importation in Brazil. J Travel Med. 2020 In press. [Links]

FUNDING:

This work was supported by a Medical Research Council and FAPESP CADDE partnership award (MR/S0195/1), FAPESP grant Nº 2018/14389-0, and a John Fell Research Fund (grant Nº 005166). NRF is supported by a Wellcome Trust and Royal Society Sir Henry Dale Fellowship (204311/Z/16/Z). DDSC is supported by the Clarendon Fund and by the Oxford University Zoology Department.

SUPPLEMENTARY MATERIAL

Table S1 Sequencing statistics for the Brazilian SARS-COV-2 genomes from this study.

Isolate	Mapped Reads	Average depth coverage	Bases covered >10x	Bases covered >25x	Reference covered (%)
SPBR1	552730	3622.14	29426	29106	96.8966
SPBR2	3461754	5117.28	29849	29845	99.5954

We gratefully acknowledge the authors, originating and submitting laboratories of the sequences from GISAID's EpiFlu™ Database on which this research is based. The list is detailed on Supplementary Table 2, which is available on GitHub (https://github.com/CADDE-CENTRE/REPOSITORY/blob/master/First%20genomes%20from%20Americas.docx). All submitters of data may be contacted directly via www.gisaid.org.

3. Implications of The First Confirmed Case In Brazil

Alfonso J. Rodriguez-Morales* Viviana Gallego,Juan Pablo Escalera-Antezana,Claudio A. Méndez,Lysien I. Zambrano,Carlos Franco-Paredes,Jose A. Suárez,Hernan D. Rodriguez-Enciso,Graciela Josefina Balbin-Ramon,Eduardo Savio-Larriera,Alejandro Risquez,Sergio Cimerman,

The spread of the Coronavirus Disease 2019 (COVID-19), caused by the Severe Acute Respiratory Syndrome Coronavirus 2 (SARS-CoV-2) [1], has been steady in Asia and other regions in the world. Latin America was an exception until February 25, 2020, when the Brazilian Ministry of Health, confirmed the first case.

This first case was a Brazilian man, 61 years-old, who travelled from February 9 to 20, 2020, to Lombardy, northern Italy, where a significant outbreak is ongoing. He arrived home on February 21, 2020 and was attended at the Hospital Albert Einstein in São Paulo, Brazil. At this institution, an initial real-time RT-PCR was positive for SARS-CoV-2 and then confirmed by the National Reference Laboratory at the Instituto Adolfo Lutz using the real-time RT-PCR protocol developed by the Institute of Virology at Charité in Berlin, Germany [2].

The established protocol also included now, as part of the Sao Paulo State Health Secretary, metagenomics and immunohistochemistry with PCR, as part of the response plan to COVID-19 outbreak in the city [3]. The patient presented with fever, dry cough, sore throat, and coryza. So far, as of February 27, the patient is well, with mild signs. He received standard precautionary care, and in the meantime, he is isolated at home [4]. Local health authorities are carrying out the identification and tracing of contacts at home, at the hospital, and on the flight. For now, other cases are under investigation in São Paulo, and other cities in Latin America. In addition to the São Paulo State Health Secretary, the Brazilian Society for Infectious Diseases have developed technical recommendations [4].

This is the first case of COVID-19 in the South American region with a population of over 640 million people [5] who have also experienced significant outbreaks of infections which were declared *Public Health Emergencies of International Concern* (PHIC), by the World Health Organization (WHO). So, it was with Zika in 2016. The Zika outbreak also began in Brazil [6]. In the current scenario, the spread of COVID-19 to other neighbouring countries is expected and is probably inevitable in the light of the arrival of suspected cases from Italy, China, and other significantly affected countries. São Paulo is the most populated city in South America, with more than 23 million people and high flight connectivity in the region (Fig. 1). Its main airport, the São Paulo-Guarulhos International Airport, is the largest in Brazil, with non-stop passenger flights scheduled to 103 destinations in 30 countries, and 52 domestic flights, connecting not only with major cities in Latin America but also with direct flights to North America, Europe, Africa and the Middle East (Dubai). There are also buses that offer a service to and from the metropolitan centres of Paraguay, Argentina, Uruguay and Bolivia. Brazil also connects with the countries of Chile, Argentina and Bolivia through some rail connections. The main seaport of Brazil is in Rio de Janeiro, where many international cruises also arrive. Thus, over the course of the next few days, a significant expansion in the region would be possible.

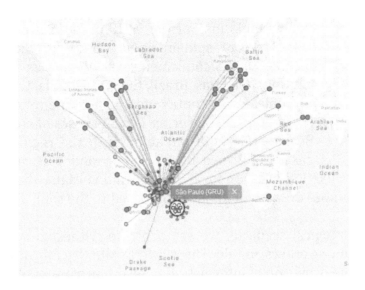

**Fig. 1:Flight connections from São Paulo's main international airport, Brazil.
Source: flightconnections.com.**

The healthcare systems in this region are already fragile [7]. Moreover, fragmentation and segmentation are ongoing challenges for most of these vulnerable systems. Multiple social and economic issues are ongoing and will impact the situation, including the massive exodus from Venezuela to many countries in the region. This human migration is associated with other infectious diseases, such as malaria or measles [8]. The burden that will be imposed on the region, if and when COVID-19 spreads, would be an additional challenge for the healthcare systems and economies in the region, as we faced with Zika and even the Chikungunya outbreaks [9]. For example, there is concern about the availability of intensive care units, that are necessary for at least 20–25% of patients hospitalized with COVID-19—also, the availability of specific diagnostic tests, particularly the real-time RT-PCR is a crucial challenge for early detection of COVID-19 importation and prevention of onward transmission. Even maybe in some countries, cases have been not diagnosed due to lack of availability of specific tests. Are Latin American healthcare systems sufficiently prepared? Probably not, but in general, this is the same in other regions of the world, such as in many parts of Asia and Africa [10]. Although most countries in Latin America are trying to step up their preparedness to detect and cope with COVID-19 outbreaks, it will be essential to intensify inter-continental and intra-continental, communication and health workforce training.

In the Latin American region, there is a large heterogeneity of political and social development, economic growth, and political capacities. For example, in the Caribbean subregion, countries such as Haiti have a low Human Development Index. In such areas, and Venezuela where a humanitarian crisis had occurred since 2019 spreading measles, diphtheria, and vector-borne diseases, such as malaria, over the region [[11], [12], [13]], the impact of a COVID-19 outbreak will be more devastating than in the more developed economies, such as Brazil or Mexico. Most of the countries in the region are remembering the lessons learned during SARS (2003) and pandemic influenza (2009). Protocols already developed during those crises, including laboratory and patient management, may prove useful in this new situation. Good communication strategies for preventive measures in the population, and in neighbouring countries in addition to Brazil, will be essential and this response should be aligned with the recommendations of the WHO.In Latin America, the Pan-American Health Organization (PAHO/WHO) recent epidemiological alert for measles shows that from January 1, 2019 to January 24, 2020, 20,430 confirmed cases of measles were reported, including 19 deaths, in 14 countries: Argentina, Bahamas, Brazil, Chile, Colombia, Costa Rica, Cuba, Curaçao, Mexico, Peru, Uruguay and Venezuela. Brazil contributed 88% of the total confirmed cases in the Americas [14]. In the first 4 weeks of 2020, a staggering 125,514 cases of measles were notified. The dengue incidence rate is 12.86 cases/100,000 inhabitants in the region for the ongoing year, including 27 deaths, 12,891 cases confirmed by laboratory and 498 cases classified as severe dengue (0.4%). Countries like Bolivia, Honduras, Mexico and Paraguay have reported an increase of double or triple the number of cases of dengue compared to the same period from the previous year [15].

In this complex epidemiological scenario, we are about to witness a syndemic [16] of measles, dengue, and COVID-19, among others, unfold. The World Health Organization (WHO) has published guidelines encouraging the provision of information to health professionals and the general public. Resources, intensified surveillance, and capacity building should be urgently prioritized in countries with a moderate risk that might be ill-prepared to detect imported cases and to limit onward transmission, as has already occurred in Brazil. [For the moment of proofs correction of this Editorial –Mar. 1, 2020–, 2 cases have been confirmed in Brazil, but also new 5 confirmed cases were also reported in Mexico (2° country that reported cases), 6 in Ecuador (3°) and 1 in Dominican Republic (4°), summarizing 14 cases in Latin America].

REFERENCES

1. Rodriguez-Morales A.J., MacGregor K., Kanagarajah S., Patel D., Schlagenhauf P. Going global - travel and the 2019 novel coronavirus. Trav Med Infect Dis. 2020;33:101578. [PMC free article] [PubMed] [Google Scholar]
2. ProMEDmail . vol. 2020. 2020. (PRO/PORT> Novo coronavírus, COVID-19 - brasil (11) (SP, ex-Itália), primeiro caso provável ProMEDmail). 20200225.27026525. [Google Scholar]
3. Sao Paulo State Health Secretary . 2020. Plan of response of the Sao Paulo state for the human infection due to novel Coronavirus - 2019nCoV. [Google Scholar]
4. da Cunha C.A., Cimerman S., Weissmann L., Chebabo A., Bellei N.C.J. Sociedade Brasileira de Infectologia; Sao Paulo, Brasil: 2020. Informativo da Sociedade Brasileira de Infectologia: primeiro caso confirmado de doença pelo novo Coronavírus (COVID-19) no Brasil – 26/02/2020. [Google Scholar]
5. Biscayart C., Angeleri P., Lloveras S., Chaves T., Schlagenhauf P., Rodriguez-Morales A.J. The next big threat to global health? 2019 novel coronavirus (2019-nCoV): what advice can we give to travellers? - interim recommendations January 2020, from the Latin-American society for Travel Medicine (SLAMVI) Trav Med Infect Dis. 2020:101567. [PMC free article] [PubMed] [Google Scholar]
6. Rodriguez-Morales A.J. Zika and microcephaly in Latin America: an emerging threat for pregnant travelers? Trav Med Infect Dis. 2016;14:5–6. [PubMed] [Google Scholar]
7. The Lancet The unfolding migrant crisis in Latin America. Lancet. 2019;394:1966. [PubMed] [Google Scholar]
8. Suárez J.A., Carreño L., Paniz-Mondolfi A.E., Marco-Canosa F.J., Freilij H., Riera J.A. Infectious diseases, social, economic and political crises, anthropogenic disasters and beyond: Venezuela 2019 – implications for public health and travel medicine. Rev Panam Enf Inf. 2018;1:73–93. [Google Scholar]
9. Cardona-Ospina J.A., Villamil-Gomez W.E., Jimenez-Canizales C.E., Castaneda-Hernandez D.M., Rodriguez-Morales A.J. Estimating the burden of disease and the economic cost attributable to chikungunya, Colombia. Trans R Soc Trop Med Hyg. 2015;109:793–802. 2014. [PubMed] [Google Scholar]
10. Gilbert M., Pullano G., Pinotti F., Valdano E., Poletto C., Boelle P.Y. Preparedness and vulnerability of African countries against importations of COVID-19: a modelling study. Lancet. 2020 doi: 10.1016/S0140-6736(20)30411-6. [PMC free article] [PubMed] [CrossRef] [Google Scholar]

11. Paniz-Mondolfi A.E., Tami A., Grillet M.E., Marquez M., Hernandez-Villena J., Escalona-Rodriguez M.A. Resurgence of vaccine-preventable diseases in Venezuela as a regional public health threat in the Americas. Emerg Infect Dis. 2019;25:625–632. [PMC free article] [PubMed] [Google Scholar]

12. Page K.R., Doocy S., Reyna Ganteaume F., Castro J.S., Spiegel P., Beyrer C. Venezuela's public health crisis: a regional emergency. Lancet. 2019;393:1254–1260. [PubMed] [Google Scholar]

13. Grillet M.E., Hernandez-Villena J.V., Llewellyn M.S., Paniz-Mondolfi A.E., Tami A., Vincenti-Gonzalez M.F. Venezuela's humanitarian crisis, resurgence of vector-borne diseases, and implications for spillover in the region. Lancet Infect Dis. 2019;19:e149–e161. [PubMed] [Google Scholar]

14. PAHO Epidemiological update measles - 24 january 2020. https://www.paho.org/hq/index.php?option=com_docman&view=download&category_slug=measles-2204&alias=51389-24-january-2020-measles-epidemiological-update-1&Itemid=270&lang=en.2020

15. PAHO Epidemiological update dengue - 7 February 2020. https://www.paho.org/hq/index.php?option=com_docman&view=download&category_slug=dengue-2217&alias=51690-7-february-2020-dengue-epidemiological-update-1&Itemid=270&lang=en.2020

16. Rodriguez-Morales A.J., Suarez J.A., Risquez A., Delgado-Noguera L., Paniz-Mondolfi A. The current syndemic in Venezuela: measles, malaria and more co-infections coupled with a breakdown of social and healthcare infrastructure. Quo vadis? Trav Med Infect Dis. 2019;27:5–8. [PubMed] [Google Scholar]

4. The Endless Challenges of Arboviral Diseases in Brazil[1]

[2]Tereza Magalhaes [1],*, Karlos Diogo M. Chalegre [2],
Cynthia Braga [3] Brian D. Foy [1]

[1] Arthropod-Borne and Infectious Diseases Laboratory (AIDL), Department of Microbiology, Immunology and Pathology (MIP), Colorado State University, Fort Collins, CO 80523-1692, USA; Brian.Foy@colostate.edu
[2] Oswaldo Cruz Institute (IOC), Oswaldo Cruz Foundation (FIOCRUZ), Vice Presidency of Production and Innovation in Health (VPPIS), Rio de Janeiro, RJ 21040-900, Brazil; diogochalegre@gmail.com
[3] Aggeu Magalhaes Institute (IAM), Oswaldo Cruz Foundation (FIOCRUZ), Department of Parasitology, Recife, PE 50670-420, Brazil; braga@cpqam.fiocruz.br
*

ABSTRACT

In this Editorial, we list and discuss some of the main challenges faced by the population and public health authorities in Brazil concerning arbovirus infections, including the occurrence of concurrent epidemics like the ongoing SARS-CoV-2/COVID-19 pandemic.

INTRODUCTION

Optimal ecological and environmental conditions support year-long breeding of mosquito vectors of arboviruses in several Brazilian States. This combined with socioeconomical factors that facilitate mosquito breeding (e.g., intermittent water supply that leads to short-term water storage in open-air artificial containers) and human exposure to mosquito bites, fosters cyclic and intense transmission of arboviruses in Brazil. In urban and peri-urban areas, the four dengue virus serotypes (DENV1-4), Zika virus (ZIKV), and chikungunya virus (CHIKV) are the most widespread and impactful mosquito-borne pathogens, all transmitted by the highly urbanized and anthropophagic *Aedes aegypti*. Arboviral diseases impose a great health burden to the population in Brazil and represent a constant challenge to health authorities. Diagnosis (are extremely complex. Point-of-care virus-specific testing is non-existent in the public and private health care sectors, and the most important diagnosis is clinical-epidemiological, upon which a case is notified to health authorities as suspected or confirmed based on the Ministry of Health case definitions (which uses clinical symptoms and blood test results, such as platelet counts). However, diseases caused by DENV, ZIKV and CHIKV can lead to similar acute symptoms that may differ only in time of onset, duration and severity [1]—thus, only well-trained, experienced physicians are more apt to correctly diagnose a patient, but even these professionals can misdiagnose without available virus-specific tests. Arboviral diseases are nationally notifiable diseases in Brazil, but in the public sector, which exclusively serves more than 70% of the Brazilian population, only a small proportion

[1] *Trop. Med. Infect. Dis.* **2020**, *5*, 75; doi:10.3390/tropicalmed5020075
[2] Correspondence: Tereza.Magalhaes@colostate.edu

of cases notified by health care units undergo confirmatory tests in public reference laboratories through virus-specific molecular or serological assays, or virus culture. For instance, among the notified dengue cases in 2020 (until April), only approximately 23% were tested in reference laboratories [2]. In addition, for DENV and ZIKV, cross-reactivity of serological assays represents a serious issue as it can lead to erroneous results [3]. Official government notifications may thus be biased by inaccurate clinical diagnosis and cross-reactive serological results, and clinical management of infections may not be appropriate if the wrong diagnosis is made. The different socioeconomic realities of Brazilian States also contribute to inconsistencies of arboviral disease notifications. The cross-reactivity between DENV and ZIKV serological assays are due to similar antigenic regions of viral proteins of these genetically related flaviviruses that can be recognized by the same antibodies. Besides being an issue in serological tests, cross-reactive DENV and ZIKV immunity can have important epidemiological implications in places where these viruses co-circulate.

For instance, in vitro, in vivo and epidemiological studies have shown that pre-existing DENV immunity can either protect or enhance ZIKV infection, and consequently impact disease development [4–6]. Other studies suggest that the atypically low dengue incidence observed after the Zika epidemics in Brazil and other Latin American countries was due, in part, to short-term DENV protection from ZIKV infections [7,8]. Importantly, this lower dengue incidence was followed by a significant increase in dengue cases [2,7]. The impact of pre-existing DENV and ZIKV immunity in further heterologous infections and, importantly, in clinical diseases, needs to be continuously assessed in endemic areas.

It is also possible that ZIKV or other arboviruses may establish sylvatic transmission cycles in Brazil, as discussed by other authors [9]. If one looks at the map of Paulista, for example, a municipality within the Recife Metropolitan Region (RMR) in Pernambuco State that was heavily affected by ZIKV and CHIKV, forested areas surround all the urban areas where the viruses cocirculated and human cases were concentrated in 2015-16 (Figure 1 and [10]). These forested areas may harbour several sylvatic mosquitoes like *Aedes albopictus*, *Haemagogus janthinomys*, and *Sabethes tarsopus* that feed on non-human primates (NHPs) and may serve as vectors of arboviruses [11]. In addition, NHPs like the common marmoset *Callithrix jacchus* are abundant in the area [12] and found near humans. Importantly, ZIKV RNA and antibodies against several arboviruses have been found in NHPs in different regions of Brazil, including marmosets [13–16]. The seriousness of an established sylvatic arbovirus transmission cycle in NHPs and sylvatic mosquitoes in Brazil is well represented by yellow fever virus (YFV), which causes sporadic spill over human outbreaks leading to hundreds of deaths. Although a few studies have found little evidence of sylvatic ZIKV transmission in Brazil [16,17], the possibility of a sylvatic cycle being established in distinct Brazilian regions and at different times cannot be excluded. Further governmental or research-related arbovirus surveillance activities should intensify monitoring of sylvatic mosquitoes, NHPs and other small mammals, as the establishment of sylvatic cycles will require changes in the design of control programs.

The ZIKV outbreaks that occurred in Brazil in 2014-16 probably ceased due to herd immunity – however, instead of disappearing, the virus is still circulating in areas that were intensely affected, like the RMR, even if at low rates. In addition, virus transmission during the outbreaks was focal across metropolitan regions, where some areas were more intensely hit than others within the same municipality [4], corroborating the notion of clustered household/community transmission of arboviruses transmitted by *Ae. aegypti*.

The low but constant circulation of ZIKV, the presence of prior virus foci with surrounding patchy areas containing higher numbers of naïve people, and the possibility of a sylvatic cycle being established in some regions increase the chances of unexpected re-emergence of the virus. It will also be important to assess the importance of sexual transmission among the sustained, low ZIKV circulation in endemic regions, as the epidemiological relevance of ZIKV sexual transmission may be higher than previously thought ([18] and Magalhaes et al., unpublished).

Escalating the problem of arboviral disease surveillance and management, concurrent outbreaks epidemics of arboviruses and non-arthropod-borne pathogens can further complicate clinical diagnosis and completely overwhelm/saturate the health care system, as we may be seeing now with the pandemic of coronavirus disease COVID-19) caused by severe acute respiratory syndrome coronavirus 2 (SARS-CoV-2). The number of notified dengue, Zika and chikungunya cases in Brazil in 2020 have reached over 660,000 by April [2], reflecting a difficult year for arboviral diseases in the country (Figure 2A). Although the true incidences of SARS-CoV-2 infections and COVID-19 cases are unknown in Brazil due to the very limited testing (currently, the Brazilian government recommends that only severe cases are tested in health clinics and hospitals), the notified numbers of infections and deaths are starting to increase, indicating a worsening epidemic scenario as of April 2020 (Figure 2B) [2].

At the moment, health care units like the local rapid-access units (Unidades de Pronto Atendimento-UPAs), which serve communities like the Paulista population (~330,000 habitants), are working with a reduced number of staff as some individuals have fallen ill and many elderly professionals or those with comorbidities are on leave due to fear of becoming infected with the virus. In a recent survey of SARS-CoV-2 antibodies among health professionals in Pernambuco State, 60% have tested positive, confirming these professionals are under very high risk of infection [19].Although the highest numbers of notified arboviral diseases seemed to have occurred in March 2020, it is very likely that case notification has dropped as a result of fewer people infected with arboviruses seeking health facilities due to the SARS-CoV-2 pandemic. In fact, it would be important to see if household mosquito transmission of arboviruses increases because of social isolation during the COVID-19 pandemic, considering the endophilic behaviour of *Ae. aegypti* (although social isolation is necessary, it is also important to assess its effects on other health factors).

The blunt reality is that health care units have been dealing with a peak in arbovirus infections and COVID-19 cases concomitantly. Besides the many troubles inherent to an overwhelmed health care system, concurrent epidemics also can complicate clinical-epidemiological diagnoses. Some studies show that dengue cases can be misdiagnosed as respiratory infections and vice-versa [20,21]. Coinfections during concurrent epidemics must also be considered as they may worsen clinical diseases. Coinfections of influenza virus and DENV have been identified in several occasions during concurrent epidemics [22–24]. Future control efforts and programs must consider concurrent epidemics as they will most likely continue to happen in the future (e.g., epidemics of DENV and new strains of influenza virus).

CONCLUSIONS

Effective management of arboviral diseases in Brazil requires confronting major challenges. The co-endemicity of multiple and related arboviruses complicates clinical-epidemiological diagnoses, clinical management and case notification, in addition to impacting the epidemiology of arboviral diseases in unclear ways. The possible establishment of sylvatic transmission cycles will represent a significant additional challenge to the development of control programs and should be constantly monitored. Epidemics like the SARS-CoV-2/COVID-19 or other respiratory pathogens/illnesses can overwhelm health care systems and further complicate clinical epidemiological diagnoses. Efforts to better control these diseases must seriously consider all these issues.

Author Contributions: Conceptualization, T.M.; investigation, T.M., K.D.M.C., C.B., B.D.F.; writing—original draft preparation, T.M., K.D.M.C., C.B., B.D.F.; writing—review and editing, T.M., K.D.M.C., C.B., B.D.F. All authors have read and agreed to the published version of the manuscript.

Funding: This research was funded by the National Institutes of Health (NIH, USA), grant number R21AI129464.

Conflicts of Interest: The authors declare no conflict of interest.

REFERENCES

1. Brito, C.A.; Cordeiro, M.T(2020).. One year after the Zika virus outbreak in Brazil: From hypotheses to evidence. *Rev. Soc. Bras. Med. Trop.* 2016, *49*, 537–543, doi:10.1590/0037-8682-0328-2016.
2. Ministério da Saúde do Brasil. Boletins Epidemiológicos. Available online: https://www.saude.gov.br/boletins-epidemiologicos (accessed on 8 May 2020).
3. Zaidi, M.B.; Cedillo-Barron, L.; Gonzalez, Y.A.M.E.; Garcia-Cordero, J.; Campos, F.D.; Namorado-Tonix, K.; Perez, F. (2020). Serological tests reveal significant cross-reactive human antibody responses to Zika and Dengue viruses in the Mexican population. *Acta Trop.* 2020, *201*, 105201, doi:10.1016/j.actatropica.2019.105201.
4. Rodriguez-Barraquer, I.; Costa, F.; Nascimento, E.J.M.; Nery, N.J.; Castanha, P.M.S.; Sacramento, G.A.; Cruz, J.; Carvalho, M.; De Olivera, D.; Hagan, J.E.; et al. (2019). Impact of preexisting dengue immunity on Zika virus emergence in a dengue endemic region. *Science* 2019, *363*, 607–610, doi:10.1126/science.aav6618.
5. Oliveira, R.A.; de Oliveira-Filho, E.F.; Fernandes, A.I.; Brito, C.A.; Marques, E.T.; Tenorio, M.C.; Gil, L.H.(2019).Previous dengue or Zika virus exposure can drive to infection enhancement or neutralisation of other flaviviruses. *Mem. Inst. Oswaldo Cruz* 2019, *114*, e190098, doi:10.1590/0074-02760190098.
6. Watanabe, S.; Tan, N.W.W.; Chan, K.W.K.; Vasudevan, S.G. (2019).Dengue Virus and Zika Virus Serological Cross-reactivity and Their Impact on Pathogenesis in Mice. *J. Infect. Dis.* 2019, *219*, 223–233, doi:10.1093/infdis/jiy482.
7. Borchering, R.K.; Huang, A.T.; Mier, Y.T.-R.L.; Rojas, D.P.; Rodriguez-Barraquer, I.; Katzelnick, L.C.; Martinez, S.D.; King, G.D.; Cinkovich, S.C.; Lessler, J.; et al. (2019).Impacts of Zika emergence in Latin America on endemic dengue transmission. *Nat. Commun.* 2019, *10*, 5730, doi:10.1038/s41467-019-13628-x.
8. Perez, F.; Llau, A.; Gutierrez, G.; Bezerra, H.; Coelho, G.; Ault, S.; Barbiratto, S.B.; de Resende, M.C.; Cerezo, L.; Kleber, G.L.; et al. (2019). The decline of dengue in the Americas in 2017: Discussion of multiple hypotheses. *Trop. Med. Int. Health* 2019, *24*, 442–453, doi:10.1111/tmi.13200.
9. Figueiredo, L.T.M. (2019).Human Urban Arboviruses Can Infect Wild Animals and Jump to Sylvatic Maintenance Cycles in South America. *Front. Cell. Infect. Microbiol.* 2019, *9*, 259, doi:10.3389/fcimb.2019.00259.
10. Magalhaes, T.; Braga, C.; Cordeiro, M.T.; Oliveira, A.L.S.; Castanha, P.M.S.; Maciel, A.P.R.; Amancio, N.M.L.; Gouveia, P.N.; Peixoto-da-Silva, V.J., Jr.; Peixoto, T.F.L.; et al. (2017).Zika virus displacement by a chikungunya outbreak in Recife, Brazil. *PLoS Negl. Trop. Dis.* 2017, *11*, e0006055, doi:10.1371/journal.pntd.0006055.
11. Aragao, N.C.; Muller, G.A.; Balbino, V.Q.; Costa Junior, C.R.; Figueiredo Junior, C.S.; Alencar, J.; Marcondes, C.B. (2010). A list of mosquito species of the Brazilian State of Pernambuco, including the first report of Haemagogus

janthinomys (Diptera: Culicidae), yellow fever vector and 14 other species (Diptera: Culicidae). *Rev. Soc. Bras. Med. Trop.* 2010, *43*, 458–459, doi:10.1590/s0037-86822010000400024.

12. Thompson, C..; Robl, N.J.; Melo, L.C.O.; Valença-Montenegro, M.M.; Valle, Y.B.M.; Oliveira, M.A.B.; Vinyard, C.J. (2013). Spatial distribution and exploitation of trees gouged by common marmosets (*Callithrix jacchus*). *Int. J. Primatol.* 2013, *34*, 65–85.

13. Terzian, A.C.B.; Zini, N.; Sacchetto, L.; Rocha, R.F.; Parra, M.C.P.; Del Sarto, J.L.; Dias, A.C.F.; Coutinho, F.; Rayra, J.; da Silva, R.A.; et al. (2018). Evidence of natural Zika virus infection in neotropical non-human primates in Brazil. *Sci. Rep.* 2018, *8*, 16034, doi:10.1038/s41598-018-34423-6.

14. Favoretto, S.R.; Araujo, D.B.; Duarte, N.F.H.; Oliveira, D.B.L.; da Crus, N.G.; Mesquita, F.; Leal, F.; Machado, R.R.G.; Gaio, F.; Oliveira, W.F.; et al.(2019). Zika Virus in Peridomestic Neotropical Primates, Northeast Brazil. *Ecohealth* 2019, *16*, 61–69, doi:10.1007/s10393-019-01394-7.

15. de Oliveira-Filho, E.F.; Oliveira, R.A.S.; Ferreira, D.R.A.; Laroque, P.O.; Pena, L.J.; Valenca-Montenegro, M.M.; Mota, R.A.; Gil, L.(2018). Seroprevalence of selected flaviviruses in free-living and captive capuchin monkeys in the state of Pernambuco, Brazil. *Transbound. Emerg. Dis.* 2018, *65*, 1094–1097, doi:10.1111/tbed.12829.

16. Moreira-Soto, A.; Carneiro, I.O.; Fischer, C.; Feldmann, M.; Kummerer, B.M.; Silva, N.S.; Santos, U.G.; Souza, B.; Liborio, F.A.; Valenca-Montenegro, M.M.; et al.(2018) Limited Evidence for Infection of Urban and Peri-urban Non-human Primates with Zika and Chikungunya Viruses in Brazil. *mSphere* 2018, *3*, doi:10.1128/mSphere.00523-17.

17. Pauvolid-Correa, A.; Goncalves Dias, H.; Marina Siqueira Maia, L.; Porfirio, G.; Oliveira Morgado, T.; Sabino-Santos, G.; Helena Santa Rita, P.; Teixeira Gomes Barreto, W.; Carvalho de Macedo, G.; Marinho Torres, J.; et al. (2019). Zika Virus Surveillance at the Human-Animal Interface in West-Central Brazil, 2017–2018. *Viruses* 2019, *11*, doi:10.3390/v11121164.

18. Rosenberg, E.S.; Doyle, K.; Munoz-Jordan, J.L.; Klein, L.; Adams, L.; Lozier, M.; Weiss, K.; Sharp, T.M.; PazBailey, G.(2019). Prevalence and Incidence of Zika Virus Infection Among Household Contacts of Patients With Zika Virus Disease, Puerto Rico, 2016–2017. *J. Infect. Dis.* 2019, *220*, 932–939, doi:10.1093/infdis/jiy689.

19. Centro de Informações Estratégicas de Vigilância em Saúde de Pernambuco (CIEVS). Available online: https://www.cievspe.com/novo-coronavirus-2019-ncov (accessed on 8 May 2020).

20. Chacon, R.; Clara, A.W.; Jara, J.; Armero, J.; Lozano, C.; El Omeiri, N.; Widdowson, M.A.; AzzizBaumgartner, E. (2015). Influenza Illness among Case-Patients Hospitalized for Suspected Dengue, El Salvador, 2012. *PLoS ONE* 2015, *10*, e0140890, doi:10.1371/journal.pone.0140890.

21. Restrepo, B.N.; Piedrahita, L.D.; Agudelo, I.Y.; Parra-Henao, G.; Osorio, J.E.(2012) Frequency and clinical features of dengue infection in a schoolchildren cohort from medellin, Colombia. *J. Trop. Med.* 2012, *2012*, 120496, doi:10.1155/2012/120496.

22. Perez, M.A.; Gordon, A.; Sanchez, F.; Narvaez, F.; Gutierrez, G.; Ortega, O.; Nunez, A.; Harris, E.; Balmaseda, A. (2010). Severe coinfections of dengue and pandemic influenza A H1N1 viruses. *Pediatr. Infect. Dis. J.* 2010, *29*, 1052–1055, doi:10.1097/INF.0b013e3181e6c69b.

23. Lopez Rodriguez, E.; Tomashek, K.M.; Gregory, C.J.; Munoz, J.; Hunsperger, E.; Lorenzi, O.D.; Irizarry, J.G.; Garcia-Gubern, C. (2010). Co-infection with dengue virus and pandemic (H1N1) 2009 virus. *Emerg. Infect. Dis.* 2010, *16*, 882–884, doi:10.3201/eid1605.091920.

24. Hussain, R.; Al-Omar, I.; Memish, Z.A. (2012). The diagnostic challenge of pandemic H1N1 2009 virus in a dengueendemic region: A case report of combined infection in Jeddah, Kingdom of Saudi Arabia. *J. Infect. Public Health* 2012, *5*, 199–202, doi:10.1016/j.jiph.2011.12.005.

5. COVID-19 and Other Viruses in Brazil: Can the New Pandemic Influence Epidemiological Records?

Haniel Soares Fernandes[1]

[1]Faculdade Estácio de Sá, Departamento de nutrição, Fortaleza, Ceará, Brasil
[1]Faculdade São Gabriel da Palha, Nutrição, metabolismo e fisiologia no esporte, Minas

Gerais, Brasil
[1]Faculdade de Economia, Administração, Atuariais e Contábeis,
Universidade Federal do Ceará, Fortaleza, Ceará, Brasil

ABSTRACT

Amid the COVID-19 pandemic, other diseases, including viruses, are still acting to the detriment of their seasonality and risk factors for contagion. For this reason, it is interesting to know the degree of impact of other viruses, mainly respiratory, in which they have similar symptoms, in diagnoses for contamination by the new coronavirus based on epidemiological surveys, via epidemiological weeks, in Brazil. To what extent there may be a hypothesis of confusion of contaminated data, harming the health system, with regard to the need for intensive care units and control of viruses, and negatively or positively implying in the control or uncontrol ling of viruses in general.

INTRODUCTION

Brazil has control of epidemiological data on the main diseases diagnosed in the country through the dissemination of weekly epidemiological bulletins, based on surveys by the Health Departments of each municipality to assess contagion projections by statistical calculations, culminating in the possible creation of health policies. public health determinants for each disease. However, with the arrival of the new coronavirus pandemic and all national precautions to avoid its peak of contagion, there may be conflicts in the health system due to the continued incidence of other viral diseases, especially respiratory diseases, in which they have symptoms similar to that cause by COVID-19 (coronavirus disease 19). The hypothesis is that the new virus may be confusing the diagnosis of the other viruses and influencing the disclosures and projections of contagions.

The New Coronavirus Pandemic

The infection by Sars-Cov-2 (Severe Acute Respiratory Syndrome Coronavirus 2), also known as COVID-19, started in mid-November 2019 in China and, spreading to other countries and continents, reached approximately 80 thousand confirmed cases until January this year, being declared a pandemic on March 11, 2020 by the World Health Organization (WHO) due to its high transmissibility power from human to human, where an infected person can transmit, on average, to six other individuals [1].

Other Viral Diseases Amid the COVID-19 Pandemic in Brazil

In addition, a recent study brought the alert from the Pan American Health Organization (PAHO / WHO) to the current scenario, including Brazil, regarding the possibility of a union, which would involve the pandemic of the new coronavirus and the increase of the incidence of arboviruses and respiratory diseases, including Dengue and Influenza, taking into account their seasonality, that is, the influence of the rainy season in the region [2].

The Ministry of Health of Brazil publishes epidemiological bulletins of contagious diseases, as well as arboviruses (Dengue, Chikungunya and Zika), based on epidemiological weeks (SE) through data recorded every 2 weeks of the year. Up to SE 15 (from the beginning of the year to the second week of April), 90,855 probable dengue cases were reported in 2018 [3], 451,685 probable dengue cases in 2019 [4] and 557,750 probable dengue cases in 2020 [5]. Counting an increase, between the same periods, of approximately 397% from 2018 to 2019 and 23% from 2019 to 2020, the latter already in the middle of the COVID-19 pandemic [1] and their respective social isolation measures in the country [6] after almost 24 thousand confirmed cases in this period [7]. However, dengue symptoms are not so similar to COVID-19 symptoms [8]. However, some respiratory diseases have similar symptoms of COVID-19 infection [9], in such a way that perhaps it can confuse the diagnosis without precise tests for correct analysis of the contagious virus [10]. In view of this, PAHO, like the Ministry of Health of Brazil, also publishes epidemiological bulletins of infectious diseases, and during SE 9 2020, the detections of influenza A (H1N1 and H3N2) and B decreased compared to the previous week. along with a smaller peak in SE 12, with inter-seasonal levels, culminating in a low activity recorded in SE 15, including the respiratory syncytial virus that did not record any records in that period [12,13].

Given the above, a recent study evaluated the increase in hospitalizations for respiratory viruses, which included influenza A (H1N1 and H3N2), B and respiratory syncytial virus, in 2020 in Brazil until the epidemiological week 12, concluding that the lack of specific information about the etiological agent of hospitalizations, in addition to the greater number of cases among the elderly during the same period in which there was an increase in contagion due to coronavirus, culminates in the hypothesis that there may be a possible detection of the current pandemic disease (COVID-19) by the system of surveillance of respiratory viruses already known, although it is not possible to prove due to the lack of elaboration of precise statistical calculations [14], taking into account the lack of an expressive number of specific tests, which could result in a better accuracy of diagnoses and, probably, minimize the effects of the pandemic [15].

CONCLUSION

In terms of problems in diagnoses and test accuracy in parallel to other common viruses in Brazil, such as Dengue and Influenza, there seems to be a correlation, not statistically elaborated, between the fall in the contagion of these diseases and the peak of contamination by COVID-19. What denotes a possible control of the incidence of arboviruses, such as dengue, and of respiratory diseases, such as influenza A, B and respiratory syncytial virus, in parallel to the increase in the number of contaminated by the new coronavirus, or a possible indication of problems to diagnose inpatient screening precisely in the midst of a pandemic panic.

REFERENCES

1. Liu, Y. Gayle, A,A., Wilder-Smith A, Rocklöv, J.(2020.)The reproductive number of COVID-19 is higher compared to SARS coronavirus. *J Travel Med.* 2020;27(2):1-6. doi:10.1093/jtm/taaa021

2. Rodriguez-Morales A.J., Gallego, V, Escalera-Antezana J.P, et al. (2020) COVID-19 in Latin America: The implications of the first confirmed case in Brazil. *Travel Med Infect Dis.* 2020;(February):101613. doi:10.1016/j.tmaid.2020.101613

3. Brasil, M. (2020). da saude. Boletim epidemiológico 15 - Arboviroses urbanas 2018. In: Vol 49. ; 2018:1-14.

4. Brasil, M. (2020). da saude. Boletim epidemiológico 15 - Arboviroses urbanas 2019. 2019:1-11.

5. Brasil M da saude. Boletim epidemiológico 15 - Arboviroses urbanas 2020. In: Vol 51. ; 2020.

6. Brasil, M. (2020). da saude. Saúde regulamenta condições de isolamento e quarentena. https://www.saude.gov.br/noticias/agencia-saude/46536-saude-regulamentacondicoes-de-isolamento-e-quarentena. Published 2020. Accessed May 1, 2020.

7. G1. Casos de coronavírus no Brasil em 13 de abril. Secretarias estaduais de saúde contabilizam 23.753 infectados em todos os estados e 1.355 mortos. https://g1.globo.com/bemestar/coronavirus/noticia/2020/04/13/casos-decoronavirus-no-brasil-em-13-de-abril.ghtml. Published 2020. Accessed May 1, 2020.

8. Halstead, S.B. Dengue. 2007. Investigation O. Clinical Signs and Symptoms Predicting Influenza Infection. 2000;160:3243-3247.

9. Yan, C.H, Faraji, F, Prajapati, D.P., Boone, C.E, DeConde, A.S. (2020). Association of chemosensory dysfunction and COVID-19 in patients presenting with influenzalike symptoms. *Int Forum Allergy Rhinol.* 2020:1-18. doi:10.1002/alr.22579

10. Ceará G do E do. Boletim epidemiológico 11 - SARG e Influenza 2020. 2020;(Quadro 1):1-8.

11. OPAS/WHO. Influenza Report EW 9/ Reporte de Influenza SE 9 - 2020. In: ; 2020:1-40.

12. OPAS/WHO. Influenza Report EW 15/ Reporte de Influenza SE 15 - 2020. In: ; 2020:1-38.

13. Niquini, R.P., Lana, R.M. (2020). COVID-19 and hospitalizations for SARI in Brazil : a comparison up to the 12th epidemiological week of 2020 COVID-19 e hospitalizações por SRAG no Brasil : uma comparação até a 12 a semana epidemiológica de 2020 COVID-19 y las hospitalizaciones por el SRA.2020;36(4):1-8. doi:10.1590/0102-311X00070120

14. Peto. J.(2020). COVID-19 mass testing facilities could end the epidemic rapidly. *BMJ.*2020;368(March):110110. doi:10.1136/bmj.m1163

CHAPTER 2

PREPARING FOR THE PANDEMIC STORM

1. Disaster Preparedness and Response In Brazil In The Face of The COVID-19 Pandemic

Karina Furtado Rodrigues[1]
http://orcid.org/0000-0001-9330-6399
Mariana Montez Carpes[1]
http://orcid.org/0000-0002-7581-2973
Carolina Gomes Raffagnato[1]
http://orcid.org/0000-0001-7426-3864

[1]Escola de Comando e Estado-Maior do Exército / Post-Graduate Program in Military Sciences (PPGCM) at the Meira Mattos Institute (IMM), Rio de Janeiro / RJ - Brazil

ABSTRACT

This article aims to understand how the National System of Protection and Civil Defence functions in response to COVID-19, with emphasis on the work of the Ministry of Health, which is the body responsible for tackling health threats. Three specific objectives were used: the first characterizes COVID-19 as a public health event that can represent a disaster; the second situates the concepts of preparedness and response in the disaster governance literature; the third identifies the jurisprudence and the functioning of disaster management in Brazil. The findings show that, despite the political decision-making tensions, the Brazilian professional bureaucracy managed to guarantee the activation of the disaster governance system related to the preparation and response phases. However, its activation was not enough to allay the crisis. The severity of the pandemic exposed flaws in the phases of disaster prevention and mitigation, as well as the lack of coordinated government response.

1. INTRODUCTION

In mid-November 2019, rumours of a "mysterious pneumonia" surfaced in Wuhan, China. On December 31, the World Health Organization (WHO) was notified of the disease (Praia Vermelha Military Observatory [OMPV], 2020a), and in the first days of January 2020, several researchers around the world had completed the RNA sequencing of the virus. There was no doubt: a new virus of the coronavirus family, SARS-CoV-2, and the respiratory disease caused by it, COVID-19, had been discovered.

Subsequently, on January 27, 2020, three events prompted WHO to change the COVID-19 global risk from moderate to high. First, the confirmation that the disease could be transmitted human to human in a sustainable manner (OMPV, 2020c). Second, on January 11, the first death by COVID-19 in China was recorded (OMPV, 2020b). Finally, the disease arrive in other countries (OMPV, 2020c). On January 30, WHO declared a Public Health Emergency of International Importance (ESPII) (OMPV, 2020d). On March 11, the organization updated the status of COVID-19 to a pandemic (OMPV, 2020e), which meant that the virus was circulating in all continents. The most important event, however, was the declaration of the ESPII in January; it conveyed the message of the risk posed by the disease on the world, indicating the need for coordinated actions to combat it. In other words, the WHO declaration was a call to States to prepare their national mechanisms for managing and responding to this biological disaster.

Although the COVID-19 pandemic was not the first in this century[1], and is still in an upward contamination curve in some countries, it has generated unprecedented impacts on society. It is not possible to determine the consequences that it will have in the medium and long terms, but in the short term, it is clear that the main challenge has been the management of the disaster (see section 3).Given this scenario, the question this article poses is how the public health crisis caused by the COVID-19 pandemic can help to understand the work of the National Civil Protection and Defense System (SINPDEC) in the preparedness and response phases of health disasters in Brazil. The general objective of this study is to understand how the system worked in response to COVID-19, with emphasis on the work of the Ministry of Health (MS), the managing body in the fight against health threats. The operationalization of this study will be undertaken by characterizing COVID-19 as a public health threat with potential to cause disaster; by verifying the concepts of preparedness and response in the disaster governance literature; and by identifying the legal provisions and the work of disaster management in Brazil. The time frame of this article begins with the first reports of atypical pneumonia in China and ends with the dismissal of the now former Minister of Health, Luiz Henrique Mandetta.

Despite the political decision-making tensions, the Brazilian professional bureaucracy was able to guarantee the activation of the system with regard to the preparedness and response phases provided in the SINPDEC. For the sake of the argument presented in this article, the assumption is that the country has a disaster governance structure that includes measures ranging from prevention to recovery of the affected areas, as described in the National Civil Protection and Defense Policy (PNPDEC). Considering that Brazil is a member of both the United Nations (UN) and the World Health Organization (WHO), it is the country's responsibility to internalize, by way of appropriate legal frameworks, the agreed international commitments. For instance, (a) the WHO recommendations of 2005 regarding the need for countries to strengthen, or establish, their pandemic preparedness and response mechanisms (see section 3); and (b) the International Health Regulations (RSI) approved at the WHO 58th World Health Assembly (see section 4).Health is not one of Brazil's strategic areas, and consequently, the country's health structure is fragile, jeopardizing its ability to react to the prevention and mitigation phases, and to the response and recovery phases of the disaster cycle[2]. This became evident upon the discontinuity of leadership in the Ministry of Health (MS) and in the political tension that marks the management of the crisis. Furthermore, the pressure to minimize the gravity of the crisis has not gone unfelt by the bureaucratic isolation of specialized health and disaster structures in Brazil.

This article is divided in seven parts, including this Introduction. The second part presents the chosen methodological tool: process tracing. The third introduces the theoretical-conceptual framework of the governance literature and the disaster management cycle. The fourth deals with the disaster governance structure of the Brazilian health system, while the fifth discusses the activation of the system to face the pandemic in Brazil. The sixth returns to the methodological choices and the theoretical-conceptual framework, inferring the challenges in the work of the SINPDEC, based on the chronological sequence in the fifth section.

Finally, in the conclusions, the findings of this article are discussed and suggestions for a follow up to this research are presented, emphasizing the assessment of the decisions made.

2. METHODOLOGY

In this article, the method chosen to operationalize the research and give meaning to its findings was process tracing. The most widespread classification of process tracing divides this methodology between testing and theory development (Checkel, 2008; George & Bennett, 2005); some authors consider the historical narrative to be a third type of process tracing (George & Bennett, 2005; Mahoney, 2015; Tannenwald, 2007) and others propose the explanation of results as the third variant of the method (Beach & Pedersen 2013).

Nevertheless, these classifications leave out a simpler, but fundamental type of process tracing: the descriptive inference, whose definition comes close to the historical narrative, but cannot be considered a synonym. The reason for this is that tests, theoretical development and historical narratives focus on the causative dimension of the phenomena to be studied. Thus, descriptive inferences would be an earlier step, in which one seeks to select and make sense of the phenomena before analyzing them.

With this methodological approach, the focus here is exclusively on the process tracing of descriptive inferences in order to understand the limitations of the handling of COVID-19 in Brazil, regardless of the adequate operation of the National Civil Protection and Defense System (SINPDEC), and the consequent triggering of the pandemic preparedness and response phases. Despite the closeness of the historical narrative to the descriptive inference, the latter allows the study of empirical cases of the present time (Bennett, 2015), yet it is not committed to demonstrating the causal nexus that link initial conditions to results. In the descriptive inferences, the method uses the surgical study of a previously defined chronological sequence of events, looking for evidence that supports or rejects the arguments defended by the research (Collier, 2011). Thus, the descriptive inferences derived from process tracing are not intended to be generalizable. They are, nonetheless, a useful variant of the method for single case studies, such as the one undertaken here.

Bennett (2015) and Collier (2011) argue in favor of the legitimacy of this type of study, despite recognizing that the notoriety of process tracing came from its ability to generate causal inferences (George & Bennett, 2010; Mahoney, 2015). However, according to Bennett (2015), descriptive inferences are a precondition - although often neglected - for causal inferences, which depend on the previous domain of the phenomenon to be analyzed. This domain derives from the vertical and systematic knowledge of the empirical case.

To clarify the differentiation and codependency between the forms of process tracing, it is necessary to characterize the causal inference. As Checkel (2006) explains well, process tracing, in its analytical form, seeks to identify the causal mechanisms of explanatory variables. This is possible because, as the name reveals, it is a process mapping methodology. Beach and Pedersen (2013) disagree with Checkel's proposition - as do George and Bennett - on the relationship between process tracing and the process as an empirical part of a historical continuum, defending that process tracing allows an analytical exercise focused on specific moments, enabling the visualization of the causal mechanism of interest (Beach & Pedersen, 2013; Beach, 2016). Given that the present article constitutes the publication of the first phase of a research agenda on disaster governance in Brazil, the focus being on the description of the events is justifiable, concomitantly with the identification of the obstacles, which will be analyzed in later phases of the research. It is also important to note the relevance of this type of process tracing beyond the academic debate on testing or generating hypotheses. Bennett (2015, p. 4) defends the application of process tracing as a methodology that helps decision makers to "make mid-course corrections with the help of process tracing, updating expected outcomes in light of new evidence on whether policies are working as planned". His observation sheds light on two valued aspects of the present research. The first deals with the characteristics of the study of public policies that assume the need to make fine adjustments to decisions while they are taking place. The second is in respect to the methodological aspect, since process tracing is not a closed model and allows the researcher to extrapolate the established chronological profile, shedding light on moments of decision making prior to the observed phenomenon whose implications materialize in the period under observation. Specifically in the case of the present research, the (non) choices made by Brazil still in the early years of the 21st century, will demonstrate the impact on the country's ability to prepare for (and respond to) a disaster like the current one. Finally, it is worth making some further observations regarding the choice of the method and the way it enables the operationalization of this research.

As George and Bennett (2005) have well observed, process tracing is a methodology that considers the complexity of the social phenomenon. Thus, the method works with the concept of equifinality, i.e., it assumes that the resulting observations of social phenomena can originate from different combinations of initial causes, being, therefore, sceptical of the existence of singular causes capable of giving meaning to social complexity. With this in mind, and returning to the debate presented in this section, this article offers a proximity to the discussion on disaster management in Brazil, focusing on the preparedness and response phases to COVID-19, without, however, denying that part of the current difficulties stem from past decisions that have undermined the prevention and mitigation phases. This article used news clippings organized by the Military Observatory of Praia Vermelha (OMPV, 2020). The collection was made based on the review of publications from the main news agencies in the world, mostly free of charge, and from the largest newspapers in Brazil[3]. In addition, the article is supported by secondary literature on disaster governance, the documentation that structures governance and international documents on health and disasters.

3. THEORETICAL-CONCEPTUAL FRAMEWORK

Pandemics such as COVID-19 can be characterized as disasters, i.e., atypical crises of large magnitude, which provoke an exhaustion of the responding agencies' individual capabilities in the country where they occur (Kiruthu, 2012).

Prognosis of this type of disaster have long existed in literature, and since the beginning of the debate the question has always been less about *whether* and more about *when* a pandemic[4] would occur (Enserink, 2004). This has been evident since 2005 when, because of the consequences of the Severe Acute Respiratory Syndrome (SARS-CoV-2), WHO put forth a series of recommendations to help countries prepare for such an event. The WHO Executive Secretariat's report, released that same year, entitled 'Strengthening pandemic influenza preparedness and response', already affirmed that this event (SARS-CoV-2) was the closest to a pandemic[5] that the world had seen since 1968[6]. In this context, and based on the logic of strategic thinking, it was pressing to strengthen (or develop) national plans and structures for a disaster management cycle.

This included ensuring the capacity to produce vaccines, guaranteeing the production of supplies and assuring the development of human capital. More recently, documents setting out general priorities for disaster preparedness, control and risk reduction- which include pandemic disasters have also been developed. This is the case of the Marco Sendai for Disaster Risk Reduction 2015-2030, written by the United Nations Office for Disaster Risk Reduction (UNDRR)[7] (Etinay, Egbu, & Murray,

2018). In this document, the Office establishes four priority actions for States: understanding disaster risks, strengthening disaster risks governance to manage those risks, investing in building resilience for risk reduction and increasing disaster preparedness; enabling an effective response and swift recovery, rehabilitation and reconstruction phases (UNDRR, 2015). The priority actions suggested by the UNDRR may take different forms depending on the type of disaster that has occurred. WHO distinguishes them into four types: natural, technological, biological and societal. Examples of natural disasters are earthquakes, tsunamis, cyclones, droughts and floods.

The technological ones are different from the first because they result from human error, such as the one that led to the nuclear accident in Fukushima, the collapsing of buildings and other structures, plane crashes and chemical spills. Examples of biological disasters are epidemics, infestations and pests. Finally, societal disasters involve conflicts or intentional acts such as terrorism and cyber attacks, among others (Do, 2019; WHO, 2011; Quarantelli, Lagadec, & Boin, 2007).

According to this classification, the COVID-19 pandemic is a biological disaster. However, it would be an oversight not to add that, although a disease may appear to be a natural phenomenon, human practices - ranging from deforestation to the indiscriminate consumption of game meat - have generated imbalance in the ecosystem, increasing the likelihood of new zoonotic[8] diseases. In addition to this, technological advancement has greatly increased the circulation of people around the world. Furthermore, there is an incidence of a societal character to the disaster in many countries, given that large portions of the population do not have access to basic sanitation and live in precarious structures that make isolation impossible, impelling them to break the isolation to maintain their livelihood (Lima, 2014). Thus, the COVID-19 pandemic could be defined as a *biological disaster with technological and societal elements actively affecting its dissemination*. This type of disaster can be called a "trans-system social rupture" (terminology suggested by Quarantelli et al., 2007), which, due to its scale, impact and information and misinformation overflow, increase the probability of social amplification of the tragedy. In other words, the perception of the crisis can be distorted given the psychological, social, institutional and cultural characteristics of the affected area. Faced with such a complex problem, disaster governance[9] and its effect on the management cycle of disasters must be considered.

In this type of governance, the assumption is that "only variety can destroy variety" (Kooiman, 1999, p. 74). This implies that the problems have multiple origins, which means that only the joint and coordinated action of various solutions and institutions can be capable of placating the problem, not just in terms of health, but also in the impacts that the pandemic brings to the economic, social and environmental dimensions of this event (Börzel, 2011; Zurita, Cook, Harms, & March, 2015). Because each type of disaster affects a different range of specialties, the initial action of a specific area often prevails. In the case of the COVID-19 pandemic, as it is fundamentally a biological disaster, the primary action comes from the area of Health. The involvement of other actors starts after the results of initial diagnosis and planning are provided by that specific area. The disaster management cycle provides guidance on the steps that must be taken in each of the phases, including the initial ones that are sustained in specific areas. This cycle is the analytical framework most used in studies on tragedies, having migrated over the 20th century from a vision focused on responding, to one that busies itself with prevention and mitigation measures (Coetzee & Niekerk, 2012). Both WHO and the National Civil Protection and Defense Policy (PNPDEC) use five phases to define the disaster cycle: prevention, mitigation, preparedness, response and recovery, as shown in Figure 1.

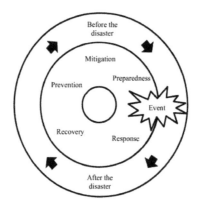

Source: Elaborated by the authors based on PNPDEC (2012) and Wisner and Adams (2002).

FIGURE 1 THE DISASTER MANAGEMENT CYCLE

The prevention, mitigation and preparedness phases entail much of what is discussed in literature regarding disaster risk management (Matyas & Pelling, 2014). Prevention focuses on permanent measures to avoid the occurrence of a disaster. These are taken by developing risk assessments and educational materials, as well as producing risk codes and zones. Mitigation, on the other hand, focuses more on creating resilience in structures and processes (Wisner & Adams, 2002).

The preparedness phase consists of actions whose objective is to minimize the human and material losses of an imminent event, to enable the first responders' immediate availability and to organize the temporary removal of people. This may include drafting national plans and legislation for disaster management, forecasting international, national and sub-national levels of coordination and collaboration, training and strengthening staff and institutions who work with first responders, and educating the population, especially in areas most at risk of being affected (Wisner & Adams, 2002).

The response, in turn, depends on all the previous phases, especially preparedness, which provides the basis for a prompt response. The following are the necessary conditions for an adequate response: availability of trained human resources, experienced leaders, adequate communication, access to transport and logistics, as well as action protocols for each type of emergency. Response actions can vary widely depending on the type of disaster. In the case of biological threats, the response time is different from that of natural and technological threats, for which the first 72 hours are decisive for the life-saving rescue of victims. In the case of infestations, pests and epidemics, the response time depends on the State's ability to contain or control the dissemination of the biological agent; therefore, the response time is extended. Finally, the recovery phase - or, according to WHO, of rehabilitation, reconstruction and recovery - consists of post emergency actions that aim the return to normality. Again, in the case of biological threats the recovery time is distinct and is directly proportional to the time required. When evaluating the preparedness and response phases, there is a follow up assessment of the structure that precedes them - those of prevention and mitigation, which generated plans and legislation relevant to disasters. In addition, adequate preparedness is a necessary-but-not-sufficient condition for the response to be effective, which justifies the relevance of the mapping proposed in the present study.

Brazil is a signatory to the UN, and as such, is one of the 196 countries in which the International Health Regulations (RSI) have been in effect since 2007, when they were approved at the 58th WHO

World Health Assembly. The text provides instructions for preventing and responding to a Public Health Emergency of International Importance (ESPII). According to the RSI, this emergency is characterized as "an extraordinary event which, under the terms of the present regulation, is determined as: (a) constituting a risk to public health for *other* States, due to the international dissemination of the disease and (b) potentially requiring a coordinated international response" (WHO, 2005, p. 9). The RSI stipulates that countries are responsible for improving the means for detecting and evaluating events that occur in their territories, classifying them in emergencies of national or international importance, and they must communicate them to WHO when there is a risk of dissemination to other countries - exactly what China did with COVID-19. In addition, countries need to define the 'National Focal Points' (PFN) for the RSI. Among its attributions are the dissemination of information to the country's administrative sectors and the consolidation of the information that was sent, including the sectors responsible for surveillance and notification, points of entry, public health services, clinics, hospitals and other public departments (WHO, 2005).

The emphasis on the specialized response agencies. Health, in the case of this article does not reduce the importance of actions aimed at disaster governance amid a plurality of other problems that arise from the same issue. This is due to the fact that there are many elements that alter the States' capacity for action in each of the phases, such as the level of bureaucratic-institutional capacity of the responding entities, the level of urbanization, the coexistence of structural problems that increase the difficulty of the response, the level of centralization/decentralization of governmental decisions, the level and way in which citizens access information, the social capital of each region and the diversity of habits and ways of living (Ahrens & Rudolph, 2006; Kiruthu, 2012; Quarantelli, Lagadec, & Boin, 2007; Rumbach, 2016; Tierney, 2012).

Therefore, albeit not the primary objective of this article, pointers and roadmaps for governance will be analyzed, based on the study of the activation of the National Civil Protection and Defense System (SINPDEC) in the preparedness and response phases (see section 5). With that in mind, the next section explores how this activation is set out in the legislation. Next, it explores how it took place in the case of the COVID-19 pandemic.

4. THE STRUCTURE OF HEALTH DISASTERS MANAGEMENT IN BRAZIL

This section describes the Brazilian structure organized by the National Civil Protection and Defense Policy (PNPDEC), which involves institutions such as the Ministry of health (MS), and institutes the National Civil Protection and Defense System (SINPDEC). This debate underlies the concept of disaster discussed in section 3 and its embodiment in the Brazilian legislation.

In accordance with the International Health Regulations (RSI) and Marco Sendai, the Brazilian legal framework, materialized in the Normative Instruction No. 2, 2016, and in the PNPDEC, supplies the definition and understanding of what is a Public Health Emergency (ESP), which at municipal and state levels, has two actions - emergency situation (SE) and state of public calamity (CP), subdivided into three hierarchical levels, according to the degree of intensity of the phenomenon.

These are (1) an event that causes damages and losses that imply a *partial* impairment of the responsiveness of the Public Power towards the affected federative entity (SE), and (2) an event that affects the *substantial* impairment of the responsiveness of the Public Power towards the affected federative entity (CP).Thus, the difference between SE and CP is the intensity and gravity of the damage caused, compared to the capacities of states and municipalities to deal with such damage (PNPDEC, 2017). As will be demonstrated in Box 1, the SE corresponds to levels I and II relative to the intensity of the event, while Level III corresponds to the CP. At the federal level, on the other hand, there is the Declaration of Public Health Emergency of National Importance (ESPIN), regulated by Decree No. 7,616, of 2011, and Ordinance No. 2,952, of the same year.

EL	CHARACTERISTICS	ACTION
Level 1 **Low Intensity**	Only Considerable human damage can be resolved with resources mobilized at the local level	SE
Level 2 **Medium Intensity**	Damages and losses bearable and surmountable by local government whose normality can be restored with the resources mobilised at the local level or complimented with the contribution of state and federal level resources affecting the capacity of the local public power to respond and manage the crisis installed	SE
Level 3 **High Intensity**	Damages and losses that cannot be overcome nor sustained by local governments action or the three spheres of SINIDEC and in some cases, international aid	CP

Source: Adapted from PNPDEC (2017).

BOX 1 CLASSIFICATION, CHARACTERISTICS AND DISASTER ACTION[10]

It is clear that the delegation of responsibilities for each entity of the federation is based on the gravity of the disaster. Depending on the magnitude of the event, the coordination of the response with other entities may be necessary due to the exhaustion of the capacities deployed. Thus, disaster management in Brazil suggests a staggered mobilization of SINPDEC actors according to how the scenario evolves.

Law No. 12,608, of 2012, instituted the National Civil Protection and Defense System (SINPDEC). This legislation, updated in 2017, created the National Civil Protection and Defense Policy (PNPDEC). Until then, the document had been called the National Civil Defense Policy, and the protection dimension was only included in this latest version. The insertion of protection in the policy indicates an effort to emphasize the prevention and mitigation phases of the disaster management cycle, even though, as seen in the case of handling COVID-19, it has not materialized into actions. The SINPDEC, like the PNPDEC, is supported by a systemic approach, assigning an inter-agency aspect to disaster governance in Brazil. ESPs - municipal, state or national are subject to compulsory notification, controlled by the Center for Strategic Information on Health Surveillance (CIEVS), an agency subordinated to the Health Surveillance Secretariat (SVS) of the MS (Ordinance No. 30, 2005). The CIEVS is responsible for searching and gathering compulsory notifications and analyzing relevant data and information. It also tracks down, monitors and coordinates the response of the ESPs in conjunction with the state and municipal health departments. In addition, the CIEVS deals with crisis by organizing the monitoring of events that present a high potential for dissemination or risks to public health.

The 2016 National Focus Points (PFN) in the RSI operation plan says that the National SVS coordinates the preparation and response of health surveillance actions within the scope of the ESPIN and ESPII, with the CIEVS responsible for its operation. Within its actions, the plan provides for detecting ESPs and adopting appropriate measures, in addition to surveillance, prevention and control of communicable diseases, among other attributions (Brasil, 2016). In addition, it gives support to states and municipalities in situations of ESP. The legal landmark for public health disaster governance in the PNPDEC is Law No. 8,080. In accordance with the PFN-RSI operation plan, "it instituted the Brazilian Universal Health System (SUS) as the single health administrator in each sphere of government (municipalities, states, Federal District and Union) and appointed the MS as its manager within the Union". The SUS has its own regulations on disaster risk management, established by the MS, setting out responsibilities, guidelines on implementation and funding of health surveillance actions, within the scope of the National Health Surveillance System and the National Sanitary Surveillance System (PNPDEC, 2017).

The *Health sector preparedness and response to disasters guide*, 2015 (Freitas, 2018), states that disaster preparedness begins long before it happens, through the elaboration and systematization of actions in the Preparedness Plan and Response (PPR). According to the PNPDEC, it is the responsibility of the National SVS to coordinate the preparedness and response of health surveillance actions regarding the ESPIN and ESPII. In order to do this, the National SVS establishes preparedness and response plans and elaborates specific contingency plans, which must be aligned with the Public Health Emergency Response Plan (PRESP), approved in 2014. The PRESP provides the guidelines for the National SVS to act in a timely, qualified and cooperative manner (Brasil, 2014; PNPDEC, 2017). The PRESP systematizes the response to public health emergencies through steps to be taken according to a decision algorithm (Annex A - PRESP). Annex A contains the organized structures for dealing with the crisis. When the CIEVS notifies a rumor, a response is made by activating the Event Monitoring Committee (CME), whose objective is to monitor events of interest to the public health. If necessary, the decision-maker can choose to set up an Emergency Health Operations Center (COES), comprised of the general coordination and departments of the appropriate SVS, whose objective is to articulate and integrate the actors involved in the response (Brasil, 2014). It is also worth highlighting some specific characteristics of the disaster caused by COVID-19.

The occurrence of epidemics, especially of unknown diseases, can issue the ESPIN (PNPDEC, 2017). Unknown diseases, such as those caused by viruses of the beta coronavirus family, affect the response protocols, given that their epidemiological patterns - rate of dissemination, morbidity and type of contamination - are still undetermined. These characteristics affect the time of preparedness and response to the disaster (see section 3), since the event results from the exhaustion of the individual capacities of the federal entities. As will be discussed in section 5, despite being aware of the characteristics in the case of this pandemic, Brazil was one of the only countries in the world not to provide a nationally coordinated response to the disaster.

5. FROM THE EMERGENCE OF THE DISEASE IN BRAZIL TO THE DISMISSAL OF MANDETTA

This section explores the activation of the system presented in section 4 in a timeline that covers the period between the first cases of atypical pneumonia in China to the dismissal of former Minister Mandetta, as a mark of administrative discontinuity. Thus, we will seek to identify which actions were taken in the activation of the structures for disaster preparedness and response provided for in SINPDEC, as well as evidences of coordination between agencies. Brazil has followed the evolution of the disease in China since December 12, 2019, through the Public Health Emergency Response Plan (PRESP), when it was still unclear whether the atypical pneumonias recorded in Wuhan were due to an unknown disease. On January 3, 2020, the Center for Strategic Information on Health Surveillance (CIEVS) requested a "rumor check" on the disease in China, the first step (preparedness phase) laid out in the PRESP that would activate the response to a health disaster. On January 10, the day after confirmation that it was a new virus, the Event Monitoring Committee (CME) was called on to monitor the outbreak of COVID-19 in the Asian country (PRESP, 2014). Six days later, the National Health Surveillance Secretariat (SVS) published the first epidemiological bulletin with information on the new pneumonia (MS, 2020a). From then on, all the eventually confirmed cases of COVID-19 in Brazil would have to be reported to the CIEVS, in order to gather data about the epidemiology of the disease and its evolution in the country. Thus, January 3 marks the beginning of the operation of the health disaster management in Brazil regarding the preparedness phase (PNPDEC, 2017). On the 22nd of the same month, one day after the WHO statement regarding the moderate global risk of COVID-19, Brazil activated the Public Health Emergency Operations Center for the New Coronavirus (COE-nCoV), to alert level I (PRESP, 2014; Croda et al., 2020).

On January 27, Brazil announced the first suspected case of infection in the country, causing COE-nCoV to change the national alert level from I to II (PRESP, 2014). On the same day, Ordinance No. 74 (National Health Surveillance Agency [Anvisa], 2020) established a Public Health Emergency Group to conduct the actions regarding the new coronavirus. On the 30th, the Interministerial Executive Group of Public Health Emergency of International Importance (GEI-ESPII) (see Decree nº 10.211, of 2020), was created and, on February 3, the Ministry of Health (MS) instituted the Declaration of Public Health Emergency of National Importance (ESPIN) (see Ordinance nº 188, of º 2020) and enforced the Decree Nº 7,616, and Ordinance Nº 2,952, both of 2011. Consequently, the COE-nCoV raised the national alert level to III in accordance with PRESP (2014).

On the same day, Decree No. 10,212 issued Article 4 in the International Health Regulations (RSI), indicating the activation of the Health Surveillance Secretariat/Ministry of Health (SVS/MS) as the National Focus Point (PFN) in the RSI in Brazil. Its greatest mission would be to represent and notify WHO of events related to the pandemic. What prompted the issuing of the ESPIN was the need to repatriate the Brazilians who were in Wuhan. Thus, on February 4, Law No. 13,979, of 2020, was passed, providing the guidelines on the quarantine period to which Brazilians repatriated from Wuhan would be subjected to when they arrived in Brazil. The confirmation of the first case of COVID-19 in Brazil, on February 26, 2020, launched a new phase of the health disaster management cycle in the country. In response to this, on March 2, the MS launched the treatment protocol for the new coronavirus (MS, 2020b). Two days later, the Oswaldo Cruz Foundation (Fiocruz) started to distribute rapid testing kits (OMPV, 2020g), demonstrating the nation's watchful eye towards the international behaviour of the virus.

As of February 29, when Brazil only had local transmission of the virus (OMPV, 2020f), a series of airspace restriction measures (OMPV, 2020f) and partial closure of national land borders (OMPV, 2020f) were adopted in an attempt to delay, albeit not able to prevent, the circulation of the virus throughout the national territory. Continuing with the implementation of the Brazilian disaster response structure, on March 16, the Federal Government established the Crisis Committee for Supervising and Monitoring the Impacts of COVID-19 to deal with the operational demands of the pandemic, such as the use of the National Public Security Funds, opening a public call for the acquisition of medical equipment considered strategic, and simplifying the process for declaring a Public Calamity (CP) in the national territory (Decree nº 10.277, of 2020). This Committee was initially not envisaged in the disaster governance, but it was established to manage the crisis within the scope of the Federal Government.

On March 20, Ordinance No. 454 (2020) declared the state of community transmission of COVID-19 in Brazil. On the same day, the Senate passed the Legislative Decree No. 6 (2020), which had been sent to Congress by the Presidency, which declared the state of CP throughout the national territory. The only national coordination action proposed by the Presidency up to that point. It is worth noting that the measure was not because of the Presidency's understanding of the need for nationally coordinated actions to tackle the pandemic; it was only taken to demonstrate their concern of incurring in actions that could be classified as a crime of responsibility - with the Decree, the Executive Branch was now allowed to spend more than what had been budgeted, and in so doing, circumvent the fiscal targets in order to fund actions to combat the pandemic. One day after the CP was issued, the Joint Operations Center for the employment of the Armed Forces in combating COVID-19 was activated. Finally, on March 31, the then Minister of Justice, Sérgio Moro, authorized the use of the National Force to combat the pandemic in the country (OMPV, 2020i). At the same time, on February 29, the same day that Brazil declared community transmission of the virus, in a statement on national television, the President minimized the possible impacts of COVID-19. This statement marked the beginning of the separation between the international recommendations and the views of the national technical bureaucracy, and what would become the Presidency's views regarding the gravity of the situation (OMPV, 2020g).

The escalation of the deterioration generated by this separation would also be reflected in the manifestations of mayors and governors in favor of the adequate treatment that the pandemic demanded, and in opposition to the stance taken by the Presidency (OMPV, 2020e; OMPV, 2020h). In the Executive Branch, however, disagreements over the most appropriate ways to manage the pandemic reached its peak with Mandetta's dismissal and his replacement by Nelson Teich, on April 17, 2020 (OMPV, 2020j), resulting in an administrative discontinuity in the management of the crisis. To understand the sequence of events, Figure 2 shows the chronology of the pandemic preparedness and response phases.

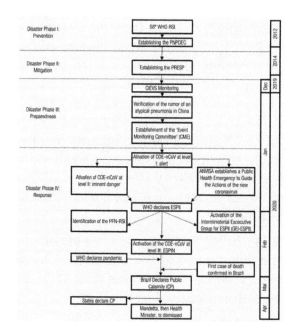

Source: Developed based on data from section 5.

FIGURE 2 CHRONOLOGY OF PREPAREDNESS AND RESPONSE TO THE

COVID-19 PANDEMIC IN BRAZIL

6. DESCRIPTIVE INFERENCES BASED ON THE CASE STUDY

This section aims to retrieve the methodological arguments introduced in section 2 regarding the relevance of the method of descriptive inferences based on the chronological sequence of the phenomenon in question. Grounded on the concepts of the disaster cycle, the presentation of the

Brazilian legal frameworks on disaster management and the chronology of the activation of the preparedness and response phases to COVID-19, this section offers some assertions stemming from the case. These assertions are not generalizable; they are only intended to serve as a guide for the future stages of this research agenda on disaster governance in Brazil. Therefore, they are proposed assertions according to the understanding of the empirical case and their scope is restricted to that case.

That aside, and considering what was set out in the previous sections, in an ESPII with strong social, economic and health impacts such as the COVID-19 pandemic, it is clear that disaster governance does not prevent the problem, but can manage it. Of course, this will depend on the mitigation of its impacts in the medium and long term, which can then provide a faster recovery in the post-crisis. Thus, the diagnoses provided from examining the Brazilian case sought to find a complex management, equal to an equally complex phenomenon. Nonetheless, what was uncovered was a situation aggravated by political decisions in an attempt to minimize the magnitude of the problem.

Since the first confirmed case of COVID-19 contamination in Brazil, a series of measures have been adopted by the SINPDEC, with the view of preparing the country to respond to the public health crisis resulting from the disease. Since the actions taken in the activation of the preparedness and response phases initially followed the WHO recommendations, the immediate response in Brazil shows an alignment between the national and international disaster governance structures.

The concomitance between international recommendations and national decisions up to that point suggests that the evaluation from the specialized technical bureaucracy prevailed, in detriment of political readings of the situation at hand. From what is presented in sections 4 and 5, it is possible to conclude that Brazil has a robust legal framework with regard to tragedies and health disasters. If disaster management structures were properly activated, why does the epidemiological curve in Brazil show such worrying results? At the time of writing this article, on July 2, 2020, the number of deaths recorded per day was 1,252, and the total number of deaths already exceeded 61,880 (COVID, 2020). Given the time limitation of the tests, the measures analyzed here referred to a still manageable context of records of contaminations and deaths. On the day that Mandetta was dismissed, there were 1,924 deaths and 30,425 infected (COVID, 2020). Therefore, the exponential growth of these numbers shows that the measures taken at the beginning of the crisis were insufficient. Therefore, the answer seems be to that the legal robustness does not necessarily translate into implementation. In spite of that, Brazil is an experienced country with a vast history in combating epidemics, not only in the most recent cases such as dengue and the zika virus, chikungunya and yellow fever, but also in prevention campaigns, such as vaccination against influenza, measles and rubella, as well as in the treatment of serious infectious diseases, such as tuberculosis. In addition, the country has a public health system that, despite cuts in funding, is considered an example of universal care in the world (Gragnolati, Lindelow, & Couttolenc, 2013).

Through the Universal Health System (SUS), expensive and prolonged treatments, such as those for tuberculosis, syphilis, leprosy and leishmaniosis, are free for all Brazilians, as well as the supply of medicines for patients with chronic diseases, such as diabetics, cardiac and immunocompromised patients. Although the MS followed international standards and recommendations in the preparation and initial response to the pandemic, a series of challenges in the sustained continuation of the response that had been outlined by the specialized bureaucracy, was quickly unveiled. The first challenge pertained to decision-making tensions on the proper way to control the contamination curve, in order to avoid the collapse of the public health system. An example of that can be found by retrieving successive presidential speeches that minimize the impacts of the disease and criticizes social isolation, under the cover of the need to maintain the national economy healthy (OMPV, 2020g).

Furthermore, by increasing the tone of the gravity of the pandemic in Brazil, the political impasse generated conflicts between the Presidency, on the one hand, and the Ministry of Health (MS) and state governments, on the other, with the last two adopting measures to flatten the contamination curve of COVID-19, regardless of the Presidency's views (OMPV, 2020g; OMPV, 2020h). The escalation of the pandemic management crisis headed by the Presidency led to the establishment of a 'Federal Government Joint Command', which, in practice, established a management structure to support the Presidency that resulted in emptying the decision-making power of the MS, reaffirming the administrative discontinuity represented by Mandetta's dismissal (Reuters, 2020).

The political and decision-making tensions arising from the positioning of the Presidency, at first, did not impact the work of the specialized health bureaucracy and inter-ministerial coordination, so there was no paralyzing decision affecting the public machinery, demonstrated by the development of inter-ministerial committees and centers, the daily press conferences of Minister Mandetta and the activation of the coordination within the scope of the PRESP and COE-nCoV, among others. Nevertheless, while the diagnosis offered here supports the thesis that the technical understanding of the activation of the preparedness and response phases to COVID-19 prevailed, it is important to consider that this scenario has suffered the consequences of the (non) made decisions in the prevention and mitigation phases. Emphasizing the aforementioned fact that health treatment is not a strategic area in Brazil, the nation faced severe challenges in obtaining testing kits, materials and supplies necessary for RT-PCR tests, as well as simple items for individual protection equipment (IPEs) and other more complex ones, such as the respirators on which critically ill patients depended (Barifouse, 2020).

The lack of human resources generated a rush for emergency courses and an ad hoc call for professionals from all health segments: dentists, veterinarians, physiotherapists and physical educators (Barifouse, 2020; Ordinance No. 639, 2020; Operation COVID-19, 2020). As mentioned before, these difficulties confirm the flaws in the phases of prevention and mitigation of the disaster cycle, with considerable room for improvement. From the study of the Brazilian case, it appears that, despite the country's experience in handling public health crises, neglect in the prevention and mitigation phases became barriers in carrying out the preparedness and response to the event, jeopardizing the structure of the entire cycle of disasters. Conversely, if Brazil had implemented the guidelines of the 58th World Health Assembly and Marco Sendai, as well as treated the health area from a strategic perspective, it would have been able to manage the preparedness and response phases as the problem required, however complex.

Likewise, the politicization of disaster management has aggravated the already fragile disaster management structure, resulting in worsening rather than in overcoming the phenomenon. Finally, the strength of the bureaucratic isolation of specialized institutions, such as the "islands of rationality and technical specialization" (Nunes, 2017), protected from political wilfulness, was challenged by the pandemic, and only resisted the prolonged friction with the Presidency to a certain extent. As a result, it is necessary to reflect on the need to create other mechanisms that shield specialized areas, especially in the case of disasters that affect the lives of all citizens.

FINAL CONSIDERATIONS

As a general objective, this article questions how the public health crisis caused by the COVID-19 pandemic helped to understand the work of the National System of Civil Defense and Protection (SINPDEC) in the phases of preparedness and response to health disasters in Brazil, with an emphasis on the role of the Ministry of Health (MS), defined as the management body in the fight against health threats. The study was limited to the period that started with the first rumours of atypical pneumonia in China, verified by the Ministry of Health, ending with the dismissal of Luiz Henrique Mandetta. The operationalization of the general objective was determined by the characterization of COVID-19 as a public health event with potential to cause disaster. It also verifies the existence of the concepts of preparedness and response in the disaster governance literature, as well as what that section entailed, the identification of legal provisions and the work of disaster management in Brazil, described in sections 4 and 5, respectively. The process tracing variant of descriptive inferences, presented in section 2, was used as a methodological support to guide research between the empirical and theoretical-conceptual universes.

Despite the political decision-making tensions, the Brazilian professional bureaucracy managed to guarantee the activation of the system regarding the preparedness and response phases in the

National Civil Protection and Defense System (SINPDEC). However, as expressed by the 4 assertions in section 6, this article concludes that the country's weakness in health is structural. This conclusion comes as a result of health treatment not being a strategic area in Brazil, which jeopardized the entire cycle of disaster management in dealing with COVID-19, deteriorating the situation identified in the response phase. Thus, the bureaucratic isolation of specialized structures in health and disasters, which could only resist the pressure to minimize the gravity of the crisis to some extent, took its toll. The dismissal of Mandetta and the consequent discontinuity of the leadership of the MS has led to this realization. This article was conceived as part of a research agenda that aims to debate these and other points concerning governance and the disaster management cycle in Brazil. The understanding of the issue, specifically in the case of COVID-19, still needs future researches that will contemplate: a methodological discussion, now using the causal variants of process tracing; an analysis of the recovery phase of the post-COVID-19 crisis management; the coordination between the federal and state levels of response; the systemic approach proposed in the National Civil Protection and Defense Policy (PNPDEC) and the practical difficulties that this entails in managing a crisis; the limits of government transparency during the phases of the disaster; disaster risk analysis versus preparedness of responders; and, finally, the debate between health disasters, zoonoses and the concept of One Health proposed by WHO.

REFERENCES

Ahrens, J., & Rudolph, P. M. (2006). The importance of governance in risk reduction and disaster management. *Journal of Contingencies and Crisis Management, 14*(4), 207-220. [Links]

Barifouse, R. (2020, 09 de março). Brasil não adota novo critério da OMS que amplia busca por casos suspeitos. Época. Recuperado de https://epoca.globo.com/brasil/coronavirus-brasil-nao-adota-novo-criterio-da-oms-que-amplia-busca-por-casos-suspeitos-24294775 [Links]

Beach, D. (2016). It's all about mechanisms-what process-tracing case studies should be tracing. *New Political Economy, 21*(5), 463-472. [Links]

Beach, D., & Pedersen, R. B. (2019). *Process-tracing methods: Foundations and guidelines.* Ann Arbor, Michigan: University of Michigan Press. [Links]

Bennett, A., & George, A. L. (1997). *Process tracing in case study research.* Washington, DC: MacArthur Program on Case Studies. [Links]

Bennett, A. (2015). Using process tracing to improve policy making: The (negative) case of the 2003 intervention in Iraq. *Security Studies, 24*(2), 228-238. [Links]

Casa Civil. (2017). *Manual de Proteção e Defesa Civil: A Política Nacional de Proteção e Defesa Civil.* Brasília, DF: Ministério da Integração Nacional. [Links]

Centro Universitário de Estudos e Pesquisas sobre Desastres. (2012). *Política Nacional de Defesa Civil.* Florianópolis, SC: Universidade Federal de Santa Catarina. [Links]

Checkel, J. T. (2006). Tracing causal mechanisms. *International Studies Review*, 8(2), 362-370. [Links]

Coetzee, C., & Van Niekerk, D. (2012). Tracking the evolution of the disaster management cycle: a general system theory approach. *Jàmbá: Journal of Disaster Risk Studies*, 4(1), 1-9. [Links]

Collier, D. (2011). Teaching process tracing: exercises and examples. *PS: Political Science and Politics, 44*(4), 823-830. [Links]

Croda et al. (2020). COVID-19 in Brazil: advantages of a socialized unified health system and preparation to contain cases. *Journal of the Brazilian Society of Tropical Medicine, 53*, e20200167. [Links]

Decreto Legislativo nº 6, de 20 de março de 2020. (2020). Reconhece, para os fins do art. 65 da Lei Complementar nº 101, de 4 de maio de 2000, a ocorrência do estado de calamidade pública, nos termos da solicitação do presidente da República encaminhada por meio da mensagem nº 93, de 18 de março de 2020. Brasília, DF: Presidência da República. [Links]

Decreto nº 10.211, de 30 de janeiro de 2020. (2020). Dispõe sobre o Grupo Executivo Interministerial de Emergência em Saúde Pública de Importância Nacional e Internacional (GEI-ESPII). Brasília, DF: Presidência da República . [Links]

Decreto nº 10.212, de 30 de janeiro de 2020. (2020). Promulga o texto revisado do Regulamento Sanitário Internacional, acordado na 58ª Assembleia Geral da Organização Mundial de Saúde, em 23 de maio de 2005. Brasília, DF: Presidência da República . [Links]

Decreto nº 10.277, de 16 de março de 2020. (2020). Institui o Comitê de Crise para Supervisão e Monitoramento dos Impactos da COVID-19. Brasília, DF: Presidência da República . [Links]

Decreto nº 7.616, de 17 de novembro de 2011. (2011). Dispõe sobre a declaração de Emergência em Saúde Pública de Importância Nacional (ESPIN) e institui a Força Nacional do Sistema Único de Saúde (FN-SUS). Brasília, DF: Presidência da República . [Links]

Dhiman, C, R., Tiwari, A. (2018). Emergence of Zoonotic Diseases in India: A Systematic Review. Medical Reports & Case Studies, 3(3), 1-8. [Links]

Do, X. B. (2019, junho). Return migration after the Fukushima Daiichi nuclear disaster: the impact of institutional and individual factors. *Disasters, 44*(3):569-595. [Links]

Enserink, M. (2004). Looking the Pandemic in the Eye. *Science, 306*(5695), 392-394. [Links]

Etinay, N., Egbu, C., & Murray, V. (2018). Building Urban Resilience for Disaster Risk Management and Disaster Risk Reduction. Procedia Engineering, *212*(2017), 575-582. [Links]

Freitas, C. M. (2018). Guia de preparação e respostas do setor saúde aos desastres. Rio de Janeiro, RJ: Fiocruz, Secretaria de Vigilância em Saúde. [Links]

George, A. L., Bennett, A., Lynn-Jones, S. M., & Miller, S. E. (2005). *Case studies and theory development in the social sciences*. Cambridge, MA: MIT Press. [Links]

Gragnolati, M., Lindelow, M., & Couttolenc, B. (2013). Twenty Years of Health System Reform in Brazil: An Assessment of the Sistema Único de Saúde. Directions in Development--Human Development. Washington, DC: World Bank. [Links]

Instrução Normativa nº 2, de 20 de dezembro de 2016. (2016). Estabelece procedimentos e critérios para a decretação de situação de emergência ou estado de calamidade pública pelos Municípios, Estados e pelo Distrito Federal, e para o reconhecimento federal das situações de anormalidade decretadas pelos entes federativos e dá outras providências. Brasília, DF: Ministério da Integração Nacional. [Links]

Kiruthu, F. (2014). Book Review: Building Resilience: Social Capital in Post Disaster Recovery. Daniel P. Aldrich. University of Chicago Press, 2012. *Governance*, 1, 169-171. [Links]

Kooiman, J. (1999). Social-Political Governance. *Public Management: An International Journal of Research and Theory*, 1(1), 67-92. [Links]

Lei 12.608, de 10 de abril de 2012. (2012). Institui a Política Nacional de Proteção e Defesa Civil (PNPDEC); dispõe sobre o Sistema Nacional de Proteção e Defesa Civil (SINPDEC) e o Conselho Nacional de Proteção e Defesa Civil (Conpdec); autoriza a criação de sistema de informações e monitoramento de desastres; altera as Leis nº 12.340, de 1º de dezembro de 2010, 10.257, de 10 de julho de 2001, 6.766, de 19 de dezembro de 1979, 8.239, de 4 de outubro de 1991, e 9.394, de 20 de dezembro de 1996; e dá outras providências. Brasília, DF. [Links]

Lei nº 12.340, de 1º de dezembro de 2010. (2010). Dispõe sobre as transferências de recursos da União aos órgãos e entidades dos Estados, Distrito Federal e Municípios para a execução de ações de prevenção em áreas de risco de desastres e de resposta e de recuperação em áreas atingidas por desastres e sobre o Fundo Nacional para Calamidades Públicas, Proteção e Defesa Civil; e dá outras providências. Brasília, DF: Presidência da República . [Links]

Lei nº 13.979, de 6 de fevereiro de 2020. (2020). Dispõe sobre as medidas para enfrentamento da emergência de saúde pública de importância internacional decorrente do coronavírus responsável pelo surto de 2019. Diário Oficial da União: seção 1, Brasília, DF: Agência Nacional de Vigilância Epidemiológica. [Links]

Lima, Y, Costa, E. (2014). Regulamento sanitário internacional: emergências em saúde pública, medidas restritivas de liberdade e liberdades individuais. *Vig Sanit Debate*, 3(1),10-18. [Links]

Mahoney, J. (2015). Process tracing and historical explanation. *Security Studies*, *24*(2), 200-218. [Links]

Matyas, David; Pelling, Mark. (2014). Positioning resilience for 2015: the role of resistance, incremental adjustment and transformation in disaster risk management policy. *Disasters*, *39*(s1), 1-19. [Links]

Ministério da Saúde. (2018). *Guia para Investigações de Surtos ou Epidemias*. Brasília, DF: Autor. Recuperado dehttps://www.saude.gov.br/images/pdf/2018/novembro/21/guia-investigacao-surtos-epidemias-web.pdf [Links]

Ministério da Saúde. (2020a). *Boletim Epidemiológico. Situação epidemiológica da febre amarela no monitoramento 2019/2020*. Brasília, DF: Secretaria de Vigilância Epidemiológica. [Links]

Ministério da Saúde. (2020b). *Protocolo de Tratamento do Novo Coronavírus (2019-nCoV)*. Brasília, DF: Autor . [Links]

Ministério da Saúde. (2020c, 30 de abril). *Painel Coronavírus*. Brasília, DF: Autor . Recuperado de https://covid.saude.gov.br/ [Links]

Ministério da Saúde. (2014). *Plano de Respostas às Emergências em Saúde Pública*. Brasília, DF: Autor . [Links]

Nunes, E. O. (2017). *A gramática política do Brasil: clientelismo, corporativismo e insulamento burocrático*. (5. Ed.). Rio de Janeiro, RJ: Garamond. [Links]

Observatório Militar da Praia Vermelha. (2020). *DQBRN e Precursores - Clipagem de Notícias*. Rio de Janeiro, RJ: Autor. Recuperado de http://ompv.eceme.eb.mil.br/masterpage_assunto.php?id=210 [Links]

Observatório Militar da Praia Vermelha. (2020a). *DQBRN e Precursores - Clipagem de Notícias - Semana 1*. Rio de Janeiro, RJ: Autor . Recuperado de http://ompv.eceme.eb.mil.br/docs/dqbrn/SEM01_31_12ate05_01.pdf [Links]

Observatório Militar da Praia Vermelha. (2020b). *DQBRN e Precursores - Clipagem de Notícias - Semana 2*. Rio de Janeiro, RJ: Autor . Recuperado de http://ompv.eceme.eb.mil.br/docs/dqbrn/SEM02_06_01ate12_01.pdf [Links]

Observatório Militar da Praia Vermelha. (2020c). *DQBRN e Precursores - Clipagem de Notícias - Semana 3*. Rio de Janeiro, RJ: Autor . Recuperado de http://ompv.eceme.eb.mil.br/docs/dqbrn/SEM03_13_01ate19_01.pdf [Links]

Observatório Militar da Praia Vermelha. (2020d). *DQBRN e Precursores - Clipagem de Notícias - Semana 5*. Rio de Janeiro, RJ: Autor . Recuperado de http://ompv.eceme.eb.mil.br/docs/dqbrn/SEM05_27_01ate02_02.pdf [Links]

Observatório Militar da Praia Vermelha. (2020e). *DQBRN e Precursores - Clipagem de Notícias - Semana 11*. Rio de Janeiro, RJ: Autor . Recuperado de http://ompv.eceme.eb.mil.br/docs/dqbrn/SEM11_09_03ate15_03.pdf [Links]

Observatório Militar da Praia Vermelha. (2020f). *DQBRN e Precursores - Clipagem de Notícias - Semana 9*. Rio de Janeiro, RJ: Autor . Recuperado de http://ompv.eceme.eb.mil.br/docs/dqbrn/SEM09_24_02ate01_03.pdf [Links]

Observatório Militar da Praia Vermelha. (2020g). *DQBRN e Precursores - Clipagem de Notícias - Semana 10*. Rio de Janeiro, RJ: Autor . Recuperado de http://ompv.eceme.eb.mil.br/docs/dqbrn/SEM10_02_03ate08_03.pdf [Links]

Observatório Militar da Praia Vermelha. (2020h). *DQBRN e Precursores - Clipagem de Notícias - Semana 12*. Rio de Janeiro, RJ: Autor . Recuperado de http://ompv.eceme.eb.mil.br/docs/dqbrn/SEM12_16_03ate22_03.pdf [Links]

Observatório Militar da Praia Vermelha. (2020i). *DQBRN e Precursores - Clipagem de Notícias - Semana 14*. Rio de Janeiro, RJ: Autor . Recuperado de http://ompv.eceme.eb.mil.br/docs/dqbrn/SEM14_30_03ate05_04.pdf [Links]

Observatório Militar da Praia Vermelha. (2020j). *DQBRN e Precursores - Clipagem de Notícias - Semana 16*. Rio de Janeiro, RJ: Autor . Recuperado de http://ompv.eceme.eb.mil.br/docs/dqbrn/SEM16_13_04ate19_04.pdf [Links]

Operação COVID-19. (2020, 30 de março). *Militares realizam treinamento em defesa nuclear, biológica, química e radiológica para operação COVID-19*. Recuperado de https://operacaocovid19.defesa.gov.br/noticias/noticia/770-militares-realizam-treinamento-em-defesa-nuclear-biologica-quimica-e-radiologica-para-operacao-COVID-19 [Links]

Organização Mundial da Saúde. (2005). *International Health Regulations* (2nd. Ed.). Geneva, Switzerland: Autor. Recuperado de http://portal.anvisa.gov.br/documents/375992/4011173/9789241580410_eng.pdf/36b8b474-c10f-4433-82d4-18a04bc5a736 [Links]

Organização Mundial da Saúde. (2020a, 21 de fevereiro). *Coronavirus disease 2019 (COVID-19)* (Situation Report, 32). Geneva, Switzerland: Autor . Recuperado de https://www.who.int/docs/default-source/coronaviruse/situation-reports/20200221-sitrep-32-COVID-19.pdf?sfvrsn=4802d089_2 [Links]

Organização Mundial da Saúde. (2011, maio). *Disaster Risk Management for Health: overview*. Geneva, Switzerland: Autor . Recuperado dehttps://www.who.int/hac/events/drm_fact_sheet_overview.pdf [Links]

Tannenwald, N. (1999). The nuclear taboo: The United States and the normative basis of nuclear non-use. *International organization, 53*(3), 433-468. [Links]

Portaria ANVISA nº 74, de 27 de janeiro de 2020. (2020). Dispõe sobre a criação de Grupo de Emergência em Saúde Pública para condução das ações referentes ao Novo Coronavírus (NCoV). Brasília, DF: Ministério da Saúde. [Links]

Portaria nº 2.952, de 14 de dezembro de 2011. (2011). Regulamenta, no âmbito do Sistema Único de Saúde (SUS), o Decreto nº 7.616, de 17 de novembro de 2011, que dispõe sobre a declaração de Emergência em Saúde Pública de Importância Nacional (ESPIN) e institui a Força Nacional do Sistema Único de Saúde (FN-SUS). Brasília, DF: Ministério da Saúde . [Links]

Portaria nº 30, de 7 de julho de 2005. (2005). Institui o Centro de Informações Estratégicas em Vigilância em Saúde, define suas atribuições, composição e coordenação. Brasília, DF: Ministério da Saúde . [Links]

Portaria nº 454, de 20 de março de 2020. (2020). Declara, em todo território nacional, o estado de transmissão comunitária do coronavírus (COVID-19). Brasília, DF: Ministério da Saúde . [Links]

Portaria nº 639, de 31 de março de 2020. (2020). Dispõe sobre a Ação Estratégica "O Brasil Conta Comigo - Profissionais da Saúde", voltada à capacitação e ao cadastramento de profissionais da área de saúde, para o enfrentamento à pandemia do coronavírus (COVID-19). Brasília, DF: Ministério da Saúde . [Links]

Portaria nº 188, de 3 de fevereiro de 2020. (2020). Declara Emergência em Saúde Pública de importância Nacional (ESPIN) em decorrência da Infecção Humana pelo novo Coronavírus (2019-nCoV). Brasília, DF. [Links]

Programa das Nações Unidas para o Desenvolvimento. (2020). Gestão de Riscos e Desastres Naturais. Brasília, DF: Autor . Recuperado dehttps://www.br.undp.org/content/brazil/pt/home/projects/risco-e-desastres.html [Links]

Programa das Nações Unidas para o Meio Ambiente. (2020, 03 de março). *Coronavirus outbreak highlights need to address threats to ecosystems and wildlife*. Recuperado de https://www.unenvironment.org/news-and-stories/story/coronavirus-outbreak-highlights-need-address-threats-ecosystems-and-wildlife [Links]

Quarantelli, E. L., Lagadec, P., & Boin, A. (2007). A heuristic approach to future disasters and crises: new, old, and in-between types. In H. Rodriguez, E L. Quarantelli, R. Dynes (Eds.), *Handbook of disaster research* (pp. 16-41). New York, NY: Springer. [Links]

Resolução nº 588, de 12 de julho de 2018. (2018). Fica instituída a Política Nacional de Vigilância em Saúde (PNVS), aprovada por meio desta resolução. Brasília, DF: Conselho Nacional de Secretarias Municipais de Saúde. [Links]

Reuters. (2020, 26 de maio). *Special Report: Bolsonaro brought in his generals to fight coronavirus. Brazil is losing the battle*. Recuperado dehttps://www.reuters.com/article/us-health-coronavirus-brazil-response-sp-idUSKBN2321DU [Links]

Rumbach, A. (2016). Decentralization and small cities: Towards more effective urban disaster governance?Habitat International, *52*(2015), 35-42. [Links]

Sabatier, P. A. (Ed.). (2007). *Theories of the Policy Process*. Boulder, Colorado: Westview Press. [Links]

Secretaria Nacional de Defesa Civil. (2007). *Política Nacional de Defesa Civil*. Brasília, DF: Ministério da Integração Nacional. [Links]

Stoker, G. (1998). Governance as theory: five propositions. *International Social Science Journal, 50*, 17-28. [Links]

Tierney, K. (2012). Disaster Governance: Social, Political, and Economic Dimensions. *Annual Review of Environment and Resources, 37*(1), 341-363. [Links]

Wisner, B, Adams, J. (2002). Environmental health in emergencies and disasters: a practical guide. Geneva, Switzerland: World Health Organization. Recuperado de https://apps.who.int/iris/handle/10665/42561 [Links]

United Nations Office for Disaster Risk Reduction. (2009). *UNISDR terminology on disaster risk reduction*. Recuperado de https://www.undrr.org/publication/2009-unisdr-terminology-disaster-risk-reduction [Links]

United Nations Office for Disaster Risk Reduction. (2015). Marco de Sendai para la Reducción del Riesgo de Desastres 2015-2030. Recuperado de https://www.preventionweb.net/files/43291_spanishsendaiframeworkfordisasterri.pdf [Links]

Zurita, M. de L. M., Cook, B., Harms, L., & March, A. (2015). Towards New Disaster Governance: Subsidiarity as a Critical Tool. *Environmental Policy and Governance*, *25*(6), 386-398. [Links]

Karina Furtado Rodrigues - Ph.D. in Administration from the Brazilian School of Public Administration and Business of the Getulio Vargas Foundation (FGV EBAPE); Professor of the Post-Graduate Program in Military Sciences (PPGCM) at the Meira Mattos Institute, in the Brazilian Army Command and General Staff College (IMM/ECEME). E-mail: karinafrodrigues@gmail.com

Mariana Montez Carpes - Ph.D. in International Relations from the University of Hamburg; Professor of the Post-Graduate Program in Military Sciences (PPGCM) at the Meira Mattos Institute, in the Brazilian Army Command and General Staff College (IMM/ECEME). E-mail: mariana.montez.carpes@gmail.com

Carolina Gomes Raffagnato - Bachelor Degree in Chemical Engineering from the Federal University of Rio de Janeiro; M.A. Student of the Post-Graduate Program in Military Sciences (PPGCM) at the Meira Mattos Institute, in the Brazilian Army Command and General Staff College (IMM/ECEME). E-mail: carolina.raffagnato@gmail.com

2. The Brazilian Healthcare System and COVID-19

The first confirmed case of COVID-19 in Brazil was reported in the city of São Paulo on February 25, 2020. By mid-June, Brazil had the second largest number of confirmed COVID-19 cases and deaths globally, with a 4.9 percent case fatality rate (CFR) as estimated by the Ministry of Health (MOH). These numbers are to be taken with caution, since recent reports point to a large degree of under-notification in cases and deaths in the country. Considering both the number of deaths and the speed of spread, Brazil is among the most exposed countries in the whole world, and the single most exposed country in the Latin America and Caribbean (LAC) region. This rapid increase in cases puts additional pressure on Brazil's Unified Health System (or Sistema Único de Saúde, SUS), the country's public health care network, which is the primary (and often only) source of care for over 75 percent of the population, especially among the poor.

The SUS, often referred to as the biggest public health care system in the world, is funded through general taxes, and offers universal access to health care at no cost at the point of delivery. The COVID-19 pandemic will pose additional pressure on a system that is already pushed to the limit and is often seen as overcrowded and unable to offer anything beyond limited access to hospital and specialist care. The SUS will not be immune from the challenges that cases per 100,000 people in the country are in the northern states of Amapá (3,241), Roraima (1,959), Amazonas (1,623), and Acre (1,395). These rates are significantly higher than those observed even in the most severely affected countries around the world.

Figure 4: COVID-19 Cases and Deaths across Brazilian States per Population as of June 25
Confirmed COVID-19 Cases per 100,000 People

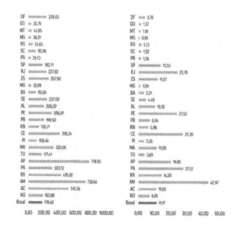

There are several reasons why the spread of the virus in Brazil's North region can be particularly problematic. Firstly, even by Brazilian standards, the region has a deficit in ICU beds, with many municipalities not having the appropriate facilities to care for patients who may fall ill due to severe complications from COVID-19 (figures 5 and 6). Secondly, states like Roraima and Amapá have large and virtually open borders with Venezuela and French Guiana, respectively, which can make it more challenging to control virus transmission from one territory to another.

Thirdly, the geography of the region imposes transportation challenges, which means that people cannot be taken easily from their municipality of residence to another where to find appropriate health care facilities. Finally, the region is home to the largest indigenous groups in the country, and indigenous people often have lower immunity to new diseases than those who live in urban areas.

Figure 5a: Intensive Care Unit Beds—
Non-SUS (per 100,000 people)

Figure 5b: Intensive Care Unit Beds—
SUS (per 100,000 people)

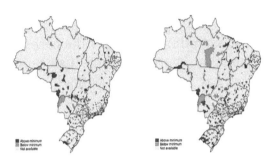

Note: "Below minimum" represents less than 10 adult ICU beds per 100,000 people. "Above minimum" represents more than 10 adult ICU beds per 100,000 people. Source: World Bank using DATASUS - February 2020.

At the outset of the pandemic, the Brazilian federal government tried to coordinate its response to the crisis with subnational governments. In fact, more than three weeks before the first case was reported in Brazil, the government issued guidance laying down a set of measures to address a public health emergency resulting from COVID-19.All states in the country were encouraged to follow and adapt the National Contingency Plan based on their infrastructure and regional characteristics. By March 20, the MOH recognized that community transmission was already taking place in Brazil. The recognition of community transmission allowed policymakers across the country to adopt non-pharmacological measures to fight the pandemic, including social distancing and quarantine.

By the end of March, most of the states and larger municipalities had implemented social distancing measures to contain the spread of the virus. While subnational authorities promoted strong containment measures in order to decrease the levels of disease transmission and prevent their local health care systems from being overwhelmed, the debate on whether to adopt a vertical or horizontal social isolation strategy remains (the former focusing on the selective isolation of groups with the highest risk of clinical severity, such as the elderly and those with chronic diseases, as well as all confirmed cases; while the latter establishes social distancing measures for the entire population). The debate over these strategies focuses on the economic and social consequences of each of them.

Despite the lack of agreement among policy makers, horizontal social isolation measures were applied in most states—although with limited adherence. As mentioned above, the highest social distancing level achieved was 62.2 percent in late March. Notwithstanding the challenges related to implementing a national response strategy, the federal government has significantly increased the level of resources allocated to the SUS to respond to the COVID-19 pandemic. By early April, the federal government had already committed R$16.7 billion in resources to states, hospitals and federal government agencies to support the response to the COVID-19 pandemic. In addition to these measures, the MOH introduced telemedicine services to allow physicians to make online consultations and to issue prescriptions electronically; increased the number of ICU beds available in the SUS network; and ramped up efforts to hire more physicians (the plan is to hire over 5,800 physicians across the country).

Both the novel coronavirus pandemic and the measures to contain its spread result in losses of livelihood. According to the World Bank's April 2020 LAC Semi-annual Report,11 containment measures such as social distancing work best when they are applied with a broad and clear focus. These measures are intended to slow the spread of the virus, also known as "flattening the curve", thus giving health care systems enough time to stagger the cases that require treatment in limited intensive care units. Yet, this results in severe economic dislocations and can threaten livelihoods. Finding the right balance between saving lives and saving livelihoods is the core challenge of the COVID-19 pandemic.

3. Is Brazil Prepared for The New Era of Infectious Disease Epidemics?

Creuza Rachel Vicente[1]

The world has been facing a new era of emerging and re-emerging infectious diseases and the century XXI possibly will be marked by frequent, complex, and impactful epidemics[1]. Nowadays, an unprecedented pandemic related to severe acute respiratory syndrome coronavirus 2 (SARS-CoV-2) is imposing social and economic losses. Preventive measures, such as travel restrictions and quarantine for entire populations, are been adopted on a global scale, and the health systems of developing and developed countries are being overwhelmed due to the increase of services demand. The health systems of all countries must be constantly prepared to deal with emerging and re-emerging infectious diseases, in an integrated cycle of preparation, response, and recovery[1]. Global health needs an efficient local response since infectious diseases present a fast spread in the globalized world. Therefore, the implementation of the International Health Regulations (IHR) by all nations, as well as the establishment of the Universal Health Coverage (UHC), are essential for dealing with this reality, as well as to achieve the Sustainable Developing Goals.

In Brazil, the Unified Health System (SUS) plays the main role in the preparation of the country for this new era. SUS has been acting in the response to the novel coronavirus disease 2019 (COVID-19) even before the identification of the first case in Latin America, with the declaration of national public health emergency[2]. Then, the Emergency Health Operations Centres for COVID-19 were activated to prepare organized and coordinated actions and advise the health sector on contingency plans and response measures to prevent the spread of the disease[2].

In 2018, Brazil scored higher than the world average on IHR all capacities thanks to its universal public health system. Nevertheless, health service provision and points of entry were detected as its main challenges[3]. Zoonotic events and the human animal interface, food safety, risk communication, national health emergency framework, and legislation and finance also may be improved to guarantee timely and effective prevention, detection, assessment, notification, reporting, and response to health risks and emergencies (**Table 1**).

Brazil presented all indicators related to health service provision below the world average, with a little functional capacity. It reached a score of 40% for management of health emergency response operation (world = 57%) and capacity for infection prevention and control and chemical and radiation decontamination (world = 56%)[3], indicating a compromised ability of response due to lack of case management and infection control[6]. The country also scored 60% for access to essential health services (world = 66%)[3], which affects the ability to prevent, detect, and control infectious disease outbreaks[6]. The improvement of this capacity is essential to provide critical services to maintain local populations healthy and safe, not only for protecting against cross-border outbreaks[7]. The indicators related to UHC (**Table 1**) demonstrate that Brazil needs to improve infectious disease control, including basic sanitation, which depends on sustained intersectoral investments. In the COVID-19 response, availability of intensive care units and mechanical ventilators are concerns regarding health service provision[2]. Core capacity requirements at all times for designated airports, ports and ground crossings, and effective public health response at

---

[1] Universidade Federal do Espírito Santo, Departamento de Medicina Social, Vitória, ES, Brasil.

points of entry, both indicators related to points of entry capacity, scored 60% in Brazil (world = 55% and 48%, respectively)[3], indicating low effectiveness on prevention and control measures at the subnational level[6]. All points of entry must be provided with the necessary capacities to deal with travellers, animals, and cargo transported since they could play a role as reservoirs or vectors for different pathogens[8]. Many viruses circulating currently in Brazil, such as SARS-CoV-2,

TABLE 1: Scores of capacities related to International Health Regulations in 2018 and Universal Health Coverage in 2017, Brazil and World.

	Brazil	World
International Health Regulations*		
Legislation and financing	93%	62%
IHR coordination and national IHR focal point functions	100%	67%
Zoonotic events and the human-animal interface	80%	63%
Food safety	80%	61%
Laboratory	100%	70%
Surveillance	100%	71%
Human resources	100%	63%
National health emergency framework	87%	59%
Health service provision	47%	60%
Risk communication	80%	57%
Points of entry	60%	52%
Chemical events	100%	50%
Radiation emergencies	100%	52
All capacities average	87%	61%
Universal Health Coverage# Index of Service Coverage¶	79%	66%
Infectious diseases control	70%	58%
Service capacity and access	99%	70%

Sources: *World Health Organization (2019)[3]; #World Health Organization (2019)[4]. ¶Index of service coverage considers reproductive, maternal, new born and child health, infectious disease control, noncommunicable diseases, and service capacity and access[5].

Zika, and Chikungunya, were imported from other countries in recent years[9]. Therefore, the National Agency of Sanitary Surveillance (ANVISA),responsible for the activities related to IHR at the Brazilian points of entry, must receive increasing investments to improve core capacities, enabling effective response. Brazil scored 80% for the indicators collaborative effort on activities to address zoonosis (world = 63%), multisectoral collaboration mechanism for food safety events (world = 61%), and capacity for emergency risk communications (world = 57)[3]. Therefore, the country has the national and subnational functional capacity to deal with diverse health events, providing preventive measures, but needs improvement to be considered dvanced and sustainable in these areas[6]. Zoonotic events and the human-animal interface are important capacities considering the emerging infectious diseases since 75% of the pathogens related to them have an animal origin[10]. The improvement of this capacity may permit to attain higher proportion zoonotic events, detecting animal reservoir, and vectors timely.

Since food may be a vehicle for various pathogens, developing food safety capacity collaborates to prevent infection outbreaks[6]. The One Health approach must be emphasized in the country's health system to address these two points. Risk communication also must be improved to reach out to communities at the local, national, and global levels, encouraging their participation.

In Brazil, management of health emergency response operation scored 60% (world = 64%) and was the only of the three indicators related to the national health emergency framework with less than 100%[3], indicating the necessity of improvement to incident management systems for public health events at the subnational level[6]. Besides, the country scored 80% for financing mechanisms and funds for the timely response to public health emergencies (world = 63%), one of the three indicators related to legislation and finance capacity[3]. This indicator is related to the availability of access to finance, which must be improved especially at the sub-national level[6].

Despite the high score in the laboratory capacity, it has been a fragile point to respond to COVID-19, with Brazilian National Laboratory Network having the insufficient capability to perform the tests necessary for dealing with the incident cases[11], particularly regarding RT-PCR[2]. Therefore, it raises the question of the overestimation of the real capacity by country self-assessment[7].Brazil must maintain a focus on enhancing the capacities related to IHR and UHC, especially those in deficit, and, at the same time, develop measures to prevent outbreaks related to emerging and re-emerging infectious diseases, targeting animals, human sentinels for spill over events, and the general human population[12]. Thus, the country will be more prepared for a globalized world marked by alterations in the environment and human behaviour, urbanization, climate change, and increased travel, factors that contribute to the challenging infectious diseases epidemics.

REFERENCES

1. Bedford, J., Farrar, J., Ihekweazu, C, Kang, G., Koopmans, M., Nkengasong, J. (2019). A new twenty-first century science for effective epidemic response. Nature. 2019;575:130-6.
2. Croda, J. Oliveira, W.K, Frutuoso, R.L, Mandetta, L.H, Baia-da-Silva, D,C, Brito-Sousa, J,D, et al.(2020). COVID-19 in Brazil: advantages of a socialized unified health system and preparation to contain cases. Rev Soc Bras Med Trop. 2020;53:e20200167.
3. World Health Organization (WHO). Electronic state parties selfassessment annual reporting tool [Internet]. Geneva: WHO; 2019 [cited 2020 Abr 10]. Available from: https://extranet.who.int/espar/#capacity-score
4. World Health Organization (WHO). Global health observatory data repository [Internet]. Geneva: WHO; 2019b [cited 2020 Abr 10]. Available from: https://apps.who.int/gho/data/view.main.INDEXOF ESSENTIALSERVICECOVERAGEREGv?lang=en
5. World Health Organization (WHO). Tracking universal health coverage: 2017 global monitoring report. Geneva: WHO; 2017. 69 p.
6. Kandel, N., Chungong, S., Omaar, A., Xing, J. (2020) Health security capacities in the context of COVID-19 outbreak: an analysis of international health regulations annual report data from 182 countries. Lancet. 2020;395(10229):1047-53.
7. Gupta, V., Kraemer, J.D., Katz, R, Jha A.K., Kerry, V.B., Sane, J, et al. (2018). Analysis of results from the joint external evaluation: examining its strength and assessing for trends among participating countries. J Glob Health. 2018;8(2):020416.
8. World Health Organization (WHO). International health regulations (2005). 3rd ed. Geneva: WHO; 2016. 74 p.
9. Findlater, A., Bogoch, II. (2018). Human mobility and the global spread of infectious diseases: a focus on air travel. Trends Parasitol. 2018;34(9):772-83.
10. Amri, H.E, Boukharta, M., Zakham, F., Ennaji, M.M. (2020). Emergence and reemergence of viral zoonotic diseases: concepts and factors of emerging and reemerging globalization of health threats. In: Ennaji MM. Emerging and reemerging viral pathogens: fundamental and basic virology aspects of human, animal and plant pathogens. London: Elsevier; 2020. p. 619-34.
11. Ministério da Saúde (MS). Boletim epidemiológico 07. Brasília: MS; 2020. 28 p.
12. Ellwanger, J.H., Kaminski, V.L, Chies, J.A.B. (2919). Emerging infectious disease prevention: where should we invest our resources and efforts? J Infect Public Health. 2019;12(3):313-6.

4. How Prepared Is Brazil To Tackle The COVID-19 Disease?

Rodrigo Martins Moreira[1], Alejandra Carolina Villa Montoya[2], Sara Line Silveria Araujo[1], Rafaela Aparecida Trindade[1], Dara da Cunha Oliveira[1], Guilherme de Oliveira Marinho[1]

Department of Environmental Engineering, Federal University of Rondônia, Brazil

Faculty of Basic Sciences and Common Areas, CBATA Group (Applied basic sciences), Tecnológico de Antioquia, Medellín, Colombia

INTRODUCTION

The emergence of new diseases such as Sars-Cov-2 is a reflection of the expansion of anthropic activities on natural ecosystems. Food insecurity is also a key problem that causes the ingestion of wild protein sources, causing imbalance and the contact of human populations with pathogens unknown by modern medicine and raising the importance of health care infrastructure [1]. The first case in Brazil was reported on February 25, 2020, in the city of São Paulo; however, to date the number of confirmed cases, until May 28, 2020 nationwide was 391 222 confirmed and of 24 512 deaths, which are underestimated values due to the lack of mass tests. As a result of the city of São Paulo being a hub for several national and international transport systems, COVID-19 reached the entire Brazilian states and South American countries.

Brazil is facing immense challenges with the arrival of COVID-19, since the vast territorial extension, high population density in some cities, wide variety of air, land and sea routes with connections to the whole world, and a health system with limited access to methodologies for virus detection and attention through intensive care [2,3] make it hard to control the epidemic, increase the number of people susceptible to infection, reduce the response capacity of medical attention and increase the risks of death. The COVID-19 epidemic has negative effects as well at the economic level, due to the large number of hospitalizations, prolonged quarantines, and closure of cities and local and global transport systems, which consequently affects the production chain, international relations and social functioning. In this context, Brazil as a developing country is particularly threatened. The lack of information about COVID-19 hinders the response capacity of health personnel, government entities and the susceptible population, leading to an exponential increase in the number of confirmed cases. In the national context,

it is necessary to analyse the factors that affect the spread of the virus, its control and infrastructure to respond to this emergency in order to identify places of risk and create strategies that allow reducing the negative impact of COVID-19. Disease mapping allow to understand and predict disease risk, considering observed cases within small regions and estimating the effect in a bigger region, according to disease characteristics [4]. Geographic Information Systems (GIS) are key tools that make it possible to prepare, store, process, retrieve, analyse and present geographic information and make appropriate decisions of response to the epidemics, being used to identify strengths and weaknesses, and thus target economic and human efforts effectively and efficaciously. In this context, this study aims to answer how prepared is Brazil to tackle the COVID-19 disease by applying the Moran's Autocorrelation Index using GIS. Confirmed cases and health equipment data were acquired from the Brazilian Ministry of Health's Tabnet DataSUS platform [5]. Vectorial data for the administrative boundaries were acquired from the Brazilian Institute of Geography and Statistics (2015).To apply spatial analysis, a technique based on the Moran's Autocorrelation Spatial Index was used, through exploratory analysis of geospatial data associated with area features, in which it was suggested as a possibility of non-spatial statistical measure of correlation [6,7]. Direct correlation is indicated by positive values, ranging from 0 to +1, and inverse correlation by values between -1 and 0, the negative ones. In which, for the purpose of obtaining the significance estimate, we try to relate the test statistic to the normal distribution or, as a method of realization without assumptions, the pseudo-significance test.

MATERIALS AND METHODS

Confirmed cases and health equipment data were acquired from the Brazilian Ministry of Health's Tabnet DataSUS platform [5]. Vectorial data for the administrative boundaries were acquired from the Brazilian Institute of Geography and Statistics (2015). To apply spatial analysis, a technique based on the Moran's Autocorrelation Spatial Index was used, through exploratory analysis of geospatial data associated with area features, in which it was suggested as a possibility of non-spatial statistical measure of correlation [6,7]. Direct correlation is indicated by positive values, ranging from 0 to +1, and inverse correlation by values between -1 and 0, the negative ones. In which, for the purpose of obtaining the significance estimate, we try to relate the test statistic to the normal distribution or, as a method of realization without assumptions, the pseudo-significance test. Thereby, we have:

(HH) high-high: Value above the mean for the unit and its neighbours, indicating the existence of clusters of high values of the analysed variable;
(LL) low-low: Value below the mean for the unit and its neighbours, indicating the existence of clusters of low values of the analysed variable;
(HL) high-low: Value above the mean for the unit and below the mean for its neighbours;
(LH) low-high: Value below the mean for the unit and above the mean for its neighbours.

Brazil is contained in South America and is the fifth largest country in territorial extension, the territory is divided into five regions, namely: North, Midwest, Northeast, Southeast and South, and is divided into 26 states and one Federal District, which results in 5570 municipalities. In Brazil, the estimated population is in the order of 210 million people [8] and a total of 391 222 confirmed cases for COVID-19 were registered from February 10th to May 25th, 2020. The results of the application of the Moran Index are presented in **Figure 1**.
The spread of the virus in the Brazilian territory may be linked to the financial market, since Brazilian foreign trade is fostered by China, which occupies the first place in the ranking of export recipients, so this is one of the countries that most sell to Brazil. Because of this evidence, China is the destination of many Brazilians.

Until May 28, 2020, southeast region was the most affected region, with 151 376- confirmed cases, the state of São Paulo was leading the number of confirmed COVID-19 cases, with approximately 89 483- infected people, and Rio de Janeiro a total of 42 398.COVID-19 symptoms are varied, but part of the infected population needs hospital care.

The gradual increase in positive cases in a short period suggests the need to supply health centres with personal protective equipment, beds, ventilators, pulmonary resuscitators, medications and other materials and equipment necessary for hospitalization, care and treatment of patients with more serious symptoms. Mattos et al. (2020) estimates that of the 20% of the population infected with SARS-CoV-2, 5% needed intensive therapy for 5 days [9]. From this scenario, it is assumed that of the 2 113 749 people sick with COVID-19 in Brazil, 422 750 will need hospital beds. The spatial autocorrelation of hospital beds in Brazil, presented values for the Global Moran Index of 0.13 ($P > 0.01$). Where 3.25% of municipalities present HH values, 4.44% present LL, 0.04% presented HL and 4.75% present LH values, as shown in **Figure 1**. HH clusters can be noticed in the southeast region. Specially around the municipality of São Paulo. Northeast and North region are present several clusters with LL and LH. In Brazil, these are the regions with lowest MHDI (municipal human development index) and highest Gini in.

Pulmonary ventilators are key for treating the COVID-19 patients. The spatial autocorrelation for pulmonary ventilators presented Global Moran Index values of 0.14 ($P > 0.01$), presented 2.59% of municipalities with HH values, 5.27% of municipalities presented LL values and 4.87% presented LH values. Clusters can be noticed in southeast and south regions. Northeast and North regions have only 10% of municipalities with HH values. The spatial autocorrelation for pulmonary reanimators presented Global Moran Index value of 0.14 ($P > 0.01$)with2.80% of municipalities with HH values, 8.07% of municipalities with LL values and 4.84% of municipalities with LH values. The majority of LL values are clustered in northeast region.

These results raise the flag of years of lack of investments regard operational and human resources infrastructure and lack of political interest in the health public services in Brazil. The mapping and autocorrelation analysis are key for displaying discrepancies in the public health sector of Brazil. Health services requires revision and funding for universalization purposes [1]. The spatial autocorrelation made possible to answer how prepare is Brazil by analysing the number of hospital beds, pulmonary ventilators and reanimators, factors that affect the dynamics of the pandemic and allow adequate decision making in the health sector. Spatial variability display that the northeast and southeast regions show less availability of health infrastructure, places where the number of people affected is enormous. North and Northeast regions are the most threatened by the COVID-19 disease regard lack of hospital infrastructure. This potentially leads to an imbalance between demand and supply, with precarious medical care for people with severe symptoms and increased deaths. This work is key for assessing the relationship between the number of people infected and health care systems, allowing decision-makers to focus efforts. Measures such as the capacity for hospital care, isolation, closure of mass transport systems and hygiene are recommended to avoid collapse of the health system.

Figure 1. Key health infrastructure indicators to assess the preparedness of a country to tackle the COVID-19. **Panel A.** Confirmed cases distributed by regions (top left). **Panel B.** The spatial autocorrelation of pulmonary ventilators (top right). **Panel C.** Number of hospital beds (bottom left). **Panel D.** Number of pulmonary reanimators (bottom right). All figures are presented in municipal scale. NS – non- significant, HH – High-High, LL – Low-Low, HL – High-Low, LH – Low-High.

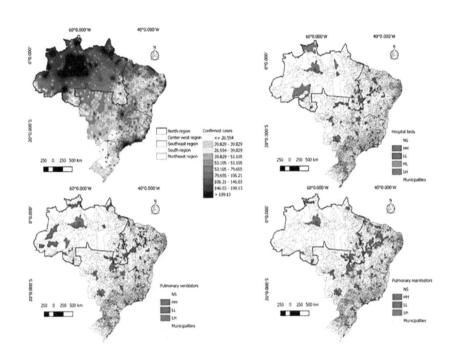

Acknowledgments: We would like to thank to the IBGE (Instituto Brasileiro de Geografia e Estatistica), Datasus and Ministry of Health (Brazil) for the data availability.

Authorship contributions: RMM formulated the argument, curated the data, developed the first draft, and coordinated continued manuscript development. ACVM was responsible literature searching, date analysis and revised the framework. SLSA, RAT, DCO, GOM collected the data and contributed to data analysis. All authors contributed to revising the manuscript and approved the final manuscript.

Competing interests: The authors completed the ICMJE Unified Competing Interest form (available upon request from the corresponding author) and declare no conflicts of interest.

REFERENCES

1 Armocida B, Formenti B, Palestra F, Ussai S, Missoni E. COVID-19: Universal health coverage now more than ever. J Glob Health. 2020;10:010350. Medline:32426119 doi:10.7189/jogh.10.010350

2 Rodriguez-Morales AJ, Pablo J, Antezana E, Rodriguez-morales AJ, Escalera-antezana JP, Mendez CA. COVID-19 in Latin America: the implications of the first confirmed case in Brazil. Travel Med Infect Dis. In press. Medline:32126292 doi:10.1016/j.tmaid.2020.101613

3 Filho TMR, Sherine F, Gomes VB, Rocha AH, Henrique J, Croda R, et al. Expected impact of COVID-19 outbreak in a major metropolitan area in Brazil. medRxiv. 2020. Available: https://www.medrxiv.org/content/10.1101/2020.03.14.200 35873v1. Accessed: 21 April 2020.

4 Zhou C, Su F, Pei T, Zhang A, Du Y, Luo B, et al. COVID-19: Challenges to GIS with Big Data. Geogr Sustain. In press. doi:10.1016/j.geosus.2020.03.005

5 Ministry of Health Brazil. DataSUS 2020. 2020. Available: http://www2.datasus.gov.br/DATASUS/index.php?area=02. Accessed: 21 April 2020.

6 José A, Luzardo R, March R, Filho C, Rubim IB. Análise espacial exploratória com o emprego do Índice de Moran. GE-Ographia. 2017;19:161-79. doi:10.22409/GEOgraphia2017.v19i40.a13807

7 Moran PA. Notes on continuous stochastic phenomena. Biometrika. 1950;37:17-23. Medline:15420245 doi:10.1093/biomet/37.1-2.17

8 Instituto Brasileiro de Geografia e Estatistica. Brasil. 2019. Available: https://www.ibge.gov.br/estatisticas/sociais/populacao/9103-estimativas-de-populacao.html?=&t=resultados. Accessed: 23 April 2020.

9 De Mattos R, Rafael R, Ii MN, Maria M, De Carvalho B, Maria H, et al. Epidemiologia, políticas públicas e pandemia de COVID-19: o que esperar no Brasil? Rev Enferm UERJ. 2020;28:49570.

Correspondence to: Rodrigo Martins Moreira Brazil 369 Amazonas St. Ji-Paraná, RO Brazil rodrigo.moreira@unir.br

5. COVID-19 In Brazil:
Advantages of A Socialized Unified Health System

[1]Julio Croda[123*] Wanderson Kleber de Oliveira[4] Rodrigo Lins Frutuoso[5] Luiz Henrique Mandetta[6] Djane Clarys Baia-da-Silva[78]
José Diego Brito-Sousa[78]
Wuelton Marcelo Monteiro[78] Marcus Vinícius Guimarães Lacerda[789]

ABSTRACT

The outbreak of new coronavirus disease 2019 (COVID-19) reported for the first time in Wuhan, China in late December 2019 have rapidly spread to other countries and it was declared on January 30, 2020 as a public health emergency of international concern (PHEIC) by the World Health Organization. Before the first COVID-19 cases were reported in Brazil, several measures have been implemented including the adjustment of legal framework to carry out isolation and quarantine. As the cases increased significantly, new measures, mainly to reduce mortality and severe cases, have also been implemented. Rapid and robust preparedness actions have been undertaken in Brazil while first cases have not yet been identified in Latin-American. The outcome of this early preparation should be analysed in future studies.

International Public Health Problems And Emergency Health Operations Centres

In the last two decades, the world has undergone important changes that impact health and the economy at individual and global levels, and these reflect directly on the public health of populations of many countries [1]. The recently emerged SARS-CoV-2 pandemic, with first cases reported in Wuhan, China in late December, 2019, quickly spread to other countries [2] and was declared by the World Health Organization (WHO) as of January 30, 2020, an Public Health Emergency of International Concern (PHEIC) [3,4]. PHEIC are extraordinary events which pose a large scale public health risk with international spreading and which, in general, require a coordinated response [5]. In Brazil, national public health emergencies (NPHE) are defined according to Brazilian Ministry of Health (MoH) as events that represent risks to public health and that occur in situations of outbreaks or epidemics (as a result of unexpected agents or reintroduction of eradicated diseases or with high severity), disasters and of lack of assistance to the population, which go beyond the response capac-

[1] Rev. Soc. Bras. Med. Trop. vol.53 Uberaba 2020 Epub Apr 17, 2020
http://dx.doi.org/10.1590/0037-8682-0167-2020

ity of the state [6]. In our current pandemic scenario, which represents an important NPHE, the promotion of actions and quick responses is necessary and Emergency Health Operations centres (EHOCs) play an important role. When necessary, EHOCs are activated and work continuously in an organizational structure by monitoring and analysing epidemiological data and field reports from various sources in order to support the decision making of managers and technicians in the definition of appropriate and timely strategies and actions for coping with such public health emergencies [7,8]. In Brazil, the health surveillance secretariat (HSS) is responsible for activating EHOCs, based on the Event Monitoring Committee's (EMC) recommendations, as well as for classifying the emergency level (zero, I, II, III) [9].

How Did Brazil Respond To COVID-19?

In the context of COVID-19 in China and the provisions of decree MH No. 2,952 of December 14, 2011 [10], NPHE was declared in Brazil on January 10, 2020. On January 22 the Brazil's MoH, via Decree No.188 [11] activated the EHOC-nCoV operations centre, with alert level 1 (no suspected cases at the time), which was coordinated by HSS. The fundamental objective of EHOC-nCoV was to respond to the SARS-CoV-2 emergency at the national level by organizing a coordinated action within the scope of UHS. In addition, EHOC-nCoV would advise states and municipalities secretaries of health and the federal government, public and private health services, agencies and companies regarding contingency plans and response measures that should be proportional and restricted to the current risks [12].

On January 27 the first suspected coronavirus case in Brazil was identified, leading to raising the alert level to level 2 (imminent risk).On January 28, the first EHOC-nCoV Epidemiologic Bulletin [13], epidemiological surveillance guideline and National Contingency Plan (NCP) for the COVID-19 with alert levels were published [13]. Epidemiological surveillance aims at guiding the National Health Surveillance System and the UHS service network to act in the identification of COVID-19 cases in order to mitigate the risks of sustained transmission and the appearance of severe cases and subsequent deaths [12]. The epidemiological surveillance and NCP are based on structured documents and evidence accumulated by other countries including China, in epidemics such as SARS-CoV, MERS-CoV and SARS-CoV-2, which had never occurred before in Brazil. However, Brazil had previous experience with other respiratory virus pandemics, such as H1N1, which started in 2009 and was responsible for 46,355 cases registered in the country until March 2010. In addition, NCP actions are based on national and state plans for surveillance and clinical management of severe acute respiratory syndrome (SARS) and flu syndrome (FS) [13].

All states in the country were encouraged to adapt the NCP based on their infrastructure and regional characteristics, as well as to provide for actions to combat the disease in their territories. It is important to highlight that the NCP is based on the information made available by WHO (based on compilation of information received by different countries) and on scientific evidence, and therefore the NCP procedures undergo necessary changes [14]. Risks should be assessed and reviewed periodically, with a view to developing scientific knowledge and adoption of locally appropriate measures [13].On January 30, COVID-19 was declared a Public Health Emergency of International Concern (PHEIC) by WHO. The Brazilian Inter-ministerial Executive Group on Public Health (IEG-PHE) was reactivated through Decree No. 10,211 (January 30). Its main attributions are i) to propose, monitor and articulate preparedness and coping measures, allocation of budgetary-financial resources to implement the necessary measures; ii) to establish guidelines for the definition of local criteria for monitoring the implementation of emergency measures and iii) to prepare reports on the public health emergency situation and disseminate to ministers [15].

Brazil declared COVID-19 a public health emergency (PHE) on February 3, and on February 6 the MoH approved the law No.13,979 [16] (Quarantine Law), with measures aimed at protecting the community and dealing with PHE resulting from SARS-CoV-2, including isolation; quarantine; compulsory notification, epidemiological study or investigation; exhumation, necropsy, cremation and corpse management; exceptional and temporary restriction on entering and leaving the country; requisition of goods and services from natural and legal persons, in which case the subsequent payment of fair compensation will be guaranteed. However, these measures can only be determined based on scientific evidence and analysis of strategic health information.

The first case of coronavirus in Brazil and in South America [17] was registered on February 26, 2020 in São Paulo. It was a 61-year-old man with a history of travel to the Lombardy region, Italy, which had reported a high number of cases and deaths. The number of cases has increased since in the territory, and several measures have now been taken. On March 13, MoH and professionals from the state health departments across the country announced recommendations to prevent the spread of the disease, as previously determined in Decree No. 356 of March 11 [18,19].

MoH recognized that community transmission was occurring across the country on March 20, as a strategic measure to ensure a collective effort by all Brazilians in order to reduce the virus transmission [20]. Implementation of nom-pharmacological measures, including physical distancing and quarantine required the determination of community transmission countrywide by the MoH. Quarantine has been controversial and must be evaluated very carefully, considering the COVID-19 epidemic progression in China, Italy and Spain.

Currently, the disease has shown an increase in the number of cases, and as of March 31, 5,933 reported cases and 206 deaths had been registered in Brazil. São Paulo has been the most affected state, with 136 deaths and 2,339 confirmed cases, followed by Rio de Janeiro with 23 deaths and 708 confirmed cases. On March 27, MoH made official (Note nº 5/2020-DAF/SCTIE/MS [21]) the use of chloroquine (CQ) and hydroxychloroquine (HCQ) in patients with severe forms of COVID-19 [22-27] The proposed protocol consists of treatment over five days, however these two drugs should be used as a complementary measure to all other types of treatment support used, such as mechanical ventilation and symptomatic medications, as well as others provided in the treatment manual [21]. Two national clinical studies to evaluate the effectiveness of the CQ use as treatment for COVID-19 infection were approved by the national research ethics committee (CONEP) [28].

Progression of Cases in Brazil and Mistakes Along the Way

The number of cases in Brazil is growing rapidly. Several measures had been taken by MoH even before the first case was registered in the country, as previously described and shown in Figure 1. It is important to note, however, that on January 27 WHO admitted a significant error associated with COVID-19 global risk assessment, which until three days earlier was considered moderate, however the disease was considered of very high risk in China, while at high regional and global levels. This may have hindered measures to implement specific international interventions in a timely manner and may have resulted in an increase in the number of cases in China and the spread of the disease to other countries, including Brazil.

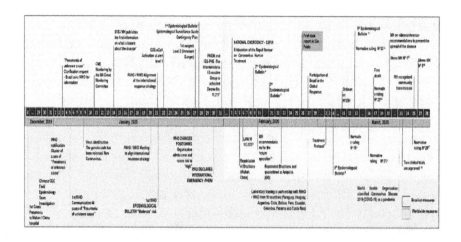

FIGURE 1: Evolution of the Coronavirus emergency and response from the Brazilian Ministry of Health (Adapted from: https://www.saude.gov.br/images/pdf/2020/fevereiro/04/Boletim-epidemiologico-SVS-04fev20.pdf)

*1st Epidemiological Bulletin: International monitoring event in Chin. (https://portalarquivos2.saude.gov.br/images/pdf/2020/janeiro/15/Boletim-epidemiologico-SVS-01.pdf)

1. http://www.planalto.gov.br/ccivil_03/_ato2019-2022/2020/lei/L13979.htm

2. http://www.planalto.gov.br/ccivil_03/_ato2019-2022/2020/decreto/D10211.htm

3. Relates to measures for dealing with the public health emergency of international importance resulting from the coronavirus responsible for the 2019 outbreak (http://www.planalto.gov.br/ccivil_03/_ato2019-2022/2020/lei/L13979).

4. https://portalarquivos2.saude.gov.br/images/pdf/2020/fevereiro/13/Boletim-epidemiologico-COEcorona-SVS-13fev20.pdf

5. https://portalarquivos2.saude.gov.br/images/pdf/2020/fevereiro/11/operacao-regresso-11fev-b.pdf

6. https://www.saude.gov.br/images/pdf/2020/fevereiro/21/2020-02-21-Boletim-Epidemiologico03.pdf

7. Treatment Protocol (https://www.arca.fiocruz.br/bitstream/icict/40195/2/Protocolo_Tratamento_Covid19.pdf)

8. https://www.saude.gov.br/images/pdf/2020/marco/04/2020-03-02-Boletim-Epidemiol--gico-04-corrigido.pdf

9. Relates to the regulation and operationalization of the provisions of Law No. 13,979, of February 6th, 2020, which establishes the measures to overcome the public health emergency of international importance resulting from the coronavirus (COVID-19) (http://www.in.gov.br/en/web/dou/-/portaria-n-356-de-11-de-marco-de-2020-247538346)

10. Establishes guidelines for the bodies and entities of the Civil Personnel System of the Federal Public Administration - SIPEC, regarding the protection measures for overcoming the public health emergency of international importance resulting from the coronavirus (COVID-19). http://www.in.gov.br/en/web/dou/-/instrucao-normativa-n-19-de-12-de-marco-de-2020-247802008)

11. https://www.saude.gov.br/images/pdf/2020/marco/24/03--ERRATA---Boletim-Epidemiologico-05.pdf

12. Amends the Normative Ruling No. 19 (http://www.in.gov.br/en/web/dou/-/instrucao-normativa-n-20-de-13-de-marco-de-2020-247887393)

13. Amends the Normative Ruling No. 19 (http://www.in.gov.br/en/web/dou/-/instrucao-normativa-n-21-de-16-de-marco-de-2020-248328867)

14. Establishes guidelines for the bodies and entities of the Civil Personnel System of the Federal Public Administration - SIPEC, regarding the protection measures to overcome the public health emergency of international importance resulting from COVID-19, related to the process of re-registering retirees, pensioners and civilian politicians (http://www.in.gov.br/en/web/dou/-/instrucao-normativa-n-22-de-17-de-marco-de-2020-248564245)

15. Memo MH Nº 114- Coronavirus and risk in patients with Hereditary Hemorrhagic Diseases (https://www.saude.gov.br/images/pdf/2020/marco/19/SEI-MS---0014038615---Nota-Informativa.pdf)

16. Two clinical trials are approved to assess the effectiveness of chloroquine in critically ill patients (https://conselho.saude.gov.br/images/BOLETIM_EP_EdEspecialCoronavirus_23marco2020.pdf)

17. Establishes guidelines for the bodies and entities of the Civil Personnel System of the Federal Public Administration - SIPEC, regarding the authorization for extraordinary service, the granting of transport assistance, night allowances and occupational allowances to public servants and employees who perform their activities remotely or who are away from their face-to-face activities, under the terms of Normative Ruling No. 19, of March 12th, 2020, and to take other measures (http://www.in.gov.br/en/web/dou/-/instrucao-normativa-n-28-de-25-de-marco-de-2020-249807751)

18. Chloroquine as an adjunct therapy in the treatment of critically-ill patients. (https://12ad4c92-89c7-4218-9e11-0ee136fa4b92.filesusr.com/ugd/3293a8_49de9bf961b846708f91cb03dfe076bc.pdf)

In this sense, Brazil has been following WHO recommendations and recent scientific evidence generated by China and Italy [29] . However, it is important to note that Brazil has distinct and peculiar characteristics, including population structure. It is a country whose population consists mainly of young adults. In addition, comorbidities and co-infections, such as diabetes, hypertension, HIV, tuberculosis, obesity, among others, are prevalent. Thus, it is potentially important that the younger population with comorbidities/co-infections are not neglected. In addition, it is important to note that fall is coming in the next days in the southern half of Brazil. During fall and winter seasons, the incidence of respiratory diseases increase (cold, flu, asthma attacks, sinusitis, pneumonia, bronchitis) and currently COVID-19 should be added to this list. Drier air and lower temperature may lead to an increase in the risk of coronavirus transmission and number of COVID-19 cases. Because symptoms of flu and SARS-CoV-2 are similar, MoH anticipated the usual free vaccination for influenza, for major risk groups, in order to help health professionals, rule out influenza in patient screening and improve diagnosis of the new virus.

Brazil's Experience with Other Health Emergencies

Brazil has already experienced other public health emergencies with diseases including polio, smallpox, cholera, H1N1 (influenza A), avian influenza, yellow fever, severe acute respiratory syndrome, and zika. Many of these emergencies marked the history of Brazilian public health policy and led to the implementation of control and eradication measures, such as for smallpox, which was eradicated in 1977. Among the most recent public health emergency diseases, the H1N1 epidemic in 2009 and the Zika epidemic in 2015-2016 are noteworthy. Both constitute an important legacy of how to deal with epidemics; the latter (Zika) demonstrated Brazil's scientific leadership due to the association of infection with cases of microcephaly [30] .

The H1N1 pandemic helped UHS improve its capacity to respond to emergencies due to respiratory syndromes (RS), an ongoing process since 2005. Currently, UHS has plans, protocols, procedures and guides for identifying, monitoring and responding to emergencies due to RS. Many recommended procedures, mainly those included in the influenza chapter of the Epidemiological Surveillance Guide, are applied in the context of suspected cases of Coronavirus [12,14] . However, the initial recommendation is to discard the most common respiratory diseases and adopt the flu treatment protocol in a timely manner to avoid serious cases and deaths from known respiratory diseases, when indicated. The UHS has the capacity and experience to respond to RS-related emergencies and currently, with the new Coronavirus protocol, it has been possible to adjust some recommendations to the specific context of the COVID-19 emergency. These adjustments are based on the information made available by WHO on a daily basis and every procedure is susceptible to the necessary changes and its adequacy may be fundamental to deal with the next pandemics that are likely to occur [14] .

In addition to that, the country counts on a decentralized network of central laboratories in each state (LACENs), with existing capacity, and a public manufacture chain of laboratory supplies for diagnostic RT-PCR, e.g., in Fiocruz (Biomanguinhos).

In case of evidence of CQ efficacy, Farmanguinhos and LQFEx are already public producers of CQ diphosphate for malaria treatment.During the Zika epidemic, Brazil led the discovery and reported the relationship between the Zika virus and the increase in cases of microcephaly. The first reports of increased cases of microcephaly occurred in the state of Pernambuco, in October, 2015 [30,32].

As soon as it was discovered by the state health departments, the MoH sent technical teams to help with the investigations and notified WHO of the situation [30]. Once the association between Zika and microcephaly in Brazil, where it occurred first, was confirmed, the first version of the plan to fight *Aedes* spp. and microcephaly was published in December 2015 [31,32]. WHO recognized Brazil's main role in this critical finding, In May 2017, a risk assessment concluded that Brazil no longer met the criteria for defining an emergency, according to WHO parameters.

COVID-19: The Way Forward

Although Brazil is attempting to implement measures to reduce the number of cases, mainly focused on physical distancing, an increase in COVID-19 cases is expected in the coming months. Several mathematical models have shown that the virus will be potentially circulating until mid-September, with an important peak of cases in April and May. Thus, there are concerns regarding availability of intensive care units (ICUs) and mechanical ventilators necessary for patients hospitalized with COVID-19 as well as the availability of specific diagnostic tests, particularly real time RT-PCR, for the early detection of COVID -19 and the prevention of subsequent transmission. RT-PCR increased capacity and serologic/RDT tests may become available soon, in part due to the private and public/academia collaboration/contribution (e.g., Farmanguinhos, Vale). Virus sequencing has been performed by sentinel sites and molecular biologists interact intensely now.

Regarding cultural differences, the use of masks is common and accepted in Asia, none existing in Latin America. This means both culturally accepted and daily routine, but also people can buy them easily there, as well as bowing more there, much more physical contact in our cultures. These differences might be decisive in the evolution of the pandemics, and also need to be addressed in social sciences protocols. Physical distancing is a measure that should be suggested early in order to flatten the epidemiological curve with the least possible economic impact. By the end of March 2020, Brazilian authorities still maintain the recommendation of physical distancing and have not implemented a lockdown through the use of security forces to prevent mass movement of people. If physical distancing is effective by limiting the public's access to essential services only, the economic impact can be mitigated while the current COVID-19 epidemic is controlled.

AFFILIATIONS

[1]Universidade Federal do Mato Grosso do Sul, Faculdade de Medicina, Campo Grande, MS, Brasil.
[2]Fundação Oswaldo Cruz, Campo Grande, MS, Brasil.
[3]Ministério da Saúde, Secretária de Vigilância em Saúde, Departamento de Imunizações e Doenças Transmissíveis, Brasília, DF, Brasil.
[4]Ministério da Saúde, Secretária de Vigilância em Saúde, Brasília, DF, Brasil.
[5]Ministério da Saúde, Departamento de Saúde Ambiental e Saúde do Trabalhador, Brasília, DF, Brasil.
[6]Ministério da Saúde, Brasília, DF, Brasil
[7]Universidade do Estado do Amazonas, Manaus, AM, Brasil.

[8]Fundação de Medicina Tropical Doutor Heitor Vieira Dourado, Manaus, AM, Brasil.
[9]Fundação Oswaldo Cruz, Instituto Leônidas & Maria Deane, Manaus, AM, Brasil.

ACKNOWLEDGEMENTS

We thank Judith Recht for the critical review of the manuscript.

REFERENCES

1. Carmo EH, Penna G, de Oliveira WK. Emergências de saúde pública: Conceito, caracterização, preparação e resposta. Estud Avancados. 2008;22(64):19-32. doi:10.1590/s0103-40142008000300003. [Links]
2. Velavan TP, Meyer CG. The COVID-19 epidemic. Trop Med Int Heal. 2020;25(3):278-280.
3. WHO/Europe. Statement on the second meeting of the International Health Regulations (2005). Emergency Committe regarding the outbreak of novel coronavirus (2019-nCov). https://www.who.int/news-room/detail/30-01-2020-statement-on-the-second-meeting-of-the-international-health-regulations-(2005)-emergency-committee-regarding-the-outbreak-of-novel-coronavirus-(2019-ncov) [Links]
4. WHO. 2019-nCoV outbreak is an emergency of international concern. January 2020. Available from: http://www.euro.who.int/en/health-topics/health-emergencies/international-health-regulations/news/news/2020/2/2019-ncov-outbreak-is-an-emergency-of-international-concern . [Links]
5. WHO/HSE/IHR/2010.4. Guidance for the Use of Annex 2 of the International Health Regulations (2005). Available from: https://www.who.int/ihr/revised_annex2_guidance.pdf?ua=1 [Links]
6. Brasil. Decreto no 7616. Dispõe sobre a declaração de Emergência em Saúde Pública de Importância Nacional - ESPIN e institui a Força Nacional do Sistema Único de Saúde - FN-SUS. Lex: Coletânea de Legislação e Jurisprudência, Distrito Federal, 2011. Available from: http://www.planalto.gov.br/ccivil_03/_Ato2011-2014/2011/Decreto/D7616.htm . Accessed March 27, 2020. [Links]
7. CDC. CDC Emergency Operations Centre |. Available from: https://www.cdc.gov/cpr/eoc.htm . Accessed March 27, 2020. [Links]
8. PAHO/WHO. Health Emergencies - Emergency Operations Centre. Available from: https://www.paho.org/disasters/index.php?option=com_content&view=article&id=642:emergency-operations-centre&Itemid=867&lang=en . Accessed March 27, 2020. [Links]
9. Brasil. Ministério da Saúde. Secretaria de Vigilância em Saúde. Departamento de Vigilância em Saúde Ambiental e Saúde do Trabalhador. Plano de Resposta às Emergências em Saúde Pública / Ministério da Saúde, Secretaria de Vigilância em Saúde, Departamento de Vigilância em Saúde Ambiental e Saúde do Trabalhador. - Brasília : Ministério da Saúde, 2014. 44 p. [Links]
10. Brasil. Portaria No 2.952, de 14 de dezembro de 2011. Regulamenta, no âmbito do Sistema Único de Saúde (SUS), o Decreto nº 7.616, de 17 de novembro de 2011, que dispõe sobre a declaração de Emergência em Saúde Pública de Importância Nacional (ESPIN) e institui a Força Nacional do Sistema Único de Saúde (FN-SUS). Available from: https://bvsms.saude.gov.br/bvs/saudelegis/gm/2011/prt2952_14_12_2011.html . Accessed March 27, 2020. [Links]
11. Brasil. Portaria No 188, de 3 de fevereiro de 2020. Declara Emergência em Saúde Pública de importância Nacional (ESPIN) em decorrência da Infecção Humana pelo novo Coronavírus (2019-nCoV). Coletânea de Legislação e Jurisprudência, Distrito Federal, 2011. Available from: http://www.in.gov.br/web/dou/-/portaria-n-188-de-3-de-fevereiro-de-2020-241408388 . Accessed March 27, 2020. [Links]
12. Ministério da Saúde. Plano de Contingência Nacional Para Infecção Humana Pelo Novo Coronavírus COVID-19. Tiragem: 1ª edição - 2020 - versão eletrônica preliminar Available from: Available from: http://bvsms.saude.gov.br/ . Accessed March 27, 2020. [Links]
13. Ministério da Saúde. Boletim Epidemiológico | Secretaria de Vigilância em Saúde | Ministério da Saúde. COE Nº 01 | Jan. 2020. Available from: https://portalarquivos2.saude.gov.br/images/pdf/2020/janeiro/28/Boletim-epidemiologico-SVS-28jan20.pdf . [Links]
14. Ministério da Saúde. Protocolo de Tratamento do Novo Coronavírus (2019-nCoV). 2020. Available from: https://portalarquivos2.saude.gov.br/images/pdf/2020/fevereiro/05/Protocolo-de-manejo-clinico-para-o-novo-coronavirus-2019-ncov.pdf . [Links]

15. Brasil. Decreto No 10.211, 30 de Janeiro de 2020. Dispõe sobre o Grupo Executivo Interministerial de Emergência em Saúde Pública de Importância Nacional e Internacional - GEI-ESPII. Available from: http://www.planalto.gov.br/ccivil_03/_ato2019-2022/2020/decreto/D10211.ht . Accessed March 27, 2020. [Links]

16. Brasil. Lei No 13.979, de 6 de fevereiro de 2020. Dispõe sobre as medidas para enfrentamento da emergência de saúde pública de importância internacional decorrente do coronavírus responsável pelo surto de 2019. Available from: http://www.planalto.gov.br/ccivil_03/_ato2019-2022/2020/lei/L13979.htm .

17. Biscayart C, Angeleri P, Lloveras S, Chaves T do SS, Schlagenhauf P, Rodríguez-Morales AJ. The next big threat to global health? 2019 novel coronavirus (2019-nCoV): What advice can we give to travellers? - Interim recommendations January 2020, from the Latin-American society for Travel Medicine (SLAMVI). Travel Med Infect Dis. 2020;33. doi:10.1016/j.tmaid.2020.101567. [Links]

18. Ministério da Saúde. Saúde anuncia orientações para evitar a disseminação do coronavírus.

19. Brasil. Portaria No 356, 11 de Março de 2020. Dispõe sobre a regulamentação e operacionalização do disposto na Lei nº 13.979, de 6 de fevereiro de 2020, que estabelece as medidas para enfrentamento da emergência de saúde pública de importância internacional decorrente do coronavírus (COVID-19). Available from: http://www.in.gov.br/en/web/dou/-/portaria-n-356-de-11-de-marco-de-2020-247538346 . Accessed March 27, 2020. [Links]

20. Ministério da Saúde. Ministério da Saúde declara transmissão comunitária nacional. Available from: https://www.saude.gov.br/noticias/agencia-saude/46568-ministerio-da-saude-declara-transmissao-comunitaria-nacional . Accessed March 27, 2020. [Links]

21. Ministério da Saúde. Cloroquina poderá ser usada em casos graves do coronavírus. Available from: Available from: https://www.saude.gov.br/noticias/agencia-saude/46601-cloroquina-podera-ser-usada-em-casos-graves-do-coronavirus . Accessed March 27, 2020. [Links]

22. Gautret P, Lagier J-C, Parola P, Hoang VT, Meddeb L, Mailhe M, Doudier B, Courjon J, Giordanengo V, Vieira VE, Dupont T, Honoré S, Colson P, Chabrière E, Scola B La, Rolain J-M, Brouqui P, Raoult D. Hydroxychloroquine and azithromycin as a treatment of COVID-19: results of an open-label non-randomized clinical trial. Int J Antimicrob Agents. March 2020:105949. doi:10.1016/j.ijantimicag.2020.105949. [Links]

23. Keyaerts E, Vijgen L, Maes P, Neyts J, Ranst M Van. In vitro inhibition of severe acute respiratory syndrome coronavirus by chloroquine. *Biochem Biophys Res Commun* . 2004;323(1):264-268. doi:10.1016/j.bbrc.2004.08.085.

24. Wang M, Cao R, Zhang L, Yang X, Liu J, Xu M, Shi Z, Hu Z, Zhong W, Xiao G. Remdesivir and chloroquine effectively inhibit the recently emerged novel coronavirus (2019-nCoV) in vitro. *Cell Res* . 2020;30(3):269-271. doi:10.1038/s41422-020-0282-0. [Links]

25. Gao J, Tian Z, Yang X. Breakthrough: Chloroquine phosphate has shown apparent efficacy in treatment of COVID-19 associated pneumonia in clinical studies. Biosci Trends. February 2020. doi:10.5582/bst.2020.01047. [Links]

26. Multicentre collaboration group of Department of Science and Technology of Guangdong Province and Health Commission of Guangdong Province for chloroquine in the treatment of novel coronavirus pneumonia [Expert Consensus on Chloroquine Phosphate for the Treatment of Novel Coronavirus Pneumonia]. Zhonghua Jie He He Hu Xi Za Zhi. 2020;43(3). doi:10.3760/CMA.J.ISSN.1001-0939.2020.03.009. [Links]

27. LCI richtlijnen. https://lci.rivm.nl/COVID-19/bijlage/behandeladvies . (Accessed on 6th March 2020). Cited March 20, 2020. [Links]

28. Brasil. Comissão Nacional de Ética em Pesquisa. Boletim Ética em Pesquisa- Relatório Semanal 01. Edição Especial Coronavirus (COVID-19

29. WHO. Clinical management of severe acute respiratory infection when novel coronavirus (nCoV) infection is suspected. Available from: Available from: https://www.who.int/publications-detail/clinical-management-of-severe-acute-respiratory-infection-when-novel-coronavirus-(ncov)-infection-is-suspected

30. Brady OJ, Osgood-Zimmerman A, Kassebaum NJ, Ray SE, De Araùjo VEM, Da Nóbrega AA, Frutuoso LCV, Lecca RCR, Stevens A, De Oliveira BZ, De Lima JM, Bogoch II, Mayaud P, Jaenisch T, Mokdad AH, Murray CJL, Hay SI, Reiner RC, Marinho F. The association between zika virus infectionand microcephaly in brazil 2015-2017: Anobservational analysis of over 4 million births. PLoS Med. 2019;16(3). doi:10.1371/journal.pmed.1002755.

31. Ministério da Saúde. Ministério da Saúde declara fim da Emergência Nacional para Zika e microcefalia.

32. Ministério da Saúde. Brasil apresenta balanço após 4 anos de epidemia do zika. Available from: https://www.saude.gov.br/noticias/agencia-saude/28347-ministerio-da-saude-declara-fim-da-emergencia-nacional-para-zika-e-microcefalia . Accessed March 27, 2020. [Links]

*Corresponding author: Julio Croda. e-mail:juliocroda@gmail.com

6.Coronavirus Disease 2019 (COVID-19) And Healthcare-Associated Infections

Rosineide Marques Ribas,* Paola Amaral de Campos,
Cristiane Silveira de Brito, and Paulo Pinto Gontijo-Filho

In lower and middle-income countries as Brazil, where there is a lack of efficient prevention and control measures, the emergence and spread of the Coronavirus Disease 2019 (COVID-19), caused by the Severe Acute Respiratory Syndrome Coronavirus 2 (SARS-CoV-2) it can be a calamity considering that initial estimates of R0. To date, the impact of development of healthcare-associated infections (HAIs) in patients with COVID-19 or vice versa is uncertain. The situation gets even more difficult given the high rate of HAIs in the country as well as lack of effective antiviral therapy and absence of vaccines against this virus, what makes current treatments for this disease are mainly focused on symptomatic and respiratory support and of rigorous implementation of public health measures.

Regarding COVID-19, two recent articles in the present journal touched the problem. Alfonso J. Rodriguez-Morales and your group [1] reported the implications of the first case of COVID-19 in the South American region. In countries like Brazil, the possibility of the experiencing of significant outbreaks of infections, which were declared Public Health Emergencies of International Concern (PHIC) by the World Health Organization (WHO) it is a reality. In the study of the Cristian Biscayart and collaborators [2] emerging and re-emerging pathogens are global challenges for public health and a matter for concerns in travellers from all over the world. But, are Brazil healthcare systems sufficiently prepared? Probably not. Its continental dimensions must be considered, with macro and micro regional differences in relation to existing hospitals and problems of assisted population and available resources. In addition, other factors such as HAI and bacterial resistance in hospitals offering tertiary care are significant problems and challenges for the treatment of patients. In our country as well as worldwide, the HAIs are the most frequent adverse event in healthcare delivery. This is well exemplified in a recently published multi-centre study, involving 28 adult ICUs in Brazil reported a high burden of HAIs in acute care hospitals with the overall prevalence of HAIs of the 51.2% [3]. It is estimated that for every 100 hospitalized patients at any given time, 7 in developed and 10 in developing countries will acquire at least one HAI. The HAI is a real endemic, ongoing problem that prolongs hospital stays, increases resistance to antimicrobials, cause increased morbidity and mortality, generating high costs for health systems.

It is also important to highlight to the role of HAI as secondary infections as well as antibiotic resistance in patients with COVID-19. A recently published by Zhou et al. [4] looked hospitalized adult inpatients in Wuhan, China, that had been diagnosed with COVID-19. Half of non-survivors (n = 27/54) experienced a secondary infection, and that all but one of them had been treated with antibiotics. Besides that, ventilator-associated pneumonia occurred in ten (31%) of 32 patients requiring invasive mechanical ventilation. This is very worrying because the countries as Brazil, that have a higher burden of antibiotic resistance and higher rates of nosocomial ventilator-associated pneumonia might be worse off if secondary bacterial infections are a common complication.

In relation to the emergence of microorganisms, some factors are also important in the epidemiology of infections in these countries, including: (1) critically ill patients in ICUs, that are often exposed to numerous invasive devices and heavy use of inappropriate empirical therapy; (2) the current social mobility, with the ease of making international air travel; (3) poor implementing of infection prevention and control practices by the lack of resources, human, both in qualitative and quantitative terms and finally not least; (4) healthcare in developing countries is affected by severe poverty, political instability and diseases that may be of lesser importance in industrialized nations; (5) microorganisms such as COVID-19 and high-risk clones of multi-resistant bacteria with better adaptation in the environment and faster dissemination capacity have a selective advantage.

The outlook today in hospitals across the country is bleak, both for viral epidemics and those associated with HAI. Regarding COVID-19, measures are being taken with protocols already developed during other crises such as SARS (2003) and pandemic influenza (2009). However, it is strongly maintained that in low and middle income countries, mainly hand hygiene is not a reality, and this is among the most efficient measures to contain microorganisms such as those reported here [5]. Regarding HAI, we will have to wait to determine what impacts the COVID-19 epidemic will leave for our health system. It is noteworthy that, although we have evolved a lot among public health issues, broad and fair access to medicines, rapid diagnoses and the development of treatments for diseases neglected appear as an important priority not only in countries like Brazil, but for the whole world.

Funding

This study was supported by Cap, CAPES and FAPEMIG.

REFERENCES

1. Rodriguez-Morales A.J., Gallego V., Escalera-Antezana J.P. COVID-19 in Latin America: the implications of the first confirmed case in Brazil. Trav Med Infect Dis. 2020 doi: 10.1016/j.tmaid.2020.101613. [CrossRef] [Google Scholar]
2. Biscayart C., Angeleri P., Lloveras S. The next big threat to global health? 2019 novel coronavirus (2019-nCoV): what advice can we give to travellers? - interim recommendations January 2020, from the Latin-American society for Travel Medicine (SLAMVI) Trav Med Infect Dis. 2020 doi: 10.1016/j.tmaid.2020.101567. [CrossRef] [Google Scholar]
3. Braga I.A., Gontijo-Filho P.P., Ribas R.M. Multi-hospital point prevalence study of healthcare-associated infections in 28 adult intensive care units in Brazil. J Hosp Infect. 2018;99(3):318–324. doi: 10.1016/j.jhin.2018.03.003. [PubMed] [CrossRef] [Google Scholar]
4. Zhou F., Yu T., Du R. Clinical course and risk factors for mortality of adult inpatients with COVID-19 in Wuhan, China: a retrospective cohort study. Lancet. 2020 doi: 10.1016/S0140-6736(20)30566-3. [CrossRef] [Google Scholar]
5. Loftusa M.J., Guitart C., Tartari E. Hand hygiene in low- and middle-income countries. Int J Infect Dis. 2019;86:25–30. doi: 10.1016/j.ijid.2019.06.002. [PubMed] [CrossRef] [Google Scholar]

CHAPTER 3

FAILURE TO
RESPOND AND CONTAIN

1. Epidemiologic And Clinical Features of Patients With COVID-19 In Brazil

Vanessa Damazio Teich[1], Sidney Klajner[1],
Felipe Augusto Santiago de Almeida[1],
Anna Carolina Batista Dantas[1], Claudia Regina Laselva[1],
Mariana Galvani Torritesi[1],
Tatiane Ramos Canero[1], Otávio Berwanger[1], Luiz Vicente Rizzo[1],
Eduardo Pontes Reis[1], Miguel Cendoroglo Neto[1]

[1] Hospital Israelita Albert Einstein, São Paulo, SP, Brazil.

ABSTRACT

Objective: This study describes epidemiological and clinical features of patients with confirmed infection by SARS-CoV-2 diagnosed and treated at *Hospital Israelita Albert Einstein*, which admitted the first patients with this condition in Brazil. **Methods:** In this retrospective, single-center study, we included all laboratory confirmed COVID-19 cases at *Hospital Israelita Albert Einstein*, São Paulo, Brazil, from February until March 2020. Demographic, clinical, laboratory and radiological data were analyzed. **Results:** A total of 510 patients with a confirmed diagnosis of COVID-19 were included in this study. Most patients were male (56.9%) with a mean age of 40 years. A history of a close contact with a positive/suspected case was reported by 61.1% of patients and 34.4% had a history of recent international travel. The most common symptoms upon presentation were fever (67.5%), nasal congestion (42.4%), cough (41.6%) and myalgia/arthralgia (36.3%). Chest computed tomography was performed in 78 (15.3%) patients, and 93.6% of those showed abnormal results. Hospitalization was required for 72 (14%) patients and 20 (27.8%) were admitted to the Intensive Care Unit. Regarding clinical treatment, the most often used medicines were intravenous antibiotics (84.7%), chloroquine (45.8%) and oseltamivir (31.9%). Invasive mechanical ventilation was required by 65% of Intensive Care Unit patients. The mean length of stay was 9 days for all patients (22 and 7 days for patients requiring or not intensive care, respectively). Only one patient (1.38%) died during follow-up. **Conclusion:** These results may be relevant for Brazil and other countries with similar characteristics, which are starting to deal with this pandemic.

INTRODUCTION

Since December 2019, several cases of pneumonia of unknown origin have been reported in Wuhan, China.[1] The pathogen was further identified as a novel RNA coronavirus, currently named as severe acute respiratory syndrome coronavirus 2 (SARSCoV-2).[2] Huang et al., reported the first cases in China, with a common clinical presentation of fever, cough, myalgia, fatigue and dyspnea, with organ dysfunction (*e.g.*, acute respiratory distress syndrome – ARDS, shock, acute cardiac and kidney injuries) and death, in severe cases.[3] Afterwards, in January 2020, the World Health Organization (WHO) declared the outbreak a Public Health Emergency of International Concern (PHEIC), and next, in March 2020, it was characterized as a pandemic.[4] As of April 7, 2020, a total of 1,429,437 cases had been reported in 184 countries and regions across all five continents, with 82,074 deaths worldwide.[5] More recently, the Chinese Center for Disease Control and Prevention published data on 72,314 patients, with 44,672 (62%) classified as confirmed cases of coronavirus disease 2019 (COVID-19). Most patients were aged 30 to 79 years (87%), with mild clinical presentation (81%; *i.e.*, non-pneumonia and mild pneumonia) and overall case-fatality rate of 2.3% (increased in elderly population, with case-fatality rate of 14.8% in those aged 80 years and older).[6]

On February 26, 2020, the first Brazilian patient had a confirmed diagnosis of COVID-19 at *Hospital Israelita Albert Einstein* (HIAE). *Hospital Israelita Albert Einstein* is a philanthropic hospital in the city of São Paulo (SP), Brazil, with twelve health care units, including a quaternary hospital with 592 beds, and four outpatient emergency care units. By the end of this study, on March 25, 2020, of 2,433 patients with confirmed COVID-19 in Brazil, 32% (769) had been diagnosed at HIAE.

Given the rapid spread of the COVID-19, clinical and epidemiological data of several countries are being published on a daily basis.[7-9] However, no studies have been reported to date presenting the characteristics of COVID-19 patients diagnosed in Brazil.

OBJECTIVE

To describe epidemiological and clinical features of patients with confirmed infection by SARS-CoV-2, diagnosed and treated at *Hospital Israelita Albert Einstein*, which admitted the first patients with this condition in Brazil.

METHODS

Study design and oversight

This was a retrospective, observational, single-center study, which included all consecutive patients with a confirmed diagnosis of COVID-19, at HIAE, between February 26, 2020 and March 25, 2020. The study was supported by an internal grant from HIAE and designed by the investigators.

The study was approved by the Research Ethics Committee of the organization, protocol number 3.921.190, CAAE: 30047620.3.0000.0071, and the National Commission for Research Ethics.

Patients

The diagnosis of the COVID-19 disease was performed according to the WHO interim guidance.[10] A confirmed case of COVID-19 was defined as a positive result of real-time reverse transcriptase polymerase chain reaction (RT-PCR) assay of nasal and pharyngeal swab specimens.[11] All cases included in the current analysis had laboratory confirmation.

Data sources

The data were obtained from patients' electronic medical records (EMR), including inpatients and outpatients with laboratory-confirmed COVID-19. Data collected included demographic, clinical, laboratorial and radiological information, and was anonymized so that patients could not be identified. Demographic characteristics included age, sex, tobacco smoking, weight and body mass index (BMI). Clinical information included medical, travel and exposure history, signs, symptoms, underlying comorbidities, continuous medication use and treatment measures (*i.e.*, antiviral therapy, steroid therapy, respiratory support and kidney replacement therapy). Laboratory assessment consisted of complete blood count, assessment of renal and liver function, and measurements of electrolytes, D-dimer, procalcitonin, lactate dehydrogenase, C-reactive protein, and creatine kinase. Radiologic abnormality was defined based on the medical report documented in the EMR. Disease duration from onset of symptoms, hospital and Intensive Care Unit (ICU) length of stay (LOS) were also documented.

Statistical analysis

Continuous variables were expressed as means with standard deviations, medians, minimum and maximum values. Categorical variables were summarized as counts and percentages. No imputation was made for missing data. All statistics are deemed to be descriptive only, considering that the cohort of patients in our study was not derived from random selection. All analyses were performed using Microsoft Excel 2013.

RESULTS

Demographic and Clinical Characteristics

Between February 26 and March 25, 2020, a total of 769 patients were diagnosed with COVID-19 at HIAE. This study included 510 (66%) patients, for whom data regarding demographics, clinical symptoms, laboratory and imaging findings were available in the EMR. The remaining 259 patients had only used the hospital laboratory facilities and were followed-up by physicians not working in our service network. A total of 34.4% had a recent international travel history and 5.7% had been at the same marriage celebration in Bahia, a state in the Northeast region of Brazil; 184 (61.1%) patients had a history of close contact either with a positive or suspected case of COVID-19. Most patients were male (56.9%) and the mean age was 40 years. Only 0.6% of patients were younger than 11 years old and 6.5% were older than 65 years.

Fever was present in only 15.6% of patients upon admission, but 67.5% had a reported history of fever, followed by nasal congestion (42.4%), cough (41.6%) and myalgia or arthralgia (36.3%). The mean duration of symptoms was 2.8 days, which was the same for patients hospitalized or not. Upon admission, the majority of patients (80.6%) had no significant changes on physical examination. Considering all included patients, 20.2% had at least one comorbidity. This rate, however, was far higher in the hospitalized group (50%) when compared with the non-hospitalized group (15.2%); the most common comorbidities were hypertension and diabetes. The distribution of patients in the Emergency Severity Index (ESI) differs between the two groups analysed, with the hospitalized group showing a higher rate of ESI 2, indicating that the initial severity was greater in this group since the onset of symptoms.

Radiologic and Laboratory Findings

The radiologic and laboratory findings upon admission showed that only 7.3% of patients were initially evaluated with chest radiographs, whereas 15.3% were submitted to computed tomography (CT). Of the radiographs performed, 24.3% had some abnormality, while 93.6% of CT scans showed abnormal results.

The most common patterns on chest CT were ground-glass opacity (84.6%) and bilateral patchy shadowing (79.5%). Upon admission, lymphocytopenia was identified in 76.3% of patients, thrombocytopenia in 25.9%, and leukopenia in 21.5%. Most patients had elevated levels of both C-reactive protein and lactate dehydrogenase. Less common findings were elevated levels of D-dimer, aspartate aminotransferase and alanine aminotransferase. The hospitalized group had more patients with higher levels of C-reactive protein, procalcitonin and lactate dehydrogenase.

The other results do not show any major difference between groups. A viral panel was collected in 146 (29%) patients, and it was positive for rhinovirus in nine cases, influenza B in two cases, and influenza A, in one case.

Treatment and Complications.

Patients had been hospitalized at HIAE by the time of the analysis. Among those, 20 patients (27.8%) required intensive care during their hospital stay; in that, 12 were referred from the emergency room to the ICU, and eight presented worsening of the clinical condition at inpatients units and were transferred to the ICU. The majority of patients received intravenous antibiotic therapy (84.7%), 45.8% received chloroquine and 31.9% oseltamivir. Oxygen therapy was necessary in 44.4% of hospitalized patients; 23.6% required mechanical ventilation (18.1% invasive and 5.6% non-invasive) and extracorporeal membrane oxygenation (ECMO) was used in only one case. Considering patients admitted to the ICU, invasive mechanical ventilation was required by 65% of them. During hospital admission, most patients were diagnosed with pneumonia (58.3%), followed by acute kidney injury (9.7%) and ARDS (8.3%). The mean LOS was 9 days; considering only patients requiring intensive care, the mean ICU LOS was 15.25 days, and the mean total LOS was 22 days, whereas for patients not admitted to the ICU, the mean LOS was 7 days. Only one patient died in this series, that is, 1.38% mortality rate.

DISCUSSION

It took 3 months from the first diagnosed case of COVID-19 in China until diagnosis of patient zero in Brazil, on February 26, 2020, at HIAE. During 16 days after the first diagnosis, all cases had a history of recent international travels. On March 11, 2020, the first case of local transmission was confirmed, also at HIAE. A relevant proportion of all patients with confirmed COVID-19 infection had been diagnosed at HIAE by the time of the analysis. The patients in our series had a mean age of 39.9 years and were mostly male (56.9%). The studies describing demographic characteristics in the infected general population showed a median age of 47 years,[7,12] and the proportion of males was 58.1% in the Chinese report[7] and 50% in the Singapore report. [12]

The respiratory symptoms were similar to those of patients described in reports from China, United States and Europe.[7,9,13] However, the mean days of symptoms was far lower in our series (2.8 days *versus* 13 days in Singapore,[12] 7 days in the United States[13] and 7 days
in China.[3] Although fever was reported by the majority of patients, it was only present in 15.6% of patients at the initial assessment at hospital, suggesting not only it might not be considered to determine severity of illness, but also that diagnostic algorithms using fever for testing may mask the total number of cases and delay diagnosis. The prevalence of chronic diseases was far higher in the hospitalized group (50%) as compared to non-hospitalized group (15.2%). This prevalence was even higher in the subgroup admitted to the ICU (80%).

The mean age of hospitalized patients was higher than non-hospitalized patients (51.8 *versus* 38.6 years) and the required hospitalization increased with age (7.8% for patients aged 12 to 49 years, 33.8% for 50 to 64 years, and 45.5% for patients older than 65 years). In this Brazilian case series, hospitalization was required for 72 (14.1%) patients, and 20 of them demanded critical care, accounting for 27.8% of total admissions, a number far greater than the Chinese series, in which only 5% required ICU.[7]

The majority of patients were admitted to the ICU because of acute hypoxemic respiratory failure that required ventilatory support. Invasive mechanical ventilation was needed in 65% of ICU patients (18.1% of total hospitalizations), whereas 20% were managed with non-invasive mechanical ventilation.

The necessity of invasive mechanical ventilation was similar to an ICU series reported from the United States (75% of Washington),[13] lower than that reported in an Italian publication (88% of Lombardy),[9] but higher than the Chinese reports (47%, 42% and 30% of Wuhan; half of these treated with extracorporeal membrane oxygenation).[3,14,15] Considering the use of non-invasive ventilation, the rate was again similar to that reported in Washington (19%)[12] and lower than the rates in China (42%, 56% and 62% of Wuhan, including patients receiving high-flow nasal cannula).[3,14,15] A total of three patients (15% of patients admitted to the ICU) developed acute kidney injury and required continuous renal replacement therapy. Among those, only one patient had chronic kidney disease. The prevalence of chronic kidney disease was 2.9% among hospitalized patients in the Chinese report,[14] and 21% among patients admitted to the ICU in the series from the United States (21%).[13

This study has important limitations. First, part of the cases had incomplete information documented in the medical records, and patient clinical history documentation was not homogeneous among all patients. This is a common limitation in retrospective observational studies, taking into account that data generation was clinically driven and not in systematic fashion. Second, since many patients remained at the hospital and the outcomes were unknown at the time of data collection, we censored the data regarding their clinical outcomes as of the time of the analysis. Third, only patients hospitalized at HIAE were included in the hospitalization group, and there is no documentation of hospital admissions outside of our service network. Finally, this study only included patients attended as outpatients or inpatients at HIAE; therefore, asymptomatic and mild cases who did not seek medical care were not considered. Hence, our study cohort may represent more severe COVID-19 cases.

CONCLUSION

To date, there is no study in Brazil reporting the characteristics of patients diagnosed with COVID-19. Brazil is the country in the south hemisphere with the highest number of confirmed cases this disease and *Hospital Israelita Albert Einstein* is the center where the first patient was diagnosed, with a representative sample of all confirmed COVID-19 cases in the country. The results presented in this study may be relevant for Brazil and other countries with similar characteristics, which are starting to deal with this pandemic.

Contribution of Authors

Data were analyzed and interpreted by the authors. All authors reviewed the manuscript and checked the exactness and completeness of data.

Authors' Information

Teich VD: http://orcid.org/0000-0002-8539-6037
Klajner S: http://orcid.org/0000-0003-4120-1047
Almeida FA: http://orcid.org/0000-0001-7131-0039
Dantas AC: http://orcid.org/0000-0001-9505-6784
Laselva CR: http://orcid.org/0000-0001-8285-9633
Torritesi MG: http://orcid.org/0000-0002-3623-6475
Canero TR: http://orcid.org/0000-0002-7399-4718
Berwanger O: http://orcid.org/0000-0002-4972-2958
Rizzo LV: http://orcid.org/0000-0001-9949-9849
Reis EP: http://orcid.org/0000-0001-5110-457X
Cendoroglo Neto M: http://orcid.org/0000-0002-8163-4392

REFERENCES

Lu H, Stratton CW, Tang YW. Outbreak of pneumonia of unknown etiology in Wuhan, China: The mystery and the miracle. J Med Virol. 2020;92(4):401-2.
Zhu N, Zhang D, Wang W, Li X, Yang B, Song J, Zhao X, Huang B, Shi W, Lu R, Niu P, Zhan F, Ma X, Wang D, Xu W, Wu G, Gao GF, Tan W; China Novel Coronavirus Investigating and Research Team. A novel coronavirus from patients with pneumonia in China, 2019. N Engl J Med. 2020;382(8):727-33.

Huang C, Wang Y, Li X, Ren L, Zhao J, Hu Y, et al. Clinical features of patients infected with 2019 novel coronavirus in Wuhan, China. Lancet. 2020;395(10223):497-506. Erratum in: Lancet. 2020 Jan 30.

World Health Organization (WHO). Coronavirus disease (COVID-19) outbreak [Internet]. Geneva: WHO; 2020 [cited 2020 July 21]. Available from: https://www.who.int/westernpacific/emergencies/COVID-19

The Johns Hopkins Coronavirus Resource Center (CRC). COVID-19 Dashboard by the Center for Systems Science and Engineering (CSSE) at Johns Hopkins University [Internet]. CRC; USA; 2020 [cited 2020 July 21]. Available from: https://coronavirus.jhu.edu/map.html

Wu Z, McGoogan JM. Characteristics of and important lessons from the coronavirus disease 2019 (COVID-19) outbreak in China: Summary of a report of 72 314 cases from the Chinese Center for Disease Control and Prevention. JAMA. 2020. Feb 24. doi: 10.1001/jama.2020.2648.

Guan WJ, Ni ZY, Hu Y, Liang WH, Ou CQ, He JX, et al. Clinical characteristics of coronavirus disease 2019 in China. N Engl J Med. 2020;382(18):1708-20.

Holshue ML, DeBolt C, Lindquist S, Lofy KH, Wiesman J, Bruce H, Spitters C, Ericson K, Wilkerson S, Tural A, Diaz G, Cohn A, Fox L, Patel A, Gerber SI, Kim L, Tong S, Lu X, Lindstrom S, Pallansch MA, Weldon WC, Biggs HM, Uyeki TM, Pillai SK; Washington State 2019-nCoV Case Investigation Team. First case of 2019 novel coronavirus in the United States. N Engl J Med. 2020;382(10):929-36.

Grasselli G, Zangrillo A, Zanella A, Antonelli M, Cabrini L, Castelli A, et al. Baseline characteristics and outcomes of 1591 patients infected with SARS-CoV-2 admitted to ICUs of the Lombardy region, Italy. JAMA. 2020; 323(16):1574-81.

World Health Organization (WHO). Clinical management of severe acute respiratory infection when novel coronavirus (2019-nCoV) infection is suspected: interim guidance [Internet]. Geneva: WHO; 2020 [cited 2020 July 21]. Available from: https://www.who.int/docs/default-source/coronaviruse/ clinical-management-of-novel-cov.pdf

Brasil. Ministério da Saúde. Centro de Operações de Emergências em Saúde Pública. Coronavirus COVID-19. Boletim Diário [Internet]. Brasília (DF):
Ministério da Saúde; 2020 [citado 2020 Jul 21]. Disponível em: https://www.saude.gov.br/images/pdf/2020/marco/29/29----COVID.pdf

Young BE, Ong SW, Kalimuddin S, Low JG, Tan SY, Loh J, Ng OT, Marimuthu K, Ang LW, Mak TM, Lau SK, Anderson DE, Chan KS, Tan TY, Ng TY, Cui L, Said Z, Kurupatham L, Chen MI, Chan M, Vasoo S, Wang LF, Tan BH, Lin RT, Lee VJ, Leo YS, Lye DC; Singapore 2019 Novel Coronavirus Outbreak Research Team. Epidemiologic features and clinical course of patients infected with SARSCoV-2 in Singapore. JAMA. 2020 Mar 3. doi: 10.1001/jama.2020.3204.

Bhatraju PK, Ghassemieh BJ, Nichols M, Kim R, Jerome KR, Nalla AK, et al. COVID-19 in critically Ill patients in the Seattle region - Case series. N Engl J Med. 2020;382(21):2012-22.

Wang D, Hu B, Hu C, Zhu F, Liu X, Zhang J, et al. Clinical characteristics of 138 hospitalized patients with 2019 novel coronavirus-infected pneumonia in Wuhan, China. JAMA. 2020 Feb 7. doi: 10.1001/jama.2020.1585.

Yang X, Yu Y, Xu J, Shu H, Xia J, Liu H, et al. Clinical course and outcomes of critically ill patients with SARS-CoV-2 pneumonia in Wuhan, China: a single-centered, retrospective, observational study. Lancet Respir Med. 2020;8(5):475-81. Erratum in: Lancet Respir Med. 2020;8(4):e26.

2. The COVID-19 Pandemic In Brazil: Chronicle of A Health Crisis Foretold[1]

[2]Guilherme Loureiro Werneck [1,2] Marilia Sá Carvalho [3]

The COVID-19 pandemic, caused by the novel coronavirus (SARS-CoV-2), has emerged as one of this century's major global health challenges. In the middle of April, just a few months after the epidemic erupted in China in late 2019, there had been more than a 2 million cases and 120,000 deaths from COVID-19 worldwide. Many more cases and deaths are predicted in the coming months. In Brazil, to date, there have been some 21,000 confirmed cases and 1,200 deaths from COVID-19. Insufficient scientific knowledge on the novel coronavirus, the fast pace of its spread, and its capacity to cause deaths in vulnerable groups have generated uncertainties on the best strategies for confronting the epidemic in different parts of the world. The challenges are even greater in Brazil, since little is known about the characteristics of COVID-19 transmission in a context of huge social inequality, with communities exposed to precarious housing and sanitation conditions, without systematic access to running water, and with widespread crowding. In a schematic, simplified approach, the response to the COVID-19 pandemic can be divided into four stages: containment, mitigation, suppression

The first stage, and recovery., containment, begins before cases are reported in a country or region. It mainly involves active tracing of inbound international passengers and their contacts, aimed at avoiding or postponing community transmission. In the current pandemic, an exemplary containment stage was essential for decreasing the pandemic's initial impact in Taiwan, Singapore, and Hong Kong, despite their proximity to China. Previous experience with the first major epidemic of severe acute respiratory syndrome (SARS) caused by coronavirus in this century (2003) may, at least partially, explain the successful containment of COVID-19 in these countries.

The second stage, mitigation, begins when there is already sustained transmission of the infection in the country. The goal is to decrease the levels of disease transmission in groups with the highest risk of clinical severity, besides, of course, isolation of positive cases. These measures, called "vertical isolation", are generally accompanied by some degree of reduction of social contact. The approach generally begins with the cancellation of large events, followed gradually by suspension of school activities, a ban on smaller events, closing of theatres, cinemas, and shopping malls, and recommendations to reduce people's circulation.

This is what has come to be called "flattening the curve" of the epidemic. A suppression stage may be necessary when the previous measures have not proven effective, either because their implementation may not have been adequate and immediate (e.g., insufficient supply of diagnostic tests to identify infective individuals at the epidemic's onset) or because the achieved reduction in

---

[1] Cad. Saúde Pública 2020; 36(5):e00068820
[2] 1 Instituto de Medicina Social, Universidade do Estado do Rio de Janeiro, Rio de Janeiro, Brasil.
2 Instituto de Estudos em Saúde Coletiva, Universidade Federal do Rio de Janeiro, Rio de Janeiro, Brasil.
3 Programa de Computação Científica, Fundação Oswaldo Cruz, Rio de Janeiro, Brasil.

transmission is insufficient to prevent the healthcare system's collapse. In the suppression stage, more radical social distancing measures are implemented in the entire population. The goal is to postpone, if possible, an explosion in the number of cases until the situation stabilizes in the healthcare system, testing procedures can be expanded, and eventually some new therapeutic or preventive tool (e.g., a vaccine) becomes available.

There are controversies [1] concerning these "horizontal isolation" measures, particularly involving their economic, social, and psychological repercussions at the population level [2].Last but not least is the recovery stage, when there are consistent signs of a downturn in the epidemic and when the number of cases becomes residual. This last stage requires society's organization for the country's social and economic restructuring, and it definitely involves government intervention.

In Brazil, the question of the most adequate strategy for the epidemic's current context, whether "vertical isolation" or "horizontal isolation", has dominated the debate in different sectors of civil society, but also among researchers and professionals directly or indirectly involved in confronting the epidemic. The debate is analogous to the dilemma of the choice between interventions based on "high-risk strategies" or "population strategies" [3].Geoffrey Rose's seminal work still influences the debate on public health interventions. Briefly, interventions based on "high-risk strategies" are targeted to reducing the disease's impact and complications in a population subset considered at highest risk. Meanwhile, the "population strategy" proposes a preventive approach for the entire population.

In chronic diseases with high prevalence, there is a preference for population-based strategies, since the benefits of preventive measures are felt not only by the highest-risk groups, but by everyone. Assuming that the health risks are distributed evenly in a population, a population-based approach would reach a larger contingent of persons accounting for the largest burden of disease at the population level [4]. Meanwhile, for communicable diseases, the high-risk focus has been proposed more frequently, since the approach targeted to the groups at greatest risk (of transmitting and/or acquiring the infection) would be more efficient for limiting transmission to the entire population [5]. Sometimes a combination of the two approaches is used.

This is the case with AIDS, with population strategies using promotion of condom use, alongside campaigns targeted to groups at increased risk such as sex workers [6].The adoption of different strategies of social distancing, vertical or horizontal, must be guided by an analysis of the situation and progression of the epidemic in a given context. Thus, from the strictly theoretical point of view, an effective "vertical isolation" strategy might be the most efficient, because it also reduces the economic and social repercussions associated with "horizontal isolation".

However, the conditions are limited for the implementation of "vertical isolation" in the current epidemic's situation in Brazil. This is partly due to the fast pace of the infection's spread and the difficulties in strict monitoring and surveillance of cases and contacts, since asymptomatic cases represent nearly 80% of infected individuals.

The limitation is also due mainly to the lack of a broad testing system starting early in the epidemic, which would have allowed early identification of infected individuals. In fact, experience in China shows that at the beginning of the epidemic, 86% of the infections were not detected, but they constituted the source of infection for 79% of the cases [7]. Not by coincidence, progress with the epidemic's control in China only occurred after the enforcement of broad and drastic social distancing measures. In countries with serious limitations in both testing capacity in the initial moments of the epidemic and coverage of care for severe patients, such as in the United States and Italy, "vertical isolation" was tried initially, but the rapid rise in the number of cases required (albeit late) the introduction of the suppression strategy via "horizontal isolation".

Similarly, in the United Kingdom, the vertical isolation strategy was initially recommended, but the evolution of the epidemic and the available projections led to a change of course, with the adoption of the suppression strategy based on horizontal isolation.

For years, the scientific community in the field of infectious diseases has warned that the emergence of new pandemics is not a question of "if", but of "when" they will occur [8].

The 21st century has witnessed various epidemics that were able to be contained at some level in time or geographically, like the two previous coronavirus epidemics (SARS and the Middle East respiratory syndrome MERS), the Ebola epidemics in Africa, and the H5N1 avian influenza epidemic. Together, they caused fewer deaths than COVID-19. The H1N1 influenza pandemic of 2009, for which there is a vaccine available, was devastating, with an estimating 150 to 575 thousand deaths from causes associated with the infection [9]. The number of deaths that will be caused by COVID-19 is unknown, but current estimates indicate that the figure may exceed 2 million, even with the implementation of early suppression measures [10].

The scenario in Brazil is uncertain, and valid and reliable estimates of the number of cases and deaths from COVID-19 are hindered by the lack of reliable data on cases and on the actual implementation of suppression measures, given the contradictory recommendations issued by government authorities. Among the regions of Brazil, preliminary studies using data on interurban mobility point to the potential paths for the epidemic's spread as a potential tool for allocating the necessary resources (already scarce) for adequate care [11]. Little is known about how the epidemic will spread in (and impact) low-income communities, a completely new scenario when compared to the countries most affected by the pandemic thus far. The COVID-19 pandemic has reached the Brazilian population in a scenario of extreme vulnerability, with high unemployment rates and severe budget cuts in social policies.

In recent years, especially since Brazilian Congress passed *Constitutional Amendment n. 95*, which places a radical ceiling on public expenditures, and with the economic policies enforced by the current Administration, there is an increasingly intense stranglehold on funding for health and research in Brazil. Precisely in such times of crisis, society appreciates the importance of a country's strong science and technology system and a unified health system that guarantees the universal right to health. The immediate decisions in the current scenario should seek to spare lives by guaranteeing quality of healthcare for severe cases. It is also crucial to minimize the economic, social, and psychological harms to the most vulnerable groups through the adoption of appropriate fiscal and social measures [12]. We Brazilians should raise our voices in defence of the Unified National Health System and demand that those currently governing the country participate in the defence of our people's lives; otherwise, those same administrators will be held accountable for promoting what is potentially one of the worst health tragedies in Brazil's history.

REFERENCES

1. Ioannidis, J.P.A. (2020). Coronavirus disease 2019: the harms of exaggerated information and nonevidence-based measures. Eur J Clin Invest 2020; 50:e13222.
2. Kissler, S.M, Tedijanto, C, Lipsitch M, Grad, Y.(2020) Social distancing strategies for curbing the COVID-19 epidemic. medRxiv 2020; 24 mar. https://www.medrxiv.org/content/10.1101/2 020.03.22.20041079v1.
3. Rose, G. (1992). The strategy of preventive medicine. Oxford/New York: Oxford University Press.
4. Chor, D., Faerstein, E. (2000). Um enfoque epidemiológico da promoção da saúde: as idéias de Geoffrey Rose. Cad Saúde Pública 2000; 16:241-4.
5. Koopman, J.S. Simon, C.P.,Riolo, C.P. (2005) When to control endemic infections by focusing on high risk groups. Epidemiology 2005; 16:621-7.

6. Chang L.W., Serwadda, D, Quinn, T.C., Wawer, M.J., Gray, R.H., Reynolds, S.J. (2013) Combination implementation for HIV prevention: moving from clinical trial evidence to population-level effects. Lancet Infect Dis 2013; 13:65-76.
7. Li R, Pei S, Chen, B., Song, Y., Zhang, T., Yang, W., (2020) et al. Substantial undocumented infection facilitates the rapid dissemination of novel coronavirus (SARS-CoV2). Science 2020; [Epub ahead of print].
8. Wolfe, N. (2011) The viral storm: the dawn of a new pandemic age. New York: Times Books
9. Dawood, F.S., Iuliano, A.D., Reed, C, Meltzer, M.I., Shay, D.K., Cheng, P-Y, et al (2012). Estimated globalmortality associated with the first 12 months of 2009 pandemic influenza A H1N1 virus circulation: a modelling study. Lancet Infect Dis 2012; 12:687-95.
10. Walker, P., Whittaker, C., Watson, O., Baguelin, M., Ainslie, K., Bhatia, S., et al.(2020) Report 12: The global impact of COVID-19 and strategies for mitigation and suppression. http://spiral.imperial. ac.uk/handle/10044/1/77735 (accessed on 03/ Apr/2020).
11. Coelho, F.C., Lana, R.M., Cruz, O.G., Codeco, C.T, Villela, D., Bastos, L.S, et al. (2020) Assessing the potential impact of COVID-19 in Brazil: mobility, morbidity and the burden on the health care system. medRxiv 2020; 26 mar. https://www. medrxiv.org/content/10.1101/2020.03.19.200 39131v2.
12. Apuzzo M, Pronczuk, M. COVID-19's economic pain is universal. But relief? Depends on where you live. The New York Times 2020; 23 mar. https://www.nytimes.com/2020/03/23/ world/europe/coronavirus-economic-reliefwages.html.

3. Estimate of Underreporting Of COVID-19 In Brazil

Leonardo Costa Ribeiro[1]
Américo Tristão Bernardes[2]

ABSTRACT

The number of COVID-19 infected people in each country is a crucial factor to determine public policies. It guides the governments to strengthen movement restrictions of people or to relieve it. The number of infected people is very important to forecast the needs of the health systems, which are collapsing in many countries. Thus, underreporting of infected people is a huge problem, since authorities do not know the real problem and act in darkness. In the present work, we discuss this subject for the Brazilian case. We take the time series of acute respiratory syndromes reported in the health public system in the last ten years and estimated the number for March/20 when the COVID-19 appeared in Brazil. Our results show a 7.7:1 rate of underreporting, meaning that the real cases in Brazil should be, at least, seven times the publicized number.

INTRODUCTION

As pointed out by the World Health Organization, by several epidemiologists and massively disseminated by the media whether in Brazil or globally, it is extremely important to know the real number of COVID-19 cases. This number informs the stage of evolution of a pandemic in each location and allows us to project its further evolution, giving to the government conditions to decide to harder containment measures or even know if it is time to relieve such measures. However, several countries have been facing great difficulties in estimating the real amount of infected people mainly due to reduced capacity for COVID-19 diagnostic tests.

Among these difficulties are absence of adequate laboratory infrastructure and qualified people, which are often not available in the appropriate quantity; difficulty in buying tests due to high international demand and low availability of suppliers; logistical difficulty in the national distribution of tests in a country of continental dimensions such as Brazil. Among the countries with population greater than 1 million people, Brazil is in the 13th position in the rank of infected reported people, but it is in the 29th position in the ranking of application of diagnostic tests. Up to 04/12/2020, 296 tests per million inhabitants have been applied (Figure 1). While the USA has applied about 8,000 tests per million inhabitants and countries like Germany and Italy have applied about 16,000 tests per million inhabitants. This statistic makes clear the low effectiveness in confirming cases of infected people by COVID-19 in Brazil. We presume that there is a large gap between the number of suspected and confirmed cases in Brazil. Therefore, there is great

[1] Professor of Departamento de Ciências Econômicas and Centro de Desenvolvimento e Planejamento Regional (CEDEPLAR) at Universidade Federal de Minas Gerais
(UFMG). E-mail: lcr@cedeplar.ufmg.br
[2] Professor of Departamento de Física at Universidade Federal de Ouro Preto (UFOP).
E-mail: atb@iceb.ufop.br

uncertainty about the actual number of cases of COVID-19 infection and, consequently, the current stage of the evolution of the pandemic in Brazil and which containment measures are necessary. Thus, it can be suspected that there is an underreporting of cases in Brazil. This was pointed out in a study by the London School of Hygiene and Tropical Medicine (LSHTM)[1] that estimated that only 11% of the actual cases of deaths were being reported, which generates a 9:1 ratio between the actual cases and those reported.

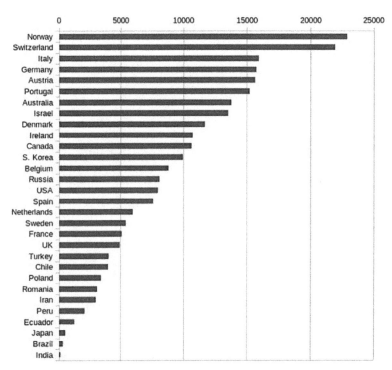

Figure 1 - COVID-19 diagnostic test ranking. 30 countries with higher number of infected people. Only countries with population greater than 1 M inhabitants have been computed. (Source: WorldoMeters[2]; Author's elaboration)

The present paper has been also developed seeking to estimate the proportion between real and confirmed cases. Different from previous studies, we do not consider only the cases of deaths, but all the cases of hospitalization in Brazil having as cause some type of acute respiratory syndrome (ARS).

DATA AND METHODOLOGY

Statistics on the number of hospitalizations in Brazil by ARS are collected by Fundação Oswaldo Cruz - Fiocruz[3] and are available on the website http://info.gripe.fiocruz.br/. The total number of new cases of hospitalization by ARS for the months from January, February, and March, from 2012 up to 2020 are shown in Table 1. Plots of temporal evolution for January, February and March were constructed in the period considered and shown in Figures 2 respectively.

---

[1] https://cmmid.github.io/topics/covid19/severity/global_cfr_estimates.html

[2] . https://www.worldometers.info/coronavirus/covid-19-testing/ accessed on 04/12/2020

[3] Fundação Oswaldo Cruz is a public institution of science and technology in health, belonging to the Ministry of Health.

TABLE 1 - Hospitalizations due to ARS

	Jan	Fev	Mar
2020	1264	1726	12508
2019	1034	1646	3305
2018	729	772	1704
2017	718	1097	1770
2016	428	787	3821
2015	669	537	1001
2014	712	572	812
2013	581	434	638
2012	302	247	468

Source: http://info.gripe.fiocruz.br/ accessed on 04/12/2020, those data can be updated by Fiocruz.

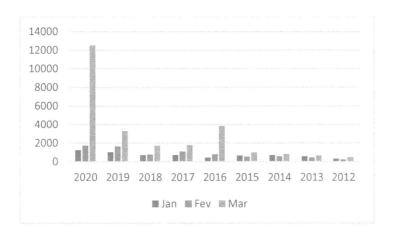

Figure 2: Total number of ARS hospitalizations as given by Fiocruz. The high number of cases in 2016 are attributed to H1N1 (Source: http://info.gripe.fiocruz.br, those data can be updated by Fiocruz; Author's elaboration)

Based on these data, a mathematical analysis of the temporal evolution of hospitalizations for each month of the period between 2012 and 2019 has been performed, and therefore, excluding the period in which the occurrence of cases of COVID-19 infection in Brazil began. This analysis identified, using the regression technique, a mathematical function that replicates, with a high degree of reliability (given by a correlation coefficient near 0.9), the typical behaviour of cases of hospitalization due to ARS. Note that this function does not intend to explain the relation of causality between the two variables, but only to be used to extrapolate data. The dotted line in Figure 3 shows the behaviour of the curve obtained with the mathematical analysis and makes clear the similarity between the modelled curve and the actual behaviour of the data. The mathematical curves obtained for each month are shown in Annex I.

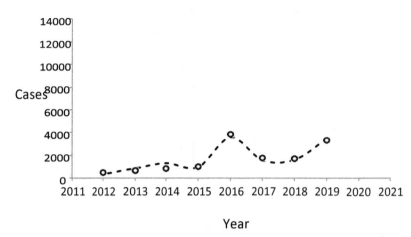

Figure 3: Hospitalizations due to ARS in Brazil in March. Circles represent real data and dotted line represents a mathematical function that matches them. (Source: http://info.gripe.fiocruz.br/ accessed on 04/12/2020, those data can be updated by Fiocruz; Author's elaboration)

Those functions allow us to use the concepts of impact analysis using time series[1]. The typical behaviour of the system obtained between 2012 and 2019 was then extrapolated to the year 2020 (by using the mathematical functions described above). This extrapolation, therefore, represents the number of cases that would be expected if the system followed its natural dynamics, that is, there was no outbreak of infection that would lead to an atypical increase in hospitalizations for ARS. It is known that, in the present moment in Brazil, there is no atypical outbreak by other viruses such as Influenza, H1N1, MERS-Cov, etc. So, we assume that an atypical increase in the cases of ARS hospitalization must then be attributed to COVID-19 infection.

RESULTS

Following this procedure, we compute the difference between the simulated data extrapolated to 2020 and the actual number of cases of hospitalization due to ARS as informed by Fiocruz:

- Cases of hospitalization due to ARS above the simulated trend for February: 404
- Cases of hospitalization due to ARS above the simulated trend for March: 9174

As we have mentioned above, this atypical behaviour would be given by hospitalizations due to COVID-19. However, the number of cases of hospitalizations for COVID-19 confirmed by the Ministry of Health are[2]:

- Cases of hospitalization due to ARS and confirmed as infection by COVID-19 in February: 1
- Cases of hospitalization due to ARS and confirmed as infection by COVID-19 in March: 1195

Therefore, we can compute the relation between atypical cases of hospitalizations and those confirmed cases of COVID-19 for March and reported by the Ministry of Health. This relation is of

---

[1] . Montgomery, D.C.; Jennings, C.L. & Kulahci, M. (eds). Introduction to Time Series Analysis and Forecasting, 2nd Ed. Hoboken, NJ: John Wiley and Sons. 2015.

[2] . https://portalarquivos.saude.gov.br/images/pdf/2020/April/03/BE6-Boletim-Especial-doCOE.pdf

9174:1195, that is, approximately 7.7:1. This means that the confirmed number of cases must be multiplied by a factor of 7.7 to obtain the actual number of infected patients in hospital conditions. This underreporting index was obtained from the number of hospitalization cases, which are severe cases. So, it is to be expected that in the general scenario, also considering the cases that do not generate hospitalization, this rate of underreporting should be even higher. Considering an optimistic scenario in which this lower notification rate is applied to all cases, Brazil would have on 04/12/2020 approximately 160 thousand cases of infection by COVID19 and not only the 21 thousand confirmed cases.

As a comparison, the proportion between confirmed cases of COVID-19 infection in the USA and cases of hospitalization due to ARS has been calculated using the information provided by the centres for Disease Control and Prevention[1]. The proportion obtained, using 03/28/2020 data, was approximately 8:1, that is, each 8 confirmed cases of COVID-19 cause hospitalization in the USA. Applying this proportion to the total number of hospitalizations for COVID-19 obtained in this study, we estimate that there are approximately 136 thousand cases, which is close to the most accurate estimate above. In conclusion, our study shows that the numbers reported by Brazilian government should be far from the real situations. In this context, manifestations of some politicians in favour of a less restrictions of people movement should be seen with enormous worrying.

Annex I

The mathematical curves obtained for each month through the regression performed:

January Cases = 67.154*Year - 134703.797 - 155.567*cos(Year + 0.104) + 47.412*cos(2* Year + 0.104) + 65.483*cos(3*Year + 0.104)

February Cases = 158.428*Year - 318551.285 - 44.433*cos(Year+0.931) +150.624*cos(2* Year +0.931) + 403.2453933*cos(3* Year +0.931)

MarchCases = 367.654*Year - 739318.297 + 473.568*cos(Year +1.667) + 995.201*cos(2* Year +1.667) + 755.105*cos(3*Year +1.667)

---

[1] https://gis.cdc.gov/grasp/COVIDNet/COVID19_3.html, accessed on 04/08/2020.

4. Floundering Power Brazil's Response To The COVID-19 Pandemic

Adriana Erthal Abdenur

Every country is facing the unprecedented challenges of the novel coronavirus pandemic, but also the magnified consequences of policy decisions made by its leaderships during the preceding years. Brazil ,a country of continental proportions that, not long ago, was widely considered to be a rising power on the global stage, is clearly floundering in its response to the spread of the virus.

This results from an accumulation of errors some of them dating back decades, but most accelerated under the right-wing government of Jair Bolsonaro. Over the past year sixteen months, Brazil has seen the relentless dismantling of institutions (including the universal health care system, called SUS) meant to protect the most vulnerable populations and the environment; repeated and frontal attacks on democracy; and the pursuit of a bewilderingly directionless foreign policy that disdains international cooperation, human rights, and climate action. All of these mistakes set the stage for a bumbling, incoherent, and ultimately, deadly lack of efficacy in responding to the coronavirus crisis. Not all is bleak. A government document released by the Ministry of Economy lists a series of measures adopted in light of the pandemic (Ministério da Economia, 2020). Those measures include: a constitutional amendment that allows detaching expenses incurred to combat COVID-19 from the federal government budget; a R\$2 billion credit line offered by the Brazilian National Development Bank (BNDES) to increase emergency capacity; expansion of the availability of medical equipment, ICU beds and telemedicine services; trade facilitation for imported goods such as personal protective equipment (PPE); and temporary social benefits to informal workers and unemployed members of low-income families. Read out of context, the list reads like a "best practices" roster of emergency responses. Indeed, many of them have been designed by well-intentioned and competent technical teams. However, standing in the way of the ultimate impact of these measures is a bewildering array of political firestorms, most of them fed by the president himself.

On the domestic front, Brazil has attained the dubious distinction of becoming one the handful of countries in the world whose health ministers were fired precisely as the spread of the virus began spiralling out of control —for the express reason that he was doing his job. Ousted Minister Luiz Henrique Mendieta, who had defended isolation measures before being fired on April 16, offered a reasonably technical leadership for the country's public health response (Lopes, 2020). Just two months into the crisis, he was replaced by Bolsonaro with a lacklustre successor, oncologist Nelson Teich, who upon taking office as Health Minister called for a "people-focused" approach yet quickly showed to be aligned with extreme right president Jair Bolsonaro's views on the pandemic: an insistence that COVID-19 is nothing more than another "little flu", and the belief that isolation policies are economic suicide.

Far from an outlier, the swift replacement of the minister mid pandemic is emblematic of a government whose empathy-challenged president, when asked to comment on the fact that Brazil had surpassed China in number of COVID-19 deaths, shot back: "So what?".

Indeed, the country's changing medical leadership is only the latest episode in the political minefield into which the coronavirus erupted. Since the first case of COVID-19 was confirmed in Brazilian territory, on February 26, the virus has contaminated over 62,000 people and killed 7,367 people in Brazil (according to official figures from May 5th, Google, 2020). This makes Brazil the sixth country with the highest number of total deaths attributed to COVID-19 (Financial Times, 2020). Yet these statistics fail to convey the true extent of the crisis. Brazil's unusually low rate of testing, the lowest among the ten countries with the highest number of cases suggests that the total cases in the country may be as much as ten times higher.

Some of the emerging evidence for this gap comes from health statistics: in many parts of the country, the number of deaths due to mystery respiratory problems is skyrocketing due to delays in diagnosis and false negative tests (Saraiva, 2020). The trend is corroborated by gravediggers in the Amazon city of Manaus, the first state capital to succumb to a collapse of the public health system; the cemetery workers report a sharp increase in burials (some of which are now being carried out in collective graves) far beyond the statistics provided by government authorities.

This chaotic scenario, and the growing knowledge that there is far more going on under the surface than the official statistics reveal, begs the question of whether there is a "Brazilian approach" to the epidemic. In fact, there are multiple Brazilian approaches being promoted by authorities —either at different levels of government or even within the same echelons, and they often clash, confusing citizens or allowing them to cherry-pick which political leader to follow in their public health recommendations. First, there has been a gap between what the president says and the messages coming out of the health ministry. While Mandetta was minister, he promoted self-isolation even as Bolsonaro continued to dismiss the gravity of the virus —sometimes during the same press conference. It quickly became clear that their messages appeal to different groups. Mandetta was shown to enjoy not only the backing of the scientific community, but also widespread popular support for his technocratic approach to the pandemic (in fact, this popularity has been cited as a key reason behind his firing) (Ceriono, 2020). Survey data indicates that most Brazilians (76%) agree with the need for isolation policies and would support the imposition of penalties for breaching quarantine (a measure that has not yet been applied) (Congresso em Foco, 2020).

Bolsonaro's anti-isolation messages, on the other hand, have appealed to groups that were essential to his election: businesspeople and key evangelical leaders (the senior military officials with which Bolsonaro has populated top posts in his government, including the vice-presidency, are reluctant to contradict him directly, but the Armed Forces have quietly adopted social distancing) (Exame, 2020).

The president's support base has shrunk considerably since the dramatic exit of Justice Minister Sergio Moro, an ex-judge who left his post leading the "Car Wash" anticorruption investigation to join the far-right government (Zafalon, 2020). Moro resigned abruptly, accusing the president of misdeeds during a carefully orchestrated press conference; among his allegations are the claim that the president attempted to politically interfere with the Federal Police, and of prioritizing personal interests over institutional ones. As a result, Brazilians have found themselves whiplashed by a series of political explosions, even as the virus rages across much of the country. Instead of harnessing his considerable powers as president of a highly centralized republic to flatten the COVID-19 curve, the president adds fuel to the fire on the political front, actively supporting and even taking part in protests that mingle demands for lifting social distancing policies with open calls for military intervention and closing down Congress and the Supreme Court. In a number of major cities, Bolsonaro's supporters have organized right-wing motorcades.

The frenzied protesters, some wrapped in the national flag or wearing the national football jersey, drive their cars, trucks and motorcycles through central streets, honking their horns (sometimes, outside hospitals treating COVID-19 patients).Although the number of people taking part in these protests is small, they tend to attract attention in the media due to displays of radicalism, including, occasionally, acts of violence (Veja, 2020). Their visibility is also bolstered in social media by the vast "army of hate" the tens of thousands of profiles (some of them bots) that carry out orchestrated vicious attacks against those who detract from the president's extreme right views. Moro followed up on his resignation by giving a deposition against Bolsonaro at the Federal Police, on May 2nd (BBC, 2020). Since then, his supporters have appeared among groups targeted by protesters, potentially signalling a schism between the hardliners *bolsonaristas* and the *lavajatistas*, as Moro's supporters are often called.

As in so many moments during this presidency, Brazilians find themselves waiting with bated breath to see if the top brass will speak out decisively so as to curb the president's increasingly frantic authoritarianism (it won't). In attacking social distancing measures, Bolsonaro wavers between different arguments. At times, he argues that isolation measures will end up causing catastrophic harm, even more than the pandemic itself. In posing a stark false dichotomy between economic growth and public health a simplistic view widely rebutted by both health specialists and economists. Bolsonaro whips up support not only among businesspeople, but also among many of those who are losing their jobs. Bolsonaro has called for "vertical isolation" (UOL, 2020), despite growing evidence that such a strategy would lead to rapid contagion and overwhelmed public health systems.

At other times, like Donald Trump promoted the belief in the efficacy of hydroxychloroquine as a silver bullet for treating COVID-19. Across these positions, Bolsonaro has eschewed scientific evidence and disdained expertise, clinging to the hopes of an easy fix that will cast him as the saviour of the economy (and thus boost his chances of re-election).

The mixed messages being issued by Brazilian authorities are not restricted to the federal government. Bolsonaro continues to face defiance and open opposition from several governors and mayors, some of whom had bandwagoned with him during the campaign and even after he assumed the presidency. The governors of the two states with the highest numbers of cases and deaths so far —João Doria, the governor of São Paulo state, and Winston Witzel, of Rio de Janeiro state implemented social distancing policies, including school system closures, and imposed relatively stringent restrictions on nonessential workers and businesses. Bolsonaro has repeatedly attacked these and other governors (such as those of the Federal District and Goiás) for their pro-isolation stances. He has threatened to reverse their policies and reopen businesses with a "flick of the pen" (*canetada*), although his ability to do so has been called into question by legal experts and political scientists (Shalders, 2020).

At the same time, some governors have circumvented the federal government by directly importing ventilators and PPE; the Northeastern state of Maranhão, for example, managed to purchase 107 ventilators and 200 thousand medical masks by routing the material via Ethiopia and submitting it to customs only once the shipment arrived in Maranhão, as opposed to the port of entry (Correio, 2020). That a state government should import humanitarian material hidden from the federal government attests confirms that the presidency has become, more often than not, a hurdle rather than a helper in combating the coronavirus.

This confusing panorama means that responses to the pandemic vary widely across the country. Some major cities have adopted stricter self-isolation measures and are scrambling to expand the number of Intensive Care Unit (ICU) beds available. Rio de Janeiro, which has the second-highest absolute number of COVID-19 cases in the country after São Paulo, opened its first field hospital in late April just as its public health system became saturated. In Manaus, the capital of the Amazonas state, the already strained health care system has already collapsed, as has the funerary system (Correio Braziliense, 2020). The remainder of the entire state of Amazonas —the largest by territory in the Union— has no ICU beds at all.

In a sad rerun of scenes that have played out in Europe and New York, in Rio de Janeiro and Belém (the capital of Pará), bodies have been shown stacked in mortuary chambers and even hospital hallways as funeral parlours, cemeteries and crematoria become overloaded (Lemos, 2020). The muddled messages sent by government authorities have had a concrete impact on the behaviour of the population. Statistics indicate a relaxation in the adherence to isolation policies in April and May, with a larger number of people in the streets of major and medium cities, including those most affected by the pandemic. In São Paulo state, for instance, whose government has established 70% isolation among citizens as the ideal threshold in order to "flatten the curve", the rate dipped to 58% during a sunny weekend in late April (Santiago, 2020).

City and state leaders bent on implementing social isolation have also faced considerable challenges stemming from the country's widespread poverty and inequality, and from the limited reach of emergency measures, some of which are marked by bureaucratic hurdles. Brazil, it bears repeating, is one of the world's most unequal countries. The country's six richest men possess the same wealth as the poorest 50% of the population, some 100 million people (Oxfam, 2019). Brazil's richest 5% have the same income as the remaining 95%. Socioeconomic inequalities also have deep racial, gender, ethnic, and regional cleavages, and widespread crime and violations by state forces generate abnormally high homicide rates compared to states of equivalent development levels. Brazil's social abysses mean that confronting the pandemic entails considerable challenges related to access to resources, institutions and services.

Social distancing has proven especially difficult to implement in the *favelas*, the densely packed urban communities that often lack adequate infrastructure, including basic sanitation, and whose residents are disproportionately employed in the informal sector (and increasingly, unemployed). For large numbers of low-income Brazilians, economic survival was a short-term concern even before the pandemic. Many millions earned so little that they have been unable to save any money or buy food stocks. According to the Brazilian Institute of Geography and Statistics (IBGE), Brazil's most deprived families spend two-thirds of their income on basic necessities: food, housing, and clothing. The economic precariousness of this low-income population —staggering even before the novel coronavirus reached Brazil, has been magnified by the pandemic.

The results are only beginning to emerge. According to one study, approximately 91 million Brazilians (around 58% of the country's adult population) defaulted on their bills in April (Ribeiro, 2020). The pandemic may yet push more millions below the poverty line and into the hunger zone. Although not all low-income Brazilians live in urban communities, these areas pose the twin challenges of dense population (which makes social distancing all but impossible in some places) and economic precariousness. Favelas and other informal settlements historically have lacked significant state presence except for repressive police force incursions. Public health services are hard to come by, and public education is severely deficient. In the absence of adequate state responses local networks of citizens have attempted to fill in the shoes of the state, for example by distributing food packets and hygiene products with donations from businesses and individuals. There have also been commendable innovations.

In Paraisopólis, a large favela in Sao Paulo, the local residents' association organized to hire doctors, emergency workers and ambulances to treat those within the community suspected of having contracted COVID-19 (Paiva Paulo, 2020). In Rio de Janeiro, the newly founded Marielle Franco Institute, a private foundation launched in 2019 in honour and memory of the late city councillor and activist assassinated in March 2018 by Rio militia, has created an interactive online map to track local initiatives to protect the favelas from the pandemic[1]. Despite being the tremendous organizing power and solidarity, such initiatives reflect, they also cast light on the state's failure in (and political unwillingness to) reach the most vulnerable populations a failure that has only been augmented by Bolsonaro's anti-poor, anti-human rights policies.

Concern is also growing for other vulnerable groups in Brazil. Indigenous peoples have already suffered violence and loss of livelihood resulting from the dismantling of institutions promoted by the Bolsonaro government. Communities in the Amazon, who had already been under attack from massive invasions of illegal miners, land grabbers, and others who have been encouraged by the president's discourse to invade protected lands in the region, are facing new threats. Given Brazil's long and tragic history of genocide against its indigenous populations, the advance of the pandemic among the country's indigenous villages including several confirmed deaths have prompted new prevention efforts by networks of indigenous communities (Quadros and Anjos, 2020). The Articulação dos Povos Indígenas do Brasil (APIB), despite facing scarce resources, little government support, and rapidly increasing food insecurity, has tried to mobilize different groups to monitor symptoms, identify cases, and facilitate access to health care for affected citizens. Yet they, too, face the considerable constraints generated through budget cuts and political persecution of civil society entities since Bolsonaro took office. Other populations in Brazil particularly susceptible to the pandemic are migrants, including refugees.

Around 264.000 Venezuelans have crossed the border into Brazil and remain in the country (Cruz, 2020), and in 2018 the government set up military-led Operação Acolhida, with the support of the UN High Commissioner for Refugees (UNHCR) and other international organizations and non-governmental organizations, to improve logistics. The operation also coordinates the process of voluntary relocation of migrants from the state of Roraima, which borders Venezuela, to other parts of Brazil. Invoking the pandemic, Brazil closed its border with Venezuela, although there have been reports that some refuge seekers are crossing back into Venezuela due to the precarious situation in Brazil, especially in Roraima, where thousands of migrants still live in temporary shelters and in the streets of Pacaraima and Boa Vista.

As of late April, there were 10 confirmed cases of COVID-19 among the refugees, and Operação Acolhida, the UN agencies, local government, and NGOs began working to expand migrant shelters. There is nonetheless growing concern about the potential impact of the pandemic among this population and its host communities. Brazil's embattled civil society has worked to boost protection of these vulnerable populations, while also working to shape pandemic responses at the national level. After Bolsonaro announced measures to support businesses, a coalition of 35 civil society groups and activists successfully pressed the government for an emergency universal income program[2]. The funds, however, have not been implemented in an agile manner; they only began to be disbursed in mid-April, and many people are finding their access blocked due to the excess of red tape. While the program accounts for female heads of household working in the informal economy by providing double that amount, policy specialists have expressed concern that the emergency

---

[1] https://www.institutomariellefranco.org/.

[2] https://www.rendabasica.org.br/.

relief will fail to reach certain categories of autonomous workers, including those in transportation, as well as the homeless and other categories.

In addition, the program's three-month duration has been criticized as being inadequate given the scope of the economic and health crisis. Although Brazil is considered to be an agricultural powerhouse, largely due to export-oriented monoculture —the sector accounted for 25% of the GDP during the past twenty years— the government's patchwork approach to the pandemic, rife with mixed messages, may contribute towards food insecurity. In addition to the challenge of feeding low income populations who have no money with which to purchase food, there may be challenges ahead in terms of distribution. Because Brazil lacks an adequate railway system, food distribution depends heavily on the class of politically powerful (but, from a public health perspective, highly exposed) truck drivers.

The Public Ministry has also sounded alarm bells that the government is allocating insufficient funds to the Food Acquisition Program, which purchases food from family farmers and encourages diversification (DiarioAM, 2020). As a result, some experts have begun ringing alarm bells about the ability of low-income populations to access adequate food, and there are already reports of residents in the favelas of São Paulo —he country's richest state in GDP per capita going hungry (Canzian, 2020). Even as the spread of the virus accelerates, the Bolsonaro government continues to take measures that erode Brazilian institutions, including those related to basic research. As in public health and environmental protection, Bolsonaro has worked to weaken public education systems, especially at the higher level, and to cut research funding. In mid-April, Bolsonaro fired the head of the Brazilian National Council for Scientific and Technological Development (CNPq), which was subjected to repeated budget cuts even before the pandemic (Saldaña, 2020). The government's disdain for research and education has even affected the work of researchers working on Covid-10, whose projects lost funding. Such moves reflect the deep distrust of knowledge and research that is not only the hallmark of the president and his supporters, but indeed their object of pride —even when faced with its fatal consequences.

On the foreign policy front, Bolsonaro offers a sui generis mix of subservience and squabbles. Here we find some breaks with Brazil's past. While its foreign policy has waxed and waned over the years, there has been remarkable continuity in some of the core principles of Brazil's diplomatic tradition. After Brazil's return to democracy in the 1980s and 90s, its foreign policy elites placed a heavy emphasis on multilateralism, universalism, and autonomy. Multilateralism was viewed to amplify Brazil's reach abroad, as well as the most effective, pacific and just channel through which to influence international affairs. When Brazilian political elites encountered what they considered to be a flaw or inadequacy in the global governance system, the strategy was to try to mend or strengthen it, not undermine the system altogether. Through universalism, on the other hand, Brazil built and maintained dialogue channels with all possible partner states, even when there were vast differences in interests, values, and aspirations. Universalism never meant homogeneity across foreign relations; Brazil always has, to some extent, played favourites, namely through the establishment of strategic partnerships, such as those with Argentina, the United States, Japan, China, India, South Africa, and the European Union. But adherence to universalism meant that Brazil could mobilize a wide array of support in multilateral fora, and that it could more easily diversify bilateral relations when the need arose. Combined, these elements (multilateralism and universalism) allowed Brazil to punch at its weight on the world scene, and sometimes even above it. The mix also allowed Brazil to pursue a degree of autonomy, that is, the political space needed to make its own decisions regarding its path to development and its role on the global stage. Not anymore. Under Bolsonaro, Brazil has mimicked Trump's impulsive disdain for the United Nations (but without the accompanying leverage) and has attacked the very notion of multilateralism, even as his government maintains the aspiration of joining the Organization for Economic Development and Cooperation (OECD). The ideal of universalism was thrown out the window as Brazil began rooting for practices it has historically rejected on principle, such as the imposition of sanctions that were not approved by the United Nations (Bolsonaro has threatened to impose sanctions on Venezuela, following the example of the United States).

Early in the presidency, Bolsonaro's foreign minister, Ernesto Araújo, sided with American foreign policy "hawks" who defended using the Brazilian Amazon as a corridor for American troops to invade Venezuela. This type of blind follow-the leader stance has not been seen in Brazil since the military dictatorship years, and it represents a direct contradiction of the principle (enshrined within the Brazilian Constitution[1]) of peaceful resolution of conflicts. Even the Armed Forces, who have invigorated on their nationalist rhetoric and sovereignty discourse, rejected the proposal as an unwise adventure. Ultimately, Bolsonaro's Chief of Staff shot down the idea publicly (Brígido, 2020). The contrast with Brazil as an international actor ten years ago could not be starker. From the (sometimes overblown) "rising power" bravado of the Lula years, when Brazil openly aspired to a permanent seat at the UN Security Council and wielded its South-South cooperation ties to deep ties to countries around the Global South, Brazil has hitched its wagon to the lopsided trio pushing for a global conservative agenda: the United States, Poland and Hungary. The country's otherwise highly professional and capable diplomatic corps, who helped lead the expansion of Brazil's embassy network to nearly every country on Earth, has been relegated to humdrum bureaucratic tasks or, at most, near-hidden attempts to provide some continuity in areas that have not been shrunk into oblivion.

It is not surprising, then, that —faced with a pandemic of historic proportions— Brazil's foreign policy has not been of much help at a time when countries compete for scarce essential supplies, such as masks and respirators. Far from it. After picking fights and hurling insults at heads of state of major partners, such as France's Emmanuel Macron, Germany's Angela Merkel and Argentina's Alberto Fernández, Bolsonaro has placed almost all of Brazil's political eggs in one basket, grovelling to his would-be kindred spirit, Donald Trump.

But the relationship, by definition, highly asymmetrical has failed to deliver the promised results (namely, a resounding endorsement by the US government for Brazil's entry into the OECD) even before the pandemic. By slamming the door in the face of established partners and neighbouring states, Bolsonaro's foreign policy has pre-empted cooperation paths that could already have been put in place had some degree of universalism been maintained, even in these cutthroat days.

Rather than spend the political capital accumulated on the global stage when the country needs it most; Bolsonaro has poured Brazil's soft power down the drain. Another case in point: China, which is not only Brazil's top trade partner, but also a fellow member of the once-promising BRICS (Brasil, Russia, India, China and South Africa) grouping. Political relations with Beijing were painstakingly mended by advisors and ministers after a series of destructive comments by Bolsonaro nearly detailed those ties. Political relations have been shaken yet again during the pandemic —this time, by Bolsonaro's third son, deputy Eduardo Bolsonaro, who has (unsurprisingly, following in the footsteps of his American idols) needled Beijing with the phrase "the Chinese virus".

In response, the Chinese ambassador to Brazil has issued a series of strongly worded messages, in an almost unheard-of display of disapproval regarding Brazilian politics (Embaixada da China no Brasil, 2020). Although the economic aspect of the bilateral relations continues for all purposes,

---

[1] http://www.planalto.gov.br/ccivil_03/ constituicao/constituicao.htm.

Agriculture Minister Teresa Cristina lead the economic dimension of those ties some private sector actors and government authorities fear that the offending comments may lead China to further react by exacting concessions in trade, or by diverting commerce to other sources of soybeans and other commodities (Jiménez, 2020). The offenses take place precisely when China. one of the world's main sources of masks, gloves, ventilators and other medical equipment being used in the pandemic— having overcome its first wave of coronavirus, embarks on a broad "mask diplomacy" offensive, offering COVID-19 assistance (primarily surgical masks, N95 respirators, protective suits, nucleic acid test kits, and ventilators) to 120 countries around the world (Mulakala, 2020). The missed opportunities, not only to receive assistance at a time of growing need, but also to contribute with the country's accumulated experience in public health are particularly glaring in Latin America and the Caribbean.

Brazil was once a leader in public health cooperation across the Global South, through an extensive South-South cooperation program (coordinated by the Brazilian Cooperation Agency of the Foreign Ministry) that covered not only bilateral projects, but also regional engagements and initiatives with multilateral organizations such as the Organization of Portuguese- Language Countries, CPLP. In great part through these efforts, Brazil developed a tradition of "health diplomacy" that draws on historic ties to public health institutes around the world (Marchiori, 2018), as well as on the idea of health as a human rights and which, over time, became a central component of Brazil's technical cooperation programs abroad. By 2017, when the program all but ground to a halt, Brazil had more than 350 completed and ongoing health projects covering a wide variety of objectives, countries, and participating institutions. Cooperation projects garnering praise in Brazil and abroad included the Human Milk Bank Program, which helped reduce mortality in the first year of life in Latin America and the Caribbean, Europe, and Africa. Such initiatives lost momentum when Bolsonaro's foreign policy even more than that of his predecessor, Michel Temer cast aside South-South cooperation, and many of those projects have since been suspended. Within Latin America and the Caribbean,

Brazil became highly proactive in the Pan American Health Organization (PAHO), which is part of the WHO system (and which has been hit by the recent US funding freeze to the WHO announced by Trump on April 14 (Mckenzie, 2020).Until Bolsonaro helped to torpedo the Union of South American States (UNASUR), which was widely associated with his left leaning predecessors, Brazil also provided the main momentum for the South American Institute in Health Governance (ISAGS), which drove Unasur's highly progressive and human rights-based Strategic Five-year Health Plan. These institutional roles and cooperation ties, built up painstakingly over decades, have been frayed by Bolsonaro's foreign policy, as well as by the dismantling of domestic institutions in charge of public health, such as Fiocruz. Other regional organizations have not provided much respite from the pandemic despite some collaborative efforts. While Mercosur, the Organization of American States (OAS) and the newly-minted and conservative-bending Prosul have announced joint efforts, these initiatives pale in comparison to the cooperation ties that could have been activated had Brazil maintained its once-robust technical cooperation program and its political role within the region. Instead, Brazil continues to scramble to implement ad hoc measures, including (ironically) hiring more than a thousand Cuban doctors a year after Bolsonaro belittled the "More Doctors" (Mais Médicos) program that brought them to Brazil in the first place —a program founded by President Dilma Rousseff to provide doctors in the interior communities of Brazil.

Bolsonaro has not bothered to hide his disdain for the United Nations, of which Brazil is a founding member. He has declared, for example, that "UN decisions don't matter for us" and vetoed the inclusion of the Sustainable Development Goals (SDGs) in the country's multi-year plan (Gullino,

2020). Araújo has gone further, referring to the United Nations as a conspiracy drawing on "Marxist" and "globalist" ideologies. As the pandemic worsens, Araújo (like his boss) has doubled down on the bunker mentality, saying that the World Health Organization (WHO) is an instrument to propagate a communist plan, which he has dubbed the "comunavirus" (Putti, 2020). Brazil's zealous alignment with the positions of the Trump government also prompted it to decline to support a UN resolution on access to medications and treatments (Chade, 2020), despite Brazil's long history of defending these causes abroad —not only at UN headquarters, but also via the TRIPS agreement.

Under attack from Brasilia, the United Nations agencies, funds and programs have maintained a low profile in the country but continue to provide valuable support to the most vulnerable populations, including refugees on the border with Venezuela.

No government on the planet has proven fully ready to tackle the immense challenge of COVID-19, but most have been willing to take on the challenge. That Brazil happens to have such an inward-looking, mixed message-giving, ignorance promoting, Trump-idolizing, Unbeaching, human-rights disdaining government in place as the pandemic strikes helps to explain the spiralling catastrophe unfolding in the country. It is now up to a motley crew of stakeholders to boost emergency measures and launch an evidence-based discussion of recovery efforts.

Technical ranks within government; Brazilian subnational governments, civil society entities; private sector actors; and cautious yet persistent foreign partners —all of these will be needed to mitigate the damage underway and to work towards a more just, democratic, dignified, and healthier Brazil in the post-pandemic world.

Adriana Erthal Abdenurl. Brazilian expert in public policy and international relations.

REFERENCES

BBC (2020): "O depoimento de Moro na PF contra Bolsonaro em meio a protestos polarizados e expectativa" (3/05/2020): https://www.bbc.com/portugu ese/brasil-52516789.

Brigido, C. (2020): "Onyx descarta participação do Brasil em eventual invasão à Venezuela", *O Globo* (2/05/20202): https://oglobo.globo.com/mu ndo/onyx-descartaparticipacao-do-brasil-emeventual-invasao-venezuela23635868.

Canzian, F. (2020): "Nas favelas, moradores passam fome e começam a sair às ruas", *Folha de S. Paulo* (28/03/2020): https://www1.folha.uol.com.br/cotidiano/2020/03/nasfavelas-moradores-passamfome-e-comecam-a-sair-asruas.shtml.

CerionI, C. (2020): "Mandetta é ministro mais popular do governo; 76% rejeitam sua demissão", *Exame* (16/04/2020):
https://exame.abril.com.br/br asil/mandetta-e-ministromais-popular-do-governo-76rejeitam-sua-demissao/.

Chade, J. (2020): "Pressionado por Trump, Brasil evita apoiar re solução da ONU contra vírus", *UOL* (21/04/2020): https://noticias.uol.com.br/col unas/jamilchade/2020/04/21/refem-detrump-brasil-rompe-suatradicao-diplomatica-durantea-pandemia.htm.

Congresso, E.F. (2020): "Datafolha: 76% dos brasileiros apoiam isolamento social contra o coronavírus" (6/04/2020):
https://congressoemfoco.uol.c om.br/saude/datafolha-76dos-brasileiros-apoiamisolamento-social-contra-ocoronavirus/.

Correio (2020): "Maranhão dribla EUA, Europa e governo Bolsonaro para comprar 107 respiradores" (14/04/2020): https://www.correio24horas.c om.br/noticia/nid/maranhaodribla-eua-europa-e-governobolsonaro-para-comprar-107respiradores/.

Correio, B. (2020): "Saiba por que Manaus entrou em rápido colapso com os casos de COVID-19" (23/04/2020): https://www.correiobraziliens e.com.br/app/noticia/brasil/20 20/04/23/internabrasil,847395/saiba-por-quemanaus-entrou-em-rapidocolapso-com-os-casos-deCOVID-19.shtml.

Cruz, I. (2020): "Como refugiados ficam vulneráveis na pandemia do coronavírus", *Nexo* (8/04/20202): https://www.nexojornal.com. br/expresso/2020/04/07/Com o-refugiados-ficamvulner%C3%A1veis-napandemia-docoronav%C3%ADrus.

Diarioam (2020): "MPF: recursos à segurança alimentar são insuficientes" (4/05/2020): https://d24am.com/claroescuro/mpf-recursos-aseguranca-alimentar-saoinsuficientes/.

Embaixada Da China No Brasil (2020): "Nota da Embaixada da China no Brasil" (20/03/2020): http://br.chinaembassy.org/por/sghds/t1758489.ht m.

Exame (2020): "Documento do exército defende isolamento social no combate ao coronavírus" (6/04/2020): https://exame.abril.com.br/br asil/documento-do-exercitodefende-isolamento-socialno-combate-ao-coronavirus/.

Financial Times (2020): "Coronavirus tracked": https://www.ft.com/content/a 26fbf7e-48f8-11ea-aeb3955839e06441.

GOOGLE (2020): "Brasil casos": https://www.google.com/sear ch?q=brasil+casos&rlz=1C5 CHFA_enBR786BR786&oq =brasil+casos+&aqs=chrome. .69i57j0.2407j0j7&sourceid= chrome&ie=UTF-8.

Gullino, D. (2019): "Bolsonaro diz que ONU está 'aparelhada' e não teme perda de voto por falta de pagamento", *O Globo* (10/12/2019): https://oglobo.globo.com/mu ndo/bolsonaro-diz-que-onuesta-aparelhada-nao-temeperda-de-voto-por-falta-depagamento-24128875.

Jiménez, C. (2020): "Provocações à China geram apreensão em plena pandemia e podem cobrar 'desconto' em exportações do Brasil", *El País* (9/04/2020): https://brasil.elpais.com/brasil /2020-04-09/provocacoes-achina-geram-apreensao-emplena-pandemia-e-podemcobrar-desconto-emexportacoes-do-brasil.html.

Lemos, M. (2020): "Coronavírus: Necrotério de hospital no Rio lota e corpos se acumulam", *UOL* (1/05/2020): https://noticias.uol.com.br/sa ude/ultimasnoticias/redacao/2020/05/01/riocamara-frigorifica-dehospital-lota-e-corpos-seacumulam-fora.htm.

Lopes, M. (2020): "Brazil's Bolsonaro fires Health Minister Mandetta after differences over coronavirus response", *Washington Post* (16/04/2020): https://www.washingtonpost. com/gdprconsent/?next_url=https%3a%2f %2fwww.washingtonpost.co m%2fworld%2fthe_americas %2fcoronavirus-brazilbolsonaro-luiz-henriquemandetta-healthminister%2f2020%2f04%2f16%2f c143a8b0-7fe0-11ea-84c2-0792d8591911_story.html.

Marchiori Buss, P. (2018): "Brazilian international cooperation in health in the era of SUS", *Ciênc. saúde coletiva* vol. 23 nº6: https://www.scielo.br/scielo.p hp?pid=S14138123201800 0601881&script =sci_arttext&tlng=en.

Mckenzie, N. (2020) PAHO hit by US funding freeze", Enews (29/04/2020): https://ewnews.com/paho-hitby-us-funding-freeze.

MINISTÉRIO DA ECONOMIA (2020): "Brazil's Policy Responses to COVID-19" (28/04/2020): https://www.gov.br/economia/pt-br/centrais-deconteudo/publicacoes/publicacoesem-outros-idiomas/covid19/COVID-19-2020-04-24brazil-policy-measures-18301.pdf/view.

Mulakala, A. (2020): "COVID-19 and China's soft power ambitions", *Devpolicy*: https://devpolicy.org/covid19-and-chinas-soft-powerambitions-20200424-2/.

OXFAM (2019): "Brazil: extreme inequality in numbers": https://www.oxfam.org/en/br azil-extreme-inequalitynumbers.

PAIVA PAULO, P. (2020): "Paraisópolis contrata médicos e ambulâncias, distribui mais de mil marmitas por dia e se une contra o coronavírus", *O Globo* (7/04/2020): https://g1.globo.com/sp/saopaulo/noticia/2020/04/07/paraisopolis-se-une-contra-ocoronavirus-contrataambulancias-medicos-edistribui-mais-de-milmarmitas-por-dia.ghtml.

PUTTI, A. (2020): "Ernesto Araújo diz que pandemia é usada para implementar o 'comunaví rus'", *Carta Capital* (22/4/2020): https://www.cartacapital.com. br/politica/ernesto-araujo-dizque-pandemia-e-usadaparaimplementar-o-comunavirus/.

Quadros, V. And Anjos, A.B. (2020): "Coronavírus de um lado, invasores de outro: como está a situação dos indígenas no Brasil", *Publica* (14/04/2020): https://apublica.org/2020/04/c oronavirus-de-um-ladoinvasores-de-outro-comoesta-a-situacao-dosindigenas-no-brasil/.

Ribeiro, G. (2020): "91 million Brazilians to default on their bills in April", *The Brazilian Report* (19/04/2020). Disponible en: https://brazilian.report/corona virus-brazil-liveblog/2020/04/19/coronavirus91-million-brazilians-defaultbills-april/.

Saldaña, P. (2020): "Governo Bolsonaro demite o presidente do CNPq, órgão de fomento à pesquisa", *Folha de S. Paulo* (17/04/2020):
https://www1.folha.uol.com.b r/educacao/2020/04/governobolsonaro-demite-opresidente-do-cnpq-orgao-defomento-a-pesquisa.shtml.

Santiago, T. (2020): "Taxa de isolamento social em SP foi de 58% no domingo; pior índice para o dia desde o início da quarentena do coronavírus",*Globo* (27/04/2020):
https://g1.globo.com/sp/saopaulo/noticia/2020/04/27/taxade-isolamento-social-em-spfoi-de-58percent-nodomingo-durante-quarentenado-coronavirus-indice-ideale-de-70percent.ghtml.

Saraiva, A. (2020): "Brazil records nearly 2,800 deaths from mystery respiratory problems", *The Brazilian Report* (23/04/2020): https://brazilian.report/corona virus-brazil-liveblog/2020/04/23/brazilrecords-nearly-2800-deathsfrom-mystery-respiratoryproblems/.

Shalders, A. (2020): "Bolsonaro diz que pode determinar abertura do comércio com 'uma canetada' semana que vem", *BBC* (2/04/2020):
https://www.bbc.com/portugu ese/brasil-52144782.

UOL (2020): "Por que isolamento vertical defendido por Bolsonaro é visto com ceticismo?" (30/03/2020):
https://noticias.uol.com.br/ult imas-noticias/agenciaestado/2020/03/30/por-queisolamento-vertical-e-vistocom-ceticismo.htm.

VEJA (2020): "Com coronavírus, 1º de Maio é marcado por protestos pequenos e virtuais" (1/05/2020):
https://veja.abril.com.br/mun do/com-coronavirus-1o-demaio-e-marcado-porprotestos-pequenos-evirtuais/.

Zafalon, M. (2020): "Temeroso das ações do governo, agronegócio reduz apoio a Bolsonaro", *Blog vaivém das commoditiesFolha de S. Paulo* (5/05/2020):
https://www1.folha.uol.com.b r/colunas/vaivem/2020/05/te meroso-das-acoes-dogoverno-agronegocio-reduzapoio-a-bolsonaro.shtml.

5. Internet Searches For Measures To Address COVID-19 In Brazil

Carlos Garcia Filho[1]
Luiza Jane Eyre de Souza Vieira[1]
Raimunda Magalhães da Silva[1]

[1]Universidade de Fortaleza, Programa de Pós-Graduação em Saúde Coletiva, Fortaleza, CE, Brazil

ABSTRACT

Objective: to describe profiles of interest of web search queries related to the COVID-19 epidemic in Brazil. **Methods:** This was a quantitative and exploratory study using Google Health Trends. We analyzed daily data of interest, defined as search probability (Pr), in 23 terms in searches performed by users connected in Brazil from January 1 to April 9, 2020. **Results:** the peak in interest (Pr=0.0651) on the theme of coronavirus occurred on March 21. Interest in use of face masks (Pr=0.0041), social distancing (Pr=0.0043) and hand hygiene with alcohol gel (Pr=0.0037) was greater than interest in respiratory etiquette (Pr=0.0010) and hand hygiene with soap and water (Pr=0.0005).**Conclusion:** The difference in interest in issues related to combating COVID-19 was substantial and can guide new strategies for disseminating health information.

INTRODUCTION

COVID-19 is a communicable disease caused by a recently discovered coronavirus (SARS-CoV-2). The virus and the disease were unknown until the outbreak in Wuhan, China, in December 2019.[1] The first confirmed case in Brazil was detected in São Paulo on February 26th,[2] and by April 8th2020, 15,927 cases and 800 deaths had been confirmed nationwide.[3] The World Health Organization (WHO) has considered COVID-19 to be a public health emergency of international concern since January 30th2020.Medication for effective treatment of the disease and vaccines to prevent SARS-CoV-2 infection are not available thus far. As such, social distancing, respiratory etiquette and hand sanitizing are recommended as measures to combat the pandemic.[2] Among these measures, it is social distancing that has had the greatest impact on the everyday lives of Brazilian people. The Federal District implemented this strategy on March 11th,[2] followed by São Paulo, Brazil's most populous state, which adopted social distancing on March 21st.[4] Other states also adhered to social distancing, but on March 24th2020, the President of the Republic used a national TV network to call for a "return to normality", going against global recommendations for fighting the epidemic.[5]The profile of queries on internet search engines is a good proxy of a population's interest, concerns and intentions regarding a given issue. Although it does not represent the opinion of the person doing the search query, it points to their tendency, since while it is not possible to know the reason for a given search query, it is possible to know its contents.[6] This is a tool that is gaining force in monitoring health conditions[7] and behaviours related to them.[9]The strategies for containing COVID-19 propagation are, for the most part, behavioural and impact the population's sociability and subsistence. It must be added that these measures have updated and renewed political and social polarization among the population. Within this context, knowing what the Brazilian population's doubts are about this subject can offer public policy makers possibilities for enhancing people's adherence to measures to contain the pandemic. The objective of this study was to describe profiles of interest of web search queries related to the COVID-19 epidemic in Brazil.

METHOD

This was a quantitative and exploratory study describing Google searches for terms related to the COVID-19 pandemic and containment measures established by the Ministry of Health. By 2018, 70% of Brazilians were accessing the internet, which is equivalent to approximately 127 million people. In the country's Southeast region, 75% of its inhabitants had access to the internet, while 64% had access in the Northeast region. In the other regions, 70% had access to the internet.[10]We analyzed 23 terms related to COVID-19 using Google Health Trends (GHT), an interface for accessing data on internet searches. GHT is free and requires access by means of an application programming interface (API; available at: https://sites.google.com/a/google.com/health-trends-api-getting-started-guide/).The GHT API provides data on internet searches since 2004, at various levels of spatial and temporal aggregation. Searches are retrieved from Google's general dataset in the form of a proportion, dividing the number of searches for a specific term in a given time interval by the total number of searches for terms in the same period. The result is multiplied by a predefined constant to facilitate its visualization. Its results therefore express the probability (Pr) of searches for a given term, referred to as *interest* in this article, standardized for the interval between 0 and 1.Daily data were retrieved on searches made by users connected in Brazil between January 1st and April 9th 2020. The Pr of each term was aggregated according to defined categories.

Overall interest in the subject was represented by the terms "coronavirus", "corona", "covid" and "sars". Interest in respiratory etiquette was represented by: 'cough', 'to cough', 'sneeze', 'to sneeze', 'handshake', 'to shake hands', 'hug', 'to hug'. For face mask use: 'mask', 'N95', 'duckbill'. For social distancing: 'quarantine', 'social isolation', 'social distancing'. For hand sanitizing with alcohol gel: 'alcohol gel', 'alcohol-based gel'. For hand sanitization with soap and water: 'soap', 'toilet soap', 'hand washing'. When choosing the terms, non-technical terms were selected, which, although imprecise, are probably the closest to the everyday language of the Brazilian population in general. The GHT API uses the Python programming language, while data organization and graph preparation was done using the R programming language.

RESULTS

Between January 1st and April 9th 2020, there was an increase in interest about the theme of coronavirus and about themes associated with behavioural measures to contain it. Figure 1 shows the P trend between some of the epidemic's landmarks in Brazil. The peak in interest (P=0.0651) in the theme occurred on March 21st, when São Paulo published its decree on social distancing.

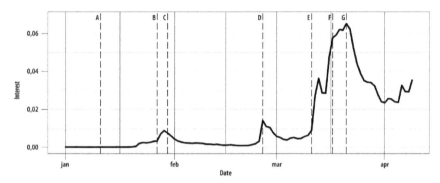

Figure 1 – Trend of probability of internet search interest in the theme of COVID-19 in Brazil, according to Google Health Trends, from January 1st to April 9th 2020Legend:A: 11/01 – 1stdeath registered in China.B: 27/01 – 1stsuspected case in Brazil (in the state of Minas Gerais).C: 30/01 – World Health Organization (WHO) declares public health emergency.D: 26/02 – 1stcase confirmed in Brazil.E: 11/03 – 1stdecree on social distancing in Brazil (Federal District).F: 17/03 – 1stdeath registered in Brazil (in São Paulo).G: 21/03 – The State of São Paulo announces decree on social distancing. Of note is the low interest (lowest P=0.0008) in the theme in the period between the epidemic being considered a public health emergency and the first confirmed case in Brazil. Consistent and sustained growth of interest in the theme can only be seen with effect from the application of social distancing measures (P=0.0273) and the first death in Brazil (P= 0.0577).In Figure 2 it can be seen that the population's interest in seeking information about pandemic containment measures showed substantial growth with effect from the first social distancing measures. Interest in the subject of face mask use (P=00041), social distancing (P=0.0043) and sanitizing hands with alcohol gel (P=0.0037) was greater than interest in the subject of respiratory etiquette (P=0.0010) and sanitizing hands with soap and water (P=0.0005).

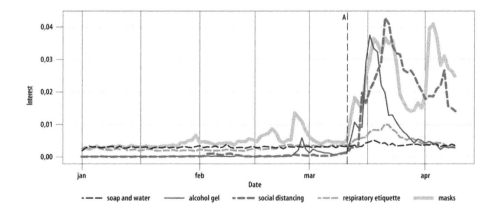

Figure 2 – Trend of probability of internet search interest in themes related to COVID-19 prevention in Brazil, according to Google Health Trends, from January 1st to April 9th 2020Legend:A: 11/03 – 1stdecree on social distancing in Brazil (Federal District).

DISCUSSION

The periods of increased interest in COVID-19 occurred after the main epidemiological landmarks of the disease in Brazil were publicized by the media. Moreover, the results suggest possible information gaps about some of the main forms of prevention. The internet search profile found during the current COVID-19 epidemic was similar to that seen during the Zika epidemic in 2015, when there was a predominance of reactive rather than proactive searches for prevention strategies.[11]

Fake news, unclear communication and divergences between the President of the Republic and the State Governors and the Minister of Health about how to deal with the epidemic[5] may have contributed to reducing the population's interest in the disease up until the end of March, as well as to the sudden and heterogeneous growth in interest in themes related to its prevention following the adoption of social distancing measures. In addition, lack of clearness in information provided by health authorities about social distancing, including absence of uniformity as to what care should be taken, can contribute to worsening the psychological impacts of quarantine.[12] Substantial and sustained growth in interest in the pandemic in Brazil occurred with effect from the first social distancing measures. It is therefore not surprising that the theme of most interest is social distancing, given its implications beyond the field of health, including its impacts on the income of informal workers and workers in precarious job situations and the need for emergency government programs targeting these segments.[13] The theme of face masks was the second most searched subject, principally after the Health Ministry recommendation regarding use of face masks by the population in general, including suggesting homemade masks and encouraging the population to share the results of this experience on social networks.[14] Substantial interest in hand sanitization using alcohol gel and low interest in hand sanitization using soap and water is relevant for questioning whether communication between health authorities and the population has been effective. It is possible that there is an information gap about an effective and low-cost behaviour for containing the pandemic.

The main limitation of this study is that is based on the probability of searching for terms, without it being possible to establish the reasons that led to the searches. Social distancing, for instance, was the most outstanding theme among the containment measures, but this study is not capable of defining whether the population does or does not support and adhere to this measure. As such, further research is needed. An example could be research into the contents of posts on social networks. The conclusion is therefore reached that there was a difference in interest in themes related to combating COVID-19, and this can guide new strategies for disseminating health information. Public health authorities can use internet search monitoring as a proxy for health information dissemination.[9]

REFERÊNCIAS

1. World Health Organization - WHO. Q&A on coronaviruses (COVID-19). Geneva: World Health Organization; 2020 [cited 2020 Apr 6]. Available from: https://www.who.int/news-room/q-a-detail/q-a-coronaviruses [Links]

2. Ministério da Saúde (BR). Secretaria de Vigilância em Saúde. Centro de Operações de Emergência em Saúde Pública. Especial: doença pelo coronavírus 2019. Bol Epidemiol [Internet]. 2020 abr [citado 2020 abr 6];7:1-28. Disponível em: https://www.saude.gov.br/images/pdf/2020/April/06/2020-04-06-BE7-Boletim-Especial-do-COE-Atualizacao-da-Avaliacao-de-Risco.pdf [Links]

3. Ministério da Saúde (BR). Painel coronavírus [Internet]. Brasília: Ministério da Saúde; 2020 [citado 2020 abr 9]. Disponível em: https://covid.saude.gov.br [Links]

4. Governo de São Paulo. Saiba quais as medidas do Governo de SP para o combate ao coronavírus [Internet]. São Paulo: Governo de São Paulo; 2020 [citado 2020 abr 8]. Disponível em: https://www.saopaulo.sp.gov.br/spnoticias/saiba-quais-as-medidas-do-governo-de-sp-para-o-combate-ao-coronavirus-2/ [Links]

5. G1. Ao menos 25 dos 27 governadores manterão restrições contra coronavírus mesmo após Bolsonaro pedir fim de isolamento [Internet]. São Paulo: G1; 2020 [citado 2020 abr 6]. Disponível em: https://g1.globo.com/politica/noticia/2020/03/25/governadoras-reagem-ao-pronunciamento-de-bolsonaro-sobre-coronavirus.ghtml [Links]

6. Stocking G, Matsa KE, Pew Research Center. Using Google trends data for research? Here are 6 questions to ask [Internet]. [S.l.]: Medium; 2017 [cited 2020 Apr 6]. Disponível em: https://medium.com/pewresearch/using-google-trends-data-for-research-here-are-6-questions-to-ask-a7097f5fb526 [Links]

7. Cervellin G, Comelli I, Lippi G. Is Google trends a reliable tool for digital epidemiology? Insights from different clinical settings. J Epidemiol Glob Health [Internet]. 2017 Dec [cited 2020 May 13];7(3);185-9. Available from: http://dx.doi.org/10.1016/j.jegh.2017.06.001 [Links]

8. Mavragani A, Ochoa G, Tsagarakis KP. Assessing the methods, tools, and statistical approaches in google trends research: systematic review: systematic review. J Med Internet Res [Internet]. 2018 Nov [cited 2020 May 13];20(11);e270. Available from: http://dx.doi.org/10.2196/jmir.9366 [Links]

9. Ayers JW, Althouse BM, Dredze M. Could behavioral medicine lead the web data revolution? JAMA [Internet]. 2014 Apr [cited 2020 May 13];311(14):1399-400. Available from: http://dx.doi.org/10.1001/jama.2014.1505 [Links]

10. Centro Regional de Estudos para o Desenvolvimento da Sociedade da Informação. C2 - indivíduos, por último acesso à Internet [Internet]. [S.l.]: Centro Regional de Estudos para o Desenvolvimento da Sociedade da Informação; 2019 [citado 2020 abr 23]. Disponível em: https://cetic.br/tics/domicilios/2018/individuos/C2/ [Links]

11. Bragazzi NL, Alicino C, Trucchi C, Paganino C, Barberis I, Martini M, et al. Global reaction to the recent outbreaks of Zika virus: insights from a big data analysis. PLoS One [Internet]. 2017 Sep [cited 2020 May 13];12(9):e0185263. Available from: https://doi.org/10.1371/journal.pone.0185263 [Links]

12. Brooks SK, Webster RK, Smith L, Woodland L, Wessely S, Greenberg N, et al. The psychological impact of quarantine and how to reduce it: rapid review of the evidence. Lancet [Internet]. 2020 Feb [cited 2020 May 13];395(10227);912-20. Available from: http://dx.doi.org/10.1016/s0140-6736(20)30460-8 [Links]

13. Parmet WE, Sinha MS. COVID-19 — the law and limits of quarantine. N Engl J Med [Internet]. 2020 Apr [cited 2020 Apr 9];382(15):e28. Available from: http://dx.doi.org/10.1056/nejmp2004211 [Links]

14. Ministério da Saúde (BR). Máscaras caseiras podem ajudar na prevenção contra o Coronavírus [Internet]. Brasília: Ministério da Saúde; 2020 [citado 2020 abr 9]. Disponível em: https://www.saude.gov.br/noticias/agencia-saude/46645-mascaras-caseiras-podem-ajudar-na-prevencao-contra-o-coronavirus [Links]

Correspondence: Carlos Garcia Filho - Av. Washington Soares, No. 1321, Edson Queiroz, Fortaleza, Ceará, Brazil. Postcode 60811-905 E-mail: cgarciafilho@gmail.com

6.Why Brazil's COVID-19 Response is Failing

Mariana Urban and Eduardo Saad-Diniz

Brazil has[1] the second highest number of confirmed COVID-19 cases in the world. The first case was identified[2] on February 25 in São Paulo, and since then, the federal government has tried to enforce new measures in all 26 states and the Federal District through federal regulation, including travel restrictions, taxes, mass layoffs, credit facilities, opening restrictions, social distancing, and financial aid. The Bolsonaro Administration, however, is sending[3] mixed signals about the severity of the outbreak in Brazil and turning a pandemic into a political debate. This posture has provoked[4] negative responses by the media, the population, and the international community, which has led[5] to some resistance by state governments to comply fully with federal guidelines.

In the early 20th century, Brazilian public figures, such as Oswaldo Cruz and Carlos Chagas, became a reference in the treatment of several outbreaks, such as malaria, yellow fever, smallpox, and—not coincidentally—Chagas[6] disease. Brazil was also a "trailblazer[7] in the HIV response," according to the World Health Organization[8] (WHO).

Furthermore, Brazil was one of the first countries outside the Organization for Economic Cooperation and Development[9] (OECD) to implement the constitutional right to universal health coverage through Sistema Único de Saúde[10]—the country's Unified Health System. Brazil's National Immunization Program[11] is known[12] worldwide, and Brazil recently led[13] research on the Zika virus.

Yet Brazil has one of the worst responses[14] to COVID-19 among all affected countries, and it is heading toward becoming the new epicenter of the pandemic. What went wrong?

Brazil now faces three different crises due to a lack of regulatory excellence: a health crisis, an economic crisis, and a political crisis. The health and economic crises were to be expected once the outbreak of the novel coronavirus began to spread throughout the world. But the political crisis in Brazil is completely homegrown.

---

[1] https://coronavirus.jhu.edu/map.html

[2] https://www.nytimes.com/2020/02/26/world/americas/brazil-italy-coronavirus.html

[3] https://www.washingtonpost.com/opinions/global-opinions/jair-bolsonaro-risks-lives-by-minimizing-the-coronavirus-pandemic/2020/04/13/6356a9be-7da6-11ea-9040-68981f488eed_story.html

[4] https://www.bbc.com/news/world-latin-america-52040205

[5] https://www.theguardian.com/world/2020/apr/01/brazil-bolsonaro-ignored-by-state-governors-amid-anger-at-handling-of-covid-19-crisis

[6] https://www.cdc.gov/parasites/chagas/index.html

[7] https://www.who.int/hiv/mediacentre/news/brazil-hiv-treatment-all-plhiv/en/

[8] https://www.who.int/

[9] https://www.oecd.org/

[10] http://www.saude.gov.br/sistema-unico-de-saude

[11] http://www.blog.saude.gov.br/index.php/entenda-o-sus/50027-programa-nacional-de-imunizacoes-pni#:~:text=O%20Programa%20Nacional%20de%20Imuniza%C3%A7%C3%B5es,a%20poliomielite%20(paralisia%20infantil)

[12] https://www.who.int/news-room/feature-stories/detail/from-warehouse-to-remote-indigenous-communities-the-journey-of-vaccines-in-brazil

[13] http://www.brazil.gov.br/about-brazil/news/2017/06/brazil-is-at-the-forefront-of-zika-research

[14] https://coronavirus.jhu.edu/data/new-cases

Despite concern[1] about the impact of the outbreak on Brazilians, particularly those living in poor communities, the response of the federal government has been plagued by disputes inside the Bolsonaro Administration. Fueled by the strong denialist rhetoric of President Jair Bolsonaro—who has referred[2] to COVID-19 as a "little flu" and refused[3] to comply with WHO guidelines—the Administration's internal disputes have delayed implementation of coherent federal regulatory measures in the health system and increased the ongoing political instability.

In contrast, the Ministry of Health[4], at that time led by Luiz Henrique Mandetta, advocated[5] a strict social distancing framework recommended by the WHO. But following his ally President Donald J. Trump, President Bolsonaro failed to take seriously the need to mitigate[6] the potential impacts of the pandemic, ignoring scientific findings that were against his beliefs and showing[7] more concern about an economic recession than the spread of the virus. The dispute inside the federal government led to Bolsonaro's dismissal[8] of Mandetta and, less than a month later, the resignation[9] of Mandetta's successor as Health Minister, Nelson Teich.

Adding to the political turmoil, Sérgio Moro—the former judge who oversaw several cases in the so-called Lava Jato, or Car Wash, investigation[10]—resigned[11] his position as justice minister due to an alleged[12] interference by President Bolsonaro in matters under the authority of the federal police and the regional head of police in Rio de Janeiro. The allegations have significantly increased[13] political instability and ignited ongoing impeachment discussions.

Resisting the minimal COVID-19 guidelines propagated by the Bolsonaro Administration, the state governors decided[14] not to comply[15] with federal regulations and guidelines. As a result, public health measures became[16] regionalized, with an ongoing dispute for needed health care resources taking place across the country. Although governors and mayors became essential leaders in the fight to contain the impact of the pandemic, the lack of federal regulation has jeopardized the effective monitoring and control of the population to contain the spread of the virus.

Federal prosecutors have launched[17] an investigation into the Rio de Janeiro state governor because of "irregularities in contracts awarded for the construction of emergency field hospitals." Other federal investigations related to states' pandemic responses have emerged[18] across the country.

---

[1] https://www.nytimes.com/pt/2020/03/31/espanol/opinion/a-maior-tragedia-do-coronavirus-pode-ser-nas-favelas-brasileiras.html

[2] https://edition.cnn.com/2020/05/23/americas/brazil-coronavirus-hospitals-intl/index.html

[3] https://www.forbes.com/sites/carlieporterfield/2020/04/10/brazils-bolsonaro-slights-social-distancing-as-coronavirus-deaths-hit-1000/#460c47b21376

[4] http://www.brazil.gov.br/government/ministers/health

[5] https://www.theguardian.com/world/2020/apr/13/brazil-bolsonaro-coronavirus-covid-19-social-distancing

[6] https://www.theguardian.com/world/2020/mar/23/brazils-jair-bolsonaro-says-coronavirus-crisis-is-a-media-trick

[7] https://www.aljazeera.com/indepth/features/deny-defy-bolsonaro-approach-coronavirus-brazil-200330181645501.html

[8] https://edition.cnn.com/2020/04/16/americas/brazil-health-minister-fired-intl/index.html

[9] https://www.nytimes.com/2020/05/15/world/americas/brazil-health-minister-bolsonaro.html

[10] https://www.theguardian.com/world/2017/jun/01/brazil-operation-car-wash-is-this-the-biggest-corruption-scandal-in-history

[11] https://www.bbc.com/news/world-latin-america-52415863

[12] https://time.com/5840854/sergio-moro-brazil-interview/

[13] https://theintercept.com/2020/04/24/bolsonaro-impeachment-moro-resigns-brazil/

[14] https://www.bloomberg.com/news/articles/2020-03-25/brazilian-state-governors-defy-bolsonaro-in-coronavirus-fight

[15] https://www1.folha.uol.com.br/equilibrioesaude/2020/06/maioria-dos-estados-ignora-protocolo-do-governo-e-nao-indica-cloroquina-para-casos-leves.shtml

[16] https://oglobo.globo.com/rio/crivella-anuncia-lockdown-parcial-com-fechamento-do-calcadao-de-campo-grande-nesta-quinta-feira-24413522

[17] https://www.washingtonpost.com/world/the_americas/brazil-obeys-court-order-to-resume-providing-full-virus-data/2020/06/09/8886f10c-aaca-11ea-a43b-be9f6494a87d_story.html

[18] https://brazilian.report/coronavirus-brazil-live-blog/2020/06/12/police-investigate-ventilators-deal-fraud-in-sao-paulo/

The regulatory measures implemented by the federal government were generally related to addressing economic impacts, implementing[1] travel and border restrictions, providing[2] financial support for businesses and some social aid programs. and increasing[3] liquidity through the Central Bank of Brazil[4]. The government has recognized[5] that the calamity in Brazil will affect compliance with the fiscal primary balance target for the year. The media have criticized several federal policies. For instance, federal tax measures have been interpreted[6] as an opportunity identified by the government to anticipate changes that were already in sight with the tax reform. The amendment[7] of labour laws has been seen[8] by some commentators as a violation of socioeconomic rights.

The federal government has also been the target[9] of critics regarding transparency of the number of confirmed COVID-19 cases and deaths. After the federal government was accused[10] of delaying daily reports, and even ceasing to report the cumulative COVID-19 numbers on the Ministry of Health website, the Brazilian Supreme Court interfered[11], determining that the government must resume full disclosure of COVID-19 cumulative data. Perhaps because of the internal instability caused by authoritarian-inspired leadership and a strong sense of moral indifference against the social and moral costs of the pandemic—or perhaps due to the restrictions that President Bolsonaro has imposed on ministers—the Brazilian Ministry of Health is not acting[12] as a protagonist in the fight against COVID-19. Following ongoing discussions[13] on chloroquine, for example, health officials became[14] much more focused on the treatment of COVID-19 instead of the prevention of the spread of the virus.

The Ministry of Health should have implemented a system of contact tracing and selective isolation, as was done[15] in Vietnam. In the United States, Massachusetts is using[16] a network of public health workers to contain the spread of the virus. Brazil has a similar program[17] in which community health agents can follow up with local health conditions and monitor diseases and risk areas in communities. But the Ministry of Health has yet to use the program so it could play a key role in containing the spread of the coronavirus.

---

[1] https://br.usembassy.gov/health-alert-march-28-2020/

[2] https://home.kpmg/xx/en/home/insights/2020/04/brazil-government-and-institution-measures-in-response-to-covid.html

[3] https://www.bcb.gov.br/en/pressdetail/2321/nota

[4] https://www.bcb.gov.br/en/

[5] https://brazilian.report/coronavirus-brazil-live-blog/2020/03/20/brazilian-senate-approves-state-of-calamity-against-covid-19/

[6] https://www.gazetadopovo.com.br/republica/a-reforma-tributaria-do-coronavirus-como-a-pandemia-mudou-e-ainda-pode-mudar-os-impostos/

[7] https://www1.folha.uol.com.br/mercado/2020/06/guedes-quer-ampliar-suspensao-de-contrato-e-corte-de-jornada-para-ate-quatro-meses.shtml

[8] https://economia.uol.com.br/noticias/redacao/2020/04/02/mp-coloca-pessoas-com-medo-para-negociarem-diz-associacao-de-magistrados.htm

[9] https://www.reuters.com/article/us-health-coronavirus-brazil/brazil-takes-down-covid-19-data-hiding-soaring-death-toll-idUSKBN23D0PW

[10] https://www.reuters.com/article/us-health-coronavirus-brazil/brazil-takes-down-covid-19-data-hiding-soaring-death-toll-idUSKBN23D0PW

[11] https://time.com/5851119/brazil-supreme-court-covid-19-data-death-toll/

[12] https://www.france24.com/en/20200620-brazil-ex-health-chief-says-ministry-lost-credibility

[13] https://www.nytimes.com/2020/06/13/world/americas/virus-brazil-bolsonaro-chloroquine.html

[14] https://www.independent.co.uk/news/world/americas/coronavirus-brazil-chloroquine-cases-deaths-bolsonaro-a9526056.html

[15] https://www.bbc.com/news/world-asia-52628283

[16] https://www.nytimes.com/2020/04/16/us/coronavirus-massachusetts-contact-tracing.html

[17] https://www.saude.gov.br/acoes-e-programas/saude-da-familia/agente-comunitario-de-saude

Analyzing Brazilian demographics is also essential to understand the high transmission rate of the coronavirus. Although Brazil has infrastructure for interstate and international travel, several regions have yet to reach a sufficient stage of development to implement[1] preventive measures, much less to maintain the social distancing of the population. For instance, almost 35 million people in Brazil have[2] no access to clean water, so they are barely able to comply with the primary recommendations to wash hands and to stay at home. The social inequalities among communities make complying with the "stay-at-home" orders impractical for disadvantaged populations.

The country's COVID-19 case numbers reflect this inequality in Brazil, considering that a significant part of the population cannot stay isolated at home and protect themselves against the virus. In addition, COVID-19 infections are now spreading[3] at a faster pace in countryside cities that have less infrastructure and resources, while the capitals are gradually reopening the economy. The federal government has implemented a regulatory framework for social assistance to provide financial aid to some retired elderly, unemployed, and underprivileged people who are registered in the social protection program, Cadastro Único Federal[4]. Despite this program, many Brazilians lack important resources. For example, almost one million people have[5] no access to electricity in the Amazon region, and about 46 million people in Brazil had[6] no internet access in 2018. With such limitations, these people face additional struggles to register for the social protection program to receive government assistance.

Another problematic factor is that many of those Brazilians who do have the financial means to comply with social distancing measures are instead taking their example from the President and ignoring all public health recommendations. As the pandemic has spread throughout Brazil, a significant proportion of Bolsonaro's supporters have joined[7] in protests against the state governors and the Federal Supreme Court—the latter for opposing[8] President Bolsonaro and reassuring the power of states and municipalities in Brazilian federalism. These protests have been supported by part of the nation's population due to misleading information spread by high levels of the federal government, which have ended up jeopardizing local efforts to contain the pandemic based on scientific data and WHO guidelines. Although President Bolsonaro appointed[9] a former military officer to serve as the Health Minister for an interim period, that position remains unfilled with a permanent Minister, even as deaths and confirmed cases continue to increase exponentially.

Even more tragically, the adverse effects of the lax regulatory framework imposed by the Bolsonaro Administration are not limited to the Brazilian borders. When governments disregard reasonable or appropriate public health measures, the moral vacuum only further increases marginalization, extreme poverty, and violence in the entire region. International bodies should take a closer look at what is happening—or, all too often, what is not happening—in Brazil that has led it to become one of the global pandemic's top victims.

---

[1] https://journals.openedition.org/echogeo/15060

[2] https://noticias.r7.com/brasil/quase-35-milhoes-de-brasileiros-nao-tem-acesso-a-agua-tratada-24092019

[3] https://www1.folha.uol.com.br/cotidiano/2020/06/onda-de-infeccoes-por-covid-19-tem-nova-aceleracao-no-interior.shtml

[4] http://www.caixa.gov.br/cadastros/cadastro-unico/Paginas/default.aspx

[5] https://www.poder360.com.br/brasil/quase-1-milhao-nao-tem-acesso-a-energia-eletrica-na-regiao-da-amazonia-legal/

[6] https://g1.globo.com/economia/tecnologia/noticia/2020/04/29/em-2018-quase-46-milhoes-de-brasileiros-ainda-nao-tinham-acesso-a-internet-aponta-ibge.ghtml#:~:text=Dados%20divulgados%20nesta%20quarta%2Dfeira,anos%20ou%20mais%20de%20idade

[7] https://www.washingtonpost.com/world/the_americas/brazil-bolsonaro-military-takeover-coronavirus/2020/05/11/935b680e-8fce-11ea-a9c0-73b93422d691_story.html

[8] http://portal.stf.jus.br/processos/detalhe.asp?incidente=5880765

[9] https://brazilian.report/coronavirus-brazil-live-blog/2020/05/19/interim-health-minister-appoints-nine-military-officers/

7. Interstate Heterogeneity And Combatting COVID-19 In Brazil

Luan Borelli, Geraldo Goes

Brazil has faced great difficulties in controlling the COVID-19 epidemic, having become the world's epicentre of the coronavirus pandemic and recently reaching 50,000 fatalities. This column argues that the great heterogeneities between states in Brazil, together with difficulties in political coordination, may have shaped these consequences. Looking at five states, it investigates whether certain differences in the states' intrinsic characteristics may have influenced the dynamics of the local epidemic. Governments may need to consider local conditions and adopt heterogeneous containment policies.

With a territory of over 3 million square miles and a population of more than 210 million, Brazil is geographically the fifth-largest country in the world and the sixth-largest in population. It encompasses a wide range of cultural, political, demographic, economic, and behavioural variations that originate from Europe to Africa. Charles Wyplosz questioned the extent to which policy reactions to COVID-19 are driven by political factors, and which are driven by other influences like history, culture, ethnic divisions, political regimes, and election laws on one hand, and the price that societies attribute of life on the other (Baldwin and Welder di Mauro 2020).

Wyplosz's question is particularly pertinent to Brazil. Given this country's social complexity, it would not be difficult to assume that Brazil would face great challenges in controlling the COVID-19 epidemic. Indeed, Brazil saw major standoffs in designing policies to combat the epidemic, with incoordination between federal and state powers over containment policies. On the one hand, the state governments defended their autonomy in implementing these policies, aiming at more severe measures, while on the other hand, the federal power, in the words of Ajzenman et al. (2020), "publicly flaunted social distancing measures and downplayed the seriousness of the disease in at least two well-publicized instances".

The impact of this lack of coordination between federal and state actions was noted on 22 May 2020 when, amid these political disputes, the WHO declared Brazil the new epicentre of the coronavirus pandemic. Wyplosz's words that "...governments' reactions will reveal the nature of their leaders and, more widely, that of societies" (Baldwin and Welder di Mauro 2020) could not be more prophetic. But is it justifiable for states to have the independence to implement their own containment policies? Are the characteristics of Brazilian individual states different to the point that epidemic dynamics differ across the country, thus justifying this state-level independence?

Remarkable Epidemic Heterogeneities In Brazil

A recent study by Hallal et al. (2020) provides insights into these questions. The study examines first-wave seroprevalence surveys of household probabilistic samples of 133 large sentinel cities in Brazil, including 25,025 participants from all 26 states and the Federal District.It finds that the seroprevalence of antibodies to SARS-CoV-2, assessed using a lateral flow rapid test, varied markedly across the cities and regions, from below 1% in most cities in the South and centre-West regions to up to 25% in the city of Breves in the Amazon (North) region.

From these findings by Hallal et al. (2020), it is possible to observe that the regions with the greatest differences in seroprevalence of SARS-CoV-2 antibodies were precisely those regions that are most heterogeneous culturally, economically, socially, and demographically. While urban metropolises in the Southeast had, on average, low prevalence of antibodies, as in the case of São Paulo (3.3%), smaller cities in the interior of the North, mainly coastal regions of the Amazon River, presented levels on average above 10%, as in the case of Tefé (19.8%). Such results suggest that regional differences in epidemic consequences may be deeply related to differing economic, cultural, and behavioural characteristics of these states. Thus, we explore the possible influence on epidemic dynamics of the different characteristics intrinsic to each state or region.

A Theoretical Investigation For Brazil

In our study (Borelli and Góes, 2020), we use the SIR-macro model (Eichenbaum et al. 2020) to investigate how differences in local characteristics may have affected epidemic dynamics and their economic consequences in five Brazilian states with the most critical epidemic situations to date, namely, São Paulo (SP), Amazonas (AM), Ceará (CE), Rio de Janeiro (RJ) and Pernambuco (PE). The SIR-macro model (Eichenbaum et al. 2020) extends the canonical SIR model (Kermack and McKendrick 1927), allowing the behaviour of economic agents to influence epidemic dynamics. In this model, economic agents can voluntarily choose to reduce their consumption and work activities to lower their chances of being infected. They can also be induced to reduce these activities through containment measures adopted by the authorities.

The dynamics of the model follow a logic similar to that by Gourinchas (2020), that flattening the infection curve inevitably accentuates the macroeconomic recession curve. Reducing the economic activities of agents reduces the severity of the epidemic on the one hand, but deepens the severity of economic recessions on the other. The model also incorporates endogenous mortality rates and probabilities of discovering effective treatments and vaccines over time. This extended framework helps the results to better mimic reality and allows us to assess the macroeconomic impact of epidemics. To incorporate into this model the differences in state characteristics, we selected nine demographic, economic, and behavioural variables that show the greatest diversity (Table 1). These data were used to capture the different forms and intensities in which infections in each state are distributed among consumption, work, and other activities.

Table 1 Main data used for model calibration for each state

Variable	São Paulo	Amazonas	Ceará	Rio de Janeiro	Pernambuco
Pre-epidemic population	45,919,049	4,144,597	9,132,078	17,264,943	9,557,071
Number of persons employed	22,782,714	1,657,700	3,764,280	7,651,617	3,602,820
Number of students	10,306,000	1,284,000	2,376,000	3,853,000	2,475,000
Average number of people per residence	2.80	3.60	3.10	2.70	2.90
Average daily hours devoted to household chores	2.06	1.44	1.87	2.04	2.02
Average daily hours worked	8.24	7.30	7.58	8.10	7.74
Average time spent in public transport (minutes)	37.15	33.95	26.60	43.07	30.52
Per capita income (BR$)	1,889	838	939	1,809	954
Imperial College's estimated IFR (%)	0.70	0.80	1.10	0.80	1.10

Note: Imperial College's estimated infection fatality rates (IFR) were used to calibrate parameters related to the endogenous mortality rates to simulate the capacity of the health systems of each state.

To assess the results, we considered two scenarios. In the first, no containment measures are adopted by the authorities. In the second, optimal containment policies are adopted. Our results indicate that in both scenarios, the states present relevant differences in their epidemic dynamics due to their heterogeneous characteristics. From a qualitative point of view, key differences are verified in:

- Peak sizes of the infected population curves;
- Moments of the epidemic progress when the peaks of infected population curves are reached;
- Depths of economic recession curves;
- Moments of the epidemic progress when economic recovery begins;
- Shares of the total pre-epidemic population that is infected by the end of the epidemic;
- Shares of the total pre-epidemic population that die by the end of the epidemic.

An overview of these differences is in Figure 3, which presents all the results for the main variables both in the scenario in which containment policies are not adopted and in the scenario in which optimal policies are adopted.

Figure 3 Epidemic progression with adoption of optimal containment policies (solid lines) and without adoption of containment policies (dotted lines)

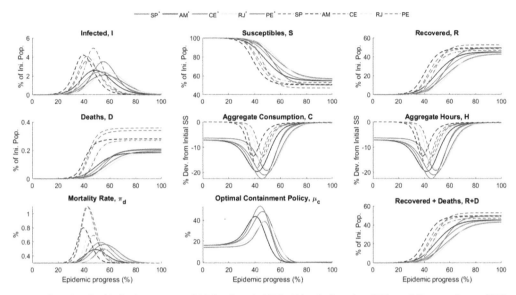

Notes: São Paulo (SP), Amazonas (AM), Ceará (CE), Rio de Janeiro (RJ) and Pernambuco (PE).

We found that states differ not only in the intensity of their local epidemics but also in their timing, a factor of great importance for the design of public containment policies. Table 2 summarises the moments in the progress of the epidemic when the main epidemic phenomena occur, showing how epidemics in states can experience different temporal dynamics.

Table 2 Moments of epidemic progress when the main peaks and valleys of the model variables occur, for each state.

Value	Scenario	São Paulo	Amazonas	Ceará	Rio de Janeiro	Pernambuco
Moment of the epidemic progress when the peak of infected population curve occurs	Without containment policy	47.33%	39.33%	42.67%	46.00%	42.00%
	Adopting optimal policy	55.33%	48.67%	56.00%	58.67%	52.67%
Moment of the epidemic progress when the peak mortality rate occurs	Without containment policy	47.33%	39.33%	42.67%	46.00%	42.00%
	Adopting optimal policy	55.33%	48.67%	56.00%	58.67%	52.67%
Moment of progress of the epidemic when the valley of recession curves occurs	Without containment policy	46.00%	38.67%	42.00%	45.33%	41.33%
	Adopting optimal policy	49.33%	42.00%	47.33%	50.67%	45.33%

Note: The moments are reported as progress percentage of the total time interval of the epidemic in each state. The beginning of the epidemic in each state is considered the moment when each state reaches the 100th infection (not necessarily the same date). This means that it would be incorrect to conclude, for example, that 'the peak in the infected population would occur first in Amazonas and then in São Paulo'. A more correct interpretation would be: 'in relation to the moment when the 100th infection occurs, the peak would occur faster in Amazonas (AM) than in São Paulo (SP)'. The observed heterogeneities between states in epidemic dynamics imply the need for heterogeneous containment policies. When optimal trajectories of containment rates are achieved, we see significant differences in the measures that should be adopted by each state. We find that trajectories vary between states in the initial severity required, the moment they must be accelerated, the extent they should be elevated, and when they should finally start to be reduced.

Table 3 Optimal containment rates for each state

State	Initially required optimal containment rate (t = 0)	Moment of progress of the epidemic when peak containment rate occurs	Peak optimal containment rate
São Paulo (SP)	14.05%	47.33%	38.76%
Amazonas (M)	16.10%	40.67%	43.68%
Ceará (CE)	16.12%	46.00%	48.35%
Rio de Janeiro (RJ)	17.78%	48.67%	39.54%
Pernambuco (PE)	15.96%	44.00%	53.40%

To illustrate the differences, note, for example, time dynamics. In Rio de Janeiro the peak of the containment rate occurs at 48.67% of the epidemic progress, while in Amazonas it is at 40.67%, a difference of 8 percentage points. Considering an average epidemic duration of one year, this difference would mean that Rio de Janeiro, relative to the moment of the 100th infection, would take approximately one month longer than Amazonas to start relaxing its containment measures.

On the intensity of optimal containment policies, while Pernambuco requires the containment rate to reach 53.40%, São Paulo needs an increase only up to 38.76%, that is, 14.64 percentage points less than in Pernambuco.

Because these containment policies are heterogeneous, the effects are also quite heterogeneous. Table 4 shows how the implications of adopting optimal policies differ across states.

Table 4 Effects of adopting optimal containment policies, by state

Variable	São Paulo	Amazonas	Ceará	Rio de Janeiro	Pernambuco
Peak infected curve reduction (Percentage points of pre-epidemic population)	1.44%	1.61%	1.54%	1.45%	1.61%
Total infections avoided by the end of the epidemic (Percentage points of pre-epidemic population)	3.19%	4.24%	4.01%	3.58%	4.04%
Peak mortality rate reduction (Percentage points)	0.20%	0.31%	0.53%	0.31%	0.51%
Saved lives (Percentage points of pre-epidemic population)	0.07%	0.10%	0.15%	0.09%	0.15%
Deepening of the macroeconomic recession curves valley (Percentage points of dev. from initial steady state)	-5.73%	-6.06%	-2.99%	-3.18%	-4.92%

Note: These numbers are obtained by calculating the difference between the results of the two scenarios.

Conclusion and Lessons For Other Countries

Qualitatively corroborating our findings with empirical evidence in the COVID-19 literature for Brazil, we conclude that the characteristics of Brazilian states may significantly affect state epidemic dynamics, making them differ substantially. From a policymaking perspective, this interstate heterogeneity implies the need for optimal containment policies that are also heterogeneous and varying in extent and duration for different states. Disregarding the importance of such heterogeneities and not taking them into account to coordinate containment policies may amplify both the severity of the economic recession and the number of infected and deaths resulting from the epidemic. This, in part, can explain Brazil's situation today and should alert any other large countries with similarly heterogeneous characteristics to the need to emphatically consider interregional heterogeneities in the fight against COVID-19.

REFERENCES

Ajzenman, N, T Cavalcanti and D Da Mata (2020), "Leaders' speech and risky behaviour during a pandemic", VoxEU.org, 2 May.

Baldwin, R, and B Weder di Mauro (2020), *Economics in the time of COVID-19*, Voxeu.org eBook, a VoxEU.org eBook, CEPR Press.

Borelli and Góes (2020), "Macroeconomics of epidemics: Interstate heterogeneity in Brazil", *Covid Economics: Vetted and Real-Time Papers* 30.

Eichenbaum, Martin S, S Rebelo and M Trabandt (2020), "The macroeconomics of epidemics", NBER Working Paper 26882.
Gourinchas, P-O (2020), "Flattening the pandemic and recession curves", in R Baldwin and B Weder di Mauro (eds.), *Mitigating the COVID economic crisis: Act fast and do whatever it takes*, a VoxEU.org eBook, CEPR Press.

Hallal, P, et al. (2020, May) "Remarkable variability in SARS-CoV-2 antibodies across Brazilian regions: Nationwide serological household survey in 27 states", medRxiv, preprint.
Kermack, W, and A McKendrick (1927), "A contribution to the mathematical theory of epidemics", *Proceedings of the Royal Society of London*, series A 115, no. 772: 700-721.

CHAPTER 4

COVID TESTING AND DIAGNOSTICS

1. information About The New Coronavirus Disease (COVID-19)

Claudio Márcio Amaral de Oliveira Lima[1]

Coronavirus is a zoonotic virus, an RNA virus in the family Coronaviridae of the order Nidovirales[1]. It is a family of viruses that cause respiratory infections, which were first isolated in 1937 and designated coronaviruses, because they have a crown-like appearance under microscopy, in 1965[2]. The types of coronavirus known to date are as follows: the alpha coronaviruses HCoV-229E and HCoV-NL63; the beta coronaviruses HCoV-OC43 and HCoV-HKU1; SARS-CoV, which causes severe acute respiratory syndrome (SARS); MERS-CoV, which causes Middle East respiratory syndrome (MERS); and SARS-CoV-2, a new coronavirus described in late 2019 after cases were reported in China[2], which causes the disease known as coronavirus disease 2019 (COVID-19).

The definitive diagnosis of COVID-19 is made by analysing respiratory samples (collected by aspiration of the airways or sputum induction). Laboratory tests to identify the virus involve the use of real-time polymerase chain reaction techniques and partial or total sequencing of the viral genome. The collection of nasopharyngeal aspirate, combined (nasal and oral) swab samples, or samples of lower respiratory tract secretions (sputum, tracheal lavage fluid, or bronchoalveolar lavage fluid) is recommended. To confirm the disease, it is necessary to perform molecular biology tests that detect viral RNA. Severe cases should be transferred to a referral hospital for isolation and treatment. Individuals with mild symptoms should be followed at the primary health care level and should be advised to self- isolate at home[1].

The clinical spectrum of coronavirus infection is quite broad, ranging from a simple cold to severe pneumonia. Clinically, COVID-19 initially presents as a flu-like syndrome. Individuals with COVID-19 usually develop signs and symptoms, such as mild respiratory illness and persistent fever, an average of 5–6 days after infection (range, 1–14 days). The fever is persistent, in contrast with the progressive decline observed in cases of influenza[1,3]. Fever may not be present in some cases, such as those occurring in patients that are very young, elderly, or immunocompromised, as well as in those that have used antipyretic medication[1].

In children, the disease appears to be relatively rare and mild, only approximately 2.4% of all reported cases occurring in individuals under 19 years of age, of whom only 2.5% and 0.2% have developed severe or critical illness, respectively[1,3].According to the Clinical Management Protocol for the New Coronavirus, disseminated by the Brazilian National Ministry of Health in February of this year[1], males and individuals over 50 years of age predominated among the first 99 patients hospitalized with pneumonia and a confirmed diagnosis of COVID-19 at a hospital in the city of Wuhan. Among those 99 patients, the main symptoms were fever (in 83%), cough (in 82%), shortness of breath (in 31%), muscle pain (in 11%), mental confusion (in 9%), headache (in 8%), sore throat (in 5%), rhinorrhoea (in 4%), chest pain (in 2%), diarrhoea (in 2%), and nausea/vomiting (in 1%). In another study, involving 41 patients diagnosed with COVID-19, lymphopenia was reported.

Evaluating data from 1,099 patients with confirmed COVID-19 in China, Guan et al.[4] observed that the mean age of the patients was 47 years and that 41.9% of the patients were female.

The primary composite outcome—defined as admission to the intensive care unit (ICU), the need for artificial ventilation, or progression to death—occurred in 67 patients (6.1%), admission to the ICU occurring in 5.0%, invasive mechanical ventilation being required in 2.3%, and death occurring in 1.4%. The most common symptoms were fever (in 43.8% at admission and 88.7% during hospitalization) and cough (in 67.8%). Diarrhoea occurred in only 3.8% of cases. Lymphopenia was present in 83.2% of patients on admission. The mean incubation period was 4 days. Patients often presented without fever and many had normal X-ray findings. Based on a study of 55,924 confirmed cases, the World Health Organization-China Joint Mission on Coronavirus Disease 2019[3] reported the most common signs and symptoms: fever (in 87.9%); dry cough (in 67.7%); fatigue (in 38.1%); sputum production (in 33.4%); dyspnoea (in 18.6%); sore throat (in 13.9%); headache (in 13.6%); myalgia or arthralgia (in 14.8%); chills (in 11.4%); nausea or vomiting (in 5%); nasal congestion (in 4.8%); diarrhoea (in 3.7%); haemoptysis (in 0.9%); and conjunctival congestion (in 0.8%).

In most cases, the disease was mild and there was complete recovery. Among patients with laboratory-confirmed COVID-19, approximately 80% had mild to moderate disease, which includes cases with and without pneumonia; 13.8% had severe disease, which includes dyspnoea, respiratory rate $\geq$ 30 breaths/min, peripheral oxygen saturation $\leq$ 93%, and arterial oxygen tension/fraction of inspired oxygen ratio < 300, with or without pulmonary infiltrate occupying more than 50% of the lung parenchyma in the first 24–48 h; and 6.1% had critical disease, which includes respiratory failure and septic shock, with or without multiple organ dysfunction/failure. Although asymptomatic infection has been reported, the proportion of truly asymptomatic cases is not well defined. The individuals most at risk of serious illness and death reportedly include people over 60 years of age, especially those with underlying conditions, such as hypertension, diabetes, cardiovascular disease, chronic respiratory disease, and cancer[1,3].

In patients with COVID-19, the CT findings most commonly reported are ground-glass opacities and areas of consolidation, sometimes with a rounded morphology and peripheral distribution. Bernheim et al.[5] evaluated pulmonary abnormalities related to the duration of the disease and reported that, on chest CT, the disease was most extensive at approximately 10 days after symptom onset. A chest X-ray is often essential for the evaluation of patients with suspected COVID-19. Immediate recognition of the disease is essential to ensure timely treatment. From a public health point of view, rapid isolation of the patient is crucial to containing this communicable disease. In the Bernheim et al. study[5], the chest CT findings of 121 patients infected with COVID-19 in China were characterized in relation to the time from the onset of symptoms to the first CT scan. The authors hypothesized that the frequency of certain CT findings would increase in parallel with an increase in the time elapsed since infection. Only the initial chest CT scans were evaluated. In 27 (22%) of the 121 patients, CT showed no changes. The remaining 94 (78%) patients had ground-glass opacities, areas of consolidation, or both. Of the 121 patients, 73 (60%) had bilateral lung disease.

None of the 121 patients had thoracic lymph node disease, pulmonary cavitation, or pulmonary nodules, and only 1 patient (1%) had pleural effusion. The time from the onset of symptoms to the first CT scan was classified as early (0–2 days; 36 patients), intermediate (3–5 days; 33 patients), or late (6–12 days; 25 patients). The frequency of ground-glass opacities and areas of consolidation was considerably lower in the early-CT group than in the intermediate-CT group and late-CT group.

Pulmonary opacities were seen in only 16 (44%) of the 36 early-CT group patients, compared with 30 (91%) of the 33 intermediate-CT group patients and 24 (96%) of the 25 late-CT group patients. Bilateral pulmonary involvement was observed in 10 (28%) of the earlyCT group patients, in 25 (76%) of the intermediate-CT group patients, and in 22 (88%) of the late-CT group patients. Linear opacities, a crazy-paving pattern, and the inverted halo sign were absent in the early-CT group but were present in the lateCT group in 5 (20%), 5 (20%), and 1 (4%) of patients, respectively. In terms of disease distribution in the axial plane, peripheral distribution was observed in 8 (22%) of the early-CT group patients, in 21 (64%) of the intermediate-CT group patients, and in 18 (72%) of the late-CT group patients. The recognition of imaging patterns based on the time since coronavirus infection is critical not only to understanding the pathophysiology and natural history of the infection but also to predicting patient progression and the development of complications. So far, the anatomopathological aspects of the disease have not been described[6]. Future studies will be able to evaluate imaging findings in patients with chronic COVID-19(5), as well as to report the pathological aspects of the infection.

REFERENCES

1. Brasil. Ministério da Saúde. Protocolo de manejo clínico para o novo-coronavírus (2019-nCoV). [cited 2020 Feb 12]. Available from: https://portalarquivos2.saude.gov.br/images/pdf/2020/fevereiro/11/protocolo-manejo-coronavirus.pdf.

2. Brasil. Ministério da Saúde. Coronavírus: o que você precisa saber e como prevenir o contágio. [cited 2020 Feb 18]. Available from: https://saude.gov. br/saude-de-a-z/coronavírus.

3. Report of the WHO-China Joint Mission on Coronavirus Disease 2019 (COVID-19). [cited 2020 Feb 25]. Available from: https://www.who.int/docs/ default-source/coronaviruse/who-china-joint-mission-on-COVID-19-finalreport.pdf.

4. Guan W, Ni Z, Hu Y, et al. Clinical characteristics of coronavirus disease 2019 in China. N Engl J Med. 2020. DOI: 10.1056/NEJMoa2002032.

5. Bernheim A, Mei X, Huang M, et al. Chest CT findings in coronavirus disease-19 (COVID-19): relationship to duration of infection. Radiology. 2020. DOI: 10.1148/radiol.2020200463.

6. Kanne JP, Little BP, Chung JH, et al. Essentials for radiologists on COVID-19: an update—Radiology Scientific Expert Panel. Radiology. 2020. DOI: 10.1148/radiol.2020200527

2. A Meta-Analysis of COVID-19 Test Accuracy In Brazil[1]

[2]Rodolfo Castro,[a,b] Paula M. Luz,[c] Mayumi D. Wakimoto,[c] Valdilea G. Veloso,[c] Beatriz Grinsztejn,[c] and Hugo Perazzo[c,*]

ABSTRACT

The accuracy of commercially available tests for COVID-19 in Brazil remains unclear. We aimed to perform a meta-analysis to describe the accuracy of available tests to detect COVID19 in Brazil. We searched at the Brazilian Health Regulatory Agency (ANVISA) online platform to describe the pooled sensitivity (Se), specificity (Sp), diagnostic odds ratio (DOR) and summary receiver operating characteristic curves (SROC) for detection of IgM/IgG antibodies and for tests using naso/oropharyngeal swabs in the random-effects models. We identified 16 tests registered, mostly rapid-tests. Pooled diagnostic accuracy measures [95%CI] were:(i) for IgM antibodies Se = 82% [76–87]; Sp = 97% [96–98]; DOR = 168 [92–305] and SROC= 0.98 [0.96–0.99]; (ii) for IgG antibodies Se = 97% [90–99]; Sp = 98% [97–99]; DOR = 1994 [385–10334] and SROC= 0.99 [0.98–1.00]; and (iii) for detection of SARS-CoV-2 by antigen or molecular assays in naso/oropharyngeal swabs Se = 97% [85–99]; Sp = 99% [77–100]; DOR = 2649 [30–233056] and SROC= 0.99 [0.98–1.00]. These tests can be helpful for emergency testing during the COVID-19 pandemic in Brazil. However, it is important to highlight the high rate of false negative results from tests which detect SARS-CoV-2 IgM antibodies in the initial course of the disease and the scarce evidence-based validation results published in Brazil. Future studies addressing the diagnostic performance of tests for COVID-19 in the Brazilian population are urgently needed.

INTRODUCTION

The World Health Organization (WHO) declared Coronavirus disease 2019 (COVID-19) as pandemic on March 11, 2020. Due to the rapid spread of severe acute respiratory syndrome coronavirus 2 (SARS-CoV-2) viruses, we are currently facing a scenario of sustained community transmission of COVID-19 worldwide.[1] Early implementation of mitigation associated with suppression strategies can drastically reduce the number of hospitalizations and deaths.[2]

Large-scale testing, rapid diagnosis and immediate isolation of cases coupled with rigorous tracking and preventive self-isolation of close contacts are essential measures to reduce the burden of the COVID-19 pandemic.[3] Therefore, tests for COVID-19 should be point-of-care, widely available, and

[1] Castro, R., Luz, P. M., Wakimoto, M. D., Veloso, V. G., Grinsztejn, B., & Perazzo, H. (2020). COVID-19: a meta-analysis of diagnostic test accuracy of commercial assays registered in Brazil. The Brazilian journal of infectious diseases : an official publication of the Brazilian Society of Infectious Diseases, 24(2), 180–187. https://doi.org/10.1016/j.bjid.2020.04.003

[2] aFundação Oswaldo Cruz (FIOCRUZ), Escola Nacional de Saúde Pública Sergio Arouca (ENSP), Rio de Janeiro, RJ, Brazil
bUniversidade Federal do Estado do Rio de Janeiro (UNIRIO), Instituto de Saúde Coletiva (ISC), Rio de Janeiro, RJ, Brazil
cFundação Oswaldo Cruz (FIOCRUZ), Instituto Nacional de Infectologia Evandro Chagas (INI), Rio de Janeiro, RJ, Brazil
Hugo Perazzo: rb.zurcoif.ini@ozzarep.oguh: moc.liamg@oguhozzarep
*Corresponding author. rb.zurcoif.ini@ozzarep.oguh: moc.liamg@oguhozzarep

implemented outside of hospital settings to prevent overwhelming the health care system as well as the risk of nosocomial transmission to other patients and healthcare workers. Results from the mathematical modelling study performed by the Imperial College of London for Brazil, the implementation of suppression strategies could save up to a million lives and prevent the collapse of the Brazilian Unified Health System (*Sistema Único de Saúde*, SUS) compared to an unmitigated strategy.[4] Though massive testing is a cornerstone to reduce the burden of COVID-19, the accuracy of commercially available tests for COVID-19 in Brazil remains unclear. The aim of this study was to perform a meta-analysis to describe the accuracy of available tests to detect COVID-19 in Brazil.

To identify the registered tests for COVID-19 diagnosis in Brazil, we performed searches on March 30, 2020 using the following terms "*COVID-19*" OR "*SARS-CoV-2*" OR "*2019-nCoV*" OR "*coronavirus*" at the Brazilian Health Regulatory Agency.[1] Data were extracted by two independent researchers to an electronic database. The identified tests were stratified according to those which detect SARS-CoV-2 immunoglobulin antibodies (IgM and/or IgG) and nucleic acid (RNA) or antigen (Ag) from SARS-CoV-2. The following data were extracted from documents uploaded by manufacturers for each registered test: test name, ANVISA registry number, type of sample, type of analysis, type of assay and data of the diagnostic value of each test as reported by the manufacturer [number of true positive (TP), false positive (FP), true negative (TN) and false negative (FN)].

Diagnostic performance for the detection of IgM and IgG antibodies was analysed separately for each test. Detection of IgM antibodies is often interpreted as an indicator of acute infection while the detection of IgG antibodies represents previous infection/immunity. Sensitivity (Se), specificity (Sp), positive predictive value (PPV), and negative predictive value (NPV) were described.

Data synthesis was performed using univariate mixed-effects logistic regression models with maximum likelihood estimation based on adaptive Gaussian quadrature using xtmelogit (midas package) from STATA for Windows (2017; StataCorp LP, College Station, TX, USA).[5] Pooled Se, Sp, positive likelihood ratio (LR+), negative likelihood ratio (LR−) and diagnostic odds ratio (DOR) are described for IgM antibodies, IgG antibodies and for tests using nasopharyngeal and/or oropharyngeal swabs for SARS-CoV-2 detection in the random-effects models. Forest plots with test-specific and overall point estimates and 95% confidence intervals (CI) were provided with Cochran's Q and I^2 heterogeneity statistics.

Summary receiver operating characteristic curves (SROC) were plotted with the presentation of a summary operating point, 95% confidence and prediction contours. A total of 16 tests for detection of COVID-19 registered in the ANVISA's online platform were identified. Out of these, 11 tests detect SARS-CoV-2 N-Protein IgM and/or IgG antibodies [nine for IgM/IgG; one for IgM and one for IgG detection] in human serum, plasma, whole blood (or finger prick samples); three detect the nucleic acid (RNA) and two detect the antigen (Ag) of SARS-CoV-2 in nasopharyngeal and/or oropharyngeal swabs. All tests considered molecular assays as the gold standard.

In addition, 11 tests are considered as point-of-care (POC) tests: nine detecting IgM/IgG antibodies in finger prick sample and two detecting SARS-CoV-2 Ag in nasopharyngeal and/or oropharyngeal swabs. A total of seven tests are imported from the following countries: China (*n*= 4), United States of America (*n*= 2), and Spain (*n*= 1) tests

---

[1] (Agência Nacional de Vigilância Sanitária, ANVISA, website: https://consultas.anvisa.gov.br/#/saude/).

For detection of IgM antibodies (eight tests; 951 samples), pooled diagnostic accuracy measures [95%CI] were: Se = 82% [76–87]; Sp = 97% [96–98]; DOR = 168 [92–305]; LR+ = 31.3 [19.7–49.7]; LR– = 0.19 [0.14–0.25] and SROC = 0.98 [0.96–0.99] (Fig. 1A and B). For detection of IgG antibodies (eight tests; 1503 samples), pooled diagnostic accuracy measures [95%CI] were: Se = 97% [90–99]; Sp = 98% [97–99]; DOR = 1994 [385–10334]; LR+ = 56.6 [30.6–104.7]; LR– = 0.03 [0.01–0.11]; and SROC = 0.99 [0.98–1.00] (Fig. 2A and B). Finally, for detection of SARS-CoV-2 by antigen or molecular assays in nasopharyngeal and/or oropharyngeal swabs (four tests; 464 samples), pooled diagnostic accuracy measures [95%CI] were: Se = 97% [85–99]; Sp = 99% [77–100]; DOR = 2649 [30–233056]; LR+ = 89.5 [3.3–2400.8]; LR– = 0.03 [0.01–0.17]; and SROC = 0.99 [0.98–1.00] (Fig. 3A and B).

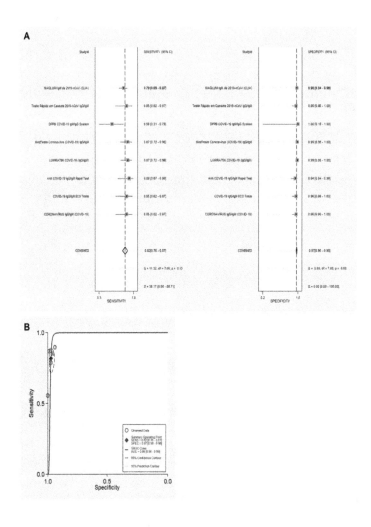

Fig. 1:Pooled diagnostic accuracy analysis (A) and summary receiver operating characteristic curve (B) of tests (*n* = 8) for detection of IgM antibodies tests against SARS-CoV-2.

115

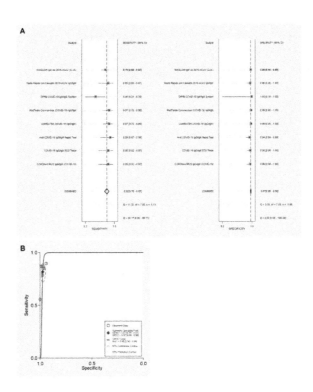

Fig. 2:Pooled diagnostic accuracy analysis (A) and summary receiver operating characteristic curve (B) of tests (*n* = 8) for detection of IgG antibodies tests against SARS-CoV-2.

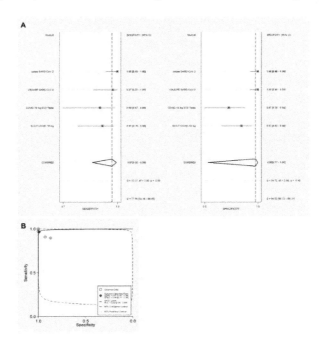

Fig. 3:Pooled diagnostic accuracy analysis (A) and summary receiver operating characteristic curve (B) of tests (*n* = 4) using nasopharyngeal and/or oropharyngeal swabs for detection of antigen or nuclei acid of SARS-CoV-2.

This meta-analysis highlighted the accuracy of tests for COVID-19 diagnosis registered by the Brazilian health authorities (ANVISA). To the best of our knowledge, this is the first study to provide pooled diagnostic accuracy of tests for COVID-19 available for clinical use in Brazil. Large scale testing is essential to tackle COVID-19 because accurate knowledge of the number of confirmed cases provides information on the spread of the virus within a population and thus on the evolution of the pandemic.

As of April 3rd 2020, the Brazilian Ministry of Health had confirmed around 9000 COVID-19 confirmed cases.[6] However, the actual number of cases is likely much higher because of limited testing. Furthermore, while we wait for effective vaccines, the knowledge of the extent of immunity in the population after the pandemic ceases depends on accurate diagnostics which will later guide the use of appropriate strategies when facing a potential second wave of COVID-19.

Since the beginning of the pandemic, medical companies and research institutes have been looking for developing and approving tests to detect current viral infection and immunity to SARS-CoV-2.[7] The diagnosis of SARS-CoV-2 infection involves collecting the correct specimen from the patient at the right time. SARS-CoV-2 detection using real-time polymerase chain reaction (PCR) test kits can be considered as the gold-standard for the diagnosis of COVID-19. However, this technique requires certified laboratories, expensive equipment and trained technicians. Rapid tests for detection of specific antibodies of SARS-CoV-2 in blood samples remain a good choice for diagnosing COVID-19. It is estimated that SARS-CoV-2 IgM antibodies can be detected in a blood sample after 3–6 days and IgG antibodies after eight days of symptoms onset.[8] Serological assays, detecting IgM/IgG antibodies, are important tests for diagnosing SARS-CoV-2 and can help understand the burden and role of asymptomatic infections. The present study showed that 10 serological tests for IgM/IgG antibodies, including nine point-of-care tests, are currently available in Brazil. These tests are simple and can provide rapid confirmation of COVID-19 confirmation while at the same time being limited due to higher rates of false-negative results when collected in the early-phase of symptoms onset. Our study reports that antigen testing and/or molecular assays using nasopharyngeal and oropharyngeal specimens had high accuracy for SARS-CoV-2 detection. in China, the rate of SARS-CoV-2 detection was higher in oropharyngeal compared to nasopharyngeal swabs during the COVID-19 outbreak.[9] Naso/oropharyngeal tests might miss early infection leading to a strategy of repeated testing since the likelihood of the SARS-CoV-2 being present in the nasopharynx increases with time.[8] In the present study, the pooled sensitivity of tests using the detection of COVID-19 IgM antibodies in blood was lower compared to antigen/molecular assay detection in nasopharyngeal/oropharyngeal swabs (82% [95%CI 76–87] vs 97% [95%CI 85–99]).

It is worth noting that for this analysis we relied on the accuracy of available tests for COVID-19 as per information provided by the manufacturers during the test registration process at ANVISA. There were no peer-reviewed publications. Moreover, data of clinical significance with regards to the diagnostic validity of each test, such as patients' characteristics or time of sample collection after the onset of symptoms, were not provided. Literature searches that included test names, dealers, or manufacturers, yielded a single paper that described the analytical performance of a molecular assay to diagnose COVID-19 in nasopharyngeal and oropharyngeal specimens.[10] Moreover, few tests have been validated with a limited number of samples (≤20), and only half of the tests included more than 150 samples in validation studies. In addition, these tests might present cross-reactivity with other coronavirus that cause respiratory diseases. Among all tests, the One Step COVID-2019 Test is said to have been tested with one of the highest study sample, $N= 596$.

However, the manufacturers did not describe accuracy for IgM and IgG assays separately in the ANVISA document leading to the exclusion of the test from the forest plot. Finally, there were few tests that clearly used similar samples for validation of different tests.

Recently, the U.S. Food and Drug Administration has granted Cellex an emergency use authorization to market a rapid antibody test for COVID-19 (Cellex qSARS-CoV-2 IgG/IgM Rapid Test), the first antibody test released during the pandemic Of 128 samples confirmed positive by reverse transcription PCR in premarket testing,[1] 120 tested positive by IgG, IgM, or both. Of 250 confirmed negative, 239 were negative by the rapid test. Moreover, the numbers translated to a positive percent agreement with RT-PCR of 93.8% (95% CI: 88.06–97.26%) and a negative percent agreement of 96.4% (95% CI: 92.26–97.78%), according to labelling.[2] In conclusion, we have reviewed the details and reported on the pooled diagnostic accuracy of different types of tests currently available to tackle COVID-19 in Brazil. A total of 16 tests currently available and registered at the Brazilian Health Regulatory Agency (ANVISA) were identified, mostly rapid tests to detect IgM and/or IgG antibodies. The pooled diagnostic accuracy of tests available in Brazil was satisfactory, and they can be helpful for emergency testing during the COVID-19 pandemic in Brazil. However, it is important to highlight that the rate of false negative results from tests which detect SARS-CoV-2 IgM antibodies, used for detection of COVID-19 in the acute phase, ranged from 10 to 44%. Furthermore, there is scarce evidence-base validation results published in Brazil. Future studies addressing the diagnostic performance of a panel of tests for COVID-19 in the Brazilian population are urgently needed.

REFERENCES

1. European Centre for Disease Prevention and Control . 2020. Novel coronavirus disease 2019 (COVID-19) pandemic: increased transmission in the EU/EEA and the UK – sixth update: European Centre for Disease Prevention and Control. Available from: https://www.ecdc.europa.eu/en/publications-data/rapid-risk-assessment-novel-coronavirus-disease-2019-COVID-19-pandemic-increased. [Google Scholar]
2. Walker P., Whittaker C., Watson O. (2020). The Global Impact of COVID-19 and Strategies for Mitigation and Suppression: Imperial College London. Available from: https://www.imperial.ac.uk/media/imperial-college/medicine/sph/ide/gida-fellowships/Imperial-College-COVID19-Global-Impact-26-03-2020v2.pdf. [CrossRef] [Google Scholar]
3. Salathe M., Althaus C.L., Neher R. (2020)COVID-19 epidemic in Switzerland: on the importance of testing, contact tracing and isolation. Swiss Med Wkly. 2020;150:w20225. [PubMed] [Google Scholar]
4. Imperial College London . 2020. The Global Impact of COVID-19 and Strategies for Mitigation and Suppression. http://www.imperial-college-covid19-global-unmitigated-mitigated-suppression-scenarios.xlsx/ [accessed 30.3.20] [Google Scholar]
5. Dwamena B. Department of Economics, Boston College; 2007. MIDAS: Stata module for meta-analytical integration of diagnostic test accuracy studies. Available from: https://ideas.repec.org/c/boc/bocode/s456880.html. [Google Scholar]
6. COVID-19 in Brazil: update of confirmed cases and deaths; 2020. https://covid.saude.gov.br/ [accessed 3.4.20].
7. Petherick A. (2020). Developing antibody tests for SARS-CoV-2. Lancet. 2020;395:1101–1102. [PMC free article] [PubMed] [Google Scholar]
8. Li Z., Yi Y., Luo X. (2020).Development and clinical application of a rapid IgM-IgG combined antibody test for SARS-CoV-2 infection diagnosis. J Med Virol. 2020 doi: 10.1002/jmv.25727. [Epub ahead of print] [PMC free article] [PubMed] [CrossRef] [Google Scholar]
9. Wang W., Xu Y., Gao R. (2020). Detection of SARS-CoV-2 in different types of clinical specimens. JAMA. 2020 doi: 10.1001/jama.2020.3786. [PMC free article] [PubMed] [CrossRef] [Google Scholar]
10. Pfefferle S., Reucher S., Norz D., Lutgehetmann M. (2020).Evaluation of a quantitative RT-PCR assay for the detection of the emerging coronavirus SARS-CoV-2 using a high throughput system. Euro Surveill. 2020;25 doi:10.2807/1560-7917.ES.2020.25.9.2000152. [PMC free article] [PubMed] [Google Scholar]

---

[1] (https://www.fda.gov/media/136622/download).
[2] (https://www.fda.gov/media/136625/download).

3. Comparison of Different Kits For SARS-CoV-2 RNA Extraction Marketed In Brazil

[1]Ana Karolina Antunes Eisen, Meriane Demoliner, Juliana Schons Gularte, Alana Witt Hansen, Karoline Schallenberger, Larissa Mallmann, Bruna Saraiva Hermann, Fágner Henrique Heldt, Paula Rodrigues de Almeida, Juliane Deise Fleck, Fernando Rosado Spilki

ABSTRACT

December 2019 marked the beginning of the greatest pandemic since Spanish Flu, the disease named COVID-19 that cause severe pneumonia. Until May 19, 2020 more than 4 million and 700 thousand cases were officially notified with about 316 thousand deaths. Etiological agent of the disease was identified as being a new coronavirus, *Severe acute respiratory syndrome-related coronavirus* (SARS-CoV-2). In this study we compared four different manual methods for RNA isolation and purification for detection of SARSCoV-2 through qRT-PCR, as well as the extraction quality itself through detection of RNAse P. Magnetic beads-based (MagMax™) and silica column-based (Biopur®) methods presented the better performances. Concerning to the mean delay in CT values when compared to MagMax™, TRIzol™, Biopur® and EasyExtract presented 0,39, 0,95 and 5,23 respectively. Agreement between positive and negative results of different methods when compared with the one with better performance MagMax™ was 94,44% for silica column-based method (Biopur®), 88,89% for phenol-chroloform-based method (TRIzol™) and 77,78% for EasyExtract. We aimed to evaluate how reliable each method is for diagnostic purposes and to propose alternatives when usual methods are not available. In this regard, magnetic beads and silica column-based methods are convenient and reliable choices and phenol-chloroform-based method could also be chosen as an alternative.

INTRODUCTION

December 2019 marked the beginning of the greatest pandemic since Spanish Flu, when the first cases of COVID-19 were identified, an atypical pneumonia of unknown origin. Infection origin was initially associated with a seafood market in Wuhan city, Hubei province, China [13]. Disease was named as COVID-19 by the World Health Organization (WHO) in a report that was published in February 22, 2020 [4]. The infection had spread rapidly through the Europe and the Americas since the first imported cases were arrived, until May 19, 2020 more than 4 million and 700 thousand cases were officially notified with about 316 thousand deaths distributed through 216 countries [5].Etiological agent of the disease was identified as being a new coronavirus originating from bats with a possible relation to a coronavirus identified in pangolins of *Manis javanica* species [2, 3, 6]. The new coronavirus was classified in the same species of the first SARS of 2003 as *Severe acute*

---

[1] Corresponding author: Ana Karolina Antunes Eisen: E-mail: akaeisen@gmail.com

respiratory syndrome-related coronavirus (SARS-CoV-2), within the subgenre *Sarbecovirus,* genre *Betacoronavirus,* subfamily *Orthocoronavirinae* and *Coronaviridae* family. Members of this viral Family are mainly spherical and have lipid envelopes with prominent proteins named Spikes, which ones give the crown appearance that inspired family name. Genome is composed by a positive single stranded RNA that measures about 26 - 31 kb and is read through 6 ORFs [7]. Besides SARS-CoV-2, six other coronavirus are already known by cause infection in humans, among them the SARS and MERS-CoV pandemic viruses that may cause severe disease and pneumonia and the other four human coronavirus (HCoV) that are causal agents of common colds OC43, 229E, HKU1 and NL63 [8,9].COVID-19 is a mainly respiratory disease that have as most common symptoms the fewer, cough, shortness of breath, fatigue and difficulty breathing, other symptoms as chills, sore throat, myalgia, loss of smell and taste may also occur with minor frequency, besides gastrointestinal manifestations as diarrhoea, nausea and vomiting. In most severe cases the disease course with severe pneumonia that usually lead to hospitalization and the need to use mechanical respirators [10-12]. Two essential measures are required to control of the pandemic while no vaccines are available: social distancing and large-scale testing of the population. Due to high infected number, even testing only symptomatic patients who looked for medical care there is still a huge sample volume to do the diagnostic. Thereby, alternative methods may be required when lack of kits and reagents would occur due to high demand, mainly in nucleic acids extraction prior to detection by quantitative reverse transcriptase polymerase chain reaction (qRT-PCR).Here we compared four different manual methods for SARS-CoV-2 RNA isolation and purification aiming detection by qRT-PCR marketed as commercial kits in Brazil.

MATERIALS AND METHODS

Methods compared in this study include magnetic beads method MagMax™ CORE Nucleic Acid Purificatioin Kit (ThermoFisher™), which was adapted for a manual procedure using magnetic racks, column-based method Mini Spin Plus Kit (Biopur®) for total nucleic acid extraction, TRIzol™ (Invitrogen™), a phenol-chloroform-based method for high quality RNA isolation and a simple fast methodology for sample preparation prior to the PCR amplification named EasyExtract (Calpro AS™). With exception of MagMax™ in which an adaption for the manual procedure, the other methods were performed exactly as described by their respective manufacturers.

SAMPLES AND CONTROLS

To compare quality of extraction methods, an inactivated Brazilian reference strain cultivated in VERO-Slam cells gently provided by Dr. Edison Durigon (Universidade de São Paulo) was used as a control, and tested pure and diluted with a dilution factor of 10, eight times into cell culture minimum essential medium (MEM), each dilution corresponded to a final sample in the performance assay. In addition to control, a set of SARS-CoV-2 positive nine clinical samples already tested in our lab was chosen based on cycle threshold value (CT), being three of each CT range in qRT-PCR for SARS-CoV-2 (allotted as low, medium and high).In order to properly compare the different methods, all final samples were aliquoted separately for each technique and freezed (ultrafreezer -80ºC) only one time before total nucleic acids/RNA extractions were done, the same attention was taken with the nucleic acids extracted before analysis by qRT-PCR.

Manual Nucleic Acid Purification By Magnetic Beads

As mentioned above, we adapted MagMax™ CORE Nucleic Acid Purificatioin Kit (ThermoFisher™) for a manual procedure using magnetic racks. Only reagents provided by the kit were used and the steps basically followed the automated ones. An initial 200 µl aliquot of each sample was mixed with 30 µl of beads mix (20 µl of magnetic beads and 10 µl of proteinase K) by pipetting up and down ten times, 700 µl of lysis-binding mix were then add and tubes were homogenized by vortexing, transferred to the magnetic rack where stayed for 1 min before supernatant removal. Five hundred microliters of Wash 1 were add to the samples, tubes were vortexed for 1 min, spinned for 10 sec at 500 rpm and then placed in the magnetic rack again for 1 min until supernatant removal, Wash 2 were used as described for Wash 1 and after supernatant removal the tubes stayed in rack with lids open to dry for 5 min. Elution buffer (90 µl) was then added to the tubes and they were homogenized in vortex for 3 min, spinned 10 sec and placed in the rack for 3 min until elute transfer to a new tube.

Detection By Quantitative Reverse Transcriptase Polymerase Chain Reaction (qRT-PCR)

Detection of SARS-CoV-2 were done with the set of primers and probe of the Charité protocol for amplification of E gene with some modifications that will be described here [13]. Reactions were done in a total volume of 20 µl, being 10 µl of 2X RT-PCR Buffer and 0,8 µl of Enzyme Mix of the AgPath-ID™ One-Step RT-PCR Reagents (ThermoFisher™), 0,8 µl of each primer and 0,4 µl of probe for E gene [13] both in a 5 µM concentration, 2,2 µl of nucleasse-free water and 5 µl of RNA sample. Amplification cycle was also adapted, starting in 50ºC during 15 min for reverse transcriptase, followed by denaturation in 95ºC for 10 min and 40 cycles in 95ºC for 15 sec and 60ºC for 45 sec. For RNAse P amplification the set of primers and probes N1 and N2 of CDC diagnostic panel [14] were used in the following conditions: 20 µl total volume being 10 µl of 2X RT-PCR Buffer and 0,8 µl of Enzyme Mix of the AgPath-ID™ One-Step RT-PCR Reagents (ThermoFisher™), 1,5 µl of primers + probe, 2,7 µl of nuclease-free water and 5 µl of RNA sample. Amplification cycle for RNAse P detection was the same described above for the E gene.

RESULTS

The method with the best performance, lower CT values to both SARS-CoV-2 or RNAse P and greater detection sensitivity of the control dilutions was the magnetic beads method MagMax™ that succeed to detect until a dilution of 10^{-8} of the control with a CT value of 38,47, all CT values to SARS-CoV-2 detection are listed in the Table 1, RNAseP detection results could be checked in the Table 2. MagMax™ and Biopur® presented the lowest CT values and TRIzol™ performed slightly better than EasyExtract.Two singularities must be mentioned, bronchoalveolar lavage sample 3539 was negative in TRIzol™ technique probably due to it's great viscosity, although it was initially diluted in MEM, which probably impaired technique execution mainly in the step of phase separation with chloroform. So, in this situation a greater dilution of the sample may be required to do this technique. When EasyExtract technique was done with the pure samples there was interference in qRT-PCR detection in control samples due to MEM coloration and in the clinical samples due to presence of inhibitors, taking into account that this method does not have a wash step. A second test was take with all the samples diluted in a 1:10 proportion, what resulted in the values utilized for comparison with the other methods and that are shown in **Table 1 and 2**, despite of one more thawn was done with the samples. Concerning to the mean delay in CT values when compared to MagMax™, TRIzol™, Biopur® and EasyExtract presented 0,39, 0,95 and 5,23 respectively. High delay in CT values of EasyExtract may impair detection in samples with low viral titer resulting in false negative results. Phenol-chloroform and silica column separation methods besides have presented few delay when compared with MagMax™ also presented similar values among itselves with 0,99 correlation. Ultimately, agreement between positive and negative results of different methods when compared with the one with better performance MagMax™ was 94,44% for silica column separation method (Biopur®), followed by 88,89% for phenol-chroloform method (TRIzol™) and 77,78% for EasyExtract. Based on these results, the better alternatives of manual extraction methods to reduce chances of false negative results in COVID-19 diagnostics are magnetic beads extraction method MagMax™ and the silica column separation method (Biopur®).

DISCUSSION

The sudden start of the current pandemic of a new coronavirus, now known as SARSCoV-2 and rapid growth in number of suspects cases took scientists all over the world to run for a sensitive, specific and reliable diagnostic method to test the growing number of victims. After the first genomes sequences were published by Chinese researchers it was possible to establish a qRT-PCR diagnostic protocol to large scale production and distribution [13, 14].With the great demand of materials and reagents some laboratories face lack of products and/or long delivery time while a growing number of patients await for a diagnostic result. Nucleic acids isolation and purification is a major step in the diagnostic of COVID-19 and although the main laboratories have this process automated, many others around the world mainly in developing countries does not have this option.

Besides of that, the already mentioned lack of products may lead automated laboratories to swift to manual process to accomplish the diagnostic requirements. In order to evaluate performance of alternative methods to the automated ones, in this study we have compared four different manual nucleic acids extraction methods for gene E SARS-CoV-2 and RNAse P detection. Being them the magnetic beads-based method MagMax™ CORE Nucleic Acid Purificatioin Kit (ThermoFisher™), column-based method Mini Spin Plus Kit (Biopur®), TRIzol™ (Invitrogen™) a phenol-chloroform based-method and the sample preparation EasyExtract.Unfortunately, besides being attractive due to fastness and low handling the EasyExtract method presented pour results, not being reliable mainly in clinical samples with low viral titers. Also, due to absence of a wash step this technique maintains the presence of inhibitors and a sample dilution may be required. Still, in emergency situations it can be used as a last resort. Phenol-chloroform-based method evaluated here presented satisfactory results, this technique possesses the advantage of allowing RNA isolation and having protective characteristics for that. Although the agreement of positive-negative results of only 88,89% comparing to MagMax™, it presented the lowest CT delay among the other techniques (0,39).Lastly, this method presents some cons given that possess a laborious and time-consuming process and requires the use of toxic, harmful and irritating reagents. With this in mind, it is still a good alternative when necessary. In this study, the silica column-based method presented results almost as good as the magnetic beads method taking into account that have a delay of 0,95 and a positive-negative agreement of 94,44%, proving itself as a good manual kit option. Both techniques have also a similar process time. Similar to our findings, another study that have compared the magnetic beads with silica column-based methods for human gut microbial community profiling obtained higher amounts of nucleic acids extracted with the magnetic beads method and greater species diversity, it also showed that manual extraction presented similar results to the automated ones when taking into account the reproducibility of microbial profiles, although it might be different for nucleic acids yields [15]. However, most studies that have done comparison of different extraction methods have used faeces samples to bacteria detection [16, 17].

CONCLUSION

In this work we have compared four different types of manual extraction methods for SARS-CoV-2 detection by qRT-PCR with clinical samples and control dilutions. We aimed to evaluate how reliable each method is for diagnostic purposes and to propose alternatives when usual methods are not available. In this regard, magnetic beads and silica column-based methods are convenient and reliable choices, phenol-chloroform-based method could also be chosen as an alternative method unlike to EasyExtract that is not a trustworthy option.

ACKNOWLEDGMENTS

We would like to thank to Coordenação de Aperfeiçoamento de Pessoal de Nível Superior – CAPES for the graduate scholarships, Financiadora de Estudos e Projetos – Finep and RedeVírus Ministério da Ciência, Tecnologia, Inovações e Comunicações – MCTIC for the research funding.

Table 1: Cycle threshold values for E gene detection of SARS-CoV-2 by different extraction methods

ID	MagMax	TRIzol	Biopur	EasyExtract
PC pure	12, 99	8,61	8,71	ND
PC -1	14,01	14,35	15,86	24,10
PC -2	17,53	21,54	23,05	22,76
PC -3	20,86	25,82	26,40	25,91
PC -4	24,43	28,00	27,98	28,90
PC -5	27,74	32,90	31,83	32,96
PC -6	30,99	36,21	34,53	35,97
PC -7	34,26	37,39	37,95	39,14
PC -8	38,47	ND	ND	37,36
6539	29,66	ND	35,90	ND
6499	33,25	32,55	33,03	ND
6842	33,69	35,38	34,97	ND
6321	ND	ND	ND	ND
6754	25,53	24,11	24,20	30,14
6928	28,75	29,08	29,67	35,57
6935	18,80	18,32	18,67	24,14
6938	20,26	20,11	18,51	27,33
6941	20,54	22,40	20,36	26,53

ID: final sample identification; PC: positive control; ND: not detected.

Table 2: Cycle threshold values for RNAse P detection of clinical samples by different extraction methods

ID	MagMax	TRIzol	Biopur	EasyExtract
6539	19,29	ND	16,25	24,43
6499	24,71	30,41	23,86	29,38
6842	26,96	31,32	27,60	32,04
6321	25,87	33,6	25,90	31,73
6754	26,24	30,97	24,14	31,17
6928	28,41	30,68	27,69	33,61
6935	27,19	30,20	24,67	32,63
6938	23,66	27,16	21,67	29,09
6941	26,66	32,44	26,30	31,48

ID: sample identification; ND: not detected

REFERENCES

1. World Health Organization (2020). Novel Coronavirus (2019-nCoV) Situation Report 1. https://www.who.int/docs/default-source/coronaviruse/situation-reports/20200121-sitrep-1-2019ncov.pdf?sfvrsn=20a99c10_4. Accessed 19 May 2020

2. Wu, F., Zhao, S., Yu, B. et al (2020). A new coronavirus associated with human respiratory disease in China. Nature 579.7798 265-269

3. Zhou, P., Yang, X.L., Wang, X.G. et al (2020). A pneumonia outbreak associated with a new coronavirus of probable bat origin. Nature 579.7798 270-273

4. World Health Organization (2020). Novel Coronavirus (2019-nCoV) Situation Report 22. https://www.who.int/docs/default-source/coronaviruse/situation-reports/20200211-sitrep-22ncov.pdf?sfvrsn=fb6d49b1_2. Accessed 17 May 2020

5. World Health Organization (2020). Novel Coronavirus (2019-nCoV) Situation Report 120. https://www.who.int/docs/default-source/coronaviruse/situation-reports/20200519-COVID-19-sitrep120.pdf?sfvrsn=515cabfb_2. Accessed 19 May 2020

6. Andersen, K.G, Rambaut, A, Lipkin, W.I. et al (2020). The proximal origin of SARS-CoV-2. Nature medicine 26.4 450-452

7. International Committee on Taxonomy of Viruses – ICTV (2011) Coronaviridae. https://talk.ictvonline.org/ictv-reports/ictv_9th_report/positive-sense-rna-viruses2011/w/posrna_viruses/222/coronaviridae. Accessed 17 May 2020

8. Drosten, C., Günter, S., Preiser, W. et al (2003). Identification of a novel coronavirus in patients with severe acute respiratory syndrome. N Engl J Med 348.20 1967-1976

9. Zaki, A.M., Boheemen, S., Bestebroer, T.M. et al (2012). Isolation of a novel coronavirus from a man with pneumonia in Saudi Arabia. N Engl J Med 367.19 1814-1820

10. Huang, C., Wang., Y, Li X et al (2020). Clinical features of patients infected with 2019 novel coronavirus in Wuhan, China. The lancet 395.10223 497-506

11. Wang, D., Hu B, Hu C et al (2020) Clinical characteristics of 138 hospitalized patients with 2019 novel coronavirus–infected pneumonia in Wuhan, China. Jama 323.11 1061-1069

12. Yan, C.H., Faraji, F., Prajapati, D.P. et al (2020) Association of chemosensory dysfunction and Covid-19 in patients presenting with influenza-like symptoms. Int Forum Allergy Rh

13. Corman, V., Bleicker, T., Brünink, S. et al (2020) Diagnostic detection of 2019-nCoV by real-time RT-PCR. World Health Organization, Jan, 17

14. Centers for Disease Control and Prevention – CDC (2020). 2019-Novel Coronavirus (2019-NCoV) Real-Time RT-PCR Diagnostic Panel https://www. fda.gov/media/134922/download

15. Lim, M.Y., Song, E.J., Kim, S.H. et al (2018). Comparison of DNA extraction methods for human gut microbial community profiling. Syst Appl Microbiol 41.2 151-157

16. Mirsepase, H., Persson, S., Struve, C et al (2014). Microbial diversity in fecal samples depends on DNA extraction method: easyMag DNA extraction compared to QIAamp DNA stool mini kit extraction. BMC Res. Notes 7.1 50

17. Persson S, de Boer, R.F., Kooistra-Smid, A.M.D. et al (2011). Five commercial DNA extraction systems tested and compared on a stool sample collection. Diagn Micr Infec Dis 69.3 240-244

4. Sensitivity and Specificity of A Rapid Test For Assessment of Exposure To SARS-Cov-2 Brazil

Lucia Campos Pellanda[1], Eliana Márcia da Ros Wendland[1], Alan John Alexander McBride [2], LucianaTovo-Rodrigues [3], Marcos Roberto Alves Ferreira [2], Odir Antônio Dellagostin [2], Mariangela Freitas daSilveira [3]. Aluísio Jardim Dornellas de Barros [3], Pedro Curi Hallal [3], Cesar Gomes Victora [3][1]

ABSTRACT

Background: While the recommended laboratory diagnosis of COVID-19 is a molecular based assay, population-based studies to determine the prevalence of COVID-19 usually use serological assays. **Objective:** To evaluate the sensitivity and specificity of a rapid diagnostic test for COVID-19 compared to quantitative reverse transcription polymerase chain reaction (qRT-PCR). **Methods:** We evaluated the sensitivity using a panel of finger prick blood samples from participants >18 years of age that had been tested for COVID-19 by qRT-PCR. For assessing specificity, we used serum samples from the 1982 Pelotas (Brazil) Birth Cohort participants collected in 2012 with no exposure to SARS-CoV-2. **Results:** The sensitivity of the test was 77.1% (95% CI 66.6 - 85.6), based upon 83 subjects who had tested positive for qRT-PCR at least 10 days before the rapid diagnostic test (RDT). Based upon 100 sera samples, specificity was 98.0% (95% CI 92.9 - 99.8). There was substantial agreement (Kappa score 0.76) between the qRT-PCR results and the RDT. **Interpretation**. The validation results are well in line with previous assessments of the test and confirm that it is sufficiently precise for epidemiological studies aimed at monitoring levels and trends of the COVID-19 pandemic.

INTRODUCTION

The COVID-19 pandemic continues to cause havoc around the world, and as of May 2nd there were 3,2362,772 confirmed cases and 239,227 fatalities reported [1]. Due to supply chain problems, many governments have opted to test only the most serious cases such that the epidemiology of the disease remains largely unknown. This has led public health experts to believe that the prevalence of COVID-19 is significantly underestimated [2,3].The laboratory reference method for detecting

[1] Affiliations
1   Community Health Department, Federal University of Health Sciences of Porto Alegre (UFCSPA), Brazil.
2   Biotechnology Department, Centre for Technological Development, Federal University of Pelotas, Brazil.
3   Post-graduate Program in Epidemiology, Federal University of Pelotas, Brazil

COVID-19 is based on real-time reverse transcriptase PCR (qRT-PCR), to detect the presence of SARS-CoV-2 in nasopharyngeal swabs collected from patients suspected to be infected [4]. While it is highly specific, there are reports of low sensitivity in the field[3,5–7]. The ability of the qRT-PCR to detect SARS-CoV-2 is dependent on the presence of the virus in the sample and this is subject to several variables, e.g. the virus must be present in the patients nasopharynx at the time of collection and the correct use of the swab [8]. The failure to meet the necessary criteria for collection can potentially result in a false negative result. This has dire consequences for public health, especially for asymptomatic individuals as they will continue to infect others as they are not aware of the risk of transmission [7], leading to the need of evaluating other diagnostic tools that could be useful in these settings.

Public health services around the world have resorted to purchasing serological assays towards overcoming the lack of availability of the standard nucleic acid tests. Given the urgent need for diagnostic tests, many regulatory agencies approved the emergency use of diagnostics based on the manufacturer's reports of diagnostic accuracy without the need for further validation [9,10]. Serological tests identify antibodies in symptomatic and asymptomatic individuals and, although of limited clinical use in diagnosis infection [11], are important in population-based studies that are necessary to estimate the seroprevalence of COVID-19. However, given the current global emergency, very few studies have evaluated the diagnostic properties of rapid diagnostic tests (RDT) in the settings where they will be used. Furthermore, there have been reports in the literature of significant discrepancies between the manufacturer's performance claims and the results from the field [4,9]. The time required for the immune system to produce detectable levels of immunoglobulins typically ranges from 5 to 10 days, but this may take longer in the case ofSARS-CoV-2 [7,12,13].

The Immunochromatographic Lateral Flow Assay (Wondfo SARS-CoV-2 Antibody Test, China)[14] used in this study detects IgG and IgM combined antibodies in blood, plasma or serum samples. This test was validated in a study performed by the manufacturer, which reported a sensitivity and specificity of 86.4 and 99.6%, respectively[14]. These tests were purchased in bulk by the Brazilian government and they were earmarked for use in population surveys and surveillance programs. An initial validation study was carried out by the National Institute for Quality Control in Health [15] using 18 qRT-PCR positive and 77 negative serum samples. The reported sensitivity was 100% (95% CI 81.50-100), while specificity was 98.7% (95% CI92.98-99.97), performance characteristics similar to those claimed by the manufacturer. However, as the RDT was to be used in a large-scale, population-based household survey of COVID-19 in the state of Rio Grande do Sul in Southern Brazil, we decided it was necessary to evaluate the RDT with an expanded panel of sera collected from the target population.

RESULTS

Volunteers were invited through newspaper and social media to participate in the RDT study; of the 95 qRT-PCR positive individuals who responded, 83 had been diagnosed 10 or more days previously and were enrolled in the study. The majority of the qRT-PCR positive participants were man (53.0%), self-reported white skin colour (96.0%), and 18 (21.7%) had at least one symptom associated with COVID-19 when tested with the RDT. The mean age for the group was 48.6 (SD = 14.4) years. In what regards the pre-COVID-19 group, 37.0% were man, 82.0% self-reported white skin colour. The mean age for the group was 30.0 (SD = 0.3) years. The sensitivity of the RDT among those previously diagnosed with COVID-19 was 77.1% (64/83) and the specificity was 98.0% in the pre-COVID-19 healthy individuals. When compared to the reference method, the RDT demonstrated substantial agreement with the qRT-PCR. As the prevalence rate of COVID-19 remains unknown, we calculated the predictive values of the RDT based on prevalence rates of 2, 4 and 10%; the PPVs ranged from 44 to 81% and the NPVs varied between 97.5 and 99.5%.

METHODS

Ethical approval. This study and the protocols used therein were approved by the National Commission on Ethics in Research (CONEP, Brasilia, DF). All participants signed an informed consent form. **Study design**. The study population included individuals (>18 yr. old) both symptomatic or asymptomatic at the time of testing and who were qRT-PCR positive for SARS-CoV-2 following the testing of nasopharyngeal swabs during March 2020. At least 10 days later (to allow for the production of anti-SARS-CoV-2 antibodies), the study participants were invited to complete a questionnaire on their COVID-19 symptoms and demographic information. A blood sample was collected by fingerstick and the RDT was carried out at the time of collection as recommended by the manufacturer. Samples from healthy individuals (n = 100) were randomly selected from a pre-COVID-19 serum collection from 3,700 individuals belonging to the 1982 Birth Cohort Study [16] and stored at the Epidemiology Research Centre, Federal University of Pelotas (UFPel, Pelotas, RS). **Sample preparation.** Fingerstick blood samples were applied directly to the RDT. Frozen serum samples were thawed at room temperature, gently shaken, and centrifuged at $10,000 \times g$ for 10 min at 4°C. A random subsample of 15 serum samples was tested by dot-blot for the presence of IgG, IgM and IgA, confirming sample integrity. **RDT procedure.** The assay used in this study was the Wondfo SARS-CoV-2 Antibody Test (Lateral Flow Method).The assays were carried out according to the manufacturers protocol: a 10 µl sample (whole blood or serum) was applied to the sample well, followed by the addition of 2-3 drops or 80µl of diluent. The test was developed for 15 minutes at room temperature and the results (positive or negative) were read by independent experienced readers blinded to the sample status. Only RDTs whose control line was positive were included in the statistical analysis. Note, while the RDT can detect both IgM and IgG antiSARS-CoV-2 antibodies, it does not discriminate between antibody types. Data analysis. Diagnostic accuracy was calculated using sensitivity and specificity, and agreement to the reference test (qRT-PCR) was assessed using Cohen's Kappa. The 95% confidence intervals for all estimates were calculated using the exact method. Statistical analyses were performed using MedCalc for Windows, version 19.2 (MedCalc Software, Ostend, Belgium).

DISCUSSION

This study reports the evaluation of an RDT using samples from confirmed COVID-19 infected individuals and a pre-COVID-19 collection from healthy individuals. While the recommended laboratory test for COVID-19 is based on qRT-PCR assay, serological assays have an important role to play in epidemiological studies of the COVID-19 pandemic. The qRT-PCR has good performance characteristics [8,15]. In controlled laboratory conditions the sensitivity and specificity were 100% and 100%, respectively [10]. Yet, it is a complex technique and there are reports that it has been difficult to implement and results from the field have been disappointing [3,5–7], with sensitivity as low as 52%[8].In addition, in Brazil there are significant problems in the supply of the kit to state central diagnostic laboratories. These shortages mean that only the most serious patients are being tested and this has made it difficult to draw any meaningful conclusions as to the transmission, prevalence and mortality rates of COVID-19.Initial reports suggest that following infection with SARS-CoV-2, the immune system takes 6-21 days to product IgM and IgG antibodies [5,7,17,18]. Indeed, the RDT manufacturer states that antibodies only become detectable 7 days after disease onset. This observation was factored into the inclusion criteria used in the current study; samples were only collected from volunteers whose qRT-PCR test had been carried out at least 10 days previously. The manufacturer of the RDT reported a sensitivity of 86.4% and a specificity of 99.6% using samples collected from 596 individuals (361 confirmed cases and 235 negative controls). In the current study, the sensitivity of the RDT was determined to be 77.1% (95% CI 66.6 - 85.6) and the specificity was 98.0% (95% CI 92.9 - 99.8).

Although the diagnostic accuracy of the current study was lower than the original study, this was not unexpected given the geographic and genetic differences between the study populations. Our results are in accordance with a validation study performed in the United States, in which the sensitivity ranged from 40% to 82% (5 and >20 days after the symptoms onset, respectively) while the specificity was 99.06% [19]. Some limitations of our study merit discussion. First, we included two different samples to study sensitivity (individuals with previous positive qRT-PCR) and specificity (sera from the Pelotas Cohort Study). Both samples are similar in percentage of self-reported skin colour, but the specificity sample was younger. Also, only the second sample is population based. Although sensitivity and specificity are intrinsic diagnostic properties of the test and theoretically do not vary with prevalence, it is important to consider that our positive sample set may not be representative of the entire spectrum of disease. However, it included both symptomatic and asymptomatic individuals at the time of testing, representing an important population regarding the need of testing. This means that the test may have even higher accuracy in more serious disease. The second limitation is inherent to the reference method. The reference method based on qRT-PCR to detect the presence of SARS-CoV-2 in nasopharyngeal swabs collected from patients suspected to have COVID-19 is highly dependent on the quality and timing of sample collection [3,5,7]. When the reference test does not present with 100% specificity or sensitivity, true results of the study test may be interpreted as false. This may happen specially when the NAAT fails to detect disease, and qRT-PCR false negatives may result in misinterpretation of a RDT positive result. It is also important to emphasize that NAATs and RDTs are designed to be used in different clinical settings, respectively, diagnosis of acute disease and population evaluation of contact with SARS-CoV-2.

While the true prevalence rate of COVID-19 remains unknown, several studies based on seroprevalence among the tested individuals have suggested that COVID-19 prevalence varies from less than 1% to 5.6% [9,20,21]. Furthermore, there are reports that the prevalence rate could be as high as 21% [22]. At a prevalence rate of 2% the PPV was 44%, meaning that just under half of the individuals with a positive RDT result will have the disease and this increased to over 81% when the prevalence rate was 10%. These are important observations and demonstrate that this RDT is suitable for a populational study to determine the levels and trends in the prevalence of COVID-19, especially when there is no need for a precise diagnosis at individual level.

Corresponding author: Lucia C Pellanda Email ellanda@ufcspa.edu.br

REFERENCES

1. Dong, E., Du, H., Gardner, L (2020). An interactive web-based dashboard to track COVID-19 in real time. Lancet Infect Dis 2020;20:533–4. https://doi.org/10.1016/S1473-3099(20)30120-1.
2. Li, R., Pei, S., Chen, B., Song, Y., Zhang, T., Yang, W., et al. (2020).Substantial undocumented infection facilitates the rapid dissemination of novel coronavirus (SARS-CoV2). Science 2020;368:489–93. https://doi.org/10.1126/science.abb3221.
3. He, X., Lau, E.H.Y., Wu, P., Deng, X., Wang, J., Hao, X., et al. (2020). Temporal dynamics in viral shedding and transmissibility of COVID-19. Nat Med 2020:1–4. https://doi.org/10.1038/s41591-020-0869-5.

4. Laboratory testing for coronavirus disease 2019 (COVID-19) in suspected human cases. 202AD.
5. Wölfel, R., Corman, V.M., Guggemos, W., Seilmaier, M., Zange, S., Müller, M.A., et al. (2020).Virological assessment of hospitalized patients with COVID-2019. Nature 2020:1–5. https://doi.org/10.1038/s41586-020-2196-x.
6. Zhang, W., Du, R.H., Li B, Zheng, X.S., Yang, X., Lou, Hu B., et al. (2020).Molecular and serological investigation of 2019-nCoV infected patients: implication of multiple shedding routes. Emerg Microbes Infect 2020;9:386–9. https://doi.org/10.1080/22221751.2020.1729071.

7. Zhao. J, Yuan Q, Wang H, Liu W, Liao X, Su Y, et al. (2020). Antibody responses to SARS-CoV-2 in patients of novel coronavirus disease 2019. Clin Infect Dis 2020. https://doi.org/10.1093/cid/ciaa344.

8. Yang .Y, Yang M, Shen C, Wang F, Yuan J, Li J, et al. (2020).Evaluating the accuracy of different respiratory specimens in the laboratory diagnosis and monitoring the viral shedding of 2019nCoV infections. MedRxiv 2020:2020.02.11.20021493. https://doi.org/10.1101/2020.02.11.20021493.
9. Rapid Risk Assessment: Coronavirus disease 2019 (COVID-19) in the EU/EEA and the UK– ninth update n.d. https://www.ecdc.europa.eu/en/publications-data/rapid-risk-assessmentcoronavirus-disease-2019-COVID-19-pandemic-ninth-update (accessed May 2, 2020).

10. ACCELERATED EMERGENCY USE AUTHORIZATION (EUA) SUMMARY Modified Thermo Fisher TaqPath COVID-19 SARS-CoV-2 Test (ORF1ab, N, and S gene detection) (Biocerna). n.d.
11. Weitz, J.S., Beckett, S.J., Coenen, A.R., Demory, D., Dominguez-Mirazo, M., Dushoff, J., et al. (2020).Intervention Serology and Interaction Substitution: Modeling the Role of "Shield Immunity" in Reducing COVID-19 Epidemic Spread. MedRxiv 2020:2020.04.01.20049767. https://doi.org/10.1101/2020.04.01.20049767.
12. Guo, L, Ren L, Yang S, Xiao M, Chang D, Yang F, et al. (2020). Clinical Infectious Diseases Clinical Infectious Diseases ® 2020;XX(XX):1-8 n.d. https://doi.org/10.1093/cid/ciaa310.
13. Long Q-X, Liu B-Z, Deng H-J, Wu G-C, Deng K, Chen Y-K, et al. (2020).Antibody responses to SARSCoV-2 in patients with COVID-19. Nat Med 2020:1–4. https://doi.org/10.1038/s41591-020-0897-
    1.
14. Wondfo SARS-CoV-2 Antibody Test(Lateral Flow Method) - wondfo n.d. https://en.wondfo.com.cn/product/wondfo-sars-cov-2-antibody-test-lateral-flow-method-2/ (accessed May 2, 2020).
15. Boletim Epidemiológico 8. Secretaria de Vigilância em Saúde. Brasília: 2020.
16. Lessa Horta, B., Gigante, D.P., Gonç Alves, H., Dos J., Motta, S., Loret De Mola, C,, et al. (2020).Cohort Profile Update: The 1982 Pelotas (Brazil) Birth Cohort Study. Int J Epidemiol 2015:441–441. https://doi.org/10.1093/ije/dyv017.

17. Liu, W., Liu L, Kou, G., Zheng, Y., Ding, Y., Ni, W., et al. (2020). Evaluation of Nucleocapsid and Spike Protein-based ELISAs for detecting antibodies against SARS-CoV-2. J Clin Microbiol 2020. https://doi.org/10.1128/JCM.00461-20.

18. Lipp, G,, Salvagno, G.L, Pegoraro, M., Militello, V., Caloi, C., Peretti, A., et al. (2020). Assessment of immune response to SARS-CoV-2 with fully automated MAGLUMI 2019-nCoV IgG and IgM chemiluminescence immunoassays. Clin Chem Lab Med 2020;0. https://doi.org/10.1515/cclm2020-0473.

19. Whitman, J.D., Hiatt, J., Mowery, C.T., Shy, B.R., Yu, R., Yamamoto, T.N., et al. (2020).Test performance evaluation of SARS-CoV-2 serological assays. MedRxiv 2020:2020.04.25.20074856. https://doi.org/10.1101/2020.04.25.20074856.
20. Bennett, S.T., Steyvers, M. ESTIMATING COVID-19 ANTIBODY SEROPREVALENCE IN SANTA CLARA COUNTY, CALIFORNIA. A RE-ANALYSIS OF BENDAVID ET AL. APREPRINT 2020. https://doi.org/10.1101/2020.04.24.20078824.
21. Silveira, M.F. et al. (2020).Repeated population-based surveys of antibodies against SARS-CoV-2 in Southern Brazil. Submitted 2020.
22. Koening, D. (2020). Evidence Mounts for Greater COVID Prevalence 2020. https://www.webmd.com/lung/news/20200424/more-data-bolsters-higher-covid-prevalence (accessed May 2, 2020).

This work started through the Data Committee created by the State of Rio Grande do Sul government to fight the COVID-19 pandemics. The tests used in the study have been provided by the Brazilian Ministry of Health. Financial support for data collection was provided by UNIMED Porto Alegre, Instituto Cultural Floresta and Instituto Serrapilheira. None of these funding sources took any part in study conceptualization, data collection, analysis or manuscript preparation, reviewing, or in the decision to submit the article for publication.

Acknowledgements

The authors thank Alessandra Dahmer, Ana Carolina de Moura, Ana Paula Palauro Goularte, Dinara Jacqueline Moura, Emerson Silveira de Brito, Indianara Franciele Porgere, Giovana Petracco de Miranda, Giovana Tavares, Giulia Souza, Luana Freese, Lara Goulart Garcia, Marilia Mesenburg, Michele Paula Pretto, Natan José Dutra Dias, Roberta Beux, Suelen Porto Basgalupp, Thayane Martins Dornelles, Tiago Fetzner and William Jones Dartora

Data Statement

Due to the sensitive nature of the questions asked in this study, survey respondents were assured raw data would remain confidential and would not be shared.
Data not available / The data that has been used is confidential

AFFILIATION

Universidade Federal de Pelotas, Brazil (Dr. Pedro C Hallal, Prof. Aluísio J D Barros, Prof. Bernardo L Horta, Prof. Mariângela F Silveira, Prof. Odir A Dellagostin,
Dr. Fernando P Hartwig, Prof. Ana B Menezes, Prof. Fernando C Barros, Prof. Cesar G
Victora), Fundação Universidade Federal de Ciências de Saúde de Porto Alegre, Brazil
(Prof. Lúcia C Pellanda, Profa Marilia A Mesenburg), Fundação Getúlio Vargas and
Universidade do Estado do Rio de Janeiro, Brazil (Prof. Claudio J Struchiner),
Universidade de São Paulo, Brazil and UniversidadeFederal de São Paulo, Brazil
(Prof. Marcelo N Burattini), Universidade de Santa Cruz do Sul, Brazil (Profa. Andréia R M Valim),Universidade de Ijuí, Brazil (Profa Evelise M Berlezi),
IMED - Passo Fundo, Brazil, (Prof. Jeovany M Mesa), Universidade do Vale do Rio dos Sinos, Brazil (Profa.
Maria Letícia R Ikeda), Universidade de Caxias do Sul, Brazil (Profa. Marina Mantesso), Universidade Federal de Santa Maria, Brazil (Profa. Marinel M Dall'Agnol), Secretaria Municipal de Saúde de Uruguaiana, Brazil (Raqueli A Bittencourt).

Universidade Federal de Pelotas, Brazil (Dr. Pedro C Hallal, Prof. Aluísio J D Barros, Prof. Bernardo L Horta, Prof. Mariângela F Silveira, Prof. Odir A Dellagostin, Dr.
Fernando P Hartwig, Prof. Ana B Menezes, Prof. Fernando C Barros, Prof. Cesar G
Victora), Fundação Universidade Federal de Ciências de Saúde de Porto Alegre, Brazil
(Prof. Lúcia C Pellanda, Profa Marilia A Mesenburg), Fundação Getúlio Vargas and
Universidade do Estado do Rio de Janeiro, Brazil (Prof. Claudio J Struchiner),
Universidade de São Paulo, Brazil and UniversidadeFederal de São Paulo, Brazil
(Prof. Marcelo N Burattini), Universidade de Santa Cruz do Sul, Brazil (Profa. Andréia R M Valim),Universidade de Ijuí, Brazil (Profa Evelise M Berlezi),
IMED - Passo Fundo, Brazil, (Prof. Jeovany M Mesa), Universidade do Vale do Rio dos Sinos, Brazil (Profa.
Maria Letícia R Ikeda), Universidade de Caxias do Sul, Brazil (Profa. Marina Mantesso), Universidade Federal de Santa Maria, Brazil (Profa. Marinel M Dall'Agnol), Secretaria Municipal de Saúde de Uruguaiana, Brazil (Raqueli A Bittencourt).

5. A Population-Based Surveys of Antibodies Against SARCOV-2 In Southern Brazil

[1]Mariângela F Silveira, Aluísio J D Barros, Bernardo L Horta, Lúcia C Pellanda, Odir A Dellagostin, Claudio J Struchiner, Marcelo N Burattini, Andréia R M Valim,Evelise M Berlezi, Jeovany M Mesa, Maria Letícia R Ikeda, Marilia A Mesenburg, Marina Mantesso,Marinel M Dall'Agnol, Raqueli A Bittencourt, Fernando P Hartwig, Ana M B Menezes, Fernando C Barros, Pedro C Hallal*[#] ,Cesar G Victora[#]

(#) Joint last authors

ABSTRACT

Population based data on COVID-19 are urgently needed for informing policy decisions, yet few such studies are available anywhere, as most surveys rely on self-selected volunteers. In the Brazilian State of Rio Grande do Sul (population 11.3 million), we are carrying out fortnightly household surveys in nine of the largest cities. Multi-stage probability sampling was used in each city to select 500 households, within which one resident was randomly chosen for testing. The Wondfo lateral flow rapid test for detecting antibodies against SARS-CoV-2 has been validated in four different settings, including our own, with pooled estimates of sensitivity (84.8%, 95% CI 81.4%;87.8%) and specificity (99.0%, 95% CI 97.8%;99.7%), which are within the acceptable range for epidemiological studies. In the first wave of the study (April 11-13), 4,188 subjects were tested, of whom two were positive (0.0477%; 95% confidence interval (CI) 0.0058%;0.1724%). In the second round (Apr 25-27) there were six positive subjects (0.1333%; 95% CI 0.0489%;0.2900%). We also tested family members of positive index cases, and nine out of 19 had positive results. Testing of reported COVID-19 cases according to RT-PCR confirmed that the test was highly sensitive under field conditions. The epidemic is at an early stage in the State, as the first case was reported on Feb 28, and by Apr 30, 50 deaths were registered. Strict lockdown measures were implemented in mid-March, and our results suggest that compliance was high, with full or near full compliance rates of 79.4% in the first and 71.7% in the second round. As far as we know, this is the only large population anywhere undergoing regular household serological surveys for COVID-19. The results show that the epidemic is at an early phase, and findings from the next rounds will allow us to document time trends and propose Public Health measures.

[1] Correspondence to: Pedro C Hallal, Marechal Deodoro 1160 – 96020-220 - Pelotas, RS, Brazil – Phone (fax): +55 53 3284-1300 - Email: prchallal@gmail.com

INTRODUCTION

Despite calls for population-based data on COVID-19, [1] there have been remarkably few household seroprevalence surveys anywhere, and none in Latin America.[2] In Rio Grande do Sul, the southernmost state in Brazil (population 11.3 million), the first case of COVID-19 was diagnosed on February 29, 2020. As of April 30, 1,466 confirmed cases (129 per 1,000,000 inhabitants) and 50 deaths had been reported [1]It is important to remark that in the state, as also in Brazil, only persons with moderate to severe symptoms had been tested, using PCR to detect SARS-Cov-2. The state and most municipal governments issued strong social distancing policies in mid-March, including closures of schools, shops and services, except for businesses deemed to be essential.

Other than studies based on convenience samples, such as individuals who volunteered to be tested, supermarket customers, or blood donors, there are few general population sample surveys in the literature. In a national study in Iceland [3], one of the three groups of participants was recruited through random sampling of the population, but only about one third of those invited were tested. In this group, 13 of 2283 persons tested positive (0.6%; 95% CI 0.3;0.9) in quantitative real-time polymerase-chain-reaction (qRT-PCR) assays. A national household study in Austria used random sampling to invite households to participate. Of the households contacted, 77% or 2,197 declared their willingness to participate, and 1,541 persons were successfully tested. Assuming two persons per household, those tested correspond to about 30% of the intended sample. The study found a prevalence of0.33% (95% CI 0.12;0.76%.) using qRT-PCR, or 5 individuals out of those tested.[4]. Smaller studies in hot spots for COVID-19 showed prevalence of 14% the German city of Gangelt[5] and 3% in the Italian village of Vò.[6]

As expected, studies based on volunteers found higher prevalence, as was the case for the first study in Iceland (0.9%)[3], the population screening in South Korea (2.1%)[7] and two studies in California: prevalence of 1.5% in Santa Clara county[8] and 4.1% in Los Angeles County.[2]

Starting on April 11-13, we set out to test the presence of antibodies against SARSCoV-2 in population-based samples of 500 individuals in each of nine sentinel cities in the state, with a total sample of 4,500. The same methodology was used in a second round in the same cities on April 25-27, and subsequent rounds are planned to take place every two weeks in order to monitor how the pandemic is evolving.

METHODS

The state of Rio Grande do Sul is divided by the National Institute of Geography and Statistics in eight intermediary regions (Figure 1). The main city in each region was selected for the study. In the main metropolitan region, we selected the State Capital, Porto Alegre, and Canoas, the second largest city in the metropolitan area. Populations ranged from 78,915 in Ijuí to 1,409,351 in Porto Alegre[3]

---

[1] (http://ti.saude.rs.gov.br/covid19/).
[2] http://publichealth.lacounty.gov/phcommon/public/media/mediapubhpdetail.cfm?prid=2328
[3] (https://cidades.ibge.gov.br/brasil/rs/panorama).

Figure 1. Location of the nine sentinel cities.

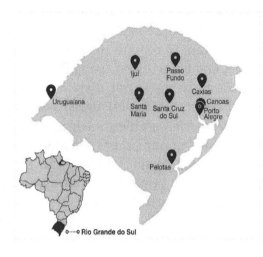

We used multistage sampling to select 50 census tracts with probability proportionate to size in each sentinel city, and 10 households at random in each tract based on census listings updated in 2019. All household members were listed at the beginning of the visit, and one individual was randomly selected through an app used for data collection. The survey waves took place on April 10-12 and 25-27.The State- wide sample of 4,500 individuals allows estimating a prevalence levels of 3%and 10% with margins of error of 0.5 and 1.0 percent points, respectively. In the first wave, interviewers had listings of 35 households in each tract. Any refusals at household level led to selection of the next household in the list, and so on until 10 households were included. In the second wave, field workers went to the house visited in the first wave, and then selected the tenth household to its right.

In case of refusal, the next household to the right side was selected. In the case of acceptance at the household level but the index individual refused to provide a sample, a second member was selected. If this person also refused, the field workers moved on to the next household in the list. Prevalence of antibodies was assessed with a rapid test using finger prick blood samples - the WONDFO SARS-CoV-2 Antibody Test (Wondfo Biotech Co., Guangzhou, China). This test detects immunoglobulins of both IgG and IgM isotypes specific to SARS-CoV-2 antigens in a lateral flow assay. The capture reagent consists of an unspecified viral antigen immobilized at a defined position on a nitrocellulose membrane. Following the introduction of the sample, a solution containing labelled detector anti-immunoglobulin monoclonal antibodies is added. If the test is valid, a control line appears on the kit's window. If this line is not visible, the test is deemed inconclusive, which is very uncommon. A positive result is triggered by binding of the detector antibody to any serum immunoglobulins immobilized on the viral antigen and is visible as a second coloured line. Two drops of blood from a pinprick are sufficient to detect the presence of antibody. Four independent validation studies are available for the rapid test.

Its sensitivity and specificity are 86.4% and 99.6% according to the manufacturer, using samples collected from 361 confirmed cases and 235 negative controls[1] The tests were purchased in bulk by the Brazilian government, being earmarked for use in population surveys and surveillance programs. An initial validation study was carried out by the National Institute for Quality Control in Health (INCQS, Oswaldo Cruz Foundation, RJ, Brazil) using 18 qRT-PCR positive and 77 negative serum samples. The reported sensitivity was 100.0% (95% confidence interval (CI) 81.5;100.0%), while specificity was 98.7% (95% CI 93.0;100.9%). Recently, Whitman and colleagues [9] evaluated 10 different lateral flow assays using as specimen plasma or serum samples from symptomatic SARSCoV-2 RT-PCR-positive individuals and 108 pre-COVID-19 negative controls. Sensitivity of the Wondfo test was 81.5% (95% CI 70.0-90.1%) among 65 patients with a positive RT-PCR 11 or more days before the test, and specificity was 99.1% (95% CI 94.9;100.0%). Of the 10 tests studied, the Wondfo test was one of the two lateral flow tests with the best performance. Lastly, we carried out our own validation study, based on 83 volunteers with a positive qRT-PCR result 10 days or more before the rapid test. This analysis showed a sensitivity of 77.1% (95% CI 66.6;85.6%).

We also analysed 100 sera samples collected in 2012 from participants of the 1982 Pelotas (Brazil) Birth Cohort Study[10] and found 98 negative results, yielding a specificity estimate of 98.0% (95% CI 93.0;99.8%). By pooling the results from the four separate validations studies, weighted by sample sizes, sensitivity is estimated at 84.8% (95% CI 81.4%;87.8%) and specificity at 99.0% (95% CI 97.8%;99.7%). Participants answered short questionnaires including sociodemographic information (sex, age, schooling and skin colour), COVID-19-related symptoms, use of health services, compliance with social distancing measures and use of masks. Field workers used tablets or smartphones to record the full interviews, register all answers, and photograph the test results. All positive or inconclusive tests were read by a second observer, as well as 20% of the negative tests. If the index subject in a household had a positive result, all other family members were invited to be tested. Interviewers were tested and found to be negative for the virus were provided with individual protection equipment that was discarded after visiting each home.

Ethical approval was obtained from the Brazilian's National Ethics Committee (process number 30415520.2.0000.5313), with written informed consent from all participants. Positive cases were reported to the state-wide COVID-19 surveillance system. The study protocol was published prior to the first wave of data collection.[11] Data will become publicly available upon request from the corresponding author 30 days after publication. In the analyses reported in the body of this article, we analysed the surveys as if it they included simple random samples from the population, using the exact binomial method for confidence intervals.

We calculated absolute and relative differences between the two survey waves regarding the prevalence of infection. P-values were calculated using Cochran's Q heterogeneity test, implemented as fixed-effects meta-regression, which also yielded confidence intervals for the differences. More complex analyses with allowances for the sampling design, population weights and corrections for the specificity and sensitivity of the rapid test, are included in the web annex. All analyses were performed using R version 3.6.1 [2] The "metafor" package was used to compare the prevalence between surveys.

---

[1] (https://en.wondfo.com.cn/product/wondfo-sars-cov-2-antibody-test-lateralflow-method-2/).
[2] (https://www.r-project.org/).

RESULTS

Out of the planned 4,500 interviews, it was possible to test 4,188 individuals in the first round. The number of tests carried out included 500 in each of five cities (Pelotas, Passo Fundo, Santa Cruz, Caxias), 396 in Porto Alegre, 332 in Canoas, 499 in Uruguaiana and 461 in Santa Maria. In the last three cities, the desired sample size was not completed due to logistic difficulties resulting from the need to complete the survey in a 3-day period. Refusals, requiring the selection of the next household in the census tract listing, ranged from 5.4% in Ijui to 26.9% in Santa Maria, with a median of 17.9% in the nine cities. In the second round, it was possible to obtain 500 interviews in each of the nine cities.

Table 1 shows the characteristics of individuals who provided blood samples. Both samples were similar in terms of sex, age, skin colour and schooling distributions. Although the nine sentinel cities are not representative of the state as a whole, the comparison shows what the samples had higher proportions of women and of older persons than the state as a whole. Young children were particularly underrepresented. Up-to-date information on schooling is not available for the State. Of the 4,188 individuals tested in the first round, 10 had inconclusive results and only two (0.0477%; 95% confidence interval (CI) 0.0058%;0.1724%) tested positive, one each in the cities of Pelotas and Uruguaiana. In the second round, there were two inconclusive results and six positive subjects (0.1333%; 95% CI 0.0489%;0.2900%).

The absolute prevalence difference between the second and first waves was equal 0.086 percent point (95% CI -0.400;0.211; P=0.181), and the ratio was equal to 2.793 (95% CI 0.564;13.831, P=0.208).Given the small numbers of subjects who tested positive, we focus the presentation on unadjusted results. The web annex provides results from more complex analyses, all of which produced results that are highly comparable to those reported here. Regarding social distancing measures, 20.6% of respondents reported leaving home on a daily basis, 58.3% leaving home occasionally for essential activities, and 21.1% staying at home all the time in the first phase, and 28.3%, 53.4% and 18.3%, respectively, in the second phase.

The households of the eight positive cases in the two phases included other 20 residents. Of these, 19 were tested; the rapid test showed nine positive, eight negative, and two inconclusive results. One positive case lived alone. Among the other seven, four had at least another positive individual in their families.

Table 1. Sociodemographic characteristics of the two samples in nine cities and of the State population.

		ROUND 1	ROUND 2	STATE POPULATION[12,13]
SEX		%	%	%
	Male	41.7	40.5	48.7
	Female	58.3	59.5	51.3
AGE				
	0-9	3.6	2.6	12.3
	10-19	5.4	5.1	12.6
	20-29	12.2	11.4	15.1
	30-39	15.3	16.9	15.1
	40-49	15.5	14.6	13.3
	50-59	17.9	17.9	12.9
	60-69	16.4	17.9	10.2
	70-79	9.4	10.2	5.7
	80+	4.3	3.4	2.9
SKIN COLOR				
	White	76.6	75.9	81.5
	Brown	15.8	16.2	13.0
	Black	6.5	6.6	5.2
	Other	1.1	1.3	0.3
EDUCATION				
	Primary or less	37.4	34.1	Not available
	Secondary	29.8	31.8	
	University or higher	32.8	34.1	

As an additional check on how the rapid test performed under field work conditions, we conducted two separate assessments. The first was during the validation study in Porto Alegre, where 83 RT-PCR positive individuals were tested in the field using the rapid test. As described in the Methods section, 64 of these had positive results with the rapid test. Second, a more limited assessment entailed asking the coordinators of field work in different cities whether they were aware of any RT-PCR positive individuals in their communities. Four persons were identified and tested, all of whom had positive results in the rapid test.

DISCUSSION

This is the first report on repeated population-based surveys for the detection of SARSCoV-2 antibodies. With two weeks interval we were able to perform antibody tests on representative samples in nine sentinel cities in Rio Grande do Sul State in Southern Brazil. Based on reported death rates by April 30, 2020, Rio Grande do Sul is one of the six states, out of 27, with the lowest mortality, of 4 per million, well below Rio de Janeiro (46 per million) or Sao Paulo (49 per million). Amazonas state (92 per million) shows the highest death rates. The national mortality rate is estimated at 26 per million.[1] Taking our present results at face value, there would be 477 cases per million inhabitants (95% confidence interval 58-1,719 cases) in the first wave, compared to 62 reported cases per million, as of April 14. According to the results of the second wave (April 25-27), there would be 1,333 cases per million inhabitants (95% CI 489;2900) compared to 128 reported cases per million as of April 30. Additional estimates, taking into account corrections for the sample design, population weighting and adjustment for sensitivity and specificity, are provided in the web annex. Important concerns have been issued about rapid serological tests, but these mostly refer to their use in making clinical decisions,[14] and on issuing "immunity passports" [15]for individuals who are assumed to have developed immunity. Both of these circumstances refer to individual-level diagnoses based on rapid tests. Use of rapid tests for population-based estimates, and particularly for monitoring trends over time, is a different issue for which rapid tests with less than perfect sensitivity and specificity may be acceptable.

The Wondfo lateral flow test used in our analyses underwent four different validation studies, being able to correctly identify 5 out of every 6 RT-PCR confirmed cases, and 99 out of 100 individuals without SARS-CoV-2 antibodies. Among 10 lateral flow tests recently assessed by Whitman and colleagues [9], it was among the two with the best performance. Our finding of positive results for 10 of 13 family members of the six index individuals who tested positive confirms that the performance of the rapid test was adequate under field conditions. The limitations of our analyses include the restriction of the sample to sentinel cities that jointly account for 31% of the state's population, while smaller towns and rural areas were not included. Second, antibody tests result in many false negatives for recent infections, particularly within the first two weeks since contagion, and thus prevalence reflects levels of infection a week or two prior to the survey, about 15 days after the first case was reported in the state.

The non-response rate at household level, estimated at 17.9%, was low compared to other population-based studies,[3,4] or to studies based on volunteers. Our samples had fewer children than expected, which was probably due to their reluctance to undergo a finger prick when randomly

---

[1] (https://covid.saude.gov.br/)

selected within the household; in these cases, a second person was randomly selected and if that person also refused the household was replaced.

Lastly, our results were at the lower range of the 95% confidence interval for the false positive rate, which in the pooled estimate from four validation studies was estimated at 1.0% (95% CI 0.3%;2.2%). In these studies, specificity was measured in frozen samples. Whitman and colleagues, in their analyses of 10 lateral flow tests, observed "moderate-to-strong positive bands in several pre-COVID-19 blood donor specimens, some of them positive by multiple assays, suggesting the possibility of non-specific binding of plasma proteins, non-specific antibodies, or cross-reactivity with other viruses."[9] Our results on family clustering show that - out of the seven index cases who lived alone - four had family members who also tested positive. These four individuals are most likely true positives, thus suggesting that up to four of the remaining index cases with positive results, out of 8,689 individuals, might represent false positive results. The test's specificity would then be equal to 99.95% (95% CI 99.88;99.99%).Our finding of low prevalence is consistent with an early phase of the pandemic, coupled with high compliance with social distancing measures, as confirmed by our own results. Such a low prevalence level is compatible with other population-based studies: 0.6% in Iceland [3] and 0.3% in Austria,[4] which is close to Northern Italy which was strongly hit by the pandemic. One should note that in both studies about 2/3 of those invited failed to participate, compared to our own non-response rate of 17.9%.

Our results are not comparable with those based on self-selected volunteers. The surveys are being partly funded by the state and national governments of Brazil. Survey results were disseminated, two days after the completion of data collection round, in press briefings with the presence of the state governor, who is making use of the information to guide stay-at-home and other policies. Results from the next rounds of our study – planned for May 8-10 and 22-23 - will allow us to follow the dynamics of the pandemic in the state, especially when social restriction measures are starting to be relaxed in most municipalities.

REFERENCES

1. Pearce, N. Vandenbroucke, J.P., VanderWeele, T.J., Greenland, S. (2020). Accurate Statistics on COVID-19 Are Essential for Policy Guidance and Decisions. American journal of public health 2020: e1-e3.
2. Barreto, M.L., Barros, A.J.D., Carvalho, M.S, et al. (2020) [What is urgent and necessary to inform policies to deal with the COVID-19 pandemic in Brazil?]. Rev Bras Epidemiol 2020; 23: e200032.
3. Gudbjartsson, D.F., Helgason, A., Jonsson, H., et al.(2020).Spread of SARS-CoV-2 in the Icelandic Population. The New England journal of medicine 2020.
4. Institute for Social Research and Consulting Ogris & Hofinger GmbH (SORA). COVID-19 Prevalence, 2020.
5. Regalado, A. (2020) Blood tests show 14% of people are now immune to COVID-19 in one town in Germany. 2020. https://www.technologyreview.com/2020/04/09/999015/blood-tests341 show-15-of-people-are-now-immune-to-COVID-19-in-one-town-in-germany/ (accessed April 27, 2020.
6. Day, M. (2020). COVID-19: identifying and isolating asymptomatic people helped eliminate virus in Italian village. BMJ 2020; 368: m1165.
7. Ministry of Health and Welfare (South Korea). Coronavirus disease 19, Repubic of South Korea. 2020. http://ncov.mohw.go.kr/en.
8. Bendavid, E., Mulaney, B., Sood, N., et al. (2020). COVID-19 Antibody Seroprevalence in Santa Clara County, California. medRxiv 2020: 2020.04.14.20062463.

9. Whitman, J.D., Hiatt, J., Mowery, C.T. et al. (2020). Test performance evaluation of SARS-CoV-2 serological assays. (unpublished) 2020.

10. Horta, B.L., Gigante, D.P., Goncalves, H., et al. (2015). Cohort profile update: the 1982 Pelotas (Brazil) Birth Cohort Study. International journal of epidemiology 2015; 44(2): 441-e.

11. Hallal, P., Horta, B., Barros. A., et al. (2020). Evolução da prevalência de infecção por COVID-19 no Rio Grande do Sul: inquéritos sorológicos seriados. . Cien Saude Colet 2020.

12. Instituto Brasileiro de Geografia e Estatística. Pesquisa nacional por amostra de domicílios : síntese de indicadores 2015. Rio de Janeiro: IBGE, 2016.

13. Instituto Brasileiro de Geografia e Estatística. Projeções da População. 2019. HTTPS://WWW.IBGE.GOV.BR/ESTATISTICAS/SOCIAIS/POPULACAO/9109-PROJECAO-DA359 POPULACAO.HTML?=&T=RESULTADOS (accessed April 30, 2020.

14. World Health Organization. Advice on the use of point-of-care immunodiagnostic tests for COVID-19. 2020. https://www.who.int/news-room/commentaries/detail/advice-on-the362 use-of-point-of-care-immunodiagnostic-tests-for-COVID-19 (accessed April 30, 2020.

15. World Health Organization. "Immunity passports" in the context of COVID-19. 2020. https://www.who.int/news-room/commentaries/detail/immunity-passports-in-the-context-of365 COVID-19 (accessed April 30, 2020.

CHAPTER 5

THE GREAT
CORONAVIRUS DENIAL

1. Brazil's Trump: Bolsonaro Is The 'Biggest Threat' To COVID Response

Martha Grevatt

On May 9,2020 The Lancet medical journal, in assessing the COVID crisis in Brazil, wrote that "perhaps the biggest threat to Brazil's COVID-19 response is its president, Jair Bolsonaro." When questioned by journalists about the country's high rate of infection, Bolsonaro had answered — this is a direct quote — "So what? What do you want me to do?"

This is a politician who takes great pride in being compared to U.S. President Donald Trump.

Now Bolsonaro's Trump-like response to the pandemic has contributed to Brazil having the second-highest number of confirmed COVID-19 cases in the world the highest being the U.S. As of June 1, almost 515,000 Brazilians are known to be infected and over 29,000 have died. Bolsonaro has also parroted Trump's denial of climate science. He has deliberately allowed climate-related fires to destroy wide swaths of the Amazon rainforest, displacing Indigenous communities and threatening the "lungs" of the planet.

None of this has endeared Bolsonaro to the Brazilian masses. On May 25, when he stepped outside his home in Brasilia to buy a hot dog from a vendor — without a face mask and deliberately flouting social distancing guidelines residents banged pots and pans and hurled insults at him: "killer," "assassin," "fascist" and "garbage." "We are in the midst of a pandemic," said Antônio Carlos Costa, an activist pastor in Rio de Janeiro. "People are dying in packed hospitals, and you don't see him shed a single tear." (Guardian, May 24)

Widespread condemnation of Bolsonaro's "so what" attitude began before the infection numbers skyrocketed. Several Brazilian scientific and human rights organizations sounded the alarm with an April 7 manifesto titled "Pact for Life and for Brazil." Organized by renowned Brazilian photojournalist Sebastião Salgado, artists, intellectuals, scientists and celebrities from around the world signed a May 3 open letter warning of a health catastrophe.

Death Toll: Legacy of Colonialism and Imperialism

Beyond Bolsonaro, Brazilians face enormous obstacles to containing the spread of the coronavirus. Poverty is widespread, with 13 million people living in crowded ghettos known as favelas, where social distancing is nearly impossible. In 2018, 19 percent of the population — almost 40 million people — were officially poor. Things like adequate food, health care and clean drinking water — needed to resist and recover from infection — are out of reach for many. This situation worsened after the illegal coup which removed President Dilma Rousseff in 2016. Hospital overcrowding has reached disastrous levels since the first cases of COVID-19 were identified.

Conditions are especially difficult for Afro-descendant and Indigenous communities — for whom Bolsonaro shares Trump's racism. Brazil's 100 million people of African ancestry, many of whom live in favelas, have higher than average poverty rates. And among Brazil's 900,000 Indigenous people, the COVID-19 death rate is twice the national average. (CNN, May 24)

On May 31, favela residents held a Black Lives Matter demonstration in Rio de Janeiro, chanting "I can't breathe" in solidarity with George Floyd. They read out the names of residents murdered by Rio's police — some 1,546 last year alone. They clashed with Bolsonaro supporters carrying what were described as neo-Nazi flags. Brazil's poverty and discrimination are not homegrown problems. They are the product of centuries of colonialism, imperialism and neo-colonialism — first imposed by the Portuguese colonialists and then by U.S. capitalists. Other countries in Latin America are in similar dire straits — and for the same reason. Going back to the 19th century's Monroe Doctrine, U.S. imperialism has viewed the conquest of Latin America as its "manifest destiny." Monroe's legacy is the rising rate of COVID-19 infection in countries like Mexico, Peru, Ecuador and Colombia, as well as Brazil .By contrast Cuba, which has been a liberated socialist country since 1959, is sending doctors all over the world to help defeat the pandemic.

2. The King is Naked': Bolsonaro & the Pandemic

Antonio Pele

The current president of Brazil, Jair Bolsonaro, has been relentlessly downplaying the dangers of the COVID-19 pandemic comparing it with a simple flue. He has claimed that the lowest social categories of the Brazilian population would be immune to diseases ("the Brazilian jumps into the sewer and doesn't get anything") [1]. Bolsonaro's main point is that the Brazilian economy cannot stop because of the pandemic. He has a two-fold argument. First, at least 40 million Brazilians need to continue to work in order to make a living. If complete lockdown is imposed, they will not be able to survive. Second, the confinement measures (similar to those

introduced in Spain, France or Italy) will eventually bring about a major economic crisis in Brazil. In this sense, according to Bolsonaro, Brazil– as one of the developed countries cannot afford the confinement/mitigations/quarantine policies undertaken by Western economies. Bolsonaro's attempts to downplay the pandemic can only be understood taking into account the economic crisis that will inevitably land on the country. Bolsonaro is already thinking about the day after the pandemic and wants to embody the one who has tried everything to save the Brazilian economy. He also wants to galvanize his electorate basis, against Brazilian State Governors who are implementing serious measures to tackle COVID-19.

It is possible to notice other elements in Bolsonaro's propaganda. On Friday 27 of March, the Brazilian government launched a TV spot called "Brazil cannot stop" ("*O Brasil não pode parar*") that urged Brazilians to keep on working while adopting basic public health measures (ie. wearing masks, washing hands) and implementing *selective* confinement measures for the most vulnerable (i.e. elderly population). A few days later, the Brazilian Supreme Court prohibited this official campaign since it was "downplaying the magnitude of the pandemic". The Court considered public resources are "scarce" and they should not be spent on public campaigns that "deceive" Brazilian public opinion. Those resources must be spent today in order to "save lives"[2]. The decision appears to manifest a biopolitics (the power to make live, and let die) as the ultimate legal framework (and not only by processes of 'normalization')[3].

On March 31st, Jair Bolsonaro made another TV address where he precisely and constantly repeated his goal during the current situation: "saving lives" ("*salvar vidas*")[4].He urged the adoption of a "Great Deal for the Preservation of Life and Employment in Brazil" (*um Gran Pacto para a Preservação da Vida e dos Empregos*). Indeed, according to Bolsonaro, "saving lives" is twofold: saving them from the pandemic and saving them from economic turmoil that is, "unemployment, violence and hunger". Therefore, Bolsonaro has drawn on the Brazilian Supreme Court 'biopolitical' observations on the imperative to "saving lives" and used it for his own political agenda. Biopolitics is absorbed within a neoliberal agenda where the lowest social categories of the Brazilian population are urged to keep on working. Foucault (and Foucauldians) have already noticed how death (and not life) is at the core of neoliberalism.

Indeed, 'competition' has now prevailed over the classical form of 'exchange'[5], resources are now understood through 'scarcity'[6], the 'psychic life' of the neoliberal subjectivities evolves around 'blaming others'[7], and 'death economies' are now everywhere, with death holding a 'positive' economic value[8]. When Bolsonaro deploys biopolitics to keep the Brazilian economy 'operative', he sacrifices the most vulnerable of the Brazilian population. The risk of becoming infected by the virus is understood through strict economic/neoliberal terms: it is less relevant than the ongoing *machine* of the Brazilian economy.

While Foucault famously noticed that (neo)liberalism is the basic framework where biopolitics can be deployed, with Bolsonaro, life is allegedly protected through its exposure to death. Bolsonaro's propaganda draws on instilling among the Brazilian public opinion, a constant awareness of the dangers that will come (i.e economic crisis) so that everyone must strive to survive and work. It is a novel form of management of the population that oscillates between the Western form of biopolitics and the genocidal expressions of necropolitics. Karsten Schubert has brilliantly referred to "populist biopolitics[1]" in order to describe how in some European countries, "members of the community shame on each other for supposedly irrational and unsolidaristic behaviour such as, for example, leaving the house or meeting with friends (...)". In Brazil, with Bolsonaro and its accomplices, the exact opposite is going on. Bolsonaro's political base, that is extremely active online, has launched messages through different digital platforms. For example:

You want quarantine and to stay home? But you need money and you want the banker to be at the bank to solve your problem! You want to buy bread? The bakery has to be open, right?! You want to stay home? But the garbage must be collected every day. Just like "populist biopolitics", 'unsolidaristic' conduct is targeted here. However, this biopolitics operates in a radically different way. Those who implement quarantine are accused of unsolidaristic conduct. Staying home equates to the exploitation of others, who are forced to provide the 'basic' needs of the Brazilian economy. One's life is guaranteed through the risk and efforts that others are obliged to cope with. One's own 'self-biopolitics' (self-quarantine, confinement, health monitoring) and the different techniques of the self that middle upper categories are used to display in time of stress (yoga, mindfulness) are brought about through the nano-necropolitics (low wages, danger to be infected by the COVID-19) of the most exploited of the Brazilian work forces. The strategy of Bolsonaro draws on shaming Brazilian society. It avoids addressing the role of the State (and public authorities) in generating a better and fairer distribution of resources (i.e. income, access to public health) for the most vulnerable.

It is a sort of 'fake' populist biopolitics. However, this 'fake biopolitics' that Bolsonaro deploys might produce a counter-effect. As mentioned above, State governors in Brazil do not follow the guidelines of the Brazilian federal government and do intend to implement effective measures against COVID-19. During each Bolsonaro's address on national TV the Brazilian population protest, "banging pots" from balconies. The fake biopolitics of Jair Bolsonaro is undermining his power. The current President of Brazil is losing his traditional allies, from the business spheres to the Brazilian military sector.

In *Society Must be Defended* Foucault wrote:

(...) let's take, if you will, the death of Franco, which is after all a very, very interesting event. It is interesting because of the symbolic values it brings into play, because the man who died has, as you know, exercised the sovereign right of life and death with great savagery, was the bloodiest of all the dictators (...) and at the moment when he himself was dying, he entered this sort of new field of power over life which consists not only in managing life, but in keeping individuals alive after they

---

[1] https://criticallegalthinking.com/2020/04/01/crying-for-repression-populist-and-democratic-biopolitics-in-times-of-covid-19/

are dead (...). And so the man who had exercised the absolute power of life and death over hundreds of thousands of people fell under the influence of a power that managed life so well, that took so little heed of death, and he didn't even realize that he was dead and was being kept alive after his death (Foucault, Society must be defended, 248-49) Foucault notices with irony how former Spanish dictator, Franco was kept 'alive' through biopolitical device, while he was not even aware of it. In relation to Bolsonaro, our biopolitical era, and the need to implement effective and genuine measures to protect the existences of the Brazilian population is quickly and surely stripping away Bolsonaro's legitimacy and power. Bolsonaro's is kept alive politically only through the display of a populist rhetoric that is designed to stimulate its deep core electorate. Simultaneously, and in a broader perspective, the need of biopolitics for the current situation has already put an end to his political life, and Bolsonaro might not be even aware of it.

"The king is naked"

Antonio Pele (Associate Professor, Law School, PUC-Rio University; Twitter: @duendeaude)

[1] https://www.bbc.com/portuguese/geral-52067247

[2] https://www.conjur.com.br/dl/liminar-barroso-proibe-campanha-brasil.pdf

[3] See Michel Foucault, *Security, Territory and Population*, Palgrave MacMillan, Lecture: 25 January 1978.

[4] https://www.youtube.com/watch?v=fy_HP3_gOoI

[5] Michel Foucault, *The Birth of Biopolitcs*, Palgrave MacMillan, p. 119.

[6] Michel Foucault, *The Order of Thing*, Routledge, p. 279.

[7] Christina Scharff, The Psychic Life of Neoliberalism: Mapping the Contours of Entrepreneurial Self, *Theory, Culture & Society*, 2016, 33(6): 107-122.

[8] Fatmir Haskaj, From Biopower to necroeconomies: Neoliberalism, biopower, and death economies, *Philosophy and Social Criticism*, 2018, 44 (10): 1148-1168

3. Jair Bolsonaro's Brazil and Coronavirus: Contesting the Incontestable

Francisca Costa Reis

Leuven Centre for Global Governance Studies
(University of Leuven).

"Brazil's President Jair Bolsonaro international norms and scientific evidence ever since he came to power, but coronavirus may be the contest he finally loses, writes Francisca Costa1 Reis"

The World Health Organization's decision on 11 March 2020 to reclassify the COVID-19 outbreak as a pandemic represented a turning point for public health systems and governments the world over. As infections soar towards 600,000 and related deaths climb beyond 25,000, states have sought to buy time and reduce the pressure on their health systems by closing schools and businesses or bringing in lockdowns and social distancing. But not all countries have followed the same path in their responses, and Brazil's reaction particularly that of its president Jair Bolsonaro has been conspicuously different.

Brazil's Reaction To COVID-19

With over 3,000 confirmed cases[2], Brazil has become one of the centres of South America's growing coronavirus crisis, yet the country's response has been patchy and uneven, revealing critical incompatibilities between the federal and state levels, not to mention Bolsonaro's personal refusal to the pandemic as a serious crisis. There are essentially two opposing camps in Brazil's response to the coronavirus outbreak: those contesting the seriousness of the issue, as personified by Bolsonaro, and those leading the country's response to the crisis, mostly state governors.

A third, middle-way group is made up of those few politicians that hope to bridge the gap between federal and state levels, such as Vice-President Hamilton Mourão. Bolsonaro's response to the reclassification of COVID-19 as a pandemic has been characterised by denial and belittling.

In various televised addresses Bolsonaro has shown little desire to mount a serious response, calling it a "little flu[3]" and attacking the media for supposed fear-mongering and sensationalism. Just days after Minister of Health Luiz Henrique Mandetta warned against the pandemic's potentially disastrous impact on Brazil's health system[4] and urged the population to respect social-distancing rules, Bolsonaro defied public-health recommendations to attend a sizeable rally of his supporters. In an attempt to take matters into their own hands[5] with the number of cases skyrocketing, cities and states like São Paulo and Rio de Janeiro have taken drastic measures, closing

---

[1] https://blogs.lse.ac.uk/latamcaribbean/2020/03/27/bolsonaros-brazil-and-coronavirus-contesting-the-incontestable/#author-info
[2] https://www.youtube.com/watch?v=VWsDcYK4STw&feature=youtu.be
[3] https://www.youtube.com/watch?v=VWsDcYK4STw&feature=youtu.be
[4] https://saude.estadao.com.br/noticias/geral,vamos-viver-umas-20-semanas-duras-diz-ministro-da-saude-sobre-novo-coronavirus,70003229311
[5] https://brazilian.report/society/2020/03/13/brazils-states-react-to-the-covid-19-outbreak/

schools and non-essential businesses in an attempt to halt the spread of the virus. These measures, which echo moves taken across the globe, have been vociferously contested by the Brazilian president, who furiously accused state governors of staging an insurrection against the federal government for their own political ends. As of late March, the President continues to urge people to go about their lives as normal[1], emphasising the need to keep the country's economy ticking over. State governors, on the other hand, have maintained their stance on the need for serious measures to fight the pandemic, pointing out that the dead cannot be resurrected[2] whereas the economy can. To complicate matters further, postures within the cabinet have also been inconsistent. Most notably, Vice-President Hamilton Mourão has emphasised[3] that the government's official position continues to require social distancing and isolation, even though Bolsonaro himself has claimed that such measures only apply to those over the age of 60.

Contesting The Incontestable: A Familiar Pattern?

While most of the world has followed the recommendations of health officials and scientists, Bolsonaro's recent behaviour and active contestation of the seriousness of this disease has done quite the opposite. While this might initially seem surprising, a closer look at Brazil's positioning vis-à-vis other global challenges reveals a familiar pattern. From the moment he took office, Bolsonaro and his cabinet have dismissed climate change as an ideological construct that suffocates the economy[4], thus ignoring a scientific consensus on the disastrous impact that this process will have for particular societies and for the planet as a whole. Prioritising the country's economic development and claiming sovereignty over its territory, Bolsonaro also encouraged deforestation while simultaneously gutting the country's environmental laws[5].In this blatant contestation of the incontestable, President Bolsonaro even went so far as to fire the head of Brazil's space agency over the institution's provision of deforestation data, an unusually direct form of rejecting scientific evidence.

Is Coronavirus One Contest Too Far For Bolsonaro?

While denying the undeniable and prioritising the economy over scientific evidence may be Bolsonaro's daily bread, contesting the seriousness of coronavirus could be a tipping point. The president's climate-change denial has sparked reactions and condemnation both inside and outside Brazil, but it comes as no surprise to Bolsonaro's core constituency, which likely agrees that the economy should come before the environment. However, reactions to the government's inaction in the face of COVID-19 seem to suggest that a tipping point could be on the horizon.

---

[1] https://www.youtube.com/watch?v=VWsDcYK4STw&feature=youtu.be
[2] https://www.bloomberg.com/news/articles/2020-03-25/brazilian-state-governors-defy-bolsonaro-in-coronavirus-fight
[3] https://www1.folha.uol.com.br/poder/2020/03/mourao-defende-isolamento-social-e-diz-que-bolsonaro-nao-se-expressou-bem.shtml
[4] https://foreignpolicy.com/2019/01/04/brazil-was-a-global-leader-on-climate-change-now-its-a-threat/
[5] https://www.theguardian.com/environment/2018/oct/09/brazils-bolsonaro-would-unleash-a-war-on-the-environment

There Have Been Three Key Developments:

Studies show that Brazilians widely support[1] the restrictive measures put in place by states to fight the pandemic. Huge pot-banging protests[2] against Bolsonaro have taken place in several cities that overwhelmingly backed Bolsonaro in the 2018 election. The idea of impeachment[3] has been floated, indicating serious discontent amongst the political class. It seems that when the lives of people are directly and visibly affected, contestation of the incontestable ceases to be sustainable. Precisely how this tipping point will ripple though Brazilian politics is difficult to predict, but Bolsonaro is finding himself increasingly alone on an island of denial as the bitter truth of coronavirus unfolds around him.

Francisca Costa Reis

Francisca Costa Reis is a doctoral researcher at the Leuven Centre for Global Governance Studies. Her research focuses on understanding the mechanisms and dynamics involved in the contestation of global norms, particularly in the case of Brazil's engagement with global norms of migration, security, and sustainable development. She is also a member of CONNECTIVITY, a research project offering a timely assessment of how differences between prominent states' conceptualisations of international norms impact upon cooperation in the international system.

---

[1] https://www.brasil247.com/brasil/maioria-da-populacao-apoia-medidas-de-contencao-contra-coronavirus-diz-datafolha
[2] https://www1.folha.uol.com.br/poder/2020/03/bolsonaro-e-alvo-do-oitavo-dia-seguido-de-panelaco-pelo-pais.shtml
[3] https://brasil.elpais.com/opiniao/2020-03-20/a-unica-saida-e-o-impeachment.html

4. Ignoring Scientific Advice During the COVID-19 Pandemic [1]

Tiago Ribeiro Duarte

One of the characteristics that analysts have attributed to the so-called "post-truth age" is an anti-science attitude and the outright downplay of scientific evidence by politicians and members of the public (Collins, Evans, and Weinel 2017; Fujimura and Holmes 2019).[2] Within this topic, the COVID-19 outbreak raises important issues for STS scholars. This highly contagious illness in a few months reached all continents. Although the death rate among the contaminated is not high in comparison to other contagious diseases, such as the Ebola, due to its transmissibility the death toll is significant and, at the moment of the writing of this op-ed, on the rise. For this reason, the World Health Organization (WHO) has urged countries that have communitarian transmission, i.e. when residents infect each other, to implement social isolation to prevent the number of cases from skyrocketing. If the coronavirus spreads too quickly, healthcare systems may collapse, being unable to treat all patients due to infrastructural limitations.

However, several national authorities were initially hesitant to take stronger measures to deal with the COVID-19 outbreak. Some of them even denied the seriousness of the coronavirus pandemic and campaigned against stringent social isolation because of the potential economic impacts of such a measure. In Brazil, around mid-March, most state governors and several municipality mayors introduced social isolation policies that allowed only what was deemed as essential activities to continue running. However, the Brazilian president Jair Bolsonaro, a far-right populist, has been ignoring scientific advice on COVID-19 and downplaying the seriousness of the pandemic to the point of beginning a political crisis by accusing state governors, mayors, and the media of hysteria, of exaggerating the coronavirus threat, and of taking measures that would seriously harm the country's economy. This is not the first time Bolsonaro shows disregard for science (Monteiro 2020).

However, during the COVID-19 pandemic, the situation is even more pressing as his actions could result in thousands of deaths in the short term. Bolsonaro defends the so-called vertical isolation, that is, putting in quarantine only people above 60 years old and other individuals who are highly vulnerable to COVID-19, such as those who have diabetes or high blood pressure, and returning the rest of the population to work. His main argument is that the economy cannot stop otherwise more people will die because of poverty and starvation than because of the pandemic.[2] He has threatened to decree the end of social isolation measures, something he was unable to do due to the Brazilian federalist political system.[3]

Following the lead of Trump, he also became a strong defender of the widespread use of chloroquine and hydroxychloroquine against COVID-19 as if they were a panacea that would save thousands of lives, even though there is no consistent scientific evidence that these drugs can have an effect

[1] Tiago Ribeiro Duarte (2020): Ignoring scientific advice during the Covid-19 pandemic: Bolsonaro's actions and discourse, Tapuya: Latin American Science, Technology and Society, DOI: 10.1080/25729861.2020.1767492

[2] I agree with critics (Jasanoff and Simmet 2017; Lynch 2020; Frickel and Rea 2020) that the term post-truth it is not conceptually accurate as it implies that there was an idyllic past in which truth prevailed in public debates, which is certainly not the case. However, as the concept has gained traction in STS debates and there is no substitute for it yet, I will use it in this paper. 2 https://www.jota.info/opiniao-e-analise/colunas/quaest-opiniao/brasil-politizou-pandemia-01042020

[3] https://oglobo.globo.com/brasil/bolsonaro-diz-cogitar-decreto-para-toda-qualquer-profissao-voltar-ao-trabalho-124336772;https://g1.globo.com/politica/noticia/2020/04/15/maioria-do-supremo-vota-a-favor-de-que-estados-e-municipios-editem-normas-sobre-isolamento.ghtml.

against the coronavirus.[1] Furthermore, on April 12th, when the pandemic was still far from reaching its peak in Brazil, Bolsonaro stated that the virus "was starting to go away."[2] He has also been to public demonstrations organized in his support a few times since the COVID-19 first infected people in Brazil. In these events, he embraced supporters and took photographs with them, disregarding all scientific advice related to social distancing and the need to avoid crowds. He also went out at other times to talk with the population, to "buy a Coca-Cola," to have an ice cream, and so on, when crowds gathered around him and he again took photographs and embraced fans.[3]Bolsonaro's actions and speeches received mixed reactions. The media was quick to point out that the president was ignoring scientific advice.

Part of the population started banging pots and pans from their windows every night to show their discontent with the president.[7] However, in several cities his supporters organized motorcades and in some cases even took to the streets to show their support for the president and to demand the end of horizontal social isolation.[4] In some occasions, shops reopened defying the quarantine policy imposed by state governors.[5] Neither Bolsonaro nor members of his entourage had any expert support to their claims. No study was presented, no data, no counter expertise was mobilized to underpin the president's position.[10] Still, he convinced part of the population that large-scale social isolation was a mistake; the coronavirus was not as bad as the media had been arguing; and that the damage to the economy due to the quarantine policy would be far worse than the impacts of the coronavirus itself. Feeling the pressure, some state governors allowed shops to reopen and social isolation diminished in the late weeks of April, in spite of the fact that the death toll due to COVID-19 in Brazil was still on the rise.[6]

In the face of far-right populist leaders such as Bolsonaro, whose discourses and actions may result in the death of thousands of people, STS scholars cannot refrain from adopting a critical position. Bolsonaro's outright neglect and downplaying of scientific evidence is not the classical type of STS case study in which subaltern people have their non-scientific expertise ignored in policymaking (Wynne 1996; Irwin 1995). As pointed out above, Bolsonaro does not have any basis on which to claim that the death toll resulting from the economic impacts of social isolation policies will be larger than that resulting from the pandemic itself if no quarantine is put in place. This claim only becomes a public fact once he utters the words and he and his supporters, be them human or robots,[7] begin

1 https://www1.folha.uol.com.br/poder/2020/04/empronunciamento-bolsonaro-defende-cloroquina-e-volta-aresponsabilizar-governadores-e-prefeitos.shtml.
2 https://www1.folha.uol.com.br/poder/2020/04/em-livecom-religiosos-bolsonaro-vai-na-contramao-deespecialistas-e-diz-que-virus-esta-indo-embora.shtml.
3 https://oglobo.globo.com/brasil/video-bolsonaro-passa-em-padaria-apos-deixar-planalto-repete-discurso-contra-isolamento-24362579;https://www1.folha.uol.com.br/poder/2020/04/bolsonarovisita-obra-de-hospital-provoca-novasaglomeracoes-e-ecriticado-por-mandetta-e-caiado.shtml; https://valor.globo.com/politica/noticia/2020/04/18/bolsonaro-causa-aglomerao-ao-comprar-picol-na-praa-dos-trs-poderes.ghtml; https://g1.globo.com/politica/noticia/2020/04/18/presenca-de-bolsonaro-provoca-aglomeracao-em-frente-ao-palacio-do-planalto.ghtml; and https://g1.globo.com/politica/noticia/2020/04/19/bolsonaro-discursa-em-manifestacao-em-brasilia-que-defendeu-intervencaomilitar.ghtml. 7 https://www1.folha.uol.com.br/poder/2020/03/bolsonaro-e-alvo-do-15o-panelaco-seguido-em-meio-a-novo-pronunciamento-na-tv.shtml.
4https://www1.folha.uol.com.br/poder/2020/03/criticadas-por-ministro-carreatas-anticonfinamento-alinhadas-combolsonaro-se-repetem-pelo-pais.shtml;https://www1.folha.uol.com.br/poder/2020/04/grupo-de-bolsonaristas-seaglomera-ignora-pandemia-ataca-doria-e-pede-reabertura-do-comercio-em-sp.shtml.
5 https://www1.folha.uol.com.br/cotidiano/2020/03/apos-falas-de-bolsonaro-circulacao-aumenta-e-parte-do-comercio-reabre-em-favelas-do-rio.shtml 10 https://www1.folha.uol.com.br/poder/2020/03/governo-bolsonaro-admite-a-estados-nao-ter-estudo-que-embaseisolamento-vertical.shtml.
6 https://exame.abril.com.br/brasil/dez-estados-ja-tomaram-medidas-para-flexibilizar-isolamento-por-covid-19/.
7 Kalil and Santini's (2020) study of social media has shown that in Twitter a significant part of those who tweet in support of Bolsonaro are "bots." In the particular instance of a call for a demonstration in support of Bolsonaro on March 15th, 2019, about 55% of the tweets were made by robots.

to share them on social media. STS has shown that "facts" are socially constructed and not sufficient for settling controversies. It has also shown that facts and values, science and politics, cannot be disentangled. However, it has never denied the importance of facts in democracies. In the case of Bolsonaro fighting against scientific advice during the COVID-19 pandemic, there are two types of facts at stake. On the one hand, scientific facts that have been collectively constructed by using an assemblage of expertise, material infrastructures, interests, i.e. a complex sociotechnical order that aims at explaining the functioning of things. On the other, we have a far-right populist leader who has no relevant expertise in economics or healthcare policy and whose statements are not based on evidence produced by any expert, be they scientific or not.

The facts here result from the "testimony" of a charismatic leader (Weber 1978), which is replicated again and again in social networks through humans and "bots" that build up an echo chamber (Nguyen forthcoming). Here we are facing a different case compared to other situations in which scientific advice was dismissed on the basis of fake controversies actively produced by denialists (Oreskes and Conway 2010; Weinel 2010). In the case at hand, there is no counter-expertise base on which Bolsonaro is relying to underpin his argument. Facts were not produced by any expert before his speeches. Rather, facts begin to circulate in social media after his speeches and gain traction with president supporters. In this case, the scientific fact-construction machinery should clearly prevail. Science is not perfect and will never be. Scientific experts make mistakes and sometimes their arrogance can be disturbing (Wynne, 1992). But it is still much better to rely on an institution that seeks to find the truth of the matter and that has mechanisms to correct itself than on the baseless testimony of a populist politician. Furthermore, science should not determine policymaking.

Rather, policymakers should take into consideration knowledge produced by scientists or other types of experts when designing policy or making decisions. In this sense, policymaking should be informed by expertise, but not determined by experts. In the case of the COVID-19, politicians and policymakers need to hear scientific advice and take responsible measures based on it. Non-scientific expertise may also contribute to policymaking, although at this point, it is not clear who the "lay experts" that should bring their expertise to the table are. Dialogue with civil society is also important to implement effective and democratic policies. However, in the context of a pandemic in which social isolation is of utmost importance, face to face participation is not possible. For this reason, alternative channels of participation need to be deployed, such as polls, meetings with civil society representatives via video conference, and so on. Brazil, during the COVID-19 pandemic, would benefit much from policies based on expertise and public dialogue. It has much to lose, however, with an authoritarian president that has very little regard for science.

REFERENCES

Collins, H., R. Evans, and M. Weinel. (2017). "STS as Science or Politics?" Social Studies of Science 47 (4): 580–586.

Frickel, S., and C. Rea. (2020). ""Drought, Hurricane, or Wildfire? Assessing the Trump Administration's Anti-Science Disaster." Engaging Science, Technology, and Society 6: 66–75.

Fujimura, J., and C. Holmes. (2019). "Staying the Course: On the Value of Social Studies of Science in Resistance to the "Post-Truth" Movement." Sociological Forum 34 (S1): 1251–1263.

Irwin, A. (1995). Citizen Science: A Study of People, Expertise and Sustainable Development. London: Routledge.

Jasanoff, S., and H. Simmet. (2017). "No Funeral Bells: Public Reason in a 'Post-Truth' Age." Social Studies of Science 47 (5): 751–770.

Kalil, I., and R. M. Santini. (2020). "Coronavírus, Pandemia, Infodemia e Política". Relatorio de pesquisa. São Paulo: FespSP/UFRJ. https://www.fespsp.org.br/store/file_source/FESPSP/Documentos/Coronavirus-e-infodemia.pdf

Lynch, M. (2020). "We have Never Been Anti-Science: Reflections on Science Wars and Post-Truth." Engaging Science, Technology, and Society 6: 49–57.

Monteiro, M. (2020). "Science is a War Zone: Some Comments on Brazil." Tapuya: Latin American Science, Technology and Society 3 (1): 4–8.

Nguyen, C. forthcoming. "Echo Chambers and Epistemic Bubbles." Episteme.

Oreskes, N., and E. Conway. (2010). Merchants of Doubt: How a Handful of Scientists Obscured the Truth on Issues from Tobacco Smoke to Global Warming. New York, NY Bloomsbury Press.

Weber, M. (1978). Economy and Society an Outline of Interpretive Sociology. Berkeley, CA: University of California Press.

Weinel, M. (2010). Technological Decision-Making Under Scientific Uncertainty: Preventing Mother-to-Child Transmission of HIV in South Africa. Unpublished PhD thesis, Cardiff University.

Wynne, B. (1992). "Misunderstood Misunderstanding: Social Identities and Public Uptake of Science." Public Understanding of Science 1 (3): 281–304.

Wynne, B. (1996). "May the Sheep Safely Graze? A Reflexive View of the Expert-Lay Knowledge Divide." In Risk, Environment and Modernity, edited by S. Lash, B. Szerszynski, and B. Wynne, 44–83. London: Sage Publications.

5. Jair Bolsonaro's Strategy of Chaos Hinders Coronavirus Response

João Nunes
Senior lecturer, University of York

Deisy Ventura
Professor in Global Health Ethics at Public Health School,
Universidade de São Paulo

Gabriela Spanghero Lotta
Professor and Researcher of Public Administration and Government,
Universidade Federal do ABC

Brazil faces a tremendous uphill struggle in its response to COVID-19, the disease associated with the new coronavirus. Already eroded by years of budget cuts,[1] the country's public health system, the Sistema Único de Saúde (SUS), has been further undermined by the president, Jair Bolsonaro. The country's public health response and political landscape have been thrown into disarray. Bolsonaro sacked his health minister, Luiz Henrique Mandetta, on April 16. He then participated in a demonstration[2] during which opposition to lockdown measures was combined with calls for a military intervention to shut down Brazil's congress and supreme court. Bolsonaro's reaction to COVID-19 is, at its heart, one of denial. On March 24, in an official national address, Bolsonaro dismissed the disease as no more than a "gripezinha" (small flu) for most people. He suggested that Brazilians have somehow acquired an immunity to disease by "diving into sewers[3]".Bolsonaro ignored and openly challenged the advice of health authorities, repeatedly clashing with Mandetta, as well as with state governors and mayors who opted to impose lockdowns. Arguing that the economy cannot stop, Bolsonaro has pushed for a return to business-as-usual, meeting crowds of supporters, going to shops and refusing to limit his own movement.

Misinformation and Politicking

But Bolsonaro has also spread misinformation about the virus. He touted a chloroquine-based[4] therapy, despite the absence of corroborating scientific evidence. He called for "a day of fast and prayer[5]" on April 5 to tackle the virus. On April 20, he knelt before an evangelical pastor[6] who declared that Brazil was free of the virus. Bolsonaro is also trying to use the pandemic for political

---

[1] https://www.conectas.org/wp/wp-content/uploads/2020/04/Urgent-Appeal-EC-95.pdf
[2] https://www.cartacapital.com.br/politica/bolsonaro-participa-de-ato-em-brasilia-e-discursa-nao-vamos-negociar-nada/
[3] https://g1.globo.com/politica/noticia/2020/03/26/brasileiro-pula-em-esgoto-e-nao-acontece-nada-diz-bolsonaro-em-alusao-a-infeccao-pelo-coronavirus.ghtml
[4] https://g1.globo.com/jornal-nacional/noticia/2020/04/08/em-pronunciamento-bolsonaro-defende-uso-da-cloroquina-para-tratamento-do-coronavirus.ghtml
[5] https://www1.folha.uol.com.br/poder/2020/04/bolsonaro-faz-chamado-para-jejum-religioso-neste-domingo-contra-coronavirus.shtml
[6] https://poligrafo.sapo.pt/fact-check/bolsonaro-ajoelhado-ouviu-pastor-evangelico-proclamar-que-o-brasil-esta-livre-do-coronavirus

gain. His followers have taken to the streets to demand the sacking of politicians who imposed lockdown. Calls for a military intervention among these supporters, and Bolsonaro's open confrontation with Brazil's legislative and judicial bodies, reveal an attempt to reinforce the executive power of the president by boosting the role of the military as political broker. This shows the radicalisation and increased militarisation of Bolsonaro's brand of populism. In early April, the ministry of health made an about-face on its coronavirus response. It moved from emphasising the need to maintain wide-ranging social distance measures, to explicitly signalling a transition to selective social distancing of vulnerable groups only – Bolsonaro's preferred solution. This revealed a creeping politicisation of the health ministry, of which Mandetta's sacking is the latest example. The Brazilian response to COVID-19 has become a terrain of political strife, which now threatens the very survival of the country's democracy.

Organised Confusion

Bolsonaro may be simply trying to weather a crisis that has revealed, once again, his own failings. He may be hoping to escape responsibility for the inevitable economic consequences of the lockdown. But some commentators have suggested[1] that there is a method behind Bolsonaro's efforts to produce confusion. The rise of "Bolsonarismo" is viewed by his supporters[2] as a war against the establishment and political correctness. Bolsonaro feeds on, and fosters, a climate of confrontation and uncertainty that helps him secure the loyalty of his base. He benefits from unsettling other forms of authority in the country, be it political or otherwise.

Since coming to power in January 2019,

Bolsonaro has led an attack on science and professional expertise[3] cutting research funds, substituting managers of research institutes with inexperienced political appointees, publicly intimidating scientists, and dismissing public universities as havens of leftist indoctrination. COVID-19 is a new phase of this ongoing war, presenting Bolsonaro with an opportunity to attack political opponents and discredit "mainstream media" and any dissent. He questions the number of reported COVID-19 deaths[4] suggesting that they have been manipulated[5] for political purposes.

His education minister, Abraham Weintraub, joined the xenophobic bandwagon by blaming China[6] for the virus. Bolsonaro's followers have accused Rede Globo, one of the country's most important media networks, of spreading alarmism and "fake news". The parallels with the US Trump administration are striking.

Populism Versus Public Health

The situation in Brazil is a reminder of the real-life consequences of politicking around science and expertise, and of populist manipulation[7]. Bolsonaro's combination of foot-dragging and political manoeuvring is costing the country precious time and many lives.

---

[1] https://piaui.folha.uol.com.br/materia/o-caos-como-metodo/
[2] http://library.fes.de/pdf-files/bueros/brasilien/14508.pdf
[3] https://www.scholarsatrisk.org/resources/free-to-think-2019/#Brazil
[4] https://catracalivre.com.br/cidadania/alguns-vao-morrer-lamento-e-a-vida-diz-bolsonaro-sobre-coronavirus/
[5] https://uk.reuters.com/article/uk-health-coronavirus-brazil/brazils-bolsonaro-questions-coronavirus-deaths-says-sorry-some-will-die-idUKKBN21E3IJ
[6] https://www.france24.com/en/20200406-brazil-minister-offends-china-with-racist-virus-tweet
[7] https://theconversation.com/are-populist-leaders-a-liability-during-covid-19-135431

His strategy of chaos produces uncertainty around COVID-19 and hampers the effectiveness of Brazil's response. The number of cases and deaths is escalating[1] with black people and other vulnerable groups taking the brunt[2] of the epidemic. In conversations we've had ourselves, frontline health workers have complained of confusing directives, inadequate training and shortages of protective equipment. In the face of the confusion, popular support for the lockdown remains high[3] although the number of Brazilians staying home is steadily decreasing[4].

This is partly because of pressure from employers for a return to work, following the lead of the federal government which backed a "Brazil cannot stop campaign" that contradicted social isolation and asked citizens to get back to work. On March 28, this campaign was banned by the judiciary. In this complex and volatile environment, Brazil's health professionals, researchers and public servants are demonstrating their dedication and excellence. Despite the uncertainty and the attacks waged by the federal government, the state and municipal levels of the SUS have shown remarkable resilience and provide a glimmer of hope.

---

[1] https://www.worldometers.info/coronavirus/country/brazil/

[2] https://www1.folha.uol.com.br/cotidiano/2020/04/coronavirus-e-mais-letal-entre-negros-no-brasil-apontam-dados-da-saude.shtml?utm_source=facebook&utm_medium=social&utm_campaign=compfb&fbclid=IwAR0BLxUsIs-ZZymzRBLqth2c-3_PajUdPC57HUkb1498jRksWfbtFS6mqR0

[3] https://oglobo.globo.com/sociedade/datafolha-quase-80-dos-brasileiros-defendem-punicoes-contra-quem-infringe-quarentena-24381609

[4] https://g1.globo.com/economia/tecnologia/noticia/2020/04/17/dados-de-localizacao-de-celulares-mostram-reducao-no-isolamento-social-no-brasil-pela-2a-semana-seguida.ghtml

6. Misinformation As A Political Weapon: COVID-19[1] And Bolsonaro In Brazil[2]

Julie Ricard [(1)], Juliano Medeiros [(2)]

With over 30,000[3] confirmed cases, Brazil is currently the country most affected by COVID-19 in Latin America and ranked 12th worldwide.

Despite all evidence, a strong rhetoric undermining risks associated to COVID-19 has been endorsed at the highest levels of the Brazilian government, making President Jair Bolsonaro the leader of the "coronavirus-denial movement"[4].To support this strategy, different forms of misinformation and disinformation[5] have been leveraged to lead a dangerous crusade against scientific and evidence-based recommendations.

Sustaining A COVID-19 Denialist Stance Through Misinformation

The spread of misinformation and disinformation, including its use by the current government, has been under investigation in Brazil since 2019 by a dedicated Parliamentary Commission[6] (created by the National Congress.

According to several testimonies collected within the scope of the investigation, it was identified that a structure linked to the office of the Presidency, nicknamed the "Office of Hatred"[7], coordinates the spread of disinformation, including defamatory messages against opponents of the President, such as prominent figures from the government[6]. In the context of the coronavirus crisis, the Commission is currently conducting a specific investigation into the online profiles spreading misinformation related to the pandemic and has identified a surge of misinformation around three major themes.

The first theme is around pseudo-scientific information about symptoms, risks and cures.

The second is regarding prevention and control measures adopted by other countries and recommended by international organizations, and their supposed 'catastrophic' collateral effects.

---

[1] A publication of the Shorenstein Centre on Media, Politics and Public Policy at Harvard University's John F. Kennedy School of Government.

[2] Affiliation: (1) Data-Pop Alliance, (2) Brasília University - Political Science Institute (IPOL / UnB)
How to cite: Ricard, J., Medeiros, J., (2020). Using misinformation as a political weapon: COVID-19 and Bolsonaro in Brazil, The Harvard Kennedy School (HKS) Misinformation Review, Volume 1, Issue 2
Received: April 12, 2020 Accepted: April 16, 2020. Published: April 17, 2020

[3] "Coronavirus COVID-19 Global Cases" by the Centre for Systems Science and Engineering (CSSE) at Johns Hopkins University (JHU), as of April 16, 2020.

[4] "The Coronavirus-Denial Movement Now Has a Leader" by Uri Friedman (The Atlantic, March 27, 2020).

[5] Respectively defined as, "information that is false, but the person who is disseminating it believes that it is true" and "information that is false, and the person who is disseminating it knows it is false", both defined as different types existing on the "spectrum of 'information disorder'". Ireton, C. and Posetti, J., 2018. Journalism, fake news & disinformation: handbook for journalism education and training. UNESCO Publishing.

[6] Comissão Parlamentar Mista de Inquérito - CPMI)

[7] "Gabinete do Ódio vira Conselho da República durante pandemia", by Agência Estado. (Correio Braziliense, March 26, 2020). [6] "Ex-aliada de Bolsonaro, Joice detalha à CPMI da Fake News como atua 'gabinete do ódio'", by Luiz Felipe Barbiéri, Fernanda Calgaro and Elisa Clavery. (G1, December 4, 2019).

The third theme focuses on attacking or promoting decision-makers or public figures in order to delegitimize those supporting social isolation measures (including state governors that have implemented quarantine, media outlets, health specialists, and even the Secretary of Health Luiz Henrique Mandetta, with whom Bolsonaro had public disagreements), and on praising those who publicly support a 'return to normality' (certain government officials and businessmen).Overall, the messages have a common intention: to minimize the severity of the disease, discredit the social isolation measures intended to mitigate the course of the disease's spread and increase the distrust of public data, as explained by Congresswoman Natália Bonavides, a member of Parliamentary Commission: "Among the fake news about the disease and the way countries and institutions are dealing with it, we identified topics such as the indication of vaccines or home remedies that would be the cure or the recipe for not contracting the virus; the statement that substances such as chloroquine or hydroxychloroquine would already have proven effectiveness; claims that there is no difference in deaths between countries that have adopted isolation or not; false news of looting or shortages due to isolation measures; about how deaths from other causes are being accounted for by coronavirus; among many others".[1]

In addition, the Brazilian news agency Lupa, which is a member of the International Fact Checking Network (IFCN)[2], compiled a collection of messages that falsely attribute "positive actions" to public figures that support the government, in order to enhance their credibility. One message showed (false) donations to fight the coronavirus by a prominent millionaire businessman (who defends the end of isolation). Another claims that General Augusto Heleno, head of the Institutional Security Office of the Presidency, was cured by the medication hydroxychloroquine, of which President Bolsonaro is a vehement advocate. To date, the Commission has not yet released evidence to conclude that the so-called Office of Hatred, or members of the Brazilian government, are directly coordinating the spread of misinformation about COVID-19. Part of the government,

in particular the President himself and his close support groups, have however sustained their denialist stance by conveying misinformation, particularly regarding the symptoms, risks, and cures of the virus, and instigating risky behaviour. Since mid-March, Bolsonaro has urged Brazilians to "return to normality" in several occasions, ignoring growing empirical evidence about the positive effects of social distancing to flatten the infection curve. He has repeatedly adopted a provocative stance, seeking to minimize the risks posed by the virus. He has engaged in risky behaviour such as breaching his quarantine order after having had contact with an infected person[3], pro-actively seeking opportunities to greet and hug supporters[4], or taking walks around the city to talk to the population or get coffee[5]. At the institutional level, the Communication Secretariat of the Presidency even launched the campaign "Brazil Cannot Stop," which was featured in official government channels for nearly an entire day (see below).

The campaign preached the end of social isolation and the reopening of businesses. Based on no scientific data or evidence, and in contradiction to the recommendations of the Brazilian Department of Health led by Luiz Henrique Mandetta, the campaign

was almost immediately suspended by the Federal Court of Rio de Janeiro and subsequently deleted. After that, the head of the Communication Secretariat, Fábio Wajngarten (who contracted COVID-19 on a trip to the United States), denied the campaign's existence.

---

[1] Natália Bonavides, Federal Congresswoman. Testimony granted to the authors on April 8, 2020.

[2] "Coronavírus: veja o que já checamos sobre a pandemia que atinge o mundo" by Equipe Lupa. (Revista Piauí, January 28, 2020).

[3] "Bolsonaro volta a descumprir quarentena e diz que há 'superdimensionamento'"by Agência Estado. (Correio Braziliense, March 16, 2020).

[4] "Após cumprimentar apoiadores, Bolsonaro diz que é o responsável caso tenha se contaminado", by Guilherme Mazui. (G1, March 16, 2020).

[5] "MPF pede multa de R$ 100 mil a Bolsonaro por descumprir decisão sobre quarentena" by João Fellet. (BBC News Brazil, March 30, 2020).

Even so, the opposition parties filed a lawsuit with the Attorney General's Office to investigate the use of official government channels for the dissemination of a campaign against World Health Organization (WHO) recommendations. According to analysts, Bolsonaro's push against social isolation is strongly motivated by mitigating, or at least dissociating himself from, the foreseen economic effects of the pandemic, as explored further ahead.

His stance has increased tensions within his own government, to the extent of triggering, on April 16, the dismissal of Secretary of Health Luiz Henrique Mandetta, who refused to adopt a denialist approach. President Bolsonaro's recurring statements about COVID-19 have become one of the main vectors of misleading content. For example, through his periodic social media live-streamed videos as well as official government channels, Bolsonaro has promoted erroneous information about the effects and cures of the virus, based on unknown data or inconclusive scientific evidence. The President has made statements such as: "90% of people infected [by COVID-19] will not feel any symptoms"[1],"if I contracted COVID-19, because of my athletic background, I wouldn't feel anything or at most the symptoms of a gentle flu[2]", or suggesting that "armoured glass protects against the virus entering a space"[3] [4]. Moreover, Bolsonaro is invoking a false certainty to promote the potential efficacy of the medication Reuquinol (hydroxychloroquine, hydroxychloroquine sulfate), urging to "apply it promptly" in severe coronavirus cases and stimulating a crusade against doctors and specialists, who are still cautious about its use for COVID-19 treatment.

In fact, a study by Prof. Didier Raoult, largely associated with the excitement about the drug, has been criticized by the scientific community as "riddled with enough methodological flaws to render its findings unreliable or misleading"[5]. The WHO is currently conducting trials for the most promising treatments, including hydroxychloroquine, but no results have been released yet[6].

These, among other statements, have triggered reactions from international stakeholders.

On March 31, the WHO publicly denied Bolsonaro's statement according to which the WHO Director-General would have argued that "informal workers had to continue working". A few days earlier, Twitter deleted two tweets from Bolsonaro's official account as part of its recent policy against COVID-19 related misinformation[7]. The tweets were related to an improvised city tour, in which the President defended the use of hydroxychloroquine and the end of social isolation.

Bolsonarist public authorities follow the President's rhetoric, such as his three children (Eduardo Bolsonaro, Federal Congressman; Flávio Bolsonaro, Senator; Carlos Bolsonaro, Councillor in Rio de Janeiro), former Secretary of Citizenship Osmar Terra; current Secretary of Environment, Ricardo Salles; current Secretary of Foreign Affairs, Ernesto Araújo, among others. On their social networks, there are posts of distorted or decontextualized information that lead to mistaken conclusions, and/or manipulated content (manipulated videos, graphics, etc.). In March, Twitter also deleted posts from the Secretary of Environment and Senator Flávio Bolsonaro. According to the Brazilian

---

[1] "Noventa por cento de nós, não teremos qualquer manifestação caso se contamine." (Official Statement from President Jair Bolsonaro, March 24, 2020), "Não vou minimizar a gripe, sem bem dizem aí os infectologistas que para 90% da população essa gripe não é quase nada". (Weekly Live with President Jair Bolsonaro, 26/03/2020)

[2] "No meu caso particular, pelo meu histórico de atleta, caso fosse contaminado pelo vírus, não precisaria me preocupar, nada sentiria, ou seria, quando muito, acometido de uma gripezinha ou resfriadinho." (Official Statement from President Jair Bolsonaro, March 24, 2020)

[3] "Fechar casa lotérica, pelo amor de Deus. Fechar casa lotérica. Inclusive o cara tá na casa lotérica, tem um vidro blindado, quer dizer, não vai passar o vírus ali. O vidro é blindado, não vai passar." (Weekly Live with President Jair Bolsonaro,

[4] /03/2020)

[5] "'This is insane!' Many scientists lament Trump's embrace of risky malaria drugs for coronavirus" by Charles Piller. (Science Mag, March 26, 2020).

[6] "WHO launches global megatrial of the four most promising coronavirus treatments" by Kai Kupferschmidt, Jon Cohen. (Science Mag, March 22, 2020).

[7] "Coronavirus: World leaders' posts deleted over fake news" (BBC News, March 31, 2020).

news agency Lupa, mentioned above, over one hundred examples of false information (ranging from misleading to fabricated content) circulating on social networks were identified, and several of those were relayed by government members mentioned above.

Nacional Populism, Dis- And Misinformation: The Case of Bolsonaro

Both Bolsonaro's campaign for office and his mandate as president since January 2019 have been marked by the recurring use of different forms of dis- and misinformation. As a campaign strategy, Bolsonaro bet on the "anti-system" rhetoric, attacking the supposed political "establishment" and invoking different types of dis- and misinformation before and during the campaign[1]. Exploring the fears and prejudices of the average voters, a pervasive social media operation involving misleading, manipulated, and fabricated content was set in motion, which leveraged to its advantage a context of rejection of traditional parties and discredit towards democratic institutions[2]. His election mirrors the process of rise of right-wing populist leaders who came to power in other countries during the past decade[3].

Bolsonaro successfully mobilized part of society against an "enemy" to be beaten (primarily the "left" or "communists", among others), normalizing discriminatory discourses, while leveraging the capillarity of social media. Several candidates in the 2018 presidential race used mass messaging services on WhatsApp (one of the most popular communication apps in Brazil) offered by the company Yacows[4] for their campaigns. Bolsonaro's campaign particularly stood out among the candidates because of its massive and orchestrated use of disinformation, and the fact that it was financed by private companies (which is currently prohibited in Brazil[5]), as shown in several investigations published by the national[6] and international media[7]. As the Folha de São Paulo newspaper has reported, the content was spread both from outside the country, as well as from Brazilian telemarketing companies. The collaboration of Steve Bannon, former vice president of Cambridge Analytica, is a strong indication that Bolsonaro's campaign has acquired databases for the distribution of messages to targeted microsegments of the electorate[8].

Since the beginning of his term, Bolsonaro has remained an agent of information disorder, leveraging his massive audience and making recurring use of bots[9]. He also uses what Giuliano Da Empoli calls "saturation of the public debate" with controversial and false statements. During this period, antiscientific theories that had no relevance in Brazil (for example, flat earth theories or negationism of climate change) have acquired strong advocates on the national level and paved the way for the dangerous equivalence between opinion and science[10].

---

[1] "Das 123 fake news encontradas por agências de checagem, 104 beneficiaram Bolsonaro", by Isabella Macedo (Congresso em Foco, October 26, 2018).

[2] "WhatsApp fake news during Brazil election 'favoured Bolsonaro'", by Daniel Avelar (The Guardian, October 30, 2019).

[3] Da Empoli, G. Os Engenheiros do Caos. São Paulo: Vestígio, 2018.

[4] "Sócio da Yacows diz que empresa fez disparos em massa para Bolsonaro, Haddad e Meirelles", by Paloma Rodrigues e Pedro Henrique Gomes. (TV Globo and G1, February 19, 2020).

[5] Because the use of databases for mass messaging financed by businessmen, Jair Bolsonaro's campaign is investigated in the Superior Electoral Court. If convicted, Bolsonaro and his deputy, retired general Hamilton Mourão, could have his victory overturned.

[6] "Empresários bancam campanha contra o PT pelo WhatsApp", by Patrícia Campos Mello. (Folha de S.Paulo, October 18, 2018).

[7] "The three types of WhatsApp users getting Brazil's Jair Bolsonaro elected", by David Nemer. (The Guardian, October 25, 2018).

[8] Amadeu, S. "Comunicação e destruição dos parâmetros de realidade". Revista Socialismo & Liberdade, nº 23, 2019, pp. 29-32.

[9] Kalil, & Santini. (2020). "Coronavírus, Pandemia, Infodemia e Política". São Paulo / Rio de Janeiro: FESPSP / UFRJ.

[10] "Terra plana, vacinas e aquecimento global: um terço dos brasileiros ainda desconfia da ciência", by Profissão Repórter. (G1, December 11, 2019).

According to Da Empoli, "behind the apparent absurdity of fake news and conspiracy theories, a very solid logic is hidden. From the point of view of populist leaders, alternative truths are not simply propaganda tools. Contrary to true information, they are a formidable vector of cohesion"[1]. That is, for national populists, the accuracy of individual facts does not matter as much as the message is tailored to speak to the feelings and sensations of the population. As a result, the defects and vices of populist leaders become instead positive qualities in the eyes of their followers and "the tensions they produce at the international level illustrate their independence, and the fake news that pervade their propaganda are the mark of their freedom of spirit"[2]. Thus, their refusal to accept and play by contemporary democratic and social standards is seen as an act of courage and a rupture with the "system" instead of simple populist pyrotechnics. This stance, however, keeps the far-right leader dependent on a vicious circle where controversies need to be constantly fuelled to keep his audience properly mobilized. This is what we have seen since the beginning of the COVID-19 crisis in Brazil.

Coronavirus Denialism:
A Risky Bet Towards Responsibility Exemption?

But why would Bolsonaro be so committed to minimizing the seriousness of the epidemic? The answer seems to go beyond pure and simple denialism. Projections by financial institutions such as Bank of America foresee a 3.5% drop in Brazilian GDP in 2020[3]. The impact of the coronavirus pandemic on Brazil's trade relations (which is dependent on commodity exports and relies on China as its main trading partner) could lead to the amplification of the social crisis that has been dragging on since 2014, when the country entered a cycle of recession and subsequent stagnation that pushed 30 million people back to poverty. According to political analysts[31], this is the main reason behind Bolsonaro's desperate attempts to minimize the urgency and severity of the pandemic. By keeping the economy running, Bolsonaro could potentially lessen the economic impacts of social isolation or exempt himself from the responsibility for the recession that looms on the horizon. In his latest official statement (April 8, 2020)[4], Bolsonaro has already shown signs that he may adopt this tactic, stating that "many measures, whether restrictive or not, are the sole responsibility of [governors and mayors]". Meanwhile, the number of cases and deaths in Brazil continues to grow exponentially, and the government's conflicting measures and statements continue to put thousands of lives at risk, particularly those of the most vulnerable[5].The stance Bolsonaro has adopted is obstructing the possibility of a nation-wide coordinated response and hindering the efforts led by the national Department of Health and (now former) Secretary Luiz Henrique Mandetta, as well as state and municipal authorities. Today, Bolsonaro is one of the only heads of state to continue denying the risks associated with COVID-19[6].

[1] Da Empoli, G. Os Engenheiros do Caos. São Paulo: Vestígio, 2019.

[2] Idem, 2019, p. 18.

[3] "Mais uma rodada de revisões, bancos veem queda de até 3,5% no PIB", by Ligia Tuon. (Revista Exame, April 3, 2020). [31] "Negacionismo no poder: Como fazer frente ao ceticismo que atinge a ciência e a política", by Tatiana Roque. (Revista Piauí, February 2020).

[4] Official Statement from President Jair Bolsonaro, April 8, 2020

[5] Carvalho, Laura & Nassif Pires, Luiza & de Lima Xavier, Laura. (2020). COVID-19 e Desigualdade no Brasil.

[6] "Jair Bolsonaro isolates himself, in the wrong way". (The Economist, April 11, 2020).

7. Brief Communication Analysis of Brazilian Presidency During COVID-19

Brazilians are torn between believing the information coming from the president or following the instructions of their governors. The president has been asking the population to return to normalcy. Governors, however, call on the population to continue in isolation at home in order to reduce the rate of community transmission of the new coronavirus. The purpose of this article is to understand the reasons that led to this predicament through a review of public statements made by the current Brazilian president from the beginning of the global COVID-19 crisis to the present moment. For this analysis, this article resorts to the theoretical framework developed by Professor Arjen Boin and his co-authors in 'The Politics of Crisis Management'[1].

After the Chinese government announced and enforced mandatory quarantine in Wuhan as a measure to contain the spread of the new coronavirus, the Brazilian president's first reaction was to rule out the possibility of 'rescuing' the country's citizens claiming the government did not have enough resources[2] to carry out such an operation. Days after the confirmation of the first official report for an individual infected by the new coronavirus in the country, the president minimized the severity[3] of this respiratory disease. After the exponential growth of cases across the country and state governors deciding to restrict the movement of people, the president launches a campaign[4] asking Brazilians to leave their homes on the grounds that responsibility for preventing the spread of this virus among the most vulnerable is up to families[5] and not the state. At the present time, the Brazilian society is unsure whether they should follow the president's requests or local authorities' recommendations.

Arjen Boin, an expert in crisis management, gives us a solid theoretical background for the assessment of the current political scenario. Boin (2016) explains that in times of crisis, people look up to authorities for information on how to proceed. These authorities reduce anxiety explaining to the population i) what is going on, ii) the reasons for so much uncertainty and iii) what needs to be done. These are the elements that substantiates strategic political communication in times of crisis. If officials fail in one of these aspects, their political decisions risk not being widely accepted. As a result, other voices are given the opportunity to interpret facts and suggest alternatives. It is in this imbroglio that Brazilians are immersed in: who to believe in?

Politicians that master strategic communication can effectively reverse the snowballing effects of crises. This effort, however, depends on authorities' credibility. This leads to the review of how authorities gain or lose trust placed upon them.

---

[1] Boin, A., Stern, E. and Sundelius, B., 2016. *The politics of crisis management: Public leadership under pressure.* Cambridge University Press.

[2] Globo 2020, *Bolsonaro diz que não traz brasileiros da China porque 'custa caro' e não há lei dequarentena,* Globo.com, viewed 1 April 2020 <https://g1.globo.com/politica/noticia/2020/01/31/bolsonaro-reune-ministros-para-avaliar-risco-do-coronavirus-e-situacao-de-brasileiros-na-china.ghtml>

[3] Benites, A., Betim, F., 2020. *Bolsonaro rompe isolamento e vai a atos contra o Congresso em meio à crise do coronavírus,* El País, viewed 1 April 2020 <https://brasil.elpais.com/brasil/2020-03-15/bolsonaro-rompe-isolamento-e-endossa-atos-contra-congresso-em-meio-a-crise-do-coronavirus.html>

[4] DW 2020. *Justiça suspende campanha "O Brasil não pode parar",* DW, viewed 1 April 2020 <https://www.dw.com/pt-br/justi%C3%A7a-suspende-campanha-o-brasil-n%C3%A3o-pode-parar/a-5294 8560>

[5] Barrucho, L., 2020. *Coronavírus: os dados que põem em xeque ideia de Bolsonaro de isolar idosos,* BBC, viewed 1 April 2020 <https://www.bbc.com/portuguese/geral-52043354>

Reputation is the first source that determines the credibility of a leader's messages. If society respects a particular leader, they are more likely to interpret verbal and nonverbal cues and, as a result, comply with determinations.

The second source from which authorities derive credibility is how they *initially respond to* an unfolding crisis. If, for example, an authority minimizes its risks at first, that action will serve as a benchmark to assess the next political moves. Authorities also need to calculate the *timing*to respond to crises. If public response is too slow, opportunities for other communication channels are opened. If it is too fast, it can be interpreted as a lack of due diligence.

The theory developed by Boin and his colleagues has served in the training of authorities around the world. They point to Jacinda Arden[1], the current Prime Minister of New Zealand, as a political figure who masters crisis management communication techniques because she clearly understands a leader's priorities in times of great uncertainty. Among them: the protection of the most vulnerable segments of society. This understanding, however, which serves as a premise for the theory of Boin and his colleagues, has been repeatedly violated by the current Brazilian president.

---

[1] 1 News 2020, *'Yes we can' Jacinda Ardern confident New Zealand can beat coronavirus pandemic,* 1 News, viewed 1 April 2020 <https://www.tvnz.co.nz/one-news/new-zealand/yes-we-can-jacinda-ardern-confident-new-zealand-beat-c oronavirus-pandemic>

CHAPTER 6

THE CROSS FERTILIZATION OF BRAZILIAN POLITICS AND COVID-19

1. Brazil in the Time of Coronavirus

Maite Conde[1]

ABSTRACT

This essay outlines and analyses the spread of the coronavirus in Brazil. In doing so it explores how the pandemic, whilst initially brought into the country by the wealthy elite, has predominantly affected the country's poor, revealing structural inequalities that encompass class, race and ethnic differences, in which the poor are not afforded the right to live. It additionally examines the response to COVID-19 by the country's far right president, Jair Messias Bolsonaro, looking at how his *laissez faire* reaction to the virus builds on a history of violence against the marginalized, especially to the country's indigenous peoples, that has not just excluded them from the nation state but at times actively and violently eradicated them.

INTRODUCTION

"So what? I'm sorry. What do you want me to do about it?" These were the words of Jair Messias Bolsonaro, Brazil's president elect, when asked by reporters about the record of 474 deaths from coronavirus on Tuesday 28 April (*Guardian* newspaper). As Bolsonaro made his remarks, newspapers and television programmes were filled with stories about the mothers, fathers, sons and daughters losing their lives to the COVID-19 pandemic. Bolsonaro's response sparked fury and was immediately condemned throughout the country. The next day the *Estado de Minas* newspaper printed the president's words on a black page beside the country's death toll that day: 5,017 (Figure 1).Social media became rife with criticism. Marcelo Freixo, leader of the left wing PSOL party, tweeted "Bolsonaro isn't just an awful politician and bad person, he's a despicable human being" (*Guardian* newspaper, 29 April 2020). Musician Nano Moura labelled Bolsonaro "a sociopath," and screenwriter Mariliz Pereira Jorge called his words "an insult" and "intolerable" (*Guardian* newspaper, 29 April 2020).Bolsonaro's flippant reply is not surprising. Since Brazil confirmed its first case of the coronavirus on 26 February, the right-wing populist leader has constantly belittled the epidemic.

He has labelled it nothing more than a "little flu;" has said that Brazilians can swim in excrement "and nothing happens;" he has rejected the media "hysteria" over its dangers; has purposefully undermined social distancing guidelines by mingling with his supporters and attending mass rallies protesting against lockdowns; and on 16 April he sacked his health minister, Luiz Henrique Mandetta, after he publicly challenged the president's behaviour.

But, in spite of Bolsonaro's denial, there is no escaping the scale of the tragedy in Brazil, which has become Latin America's deadliest hotspot for COVID-19 and it is projected to become the next global

---

[1] Department of Spanish and Portuguese, University of Cambridge.
E-mail: mc534@cam.ac.uk   *Geopolítica(s)* 11(Especial) 2020: 239-249

pandemic epicentre. At the time of writing, the country has reported more cases (135,106) and more confirmed deaths (9,146) than any of its South American neighbour, and researchers at Imperial College London estimate that Brazil's transmission rate will this week have been the highest in the world. The vertiginous rise in the numbers of confirmed cases has sparked an intense national debate about the extreme class, race and social inequalities in one of the most economically lopsided societies on earth; it has also shed light on the country's historical structural violence and how it is being revived today.

Figure 1. Front-page of *Estado de Minas* newspaper (29 April 2020)

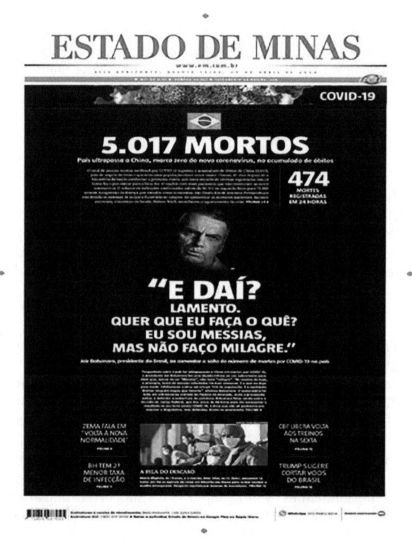

Source: *Estado de Minas*, 29 April 2020. Retrieved from https://www.em.com.br/app/noticia/capa-dodia/2020/04/29/noticia-capa-do-dia,1142827/confira-a-capa-do-jornal-estado-de-minas-do-dia-29-04-2020.shtml

Class, Race and COVID-19: The Rich Contaminate Brazil. The Poor Suffer

The first wave of cases in Brazil was primarily in the country's largely white elite, those who had travelled abroad where they exposed themselves to the virus and could then treat themselves in private hospitals. In March, for instance, descendants from Brazil's former royal family, the Braganças, gathered in a mansion in Ipanema to toast the engagement of 31-year-old Pedro Alberto de Orléans e Bragança – the great-great-great grandson of Brazil's last emperor and his 26-year-old partner, Alessandra Fragoso Pires. Guests included Pires's mother and stepfather who had jetted in from their home in London and others from Belgium, Italy and the United States. More than half of the 70 people at the lunch subsequently tested positive for COVID-19, including the bride's father and grandfather, and the groom's aunt. Shortly afterwards, in April, at Rio de Janeiro's country club, which was founded in 1916 and has been frequented since by the elite of *cariocan* society, 60 of its 850 globe-trotting members had been struck down with COVID-19. That same month, Brazil's Health Ministry estimated that 60% of suspected cases of coronavirus were people who had travelled to Europe and the USA, where the pandemic was raging.

But, while COVID-19 was introduced by Brazil's jet set elite, it is now the poor and mostly black masses, that is the 14 million Brazilians who live in favelas and urban peripheries, who are suffering the most, without the luxury of being able to self-isolate at home or to resort to expensive private hospitals. One of the country's first recorded deaths was that of Cleonice Gonçalves, a 63-year old domestic worker. She fell ill suddenly while working at an apartment in the exclusive Rio neighbourhood of Leblon, where she was reportedly infected by her wealthy employer who had recently returned from holiday in Italy. Gonçalves' family called a taxi for her when they learned of her condition. It took the domestic labourer two hours of traveling through twisting roads to reach her home in the small town of Miguel Pereira. At 6pm she checked into the local hospital and by the following afternoon she was dead. According to four state and local officials, her boss had been feeling ill and had tested positive for coronavirus but did not inform

Gonçalves, Who Had Worked For The Family For Decades.

For the black feminist intellectual Djamila Ribeiro writing in the *Folha de São Paulo* newspaper, this particular case exemplifies the precarious state of Brazil's poor. "It goes without saying' she notes, "that the most vulnerable will be the most affected. These are structural issues" (19 March, 2020).Indeed, while the coronavirus was imported by the Brazilian elite vacationing in Europe it soon began to ravage the country's poor, ripping through favelas and urban peripheries where inhabitants suffer from a lack of running water, septic systems and health care facilities making the disease hard to control. On 27 March, for instance, Rio's elite neighbourhoods of Leblon, Copacabana and Barra da Tijuca reported 190 confirmed cases of COVID-19.In contrast, the city's low-income areas of Campo Grande, Bangu and Irajá reported only eight cases. All of this changed rapidly. Just a week later those poorer neighbourhoods reported 66 cases and today the numbers are in the hundreds, although experts state that the real rate of cases in poorer areas is undoubtedly far higher than reported due to a lack of testing. Rio's secretary of health Edmar Santos, who was himself diagnosed with COVID-19 in early April admitted that underreporting and testing amongst the poor means that official figures do not capture the scale of the crisis.[1] Poor Brazilians are also more likely to die if infected, due to higher levels of pre-existing conditions and less access to healthcare. Epidemiologist Keny Colares noted that most low-income patients were showing up at hospitals days after they should have sought medical attention, leading to greater fatalities.

In Rio's exclusive neighbourhood Leblon, for example, just 2.4% of confirmed cases have resulted in deaths, roughly in line with global trends and suggesting a relatively accurate picture of infection numbers. In Irajá, meanwhile, the death rate is 16%, while in São Paulo's favela Brasilandia, it is a staggering 52%.

While state governors and health officials, like Santos, have implemented social distancing and lockdown measures, few of those living in poor neighbourhoods are adhering to quarantine measures, with life continuing more or less as usual. Shops and bars are bustling and the poor, who tend to work in the informal economy, are continuing to go to work. All of this has been intensified by the confusing messages regarding the virus. Bolsonaro's anti-scientific stance has made many people ignore state measures. Indeed, despite the rising death toll Bolsonaro has pushed to restart the economy, describing shelter-in-place policies as a poison that could kill more via unemployment and hunger than the virus. This situation has led gangs and drug traffickers to enforce their own curfews in favelas, amid growing fears of the impact the virus will have on its poor citizens. Gang members in the *Cidade de deus* favela in western Rio, for example, have ordered residents to remain indoors after 8pm. A video recorded in the favela and circulated on social media includes a loudspeaker broadcasting the alert that "anyone found walking around outside will be punished."

A report in the Rio newspaper *Extra* stated that gang members with loudhailers were moving around the *Cidade de deus* telling its 40,000 residents "we are imposing a curfew because nobody is taking coronavirus seriously. It's best to stay at home" (*Extra* newspaper, 24 March, 2020).

Cidade de deus' gangsters are not the only outlaws attacking the coronavirus in Rio's densely populated favelas, which are home to about two of the city's seven million residents. In Rio's *Morro dos Prazeres*, gang members have told residents only to circulate in groups of two, while in *Rocinha*, one of Latin America's biggest favelas, traffickers have also decreed a curfew after 8.30 pm promising reprisals for those who do not conform. In *Santa Marta*, a favela that sits in the shadow of Rio's Christ the Redeemer statue, traffickers have been handing out soap and have placed signs near a public water fountain at the community's entrance asking people to "Please wash your hands before entering the favela." Meanwhile, in some sections of the *Complexo da Maré*, a sprawling favela near Rio's international airport, traffickers have told shops and churches to reduce their operating hours.

Other favelas in which curfews have been imposed include *Pavão-Pavãozinho* in Copacabana, *Cantagalo* in Ipanema, and *Vidigal*. Inhabitants of these neighbourhoods are staying indoors for fear of the coronavirus and of the gangs' orders and threats. One *Cidade de deus* resident noted, however, "the traffickers are doing this because the government is absent. The authorities are blind to us." All of this highlights what Alba Zaluar and Marcos Alvito (1998) refer to as the 'dualism' or 'duality' in Brazil's cities, that is, a polarization between the formal and informal urban space caused by the absence of the state in peripheral areas. For Zuenir Ventura (1998), this polarity has created 'divided' or 'broken' cities, which results from varied and complex forms of state policy failure and results in a form of social and racial apartheid and exclusion.

---

[1] He believes that Rio, with a population of 17 million, has more than 15 times the official figure. A study published in Globo newspaper suggested the national figures were being similarly underestimated, with more than 1.2m likely infections, compared with the official figure of under 74,000. That would mean Brazil had more cases than the United States, so far the country worst hit by the pandemic, which has about 1 million.

Indeed, Edmund Ruge, a Rio-based editor for the RioOnWatch news site which covers the favelas, has said the imposition of curfews by gangs speaks to the Brazilian state's longstanding neglect of such areas.

Faced with this neglect, favela activists have been scrambling to respond to the coronavirus crisis with food donations and awareness campaigns, and projects such as #COVID19NasFavelas. In *Cidade de Deus*, the *Frente CDD* has also been working to raise awareness in the community, as have communicators in Rio's *Complexo Alemão* favela, by creating banners, speaking face-to-face with people and handing out leaflets emphasizing the need to stop the spread of coronavirus. Favelas in other cities around the country have seen similar initiatives. In São Paulo, the website *Peripheria em movimento* created a podcast *Pandemia sem neurose* to provide information.

In Heliópolis, São Paulo's largest favela, the Union of Residents and Associations has been holding collections for food and hygiene items. They also conducted an online survey on the impacts of coronavirus on the favela between 27 and 29 March. The 653 responses clearly illustrate the economic implications: 68 per cent of families living in Heliópolis have lost some of their monthly income since the virus restrictions were put in place. Of these, 19 per cent have lost their entire income.

The union directly deals with local concerns, something that is also evident in the *Laboratorio de jovens comunicadores* (Laboratory of Young Communicators) in the periphery of the city of Belém. This group was hastily formed in March to monitor official communication and amplify the concerns of the neighbourhood in the context of the pandemic, producing information designed for local realities. Teacher Lilia Melo who coordinates the project, emphasizes the importance of the local communicators at this time. "We're taking advantage of our network to offer guidance on prevention and combat of the virus for young people in a language they understand. We realised that there are some young people in the neighbourhood who still haven't realised how serious this is. Because of their reality, the difficulties they face, they tend to mock the recommendations from the state and federal governments, which don't speak to the reality of the periphery" (*Latin American Bureau*, 10 May 2020) she says. This question of language also arose for filmmaker Yane Mendes, who decided to adapt the official Ministry of Health information for the 2,500 residents of the Totó favela, in Recife, the capital of the state of Pernambuco. Concerned by the city government's failure to provide informative material on the prevention of coronavirus, she went looking for posters.

Dissatisfied with the dry official communication, Yane made her own posters and put them up next to the official ones – effectively translating them.

Other local groups have made efforts to directly engage with state authorities. On March 23, The Rocinha Residents Association sent a letter signed by representatives of different favelas to Rio's governor Wilson Witzel, outlining seventeen proposals to combat the pandemic. These included providing food baskets to favela residents, especially the elderly; distributing basic hygiene kits, including hand sanitizer and protective equipment, to families living in favelas; the resumption of Community Health Agents in favelas; the immediate suspension of all evictions, judicial or extrajudicial, in favelas; exemption from electricity payments and guaranteed attention for severe cases amongst favela residents by increasing the number of beds in private and public hospitals and renting empty hotels. As of today, these proposals have yet to be implemented.

If the spread of COVID-19 has exposed the vulnerability of Brazil's urban poor, it has also highlighted the extent to which the death of a part of the country's population can be included in calculations and political managements, what Achille Mbembe (2019) calls necropolitics, which entails the right to expose people (including a country's own citizens) to death. This necropolitical approach is clearly at the heart of Bolsonaro's *laissez faire* attitude to COVID-19, evident on 21 March when, referring to the certainty of a rise in coronavirus-related deaths especially amongst the poor, he noted "Will some die? Yes, some people will die. I am sorry. This is life. We do not close car factories due to the fact that there are traffic accidents" (*Wired*, 7 May 2020).

Necropolitics has of course always been part of the DNA of Brazilian society and its divided cities. In 2017, more than 150,000 Brazilians died from poor medical health and 50,000 from lack of access to health care. 35 million lack access to running water. And in favelas, inhabitants are routinely killed because of police interventions. In 2019, for instance, 1,810 residents in Rio alone died as a result of police crackdowns. Brazil has always had an unequal distribution of the opportunity to live and die. Bolsonaro's words, therefore, and his attitude to the coronavirus, much like that of the country's elite who imported and transmitted it, are part of decades of social segregation and attacks on the country's precarious populations, especially its black population. Brazil's COVID-19 crisis is in this sense, a crisis of sovereignty, revealing the absence of the state, which fails to provide health, that is to sustain the life, of *all* of its citizens.

Coronavirus and Brazil's Indigenous Peoples: Building on a History of Exclusion and Extermination

It is not just Brazil's urban poor who are disproportionately threatened and suffering from COVID-19. Indigenous communities in the Amazon region are also in danger of being 'wiped out' by the coronavirus, according to health experts. Respiratory illnesses, like those that develop from the influenza virus, are already the main cause of death for native communities and COVID-19 is now encroaching on the indigenous. By April the coronavirus had reached indigenous territories in the Amazon basin that are the size of France and Spain combined and April 13 saw the first victim of COVID-19, a 15-year-old boy, member of the Yanomani community. Since then a further three further members of the Yanomani have died.For Dr Sofia Mendoça, a researcher at the Federal University of São Paulo (Unifesp) "there is an incredible risk of spreading the virus across the native communities and exterminating them" (Qtd. in *BBC Brazil News*, 6 April 2020). She believes that coronavirus would have a similar impact to previous outbreaks of highly contagious diseases like measles. In the 1960s, a measles epidemic among the Yanomami community killed nearly 9% of those infected. As with the urban periphery, many indigenous communities lack the means to reduce the contagion, like hand sanitizer and water and soap. People too live in close proximity with each other, sharing utensils which will help the disease spread quickly. Indigenous peoples also live in areas where there is limited access to health care.

There is little expectation or hope that the state will intervene and help the indigenous communities fight against coronavirus. Over the years Bolsonaro has made numerous racist remarks about indigenous people. On April 12, 1998, he declared that it was "a shame that the Brazilian cavalry has not been as efficient as the Americans who exterminated the Indians" (qtd.in *Correio Brasiliense* Newspaper, April 12 1998).

On February 8, 2018 he stated that if he became president "there will not be a centimetre more of indigenous land" (qtd. in *Dourados Matto Grosso do Sul* Newspaper) later correcting himself to say that he meant not one millimetre (qtd. in *Globo* Newspaper, August 3, 2018); on January 23, 2020 he said, "the Indians are evolving, more and more they are human beings like us" (qtd. in *OUL Notícias*); and on 24 January 2018 he declared at a speech that indigenous peoples, as well as Afro-

Brazilians are "not fit for anything, not even procreating." Bolsonaro's words clearly signal overt discrimination; they also point to a history of exclusion and difference to indigenous communities in Brazil, which have long been considered outsiders to the nation.

From the start of the First Republic (1889-1930), Brazil's indigenous peoples were viewed as pariahs and non-citizens of the nation state. The spiritual conquest of the New World followed the logic of cleansing and persecution against indigenes on religious grounds. Modern nationalism built on this, culturally and economically, and in Brazil, the subjugation of Indians was reformulated according to the needs of the modern nation of order and progress, which either sought to exterminate communities or 'assimilate' them as workers. In the early 1900s, anthropologist Hermann von Ihering argued that Indians were incapable of learning and that they were "indolent and indifferent and would not make a minimum contribution to our culture and progress" (Andermann, 2007, p.69). In his 1905 article "Anthropology in the State of São Paulo," Ihe ring even went as far as recommending the extermination of the state's Amerindian population, writing "

The Indians of the state of São Paulo do not represent an element of labour and progress.

As in other states of Brazil, no serious and continuous work can be expected from civilized Indians, and they are an obstacle for colonizing the back land regions they presently occupy, it seems there is no other means at hand than to eliminate them" (*ibidem*.). The scientist ended another article by noting that "it is worth registering here what the American general Custer said: the only good Indian is a dead Indian" (Diacon, 2004, p.124).

Ihering's racism echoed discussions about the racial inferiority of the indigenes put forward by other intellectuals at the time. In 1911, physician and pioneering eugenicist Afranio Peixoto wrote of the inevitable disappearance of the "subhuman races" of indigenes; and historian Silvio Romero critiqued indigenous populations, who he regarded as "the lowest race on the ethnographic scale" (*ibid.*, p.123). Viewing indigenous peoples as sub-races, Romero insisted on

a break with Indianism and its object as a precondition for Brazil's progress. He criticized the indo-mania that had turned Brazil into a self-indulgent, backward nation, idealizing an indigenous population that was among the least developed in the world (Andermann, 2007, p.94). Bolsonaro's recent statements eerily echo these historical proclamations and critiques which have placed the indigenes as "alien to modernity," to cite Jean Franco (2013, p.45). His words are clearly the result of decades, even centuries, of a discourse of discrimination. Although we should not conflate the effects of ethnic and gender identity, Judith Butler's assertion (1990) in reference to gender that the epistemological mode of appropriation, instrumentality and belong to a strategy of domination that pits the I against the Other, which is in turn sedimented through a discourse of repetition can be applied to ethnic difference in Brazil.

The consequences of indigenous difference, it's supposed otherness to the modern, was often carried to violent fruition. In the late 1800s and early 1900s, rubber tappers and local agricultural *caudilhos* in the Amazon basin frequently attacked the natives in an effort to expropriate their lands or their labour. In the early 1820s, for instance, a six-year battle against the western Bororo on the eastern side of the Paraguay river, led by influential landowner and military officer João Carlos Pereira Leite, left 450 Bororo dead and 50 imprisoned. These prisoners, later deemed to be 'pacified,' were assimilated as forced labour on Leite's farm. In the late nineteenth century, the provincial government of Mato Grosso founded two military settlements near the São Lourenço river in order to integrate the Bororo communities. Lacking an effective integration system, the settlements degenerated: drunkenness, sex and fighting led to fierce clashes between Indians and soldiers. Far from alien, the indigenous peoples in Brazil have had a long history of contact with 'outsiders,' which has been violent and assimilationist.

This history is prescient today and not just discursively. Since taking office Bolsonaro has avowed open season on the Amazon rainforest, pledging to take land away from indigenous communities. On February 5, 2020 the president presented a bill to Congress to regulate mining, hydroelectric power projects and other commercial enterprises in Indigenous territories. The bill effectively invites encroachment on and deforestation of Indigenous lands, giving carte blanche to cattle ranches and rogue loggers.[1]

The result is that indigenous people have been threatened, attacked and, according to community leaders, murdered by people engaged in deforestation. The bill comes as no surprise, given Bolsonaro's dismissiveness of indigenous peoples and their rights. Today these attitudes are being revamped in the context of the coronavirus, with the pandemic being used to usher in laws that will lead to increased occupation of indigenous lands and deforestation in the Amazon, amid warning by campaigners that further environmental disruption could lead to new pandemics in the area.

Indeed, while the crisis has seen most industries grind to a halt, government data suggests that deforestation in Brazil's Amazon rose 30% in March compared to the period last year, with the most recent data suggesting the trend has continued in April. There has also been an increase in forays into indigenous lands by miners and land-grabbers as civil and official protection efforts are scaled back for fear of infection. With the cuts to protection there is nothing to protect the indigenous from pandemics brought in from outsiders. In a recent open letter to Brazil's president, photographer Sebastião Salgado and a global coalition of artists and celebrities warned that the pandemic meant that indigenous communities in the Amazon faced an extreme threat to their survival. "Five centuries ago, these ethnic groups were decimated by diseases brought by European colonizers (...). Now, with this new scourge spreading rapidly across. Brazil [they] may disappear completely since they have no means of combatting COVID-19," they wrote.[2] Indigenous peoples are attempting to combat the spread of coronavirus.

Some communities have split into smaller groups and are seeking refuge inside the forest, repeating mechanisms they used to avoid extinctions during past epidemics. The virus though has already made incursions into the area and Manaus, the capital of Amazonas and the state where part of the Yanomani reserve is located, is by far the worst city in Brazil so far hit by COVID-19. The coronavirus appears to have reached the isolated, riverside metropolis of more than 2 million people on March 11, imported by a 49-year-old woman who had flown in from London. Six weeks later it had taken a terrible toll, with more than 100 people dying each day. This month the city expects to bury 4,500 people. With so many fatalities authorities are performing night-time burials and funeral homes have run out of coffins. In Parque Tarumã, Manaus' biggest cemetery, excavators carved out mass graves called *trincheiras* (trenches)

in which the dead were stacked in three-mile piles.[5] Emergency and health services in Manaus are also buckling under the strain with ambulances roaming the city for hours in search of hospitals to admit the ill they have collected. Videos have emerged of hospitals showing corridors lined with corpses shrouded in body bags and in one an unconscious patient is seen with his head wrapped inside a ventilator hood improvised from a large plastic bag.

---

[1] Deforestation in Indigenous land in the Amazon increased 65 percent from August 2018 to July 2019, according to INPE. The Indigenist Missionary Council (CIMI), a nonprofit organization, reported that from January through September 2019 there were 160 incursions into Brazil's indigenous land by people engaged in illegal mining, logging, and land grabs.

[2] The open letter was published virtually, see:
https://secure.avaaz.org/po/community_petitions/presidente_do_brasil_e_aos_lideres_do_legislativo_ajude_
a_proteger_os_povos_indigenas_da_amazonia_do_covid19/?cZZUvqb&utm_source=sharetools&utm_mediu m=copy&utm_campaign=petition-994813-ajude_a_proteger_os_povos_indigenas_da_amazonia_do_covid19&utm_term=ZZUvqb%2Bpo [5] This occurred until a revolt from mourning families saw the practice halted.

There is a shortage of mechanical ventilators, of oxygen, staff and stretchers. There are a number of reasons for the intensity of the catastrophe in Manaus. The virus struck at the end of the rainy season when respiratory illnesses are rife, and hospitals already stretched. The city's underfunded health system was also poorly equipped and doctors and other medical workers began contracting the disease themselves. Many also believe that corruption and the government's failure to implement containment measures is also to blame.

It took 10 days after the first case was confirmed, on 23 March, for the state governor, Wilson Lima, to declare a state of emergency, ordering non-essential businesses to close. Yet even with the rising numbers of fatalities, social distancing is being ignored with people refusing to remain at home. The city's mayor, Arthur Virgilio, has pleaded for people to take the virus seriously but has blamed Bolsonaro. "It saddens me to know these lives could have been saved and weren't saved, in part because Brazil's leader said it was OK to go out" (qtd. in *Guardian* newspaper, 30 April, 2020). Virgilio has accused Bolsonaro of offering Brazil's citizens a false and dangerous choice between "freedom" and the "prison of social isolation." "He is offering freedom but it is a false freedom that could represent a kind of genocide," he said (Qtd. in *Guardian* Newspaper, 30 April, 2020). Rio-based writer, Pedro Doria, believes the coronavirus' spread throughout the country's marginalised could carry a heavy political price for president Bolsonaro, whose call for a relaxing of containment measures is an attempt to ingratiate himself with the poor.

"What is hurting people in the favelas is the economy. So, right now Bolsonaro is making lots of sense to them," Doria said. But he believes that attitudes will change "the moment people we know start dying. (…). People will not forget that he said it was OK to go out on the streets" (qtd. in *Guardian* newspaper, 25 April, 2020).Public backlash, at least amongst the middle classes, has indeed intensified, with nightly *panelaço* protests across Brazil's major cities, where dissenters express their dissatisfaction with Bolsonaro by pummelling saucepans from windows and balconies. In spite of these protests Bolsonaro has not altered his message. While state mayors and governors have declared quarantines and lockdowns in major cities, the president has decried these arguing that life must go on as normal. On Sunday 3 May, he stirred up street protests in Brazilian cities against lockdown measures in defiance of his own health ministry's appeals for citizens to stay at home. This when the numbers of deaths had risen to well over 7,000.

REFERENCES

Andermann, J. (2007). *The Optic of the State: Visuality and Power in Argentina and Brazil*. Pittsburgh: University of Pittsburgh Press.

Butler, J. (1990). *Gender Trouble. Feminism and the Subversion of Identity*. New York: Routledge.

Diacon, T. A. (2004). *Stringing Together a Nation: Cândido Mariano da Silva Rondon and the Construction of a Modern Brazil, 1906-1930*. Durham, NC: Duke University Press.

Franco, J. (2013). *Cruel Modernity*. Durham, NC: Duke University Press.

Mbembe, A. (2019). *Necropolitics*. Durham, NC: Duke University Press.

Ventura, Z. (1994). *Cidade partida*. Rio de Janeiro: Companhia das letras.

Zaluar, A., & Alvito, M. (1998). *Um século de favela*. Rio de Janeiro: FGV Editora.

2. The Perfect COVID-19 Storm in Brazil

Eduardo José Grin & Fundação Getúlio Vargas

ABSTRACT

The analysis focuses on the multifaceted impact of the coronavirus pandemic in Brazil. Besides its health and socioeconomic consequences, the pandemic has also accelerated and deepened other crises evolving for a long time, explicitly concerning intergovernmental relations and public policy management. One of the arguments is that the actions of the current government to deal with COVID-19 are detrimental to the cooperative type of federalism that is in place in Brazil in the last thirty years.

INTRODUCTION

The pandemic hits Brazil at a juncture in which several crises that have been ongoing for a long time now converge: political-institutional, public policy management, economic and social. However, COVID-19 exposed and intensified the effects underway in other dimensions on a much larger scale, and it is essential to comment on its connections and impacts in the country. Facing the pandemic, given its multiple effects, is a wicked problem (Peters,2017). Still, the country's current government is far from retaining the capacity and political will to deal with the complexity that the issue deserves. The political and institutional dilemma is related to the challenges to democratic normality that have been increasing in recent years, especially after the election of Bolsonaro in 2018. The COVID-19 virus served as a backdrop to encourage authoritarian measures by the current government, such as the issuing of provisional measures, reducing the government's legal responsibility to respond to requests for information.

Yet, the most recent initiatives have been promptly rejected by the Judiciary. Among them was an attempt to change the Access to Information Law concerning the ban on the "Brazil cannot stop" campaign. Also rejected was the request to extend the validity of provisional measures in the face of crisis caused by COVID-19.The decree of the State of Emergency has been closely monitored by the National Congress (Grin, 2020). The pandemic only accelerated and deepened the challenges, as the president decided to confront or minimize the role of horizontal control of political institutions such as the Supreme Federal Court and the National Congress, as well as vertical control based on the constitutional autonomy of states and municipalities (Abrucio et al. 2020).

The current government is based on a view of politics in which opponents are enemies (Schmitt 1991) instead of political antagonists, which supports an imperial view of governmental conduct. "I am the Constitution" summarizes this stance of political power. The battle with the pandemic exposed this authoritarian project of power. The president has suffered defeats in the Supreme Court when it recognized that states and municipalities have constitutional competence to decide about social isolation. More recently, another judicial decision forced the government to resume the release of accumulated data on the pandemic. In the National Congress, the government also suffered defeats in the model of financial aid to states and municipalities and the monetary value and rules of the emergency aid for the informal and unemployed population. In the vertical area, the president understands that he has the power to define actions unilaterally. COVID-19 is a complex intergovernmental problem (Paquet and Schertzer 2020). Thus, what was expected from the central sphere was the capacity for federative coordination. Yet the choice has been a confrontation with subnational entities. Conflicts and intergovernmental incoordination have been two elements that strongly reduce the effectiveness of actions against COVID-19. Brazil is facing the new coronavirus through two conflicting conceptions of federalism. On the one hand, there is a cooperative model (Agranoff, 2007), built thirty years ago starting with the 1988 Constitution. On the other hand, there is a new model proposed by Bolsonaro: "More Brazil and Less Brasilia." It is similar to the dualist view (Loughlin, Kincaid, and Sweden 2013) defended by Trump. It aims to reduce the Federal Government's action supporting public policies. The Federal COVID-19 Crisis Committee, without state and municipal representation, illustrates this conception of radicalized dualistic federalism with centralized command. At the same time, governors' reaction to sustain their initiatives and defend SUS (the universal health care system) is positive for federalism (Abrucio et al. 2020). In public policy management, the State is no longer an open space for social participation and becomes a producer of centralized commands.

The disarticulation of government action in the fight against COVID-19 in education, social assistance, and health shows the consequences of this conception, which believes it is possible to govern centrally and disregard society and the federation. Denying the logic of politics and public policies makes the country walk many democratic steps backward and takes a heavy toll on reconstruction. The most evident example in this direction is the dismantling that has been carried out at the Ministry of Health in full combat against COVID-19.

The peak of this process occurred with the Ministry of Health accused states of lying about the deaths from the pandemic and failing to inform about the number of victims and of those infected with the previous periodicity, which throws into suspicion the entire cooperative model of SUS (Franzese, 2010). The denial of politics as a way of mediating interests, as well as of actors constituted for this mission through political parties and the congress, delegitimizes democracy. Public policies are also victims of this exclusive view because, since 1988, forums for dialogue between government and society have been established (Grin and Andrade 2020).Besides, all cooperative logic that guided intergovernmental coordination, through arenas of dialogue and federative negotiation between the Union, states, and municipalities, has been disarticulated and disallowed as an interlocutor with technical and political legitimacy. This deconstruction process had been underway since 2019, but the fight against the pandemic uncovered and accelerated this dualist, centralized, and exclusive view of the federal government.

The institutional construction effort of the Brazilian federation to consolidate forums for intergovernmental cooperation is being severely weakened. Similar criticisms can be made for other strategic areas of the welfare state. Concerning education, the National High School Exam is not being formulated in conjunction with the Council of State Secretaries of Education. Regarding social assistance, the implementation of emergency measures to serve the most vulnerable population did not consider public facilities in the municipalities. The most likely effect of the dualistic federalism of Bolsonaro government, as Covid19 has shown, will be the weakening of the cooperative model. In the economic field, the arrival of the pandemic exacerbated the country's weakness, as the virus arrived at a moment of a fragile recovery and with a contingent of around 12 million unemployed people, besides the underemployed population.

The inability to generate new jobs, associated with the escalation of the political and institutional crisis, was exacerbated by the pandemic. Its effects on the economy will be profound and should generate a shrinkage of more than 5% this year, according to a study by Economic Commission for Latin American (2020). Political instability and pandemic will be a combination with intense effects on the economy, so the country is likely to face the worst economic recession in its history. Recovery will be slow, as the decline in economic activity and the resumption of employment will be slow. The pandemic did not create the economic crisis, but given its weakness, COVID-19 arrived unexpectedly and augmented the seriousness of the problem. Since 2014, the informal labour market has grown, but even that possibility has not reached the poorest. The pandemic will worsen this situation, and extreme poverty is expected to increase. The social crisis was already deep in Brazil and had been intensifying since 2015, with the expansion of unemployment and the growth of poverty being two indicators that callously exemplify this reality. For millions, the economic crisis with its slow recovery has left the poorest 40% even Middle Atlantic Review of Latin American Studies worse off than before COVID-19. Almost a third of the population (66.3 million people) lives in families where more than half of the income comes from unprotected sources of work (Muñoz, 2020).

The most dramatic social effect of COVID-19 in the short term will be the disproportionate increase in the number of infected and dead within the most vulnerable population. At the most immediate level, the main ones affected by the deaths caused by the pandemic are poor and black people living on the outskirts of large cities. After the health crisis, its most pronounced effect will be the intensification of social inequality and income concentration, since the most disadvantaged sectors will be those with more significant difficulties in economic reintegration, apart from educational, family, and health consequences. COVID-19 did not create the problems the country is facing since 2015, and that has become more acute in the Bolsonaro government. However, the perfect storm has formed in this juncture. The health crisis outcome is still not entirely predictable, although the country is moving quickly to increase its deaths that are at levels like those of the United States. However, the pandemic highlighted the country's political, social, and economic dramas. The horizon still shows only many clouds, and there is no sign of optimism.

REFERENCES

Abrucio, Fernando Luiz et al.2020 "Combate à COVID-19 sob o federalismo bolsonarista: um caso de descoordenação intergovernamental". Revista de Administração Pública (article in submission).

Agranoff, Robert 2007 "Intergovernmental Policy Management: Cooperative Practices in Federal Systems." In The Dynamics of Federalism in National and Supranational Political Systems, edited by Michael A. Pagano and Robert Leonardi, 248–284. New York: Palgrave Macmillan.

LAS rin – The Perfect COVID-19 Storm in Brazil Economic Commission for Latin America 2020 "Pandemia de COVID-19 levará à maior contração da atividade econômica na história da região: cairá -5,3% em 2020." Available on: https://www.cepal.org/ptbr/comunicados/pandemia-COVID-19-levara-maior-contracao-atividade-economica-historiaregiao-caira-53. Access: 13 Jun. 2020.

Franzese, Cibele 2010 Federalismo cooperativo no Brasil: da Constituição de 1988 à constituição dos sistemas de políticas públicas. São Paulo: EAESP.

Grin, Eduardo José 2020 "COVID-19 también puede infectar y matar la democracia." Diálogo Político. Available on: https://dialogopolitico.org/agenda/COVID-19-tambien-puede-infectar-y-matar-lademocracia/. Access: 13 Jun. 2020.

Grin, Eduardo José, and Lilian Furquim Andrade 2020 "A Constituição sou eu, e daí?" Jornal O Nexo.

Loughlin, John, John Kincaid, and Wilfried Sweden 2013 Handbook of Regionalism & Federalism. London and New York: Routledge Taylor & Francis Group.

Muñoz, Rafael 2020 "Novos números mostram por que é crucial proteger os mais pobres na crise da COVID-19." Paquet, Mireille, and Robert Schertzer 2020 "COVID-19 as a Complex Intergovernmental Problem." Canadian Journal of Political Science, 14 April: 1–5. doi: 10.1017/S0008423920000281

Peters, Brainard Guy 2017 "What Is So Wicked about Wicked Problems? A Conceptual Analysis and a Research Program." Policy and Society 36 (3): 385–96.

Schmitt, Carl 1991 El concepto de lo político. Madrid: Alianza Universid

3. Bolsonaro, COVID-19, and the Crisis of Brazilian Democracy

Márcia Cury is a Senior Research Fellow at COHA

The Brazilian President Jair Bolsonaro's statements are at first shocking, leaving one wondering what he really means. But they are not surprising in the context of the paranoid rhetoric that has always characterized his administration. Since the start of the Coronavirus pandemic that is ravaging the world, for which the World Health Organization (WHO) has established preventive measures, the President of Brazil stands out for his public statements refusing to take any precautions. Contrary to all predictions of the consequences of infection, Bolsonaro insists on minimizing the risks posed by the virus and defies social distancing guidelines. He calls the disease a "fantasy" and "hysteria" whipped up by the media.[1] Jair Bolsonaro's remarks and inaction fit into his pattern of political practices. But in the middle of an unprecedented crisis, his behaviour is sounding alarm bells about the near term social and political fallout.

Bolsonaro the Science Denier

Jair Bolsonaro has never been the centre of attention for implementing important projects during his long political career, but rather for his cavalier attitude towards dictatorship, racism, homophobia, and gender equality, which are sensitive subjects in such an unequal and violent society as that of Brazil. A denial of science guides most of his speeches on a wide variety of topics, and this has been no different during the pandemic. He first showed this irresponsible approach when he said on national TV that he opposed the preventive measures instituted by the governors and mayors. He criticized the social distancing guidelines by saying that unemployment might have a worse impact on society.[2] According to Bolsonaro, people should live their lives normally because it will only be possible to create "antibodies and a barrier" to the disease if some people get infected.[3] His public appearances, during which his followers gather in the streets to greet him, have also been common and drawn the attention of the international press. The ProSul hemispheric[4] meeting held by video conference on March 16, 2020, convened to discuss joint measures to confront the pandemic, was marked by the absence of the Brazilian president. At this important event, the country was represented by Foreign Minister Ernesto Araújo. In another display of his lack of commitment to mitigation efforts, Bolsonaro skipped the meeting of heads of the Judicial, Legislative, and Executive Branches of the Government of Brazil to establish common objectives for fighting the spread of the virus in the country. Instead, Luiz Henrique Mandetta, the Minister of Health, represented the Executive Branch.

In recent weeks Bolsonaro's image has suffered as people begin to question his capacity to handle the crisis, including high-ranking public officials who have publicly expressed disagreement with his approach to containing the virus. The population is caught up in public confrontations between the Minister of Health, who defends social distancing policies, and the statements and practices of Jair Bolsonaro, who constantly questions the seriousness of the pandemic. This divergence of opinion has rattled the President's legitimacy, even among military officers, who, for a time, backed the Minister of Health when the President threatened to fire him. The growing breach, however, came to head on Thursday April 16, when President Bolsonaro fired his minister, Luiz Henrique Mandetta.[5] The conflicting messages emanating from the chief executive and his health minister have led the population to pay less attention to mitigation measures and relax social distancing. Another controversy revolves around the President's public advocacy for increasing production of hydroxychloroquine to treat COVID-19 patients. Bolsonaro has promoted this drug on radio and TV, although it is still the subject of research and debate among doctors and scientists as to whether it really is an effective treatment for the virus.[6]

Echoing Trump's Controversial Strategy

It is striking that, just like U.S. President Donald Trump, Bolsonaro is using the pandemic to fuel his unrelenting ideological war. In the context of an unprecedented crisis, this is jeopardizing the economy and the country's fragile democratic stability. The Brazilian president continues to act as if this were a political campaign and all he needs to do is whip up his base. Now he is trapped by economic indicators that are no longer showing signs of strong growth.

The pandemic can transform this precarious economic slowdown into a crisis. Added to this is his constant preoccupation with remaining in power and his dream of re-election. Taking his usual stance of someone who has no concept of the responsibility inherent in his position, Bolsonaro reverts to anti-establishment discourse, a persecution complex, and extremist ideas to exacerbate the conflict, in a desperate attempt to hang onto the support of his base as well as his authority—both of which are increasingly fragile. The show put on by Bolsonaro and his ideological promoters is a peculiar relaunching of an imaginary Cold War scenario in which the pandemic is supposedly just hysteria mounted by the opposition for political gain. For example, the president used primarily social media to spread fake news stories of shortages at a food distribution centre in Minas Gerais, supposedly caused by the stay-at-home policy.

The story was immediately refuted and Bolsonaro took down his posts.[7] A war of words can be costly for the economy. His most recent attacks were aimed at China, the country's top trading partner. The President's son and federal lawmaker, Eduardo Bolsonaro (whom the President is thinking of appointing ambassador to the U.S.), and the Minister of Education, Abraham Weintraub, went on Twitter to blame China for spreading the virus, insinuating that the country is profiting financially from the pandemic. The last tweet, which the Minister has since deleted, prompted a reply from the Chinese embassy in Brazil. Ill will has been sown and people now fear a breakdown in trade relations between the two countries, to the inevitable detriment of Brazil.[8]

An Irrational Fear Of "Socialism" Hamstrings Government Aid

Domestically, the conservative tone of Bonsonaro's political agenda is in step with the various social sectors that make up his base. But now, the dystopian reign of the Bolsonaro family has found faith to be a useful tool. He recently called upon the population to fast in response to the pandemic, clearly a move meant to stir his faithful followers, including many Evangelicals. However, this pandemic affects all sectors of the country and will likely cost many lives. The most vulnerable people face uncertainty and have already lost income due to the crisis.[9] This is especially true in a country in which a sizable number of workers have informal jobs, without any social security protections. The anti-government ideology so fiercely preached by the President and his team, despite the urgent hunger people are facing, has him refusing to believe the facts and figures in front of him.

The President's other son, Rio de Janeiro Council Member Carlos Bolsonaro, says that any state intervention would be a sign that the country is "moving toward socialism," because with the economy paralyzed, people would be dependent on the State "even to eat."[10] And Rubem Novaes, president of the country's main public bank, Banco do Brasil, says we must resist state intervention because later it will be hard to dismantle "the welfare state."[11] It was only after pressure from the public and the National Congress that Bolsonaro's proposal to allow employers freedom to lay off workers and suspend labour contracts was rolled back.

The Legislative Branch has ensured that families losing their incomes and livelihoods will receive some government compensation. The government will pay them the equivalent of US$ 120, not the mere US$ 40 per month initially proposed by Paulo Guedes, the ultra-neoliberal Minister of Finance. The Provisional Measure now includes an up to 70% wage reduction for up to 90 days and the suspension of labour contracts for up to two months. These wage losses will be offset by an extension of unemployment insurance which already exists in the country to help workers who lose their jobs in the formal economy. What is happening now in Brazil is a crisis that includes public health issues, a financial emergency, and political uncertainty.

The public's apprehension and dissatisfaction can now be heard in the pots-and-pans protests against Bolsonaro that make up the soundtrack of Brazilian nights. But just as part of society is beginning to make its dissatisfaction with the President heard, there is fear over what comes next as Bolsonaro becomes isolated. The blow to his legitimacy also threatens Brazilian democracy. What we are currently witnessing, while not a complete reversal of civilian control over the armed forces as required for a democratic system, is at least a relativization of it. The Executive Branch, through the office of the Vice-President and eight of the 22 Cabinet Ministers, is full of people whose names are embellished with military titles.

Their actions are imbued with nostalgia for the country's dictatorial past. And a policy of military officers not engaging in politics is giving way to the politicization of the military, sometimes in direct confrontation with democratic institutions such as when General Augusto Heleno called the National Congress "blackmailers."[12] In the case of the breach between the Minister of Health and the President, however, Bolsonaro has won the day, at least for now. During the pandemic crisis Bolsonaro will continue to be Bolsonaro. That is no surprise from a leader who got elected by taking conservative and authoritarian discourse to new heights, in an atmosphere of widespread "fake news." But this is a precarious moment. It has been demonstrated that the scenario of a society in isolation, with people focused on protecting lives and fearing the impacts of a crisis, is primed for political manipulation. And the danger is even more real when it goes beyond the paranoia and irresponsible actions of a joking president, to include control by other institutional actors. In such a context one may imagine the possibility of the military co-governing. These are people who represent a recent authoritarian past, and who present themselves as the new salvation for a country "that has lost its way." This situation demands that we remain vigilant, to ensure the survival of Brazil's fragile democracy.

REFERENCES

[1] "Em evento esvaziado nos EUA, Bolsonaro nega crise e diz que problemas na bolsa acontecem",https://www1.folha.uol.com.br/mercado/2020/03/em-evento-esvaziado-nos-eua-bolsonaro-nega-crise-e-diz-que-problemas-na-bolsa-acontecem.shtml

[2] "Pronunciamento do Senhor Presidente da República, Jair Bolsonaro, em cadeia de rádio e televisão", https://www.gov.br/planalto/pt-br/acompanhe-o-planalto/pronunciamentos/pronunciamento-em-cadeia-de-radio-e-televisao-do-senhor-presidente-da-republica-jair-bolsonaro

[3] "Exclusivo!, Jair Bolsonaro fala que 'coronavírus' é 'histeria' e conta que vai fazer festa de aniversário", https://www.tupi.fm/brasil/exclusivo-jair-bolsonaro-fala-que-coronovirus-e-histeria-e-conta-que-vai-fazer-festa-de-aniversario/

[4] Prosul is a conservative forum that groups right-wing governments of the Americas

[5] AP News. April 16, 2020. https://apnews.com/26dc693cc9777da62e2b609e97ae57f8?utm_campaign=SocialFlow&utm_source=Twitter&utm_medium=AP

[6] "Pronunciamento do Senhor Presidente da República, Jair Bolsonaro, em cadeia de rádio e televisão", https://www.gov.br/planalto/pt-br/acompanhe-o-planalto/pronunciamentos/pronunciamento-do-senhor-presidente-da-republica-jair-bolsonaro-em-cadeia-de-radio-e-televisao-4

[7] "Bolsonaro publica vídeo falso sobre desabastecimento e depois apaga", https://www.agazeta.com.br/brasil/bolsonaro-publica-video-falso-sobre-desabastecimento-e-depois-apaga-0420

[8] "Eduardo Bolsonaro culpa China pelo coronavírus e Embaixada responde: 'contraiu vírus mental', https://www.cartacapital.com.br/carta-capital/eduardo-bolsonaro-culpa-china-pelo-coronavirus-e-embaixada-responde-contraiu-virus-mental/ https://twitter.com/BolsonaroSP/status/1240286560953815040 ; https://twitter.com/EmbaixadaChina/status/1247001670808154113

[9] "Efeitos econômicos negativos da crise do Corona vírus tendem a afetar mais a renda dos mais pobres", https://ideas.repec.org/p/cdp/tecnot/tn003.html

[10] "Partimos para o socialismo", diz Carlos Bolsonaro sobre crise do coronavírus", https://www.cartacapital.com.br/Politica/partimos-para-o-socialismo-diz-carlos-bolsonaro-sobre-crise-do-coronavirus/ https://twitter.com/carlosbolsonaro/status/1245323223459409920

[11] "Caiam na real: governadores e prefeitos oferecem esmolas com dinheiro alheio, diz Presidente do BB", https://politica.estadao.com.br/noticias/geral,caiam-na-real-governadores-e-prefeitos-oferecem-esmolas-com-dinheiro-alheio-diz-presidente-do-bb,70003257728

[12] "General Heleno diz que Congresso faz chantagem para ficar com R$30 bi do orçamento", https://www1.folha.uol.com.br/mercado/2020/02/general-heleno-diz-que-bolsonaro-e-alvo-de-parlamentarismo-branco-na-discussao-sobre-orcamento.shtml https://twitter.com/gen_heleno/status/1230150789928230912?ref_src=twsrc%5Etfw%7Ctwcamp%5Etweetembed%7Ctwterm%5E1230150789928230912&ref_url=https%3A%2F%2Fwww1.folha.uol.com.br%2Fmercado%2F2020%2F02%2Fgeneral-heleno-diz-que-bolsonaro-e-alvo-de-parlamentarismo-branco-na-discussao-sobre-orcamento.shtml

4. Brazil And COVID-19:
The President Against The Federation

Gilberto M. A. Rodrigues,

Gilberto M. A. Rodrigues, PhD in social sciences, is professor and head of the Graduate Program in International Relations at the Federal University of ABC (UFABC). Co-coordinator of Nucleus for the Study of Federalism and Local Government.

Vanessa Elias de Oliveira,

Vanessa Elias de Oliveira, PhD in Political Science, is professor and head of the Graduate Program in Public Policy at the UFABC. Co-coordinator of Nucleus for the Study of Federalism and Local Government.

In a severe editorial, the prestigious journal The Lancet (vol.395, May 9th) said "perhaps the biggest threat to Brazil's COVID-19 response is its President, Jair Bolsonaro". A far-right politician, scientific denier, since taking office in Jan. 2019 Bolsonaro has opened a daily fight against the Congress and the Supreme Court, showing a clear resistance to deal with the checks and balances system and democratic institutions. With the advance of COVID-19 in the country, the President strongly criticized the World Health Organization (WHO) and has opened a new fight against state governors and mayors.

Brazil Administrative Divisions (States)

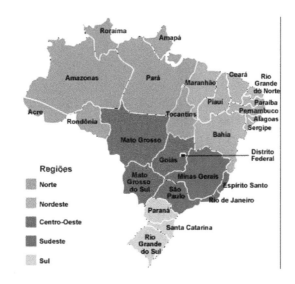

Brazil's Public Health System B

Brazil's public health system is universal and free of charge. It follows the federative logic of concurrency where municipalities focus on primary attention policies, states focus on middle complexity and the union focuses on high complex policies, together with sanitary and epidemic guidelines and the general coordination through national intergovernmental committees. The ministry of health (which holds one of the biggest parts of the national budget) concentrates huge resources and defines many of health guidelines.

The President Faces Federative Limits In The Pandemic

President Bolsonaro's rhetoric and actions denying evidence of the threats brought by the COVID-19 pandemic are based on his political and ideological visions that favour his political stakeholders and supporters. In fact, he follows President Trump in many issues and also in his methodology to create noise, confusion and "irrational conflicts" not only targeting his opponents but also democratic institutions.

In this sense, the president's attacks against governors and mayors are part of a big picture of his controversial presidency. Governors in general, as well as most of the mayors of the biggest municipalities, have been following the WHO/PAHO's guidelines and recommendations in a very responsible manner. Social isolation measures have been implemented by them in different ways, levels and time frames. In a political fight against them, the President tried to block those measures, citing economic and freedom of mobility reasons. In April 2020, the conflict reached the Supreme Court, which issued a landmark decision stating that states and municipalities have constitutional autonomy to regulate and implement health measures regarding the pandemic. On the one hand this Court's decision contradicted its own precedents in other issues that used to benefit the union's position and on the other hand the Court was coherent with its tradition in standing up for human rights in a broad sense. However, the President has not accepted losing the case in the Supreme Court and remains defiant against governors and mayors, calling his supporters to stand against them and boycott social isolation. He dismissed his minister of health, Luiz Mandetta, who was in line with the WHO/PAHO's recommendations and granted national support for isolation measures. He was succeeded by Nelson Teich, who had no experience in public health and accepted a new staff composed by military officials imposed by the President – who has been militarizing public administration in many other fields. Moreover, the President issued a decree (without consultation with Mr. Teich) including other services than supermarkets and pharmacies as essential activities allowed to be opened. But governors and mayors declared they will ignore it. After that, with less than one month in office, Mr. Teich left the Ministry; the vice-minister, general Pazuello, temporarily substituted him.

Intergovernmental Relations And Subnational Responses To COVID-19

Facing such a controversial and non-cooperative President in the middle of a devastating pandemic, governors have increased cooperation among themselves. States from the Northeast Region (the poorest and most vulnerable region), through the Northeast Consortium has created a Scientific Committee for Combating Coronavirus, coordinating actions to buy equipment and COVID-19 tests directly from other countries and international companies. They are acting under high pressure of few hospital beds due to the growing of COVID-19 infected persons needing intensive treatment, but they cannot count on the federal government support. Not surprisingly, the President is trying to wash his hands, accusing governors and mayors of blocking the country's economic development, which he will be required to coordinate in the inevitable recession after the pandemic.

The only positive federal measure approved by the Congress is the minimum wage for vulnerable people during the pandemic. But even such a good policy has been badly managed by the union due to the lack of its cooperation with states and municipalities to implement it. Unexpectedly, the presidential fight against the federation is creating a positive outcome for the Brazilian federal system: new horizontal intergovernmental relations have been strengthening subnational autonomy and decentralization. A broad recognition that states and municipalities are doing the right thing is spreading both national and internationally. The Brazilian federation will be not the same after the COVID-19 pandemic.

5. Brazil's War On COVID-19:
Crisis, Not Conflict—Doctors, Not Generals

Matheus Hoffmann Pfrimer[1]
Federal University of Goias, Brazil´

Ricardo Barbosa Jr
University of Calgary, Canada

ABSTRACT

This commentary first documents the ways in which President Jair Bolsonaro's administration has evoked securitized discursive strategies that frame Brazil's national response to COVID-19 as a matter of defence instead of public health. We then ask: What does it mean to talk about the virus and the ways to address it through war-framings? We argue that the Bolsonaro administration has framed the COVID-19 pandemic as an extra-territorial threat in an effort to create internal stability while failing to handle the matter effectively. Such politically motivated spatial framings inhibit an effective response in Brazil and pose a severe threat to public health. Once COVID-19 becomes securitized, the response is framed by the military bureaucracy rather than public health authorities, resulting in dangerous consequences.

INTRODUCTION

In this commentary, we present our deconstructions of the Bolsonaro administration's evolving COVID19 public agenda through an analysis of political discourse and recent COVID-19 media coverage. Klotz and Lynch (2014: 95) argue that: 'Public discourse ...may provide better evidence for the articulation of interests because it reveals normative rationales for policy ...it necessarily conceptualizes language as actions, not simply as evidence'. Our conceptual contribution lies in demonstrating how security discourse mobilizes different perceptions of threat—known and unknown—to constitute a shared national identity and prioritize military responses. Put differently, military jargon shapes spatial security imaginaries in order to depict the COVID-19 pandemic as war abroad to project a sense of internal stability at home.

First Deny: Mishandling the COVID19 outbreak

Bolsonaro's initial response to COVID-19 consisted of downplaying the outbreak to reduce potential economic fallout, which led to a delay in effective response in Brazil. Days before the World Health Organization categorized COVID-19 as a pandemic on 11 March, Bolsonaro mocked the virus. The

---

[1] Corresponding author:
Ricardo Barbosa Jr, Department of Geography, University of Calgary, 2500 University Drive NW, Calgary T2N 1N4, Alberta, Canada.
Email: ricardo.barbosajr@ucalgary.ca

president announced that concerns 'were being overstated' and that 'other flu have killed more'. Then, a day later, amidst speculation that Bolsonaro himself was infected, the president addressed the country in a live stream while wearing a mask since he had come in contact with multiple staffers that tested positive. Bolsonaro's inconsistent position on, and confused handling of, the 15 March pro-government demonstrations further exemplifies the extent to which COVID-19 has been mishandled in Brazil. To begin with, the president shared a video calling for demonstrations against Congress and the Supreme Court in favour of the Military, and later even summoned supporters through official state outlets. Bolsonaro then stated that demonstrations needed to be reconsidered, but he failed to establish concrete measures. On 15 March, while supporters assembled across Brazil against public health guidelines, including those of Bolsonaro's health minister (who was later fired), the president, who was still suspected to be infected, went out to embrace progovernment demonstrators

in Brasilia. When facing backlash, Bolsonaro insisted that he had stated demonstrators should stay home and lied about the video's date. Mishandling grew as the president minimized the symptoms of high-ranking officials with COVID-19 and continued to call the virus a 'little flu'.

Then Securitize: Mismanaging The COVID-19 Pandemic

With time, Bolsonaro's administration began to manage the pandemic through the lens of friend or-foe (Fidler, 2014). Bolsonaro's cabinet, one third of which are military officials, openly stated in a COVID-19 press release that Brazil is at 'war' and must 'combat' an 'invisible enemy' (TV BrasilGov, 2020). War-framings position 'friends' like healthcare workers and hospital staff as 'soldiers going to the battlefront' against named and unnamed 'foes' (TV BrasilGov, 2020).

Military framings have directed the Bolsonaro administration's messaging and response to COVID-19 from the beginning. As the defence minister put it: 'this is a war...with an invisible enemy ...and when there is a war, Brazil and Brazilians can rely on the Armed Forces' (Record News, 2020). He went on to claim: 'the first operation concerning the coronavirus was the rescue of our Brazilians who were in Wuhan, and the Armed Forces, along with other ministries, was present' (Record News, 2020). Herein, Brazil's opening response to COVID-19 was a military operation to 'rescue' Brazilians from Wuhan province in an Armed Forces aircraft and take them to an Air Force base for 15 days of quarantine. The heavily militarized affair featured a recorded message of Bolsonaro stating: 'You have just entered Brazilian airspace. Welcome back to your country, our Brazil. No one was left behind. We are a single people, a single race. We are brothers. Our Armed Forces, the Ministries of Foreign Affairs and Health, Congress and Senate, as well as Anvisa [the National Sanitary Surveillance Agency], have worked tirelessly so that this mission could be crowned a success' (Poder360, 2020).

Bolsonaro's recording illustrates how the administration framed the effort to repatriate Brazilians in Wuhan through a nationalistic repertoire, while also placing the Armed Forces first and public health authorities second. The repatriation efforts' messaging focused on the urgency of removing Brazilian nationals from China and was widely disseminated by Brazilian media as a 'rescue' from 'enemy territory'. The Bolsonaro administration's response to COVID-19 has involved aligning specific foreign enemies abroad—China and Venezuela—with the so-called 'invisible enemy'.

As Bolsonaro put it, response measures consisted of 'closing the borders, in particular the one that causes us great worry, with Venezuela' (TV BrasilGov, 2020), with which Brazil closed its frontiers first without any public health reason. When Chinese flights became restricted without holding other infected countries to the same criteria, China was tacitly framed as a foe. This progressed into COVID-19 being referred to as the 'Chinese virus', which became part of the national debate when Eduardo Bolsonaro, the president's son and a Congressman, retweeted a far-right thread blaming China for COVID-19 (BolsonaroSP,2020). Brazil's leading trade partner is attacked here in an attempt to deflect attention from the administration's mismanagement of COVID-19. On 23 March, President Bolsonaro's Chief of Staff, General Braga Netto, was placed in charge of 'centralizing' and 'coordinating' COVID-19 actions. In this, COVID-19 security discourse became security practice. Later that same day, the general spoke alongside the health minister, who, until then, was in charge of all federal government communication on COVID-19. In such a way, discussing COVID-19 in terms of war has literally led defence authorities to be in charge of handling the pandemic instead of public health authorities.

'War' against a not-so-invisible 'enemy'

We can convey the utmost gravity of the COVID-19 pandemic without war-framings (Ingram, 2005). A 'conflict' implies an enemy threat that ought to be left to the preserve of an empowered few and handled in secret (Buzan et al., 1998). By contrast, a 'crisis' demands urgency and priority without restricting participation, thereby allowing for broad open engagement, diversified expertise, and transparency (Kay and Williams, 2009). A conflict anticipates an enemy's defeat, whereas no party need be defeated in a crisis. Beyond 'combating' the COVID-19 pandemic, we must take care not to depict specific Others as 'enemies'. Yet, the question remains: In what ways and to what extent does Bolsonaro's administration benefit from securitizing COVID-19?

Bolsonaro's administration first portrayed the COVID-19 pandemic as an 'invisible enemy', seeking to justify the government's non-active role concerning public health. These statements allude to Donald Rumsfeld's speech on the 'unknown unknowns' made while serving as US President George W Bush's Secretary of Defence. The very idea that there is an 'invisible enemy' or an 'unknown known' instantiates the need for a national enemy in order to pursue internal cohesion and legitimize the administration's militaristic measures. Subsequently, COVID-19 has been portrayed as a not-so-invisible enemy aligned with specific ideological foreign enemies. In naming and attacking these perceived enemies, Bolsonaro's administration has framed the COVID-19 threat as an external Other (Bashford, 2014), to create a sense of immediate detachment from danger.

The tacit implication is that 'everything is fine' in the homeland, diverting the focus from internal problems and the ineffective response to COVID-19.This rhetorical trajectory is a means of framing COVID-19 in terms of the imaginative geographies of war (Gregory, 2010) when the domain of public health ought to be prioritized instead (Kay and Williams, 2009). Such a device enables political actors to stabilize the representations of an 'unknown' threat in terms of nationalistic and territorial discourse. Evoking military jargon spreads a sense of 'geopolitical anxiety' to replace 'pandemic anxiety' (Ingram, 2008), which instigates a need for national cohesion to face such an 'unknown' threat. These securitized discursive framings have enabled Bolsonaro's administration to reframe the 'unknown known'. Imaginative geographies stabilize the perception of threat through a referential enemy and location—in this case, China and Venezuela.

Such an attempt to project stability is only possible by framing the COVID-19 pandemic as a conflict, imperilling a matter of public health by envisioning it through the lens of war.

Whereas the imaginative geographies of COVID-19 in Brazil situate the threat abroad, discourses of shared territory and 'race' produce proximity by referencing a collective identity, as portrayed in Bolsonaro's recording played to Brazilians 'rescued' from Wuhan.

This becomes particularly strategic in a moment of strong criticism of the administration's handling of the pandemic. Klotz and Lynch (2014: 83) emphasize how identity and security imaginaries are intertwined, since 'identities imply subject positions which empower certain speakers to define collective interests'. In this, the Bolsonaro administration's effort to securitize COVID-19 discourse and response can be interpreted as an attempt to bring a sense of domestic peace and economic stability. Yet efforts to depict a peaceful homeland are only possible by portraying turmoil abroad.

CONCLUSION

By drawing attention to the dangers of discussing COVID-19 through war-framings, our intervention analyses how and why national governments like the Bolsonaro administration in Brazil benefit from evoking security discourse during a pandemic. The point we have made is that COVID-19 messaging is crucial because it has implications for how we respond to the pandemic. We advocate that Brazil's national response to COVID-19 be framed as a crisis, not as a conflict. In more direct terms, we contend that doctors and public health authorities—not generals—ought to oversee Brazil's response to COVID-19. More so, this commentary serves as a warning that a lack of effective medical response may lead to the perceived need for a militaristic response. While Sevcenko (1984) suggests that 'the health authority [is] practically indissociable from the police authority', Brazil's response to COVID-19 underscores the need for scholars to critically examine how public health crises are unnecessarily framed through the rhetoric of war to serve militaristic agendas.

REFERENCES

Bashford, A. (ed) (2014) Medicine at the Border: Disease, Globalisation and Security, 1850 to the Present. Basingstoke: Palgrave Macmillan.

Bolsonaro,S.P. (2020) 18 March 2020. Available at: https:// twitter.com/BolsonaroSP/status/1240286560953 815040 (accessed 25 March 2020).

Buzan, B. Wæver, O. and De Wilde, J.(1998) Security: A New Framework for Analysis. Boulder: Lynne Rienner Publishers.

Fidler, D.P. (2014) Biosecurity: Friend or foe for public health governance? In: Bashford A (ed) Medicine at the Border: Disease, Globalisation, and Security, 1850 to the Present. Basingstoke: Palgrave Macmillan, pp. 196–218.

Gregory, D. (2010) War and peace. Transactions of the Institute of British Geographers 35(2): 154–186.

Ingram, A. (2005) The new geopolitics of disease: between global health and global security. Geopolitics 10(3): 522–545.

Ingram, A. (2008) Pandemic anxiety and global health security. In: Pain R and Smith SJ (eds) Fear: Critical Geopolitics and Everyday Life. Hampshire: Ashgate, pp. 75–86.

Kay, A. and Williams, O.D (eds) (2009) Global Health Governance: Crisis, Institutions, and Political Economy. Hampshire: Palgrave Macmillan.

Klotz, A. and Lynch, C.M. (2014) Strategies for Research in Constructivist International Relations. New York: Routledge.

Poder360 (2020) Bolsonaro da boas-vindas a repatriados´ da China. 9 February 2020. Available at: https://www. youtube.com/watch?v¼gvGrPAZYm6U (accessed 25 March 2020).

Record News (2020) "E uma guerra", diz ministro da´ Defesa sobre coronavı´rus. 18 March 2020. Available at: https://www.youtube.com/watch?v¼05ifnLCiw-0 (accessed 25 March 2020).

Sevcenko N (1984) A Revolta Da Vacina: Mentes Insanas Em Corpos Rebeldes. Sa˜o Paulo: Brasiliense.

TV BrasilGov (2020) Presidente da Repu´blica, Jair Bolsonaro, realiza coletiva sobre o coronavı´rus. 18 March 2020. Available at: https://www.youtube.com/ watch?v¼lhltNqinvm4 (accessed 25 March 2020).

6. Fear of Death And Polarization: Political Consequences Of The COVID-19 Pandemic

Carlos Pereira [1] Amanda Medeiros [1] Frederico Bertholini [2] [1] Fundação Getulio Vargas / Brazilian School of Public and Business Administration, Rio de Janeiro / RJ – Brazil [2] Universida de Brasília / Institute of Political Science, Brasília / DF – Brazil

Humanity has always been tormented with the end of existence. On some occasions, such as the current COVID-19 pandemic, this affliction is pronounced. To what extent can fear of death alter individuals' political perceptions and beliefs? It is in this context of uncertainties and fears that we investigate how Brazilian society has been evaluating its leaders, especially concerning the policy of social distancing. The COVID-19 pandemic changed the axes of political polarization. On the one hand, governors, mayors, and legislators are concerned about the risks of a collapse of the health system. On the other, President Jair Bolsonaro focused primarily on the negative economic consequences of the pandemic. Through an opinion poll, we identified that "fear of death" diminished the ideological polarization that has existed in Brazil since Jair Bolsonaro's election. Contrary to what many expected, voters who identified themselves as right-wing and center-right supposedly, the core of Bolsonaro's voters refused to follow the president's recommendation of relaxing social distancing policies and considered his performance inappropriate during the pandemic. We also show that different income levels did not influence this change in behaviour.

1. INTRODUCTION

The epilogue above is the initial dialogue between Death and Antonius Block, a knight who returns from the Crusades in the Middle Ages and finds his homeland completely devastated by the black plague. The central theme of the Seventh Seal, Ingmar Bergman's masterpiece, is the fear of death. When the knight faces Death, he proposes a deal: a game of chess. While playing, the man gains time, because he knows that it would not be possible to win, since Death is inevitable, which is why it is impossible to escape his destiny. So the best way out would be to postpone it as much as possible. The COVID-19 pandemic was an exogenous shock of great magnitude, equivalent to the displacement of tectonic plates. Actors and political leaders had extreme reactions not only in Brazil but in several countries around the world. On the one hand, those most concerned with the speed of contagion, the severity of the disease, and the risk of death have followed the recommendations of the World Health Organization (WHO), which advises social distancing, even in the face of the negative consequences for the economy. In the countries that presented cases of the disease, almost all leaders of countries that have presented cases of the disease have adopted social distancing measures.

This has also been the case, for example, with governors, mayors, and main legislative leaders in Brazil. On the other hand, some countries have witnessed segments of the population and some governments minimizing the pandemic's virulence and consequences for health, concerned about the adverse economic effects generated by social distancing measures.[1] The Brazilian president, Jair Bolsonaro, is one of the main supporters of this strategy. Along with presidents of Nicaragua, Daniel Ortega; Belarus, Alexander Lukashenko; and Turkmenistan, Gurbanguly Berdimuhamedow, have refused to enact measures of social distancing. At the beginning of the pandemic, the presidents of the United States, Donald Trump; Mexico, López Obrador; Russia, Vladimir Putin; and the Italian Prime Minister, Giuseppe Conte, were also reluctant to support social distancing, but ended up changing their position and started to advocate that the population stay at home.

According to Kingstone and Power (2017), there has been a strong increase in political polarization in Brazil since 2013, triggered by nationwide mass demonstrations that occurred that year. For Hunter and Power (2019), the increasing polarization was visible throughout all social strata, including the vulnerable population and the political and economic elite, and it took over the country during the 2018 elections. At that time, the number of voters who chose a candidate from one of the poles approached that of those who expressed a strong dislike for the opposing candidate.

One of the poles was represented by the Workers' Party (PT), standing for the traditional politics eroded by successive corruption scandals. The other pole was Bolsonaro, who adopted the notion of "*antipetismo*" (AntiPT) (Bello, 2019; Samuels & Zucco, 2018) and grasped the expectations of another social group and promised to deliver "new politics" based on anti-establishment.

This game of polarized groups was in relative "balance" until the COVID-19 pandemic, with each group becoming stronger based on the radical opposition of political identities and preferences. The groups did not dialogue with each other and tended to consume information that only reinforced their previous beliefs. At the same time, they rejected any information that contradicted previous values, so they did not access information that could put their respective "comfort zones" at risk. Could it be possible to imagine a change in the axis of political polarization in Brazil, bringing together voters who were once located at opposite poles? Can fear of death bring new axes of polarization to emerge beyond the clash between left and right-wing?

This study addresses these questions through an opinion poll that explored people's position regarding social distancing measures, and their evaluation about the president and the governors in conducting the COVID-19 containment policy. The main hypothesis is that the pandemic has altered the axes of political polarization in the country, bringing together the ideological poles. In other words, COVID-19 caused significant segments of voters to change their political perception due to their "fear of death." The results confirm that a significant portion of voters self-identified as center-right and right wing support the social distancing policy, in the opposite direction to the position defended by President Bolsonaro, changing the terms of polarization in the country and

---

[1] The dichotomy between 'preserving health' versus 'preserving economy,' although factually false as demonstrated by experts such as Martins (2020) and Pereira (2020), permeates the political discourses of those who oppose social distancing. For Ajzenman, Cavalcanti, and Da Mata (2020), the political discourses based on this false dichotomy can greatly affect the success of social distancing measures.

suggesting its decrease.[1] Such voters also positively evaluate the performance of the governors of their respective states and negatively that of the president during the pandemic.

In addition, the low-income sectors, in theory more vulnerable, did not present systematic opposition to the social distancing policy when compared to people belonging to other income groups.

This research brings empirical and theoretical contributions on the role and limits of ideology and identity affinity in shaping political behaviour in polarized environments. Ideology, which is part of a person's identity (Huddy, 2001; Iborra, 2005; Teles, 2009), works as a cognitive and protective shortcut, facilitating that those who share beliefs and values make similar choices (Huckfeldt et al., 1999). We argue that in extreme situations – for example, when the lives of people and their loved ones are at risk, ideological and identity values may cease to be crucial to making choices. In other words, identities or ideologies become malleable and susceptible to adjustments and changes. Extreme situations can create problems for those who belong to a certain group, because sometimes the natural choice, 'natural' according to the ideology that is part of their identity and keeps them linked to a group, may represent a threat to their own lives. The next section presents our theory based on a critical dialogue with the literature on populism and identity. The third section describes the methodology and descriptive statistics. In the fourth and fifth sections, we present the main results of the research. In the final section, we conclude the article, highlighting the main findings.

2. POPULISM OF IDENTITY

The combination of a serious economic crisis and daily exposure to successive corruption scandals generated, of a large part of the Brazilian voters, the perception of politics as something dirty.

By directly associating the specific style of coalitional presidentialism practiced by the Workers Party (PT) governments with corruption, Bolsonaro fed the electorate with a kind of aversion to politics itself, thus filling an open space for the populists' emergence (Bakker, Rooduijn, & Schumacher, 2016; Busby, Gubler, & Hawkins, 2019; Hawkins, Kaltwasser, & Andreadis, 2020). President Bolsonaro sought to fulfill the expectations of "cleansing" Brazilian politics by building a platform that was initially anti-PT, but essentially anti-party, defending the idea that all acronyms and their members would be equally part of a corrupt elite. The electoral viability of this belief occurs through the identity framework that denies the institutions and praises the direct connection between the political leader and the voters. The background of this ideology/identity is the myth-making process and the homogenization of the categories "elites" and "people," identified as antagonistic (Bos et al., 2020; Mudde, 2004; Mudde & Kaltwasser, 2012). Once elected, Bolsonaro refused to build a coalition and chose to govern as a minority. To circumvent this fragility, he sought to establish direct connections with voters, adopting a kind of plebiscitary presidentialism (Conaghan, 2008).

In Congress, he worked by forming cyclical majorities to vote aligned with the executive branch's preferences, constraining legislators through pressure from public opinion. By adopting this strategy, which Kernell (2006) classifies as "going public," Bolsonaro governed in a permanent campaign of polarization. The conspiratorial tone has been a fundamental part of this government crusade against indefinite enemies that emerge every day (Kovic & Caspar, 2019).

---

[1] Not opposing social distancing, however, does not necessarily mean resigning support for the president or that these voters would be opposing Bolsonaro in all his policies or dimensions. We would like to thank RAP reviewers for pointing out this nuance.

The systematic denial of traditional instruments of government left Bolsonaro little alternative, before and during the pandemic. The uninterrupted and radical mobilization of his most loyal voters continued to be the standard model of the president's governance.

His 'plebiscitary populism' became a strategy for strengthening identity and protecting the core of his constituency of voters. As mentioned before, ideology is part of an individual's identity and an element that connects people into groups (Huddy, 2001). Insofar as people who share the same ideology see each other as peers (Mullen, Dovidio, Craig, & Copper, 1992) and form groups, it is painful to diverge from the group's political orientation, especially diverging from its main leader. For this reason, people are likely to use their ideological and identity positions as protective lenses that reduce the chances of reevaluating the group's values. The literature on motivated reasoning suggests that group members interpret information in a way that benefits the group (Bisgaard, 2015; Bolsen, Druckman, & Cook, 2014; Leeper & Slothuus, 2014) to reduce the pain generated by information updates that contradict the values on which they rely. Thus, when realizing that a particular position is shared by the community to which they belong, it is expected that its members develop their own narrative structures as a defense mechanism for that position (Bolsen et al., 2014).

Feelings of attachment generate loyalty to the members of each group and feelings of security and prestige. However, individuals who do not belong to a group develop hostility and aversion to the values and beliefs of this group, considered rival and, potentially, enemies. The intrinsic importance of sharing identities and reciprocal loyalties can be perceived among individuals who belong to a group (in-group), and a distancing of individuals who would be outside that group (out-group), leading to biases in favor of their own group and contrary to the rival (Hameleers, 2016).

The ideology and sense of belonging to a particular group can create a state of blindness in which its members tend to disregard factual information when they contradict the group's identity values (Druckman & Bolsen, 2011). In addition, the ideological congruence between individuals and the leader of the community they belong can have a dazzling effect, leaving members refractory to arguments and allegations contrary to the group's identity values. Thus, the group members would be more likely to consider false any claim contrary to the group's dominant beliefs. Therefore, people would tend to reach conclusions that confirm their identity/ ideological bias. However, supporting such distorted conclusions requires minimally reasonable justifications (Kunda, 1990). Some events, however, have such an influence on the lives of individuals that even members of strong identity groups can have their beliefs shaken. The identity/ideology may no longer be sufficient to justify the individual's alignment with the group (Kunda, 1990; Mazar et al., 2008).

It is precisely in these moments that identities become malleable and susceptible to changes. The costs of change, therefore, decrease significantly, and the chances of some members going astray when considering other identity alternatives increase.

3. METHODOLOGY AND DESCRIPTIVE STATISTICS

To study the perception of Brazilians regarding the social distancing policy and the performance of politicians during the pandemic, with the support of the newspaper *O Estado de S. Paulo*, we conducted an opinion poll between March 28 and April 4, 2020. The questionnaire was released on social networks, especially WhatsApp, and 8,168 responses, were collected. After checking the average response time, we excluded questionnaires that were less than 120 and more than 960 seconds long. We also excluded from the sample those with repeated IP numbers. The final sample was 7,848 valid responses and included the participation of respondents from all Brazilian states, with a greater concentration in São Paulo (44%), Minas Gerais (7%), and Rio de Janeiro (6%).

Of the 7,848 respondents, 50.2% were female and 49.8% male. In terms of income profile, 13.5% earned up to three minimum wages; 14.6%, up to five minimum wages; 22.5%, between three and five minimum wages; 36.3% have an income greater than 10 thousand reais; and 12% preferred not to respond. As for the age profile, 5% were between 18 and 24 years old; 16%, between 25 and 34; 20%, between 35-44 and 45-55; 27% between 55 and 65; and 10%, over 65.

Around 32% of the respondents classified themselves as being in a COVID-19 risk group, 18% knew someone who had the disease in the severe stage, and 7% knew someone who died. In terms of ideological profile, 37.1% declared themselves as someone in the 'center;' 30.1%, as center-left and left-wing; and 32.8%, as center-right and right-wing. With regard to the economic consequences of social distancing measures, 37% reported that they could cause enormous or total financial loss for their professional activity, and 32% believe that social distancing will not cause financial damage to their professional activity.[1] We did not use a probabilistic approach for the selection of the sample and chose not to perform any post-stratification in view of the potential risks of introducing bias for unobservable or unmeasured variables.

There are, therefore, limits regarding generalization for the population, especially of univariate or bivariate descriptive results, without the inclusion of additional control variables. In addition, the main demographic variables were well balanced in relation to the population, and those with over-representation of a group – the wealthiest in income and residents of the state of São Paulo – were not relevant predictors. Respondents were invited to participate in research on perception and behaviour in relation to the coronavirus. After consent, everyone responded on: (1) the situation in which they were in relation to social distancing; the financial losses resulting from staying in the situation; the social distancing measures that had been implemented by the state government and the president; if they knew someone infected with COVID-19; (2) who they believed were the authority responsible for pandemic control in Brazil; (3) how they evaluated the actions implemented to control the pandemic by the governors and the president; (4) the degree of agreement with the social distancing policy and how willing they were to follow it; (5) socio-demographic aspects. The questions were multiple-choice, respondents chose a single option, and the results were presented on a Likert scale. The confidence interval calculated for all means was 95%.

To measure the variation of complying with social distancing policies among respondents, with regard to the expected economic damage from the pandemic, and exposure of acquaintances to varying degrees of the virus effects, we used a set of linear regressions with robust standard errors and ordinal logistic regressions. All the details about the data sets and material for replicating the analyses of this work can be found in the supplementary material.

4. PANDEMIC AND IDEOLOGY

The study sought to understand the political impact of the pandemic based on how the populations' ideological preferences are connected to their evaluation of President Bolsonaro's and the state governors' performance during the pandemic, especially with regard to social distancing and how long the restrictions that aimed to promote social distancing would be in place. The choice for these

---

[1] All descriptive statistics are available in Table 2, located in the supplementary material in the following link: https://dataverse.harvard. edu/dataset.xhtml?persistentId=doi:10.7910/DVN/SUN4KZ.

aspects intended to identify whether clear and polarized ideological inclinations were aligned with the proposed solutions to face the pandemic in Brazil, or whether political polarization has lessened in view of the risks of contracting the disease with varying degrees of severity.

The first point to be highlighted is that the respondents who considered themselves as left-wing, center-left, and center disagree homogeneously with Bolsonaro and support the governors. On the other hand, respondents from the center-right and right-wing, supposedly the core of the president's voters, differ considerably over the evaluation about the support, showing a break in a supposedly previous unity (Figure 1). A greater proportion of these voters (56%) remained aligned with the president, but 40% disapproved of his performance in the pandemic, while 5% were indifferent. The division right-wing and center-right voters was more evident in the assessment of the performance of governors, in which the majority (60%) agreed, a smaller portion disagreed (35%), and 5% were indifferent.

Fig 1 Assessment Of The President And Governors (Per Ideology)

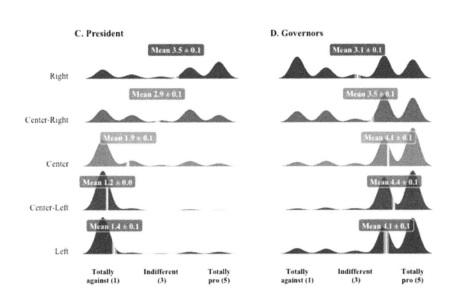

Source: Research data.

The results indicate that the diametrically opposite way in which Bolsonaro – minimizing the severity of the disease and highlighting the negative economic impacts that the social distancing policy potentially brings – and the governors – prioritizing social distancing policies to reduce the speed of contagion – reacted to the pandemic redesigned the previous political polarization. A considerable part of the individuals who supported the president went to the opposite pole, breaking the bi-modal pattern, characteristic of polarized scenarios (Bello, 2019). This does not necessarily mean that people have completely changed the lens through which they view the world or their political ideology/ identity. It shows, however, that the pandemic may have repositioned the main axis of polarization between those who identify themselves as right-wing and center-right, moving it beyond the simple direct antagonism toward the left-wing.

Fig 2 Assessment of Social Distancing (Per Ideology)

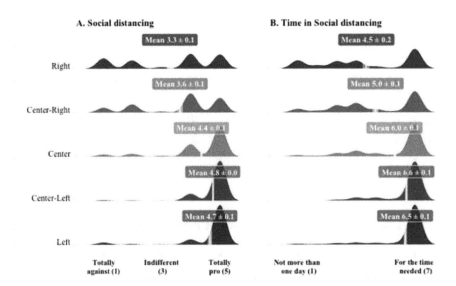

This alternative pattern of preference distribution becomes clear when we cross the respondents' position in relation to the social distancing policy, with their respective political-ideological positions (Figure 2). Left-wing, center-left, and center respondents are largely in favour of social distancing for as long as necessary. However, a considerable portion of voters who call themselves center-right and right-wing is also in favour of this policy, contrary to the president's position and recommendation to relax social distancing measures. The results suggest that, in addition to the pre-existing ideological antagonism, most of the right-wing supporters do not agree with the president's view on social distancing. It is essential, therefore, to understand the elements that determine the change in the polarization axis (which occurs fundamentally among voters from the right-wing and center-right).

8. A DIVIDED RIGHT-WING: IS SOCIAL DISTANCING ONLY FOR THE RICH?

The interpretation that the adoption of social distancing is supported mainly by those with sufficient financial resources to remain comfortably in quarantine has gained strength. The assumption, reinforced by Bolsonaro, is that it would be more viable for the higher-income social group to prioritize health care and consider the economic problems generated by the pandemic as secondary. Meanwhile, families in a more vulnerable economic situation would need to return to work and would thus be more resistant to maintaining social distancing (Jorge, 2020).

Figure 3 Position on Social Distancing (Per Income, In Minimum Wages – MW)

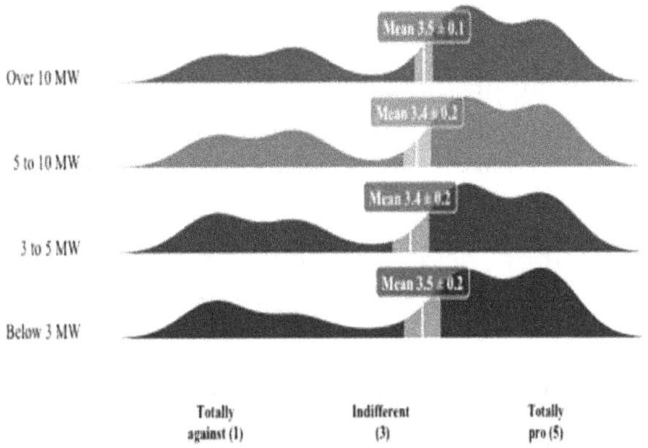

Source: Research data.

In order to verify this argument, we tested whether the apparent antagonism toward social distancing is based on income differences. Figure 3 shows that, contrary to the expectation that people with different incomes (analyzed in groups) should exhibit different patterns of support for the policy, there was no such statistical distinction. Therefore, at least until the week in which the data were collected, society was not divided by income. The poorest and the richest mostly support social distancing and oppose the president's recommendation to return to work.

For people in the upper strata, the reasoning is clear. Since they have the means to protect their income, social distancing would have a lesser cost. But what about the poorest? How is their preference for social distancing explained? We believe that the argument that those most in need would be more opposed to the policy confuses 'preferences' and 'decisions.' The data show that, for most of them, staying at home is strictly preferable to going to work. However, as the federal executive does not credibly show signs that it is committed to offering economic support, individuals observe such signs and establish a set of beliefs about the likelihood of receiving support. In this scenario, low-income people can act strategically and choose, in a rational way, to resume professional activities. However, this does not mean a sincere preference for breaking social distancing.

As Shah, Shah, Mullainathan, and Shafir (2012) suggest, scarcity changes the way people allocate their attention, causing them to become more deeply involved in some problems while neglecting others. Thus, scarcity in any of its forms of manifestation – hunger, loneliness, lack of time, and poverty – would gain our attention, self-control, and long-term planning capacity, directing the focus to the most immediate object missing. This is the situation of the poorest in the pandemic. Faced with the threat of death, they prefer to stop working and practice social distancing. However, the lack of resources for food and housing takes the focus away from social distancing and leads them to act in order to supply the most immediate needs.

6. FEAR OF DEATH BRINGS THE POLES TOGETHER

The behaviour of right-wing and center-right voters in relation to social distancing is revealing, particularly taking into account the proximity to people (friends, relatives, etc.) who were infected and developed COVID-19 with varying degrees of severity. Figure 4 shows that the greater the severity of the disease in their acquaintances, the greater the spectrum of "fear of death," and the higher the support for social distancing, for as long as needed.

Figure 4 Assessment of Social Distancing Per Proximity With Infected Persons (Only Right-Wing And Centre-Right)

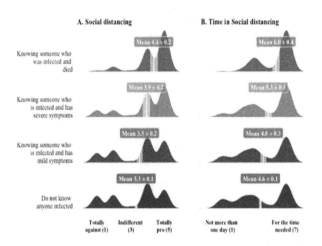

Figure 5 Assessment of Politicians Per Proximity With Infected Persons (Only Right-Wing And Center-Right)

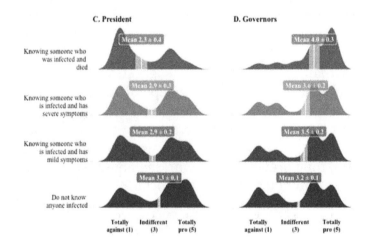

Source: Research data.

The effect of proximity to the risk of death associated with COVID-19 is also seen in the respondents' evaluation of the performance of the president and governors. The greater the exposure to the risks of the virus, the less people agree with Bolsonaro and more with the governors (Figure 5). This is evidence that reinforces the hypothesis that the identity bonds between right-wing and center-right voters and Bolsonaro became more malleable the closer these voters are to people who developed the disease, especially if they know someone who dies from it. Thus, given the weakening of identity connections, the costs of changing the position of these voters in relation to the government have decreased.

As observed before, the income did not affect the respondents' support for social distancing measures. But what about the economic loss they may generate? Figure 6 shows the distribution of the different levels of economic loss as a result of supporting the president's recommendation to make social distancing more flexible, correlated with the knowledge of people infected with COVID-19, and their respective degrees of severity. Although there is a negative relationship between expected economic loss and support for social distancing, levels of proximity to the disease make a difference in this relationship. For those who do not know infected people, the greater the economic impact, the less support for social distancing. However, among those who know people who have died, this variation does not occur. In other words, the seriousness of the contamination that can cause death leads people to minimize the potential economic losses. The fear of death seems to not only bring together ideologically opposed poles, but also different social classes and people who are experiencing different levels of economic

Figure 6: Relationship Between Social Distancing And The Potential Economic Effects (Per Proximity With Infected Persons)

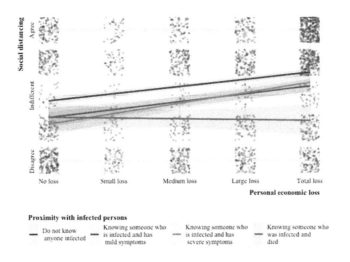

loss as a result of the policy. The results are also consistent for supporting the president in the opposite direction to supporting social distancing and governors.

Simply put, it is possible to identify two groups of Bolsonaro supporters: the group based on identity and the 'pragmatists.' The first one is organic and formed by people who believe in the president's political project. In order to remain cohesive, and keep offering basic and secure social support, this group needs to be constantly fed with populist and polarized agendas. The second group, on the other hand, supports the president, believing that his government has the capacity to meet the group's agenda, which includes liberal economic policies, combating corruption, and containing the Worker's Party.[1]The group of Bolsonaro's electorate considered as 'pragmatists,' was already withdrawing their support to the president due to his belligerent attitudes and because he did not seem to meet their expectations. While he radicalized on issues related to the environment, gender, minorities, foreign policy, education and culture, his right-wing voters were willing to continue to support him, since they believed their individual short-term risks of loss were low. However, when the president took a stand against the policy of social distancing, with the aim of mitigating economic consequences, the respondents interpreted that this position posed risks to their own lives and that of loved ones, generating real risks in the short term. The effects of Figure 6 can also be identified by means of linear estimation. The dependent variable is supporting the social distancing policy. We estimated, only for respondents who called themselves right-wing and center-right, different models of the relationship between exposure to COVID-19 and social distancing. Our preferred estimation is expressed as:

$$social\ distancing = \alpha + \beta_1\ covid + \beta_2\ loss\_dummy + \beta_3\ sex + \beta_4\ age + \beta_5\ income + \beta_6\ (covid * loss\_dummy) + \epsilon$$

The explanatory variables of the tested models are: 1) "fear of death" proxies (variable called 'covid' in our model), measured by the proximity of respondents to people contaminated by COVID-19 and their different degrees of severity ('do not know,' 'mild,' 'severe,' and 'death'); and 2) expectation of economic loss due to social distancing, measured by a Likert scale from 1 to 5. As control variables, we included the different income, sex, and age groups – people over 45 years old, as it was from that age group that we found a greater variance in preferences. In addition, in some of the models, we included interactions between "fear of death" and "economic loss."We operate the 'covid' variable in two different ways: as a quantitative variable (covid num) and as an ordinal qualitative variable (covid), with four levels. The loss variable was operationalized as a dummy (loss dummy) because only the category of total loss shows a difference in the average support for social distancing in relation to the others. Table 1 shows the results of the estimates with robust standard errors.

---

[1] Although our data do not allow us to test this assumption directly, it finds relative theoretical and empirical support in the literature on cultural wars (Hunter, 1991; Laclau, 2013; Lakoff, 1996). Specifically in the Brazilian context, data from interviews collected during the demonstrations of March 25 and 31, 2017, by Gallego, Ortellado, and Moretto (2017), suggest that the biggest factors uniting the group of 'pragmatists,' self-declared right-wing and conservatives, were the 'anti-corruption' debate and the discourse 'anti-PT.' The voters in this group, however, did not show unity around a moral agenda, which indicates a less obvious coordination, but consistent with the existence of a subgroup with more progressive moral values; another subgroup more conservative punitive; and a third, with a conservative religious profile. Such agendas can be observed in research conducted by Datafolha in October 2018 among the reasons for voting for Bolsonaro. A desire for political renewal and anti-PT brought together 55% of the motivations for voting for the candidate, while reasons linked to the candidate's personal image and values m ade up 13% of his voters.

TABLE 1 EXPLANATORY MODEL OF THE PREFERENCE FOR SOCIAL DISTANCING

	Model 1	Model 2	Model 3	Model 4
Covid_num	0,22 *** (0,03)		0,20 *** (0,03)	
Loss_dummy	-0,73 *** (0,07)	-0,81 *** (0,08)	-0,71 *** (0,07)	-0,80 *** (0,08)
Covid_num: Loss_dummy	0,14 * (0,06)		0,16 * (0,06)	
Covid Mild		0,22 * (0,09)		0,16 (0,09)
Covid Severe		0,47 *** (0,12)		0,42 *** (0,12)
Covid Death		0,87 *** (0,11)		0,81 *** (0,11)
Covid Mild: Loss_dummy		0,10 (0,18)		0,13 (0,18)
Covid Severe: Loss_dummy		0,43 * (0,21)		0,48 * (0,21)
Covid Death: Loss_dummy		0,52 (0,35)		0,56 (0,33)
Sex Male			-0,53 *** (0,06)	-0,54 *** (0,06)
Income 3 to 5 MW			-0,08 (0,11)	-0,08 (0,11)
Income 5 to 10 MW			-0,07 (0,10)	-0,06 (0,10)
Income over 10 MW			-0,01 (0,09)	0,01 (0,09)
Age			-0,27 *** (0,06)	-0,27 *** (0,06)
N	2126	2126	2126	2126
R2	0,09	0,09	0,13	0,14

All continuous predictors are centered on the mean and resized to 1 standard deviation. Standard errors are heteroskedasticity-consistent. *** p < 0,001; ** p < 0,01; * p < 0,05.
Source: Research data.

Table 1 and Figure 7 show that our hypothesis has been confirmed. The degree of proximity to someone contaminated by COVID-19 increases the chances of supporting social distancing, i.e., the support increases with the perception of proximity to the risk of death. In other words, the fear of death brought about by the pandemic is strong enough to weaken the identity/ideological ties between this group of voters and the president to the extent that these voters contradict their leader and consistently support social distancing. Keeping the other variables constant,

it is possible to infer that those who know someone who died from COVID-19 agree with the social distancing policy at a level of 19.20% higher than those who do not know people infected by the virus. As we have shown, the different income groups have no significant statistical impact on social distancing. However, those with expectations of economic loss, older people, and men tend to support social distancing less.[1]

Figure 7 Explanatory Models of Preference For Social Distancing

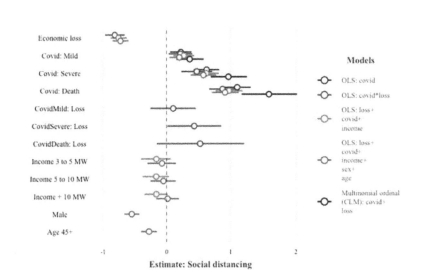

Source: Research data.

7. CONCLUSION

Severe crises, such as wars or pandemics, may be unique opportunities for government leaders willing to leave a legacy, to show their capacity to unite and lead the country against a common enemy. Bolsonaro, however, seems unable to leave behind the obstacles he created, himself, when he decided to rule as a minority without a coalition government. For the president, this was a missed opportunity. The results confirm he was one of the few world leaders who lost support and popularity with voters (see Figure 8 in the supplementary material).

Even though he was put down for preferring to implement a perpetual polarized campaign, the president had been able to maintain the popularity and political support of a significant portion of

---

[1] Additional specifications and information for replicating regressions can be found in the supplementary material (https://dataverse. harvard.edu/dataset.xhtml?persistentId=doi:10.7910/DVN/SUN4KZ).

the population. However, by emphasizing the negative impacts of social distancing on the economy and, at the same time, minimizing the risks of contagion and seriousness of the pandemic, even the significant portion of voters who were aligned with the government based on identity and ideology, decided to withdraw their support. Bolsonaro did not realize that the population's fear of losing lives with the new coronavirus outweighs the risks of economic crisis, as he did not realize that people tend to discount the future. In other words, today's concerns are always greater than those to come. Bolsonaro contradicted the population's desires, and signs of rejection among followers began to appear. The protests, inquiries about the president's interference in government control agencies, and the various requests for impeachment are evidence of this rejection. Our research revealed that as the individuals in the sample became aware of fatal victims among their acquaintances, their perceptions changed. They became more favourable of social distancing and willing to follow such policy for longer. Also, the respondents evaluated the president's performance as 'worse' and the governors' as 'better.' Thus, the identity connections between the group and its leader became malleable and fragile.

It is worth noting that this study collected the data analyzed amidst the pandemic, in a period of high transmission, and many deaths. On the one hand, we were able to capture the feeling of "fear of death" and its influence on political behaviour. On the other, this feeling may have inflated people's reactions, which could represent a limitation. In addition, the lack of probabilistic sample design limits the generalization of the findings. While recognizing the research limitations, its results offer relevant insights. The study suggests that political leaders who put effort into fighting the pandemic may obtain greater benefits than those more concerned with preventing economic downturn. The group recognized as right-wing was divided, but not because of income. The polarization reduces as the risk of death becomes more present. The fear of death is so intense that it relativizes and overcomes the losses of identity related to the ideology

REFERENCES

Ajzenman, N., Cavalcanti, T., & Da Mata, D. (2020, April 22). More than words: Leaders' speech and risky behavior during a pandemic. *SSRN*.
Retrieved from https://papers.ssrn.com/sol3/papers.
cfm?abstract_id=3582908

Bakker, B., Rooduijn, M., & Schumacher, G. (2016). The Psychological Roots of Populist Voting: Evidence from the United States, the Netherlands and Germany. *European Journal of Political Research, 55*(2), 1-58.

Bello, A. (2019). *Origens, causas e consequências da polarização política*. Brasília, DF: Universidade de Brasília.

Bisgaard, M. (2015). Bias will find a way: economic perceptions, attributions of blame, and partisanmotivated reasoning during crisis. *The Journal of Politics, 77*(3), 849-860.

Bos, L., Schemer, C., Corbu, N., Hameleers, M., Andreadis, I., Schulz, A., ... Fawzi, N. (2020). The effects of populism as a social identity frame on persuasion and mobilisation: evidence from a 15-country experiment. *European Journal of Political Research, 59*(1), 3-24.

Bolsen, T., Druckman, J. N., & Cook, F. L. (2014). The influence of partisan motivated reasoning on public opinion. *Political Behavior, 36*(2), 235-262.

Busby, E. C., Gubler, J. R., & Hawkins, K. A. (2019). Framing and blame attribution in populist rhetoric. *The Journal of Politics, 81*(2), 616-630.

Conaghan, C. M. (2008). Ecuador: Correa's plebiscitary presidency. *Journal of Democracy, 19*(2), 46-60.

Druckman, J. N., & Bolsen, T. (2011). Framing, motivated reasoning, and opinions about emergent technologies. *Journal of Communication, 61*(4), 659-688.

Hameleers, M., Bos, L., & Vreese, C. H. (2017). "They did it": The effects of emotionalized blame attribution in populist communication. *Communication Research, 44*(6), 870-900.

Hawkins, K. A., Kaltwasser, C. R., & Andreadis, I. (2020, April). The Activation of Populist Attitudes. *Government and Opposition*, *55*(2), 283-307.

Huckfeldt, R., Levine, J., Morgan, W., & Sprague, J. (1999). Accessibility and the political utility of partisan and ideological orientations. *American Journal of Political Science*, *43*(3), 888-911.

Huddy, L. (2001). From social to political identity: a critical examination of social identity theory. *Political Psychology*, *22*(1), 127-156.

Hunter, W., & Power, T. J. (2019). Bolsonaro and Brazil's illiberal backlash. *Journal of Democracy*, *30*(1), 68-82.

Iborra, A. (2005). Beyond identity and ideology: processes of transcendence associated with the experience of conversion. *Culture and Psychology*, *11*(1), 89-100.

Jorge, M. P. (2020). *Quarenta é coisa de rico?*. Retrieved from https://www.youtube.com/ watch?v=KRcNNWHM2EY

Kernell, S. (2006). *Going public: new strategies of presidential leadership*. Washington, DC: CQ Press.

Kingstone, P., & Power, T. J. (2017). *Democratic Brazil divided*. Pittsburgh, Pennsylvania: University of Pittsburgh Press.

Kovic, M., & Caspar, C. (2019, January 11). *Motivated cognition, conspiratorial epistemology, and bullshit: a model of post-factual political discourse politics*. Retrieved from https://doi.org/10.31235/ osf.io/bnv2m

Kunda, Z. (1990). The case for motivated reasoning. *Psychological Bulletin*, *108*(3), 480-498.

Leeper, T. J., & Slothuus, R. (2014). Political parties, motivated reasoning, and public opinion formation. *Political Psychology*, *35*(S1), 129-156.

Martins, P. (2020, April 24). Painel debate falso dilema entre salvar a economia ou a saúde durante a pandemia. *ABRASCO*. Retrieved from https://www. abrasco.org.br/site/sem-categoria/painel-debatefalso-dilema-entre-salvar-a-economia-ou-a-saudedurante-a-pandemia/47292/

Mazar, N., Amir, O., & Ariely, D. (2008). The dishonesty of honest people: a theory of self-concept maintenance. *Journal of Marketing Research*, *155*(6), 633-644.

Mudde, C. (2004). The Populist Zeitgeist. *Government and Opposition*, *39*(4), 541-563.

Mudde, C., & Kaltwasser, C. R. (2012). Exclusionary vs. Inclusionary Populism: Comparing Contemporary Europe and Latin America. *Government and Opposition*, *48*(2), 147-174.

Mullen, B., Dovidio, J. F., Craig, J., & Copper, C. (1992). In-group out-group differences in social projection. *Journal of Experimental Social Psychology*, *28*(5), 422-440.

Pereira, F. (2020, May 08). "Não é o isolamento que afeta a economia, é a pandemia", diz Meirelles. *UOL*. Retrieved from https://economia.uol.com.br/noticias/ redacao/2020/05/08/nao-e-o-isolamento-que-afetaa-economia-e-a-pandemia-diz-meirelles.htm Samuels, D., & Zucco, C. (2018) *Partisans, antipartisans and nonpartisans: voting behavior in Brazil*. Cambridge, UK: Cambridge University Press.

Shah, A. K., Mullainathan, S., & Shafir, E. (2012). Some consequences of having too little. *Science*, *338*(6107), 682-685.

Teles, C. D. P. (2009). Linguagem escolar e a construção da identidade e consciência racial da criança negra na educação infantil. *Anagrama – Revista Científica Interdisciplinar da Graduação*, *1*(4), 1-14.

AUTHORS

Carlos Pereira https://orcid.org/0000-0002-8978-1493 Ph.D. in Political Science; Full Professor at the Brazilian School of Public and Business Administration at Fundação Getulio Vargas (FGV EBAPE). E-mail: carlos.pereira@fgv.br

Amanda Medeiros https://orcid.org/0000-0002-0008-3905 Ph.D. in Administration; Professor at the Brazilian School of Public and Business Administration at Fundação Getulio Vargas (FGV EBAPE). E-mail: amanda.medeiros@fgv.br

Frederico Bertholini https://orcid.org/0000-0002-2480-739X Ph.D. in Administration; Adjunct Professor at the Institute of Political Science of the University of Brasília (IPOL/UNB). E-mail: frederico.bertholini@unb.br

CHAPTER 7

BRAZILIAN HEALTH CARE DISPARATIES EXPOSED

1. The Management of COVID-19 in Brazil: Implications for Human Rights & Public Health

[1]Erick da Luz Scherf,

Marcos V. V. D. Silva, and Janaina S. Fachini[1].

ABSTRACT

The objective of this article is to explore how the COVID-19 pandemic has been managed in Brazil, especially through the analysis of the actions and inactions of the Brazilian president Jair Bolsonaro related to the complete denial of the global threat that the new coronavirus represents, seeking to demonstrate its major impacts on human rights and public health in the country. Our main conclusions were that: (i) since the election of Bolsonaro in 2018, Brazilian politics have been entrenched with a neoliberal spirit marked by illiberal notions that have compromised Brazil's democracy and rights regime; (ii) since 2016, the Brazilian Unified Health System (SUS) has been subjected to a privatizing logic guided by market rules and exploitation of health as a source of profits, which represents a serious threat to the right to health in the country as a result of the first; (iii) by not making sufficient efforts to safeguard the lives of Brazilians or to strengthen public health institutions in the middle of the new coronavirus pandemic, the Brazilian State is violating the rights to life and health by omission; (iv) ultimately, it was demonstrated that Bolsonaro has worked unceasingly to bulldoze anti-COVID-19 efforts in Brazil and how it can be better explained through the concept of necro politics.

INTRODUCTION

The objective of this article is to explore how the COVID-19 pandemic has been managed in Brazil, especially through the analysis of the actions and inactions of the Brazilian president Jair Bolsonaro related to the complete denial of the global threat that the new coronavirus represents, seeking to demonstrate its major impacts on human rights and public health agendas in the country. The research was built upon an inductive approach, with a qualitative and exploratory design, based mostly on literature review and theoretical analysis and inquiry. Thus far, the new coronavirus pandemic has affected more than 100 countries, infecting almost three million people worldwide and leading to more than two hundred thousand deaths and counting[1], while these numbers are likely to be underreported: as "there is a well-documented shortage of the tests worldwide" [2], making it harder to screen /detect who carries the virus and who does not. Even though the high rate of the infection spread and the significant number of fatalities due to COVID-19 is a largely acknowledged fact amongst the scientific community[3], it does not translate automatically into a

---

[1] Please address any correspondence to Erick da Luz Scherf. Email: erickscherf@gmail.com

convergence of health policies worldwide in order to stop the spread of the virus. Differently, we have witnessed divergent political responses to the virus spread around the world.

This is so because, diseases, especially infectious diseases, are not apolitical, *i.e.* they are also vulnerable to the influence of the political game and political ideologies and agendas. Infectious diseases such as COVID-19 can be instrumentalized by politicians and political institutions to generate anxiety and insecurity for political means, distorting public health priorities[4]. Thus, even though we still are on earlier stages of the fight against the new coronavirus, it became very clear that the virus is a political problem, not just a health problem.[5] Nic Cheeseman stated that "the coronavirus pandemic might not disrupt politics in wealthy Western democracies, but it is likely to unleash political instability [...] in developing countries already suffering from an economic crisis".[6] Brazil is already experiencing this, as president Jair Bolsonaro is battling to gain political support to his actions and to maintain his allies in Congress and society. Therefore, as suggested by The Lancet's latest editorial on the new coronavirus in Brazil, the biggest threat to the country's COVID-19 response may be its president, Jair Bolsonaro[7].

Bolsonaro has constantly denied the deadly effects of the new coronavirus, undermining the pandemic and the opinions of health experts, calling self-isolation 'mass confinement' and COVID-19 a 'little cold'[8]. Unfortunately, these political shenanigans are resulting in the death-by-neglect of thousands of people in Brazil today. The intention is to argue that these actions of complete disregard for public health and putting business interests over public safety[9] do not come as a surprise for us. It is all part of a political project, sponsored by neoliberal ideas, that intend to exempt the state from its moral and legal obligations of guaranteeing the survival and quality of life of its people by ripping them off of their most fundamental rights, including - but not limited to – the right to life and the right to health. The contribution of this article is related to the expansion of the literature on human rights and politics, especially regarding the challenges that human rights face in front of public health crisis and exacerbated neoliberal ideologies. The article also contributes to the discussion around the politization of human rights during a pandemic, through the analysis of the recent (and ongoing) Brazilian experience in dealing with the new coronavirus pandemic.

Neoliberalism and Human Rights in Contemporary Brazilian Politics

Neoliberalism is not a finished concept, on the contrary, it is a widely contested one. With that being said, it is not our intention to review all the literature on the meaning and consequences of neoliberalism, as many other important works have already done so, from a wide range of disciplines[10]. Instead, the practical forms of neoliberalism in contemporary Brazilian politics should be explored, in contrast to its original theoretical formulations, to make sense of the current events that are taking place in Brazil, especially regarding the new coronavirus pandemic management (or lack thereof) and its implications to Brazilian society. Because as well pointed out by Harvey[11], neoliberalism and the role of the state in the neoliberal theory is easier to define, the hard part is characterizing the practice of neoliberalism: as "[...] the neoliberal state may be an unstable and contradictory political form."[12]

Neoliberalism does not translate into one single concept, instead, it is a polysemic concept with multiple referents[13], however, there may be a set of core principles that underline neoliberalism both as a theoretical and political movement, which encompass, among others, ideas of free markets, free trade and individual liberties, as well as a limited role of the state in regulating peoples' lives and the economy[14]. Neoliberalism had succeeded in the 1980s in defining the world's economic and political agenda for the next quarter century[15], and it has played a seminal role on the economic agenda of Latin American countries (including Brazil). Nonetheless, since 2000 Latin America experienced a major setback against neoliberal prescriptions, leading to what some authors have called "post-neoliberal" regimes[16], marked by the election of leftist leaders in Brazil, Argentina, Venezuela, Ecuador, Uruguay, Bolivia, and Chile. In Brazil, that was the case for more than a decade - from 2003 to 2015 - during the administrations of the Worker's Party (PT), when the neoliberal project was not completely abandoned[17], but ideals of social welfare, labour rights and concerns for the political autonomy of the working and lower classes prevailed at that moment.[18]

Despite the ups and downs of neoliberal policies in Brazil, up until the election of the current Brazilian president, Jair Bolsonaro, neoliberal ideologies in Latin America were marked by trends of privatization, marketization, commodification, and deregulation[19], but not necessarily by a complete abandonment of the fundamental roles of the state. According to Harvey, the neoliberal state should, in theory, guarantee at least the rule of law and some idea of constitutionality[20]. Our judgment is that, after the *coup d'état* that took place in Brazil in 2016, an unprecedented and twisted neoliberal agenda has entrenched Brazilian politics accompanied by conservatism and authoritarianism, especially after the election of former-Congressman Jair Bolsonaro. This "new" neoliberal wave, marked by illiberal notions, has compromised Brazil's young (and fragile) democracy and rights regime[21], with terrible consequences especially on social and public health services[22].

Liberal Neoliberalism and the Downfall of Human Rights under Bolsonaro's Administration

Brazil is now democratic society that has consolidated the internalization/implementation of human rights norms. Even though the transition from a military dictatorship[23] (that lasted twenty-one years) to a constitutional democracy was not smooth or flawless [24], in the decades following the downfall of the military rule and the rise of the rule of law, Brazil experienced positive changes regarding the expansion of social movements and areas including education, the role of women, race relations, and public health advanced considerably during this time[25].

However, this scenario of hope for democratic progress in Brazilian politics would change drastically in august 2016, when members of Congress performed a coup d'état, which interrupted the administration of Dilma Roussef, Brazil's first female president who in theory should have governed until 2018. The impeachment that removed Dilma from office, was influenced by misogynist [26], conservative sectors of Brazilian society [27], as well as by a geopolitical project entrenched with neoliberal ideals [28].

Since then, we have witnessed the rise of authoritarian neoliberalism: and "its main signposts are the freezing of public investment in social programs, including education, healthcare and infrastructure (2016); the obliteration of labour rights (2017); the denationalization and privatization of the economy (2018); and restricting access to pensions and social security ongoing."[29], alongside the emergence of Evangelical neoconservatism and populist leaderships in Brazilian politics [30]. Nonetheless, things are never so bad they can't be made worse. In 2018, former Congressperson Jair Bolsonaro was elected president. The election of Bolsonaro was rooted in hate speech [31], fake news [32], and in extremist and populist mobilization[33]. The election of a far-right, populist, and anti-democratic leader in Brazil - combined with the advancement of exacerbated neoliberal policies - can led to the decay of democratic institutions and to massive human rights violations: Bolsonaro is an extremist who has promised harsh security and policing and a clamp-down on all forms of liberalism. The regime's hatred is particularly focused against feminists and gay activists. Bolsonaro's neoliberal economic policies are backed up by a rhetoric of hate and by violence. The police and militias now have a license to kill and have started doing so on the streets[34].Since democratization in the late 1980s, Brazil has never had a leader so openly and publicly against democratic institutions and political plurality. Bolsonaro cultivates and instigates a feeling of nostalgia for the 1964–85 military regime that killed and tortured hundreds of people deemed "enemies of the state", and he has also spoken many times against human rights activism and activists[35]

The consequences are terrible: since he took office, several human rights violations have taken place due to his actions or omissions. The Human Rights Watch (HRW) World Report of 2020, in its section about Brazil, scrutinizes Bolsonaro's first year in office and his embracing of an "anti-rights" agenda[36]. According to the HRW[37], among other violations, the Bolsonaro administration has (i) encouraged police to take on extrajudicial killings; (ii) incentivized illegal fires on the Amazon rainforest; (iii) sought to restrict the rights of LGBT+ people; (iv) and has attempted several times against freedom of expression and association. Most recently, the president has made several moves in order to sabotage anti-COVID-19 efforts[38], the reasons for this behaviour and its impacts on human rights and public health shall be explored going forward.

The New Coronavirus Pandemic: Implications for Human Rights and Public Health in Brazil

If human rights are going downhill in contemporary Brazil due to authoritarianism and neoliberal movements, as past explored, the current COVID-19 pandemic comes as a major threat to human rights and public health in the country. As well put by Yamin and Habibi: "we should have learned by now that human rights protections cannot be an afterthought in epidemics"[39], thus, anyone interested in researching about the coronavirus outbreak should bear in mind of the implications it might have on human rights protection efforts. Human rights are usually the first casualty in natural calamities or armed conflicts; therefore, state of emergency can sometimes be used as a pretext for abuses, especially in authoritarian contexts[40]. In Brazil, our public and universal healthcare system called *Sistema Único de Saúde* (Unified Health System), better known by the acronym SUS, has been constantly threatened, maybe since its creation in 1989. However, since 2016, it has been subjected to a privatizing logic guided by market rules and exploitation of health as a source of profits[41].

The nightmare started with Constitutional Amendment 95, an Act that froze all federal expenditures with public services (such as health and education) for twenty years. Freezing resources is the same as freezing services, thus, this Amendment put SUS at checkmate.

After three decades, SUS had made considerable progress towards Universal Health Coverage (UHC) and in implementing the right to health for everyone[42]. However, the combination of economic recession, political crisis and austerity policies has implicated in serious damages for both the System and for the implementation of the right to health in Brazil. Although flawed, SUS has provided quality healthcare to millions of people, especially the poor, who were previously denied access even to basic care[43].

With the pandemic, SUS in undergoing even bigger threats: only ten per cent of Brazilian municipalities have intensive care beds and the entire System does not even have half the number of hospital beds recommended by the World Health Organization[44]. Alongside that, the country is in shortage of masks and respirators, which facilitates the spread of the virus and compromises the capacity of SUS to deliver healthcare assistance to all people infected with COVID-19. Thus, our "[...] *weakened health system is not coping and is failing to protect the rights to life and health of millions of Brazilians who are seriously at risk*".[45] According to a study developed by public health researchers in Imperial College (London), Brazil has the highest rate of Coronavirus contagion among 48 countries[46], therefore, we are at a greater risk of possible overload in our health system. Even before being aware of this fact, they projected that in the absence of interventions, COVID-19 could lead up to one million deaths in Brazil[47]. Therefore, when the federal government, especially the president, do not take any actions in order to stop the spread of the virus and to increase and strengthen both the human and material resources of our public health system, they are clearly violating a set of previously established human rights, especially the rights to life and health.

If SUS collapses, and it has already done so in many Brazilian states that have already ran out of intensive care beds (so far: Rio de Janeiro (Capital), Distrito Federal, São Paulo (Capital), Ceará, Amazonas, and Pernambuco), not only lives will be lost in the present, the number of deaths will probably be used in the future as a scapegoat to question the efficacy and *raison d'être* of the System. Politicians engaged to the neoliberal project in Brazil, especially Jair Bolsonaro, can use the collapse of SUS as a trump to bring forward measures of privatization and marketization, in order to guarantee even less budgetary participation of the state in the System's maintenance. The collapse of SUS can seriously jeopardize the right to the highest attainable standard of health in Brazil, and it also may result in a drastic reduction in universal health coverage (UHC) in the country.

The Evolution of COVID-19 in Brazil: Responses and Lack of Responsiveness

Responses to the new coronavirus in Brazil have been far from coherent so far, varying a lot according to different levels of public administration in the country. Thus, in line with this article's aim, this section intends to shine a light on the evolution of COVID-19 and its responses (or lack thereof) coming from the president himself, the Ministry of Health, the federal administration and other important political actors. Even before SARS-CoV-2 had officially "arrived" in the country, the Brazilian Ministry of Health (hereinafter "MoH") created a Joint Ministerial Working Group on a Public Health Emergency of National and International Concern to monitor the situation and establish protocols for surveillance of the new coronavirus[48]. These protocols established measures for adequate screening and treatment of people possibly infected by the virus.

On the other hand, since the beginning of the anti-COVID-19 efforts in Brazil, Jair Bolsonaro has made a mockery of the virus and of the public health professionals working to prevent greater dissemination: "since the beginning of the crisis, Bolsonaro has minimized the gravity of COVID-19, comparing it to a 'little flu' or a 'cold', calling it a 'fantasy' promoted by the media"[49]. He has also labelled preventive measures like social distancing and lockdown/quarantine 'hysterical'.

The MoH had adopted serious and responsible prophylactic measures related to COVID-19 before the first case was even registered in the country, as demonstrated by a joint research recently published in the Journal of the Brazilian Association of Tropical Medicine by professors and members of the Ministry itself[50]. According to them, Brazil had certain advantages in containing the number of cases due to its socialized unified health system[51] (SUS). However, as demonstrated before, SUS did not have at that time (and it still does not have) enough resources to deal with the pandemic if non-medical interventions like quarantine were not taken.

Thus, in early February the Congress passed bill no. 13,979, that established some measures that could be adopted to face the public health emergency, like isolation, quarantine and restriction of travels[52].Nonetheless, despite such efforts from the MoH and from Congress, Brazil's surveillance structure depended mostly on SUS, and at a time in which cutbacks in funding for the System and for health research are in effect, the country's capacity for early detection and response was seriously undermined[53]. As pointed out by Ventura: "in an extremely adverse political context for Brazilian public health, debased by successive budget cuts and suffering competition from religious fundamentalism and negation in relation to science, SUS remains the main axis of response to emergencies"[54].

On February 26 Brazil registered its first case of coronavirus, a man who had recently travelled for work to Italy during the explosion of cases in the European country[55]. The case was isolated rapidly and up until early March, there was no sustained transmission detected in the country, which led public health researchers to believe that there were possibilities of interrupting the coronavirus epidemic in Brazil[56]. However, things did not go as planned. On March 20, the MoH acknowledged the existence of community/sustained transmission of the virus throughout the national territory[57], and since then, the number of registered cases has grown exponentially (see Figure 1).In result of that, many state governors in Brazil, by late March 2020, declared a state of emergency and/or installed quarantine/lockdown measures on their territories. That was the case in the states of São Paulo, Rio de Janeiro, Espírito Santo, Pará and Santa Catarina (among others)[58]. They were severely scolded by President Jair Bolsonaro - even retaliated at times – who encouraged them to let go of these measures and even threatened to cut federal funds destined to combat the new coronavirus in the states[59].

Figure 1. Linear evolution of coronavirus cases in Brazil

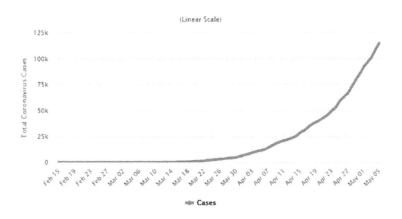

Source: Worldometer, "Brazil, Coronavirus Cases" (May 2020). Available at https://www.worldometers.info/coronavirus/country/brazil/.

At the same time, Bolsonaro launched a national campaign called *"O Brasil Não Pode Parar"* ("Brazil Cannot Stop", in English), sponsored by the Secretariat of Social Communication of the Presidency of the Republic (also known as SECOM): the campaign called Brazilians to ignore governors' orders and return to work, signalling that COVID-19 did not pose a serious threat to the health of the population[60]. Thankfully, the campaign did not hit national television because the Brazilian Supreme Court found it to violate the Constitution[61].

On March 15, Bolsonaro ignored health protocols and joined protesters in Brasília that were demanding the closure of Brazil's Congress and Supreme Court. After this episode, Bolsonaro participated on others anti-lockdown rallies[62]. Later on, on April 16, the president fired Health Minister Luiz Henrique Mandetta in the midst of the coronavirus (political and public health) crisis. Former-minister Mandetta repeatedly advocated a science-based approach to the COVID-19 pandemic that included social distancing measures and quarantines, thus, his positions weren't aligned with Bolsonaro's political project[63]. In addition, when the country registered an alarming number of deaths on late April (around five thousand, even more than China), Bolsonaro told reporters 'So what? 'What do you want me to do?', when they asked him about the record deaths that day[64]. In less than a month after stepping up into the office of the MoH, the new Health Minister Nelson Teich chose to resign, because he did not want to approve Bolsonaro's change in the protocol regulating the use of chloroquine as treatment for COVID-19[65].

He was replaced for Eduardo Pazuello, an active duty army general who is not a physician and has no experience whatsoever with public health services[66], and alongside him, twelve other military men were assigned to the MoH cabinet. Such political move made by Bolsonaro most certainly represents a clear militarization of public health in the middle of the new coronavirus pandemic. In sum, Bolsonaro has worked unceasingly to bulldoze anti-COVID-19 efforts delivered by the MoH, by health professionals, and by state governors in Brazil. Since the very begging of the pandemic, when preventive measures could have saved thousands of lives, Bolsonaro minimized the deadly effect of the virus and encouraged people to move on with their lives, urging them to not follow social distancing and quarantine measures. Such actions (and omissions) are in clear violation of human rights norms.

Ifas stated on the UN report on COVID-19 and human rights - "all States have a duty to protect human life, including by addressing the general conditions in society that give rise to direct threats to life"[67], Bolsonaro is clearly violating the right to life of thousands of Brazilians, since the federal administration has done nothing to effectively combat the spread of the virus, while the president has constantly urged people to ignore social distancing and quarantine measures (crucial to stop dissemination). In addition, by not providing SUS with enough resources to battle COVID-19, leading to a possible collapse of the system, the Brazilian government is jeopardizing the right to the highest attainable standard of health in Brazil, as underinvestment in health systems can weaken the ability to respond to the pandemic as well as provide other essential health services[68].

In international law, international responsibility in these cases is attributed to the State, not to governmental agents (such as president Bolsonaro), as the illegal actions or inactions were done under actual or apparent authority of the State[69]. By not making sufficient efforts to safeguard the lives of Brazilians or to strengthen public health institutions in the middle of the new coronavirus pandemic, the Brazilian State is violating the rights to life and health by omission: "we can talk about human rights violations by omission when the state fails to meet its responsibilities to effectively implement these rights or to protect them [...]

In these cases there are facts that clearly demonstrate that the state or its organs already knew of the risks and did not act in a diligent way to prevent the negative effects"[70] (see Figure 2).

Figure 2. State responsibility for human rights violations by omission amidst the COVID-19 pandemic.

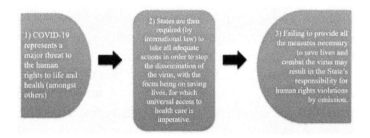

Elaborated by the authors. Sources: United Nations, "COVID-19 and Human Rights: We are all in this together" (April 2020). Available at https://unsdg.un.org/sites/default/files/202004/COVID-19-and-Human-Rights.pdf.; Soto, Marcela Barón, and Alejandro Gómez Velásquez, "An Approach to the State Responsibility by an Omission in the Inter–American Court of Human Rights Jurisprudence". *Revista CES Derecho* 6, no. 1 (2015), pp. 3-17.

In emergency times such as the one we are experiencing now, it can be pretty hard to achieve accountability for human rights violations though, especially in authoritarian contexts like the Brazilian one. So far, other branches of government like the Congress or the Judiciary, have done virtually nothing to remediate the president's actions or obligate him to follow public health protocols. Uncoordinated responses at the state and municipal levels were also insufficient to control the national health emergency generated by the new coronavirus. In addition, on May 14th, the president edited a Provisional Measure which exempted public agents from criminal liability related to actions or omissions performed in detriment of the COVID-19 pandemic[71]. We propose that the concept of necropolitics, sponsored by Achille Mbembe, is very useful when trying to understand this lack of actions by the federal administration in order to stop dissemination of the virus and provide health care for all. Aligned with neoliberal policies, the politics of death speaks directly to the president's and government agencies' inaction in face of COVID-19, which contributes to the discussion around the politization of human rights in times of coronavirus.

Understanding Necropolitics, Neoliberal Policies and Death

According to Mbembe, exercising sovereignty means exercising control over mortality and defining life as the implantation and manifestation of power[72]. Peoples' lives are then subjugated to the sovereign power and not otherwise. Thus, when Jair Bolsonaro (president of the Republic and ultimate representation of sovereignty in the country) urges people to come back to work and follow their "normal" lives/routines which results in accelerating the spread of the virus – he is simply trying to regain sovereign power: he is the one who chooses who can live and who can die. As explained by Mbembe, this type of sovereignty is not expressed by classical definitions we can find in political science textbooks, because the goal of the politics of death is the widespread instrumentalization of human existence and the material destruction of human bodies and populations[73].

Necropolitics is the ultimate result of the mix between neoliberal policies and illiberal mindset and actions in Brazil. Neoliberalism with authoritarian traces, paved the way for the construction of perfect 'death-worlds' in contemporary Brazil, especially in the middle of a public health crisis.

The lack of actions in battling the virus is intimately related to the neoliberal project, which (tries to) exempt the State from performing its most fundamental roles. As well described by professor Lee: "COVID-19 has highlighted a long-term failure among some states to sustain public health, to sustain life, through their commitment to neoliberal agendas to end state welfare in favour of privatization"[74], which results from a necropolitical approach to the lives of citizens and non-citizens[75].In the midst of the new coronavirus pandemic in Brazil, Bolsonaro saw an opportunity to speed up the realization of the neoliberal project in the country, without being blamed for it.

The aggressive spread of COVID-19 threatens to decimate vulnerable communities in Brazil[76], as marginalized citizens, *e.g.*, those who are sexual/racial minorities, people of colour, homeless, those who live in the *favelas* and/or in extreme poverty, or are imprisoned, are the ones most likely to die due to COVID-19 because they have little or almost no access to health care, to basic hygiene measures and adequate housing[77]. In general, no efforts have been taken to protect these vulnerable populations, even though the COVID-19 outbreak in Brazil has exacerbated the vulnerability of the least protected in our society. They are also the ones who depend the most on social services and public health institutions, therefore, if they die, the state saves money and no longer shares responsibility for their lives: it's a genocidal and criminal behaviour that is likely to go unpunished. If neoliberalism in itself accelerates the death of people (especially of those marginalized and/or dependent upon the state to survive) by generating poverty, inequality and privatization of essential services[78], contemporary forms of authoritarianism and necropolitics make sure no one questions these deaths, by making them look like a result of an external factor other than the state actions (or inactions in this case), by lying and manipulating the public opinion.

Thus, Bolsonaro and the federal administration act in the position of a death commissioners, executing Brazilians not by shooting them or throwing them into gas chambers, they have taken another easier route: bulldozing anti-COVID-19 efforts, sacrificing Brazil's public health system, and urging people to go back to their 'normal lives', directly and indirectly violating a set of previously stablished human rights, including but not limited to the rights to life and to the enjoyment of the highest attainable standard of health. On May 5th, when around eight thousand people died in Brazil, the president said that the worst part of this crisis was over[79]. On May 19th, the number of deaths due to COVID-19 in the country reached around eighteen thousand.

The question of how can we escape from this death machine

(composed by neoliberalism, authoritarianism and necropolitics as gears) is yet to be answered. What is known for sure is that the lives and rights of thousands of Brazilians are at great risk of extinction not solely because of the new coronavirus pandemic, but mostly due to the deadly and reckless actions taken by the president and his supporters.

CONCLUSION

After the coup d'état that took place in Brazil in 2016 - an unprecedented and twisted neoliberal agenda has entrenched Brazilian politics accompanied by conservatism and authoritarianism. This is what we called "illiberal neoliberalism": a set of mixed policies that took place after the election of current president Jair Bolsonaro which paved the way for democratic decay and human rights suppression. We demonstrated how the emergence of the new coronavirus pandemic in Brazil actually worsened this scenario. Suffering from austerity measures and cutbacks in federal funding especially after 2016, Brazil's Unified Health System (SUS) was severely injured, not being able to cope with the current COVID-19 emergency in the country, which represents a serious threat to the rights to health and life, and to public health more generally. Moreover, we also found that other sets of rights have also been violated amid the pandemic, which could be subject of further research. On top of that, we described the evolution of the new coronavirus in Brazil and what has been done about it thus far. In sum, our findings were that President Jair Bolsonaro has unceasingly tried to jeopardize anti-COVID-19 efforts delivered by the Ministry of Health, by health professionals, and by other public health actors in the country.

Since the very begging of the pandemic, Bolsonaro minimized the deadly effects of the virus and encouraged people to not follow scientific recommendations of quarantine and social distancing. Therefore, by not making sufficient efforts to safeguard the lives of Brazilians or to strengthen public health institutions in the middle of the new coronavirus pandemic, the Brazilian State is violating the rights to life and health by omission. The president's actions and inactions have great impact on the capacity of SUS to manage the new coronavirus outbreak in Brazil, leading to a possible breakdown of the country's entire public health system that was a major tool for implementing the right to health and universal health coverage. Ultimately, we argued that the concept of necropolitics is a powerful theoretical tool that can help us explain why Bolsonaro and his administration are bulldozing anti-COVID-19 efforts as a means to achieve political goals.

REFERENCES

1. Coronavirus Resource Centre, "COVID-19 Dashboard by the Centre for Systems Science and Engineering (CSSE) at Johns Hopkins University", Johns Hopkins University & Medicine (2020). Available at https://coronavirus.jhu.edu/map.html.By the time this article is published, this data will likely be outdated, please refer to the John Hopkins University's data platform (above cited) in order to keep track of the new coronavirus evolution around the globe.

2. Kuenssberg, Laura, "Coronavirus: Lack of Testing Becomes Political Problem." *BBC News* (April 1, 2020). Available at https://www.bbc.com/news/uk-politics-52118781, para. 7.

3. Nesteruk, I. (2020) "Statistics-Based Predictions of Coronavirus Epidemic Spreading in Mainland China." *Innovative Biosystems and Bioengineering* 4/1pp. 13–18.

4. Koplan, J. P., and Mcpheeters, M. (2004); "Plagues, Public Health, and Politics." *Emerging Infectious Diseases* 10/11, pp. 2039–43.

5. Candaele, Kelly, "Coronavirus is a political problem, not just a health problem. Remember that when you vote." *The Guardian* (March 19, 2020). Available at https://www.theguardian.com/commentisfree/2020/mar/19/coronavirus-political-problemhealth-voting-elections.

6. Cheeseman, Nic, "The Coronavirus Could Topple Governments Around the World." *Foreign Policy* (March 31, 2020). Available at https://foreignpolicy.com/2020/03/31/coronavirus-regimechange-could-topple-governments-around-the-world/, para. 1.

7. See: The Lancet (Editorial), "COVID-19 in Brazil: "So what?"". *The Lancet* 395/10235 (May 2020), pp. 1461.

8. Pinheiro-Machado, Rosana, "Bolsonaro Is Endangering Brazil. He Must Be Impeached." *The Washington Post* (March 29, 2020). Available at https://www.washingtonpost.com/opinions/2020/03/29/bolsonaro-is-endangering-brazil-hemust-be-impeached/.

9. Phillips, Tom, "Brazilian Left Demands Bolsonaro Resign over Coronavirus Response." *The Guardian* (March 30, 2020). Available at https://www.theguardian.com/world/2020/mar/30/tpcaptain-corona.

10. *E.g.*, Harvey, D., *A Brief History of Neoliberalism* (NY: OUP, 2005); Steger, Manfred B., and Ravi K. Roy, *Neoliberalism: a Very Short Introduction* (Oxford: OUP, 2010); Davies, William, "Neoliberalism: A Bibliographic Review." *Theory, Culture & Society* 31/7-8 (2014), pp. 309–17; among others.

11. Harvey, D., *A Brief History of Neoliberalism* (NY: OUP, 2005).

12. Ibid., p. 64.

13. Ganti, Tejaswini, "Neoliberalism." *Annual Review of Anthropology* 43/1 (2014), pp. 89– 104, p. 89.

14. Steger, Manfred B., and Ravi K. Roy, *Neoliberalism: a Very Short Introduction* (Oxford: OUP, 2010).

15. Ibid.

16. Ruckert, Arne, Laura Macdonald, and Kristina R. Proulx, "Post-Neoliberalism in Latin America: A Conceptual Review". *Third World Quarterly* 38/7 (2016), pp. 1583-1602.

17. Ibid.

18. Guidry, John A., "Not Just Another Labor Party: The Workers' Party and Democracy In Brazil". *Labor Studies Journal* 28/1 (2003), pp. 83-108; Fortes, A., and John D. French, "'Another World Is Possible': The Rise of the Brazilian Workers' Party and the Prospects for Lula's Government". *Labor: Studies in Working-Class History of the Americas* 2/3 (2005), pp. 13-31.

19. Ruckert and Proulx., "Post-Neoliberalism in Latin America: A Conceptual Review".

20. Harvey (see note 11).

21. Hunter, Wendy, and Timothy J. Power, "Bolsonaro and Brazil's Illiberal Backlash". *Journal of Democracy* 30/1 (2019), pp. 68-82.

22. Santana, Joana Valente, Cristiane Bonfim Fernandez, and Benedito de Jesus Pinheiro Ferreira, "Neoliberalism, Reduction of Social Rights, and Social Services in Brazil". *Journal of Human Rights and Social Work* 3/3 (2018), pp. 128-137.

23. See Napolitano, Marcos, "The Brazilian Military Regime, 1964–1985". *Oxford Research Encyclopedia ofLatin American History*, 2018. Available at https://doi.org/10.1093/acrefore/9780199366439.013.413.

24. O'Donnell, Guillermo, "Challenges to Democratization in Brazil". *World Policy Journal* 5/2 (2020), pp. 281-300.

25. Skidmore, Thomas E., *Brazil: Five Centuries of Change* (NY: OUP, 2009).

26. Possenti, Sírio. "Misogyny as a Condition of the 2016 Coup in Brazil". *Discurso & Sociedad* 12/3 (2020), pp. 581-593.

27. Braz, Marcelo, "The coup in democratic illusions and the rise of reactionary conservatism." *Serv. Soc. Soc.* 128 (2017), pp. 85-103.

28. Santana, Carlos Henrique Vieira, "The Geopolitics of the Brazilian Coup D'état and its Consequences". *Transcience* 9/1 (2018), pp. 75-110.

29. Bogliolo, Luís, "Law, Neoliberal Authoritarianism, and the Brazilian Crisis". *TWAIL Review* 7 (2019), pp. 1-9.

30. Cowan, Benjamin Arthur, "A Hemispheric Moral Majority: Brazil and the Transnational Construction of the New Right". *Revista Brasileira de Política Internacional* 61/2 (2018), pp. 125.

31. Cioccari, Deysi, and Simonetta Persichetti, "Armas, Ódio, Medo e Espetáculo em Jair Bolsonaro (Guns, Hatred, Fear and Spectacle in Jair Bolsonaro)". *Revista Alterjor* 18/2 (2018), pp. 201-214.

32. Chagas-Bastos, Fabrício H. "Political Realignment in Brazil: Jair Bolsonaro and the Right Turn". *Revista de Estudios Sociales* 69 (2019), pp. 92-100.

33. Souza, Marcelo Lopes de, "The Land of the Past? Neo-Populism, Neo-Fascism, and the Failure of the Left in Brazil". *Political Geography* Online first (2020), 1-2. Available at https://doi.org/10.1016/j.polgeo.2020.102186.

34. Sovik, Liv, "Brazil, now." *Soundings: A journal of politics and culture* 71/71 (2019), pp. 140-159.

35. Hunter and Power (see note 21).

36. Human Rights Watch, "Brazil: Events of 2019" (2020).

37. Ibid.

38. Human Rights Watch, "Brazil: Bolsonaro Sabotages Anti-COVID-19 Efforts" (April 10, 2020). Available at https://www.hrw.org/news/2020/04/10/brazil-bolsonaro-sabotages-antiCOVID-19-efforts.

39. Yamin, Alicia Ely, and Roojin Habibi, "Human Rights and Coronavirus: What's at Stake for Truth, Trust, and Democracy?". *Health and Human Rights Journal* (2020). Available at https://www.hhrjournal.org/2020/03/human-rights-and-corona-virus-whats-at-stake-for-truthtrust-and-democracy/.

40. Ponta, Adina, "Human Rights Law in the Time of the Coronavirus". *American Society of International Law Insights* 24/5 (2020). Available at https://www.asil.org/insights/volume/24/issue/5/human-rights-law-time-coronavirus.

41. Bravo, Maria Inês Souza, Elaine Junger Pelaez, and Juliana Souza Bravo de Menezes, "Health in Temer and Bolsonaro Governments: Struggles and Resistances". *SER Social* 22/46 (2020), pp. 191-209.

42. Massuda, Adriano *et al.*, "The Brazilian Health System at Crossroads: Progress, Crisis and Resilience". *BMJ Global Health* 3/4 (2018), pp. 1-8.

43. Jurberg, Claudia, "Flawed but fair: Brazil's health system reaches out to the poor". *Bulletin of the World Health Organization* 86/4 (2008), pp. 248-249.

44. Bohoslavsky, Juan Pablo, and Philip Alston, "COVID-19: Brazil's irresponsible economic and social policies put millions of lives at risk, UN experts say" (2020).

45. Ibid. Our italics.

46. Pinto, Ana Estela de Sousa, "Brazil Has the Highest Rate of Coronavirus Contagion in the World, Says Study". *Folha de S.Paulo* (April 30, 2020). Available at https://www1.folha.uol.com.br/internacional/en/scienceandhealth/2020/04/brazil-has-thehighest-rate-of-coronavirus-contagion-in-the-world-says-study.shtml.

47. Elsland, Sabine L. van, and Ryan O'Hare, "Coronavirus pandemic could have caused 40 million deaths if left unchecked". *Imperial College London News* (March 26, 2020). Available at https://www.imperial.ac.uk/news/196496/coronavirus-pandemic-could-have-caused-40/.

48. Raquel Martins Lana et al., "The novel coronavirus (SARS-CoV-2) emergency and the role of timely and effective national health surveillance". *Reports in Public Health* 36/3 (2020), pp. 15.

49. Human Rights Watch (see note 38), para. 11.

50. Julio Croda et al., "COVID-19 in Brazil: advantages of a socialized unified health system and preparation to contain cases", *Revista da Sociedade Brasileira de Medicina Tropical* 53 (April 2020), pp. 1-6.

51. Ibid.

52. Presidência da República, LEI Nº 13.979, DE 6 DE FEVEREIRO DE 2020: Dispõe sobre as medidas para enfrentamento da emergência de saúde pública de importância internacional decorrente do coronavírus responsável pelo surto de 2019 [Brazil's legislation on measures to combat the threat represented by the new coronavirus]. (Brasília: Presidência da República, 2020). 53 Lana et al. (see note 48).

53. Deisy de Freitas Lima Ventura, Fernando Mussa Abujamra Aith and Danielle Hanna

54. Rached, "The emergency of the new coronavirus and the "quarantine law" in Brazil", *Direito & Práxis* Ahead of Print (2020), pp. 1-36. Available at https://www.e-publicacoes.uerj.br/index.php/revistaceaju/article/view/49180.p. 30

55. Folha de S.Paulo (Editorial), "Brazil Confirms First Coronavirus Case", *Folha de S.Paulo*, (Feb 26, 2020). Available at https://www1.folha.uol.com.br/internacional/en/scienceandhealth/2020/02/brazil-confirms-firstcoronavirus-case.shtml.

56. Silva, Antônio Augusto Moura da, "On the possibility of interrupting the coronavirus (COVID-19) epidemic based on the best available scientific evidence". *Revista Brasileira de Epidemiologia* 23 (2020), pp. 1-3.

57. MoH, "Ministério da Saúde declara transmissão comunitária nacional [Ministry of Health declares national sustained transmission]." *Agência Saúde* (March 20, 2020).

58. Shalders, André, "Coronavírus: quem pode decidir sobre a quarentena dos brasileiros: Bolsonaro ou governadores? [Coronavirus: who can decide about the quarantine of Brazilians: Bolsonaro or the governors?]". *BBC News Brasil* (March 26, 2020). https://www.bbc.com/portuguese/brasil-52044708.

59. Ibid.

60. Kalil, Isabela, and R. Marie Santini, "Coronavírus, Pandemia, Infodemia e Política. [Coronavirus, Pandemic, Infodemic and Politics]" FESPSP/UFRJ (April 2020).

61. Notícias STF (Editorial), "Ministro suspende veiculação de campanha contra medidas de distanciamento social [Supreme Court justice suspends campaign against social distancing measures]". *Notícias STF* (March 31, 2020).

62. BBC News (Editorial). "Coronavirus: Brazil's Bolsonaro joins anti-lockdown protests". *BBC News* (April 20, 2020).

63. Fishman, Andrew, "Brazil's Jair Bolsonaro, the world's most powerful coronavirus denier, just fired the health minister who disagreed with him". *The Intercept* (April 16, 2020

64. Phillips, Tom, "'So what?': Bolsonaro shrugs off brazil's rising coronavirus death toll". *The Guardian* (April 29, 2020).

65. Phillips, Dom, "Brazil Loses Second Health Minister in Less than a Month as COVID-19 Deaths Rise". *The Guardian* (May 15, 2020). Available at https://www.theguardian.com/world/2020/may/15/brazil-health-minister-nelson-teich-resigns.

66. Reuters (Editorial), "Bolsonaro Says Brazil to Issue New Chloroquine Protocol on Wednesday". *Reuters* (May 19, 2020). https://www.reuters.com/article/us-health-coronavirusbrazil-bolsonaro/bolsonaro-says-brazil-to-issue-new-chloro-quine-protocol-on-wednesdayidUSKBN22V39L.

67. United Nations, "COVID-19 and Human Rights: We are all in this together" (April 2020).

68. Ibid.

69. Christenson, Gordon A., "Attributing Acts of Omission to the State". *Michigan Journal of International Law* 12, no. 2 (1991), pp. 312-370.

70. Soto, Marcela Barón, and Alejandro Gómez Velásquez, "An Approach to the State Responsibility by an Omission in the Inter–American Court of Human Rights Jurisprudence". *Revista CES Derecho* 6, no. 1 (2015), pp. 3-17, p. 8.

71. Presidência da República, MEDIDA PROVISÓRIA Nº 966, DE 13 DE MAIO DE 2020: Dispõe sobre a responsabilização de agentes públicos por ação e omissão em atos relacionados com a pandemia da COVID-19 [Brazilian Provisional Measure on responsibilities of public agents in the COVID-19 pandemic] (Brasília: Presidência da República, 2020).

72. Achille Mbembe, *Necropolitics* (Durham: Duke University Press, 2019).

73. Ibid.

74. Lee, Christopher J., "The Necropolitics of COVID-19". *Africa is a Country* (April 2020). Available at https://africasacoun-try.com/2020/04/the-necropolitics-of-COVID-19, para. 4.

75. Ibid.

76. World Vision (Editorial). "COVID-19 Threatens to Decimate Most Vulnerable Groups in Brazil". *World Vision International* (May 2020).

77. See: Regional Risk Communication and Community Engagement (RCCE) Working Group, "COVID-19: How to include marginalized and vulnerable people in risk communication and community engagement" (2020). Available at https://re-liefweb.int/sites/reliefweb.int/files/resources/COVID19_CommunityEngagement_130320.pdf.

78. Gefaell, Clara Valverde. *De la necropolítica neoliberal a la empatía radical [From neoliberal necropolitics to radical empathy]* (Barcelona: Icaria, 2015).

79. Phillips, Dom, "Brazil: largest rise in COVID-19 deaths follows Bolsonaro 'worst is over' claim". *The Guardian* (May 6, 2020). Available at https://www.theguardian.com/world/2020/may/06/brazil-coronavirus-deaths-COVID-19bolsonaro.

2. Political Struggles for A Universal Health System In Brazil: Successes and Limits in Reducing Inequalities [1]

Cristiani Vieira Machado[1*] and Gulnar Azevedo e Silva[2]

ABSTRACT

Background: Brazil is a population of high/middle-income country, characterized by deep economic and social inequalities. Like most other Latin American nations, Brazil constructed a health system that included, on the one hand, public health programs and, on the other, social insurance healthcare for those working in the formal sector. This study analyses the political struggles surrounding the implementation of a universal health system from the mid-1980s to the present, and their effects on health indicators, that focus on the relevant international and national contexts, political agendas, government orientations and actors. **Main text:** In the 1980s, against the backdrop of economic crisis and democratization, Brazil's health reform movement proposed a Unified Health System (SUS), which was incorporated into the 1988 Constitution. The combination of a democratic system with opportunities for interaction between various developmental and social agendas and actors has played a key role in shaping health policy since then. However, the expansion of public services has been hampered by insufficient public funding and by the strengthening of the private sector, subsidized by the state. Private enterprises have expanded their markets and political influence, in a process that has accelerated in recent years. Despite these obstacles, SUS has produced significant health-status improvements and some reductions in Brazil's vast health inequalities.

Conclusions: We found that a combination of long-term structural and contingent factors, international agendas and interests, as well as domestic political struggles, explains the advances and obstacles to building a universal system in an economically important yet unequal peripheral country. Further consolidation of SUS and reduction of health inequalities hinge on the uncertain prospects for democracy and national development, on enlarging the political coalition to support a public and universal health system, and on strengthening the state's ability to regulate the private sector.

BACKGROUND

Brazil is a territorially vast, populous, high/medium-income federal republic in the periphery of global capitalism, widely recognized as one of the world's most unequal countries. Its economic and social inequalities are evident in epidemiological data, access to and outcomes from the health system, across regions and demographic groups [1].

Like other Latin American countries, Brazil's health system during most of the twentieth century was characterized by public health programs that focused on the control of specific infectious diseases, combined with medical assistance services intended for urban workers in the formal

---

[1] Machado and Silva Globalization and Health 2019, 15(Suppl 1):77

sector, according to a logic of social insurance. Between the 1930s and 1980s, the country underwent a process of state-induced industrialization that emphasized import substitution, and an accompanying process of rapid urbanization. Significant demographic changes occurred, due to declining mortality and fertility and increasing life expectancy.

Health indices showed an epidemiological transition characterized by a rise in cardiovascular illnesses, cancer diseases, and external causes (violence and accidents), accompanied by the persistence of older infectious diseases (tuberculosis, Hansen's disease) and the emergence of others [2].The expansion of pension systems and access to public health services took place mainly under authoritarian governments, with limited social participation. From the 1960s, there were increasing state incentives for the private sector, with a strengthening of the corporate health-care industry over the ensuing decades.

This occurred both through the contracting of private health services mainly hospitals by social insurance institutions and through fiscal incentives for businesses to offer private health plans to their employees [3, 4] Amidst economic crisis and democratization in the 1980s, Brazil underwent a process of healthcare reform that culminated in the recognition of health care as a right of citizenship and the creation of the public, universal Unified Health System (SUS) enshrined in the Constitution of 1988. This system was to be tax-funded, comprehensive and universally accessible to all Brazilians, free of charge, regardless of their economic or social status. Brazil was the only Latin American country to propose a universalistic health reform in the 1980s, but implementation proved difficult in the following decades. What political factors led to the introduction of a universal health system in Brazil, in contrast to the predominant neoliberal international trends in healthcare reform elsewhere in Latin America?

In the face of a strong private sector, which were the political forces that supported or resisted making SUS a truly universal system over the following decades? In a context of deep social inequalities, has SUS served to reduce health inequalities? This paper analyses the political struggles over the implementation of a universal health system since the mid-1980s and their effects on selected health indicators in Brazil, during three decades of democratic rule. While recognizing the importance of the structural determinants of health policies, it focuses on the political factors (actors, agendas, power relations, interests) that enable or pose limits to ensuring health as a right of citizenship in a populous, middle-income and unequal Latin American country.

The policy analysis comprises three moments democratic transition and healthcare reform (1985–1989); the political struggle over SUS in the democratic period (1990–2015); and political crisis, democratic instability, and threats to SUS (2016–2018). Finally, we present some selected health indicators and discuss the achievements and limits in building a universal health system in Brazil.

Democratic transition and healthcare reform (1985–1989) Starting in the late 1970s and early 1980s, the international debate surrounding the crisis of the nation-state and the neoliberal agenda began to reverberate in Latin America. Some countries, like Mexico and Chile, were influenced by early neoliberal economic reforms, also with effects on their health policies [5].

While other countries in the region were moving toward a neoliberal model, Brazil took a somewhat different path. During these years, it experienced a serious economic crisis, criticisms of the model of import substitution industrialization (ISI), and a movement toward democratization after nearly two decades of military dictatorship. Brazil also experienced intense social mobilization in favour of progressive reforms. It was in this context that the movement for healthcare reform emerged, seeking to transform a health system that was segmented, fragmented, inefficient, and oriented toward privileging the private sector while excluding most of the population.

The healthcare movement brought together various groups seeking to construct an agenda for reform of this sector. Key groups involved included academics at university departments of preventive medicine or public health, administrators, and experts from the federal Ministry of Health and from the health bodies connected to the Ministry of Social Security, and health professionals, among others. These years also witnessed the formation of the Brazilian Centre for Health Studies (CEBES), the Brazilian Postgraduate Association in Collective Health (ABRASCO), and national councils of state and municipal secretaries of health.

These healthcare professionals joined with other social movements, including community-based movements associated with the Catholic Church and progressive politicians to construct a reform agenda [6, 7]. Successful experiences with reorganizing health care systems at the local level, along with the presence of progressive public health officials in national posts, set the stage for gradual transformations in healthcare institutions, even as a national reform agenda was created, based on the recognition of health as a right of citizenship. During a 1979 symposium in the Chamber of Deputies (the lower house of Congress), CEBES presented a paper focusing on the relationship between democracy and health [8].

After nearly two decades, gubernatorial elections were held in 1982, and elections for mayors of state capitals and cities designated as "national security" zones in 1985. Also, in 1985, Congress indirectly elected the first civilian president since 1964. With the death of the President-elect before his inauguration, the Vice President-elect took office and assembled a broad coalition government.

In 1986 the Eighth National Health Conference brought together over 4000 participants from across the country academics, administrators, health professionals, social movements, and ordinary citizens who advocated for the strengthening of the public system and for the designation of health as a right. The conference led to the formation of the National Committee for Health Care Reform, which elaborated a reform proposal that was presented to the 1987–1988 National Constitutional Convention. Brazil already had an important private health sector, with private hospitals contracted by public social security institutions, as well as a growing sector of private health insurance plans. These groups pressured legislators to avoid proposals that could result in a radical shift toward state control and the imposition of constraints on the private sector [9].

The 1988 Constitution recognized health as a universal right that the state was required to provide, guaranteed by broad social and economic policies. It also institutionalized the concept of "social security" comprising health, pensions, and social assistance and the Unified Health System (SUS), a public, universal system intended to ensure comprehensive health care for the population.

The Constitution affirmed the complementarity of the private sector, with priority for philanthropic and non-profit institutions. It also stated that health care would be "open for private investment," thus retaining openings for expansion of the private system, even as it failed to address important questions regarding public financing of healthcare. The global transformations of the 1970s and 1980s affected Brazil, with implications both economic (economic crisis, the exhaustion of ISI) and political (democratization). However, the national context better explains social changes, including in health care.

The international agenda of neoliberal reforms did not have the same impact on Brazil in the 1980s as elsewhere in Latin America. The temporal sequence of two processes democratization and economic liberalization and the promulgation of a comprehensive Constitution served to shield Brazilian social policies from the neoliberal reforms: they would begin later, in a less aggressive and more pragmatic form [10]. The return to democracy in the 1980s created an atmosphere conducive to mobilization for universal healthcare reform, with the support of state and local governments and legislators. The inauguration of a civilian president and the calling of a National Constitutional

Assembly, amidst a climate of intense debates over the future of the country, played a significant role in enabling the creation of SUS, a system inspired by the experiences of other countries, like the United Kingdom's National Health Service (NHS) and Italy's healthcare reform. On the other hand, several key political actors were not on board with the SUS agenda. For example, the businesspeople who controlled the private sector sought to protect their market share. The labour movement expressed inconsistent positions regarding the conflict between weakening workers' access to healthcare and universalizing the system; they also lobbied employers to provide private plans. For their part, although medical doctors rarely oppose SUS directly, and the organizations representing them espoused a range of positions, their responses to its agenda were motivated primarily by their collective professional interests. Over the following decades, these conflicts of interests and projects would surface forcefully. Two aspects restrictions on public financing, and the nature of public private healthcare relations emerged with the difficulties in constructing a universal public system capable of helping to overcome the fragmentation of the system and reduce healthcare inequalities.

Political Struggle Over SUS in The Democratic Period (1990–2015)

Like other Latin American countries in the 1990s Brazil adopted neoliberal reforms that involved economic opening, the reining-in of public spending, reduction of the size of the state apparatus, and privatizations of state enterprises. This agenda was launched by the liberal government of Fernando Collor (1990–1992). It slowed down under the transitional government of Itamar Franco (1992–1994), who took office after Collor resigned amidst a process of impeachment; and was taken up again, with new contours, during the two terms of Fernando Henrique Cardoso (1995–1998; 1999–2002).

Also influential in Latin America were healthcare reform proposals promoted by international agencies, among them the World Bank [11]. Their recommendations included the separation of funding from the provision of services; the establishment of cost-effective basic service packages; and focusing state action on the poorest citizens. In Brazil, the struggle for the creation of SUS, combined with the constitutional guarantee of health as a right, prevented the direct adoption of specific World Bank health proposals. However, the subsequent trajectory of health policy made clear the inherent tensions between a free, universal healthcare system like SUS and state-driven market reforms. The former was promoted mainly by the public health system and civil society actors; the latter was defended by government economic authorities (Ministers of Finance and Planning and Budget) and by the owners of private health enterprises, wishing to expand their share of the market. Among those advocating the expansion of the public system, a coalition coalesced around the development of a legal-institutional framework, which, in addition to the broad principles of universality and comprehensive care, envisioned federative cooperation and social participation in policy-making.

Intergovernmental health commissions were formed at the national and state levels to negotiate the decentralization of power and allocation of resources to state and local governments.

In addition, Brazil created health councils at the federal, state (26 states plus the Federal District), and local (over 5000 municipalities) levels that included administrators, providers, professionals, and users of the system.

Decentralization, the health councils, and the expansion of public services increased the number of actors with a stake in defending SUS—administrators and experts from all three levels of government, social movements, and users. Also important were the social groups, at times working with international actors, that came together to propose specific policies based on the SUS principles of universal coverage and comprehensive care. For example, mental healthcare reformers emphasized the implementation of innovative services and programs, such as the expansion of Psychosocial Community Centres and the Return Home program to deinstitutionalize long-stay patients. Their attempts at asylum closure clashed with the interests of private providers [12]. Another example was the policy offering comprehensive care to people with HIV/AIDS, with a focus on prevention and providing new treatments that were emerging in the 1990s. Collaboration involving civil society, experts, healthcare professionals, and the judicial system was central to the development of a policy that guaranteed access to treatment. By ensuring public access to expensive drugs protected by patents, Brazil's HIV/AIDS policy put the country in the spotlight of global debates and negotiations on intellectual property and the right to health in developing countries [13].

A third example concerned policies related to the control of tobacco, in which Brazil took a pioneering role through a series of initiatives in the 1990s to regulate advertising and use. These initiatives placed Brazil at the forefront of international discussions surrounding the formation of the UN Framework Convention on Tobacco Control, established in 2003 [14]. Yet another innovative policy that gained international recognition was the Family Health Program initiated in 1994, noteworthy for its emphasis on primary care and the way it brought together a range of actors in support of expanding access and changes to the healthcare model. The program was designed in accordance with the core SUS principles of universality and comprehensiveness, further expanded with incremental innovations under various governments. Ultimately, it came to cover much of the country over the next two decades, gaining international recognition for its comprehensiveness and cost-effectiveness [15].

However, implementation of a universal system in Brazil was rendered difficult due to the market-oriented reform agenda adopted by the federal government and various states, which imposed restrictions on public funding and the expansion in the healthcare professionals and supplies needed for a public, universal healthcare system. The struggle to stabilize and increase public funding mobilized actors from across the healthcare system—federal health ministers, state and health secretaries, healthcare professionals, groups of users— throughout the decade. Attempts to create a specific tax on financial transactions in 1996 and a constitutional amendment (approved only in 2000) helped to stabilize the system. but were not enough to guarantee a meaningful increase in state support for healthcare.

Thus, from the beginning, the expansion of SUS services and coverage took place under adverse financial conditions. The system remained dependent on contracting private services, which continued to play an important role in hospital, diagnostic, and therapeutic services. New public–private linkages appeared, such as outsourcing and the contracting of "social organizations" to provide certain services within public facilities—first in hospitals, then in specialized clinics, and eventually even in primary healthcare services. The boundaries between public and private spheres became less clear, favouring the transfer of resources from the state to the private services and organizations.

The private insurance sector continued to grow, lobbying governments for its own interests. In keeping with other attempts at regulation by the Ministry of Health, in 1998 Congress passed a Health Insurance Plan Law, and in 2000 a national agency was created to regulate private health plans [16].In the 2000s, several important countries in Latin America experienced a political "left turn," [17], stemming, in part, from widespread dissatisfaction with the effects of the neoliberal reforms of the preceding decades. Progressive governments implemented policies expanding the state's role in the economic and social realms, achieving reductions in inequality. By the middle of the decade, the commodities boom had come to play an important role in contributing to such policies, but they were also a result of the political orientation of Latin American governments.

The "left turn" came to Brazil in 2002, with the election to the presidency of Luis Inácio Lula da Silva, a former metal workers' union leader and founder of the Workers' Party (PT).

During Lula's two terms (2003– 2006; 2007–2010), economic tensions persisted between the promotion of austerity and attempts to resume a developmentalist agenda, especially during the second term. These tensions were exacerbated during the government of his successor, also from the PT, Brazil's first female president, Dilma Rousseff (2011–2014; 2015–May 2016). She had to govern in a less favourable economic context, with the end of the commodities boom, and in the face of formidable political opposition, which culminated in her impeachment and removal from office in 2016, charged with utilizing illegal budgetary measures. The labour policy of the PT governments focused on attempts to formalize labour relations and increase the real value of the minimum wage. Changes in foreign policy prioritized creating a new international geopolitical alignment, with an emphasis on South–South cooperation with South American and African countries, also in healthcare.

In social policy, the Lula and Dilma presidencies expanded conditional cash-transfer programs, in keeping with the poverty-fighting agenda across Latin America. They also worked to expand rights for socially vulnerable groups (women, Afro-Brazilians, LGBTIQ+ people, indigenous people, and rural communities descended from escaped enslaved people). Their education policy features the expansion of access to federal and private universities, with publicly-funded scholarships. The link between economic and social policy stimulated a certain dynamization of the internal market and helped reduce poverty and income inequalities, although they remained high. The commodities boom during Lula's second term enabled the expansion of social investment and reduction in inequality to occur with only limited resistance.

Even amidst the global economic recession of 2009, social spending in Brazil exhibited counter-cyclical behaviour. Especially during Lula's second term, the focus on "social-developmentalism" manifested itself in healthcare policy, through debates on the relation between healthcare and development, and initiatives to incentivize the domestic production of medication and medical supplies, both outlined in SUS priorities. Under the Lula and Dilma governments, new health programs were created, along with incremental policy innovations that enabled the expansion of access in areas like oral health, urgent care, access to medication, without particularly radical changes.

Noteworthy was the progressive increase of primary-care coverage, through the 1994 Family Health Strategy, along with the incorporation of other healthcare professionals to the network of primary-care teams of doctors, nursing professionals, and community health workers [18].

The coalition of actors defending SUS remained the same—administrators from all three levels of government, experts, and professionals, allied with groups of users and members of the judicial system. A caveat is in order concerning doctors, who usually practice in both the public and private systems. Throughout the period studied here, doctors joined together to defend their collective interests career, autonomy, remuneration whether engaged in dialogue with public authorities or in their negotiations with private providers and healthcare corporations.

Under Dilma's government, the "More Doctors" program aimed at hiring doctors to practice in poorly-served regions and communities, creating new degree programs in Medicine, and instituting curricular changes unleashed conflicts with the medical profession. The principal reason was the contracting of foreign doctors without requiring that they revalidate their diplomas with the Federal Council of Medicine: this was perceived as showing lack of respect for the principle of professional self-regulation, and as a threat to the labour market for Brazilian doctors. The contracting of Cuban doctors, via an accord mediated by the Pan-American Health Organization [19], encountered particularly strong opposition. Also criticized was the hasty creation of degree programs without adequate quality control. Regarding public funding, there was significant mobilization throughout this period. During Dilma's government, the "Health Plus 10" movement sought to ensure that 10% of gross federal tax revenues would be reserved for healthcare. However, the legislative measures for funding healthcare were inadequate, and the difficulties with funding the public system remained. The private sector continued to expand dynamically, diversifying its economic and political strategies.

The process of financialization accelerated, via business mergers, new financial market strategies, and the growing penetration by foreign corporations of Brazilian markets [20], despite constitutional restrictions on foreign capital in this field. In the political realm, healthcare corporations reorganized themselves, with new representative organizations, heightened lobbying of Congress, and financial contributions to executive and legislative electoral campaigns.

The state agency created in 2000 to regulate private health plans has focused on regulating contracts, systematizing information, and organizing the market—but never on restricting the growth of the private sector. To the contrary, it has frequently had directors from the very sector they are supposed to regulate. In December 2014, two months after elections that brought a second term for Dilma Rousseff, the President issued an executive order authorizing the entry of foreign capital in the field of healthcare, including service provision, which was prohibited by the 1988 Constitution. Despite protests from various pro-SUS organizations which held that this was unconstitutional, in 2015 Congress passed the executive order into law. This legal change led to an expansion in the role of foreign healthcare corporations in Brazil and their subsequent alliance with the large philanthropic hospitals and agencies seeking to regulate private healthcare plans.

This constituted yet another of the growing concessions the President made to the corporate sector, in the face of congressional opposition due to decreasing economic growth and overall lack of governability. In summary, various policy agendas and actors influenced Brazil's health policy between 1990 and 2015. The political coalition in defence of SUS involved mainly sectoral actors, health authorities, officials, professionals and academics that became more diversified as the public services were expanded; new actors also became relevant, with some public prosecutors and new social movements. On the other hand, each Presidential coalition in this period involved alliances with conservative groups, and the economic authorities favoured market-oriented reforms that were detrimental to SUS expansion and funding. Health enterprises became more dynamic and international, and intensified political lobbying. Finally, unions and doctors' organizations tended to focus on their specific group interests.

Political Crisis, Democratic Instability, And Threats To SUS (2016–2018)

Throughout 2015, the political crisis in Brazil intensified, aggravated by a national economic crisis. The Vice President, Michel Temer, engineered the impeachment of President Rousseff and launched a neoliberal reform package to placate the "markets." With the support of corporate elites, politicians, and the media, the process culminated in Rousseff's suspension from the presidency in May 2016, following controversial accusations of illegal budgetary measures—and her definitive removal from office by the Senate in August 2016. A new era began for Brazil, one in which new political actors took centre stage, with threats to social policy, the healthcare system, and democracy itself. The impeachment has been called a "parliamentary coup," supported by the judiciary and the media and aimed at removing the PT from power, after its four consecutive victories in presidential elections [21]. The imprisonment of Lula da Silva in 2018 on allegations of corruption was supported by evidence that was shaky at best, but it succeeded in impeding him from running for President, and in so doing offered more support for the argument that Brazilian democracy is under attack.

Further indications of the fragility of Brazil's democratic pact came with the rapid adoption of a reform agenda that voters had not approved when they voted for Dilma in 2014. Soon after assuming the Presidency, Temer began to implement neoliberal measures, with an emphasis on economic austerity, reduction of the size of the state apparatus, changes to the then-current social pact, and market incentives. Within the executive branch, he promoted a drastic reduction in the number of cabinet ministries by merging some key ministries and abolishing others. Working with Brazil's most conservative Congress in half a century and supported by the corporate elite, Temer signed a labour reform bill which loosened rules regulating labour and restricted worker rights. His government also gained approval of a constitutional amendment that froze social spending for 20 years, except for inflation increases, seriously harming education, social assistance, and healthcare [22]. The shift in the government's orientation was also evident in healthcare policy. Temer selected as his Minister of Health Ricardo Barros, a legislator with ties to private health insurance corporations, who defended austerity and criticized both the constitutional enshrinement of social security and SUS. Barros advocated the expansion of private health plans and created a commission to develop a proposal for "accessible private health plans," that is, low-cost, state-subsidized private plans for low income Brazilians. Accomplishing would have required slacking the requirements of the 1998 Health Insurance Plan Law's minimum operating criteria for private health insurance plans and consumer rights. After some amendments to the proposal, regulatory measures favourable to private healthcare corporations were adopted. Changes were also made to key policies covering, inter alia, primary care and mental health, which specialists have criticized for conflicting with SUS guidelines or representing setbacks to the previous model of healthcare. The sum of the Temer government's economic and social austerity measures 2016–2018 has already brought repercussions for several health indicators, as shown below (Figure 1 and Figure 2).

Universal Health System and Health Inequalities: Achievements and Limits

Since the Constitution of 1988, the recognition of health as a right of citizenship and the struggles for SUS implementation have resulted in important achievements in healthcare access and health status. Moreover, the nationwide expansion of public health programs and health services to new areas and vulnerable social groups has helped to reduce inequalities across regions and among social groups. There was a massive expansion of health care from 1990 to 2017, comprising both public and private facilities. The most remarkable increases were in basic health services (health centres, health posts, family health units), more than 99% of which are public. This has meant improvements in access to publicly provided primary health care. Private practices and polyclinics have also expanded, most of them contracted by private health insurance plans or paid out-of-pocket by clients. As to hospitals, many municipal facilities were opened, but private units are still predominant, most of them providing services exclusively for SUS or for both SUS and the private sector. Diagnosis and therapy support service units are mainly private as well, generally providing services for the private sector or for both the private sector and SUS [23].

All this shows how the public and the private healthcare organizations and services in Brazil are deeply interconnected. Expansion of primary healthcare coverage expansion, especially through the Family Health Strategy, has been important nationwide (Fig. 1). This has been more accentuated in economically less-developed regions, particularly among low-income groups [24], with some redistributive effect for federal resources [25]. Many positive outcomes of SUS have been reported, including progressive increases in immunization coverage for a range of diseases and lower rates of preventable hospitalizations [26]. Concerning health status, several studies have noted how SUS has promoted positive health results.

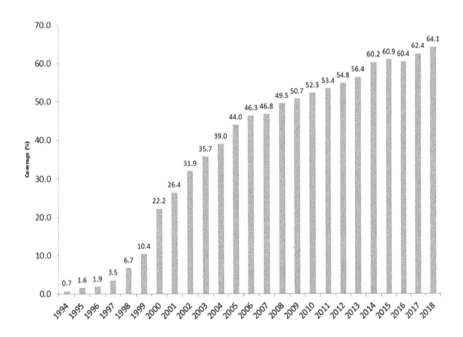

Coverage (%) of Family Health Strategy: Brazil, 1994–2018. Source: Elaborated by the authors. Data from: Basic Health Care Department, Ministry of Health, Brazil (DAB/SAS/MS). From 2002 to 2018. Data available at: http://sage.saude.gov.br/#. Accessed: 07 Set 2019

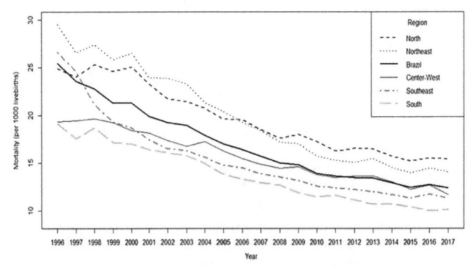

Infant mortality trends: Brazil and its regions, 1996–2017. Source: Elaborated by the authors. Data from: Brazil, Ministry of Health: http://datasus.saude.gov.br/informacoes-de-saude/tabnet/estatisticas-vitais. Accessed 15 Oct 2018

These include decreases in overall mortality rates, in infant and child morbidity and mortality, in maternal mortality [27], in mortality due to infectious diseases (especially vaccine-preventable diseases, diarrhoea, and respiratory infections) [28], and even in mortality due to some cardiovascular and chronic respiratory diseases [29]. These impressive results can be attributed, in part, to specific programs implemented during the period under study here. For instance, child malnutrition fell sharply; the prevalence of smoking among adults dropped from around 35% in 1989 to 15% in 2012 due to tobacco-control policies; and the incidence of HIV infection has fallen, although recent trends may be worrisome [29]. Similarly, decreases have been reported in inequalities in many health indicators across regions and states. Many of the states that presented the worst mortality indicators in 1990—especially those from the Northeast region—experienced the most significant improvements. For instance, regarding mortality rates for children under five years, the gap between the states with the highest and the lowest levels was almost halved—from a 4.9-fold difference to a 2.5-fold one between 1990 and 2015 [29]. There was an important decline in infant mortality rates across all regions between 1996 and 2015, but most prominently in the Northeast. Then, however, in the wake of the economic recession and the impeachment of Rousseff in 2016, infant mortality rates increased in all regions of the country, except for the highly developed South (Fig. 2). From 1996 to 2015 infant mortality was statically descendent in Brazil as a whole (β = − 0.65, p < 0.001) and in all the five regions, varying from Centre-West (β = − 0.41 p < 0.001) to Northeast Region (β = − 0.83, p < 0.001). In 2016 there was a minor increase (from 12.4 to 12.7 per 1000 live births overall), with the greatest increases occurring in the Northeast and Centre-West regions (3.4 and 3.6%, respectively). Again, the sole exception was in the South region, where infant mortality rates continued to fall. Many deaths in 2016 occurred during the post neonatal period (after the first 28 days of life), with diarrhoea as the primary cause [30]. In 2017 the rates tended to remain stable with exception of Centre-West, where there was a clear decrease. These oscillations in infant mortality trends may indicate that living standards in the country are falling, particularly among the poor, who have been severely affected by the austerity measures implemented since 2016. Also, other sensitive health indicators have shown a recent increase: for example, violence-related mortality in the 15–24 age range [30].

A recent micro-simulation study compared projections of under-five child mortality rates in two different scenarios. The first assumed reductions in the coverage of Bolsa Família (Brazil's conditional cash transfer social welfare program) and the Family Health program due to fiscal austerity; the second scenario hypothesized the maintenance of existing levels of social protection. The authors concluded that the implementation of fiscal austerity measures in Brazil could be held responsible for substantively higher childhood morbidity and mortality [31]. Regarding life expectancy, although a significant decrease occurred during this period, there was considerable variation among geographic regions. In 2013, life expectancy at birth for children born in the richest regions was 76.9 years, as against 71.5 in the least developed regions [32].

In summary, due in part to the implementation of SUS, Brazil witnessed important health advances, which can still be observed across regions and socioeconomic categories. However, the highest rates of illness are still found in the North and Northeast regions, the country's poorest [33]. Further progress in reducing health inequalities has been obstructed by structural inequities, as well as political decisions that have limited the reach of public funding and promoted the increase of private sector involvement. As Fig. 3 shows, although total health expenditures as a proportion of GDP increased from 1995 to 2015, private expenditures remained above 50% of total expenditures throughout the period. The greatest proportion of expenditure on private healthcare concerns payments for private insurance plans, which increased during this period. By 2017, close to one-fourth of Brazil's population—over 47 million people—was covered by private plans, although with regional variations, as shown in Fig. 4. With expansion of SUS and the private insurance sector, out-of-pocket expenditures fell, but remained high, particularly for prescription drugs.

DISCUSSION

The construction of a universal health system in Brazil over the past three decades has been unique in Latin America. The country's universalist health reform began in the 1980s, as other national health systems were suffering the effects of neoliberal reforms.

Democratization created an environment in which political actors dedicated to the defence of health as a citizenship right managed to occupy strategic spaces, from which they influenced policy as well as the 1988 Constitution. In the ensuing decades, under democratic governments, political struggles over a universal health system facilitated the expansion of the public system, with subsequent improvements in health outcomes and some reduction in regional inequalities, when assessed by selected health indicators. Nevertheless, Brazil still has severe health inequalities [34], due to in part to structural factors, such as the country's position in the global economy, its own historical particularities, and the characteristics of its systems of social protection and healthcare.

However, political variables must also be taken into consideration in explaining the persistence of social inequalities that manifest themselves strongly in the area of health. In their comparative study of Latin American social policies, Huber and Stephens [35] have shown that democracy was an important factor in explaining the redistributive or non-redistributive nature of social policies. They argue, however, that in the case of Latin America time does matter: longer periods of democratic stability are necessary—estimated at 20–25 years, at a minimum—to identify clearly the effects of social policies on the reduction of inequalities. This occurs, they explain, because democratic stability is a fundamental requirement for new social groups to gain access to power.

These groups, through representation or direct participation, are able to influence social policies not merely by expanding them, but by promoting policies aimed at reducing the gaps between rich and poor across various dimensions. Our examination of the case of the Brazilian health system corroborates Huber and Stephens' argument. The return to democracy proved fundamental in mobilizing societal actors in defence of the constitutional recognition of health as a right, as well for the construction of an institutional framework for SUS.

The period of democratic stability between 1988 and 2015 facilitated the expansion of universalist health policies and services, improvements in health conditions and even some reduction in health inequalities, as has been internationally recognized [34].

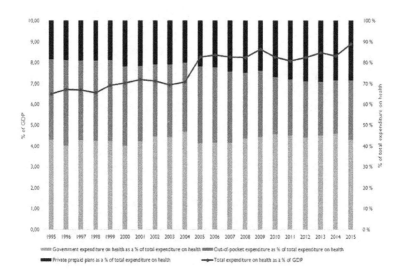

Health expenditures as % of GDP and public–private participation. Brazil, 1995–2015. Source: Elaborated by the authors. Data from World Health Organization. Global Health Observatory. Data Repository. Available at: http://apps.who.int/gho/data/ node.home. Accessed: Oct 2018

This period was also marked by moments of economic crisis, reductions in public spending, and measures aimed at facilitating expansion of the private healthcare market. Still, conflicting agendas and interests notwithstanding, we can note incremental advances in living standards and the reduction of health inequalities. The positive health outcomes registered are also consistent with the findings of a recent observational study which explored the relationships between democratic experience, adult health, and cause-specific mortality in 170 countries, 1980–2016 [36]. Comparing countries with different political regimes, the authors concluded that democracies are more likely than autocracies to lead to health gains for mortality causes requiring healthcare delivery infrastructure, such as cardiovascular diseases and transport injuries. From 2016, the new political climate surrounding the controversial presidential impeachment, supported by a neoconservative, neoliberal coalition, with democracy under threat, made possible the accelerated adoption of economic austerity and regressive social reforms. In only a short time, it was possible to observe worsening social indicators, such as rates of poverty and extreme poverty, along with stagnation in the reduction of social inequalities that had occurred between 1990 and 2014 [37].and resistance to these reforms.

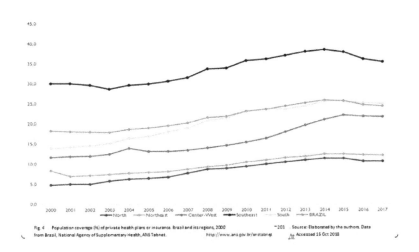

Fig. 4 Population coverage (%) of private health plans or insurance. Brazil and its regions, 2000 – 201 . Source: Elaborated by the authors. Data from Brazil, National Agency of Supplementary Health, ANS Tabnet. http://www.ans.gov.br/anstabnet. Accessed 15 Oct 2018

Population coverage (%) of private health plans or insurance. Brazil and its regions, 2000–2017. Source: Elaborated by the authors. Data from Brazil, National Agency of Supplementary Health, ANS Tabnet. http://www.ans.gov.br/anstabnet/#. Accessed 15 Oct 2018

The second level is that of the health sector itself. The political coalitions that influence health policy have changed: the broad political coalition that defended the right to health in the 1980s, which had included academics, health professionals, bureaucrats, social movements and 'centre' politicians, did not survive. Although the political support to SUS was maintained among health workers, government coalitions involved alliances with conservative sectors and adopted market-oriented reforms detrimental to the public system, and the private health industry became stronger. The adverse post-2016 context exacerbated pre-existing contradictions in the Brazilian health system. The most notable of these was the co-existence of a universal public system with a vigorous and dynamic private sector, which preyed upon SUS by competing with it for state resources and clients, while prioritizing profit. Remedying this situation would require intense social mobilization in defence of the public, universal SUS, and strengthened regulation of the private sector, aimed at containing its growth and subordinating it to the public interest.

In today's unfavourable global political context, with regressive attacks on social protection in various capitalist countries, it is essential to reflect on the possibilities and limits of political agency for the promotion of social welfare [38]. As Deaton has noted, worldwide improvements in health conditions at certain historical moments have not eliminated the immense gaps between or within rich and poor countries [39]. Brazil's health sector was not immune to the adverse political and economic context. Health indicators—such as infant mortality due to preventable causes, like diarrhoea—that had shown continuous improvement since the creation of SUS stagnated or worsened. Although these changes are recent and merit closer study, they would indicate that the advances made possible by SUS have not been entirely sustainable in the face of an adverse economic model.

Over the three decades of SUS implementation, on the heels of a situation characterized by deep poverty and inequality, gradual advances were facilitated by the promulgation of the 1988 Constitution and the intense mobilization of the health sector in support of a universalist agenda, putting pressure on democratically elected governments. Lately, however, with political instability and new threats to the social democratic pact of the 1988 Constitution, Brazil has experienced rapid setbacks that have affected the most vulnerable. Alongside recent developments, it is important to recognize the political struggles over conflicting agendas that occurred throughout the period when SUS was being implemented.

These contradictions manifested themselves most strongly in connection with financing, and the relationship between the public system and private sector. Public financing was never sufficient for achieving the goal of a universal system that would reduce social inequalities. The dynamism of the private sector was a pre-SUS legacy, but also a result of international and domestic health insurance companies adopting new business and lobbying strategies to expand their markets and increase profits. In the relationship between the state and health markets, the incentives granted by the former to the latter predominated, abetted by the weakness of regulatory policies. The political determinants of health inequalities exist on two interrelated levels. The first level concerns the general inequalities of Brazilian society, which, to be modified, would require structural changes in the pattern of development, in turn requiring political consensus on the need to redistribute power and wealth. Such a consensus appears unlikely in the face of the recent rightist consolidation of power: first, after the 2016 impeachment, when Michel Temer assumed the presidency, and then with the 2018 election of the far-right ex-military officer Jair Bolsonaro and an ultraconservative Congress. As of 2019 it seems highly likely that neoliberal policies of economic austerity, combined with continuing uncertainty about the future of Brazilian democracy, will condition the possibilities for social mobilization

CONCLUSIONS

A combination of long-term structural and contingent factors, international agendas and interests, as well as domestic political struggles, can explain the advances and obstacles to building a universal system in Brazil, an economically important yet unequal peripheral country. Democracy and political mobilization were essential to implementation of its Unified Health System (SUS) and consequent improvements in health conditions. However, obstacles to structural change persisted, with sustained effects on health inequalities. Further consolidation of SUS and reduction of health inequalities hinge on the uncertain future of Brazil's democracy and national development project, on enlarging the political coalition to support a public and universal health system, and on strengthening the state's ability to regulate the private sector. This analysis of the Brazilian case shows that reducing health inequalities in the face of the dynamics of the global capitalist economy is a major challenge, and one in which politics plays a defining role.

Abbreviations
ABRASCO: Brazilian Postgraduate Association in Collective Health;
AIDS: Acquired Immune Deficiency Syndrome; CEBES: Brazilian Centre for
Health Studies; HIV: Human Immunodeficiency Virus; ISI: Import Substitution
Industrialization; LGBTIQ+: Lesbian, Gay, Bisexual, Transgender, Intersex and
Queer; NHS: National Health Service; PT: Worker's Party; SUS: Unified Health System; UN: United Nations

Acknowledgements
The authors acknowledge the National Council for Scientific and Technological Development – CNPq-Brazil for funding, and the participants of the conference "The Political Origins of Health Inequities and Universal Health Coverage", organized by The Independent Panel on Global Governance for Health and held in November 2018 in Oslo, Norway.About this supplement

This article has been published as part of Globalization and Health, Volume 15 Supplement 1, 2019: Proceedings from the Conference on Political Determinants of Health Inequities and Universal Health Coverage. The full contents of the supplement are available online at https://globalizationandhealth. biomedcentral.com/articles/supplements/volume-15-supplement-1.

Authors' Contributions

CVM organized and analyzed the official documents and wrote the first draft of the manuscript. GAS was a major contributor in analyzing the datasets and in writing the Discussion and Conclusion sections. Both authors read and approved the final manuscript.

Funding

Both authors are supported by research productivity scholarships from the National Council for Scientific and Technological Development – CNPq-Brazil. Publication costs are covered by the Independent Panel on Global Governance for Health, an initiative funded by the University of Oslo.

Availability of Data and Materials

The datasets analysed during the current study are available in open access repositories, as quoted and listed in the 'References' section or below the Figures.
Ethical approval and consent to participate
The study was approved by the ethics committee of Sergio Arouca National School of Public Health/Oswaldo Cruz Foundation (n. 2.466.951).

Author Details

 Sergio Arouca National School of Public Health, Oswaldo Cruz Foundation, Rio de Janeiro, Brazil.
2Social Medicine Institute, State University of Rio de Janeiro, Rio de Janeiro, Brazil.

REFERENCES

1. Landmann-Szwarcwald C, Macincko, J. (2016). A panorama of health inequalities in Brazil. Int J Equity Health. 2016;15:174.
2. Araújo, J.D. (2012) Polarização epidemiológica no Brasil. Epidemiol Serv Saúde. 2012; 21(4):533–8.
3. Oliveira, J.A.A., Teixeira, S.F. (Im)Previdência Social: 60 anos de história da previdência no Brasil. 2ª ed. Petrópolis: Vozes..
4. Cordeiro, H. (1984) As empresas médicas: as transformações capitalistas na prática médica. Rio de Janeiro: Edições Graal.
5. Teichman, J.A.(2001).The politics of freeing Markets in Latin America: Chile, Argentina and Mexico. Chapel Hill: University of North Carolina Press.
6. Escorel, S. (1999). Reviravolta na Saúde. Origem e articulação do movimento sanitário. Rio de Janeiro: Editora Fiocruz.
7. Paim, J.S.(2008) Reforma Sanitária Brasileira: contribuição e crítica. Salvador: Edufba. Rio de Janeiro: Editora Fiocruz.
8. Cebes. A Questão Democrática na Área da Saúde. Documento apresentado pelo Cebes – Nacional no 1° Simpósio sobre Política Nacional de Saúde na Câmara Federal – Outubro de 1979. http://cebes. org.br/site/wp-content/uploads/2015/10/Cebes_Sa%C3%BAde-eDemocracia.pdf Accessed 15 Oct 2018.
9. Rodriguez, N.E. (2003). Saúde: promessas e limites da Constituição. Rio de Janeiro: Editora Fiocruz; 2003.
10. Fanelli, J,M. editor.(2007) Understanding market reforms in Latin America. New York: Palgrave Macmillan.
11. World Bank. World Development Report. Investing in health. https:// openknowledgeworldbankorg/handle/10986/5976 Accessed. 1993;(18 Oct 2018).
12. Borges CF, Baptista TWF. O modelo assistencial em saúde mental no Brasil: a trajetória da construção política de 1990 a 2004. Cad Saúde Pública. 2008; 24(2):456–68.
13. Greco, D.B, Simao M. (2007) Brazilian policy of universal access to AIDS treatment: sustainability challenges and perspectives. AIDS. 2007;21(suppl 4):S37–45.
14. Portes, L.H. et al. Tobacco control policies in Brazil: A 30-year assessment. Ciênc. saúde coletiva [internet]. 2018 June [cited 2019 Jan 06]; 23(6): 1837–1848.
15. Harris M. Brazil's Family Health Programme BMJ. 2010;341:c4945.
16. Machado, C.V., Lima, L.D., Baptista, T.W.F. (2017) Políticas de saúde no Brasil em tempos contraditórios: caminhos e tropeços na construção de um sistema universal. Cad. Saúde Pública. 2017; 33(Supl2):e00129616.
17. Levitsky, S, Roberts, R.M, editors. (2011).The resurgence of the Latin American left. Baltimore, MD: John Hopkins University Press.
18. Machado, C.V, Baptista, T.W.F, Lima, L.D. (2012) Políticas de Saúde no Brasil: continuidades e mudanças. Rio de Janeiro: Editora Fiocruz..
19. Molina. J, Tasca R, Suárez. J., Kemper, E.S. (2017) More doctors Programme and the strengthening of primary health Care in Brazil: reflections from the monitoring and evaluation of the more doctors cooperation project. Qual Prim Care. 2017;25(2):50–4.
20. Bahia L, Scheffer M, Tavares LR, Braga I.F. (2016). From health plan companies to international insurance companies: changes in the accumulation regime and repercussions on the healthcare system in Brazil. Cad Saúde Pública 2016;32(Supl2): e00154015.
21. Santos, W.G. (2017). A democracia impedida: o Brasil no século XXI. Rio de Janeiro: FGV.
22. Santos, I.S., Vieira, F.S. (2018) The right to healthcare and fiscal austerity: the Brazilian case from an international perspective. Ciênc saúde coletiva. 2018;23(7):2303–14.
23. Viacava F, Oliveira, R.A.D,, Carvalho, C.C., Laguardia J, Bellido J.G. (2018). SUS: supply, access to and use of health services over the last 30 years. Ciênc. saúde coletiva. 2018;23(6):1751–62.
24. Paim, J.S, et al. (2017) The Brazilian health system: history, advances, and challenges. Lancet. 2011;377:1778–97.
25. Machado, C.V, Lima, L.D, Andrade, C.L.T. 9 (2014). Federal funding of health policy in Brazil: trends and challenges. Cad. Saúde Pública. 2014;30:187–200.
26. Macinko J, et al. (2010). Major expansion of primary care in Brazil linked to decline in unnecessary hospitalization. Health Aff. 2010;29(12):2149–60.
27. Leal, M.C, et al. (2018). Reproductive, maternal, neonatal and child health in the 30 years since the creation of the unified health system (SUS). Ciênc saúde coletiva. 2018;23(6):1915–28.
28. Teixeira, M.G, et al. (2018). The achievements of the SUS in tackling the communicable diseases. Ciência saúde coletiva. 2018;23(6):1819–28.
29. Souza, M.F.M, Malta, D.C., França, E.B., Barreto, M.L. (2018) Changes in health and disease in Brazil and its states in the 30 years since the unified healthcare system (SUS) was created. Ciência saúde coletiva. 2018;23(6):1737–50.
30. ABRASCO. Especial Abrasco sobre o aumento da mortalidade infantil e materna no Brasil. 31-08-2018. <https://www.abrasco.org.br/site/outrasnoticias/institucional/especial-abrasco-sobre-o-aumento-da-mortalidadeinfantil-e-materna-no-brasil/36777/>. Accessed 18 Oct 2018.
31. Rasella, D., Basu, S., Hone, T., Paes-Sousa, R., Ocké-Reis, C.O, Millett, C. (2018). Child morbidity and mortality associated with alternative policy responses to the economic crisis in Brazil: a nationwide microsimulation study. PLoS Med. 2018;15(5):e1002570.

32. Szwarcwald, C.L, Souza Júnior, P.R.B., Marques, A.P, Almeida, W.S., Montilla, D,E.R. (2016). Inequalities in healthy life expectancy by Brazilian geographic regions: findings from the National Health Survey, 2013. Int J Equity Health. 2016; 15(1):141.

33. Marinho F, de Azeredo Passos V.M,, Carvalho Malta. D., Barboza França E, Abreu, D.M.X., Araújo, V.E.M, et al. (2018). Burden of disease in Brazil, 1990–2016: a systematic subnational analysis for the global burden of disease study 2016. Lancet. 2018;392(10149):760–75.

34. Marmot, M. (2012). Brazil: rapid progress and the challenge of inequality. Int J Equity Health. 2016;15:177.

35. Huber, E., Stephens, J.D. (2012) Democracy and the left: social policy and inequality in Latin America: University of Chicago Press.

36. Bollyky, T.J., Templin, T., Cohen, M., Schoder, D., Dieleman, J.L, Wigley, S. (2019) The relationships between democratic experience, adult health, and causespecific mortality in 170 countries between 1980 and 2016: an observational analysis. Lancet. 2019;393:1628–40.

37. Dweck, E, Silveira, F., Rossi, P. 9 (2018) Austeridade e desigualdade social no Brasil. In: Rossi P, Dweck E, Oliveira ALM, editors. Economia para Poucos. São Paulo: Autonomia Literária; 2018.

38. Evans P. Sustaining social protection and provision: the front line in the battle for the good society. Ciênc. saúde coletiva. 2018;23(7):2081–4.

39. Deaton, A. (2013) The great escape: health, wealth and the origins of inequality. Princeton, NJ: Princeton University Press.

3.(Un)Equitable Distribution of Health Resources and The Judicialization of Healthcare: 10 Years of Experience In Brazil[1]

Luciana de Melo Nunes[2] Lopes[1]*, Francisco de Assis Acurcio[2], Semíramis Domingues Diniz[1], Tiago Lopes Coelho[1]
Eli Iola Gurgel Andrade[1]

ABSTRACT

Background: Equity has been acknowledged as a required principle for the fulfilment of the universal right to health once it seeks to tackle avoidable and unfair inequalities among individuals. In Brazil, a country marked by iniquities, this principle was adopted in the Brazilian National Health System (SUS) organization. But the phenomenon known as judicialization of healthcare, anchored in the argument of universality of the right, has been consolidated as a health policy parallel to the SUS. The analysis of lawsuits distribution according to their beneficiaries' socio-economic profile can contribute to the verification of the judicialization's potential for reducing inequalities, thus becoming an auxiliary activity in the fulfilment of the universal and egalitarian right to health. This study aimed to assess what socioeconomic factors are associated to municipalities that had larger numbers of beneficiaries from lawsuits in health in the state of Minas Gerais, Brazil, from 1999 to 2009.

Methods: It is a descriptive quantitative study of the residence municipalities of beneficiaries registered in database regarding all deferred lawsuits against the state of Minas Gerais from 1999 to 2009. The verification of cities' socio-economic profile was performed based on information of the Brazilian Institute of Geography and Statistics' 2010 Demographic Census and on indexes derived from it. The variables studied for each municipality were: number of beneficiaries; resident population; Social Vulnerability Index (IVS); and Municipal Human Development Index (IDHm). Descriptive and statistical analysis were used to verify factors associated with a larger number of beneficiaries in a municipality.

Results: Out of 853 municipalities in Minas Gerais, 399 were registered as residence of at least one of the 6.906 beneficiaries of studied lawsuits. The residence non-information index was 11,5%. The minimum number of identified beneficiaries living in a municipality was 1 (one) while the maximum was 1920. The binary logistic regression revealed that high and very high IDHm (OR = 3045; IC = 1773-5228), IVS below 0.323 (OR = 2044; IC = 1099- 3800) and

---

[1] Lopes et al. International Journal for Equity in Health   (2019) 18:10

[2] * Correspondence: lucianamnlopes@gmail.com

1Faculty of Medicine, Federal University of Minas Gerais, 190 Professor Alfredo Balena Avenue, Santa Efigênia, Belo Horizonte, Minas Gerais 30130-100, Brazil

Full list of author information is available at the end of the article

population size above 14.661 inhabitants (OR = 6162; IC = 3733-10,171) are statistically associated to a greater number of beneficiaries of lawsuits in health within a municipality.

Conclusions: The judicialization of health care in Minas Gerais, from 1999 to 2009, didn't reach the most vulnerable municipalities. On the contrary, it favoured a concentration of health resources in municipalities with better socioeconomic profiles. The register of all beneficiaries' municipalities of residence as well as individual socioeconomic data can contribute to a more conclusive analysis. Nevertheless, in general, the results of this study suggest that the judicial health policy conducted from 1999 to 2009 was not an auxiliary tool for the fulfilment of an equitable right to health in Minas Gerais. Keywords: Judicialization of healthcare, Public health, Health policy, Health equity

BACKGROUND

The fundamental right to health was established in Brazil by the Federal Constitution of 1988, which declared health as a universal right and a State duty [1]. To ensure the right to health, the Brazilian Constitution created the Brazilian National Health System (SUS), based on the principles of universality, comprehensiveness and equity [1, 2]. SUS' legal framework expressly recognizes the social determination of the health-disease process, which points to the importance of assuming our social organization structure as a decisive aspect for the fulfilment of the right to health [3]. Appreciating concrete aspects of Brazil's reality, Victora [4] points that the creation of SUS is considered one of the main causes of health status evolution of the Brazilian population [4, 5].

From 1990 to 2007, child mortality rate declined 58% and life expectancy rose from 66,6 years in 1990 to 72,8 years in 2008 [5]. However, parallel to the Brazilian public health system development process, citizens began to seek the assurance of the constitutional right to health, especially regarding the access to medicines, via the Judiciary [2, 6]. This phenomenon of suing SUS to request free access to health services and goods has been called "the judicialization of healthcare". It has exponentially grown over the last two decades, becoming object of attention of several social actors [7]. Although Brazil is the most notorious country in studies and publications regarding the judicialization of healthcare [8], it has also been intensified in other places [8, 9]. In Latin America, the Judiciary has increasingly assumed the role of interpreting and protecting the human rights and has even obliged governments to redefine health policy priorities. Within the region, individual lawsuits are the large majority and judicial decisions are usually favourable to health claims without further investigation about their impact on the health policy as a whole [8].

The expenditure with judicial health demands in Brazil have grown and significantly impacted on the organization of SUS [10–13]. From 2008 to 2015, the Federal public expenditure on complying with judicial health decisions rose 1006% [13]. These unscheduled expenditures generate administrative challenges that, according to experts, potentially enlarge access to healthcare inequities [8, 11, 12] due the redirection of health resources regardless of the priorities of public health [12].Assuming that 1) health resources distribution is decisive for establishing an equitable policy [14] and 2) the judicialization of healthcare interferes in the redistribution of health resources [10, 11, 13, 15], it becomes essential to investigate if the set of judicial decisions on health has favoured a concentration or a deconcentration of health resources. Have places with better socioeconomic conditions been benefited from the judicialization of healthcare?

This study aims to assess what socioeconomic factors are associated to municipalities that had larger numbers of beneficiaries from lawsuits in health in the state of Minas Gerais, Brazil, from 1999 to 2009.

METHODS

This is a quantitative descriptive study based on registers of the 6.112 deferred lawsuits sued against the Health Secretary of the State of Minas Gerais, Brazil, in the period of October of 1999 to October of 2009. The database was built by the Federal University of Minas Gerais' Research Group in Health Economics (GPES/UFMG) from the information provided by the state of Minas Gerais. The variables registered in the database are about the lawsuit (number, date, court, kind of lawsuit, etc.), the beneficiary (municipality of residence, gender, profession, age, etc.), the author (if public defence, prosecution service, etc.), the judicial representative (kind, professional register, etc.), the defendant (government sphere), the medical care (information of health professionals, prescriptions, diagnostics, etc.), the drug (name, concentration, dosage, insertion in SUS' official list, etc.) and about the procedures and materials (name, quantity, etc.).

This database has been updated but, due to the extensive number of lawsuits to be explored, robust information after 2009 is not available yet. To conduct this study, all beneficiaries' municipalities of residence were considered. The verification of the municipalities' socioeconomic conditions was based on information of the Brazilian Institute of Geography and Statistics' (IBGE) 2010 Demographic Census and on two indexes derived from it that were defined and disclosed by the Institute of Research in Applied Economics (IPEA) of Brazil. The dependent variable analysed for each municipality was the number of beneficiaries of lawsuits in health from 1999 to 2009 while the independent variables were: the resident population in 2010, the Social Vulnerability Index (IVS) 2010 and the Municipal Human Development Index (IDHm) 2010. Detailed information about the two indexes disclosed by IPEA are provided below:

The IDHm aims to adapt the global IDH methodology to Brazilian municipalities. It is composed by the same three components of IDH: longevity (measured by life expectancy at birth), education (measured by adult population schooling and young population school flow) and income (measured by per capita income). The IDHm, which ranges from 0 to 1, enables the comparison of Brazilian municipalities over time and facilitates the orientation of interventions to improve municipalities' socioeconomic conditions. The range of municipal human development measured by the index is: very low (0–0,499), low (0,500-0,599), medium (0,600-0,699), high (0,700-0,799) and very high (0,800–1) [16]. The IVS is an index built to complement the IDHm and to identify overlaps of social exclusion and vulnerability indicative situations in a given territory. It is composed by three dimensions that represent state provisions assets whose deprivation negatively impacts on population welfare conditions and that are measured by sixteen indicators set.

The three dimensions are: urban infrastructure (measured by indicators related to water and sewage supply, to garbage collection and to travel time from home to labour), human capital (measured by indicators related to child mortality rate, to young population school flow, to adult population schooling and to young mothers proportion) and income and labour (measured by indicators related to the per capita household income, to unemployment, to informal occupation, to financial dependence on the elderly and to people from 10 to 14 years activity). Thus, the IVS aims to be an indicative of goods and services provision failures by the Brazilian State. It is available for all geographic levels: country, regions, states and municipalities. The range of social vulnerability measured by the index is: very low (0–0,200), low (0,201-0,300), medium (0,301-0,400), high (0,401-0,500) and very high (0,501–1) [17].

The names of municipalities were validated and those that could not be safely related to an existing municipality were excluded from the study. To assess the (de)concentration of health and, therefore, the equity degree achieved by the set of lawsuits in health in Minas Gerais, descriptive and statistical analysis were conducted. To identify the general profile of all municipalities that had residents who benefited from lawsuits in health in Minas Gerais, central tendency measures (mean and median) were used for the description of quantitative variables as well as the standard deviation, the minimum and maximum and the percentiles 25 and 75. Relative and absolute frequency were used for the description of the following adopted categorical variables: number of beneficiaries (1–2/above 3), municipality's populational size (below median/above median), IVS (less vulnerable = below percentile 75/more vulnerable = above percentile 75) and IDHm (high-very high/low-medium). To verify what factors were associated with a larger number of beneficiaries of lawsuits in health in a municipality, a binary logistic regression was conducted between the dependent categorical variable (number of beneficiaries) and the independent ones. Odds Ratios (OR) with the corresponding 95% Confidence Interval (CI) were used to show the strength of associations, and variables with P-values of < 0.05 were considered statistically significant. The analysis was made by the software SPSS Statistics Base Screenshot 22.0. IVS 2010 and IDHm 2010 maps were collected from IPEA's Social Vulnerability Atlas website and a map marking the main municipalities benefited from the judicialization of health care in Minas Gerais, from 1999 to 2009, was built with TabWin software.

RESULTS

Out of the 853 Minas Gerais' municipalities, 399 were registered as residence of at least one of the 6.906 lawsuits beneficiaries in the state from 1999 to 2009. These 399 municipalities concentrated 82,90% of Minas Gerais' population in 2010. The proportion of lack of information about the beneficiary's municipality of residence within lawsuits was of 11,5%. The descriptive analysis of the dependent and independent variables revealed the general profile of the 399 municipalities. The minimum number of identified beneficiaries living in a municipality was 1 (one) while the maximum was 1920. The smallest population size was 1210 inhabitants and the largest one was 2,375,151. The IVS fluctuated from very high to very low and the IDHm varied from low to very high. While the mean number of inhabitants was 40,719.92, 50% of the municipalities had a population up to 14,661 people. Absolute and relative frequencies calculated for dependent and independent categorical variables indicated that 51.9% of the 399 municipalities had 1 or 2 residents that benefited from lawsuits in health, 298 of them showed IVS below 0.323 and 44.4% of them exhibited IDHm high or very high.Table 1 provides detailed information about the descriptive analysis. The binary logistic regression revealed that high and very high IDHm (OR = 3045; IC = 1773-5228), IVS below 0.323 (OR = 2044; IC = 1099- 3800) and populational size above 14.661 inhabitants (OR = 6162; IC = 3733-10,171) are statistically associated to a greater number of beneficiaries of lawsuits in health within a municipality. Table 2 displays the findings of the statistical analysis. Maps of Minas Gerais concerning the IVS 2010 and the IDHm 2010 were compared to a map of the state where the 192 municipalities with number of beneficiaries of the judicialization of healthcare over than 2 are marked (Fig. 1).

DISCUSSION

In societies marked by inequities, as the Brazilian one, health protection necessarily passes through its social determinant's discussion, once there is convincing evidence of association between a population's diseases distribution and its socioeconomic conditions [4, 18, 19]. Therefore, according to Duarte [14], in the impossibility of redistributing diseases among populations, health actions that are proposed to be equitable must seek to attenuate factors that contribute to health inequities.

Table 1 Descriptive analysis of characteristics of the 399 municipalities that had at least 1 beneficiary from lawsuits in health in Minas Gerais from 1999 to 2009

Variables	n	%
Number of beneficiaries 1999–2009		
1–2	207	51.9
> 3	192	48.1
Mean (SD)	15.25 (102.78)	–
Median	2	–
Min – Max	1–1,920	–
Percentile 25	1	–
Percentile 75	6	–
Resident population 2010		
0–14,661	200	50.1
> 14,661	199	49.9
Mean (SD)	40,719.42 (134,843.954)	–
Median	14,661	–
Min – Max	1,210–2,375,151	–
Percentile 25	7,173	–
Percentile 75	31,883	–
IVS 2010 0–0.322	298	74.7
> 0.323	101	25.3
Mean (SD)	0.2863 (0.0785)	–
Median	0.271	–
Min – Max	0.158–0.56	–
Percentile 25	0.229	–
Percentile 75	0.324	–
IDHm 2010 high – very high	177	44.4
low – medium	222	55.6
Mean (SD)	0.69024 (0.0785)	–
Median	0.693	–
Min – Max	0.536–0.813	–
Percentile 25	0.661	–
Percentile 75	0.723	–

Source: GPES/UFMG's Judicialization of Health Care 1999–2009 Database; IPEA's Social Vulnerability Atlas 2010; prepared by the authors

Vieira-da-Silva and Almeida Filho [18] point that the State can formulate policies that are promoters of more or less equity. So, the Judiciary, as part of the State, when proposing itself as an auxiliary force for the fulfilment of the constitutional right to health, must also be alert to the health outcomes achieved by its set of decisions. In this study, complex socioeconomic evaluation indexes and descriptive and statistical analysis were adopted to substantiate the investigation about the judicialization of healthcare effects over equity. It was observed, then, that most citizens benefited by the phenomenon from 1999 to 2009, in Minas Gerais, lived in municipalities that registered better socioeconomic conditions. A statistically significative association was observed between larger number of beneficiaries of a municipality and a high or very high municipal human development, a larger municipal populational size and a lower municipal social vulnerability.

It suggests, therefore, that the set of judicial decisions in health, opposed to the principle of equity, had favoured a concentration of health resources in these municipalities for the first ten years of experience with the judicialization of healthcare phenomenon in Minas Gerais.

Furthermore, the comparison of the IVS 2010 map, the IDHm 2010 map and the map with marked municipalities with number of beneficiaries above 3 suggests that, in the studied period, the judicial performance in Minas Gerais could not reach and benefit citizens living in municipalities where interventions of the State were most needed. These outcomes are alike the data presented by Ferraz [20] in a study published in 2011 which points out that there was a concentration of lawsuits in the richest cities and states of Brazil – 93,3% of the litigation was located within the 8 states with the highest IDH (above 0,8). Ferraz [20] suggests this result can be explained by the inequity of access to courts and good lawyers. The author reflects that, for example, for every individual lawsuit demanding access to a medicine, there may be a great number of unrepresented non-litigant interested parties. Thus, limited health resources have been reallocated in favour of few privileged individuals even if their needs are not considered public health priorities [20].Brinks and Forbath [21] reflect that the Brazilian State has always favoured privileged groups and hasn't addressed structural issues to overcome historical inequalities. Therefore, it is not a surprise to figure out that the judicial intervention has also failed to benefit the unprivileged Brazilians.

The distributive justice notion, usually associated with equity, prescribes that primary social goods, as opportunities and wealth, should be equally distributed among society. Once verified the market failure in distributing social wealth in an egalitarian way, the State would intervene to correct this mistake. In order to ensure equity, the State could even adopt a positive discrimination in favour of disadvantaged groups [14, 18, 22, 23]. Thus, from the results found in this study, it arises a hypothesis of a contrary positive discrimination tendency - in favour of advantaged groups - within the scope of the judicialization of health care.

**able 2 Statistical analysis of socioeconomic factors associated to
a number of beneficiaries of lawsuits in health above 3 in a municipality**

Variable	Categorization	B	OR	IC 95%	p-value
IDHm	High-very high	1.113	3.045	1.773–5.228	< 0.001
	Medium-low		1		
IVS	0–0.322	0.715	2.044	1.099–3.800	0.024
	> 0.323		1		
Resident population	> 14.661 inh.	1.818	6.162	3.733–10.171	< 0.001
	0–14.661 inh.		1		

Source: GPES/UFMG's Judicialization of Health Care 1999–2009 Database; IPEA's Social Vulnerability Atlas 2010; prepared by the authors

As well as the distributive justice notion assigns the State the attribution of correcting market failures [14, 18, 22, 23], the justification for judicial intervention in the political field lies in an argument of public policies failures necessity of correction [24, 25]. So, since the IVS index aims to signal state failures to provide essential goods and services for the Brazilian population well-being, comparing the IVS and the judicialization of healthcare maps raises also a questioning about the adequacy of judicial performance in health for the corrective function proposed by it.

When thinking about equity and distributive justice, another point has to be discussed from this study's results.

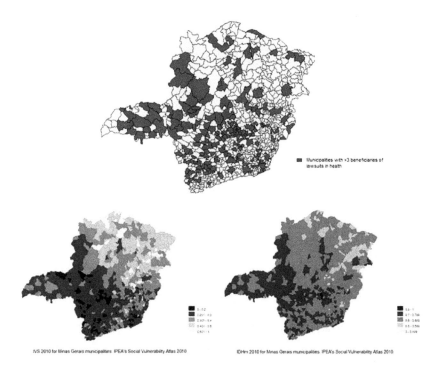

As meeting the judicial demands against SUS. requires public resources from a common budget for financing all health actions and services offered by the Brazilian public health system [15], the concentration of lawsuits beneficiaries in municipalities with better socioeconomic conditions doubly suggests damage to equity: the judicial performance set would not only be benefiting advantaged groups but would also be potentially harming disadvantaged groups by determining reallocation of health resources in order to comply with court orders. Once SUS' organization is decentralized and all government spheres are responsible for ensuring the right to health [26], states and municipalities consist in gateways for the judicialization of health care that are closer to the population, what makes it difficult to identify a national level overview of the phenomenon. Being municipalities the federated entity with lower income, the financial impact of the judicialization of health care may be more significant: in 2013, while the budget to purchase basic medicines for the entire population of Tubarão - state of Paraná - was about US$ 279,288, the municipality spent US$ 280,467 on the attendance of health judicial sentences [22].

Duarte [14] indicates that, among the factors that determine the equity degree within a health system, the way of distributing financial resources is one of the most important. Therefore, this impact of the judicialization of health care on health resources distribution must be deeply investigated, once, according to Achoki and Lesego [27], health financing changes have intended and unintended consequences that can negatively affect health outcomes when they are not holistically appreciated.

However, the configuration of the judicialization of healthcare phenomenon which has been consolidated in Brazil, through individual demands for access to health technologies - especially medicines [8, 11, 12, 20, 21, 28], makes it difficult for the Judiciary to evaluate collective results of its decisions. This conformation of the judicialization of healthcare also meets Fortes' [24] say that in late capitalism societies, citizens' individual yearnings tend to overlap collective interests, what hinders an effective implementation of equity principle. Thus, we wonder about the possibility of achieving an equitable judicial performance in health when it is based on individual demands. According to Brinks and Forbath [21, 28], different courts' interventions forms have different effects on politics. There are lawsuits challenging political issues of structural nature, on the contrary of individual demands, but Flood and Gross [9] point that courts are more conservative in intervening in them, despite being quite open to individual demands in some countries, like Brazil. In this country, for example, the Judiciary has been provoked to manifest about the constitutionality of the Constitutional Amendment 95/2016 (EC 95/16) that froze public expenditure for 20 years, including in health - what has been considered highly harmful to SUS by specialists [29, 30]. Without facing improper financial restrictions due to EC 95/16, the judicialization of health care will fight for resources of an already reduced budget, increasing probabilities of damage to equity by a judicial performance centred on individual demands. Other countries, however, have experienced other conformation of the judicialization of health care phenomenon [21, 28, 31]. The Colombian Judiciary, for example, after having extensively experienced individual demands and conflicted with the executive branch [28], started addressing what Garavito [31] called "structural demands" and could figure out the process of fulfilment of economic and social rights in a broader way. Having seriously considered the budgetary issues, the Colombian Judiciary invited interested parties to discuss the health system funding, what resulted in a completely and more equitable restructure of the public health system [28, 31]. From the perspective of structural cases, it is possible that equity issues in health become more evident and that judicial intervention become more assertive and capable of helping to ensure access to health goods and services without distributive distortions.

According to Brinks and Forbath [21], the activity of litigating social and economic rights is relatively new, and we are only starting to understand its real effects. There may be some indirect positive political consequences of litigation even individual ones [21, 28] that are difficult to assess. However, looking at the Brazilian experience in comparison with other countries as Colombia, and recognizing that an equitable assurance of the right to health passes through its social determinants coping [3, 4, 6, 24], we consider it more reasonable to think (and to suggest) that the judicialization of healthcare, once presented as a corrective tool for health public policies failures, should be driven to structural issues of collective effects that hold up the maintenance of diseases and social goods uneven distribution among society - for example issues regarding health systems financing and intellectual property of litigated technologies. When anchored in its observed conformation from 1999 to 2009 in the state of Minas Gerais, Brazil, the judicialization of healthcare, as partly demonstrated in this study, does not seem to be an auxiliary activity for the fulfilment of an equitable right to health. Lack of records about all beneficiaries' municipality of residence and about beneficiaries' individual socioeconomic conditions account for limitations of this study. However, we consider the investigation methodology suitable to substantiate the developed discussion.

CONCLUSIONS

The study points that the judicialization of healthcare in Minas Gerais, Brazil, from 1999 to 2009 did not reach municipalities where State intervention necessity was more evident. On the contrary, the phenomenon favoured a concentration of health resources in places with better socioeconomic profiles. Quality records about all beneficiaries' municipality of residence and their individual socioeconomic conditions are important for more conclusive analysis. However, despite study limitations, we believe the results to be sufficient indication that the judicialization of healthcare in Minas Gerais, from 1999 to 2009, was not an auxiliary tool for the fulfilment of an equitable right to health. New longer-term studies – including qualitative ones must be conducted to assess not only the direct but also the indirect effects of the judicialization of healthcare on the distribution of health resources in Brazil and other countries. From the findings of this investigation, we question the judicial performance suitability for its proposed corrective function as its possibility to assist in the assurance of an equitable right to health from individual demands. However, looking at the experience of other countries as Colombia, we ponder that when states fail to ensure equitable public policies, structural litigation may be an opportunity for the Judiciary to help addressing issues that affect the distribution of social goods and public services among society. The Brazilian Judiciary has been provoked to intervene in structural issues that limit SUS' capacity to fulfil a comprehensive, universal and equitable right to health. The judicial questioning of the constitutionality of the EC 95/16 is one of the main examples in this sense. Nonetheless, the Constitutional Court does not seem ready – or willing – to start addressing core issues that prevent Brazil from managing its marked social inequalities.

Abbreviations
EC 95/16: Constitutional Amendment 95/2015; SUS: Brazilian National Health Service

Acknowledgements

We thank Laura Monteiro de Castro Moreira for helping us with TabWin and CNPq, FAPEMIG and CAPES for financially supporting this research.

Funding

The Research Projects "Lawsuits impact on the National Pharmaceutical Assistance Policy: management of clinic and medicalization of justice" and "Analysis of budget impact on Brazilian National Health Service (SUS) by incorporation of most litigated medicines in pharmaceutical assistance programs" were funded by the National Council for Scientific and Technologial Development (CNPq) and the Foundation for Research Support of Minas Gerais (FAPEMIG), respectively. The Brazilian Federal Agency for Support and Evaluation of Graduate Education (CAPES) has also played an important role by funding the master's degree scholarship for the main author of this research. The funders did not interfere in any aspects of the research projects.

Availability of data and materials

The Datasets regarding IVS and IDHm indexes analysed during the current study are available in the Social Vulnerability Atlas repository, http:// ivs.ipea.gov.br/index.php/pt/. The database regarding heath lawsuits in Minas Gerais analysed during the current study is not publicly available due it contains personal information from beneficiaries but are available from the corresponding author on reasonable request.

Ethics approval and consent to participate

This study integrates the Research Project "Lawsuits impact on the National Pharmaceutical Assistance Policy: management of clinic and medicalization of justice" followed by "Analysis of budget impact on Brazilian National Health Service (SUS) by incorporation of most litigated medicines in pharmaceutical assistance programs" approved by the Federal University of Minas Gerais' Ethics Comittee (reference number 292/2008).

REFERENCES

1. Brasil. Constituição da República Federativa do Brasil. Brasilia: Senado Federal; 1988.
2. Balestra, N.O.(2015). A jurisprudência dos Tribunais Superiores e o Direito à Saúde – evolução rumo à racionalidade. Rev Dir Sanit. 2015;16(1): 87–111.
3. Araujo, I.M.M. (2016). Direito à saúde: aspecto do modelo neodesenvolvimentista brasileiro e da privatização da saúde. Rev Dir Sanit. 2015;16(1):128–45.
4. Victora, C.(2016). Socioeconomic inequalities in health: reflections on the academic production from Brazil. Int J Equity Health. 2016;15(164).
5. Paim, J, et al. (2011). The Brazilian health system: history, advances, and challenges. Lancet. 2011;377(9779):1778–97.
6. Machado, F.R.S. (2008), Contribuições ao debate da judicialização da saúde no Brasil. Rev Dir Sanit. 2008;9(2):73–91.
7. Oliveira, L.C.F, Assis., M.M.A, Barboni, A.R. (2010).. Assistência Farmacêutica no Sistema Único de Saúde: da Política Nacional de Medicamentos à Atenção Básica à Saúde. Ciênc. Saúde Coletiva. 2010;15(supl.3):3561–7.

8. Vargas-Peláez, C.M. et al. (2014). Right to health, essential medicines, and lawsuits for access to medicines – a scoping study. Soc Sci Med. 2014;121:48–55.

9. Flood, C.M., Gross, A. (2017). Litigating the right to health: what can we learn from a comparative law and health care systems approach. Health Hum Rights. 2017;16(2):62–72.

10. Bittencourt, G.B. (2016). O "estado da arte" da produção acadêmica sobre o fenômeno da judicialização da saúde no Brasil. Cad Ibero-Amer Dir Sanit. 2016;5(1):102–21.

11. Catanheide, I.D, Lisboa, E.S., Souza, L.E.P.F. (2016).Características da judicialização do acesso a medicamentos no Brasil: uma revisão sistemática. Physis. 2016; 26(4):1335–56.

12. Machado, M.A.A, (2011). et al. Judicialização do acesso a medicamentos no Estado de Minas Gerais, Brasil. Rev Saúde Pública. 2011;45(3):590–8.

13. David, G, Andrelino A, Beghin N. (2000). Direito a medicamentos: avaliação das despesas com medicamentos no âmbito federal do Sistema Único de Saúde entre 2008 e 2015 [Internet]. 2016. Available from: http://portalarquivos2.saude.gov.br/images/pdf/2017/maio/17/Livro-Direito-amedicamentos-Avalia----o-das-despesas-INESC--2016.pdf.

14. Duarte, C.M.R. (2000).Equidade na legislação: um princípio do sistema de saúde brasileiro? Cien Saude Colet. 2000;5(2):443–63.

15. Guimarães, R.(2014). Incorporação tecnológica no SUS: o problema e seus desafios. Cien Saude Colet. 2014;19(12):4899–908.

16. Atlas do Desenvolvimento Humano no Brasil. O IDHm [Internet]. Available from: <http://www.atlasbrasil.org.br/2013/pt/o_atlas/idhm/>.

17. IPEA. Atlas da vulnerabilidade social nos municípios brasileiros [Internet]. 2015. Available from: <http://ivs.ipea.gov.br/images/publicacoes/Ivs/ publicacao_atlas_ivs.pdf>.

18. Viera-da-Silva L.M., Almeida Filho. N. (2015). Equidade em saúde: uma análise crítica de conceitos. Cad. Saude Publica. 2009;25(supl.2):S2217–S226.

19. Andrade, E.I.G, (2008). et al. A judicialização da saúde e a política nacional de assistência farmacêutica no Brasil: gestão da clínica e medicalização da justiça. Rev Med Minas Gerais. 2008;18(4):46–50.

20. Ferraz, O.LM. (2010). Harming the poor through social rights litigation: lessons from Brazil. Texas Law Review. 2010;2008(89):1643–68.

21. Brinks, D.M., Forbath, W. (2011). Commentary: social and economic rights in Latin America: constitutional courts and the prospects for pro-poor interventions. Texas Law Review. 2011;89:1943–55.

22. Chieffi, A.L, Barata, R.B. (2009). Judicialização da política pública de assistência farmacêutica e eqüidade. Cad Saúde Publica. 2009;25(8):1839–49.

23. Helena, E.Z.S. (2008) Justiça Distributiva na Teoria da Justiça como Equidade de John Rawls. Revista de Informação Legislativa. 2008;45(128):337–46.

24. Fortes, P.A.C. (2008) Orientações bioéticas de justiça distributiva aplicada às ações e aos sistemas de saúde. Revista Bioética. 2008;16(1):25–39.

25. Castro, M.F. (1997). O Supremo Tribunal Federal e a judicialização da política. Revista Brasileira de Ciências Sociais. 1997; 1(34).

26. Brasil. Lei N° 8.080, de 19 de setembro de 1990. Dispõe sobre as condições para a promoção, proteção e recuperação da saúde, a organização e o funcionamento dos serviços correspondentes e dá outras providências. Brasilia: Presidência da República; 1990.

27. Achoki, L, Lesego, A. (2017). The imperative for systems thinking to promote access to medicines, efficient delivery, and cost-effectiveness when implementing health financing reforms: a qualitative study. Int J Equity Health. 2017;16(53).

28. Brinks, D.M., Forbath, W. (2013).The role of courts and constitutions in the new politics of welfare in Latin America. In: Peerenboom R, Ginsburg T, editors. Law and development of middle-income countries: avoiding the middleincome trap. New York: Cambridge University Press; 2013. p. 221–45.

29. Fiocruz. Fiocruz divulga carta A PEC 241 e os impactos sobre os direitos sociais, a saúde e a vida [Internet]. 2016. Available from: <https://portal. fiocruz.br/pt-br/content/fiocruz-divulga-carta-pec-241-e-os-impactos-sobredireitos-sociais-saude-e-vida>.

30. Chaves, G.C., Britto, W.G., Vieira, M.F. (2017). Tratado de livre comércio União EuropeiaMercosul: estudo de impacto de medidas TRIPS-plus nas compras públicas de medicamentos no Brasil [Internet]. 2017. Available from:

31. Garavito CR. El Activismo Dialógico y el Impacto de los Fallos sobre Derechos Sociales. Revista Argentina de Teoría Jurídica. 2013;14:1–27.

Health System Collapse 45 Days After The Detection Of COVID-19 In Ceará, Northeast Brazil: A Preliminary Analysis[1]

[2]Daniele Rocha Queiros Lemos[1] Sarah Mendes D'Angelo[23]
Luis Arthur Brasil Gadelha Farias[34] Magda Moura Almeida[23] Ricristhi Gonçalves Gomes[2]
Geovana Praça Pinto[1] Josafa Nascimento Cavalcante Filho[2] Levi Ximenes Feijão[2] Ana Rita Paulo Cardoso[2] Thaisy Brasil Ricarte Lima[2]Pâmela Maria Costa Linhares[23]
Liana Perdigão Mello[5] Tania Mara Coelho[34] Luciano Pamplona de Góes Cavalcanti[13]

ABSTRACT

Introduction: COVID-19 emerged in late 2019 and quickly became a serious public health problem worldwide. This study aim to describe the epidemiological course of cases and deaths due to COVID-19 and their impact on hospital bed occupancy rates in the first 45 days of the epidemic in the state of Ceará, Northeastern Brazil. **Methods:** The study used an ecological design with data gathered from multiple government and health care sources. Data were analyzed using Epi Info software. **Results:** The first cases were confirmed on March 15, 2020. After 45 days, 37,268 cases reported in 85.9% of Ceará's municipalities, with 1,019 deaths. Laboratory test positivity reached 84.8% at the end of April, a period in which more than 700 daily tests were processed. The average age of cases was 67 (<1 - 101) years, most occurred in a hospital environment (91.9%), and 58% required hospitalization in an ICU bed. The average time between the onset of symptoms and death was 18 (1 - 56) days. Patients who died in the hospital had spent an average of six (0 - 40) days hospitalized. Across Ceará, the bed occupancy rate reached 71.3% in the wards and 80.5% in the ICU. **Conclusions:** The first 45 days of the COVID-19 epidemic in Ceará revealed a large number of cases and deaths, spreading initially among the population with a high socioeconomic status. Despite the efforts by the health services and social isolation measures the health system still collapsed.

INTRODUCTION

The novel coronavirus SARS-CoV-2, the etiological agent of COVID-19, emerged in Wuhan, China in December 2019 and quickly spread to other countries[1,2]. Due to the rapid increase in the number of

[1] Rev. Soc. Bras. Med. Trop. vol.53 Uberaba 2020 Epub July 03, 2020
[2] 1Centro Universitário Christus, Faculdade de Medicina, Fortaleza, CE, Brasil.
2Secretaria de Saúde do Estado do Ceará, Fortaleza, CE, Brasil.
3Universidade Federal do Ceará, Faculdade de Medicina, Fortaleza, CE, Brasil.
4Hospital São José de Doenças Infecciosas, Fortaleza, CE, Brasil.
5Laboratório Central de Saúde Pública do Ceará, Fortaleza, CE, Brasil.

cases, on March 11, 2020, the World Health Organization (WHO) declared it to be a pandemic[3]. One month after the declaration, more than two million people worldwide had been infected and 135,000 deaths had been registered across 213 countries[4]. Worldwide, health systems faced the need to adapt to a critical overload on services, and a shortage of health care professionals and personal protective equipment[5,6]. In Brazil, the first case of COVID-19 was confirmed on February 26, 2020, and the first death on March 17, both in the state of São Paulo[7]. Community transmission was officially recognized in Brazil on March 20, 2020[8]. Through May 5, 2020, there were more than 110,000 confirmed cases and approximately 8,000 deaths, with a mortality rate of 6.9%. The three most affected states were São Paulo (34,053 deaths), Rio de Janeiro (12,391 deaths), and Ceará (11,470 deaths)[9].

The state of Ceará in Northeast Brazil was one of the first to confirm sustained transmission. Within 45 days of confirmation of its first case, Ceará had registered the third highest number of deaths in the country. The exponential increase in cases and deaths imposed a series of challenges to meet the demand for care, with a real possibility of a collapse of the health services system. The Brazilian government enacted social isolation regulations on March 19 (Decree 33,519) and a lockdown on May 8 (Decree 33,547). Considerable effort was put into expanding the capacity of emergency services, emergency department care, and laboratory testing, as well as the increasing the number of intensive care (ICU) beds[10]. We describe the epidemiological scenario of cases and deaths from COVID-19 and their impact on hospital bed occupancy rate in the first 45 days (February 17 to April 27, 2020) of the epidemic in Ceará, Northeastern Brazil.

METHODS

Study Type

The study used an ecological design to compare confirmed COVID-19 cases and deaths to bed occupancy rates in Ceará. In addition, we describe the actions implemented during the first 45 days of the epidemic.

Data sources

1. REDCap - Database in which all suspected and confirmed cases of COVID-19 were recorded from the beginning of the epidemic until April 27, 2020 (45 days after the first known case occurred).
2. SIVEP - Gripe - The National Influenza Epidemiological Surveillance Information System that records all cases of severe respiratory infections and related deaths.
3. e-SUS Notifica - A system developed specifically to meet the high demand for notifications of COVID-19, recording mild and moderate cases of the disease that have undergone laboratory investigation.
4. Ceará state civil registry - The number and cause of verified deaths.
5. Central Laboratory of Public Health of Ceará - Confirmatory laboratory testing results.
6. Unified Health System, Ceará Regulation Centre - Hospital admissions.

Cases Definitions

We followed the case definitions below for suspected cases of COVID-19:

1) An acute respiratory condition characterized by a fever or feverish sensation, even if only reported, accompanied by cough OR sore throat OR runny nose OR breathing difficulty. In the case of children, nasal obstruction was also acceptable in the absence of another specific diagnosis. In the case of the elderly, a reported or diagnosed fever was optional. 2) Specific worsening criteria such as syncope, mental confusion, excessive sleepiness, irritability, and loss of appetite. 3) Dyspnoea / respiratory discomfort OR persistent pressure in the chest OR O2 saturation less than 95% in room air OR bluish colour of the lips or face. 4) In children, in addition to the previous items, nasal flaring, cyanosis, intercostal circulation, dehydration, or lack of appetite. We followed the case definitions below for a confirmed case of COVID-19: a suspected case with molecular biology (RT-PCR in real time) detection of the SARS-CoV-2 virus OR a positive immunological test for antibody detection (rapid or classic serology) OR a history of close or home contact with a laboratory-confirmed case for COVID-19 within seven days before the onset of symptoms, and for which it was not possible to perform laboratory testing.

Study Variables And Data Analysis

The variables used in this study were sex, age group, date of onset of symptoms, whether the subject had been hospitalized, place of hospitalization (public or private), date of hospitalization, the time between first symptoms and hospitalization, whether the patient had been admitted to an intensive care unit, the time between the first symptoms and admission to the intensive care unit, laboratory diagnosis, outcome (discharged with resolved symptoms or death), date and place of death (if occurred), municipality of residence, pre-admission signs and symptoms, the ward occupancy rate, and the number (total and occupied) of ICU beds on the day the patient was admitted. All data were analysed using Epi Info software version 7.0 (U.S. Centres for Disease Control and Prevention, Atlanta, Georgia).

Ethical Aspects

All ethical principles provided for in the Resolution of the National Health Council (CNS-translated) No. 466, of December 12, 2012, were respected. The study design was approved by the State Secretariat of Health of Ceará.

RESULTS

The first confirmed cases of COVID-19 in Ceará were diagnosed on March 15, 2020, with onsets of symptoms on the 10th (two cases) and the 11th (one case). Within 45 days of the country's first known case, 37,268 cases had been confirmed in 85.9% of Brazil's 184 municipalities (Figures 1 and Figure 2). Of the confirmed cases, 7,833 (21.0%) were laboratory-confirmed, another 20,791 were under investigation and 1,019 were confirmed COVID-19-related deaths. Epidemic week 20 had the highest number of reported cases and the peak of deaths.

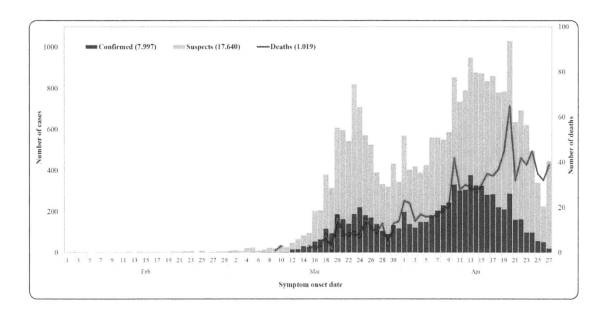

FIGURE 1: Number and temporal distribution of COVID-19 cases, by epidemiological week of symptom onset. Ceará, Brazil, 2020.

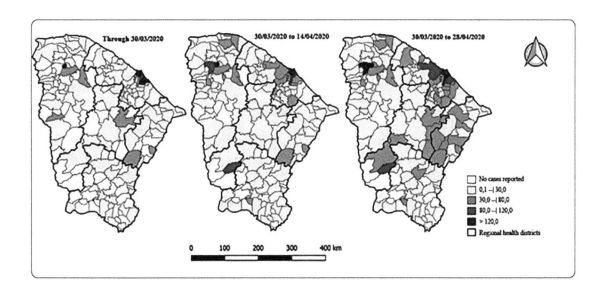

FIGURE 2: Spatial distribution of municipalities with confirmed COVID-19 cases in the first 45 days of the epidemic, by epidemiological week. Ceará, Brazil, 2020.

The distribution of cases was initially the most widespread in Fortaleza, Ceará's capital city, later overtaken by metropolitan municipalities in which the highest incidences were identified (over 120 cases per 100,000 inhabitants). The virus also spread through municipalities in the Northern region, which also had incidences above 120 cases per 100,000 inhabitants. During the 45-day period, the Central Laboratory of Public Health of Ceará (LACEN-CE) processed more than 15,000 molecular biology exams, reaching 738 tests in a single day (April 27). The lowest positive rate among the examinations was registered on March 21 (15.4%) and the highest on April 26 (84.8%). In the first 15 days, the average positivity was 21.9%, increasing to 46.2% and 73.6% over the next 15 and 30 days, respectively (Figure 3).

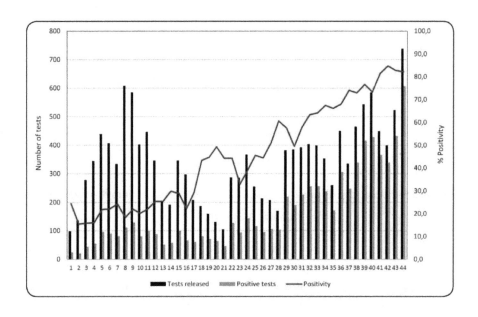

FIGURE 3: Number of tests and positivity of COVID-19 tests performed during the first 45 days of the epidemic. Ceará, Brazil, 2020.

The first death in Ceará was confirmed on March 23; within four days another 10 had been confirmed. Ten days after that, 57 more deaths had been confirmed. Subsequently, the number of confirmed deaths doubled approximately every seven days, reaching the highest single day occurrence on May 1st (53 deaths). Females made up a higher percentage than males of reported and confirmed cases (54.7%) but deaths occurred in a greater proportion in males (58.1%) (Table 1). The same pattern occurred in age groups where a predominance of cases were in people aged 20 to 59 years (70.3%), but the percentage of deaths was highest for those over 70 years of age (52.9%).

TABLE 1: Demographic and medical characteristics of COVID-19 cases and deaths in the first 45 days of the epidemic. Ceará, Brazil, 2020.

Variables	Notified		Confirmed		Deaths	
	N	%	N	%	N	%
Gender						
Male	16 874	45.3	3 666	46.8	592	58.1
Female	20 332	54.7	4 167	53.2	427	41.9
Age group						
< 1 year	570	1.5	67	0.9	0	0.0
1- 9 years	1 274	3.4	93	1.2	3	0.3
10- 19 years	1 097	2.9	134	1,7	2	0.2
20-59 years	26 031	70.3	5 492	70.1	287	28.2
60-69 years	3 727	10.1	945	12.1	188	18.4
> 70 years	4 313	11.7	1 091	13.9	539	52.9
Needed hospitalization						
Yes	2 647	7.1	1 288	16.4	878	91.9
No	34 621	92.9	6 545	83.5	77	8.1
Hospitalization in the Intensive Care Unit (ICU)						
Yes	777	2,1	499	6.4	473	58.0
No	36 491	97.9	7 334	93.6	342	42.0

The average age of the cases that progressed to death was 67 (1-101) years old, with more than half (52.9%) occurring in people over 69 years old (Table 1). The main symptoms reported among these cases were dyspnoea (86.0%), fever (85.2%), cough (84.7%), respiratory distress (77.1%), sore throat (21.5%), diarrhoea (14.1%), and vomiting (7.5%). The most common comorbidities were heart disease (66.5%) and diabetes (58.3%). Most deaths occurred in a hospital setting (91.9%), more than one-half required ICU bed hospitalization (58.0%), and 480 (53.9%) needed ventilator support. The average time between the onset of symptoms and death was 18 (1-56) days. The cases that evolved to death took 6 (0 - 40) days to be hospitalized and among those who were hospitalized, the average time in bed was 8 (1 - 49) days Considering the public hospital network in Ceará, on the 45th day of the epidemic COVID-19 patients occupied 655 ward beds, 421 ICU beds, and 376 beds with respirators. This represented 71.3% (23.8%-100.0%) of all ward beds, 80.5% (40.0%-100.0%) of all ICU beds, and 74.9% (40.0%-100.0%) of beds with mechanical ventilation (Table 2).

TABLE 2: Evaluation of bed use 45 days after the first confirmed case of COVID-19 in Ceará, in 2020.

Health Unit	Infirmary			ICU			Mechanical Ventilation		
	N	Occupied	%*	N	Occupied	%	N	Occupied	%
Hospital Leonardo da Vinci	66	61	92.4	115	83	72.2	74	66	89.2
Hospital Geral de Fortaleza	111	76	68.5	51	46	90.2	49	49	100.0
Hospital Geral Dr César Cals	24	22	91.7	10	10	100.0	10	9	90.0
Hospital São José	82	61	74.4	8	8	100.0	27	22	81.5
Hospital de Messejana	56	56	100.0	59	57	96.6	57	45	78.9
Hospital Infantil Albert Sabin	42	31	73.8	8	8	100.0	8	7	87.5
Hospital Abelardo Gadelha (Caucaia)	26	21	80.8	12	12	100.0	12	10	83.3
Hospital MM (Maracanaú)	13	9	69.2	5	2	40.0	5	2	40.0
Hospital São Vicente de Paula (Itapipoca)	11	9	81.8	10	10	100.0	8	8	100.0
Hospital Batista	124	88	71.0	7	3	42.9	3	2	66.7
Hospital Regional Norte (Sobral)	25	24	96.0	36	25	69.4	23	15	65.2
Hospital Regional SC (Quixeramobim)	33	17	51.5	30	27	90.0	30	19	63.3
Hospital Regional do Cariri (Juazeiro)	21	5	23.8	35	22	62.9	35	18	51.4
Hospital São Vicente (Iguatu)	21	5	23.8	35	22	62.9	35	18	51.4
Total	**655**	**485**	**74.0**	**421**	**335**	**79.6**	**376**	**290**	**77.1**

DISCUSSION

The first 45 days of the COVID-19 epidemic in Ceará showed an explosion in the number of cases and deaths, reaching more than 1,000 confirmed deaths. In the first days after the detection of the first cases, infections spread most rapidly in the city of Fortaleza and municipalities with higher HDI, mainly among users of the supplementary health network. In the following month, infections began to spread to the interior of the state, reaching the periphery of large cities and the most vulnerable social and economic populations. These populations have a higher prevalence of comorbidities, and often have living situations that make effective social isolation unfeasible[11]. This likely contributed to the early exponential increase in the number of cases and deaths.

The symptoms described in this study were similar to those reported for the pandemic for other countries[12]. Our findings show a predominance of male deaths, as was also reported in China[13]. A recent survey of more than 2,000 people in Ceará showed that a significant percentage of females perceive themselves to be at risk of COVID-19, while males reported greater difficulty adhering to social isolation practices[14]. These observations could, in part, explain our findings. At the beginning of the epidemic, due to concerns about the simultaneous increase of seasonal influenza and the possibility of a new dengue epidemic, the Ceará health department advised that medical care should only be sought for severe symptoms such as shortness of breath, difficulty breathing, or cognitive impairment[15,16]. This initial guidance, together with fears in the population of acquiring infection from attending a health facility, probably contributed to the increase in the number of home deaths. By the beginning of April, there were widespread notices by the Ceará health department that everyone, especially those with known risk factors, should seek basic care at the first sign of symptoms. This change reduced the number of home deaths, but also generated a large demand for basic health centres, contributing to the collapse of the outpatient care network.

This study had several limitations. We relied on secondary databases from local surveillance systems. Further, not all cases with laboratory confirmation were by RT-PCR, but those limitations don't invalidate the results. The Brazilian Ministry of Health published Decree 10.211 at the end of

January, reactivating the Inter-ministerial Executive Group on Public Health Emergency of National and International Importance (GEI-ESPII). Among other duties, the GEI-ESPII is responsible for implementing preparation measures and the official health surveillance response to the COVID-19 epidemic[17,18]. It is noteworthy that despite extensive efforts by health services, social isolation measures were not effective in reducing the speed of disease spread to the pace at which the health care network was expanding. This imbalance led to the collapse of the health system[19,20]. Development and implementation of effective health service responses to COVID-19 has been challenging, especially in poor countries[21]. In this scenario, it is essential to identify effective drugs for early stages of the disease and to develop an efficient vaccine[22].

ACKNOWLEDGEMENTS

LPGC is recipient of a fellowship for research productivity granted by the Brazilian National Council for Scientific and Technological Development (CNPq/Brazil).

REFERENCES

1. Zhu N, Zhang D, Wang W, Li X, Yang B, Song J, et al. A novel coronavirus from patients with pneumonia in China, 2019. N Engl J Med. 2020;382:727-33. [Links]

2. Holshue ML, DeBolt C, Lindquist S, Lofy KH, Wiesman J, Bruce H, et al. First case of 2019 novel coronavirus in the United States. N Engl J Med 2020;382:929-36. [Links]

3. World Health Organization (WHO). Coronavirus disease (COVID-19) . Situation Report - 51. Geneva: WHO; 2020. 9 p. [Links]

4. World Health Organization (WHO). Coronavirus disease (COVID-19) Situation Report - 101. Geneva: WHO ; 2020. 12 p. [Links]

5. Armocida B, Formenti B, Ussai S, Palestra F, Missoni E. The Italian health system and the COVID-19 challenge. Lancet Public Health. 2020; S2468-2667(20)30074-8. [Links]

6. Frank A, Fatke B, Frank W, Förstl H, Hölzle P. Depression, Dependence and Prices of the COVID-19-Crisis. Brain Behav Immun. 2020; S0889-1591(20)30642-5. [Links]

7. Oliveira WK, Duarte E, França GVA, Garcia LP. How Brazil can hold back COVID-19. Epidemiol Serv Saude. 2020;29(2):e2020044. [Links]

8. Diário oficial da União. Brasil. Portaria Nº 454, 20 de março de 2020. Declara, em todo o território nacional, o estado de transmissão comunitária do coronavírus (COVID-19). [acessed at May, 05th 2020]. Available at: http://www.in.gov.br/en/web/dou/-/portaria-n-454-de-20-de-marco-de-2020-249091587. [Links]

9. Ministério da Saúde (MS). Secretaria de Vigilância em Saúde. Sistema Nacional de Vigilância em Saúde - 15 Boletim epidemiológico especial COE COVID-19: Brasilia. 2020. 68 p. [Links]

10. Diário oficial do estado. Ceará. Decreto Nº33.519, de 19 de março de 2020. Intensifica as medidas para enfrentamento da infecção humana pelo novo coronavírus [Internet]. Editoração casa civil. [acessed at May, 05th 2020]. Available at: https://www.cge.ce.gov.br/wp-content/uploads/sites/20/2020/03/Decreto-n.-33.519-de-19-de-mar%C3%A7o-de-2020.-Intensifica-as-medidas-para-enfrentamento-da-infec%C3%A7%C3%A3o-humana-pelo-novo-coronavirus.pdf [Links]

11. Rodrigues-Junior AL, Ruffino-Netto A, Castilho EA. Distribuição espacial do índice de desenvolvimento humano, da infecção pelo HIV e da comorbidade AIDS-tuberculose: Brasil, 1982 - 2007. Rev. Bras. Epidemiol.2014;17(2):204-215. [Links]

12. Aggarwal S, Garcia-Telles N, Aggarwal G, Lavie C, Lippi G, Henry BM. Clinical features, laboratory characteristics, and outcomes of patients hospitalized with coronavirus disease 2019 (COVID-19): Early report from the United States. Diagnosis (Berl). 2020;26;7(2):91-96. [Links]

13. Lai CC, Shih TP, Ko WC, Tang HJ, Hsueh PR. Severe acute respiratory syndrome coronavirus 2 (sars-cov-2) and corona virus disease-2019 (COVID-19): the epidemic and the challenges. Int. J. Antimicrob. Agents. 2020;105924. [Links]

14. Lima DLF, Dias AA, Rabelo RS, Cruz ID, Costa SC, Nigri FMN, et al. COVID-19 in the State of Ceará: behaviours and beliefs in the arrival of the pandemic. Cien Saude Colet. 2020;25(5):1575-1586. [Links]

15. Cimerman S, Chebabo E, Cunha CA, Rodriguez-Morales AJ. Deep impact of COVID-19 in the healthcare of Latin America: the case of Brazil. Braz J Infect Dis. 2020;24(2):93-95. [Links]

16. Diaz-Quijano FA, Rodriguez-Morales AJ, Waldman AE. Translating transmissibility measures into recommendations for coronavirus prevention. Rev Saude Publica. 2020;54:43. [Links]

17. Croda J, Oliveira WK, Frutuoso RL, Mandetta LH, Baia-da-Silva DC, Brito-Sousa JD, et al. COVID-19 in Brazil: advantages of a socialized unified health system and preparation to contain cases. Rev Soc Bras Med Trop. 2020;53:e20200167. [Links]

18. Brazil. Presidência da República. Secretaria Geral. DECRETO Nº 10.211, DE 30 DE JANEIRO DE 2020. Dispõe sobre o Grupo Executivo Interministerial de Emergência em Saúde Pública de Importância Nacional e Internacional - GEI-ESPII. [acessed at May, 05th 2020]. Available at: http://www.planalto.gov.br/ccivil_03/_ato2019-2022/2020/decreto/D10211.htm [Links]

19. Garcia LP, Duarte E. Intervenções não farmacológicas para o enfrentamento à epidemia da COVID-19 no Brasil. Epidemiol Serv Saúde. 2020;29(2). [Links]

20. Bastos SB, Cajueiro DO. Modeling and forecasting the COVID-19 pandemic in Brazil. 2020; arXiv:2003.14288 [q-bio.PE]. Available at: https://arxiv.org/abs/2003.14288v1. [Links]

21. Velavan TP, Meyer CG. The COVID-19 epidemic. Trop Med Int Health. 2020 Mar;25(3):278-280. [Links]

22. Rothan A, Byrareddy SN. The Epidemiology and Pathogenesis of Coronavirus Disease (COVID-19) Outbreak. J Autoimmun. 2020;109:102433. [Links]

Received: June 04, 2020; Accepted: June 19, 2020

Corresponding author: Luciano Pamplona de Góes Cavalcanti. **e-mail:**pamplona.luciano@gmail.com

Authors' contributions: DRQL, SMD, LABGF, MMA, RGG, GPP, JNCF, LXF, ARPC, TBRL, PMCL, LPM, TMC, LPGC: Conception and design of the study, acquisition of data; **DRQL, SMD, LABGF, MMA, RGG, GPP, JNCF, LXF, ARPC, TBRL, PMCL, LPM, TMC, LPGC:** Conception and design of the study, analysis and interpretation of data, final approval of submitted manuscript; **DRQL, SMD, LABGF, MMA, RGG, GPP, JNCF, LXF, ARPC, TBRL, PMCL, LPM, TMC, LPGC:** Conception and design of the study, analysis and interpretation of data.

4. Aging And Inequalities: Social Protection Policies For Older Adults During The COVID-19 Pandemic In Brazil

[1]Alexandre Kalache[1] Alexandre da Silva[1] Karla Cristina Giacomin[1]
Kenio Costa de Lima[2] Luiz Roberto Ramos[3]
Marilia Louvison[1] Renato Veras[2]

The COVID-19 pandemic represents a challenge for the entire world, particularly low and middle income countries, An Imperial College, London study[1] highlighted the global nature of the crisis. Firm and coordinated action by governments, centred on social isolation for the entire population, could save millions of lives worldwide. While not disregarding the socioeconomic impact, emergency decisions must primarily consider the lives of **everyone**, despite the immediate economic interests. In Brazil, more than 80% of older adults depend exclusively on the National Health Service (or SUS) for their healthcare. This percentage is even higher among Afro-Brazilians[2] and the poor. The SUS has suffered severe budget cuts for years, and even before the pandemic, much of its equipment was already on the verge of collapse due to excess demand. The inequality is striking - as journalist Flavia de Oliveira has said, "The COVID-19 crisis did not create the country's ills. It exposed them"[3].

There is an urgent need to reverse policies that have led to the dismantling of the SUS, especially in Primary Care. The predictable increase in mortality from other causes due to overcrowding and the need to prioritize hospital services for patients with COVID-19 is also a worry; as is the lack of testing, resulting in an underestimating of the problem; and the shortage of respirators and personal protective equipment's (PPE's), putting the infrastructure and workforce at risk in order to support the growing need for services.

The profile of the Covid 19 pandemic in Brazil differs from that of other countries:

- it is younger, as long before the age of 60, adults suffer comorbidities that place them in the high-risk group;
- it is much "darker", as among the poorest of the poor are Afro-Brazilians. Questions of race and ethnicity are imperative - including indigenous populations, immigrants and nomadic peoples. Without this information, hitherto absent from epidemiological bulletins, strategies to tackle the crisis cannot be properly targeted;
- it affects women more, through the greater risks faced by the most exposed health professionals, the prevalence of informal work amongst women, their role as providers of food and care for their families, and increased domestic violence;
- it is even more age based, as economic choices determine the exclusion of older people from health services;

[1] 1Centro Internacional de Longevidade (ILC-Brasil). Rio de Janeiro, RJ, Brasil.
2Revista Brasileira de Geriatria e Gerontologia (RBGG). Rio de Janeiro, RJ, Brasil.
3Diretor do Centro de Estudos do Envelhecimento, Escola Paulista de Medicina / UNIFESP. São Paulo, SP, Brasil

- it is elitist, as the poorest Brazilians are deprived of access to diagnosis and treatment, wherever they live;
- it brings more suffering, given the complete lack of palliative care in the public network.

People grow old badly and early in Brazil. Thus, deaths by COVID-19 do not only reflect the age composition of the country, but above all the fact that there have never been policies for active and healthy aging, centred on the promotion of health, lifelong learning, citizen participation and the protection of the most vulnerable[4]. Therefore, the current crisis demands intergenerational and interdisciplinary solidarity from everyone. Like other countries, Brazil's response to the pandemic was "too little, too late"[5].

Millions of Brazilians have failed to follow the preventive guidelines, not because they do not want to, but because they cannot: social exclusion and structural discrimination deny them full access to their rights. Constitutional Amendment 95 further reduced resources, from health promotion to prevention, from primary care to hospital services; from sanitation conditions to care for the most dependent - all of which have been affected by severe cuts to the social policies budget. What responses are being offered to protect older adults living in long-term care facilities for the elderly (LTCFs)? How are the professionals working in these facilities being cared for and protected? How can organizational flows to referral services be guaranteed? What urgent measures can be adopted to prevent the foreseeable deaths in these institutions?

It is vital that we recognize the existence of these problems, and understand that deficiencies in gerontological knowledge make them worse[6]. Policies to combat the pandemic must consider the evidence accumulated by those who study aging in order to develop guidelines aimed at the needs of institutionalized older adults and the most vulnerable, considering the limitations of the formal services infrastructure and the absence of integrated care. That is why the ABRASCO (or Brazilian Association of Collective Health) Thematic Group (TG) on Aging and Public Health[5] has been working on reflections and proposals that can broaden our response to the serious health and political crisis that Brazil is facing. The absolute priority is the protection of the population as a whole, and in particular older adults, through social isolation aimed at flattening the epidemic curve and thus preventing the collapse of public and private health systems. We call for the urgent strengthening of primary health care policies, the creation of remote monitoring strategies, the guarantee of survival and protective equipment, the offering of concrete guidance and support for LTCFs, care for homeless older adults, support for older adults who care for other older people or who still depend on casual labour for their livelihood, as well as the assurance of a humanitarian approach and palliative care, when necessary. Public policies need to be created with people, not for people. Our older adults' rights councils have been severely weakened over the past year, in particular the National Council, which has little dialogue with civil society[7]. Once again, this TG warns: failure to consider the scientific evidence and WHO recommendations for the adoption of horizontal isolation will lead to an abject, inhuman, indefensible gerontocide. As part of the understanding that public policies are created with people and not for people, the *Revista Brasileira de Geriatria e Gerontologia* (the *Brazilian Journal of Geriatrics and Gerontology*), in its thematic issue on public policies constructed with older adults, invites submissions of scientific articles focusing on the public protection of the lives of older people.

REFERENCES

1. Walker GT, Whittaker C, Watson O, Baguelin Mark, Ainslie KEC, Bhatia S, et al. The Global impact of COVID-19 and strategies for mitigation and suppression [Internet]. London: Imperial College London; 2020 [acesso em 26 mar. 2020]. Disponível em: https://www.imperial.ac.uk/media/imperial-college/medicine/sph/ide/gida-fellowships/Imperial-College-COVID19-Global-Impact-26-03-2020.pdf [Links]

2. Werneck J. Racismo institucional e saúde da população negra. Saúde Soc [Internet]. 2016 [acesso em 20 mar. 2020];25(3):535-49. Disponível em: http://www.scielo.br/scielo.php?script=sci_arttext&pid=S0104-12902016000300535&lng=pt&tlng=pt [Links]

3. Oliveira F. Vocês que lutem! O Globo (Rio de Janeiro). 24 abr. 2020: Opinião. [Links]

4. Kalache A. Envelhecimento ativo: um marco político em resposta à revolução da longevidade. Rio de Janeiro: Centro Internacional de Longevidade Brasil; 2015. [Links]

5. The Lancet. COVID-19: too little, too late? Lancet [Internet]. 2020 [acesso em 06 mar. 2020];395(10226):1-2. PubMed; PMID: 32145772. Disponível em: https://www.ncbi.nlm.nih.gov/pmc/articles/PMC7135007/ [Links]

6. Lloyd-Sherlock PR, Ebrahim S, Geffen L, Mckee M. Bearing the brunt of COVID-19: older people in low and middle income countries. Br Med J. 2020;368:1-2. [Links]

7. Associação Brasileira de Saúde Coletiva. Pandemia da COVID-19 e um Brasil de desigualdades: populações vulneráveis e o risco de um genocídio relacionado à idade [Internet]. Rio de Janeiro: ABRASCO; 2020 [acesso em 01 abr. 2020]. Disponível em: https://www.abrasco.org.br/site/gtenvelhecimentoesaudecoletiva/2020/03/31/pandemia-do-COVID-19-e-um-brasil-de-desigualdades-populacoes-vulneraveis-e-o-risco-de-um-genocidio-relacionado-a-idade/ [Links]

8. Brasil. Centro Internacional de Longevidade. Carta aberta Conselho Nacional dos Direitos da Pessoa Idosa - CNDI [Internet]. Rio de Janeiro: ILC-Brasil; 2020 [acesso em 01 abr. 2020]. Disponível em: http://ilcbrazil.org/portugues/noticias/carta-aberta-ao-conselho-nacional-dos-direitos-da-pessoa-idosa-cndi/ [Links]

5. Geographic Access To COVID-19 Healthcare In Brazil Using A Balanced Float Catchment Area Approach

Rafael H. M. Pereira[*]

Carlos Kauê Vieira Braga

Luciana Mendes Servo

Institute for Applied Economic Research - Ipea, Brazil

Bernardo Serra

Institute for Transport Policy & Development - ITDP Brazil, Brazil

Pedro Amaral

Universidade Federal de Minas Gerais (UFMG), Brazil

Nelson Gouveia

University of São Paulo Medical School (FMUSP), Brazil

Antonio Paez

McMaster University, Canada

ABSTRACT

The rapid spread of the new coronavirus across the world has raised concerns about the responsiveness of cities and healthcare systems during pandemics. Recent studies try to model how the number of COVID19 infections will likely grow and impact the demand for hospitalization services at national and regional levels. However, less attention has been paid to the geographic access to COVID-19 healthcare services and to the response capacity of hospitals at the local level, particularly in urban areas in the Global South. This paper shows how transport accessibility analysis can provide actionable information to help improve healthcare coverage and responsiveness. It analyses accessibility to COVID-19 healthcare at high spatial resolution in the 20 largest cities of Brazil. Using network-distance metrics, we estimate the vulnerable population living in areas with poor access to healthcare facilities that could either screen or hospitalize COVID-19 patients. We then use a new balanced floating catchment area (BFCA) indicator to estimate spatial, income and racial inequalities in access to hospitals with intensive care unit (ICU) beds and mechanical ventilators while taking into account congestion effects. Based on this analysis, we identify substantial social and spatial inequalities in access to health services during the pandemic. The availability of ICU equipment varies considerably between cities and it is substantially lower among black and poor communities. The study maps territorial inequalities in healthcare access and reflects on different policy lessons that can be learned for other countries based on the Brazilian case.

1. INTRODUCTION

The global outbreak of the new coronavirus (SARS-CoV-2) has raised serious concerns about the responsiveness of healthcare systems and particularly about how vulnerable population groups might be affected (Lancet, 2020; WHO, 2020). A rapidly growing body of research has emerged to model how the number of COVID-19 infections will likely grow and impact the demand for hospitalization services globally (Petropoulos & Makridakis, 2020; Walter et al, 2020) and at the national level (Arenas et al., 2020; Moghadas et al., 2020; Paez, 2020; Paez et al., n.d.; Wu, Leung, & Leung, 2020). However, less attention has been paid to the geographic access to COVID-19 healthcare services and to the response capacity of hospitals at the local level in urban areas, despite the potential relationships between accessibility to healthcare resources and mortality (Ji, Ma, Peppelenbosch, & Pan, 2020). Early work by Ji et al. (2020) and Rader et al. (2020), for example, considered resources at the provincial level in China and at the county level in the USA, but we are not aware of studies that investigate the issue of resource allocation at higher spatial resolutions, particularly in the context of Latin America, where the epicentre of the pandemic shifted in June, 2020.

The goal of this study is to present estimates of geographic accessibility to COVID-19 healthcare at high spatial resolution in the 20 largest cities of Brazil. Healthcare services in Brazil are known to be unevenly distributed across the country and also within cities (Amaral et al., 2017). In this context, it is crucial to map where vulnerable social groups confront poor accessibility to health services. Similarly, it becomes paramount to identify which healthcare facilities are likely to face surges in demand due to the need to hospitalize severely ill patients. In this paper we combine traditional and novel accessibility metrics to address these questions. Using network distance metrics, we first estimate the number of vulnerable people living in areas with poor access to inpatient or outpatient facilities able to provide care for patients with suspected or confirmed cases of COVID-19. Next, we use a new balanced floating catchment area method (BFCA) proposed by (Paez, Higgins, & Vivona, 2019) to analyze levels of access to hospitals that could treat patients with severe symptoms of COVID-19, taking into account healthcare system capacity and competition effects for ICU beds with mechanical ventilators.

The results of this research are useful to identify, in the 20 cities examined, a population of approximately 1.6 million people who live more than 5 km away from a healthcare facility equipped to treat severe cases of COVID-19. Furthermore, although overall the average number of intensive care units (ICU)beds with ventilators is 1.06 per 10 thousand inhabitants, there are large variations in this level of service, both between and within cities. In particular, we find that the accessibility to ICU resources is substantially lower in black and poor communities. This creates a worrying scenario given the strong potential for propagation of COVID-19 combined with poor health outcomes. The study maps territorial inequalities in healthcare access and reflects on different policies that could be adopted to address them. The remainder of this paper is as follows. The next section provides relevant background information regarding the evolution of the COVID-19 pandemic in Brazil and accessibility analysis. This is followed by a discussion of the data and methods used in this research. Then, the results of the empirical analysis are presented and discussed. And finally, we offer some concluding remarks, including policy implications and directions for future research.

2. BACKGROUND

2.1 COVID-19 in Brazil

The first confirmed case of COVID-19 in Latin America was in late February 2020, in Brazil. The affected person was a man from São Paulo who had travelled that month to Italy. This case was typical of the beginning of the epidemic in Brazil, with other early cases of the disease imported via international flights coming mostly from Italy and the United States (Candido et al., 2020). At that early stage, the then-Minister of Health noted that it would remain to be seen how the virus behaved in a tropical country in the middle of summer. While there is evidence that incidence of the disease is lower at higher temperatures (Paez et al., 2020), it is now clear that the disease can be devastating during summer too: as early of July, less than five months after the first confirmed case of the COVID-19 in Brazil, over 1.8 million cases have been confirmed, and over 70 thousand deaths have been attributed to the disease, 45% of which concentrated in the 20 largest cities of the country. By early June, Brazil had become, after the United States, the country with the highest number of cases of COVID-19 in the world.

The earliest cases of COVID-19 in Brazil were concentrated among middle and upper class people (Souza et al., 2020). In Brazil's mixed health care system, these segments of the population typically can afford to pay for healthcare or use health services intermediated by private health insurance. This is not the case for lower-income groups, who are largely dependent on the public health system in Brazil, and among whom community transmission rapidly increased the number of infections. This development is particularly worrisome as low-income groups in the country also typically live in less developed urban areas with poor transport services and poor access to health, education, and employment opportunities (Pereira, Braga, Serra, & Nadalin, 2019).

Previous research, in fact, has identified important spatial gaps in accessibility to emergency services in Brazil (Rocha et al., 2017). To further complicate matters, other research has linked poor accessibility to higher pneumonia mortality (Zaman et al., 2014).

Given the rapid growth of COVID-19 in Brazil, it is important to map the potential stress on the country's healthcare system. Preliminary reports already show an unusual increase in the numbers of admissions to hospitals due to suspected COVID-19 infections (InfoGripe, 2020). These studies raise serious concerns about the overload the pandemic can generate to the public Unified Health System (Sistema Único de Saúde - SUS), which already started showing signs of collapse similar to those observed in Italy and Spain (Grasselli, Pesenti, & Cecconi, 2020; LegidoQuigley et al., 2020). The work of Noronha et al. (2020), for example, presented a simulation of nationwide spread of the new coronavirus and analyzed the supply and demand for ICU beds with ventilators, broken down by health regions. They found that even in an optimistic scenario, of an infection level of 0.1% in the first month, roughly half of the nation's health regions would face a grave deficit of ICU beds to meet demand for admission of patients with severe cases of COVID19. Similar regional modelling studies conducted by Coelho et al (2020) and Castro et al (2020) suggest the pressure on the health system is more likely to reach critical levels in large urban centres, where the number of confirmed cases is higher.In this context, there is still a lack of studies that look at the COVID-19 healthcare provision at the city level, particularly at what actionable insights can be drawn from analysis of vulnerable groups and their access to health services in high spatial resolution. The looming crisis faced by the health system due to the COVID-19 requires many emergency actions.

For this purpose, it is essential for healthcare planners to have a diagnosis of the areas of cities with less access to health services and equipment, and to identify the hospitals that might suffer overloaded demand for admissions.

2.2 Healthcare Accessibility

One of the most commonly used indicators to measure geographic access to healthcare is the shortest distance/travel time to the closest facility (Geurs & van Wee, 2004; Neutens, 2015). This indicator is widely used in part because it is relatively simple to calculate and straightforward to interpret, and thus easily communicated to policy makers. A well-known limitation of this indicator, however, is that it overlooks competition effects since it does not account for potential population demand nor for the levels of service supply. Another popular approach to measure access to healthcare is the family of Floating Catchment Area (FCA) methods (Matthews et al., 2019). A key advantage of this family of indicators is that it accounts for capacity restrictions, local competition effects as well as cross border healthcare-seeking behaviour (Neutens, 2015).

The common rationale underlying FCA methods is to calculate accessibility levels in sequential steps. This first step is to calculate the provider-to-population ratio (PPR) of each health facility as a ratio between its service supply (e.g. number of ICU beds) and its potential service demand given by the population that falls within some catchment area. The second step is to calculate accessibility levels of each population centre by aggregating the PPR of every healthcare provider that is accessible from each population centre. The first indicator of this sort is the two-step floating catchment area (2SFCA), proposed in the early 2000s (Luo & Wang, 2003; Radke & Mu, 2000). Since then, multiple authors have proposed incremental improvements to the basic model in order to incorporate more sophisticated impedance functions (Dai, 2010; Luo & Qi, 2009), to consider suboptimal configurations of health systems (Delamater, 2013) and to account for spatially adaptive floating catchments (Matthews et al., 2019; Matthew R. McGrail & Humphreys, 2009) and trip-chaining behaviour (Fransen, Neutens, De Maeyer, & Deruyter, 2015).

A fundamental limitation of FCA methods is that they overestimate both service demand and supply, which can generate misleading accessibility estimates (Delamater, 2013; Paez et al., 2019; Wan, Zou, & Sternberg, 2012). Demand inflation occurs when populations that fall within the overlap of catchment areas are counted more than once as potential demand for multiple facilities. Supply inflation, on the other hand, happens when the level of service of a healthcare unit is simultaneously allocated to multiple population centres (Paez et al., 2019). Until recently, two approaches had been proposed to address this issue. Wan et al. (2012) introduced the ThreeStep Float Catchment Area (3SFCA), which deflates demand by introducing an initial step that splits the potential demand of a population centre over multiple health facilities proportional to transport costs/distances. Meanwhile, Delamater (2013) proposed the Modified Two-Step Floating Catchment Area (M2SFCA), which deflates the supply side by increasing the friction of distance in a way that allocates levels of service more locally. Nonetheless, both methods only partially fix the inflation problem, as they compound the effects of impedance functions to address either demand inflation (3SFCA) or supply inflation (M2SFCA).

To overcome this limitation, Paez et al. (2019) recently introduced a new indicator to the FCA family, which we term here as the Balanced Float Catchment Area (BFCA). The new BFCA uses a standardized impedance matrix to generate proportional allocation of demand and level of service, fixing both demand and supply inflation issues in FCA calculations. The result is a more intuitive measure of accessibility that 1) accounts for competition effects, 2) provides a local version of the provider-to-population ratio (PPR) that is interpreted similarly to a regional PPR; and 3) preserves system-wide population and level of service, overcoming inflation issues. Estimating accessibility during a pandemic is an idoneous application of this method because congestion over the short term is one of the fundamental issues to address. Therefore, the analysis must account accurately for competition for scarce resources, if policy interventions are to have any hope of addressing shortfalls effectively.

4. DATA AND METHODS

4.1 Data

Accessibility to health facilities is estimated using data generated by the Access to Opportunities Project (Pereira et al, 2019)[1]. The method combines data from national household surveys, administrative records of the federal and municipal governments, along with satellite images and collaborative mapping data to estimate accessibility at high spatial resolution on a hexagonal grid with size of 357 meters (short diagonal), approximately the size of a typical city block. Original sociodemographic data comes from the 2010 population census conducted by the Brazilian Institute of Geography and Statistics (IBGE). These data are aggregated in a hexagonal grid using dissymmetric interpolation in two steps, as follows. Data on population count, income, race and age distribution are gathered at the census tract level. Population counts are then updated based on municipal-level demographic projections for 2020, published by Freire et al. (2020). The total projected population of each city in 2020 was distributed across census tracts assuming that the relative distribution of the population by district and age cohort of each sector remained constant between 2010 and 2020. We then use dissymmetric interpolation to pass information from census tracts to a finer regular grid of 200 meters with population count data considering aerial intersection and population sizes. Finally, these data are reaggregated from the regular grid to the hexagonal grid. Data on healthcare facilities associated with the SUS, as registered in the National Registry of Health Facilities (CNES), at the end of 2019 were geocoded and made publicly available by Pereira et al. (2019). For this paper, these data were complemented with updated information from the CNES for February 2020 about the number of adult ICU beds and ventilators in each healthcare facility. We also included geolocated data on 30 field hospitals and reactivated hospitals in 15 cities up to April 2, 2020. The functioning of these hospitals has eased demand on other hospitals and expanded the capillarity of the health system, by adding a total of 868 beds in ICUs, ITCs and semi-intensive or semi-critical care units. Finally, we used collaborative mapping data from OpenStreetMap and data on terrain from satellite images (JAXA, 2011). These data were processed with Open Trip Planner, an open routing algorithm for multimodal transport networks, to generate the door-to-door travel times between all the hexagon pairs in each city.

---

[1] More information about the Access to Opportunities Project and its databases are available at: https://www.ipea.gov.br/acessooportunidades/en/.

4.2 METHODS

The analysis presented in the paper is divided in two parts. In the first part, we estimate for Brazil's 20 largest cities the number and living places of vulnerable populations who: (a) cannot access within 30 minutes on foot an establishment associated with the SUS that can perform triage and refer patients suspected of COVID-19 infection for hospitalization; and (b) live further than 5 Km from a hospital with capacity to admit patients suffering from SARS with adult ICU beds and ventilators. Vulnerable population groups were defined as people above 50 years old with lower income (in the bottom half of the income distribution). This criteria was chosen because the resulting group includes people who: 1) are at greater vulnerability to COVID-19 infection due to their age; 2)are more dependent on the public health system; and 3) tend to face greater difficulties of urban mobility and access to health services[1].All time and distance thresholds were chosen as a first exploratory analysis following the official recommendation from the Health Ministry and local officials (state and municipal), who recommend that people with suspected COVID-19 infection stay at home if the symptoms are mild or go to the nearest health unit for an initial interview (anamnesis) and notification of the surveillance team (Brasil, 2020b). Patients with severe symptoms should be referred for admission to hospitals in general wards or ICUs (ibid.). In Brazil, the typical pattern is for people to use hospitals as entry points for daily health services and emergency care (ibid). Following clinical management and fast track service protocols (Brasil, 2020a, 2020b), this analysis included those primary health service facilities with capabilities to screen patients suspected of COVID-19, refer patients to specialized services, as well as facilities with more advanced service levels, such as emergency care centres, first aid posts and hospitals[2].Accessibility levels by public transportation were not considered because the use of collective transportation is not recommended for people with symptoms of COVID-19. Besides this, various cities saw a drop of over 70% in the supply of transit services as a response to isolation measures (NTU, 2020). This reduction makes public transport services less reliable and also more hazardous for contagion due to the large agglomeration of people at stops/stations and aboard vehicles. In the second part of the analysis we look at access to health services while taking into account healthcare system capacity and competition effects. In this part we focus on access to those facilities that could provide hospitalization in ICUs to support patients with COVID-19.

This analysis estimates provider-to-population ratios from both origin and destination perspectives. We calculated (1) for each hexagonal cell the number of accessible ICU beds with ventilators, and (2) for each hospital the ratio between the number of adult ICU beds with ventilators available and the population of the corresponding catchment area. Here we use the balanced float catchment area (BFCA) to calculate component (1) and a partial version using the

---

[1] Ideally, it would be important also to consider the population with comorbidities, such as hypertension, diabetes and cardiovascular or respiratory diseases, because people with these profiles are at greater risk of COVID-19 infection, with greater severity and lethality (Guan et al., 2020; Yang et al., 2020). However, data with this level of detail are not yet available.

[2] The following types of healthcare units for first-response services and triage were considered: community health posts, basic health centres/units, polyclinics, general hospitals, specialized hospitals, mixed care units, general first aid posts, specialized first aid posts, and units for indigenous health response. As established by the Management Protocol for the New Coronavirus (*Protocolo de Manejo para o Novo Coronavirus*), "All patients who seek health services (Primary Health Response Units, Emergency Care Units, First Aid Posts, Mobile Pre-Hospital Service Units and Hospitals), must be submitted to clinical triage that includes early recognition of suspected cases, and if necessary, immediate referral of the patient to an area separated from those that contain respiratory and hand hygiene supplies" (free translation from Ministério da Saúde, 2020b).

first two steps of BFCA to calculate component (2). There are generally two approaches to implement accessibility measures: positive and normative.

The first one considers the willingness of people to travel whereas the latter captures a norm to be satisfied (Páez, Scott, & Morency, 2012).

In practice, the difference between positive and normative accessibility is the definition of the impedance function. In this study we consider both approaches. In the first part of the empirical analysis we consider a normative implementation with a threshold of 30 minutes travel time based on research by McGrail et al. (2015). This threshold was chosen with a policy assumption that tries to minimize the distance that patients travel as a way to reduce contagion risks for others. In the second part of the analysis, we calculated accessibility considering as a threshold the maximum distance to the nearest hospital in each city. This threshold can be interpreted as the minimum necessary distance that guarantees that every person can reach at least one hospital, and is normatively in line with the recommendation from the Ministry of Health (Ministério da Saúde, 2020b) that suspected cases should visit their nearest hospital. Because this treatment of patients with SARS often requires combined availability of ICU beds and mechanical ventilators, we only considered the joint availability of bed/ventilator. Thus, in the case of a hospital with 30 adult ICU beds but only 20 ventilators, we considered only 20 beds (one ventilator per bed).

As a rule, however, there are more ventilators than ICU beds. For ICU beds in field hospitals, we assumed there was at least one ventilator available per bed. A limitation of this method is that it considered the ICU beds and ventilators that are in use, but these might not be the appropriate models for long use as in COVID-19 cases. Another limitation is that we analysed the attendance capacity of the public healthcare system focusing only on the number of adult ICU beds and ventilators. Other studies should also consider restrictions imposed by the availability of healthcare professionals to staff ICUs when the data is available.

Another limitation of the method is that our analyses are restricted to the population and supply of services within cities. This generates two effects. The first is the tendency to underestimate the level of access to services by people who live near the border between two cities, since they could possibly access hospitals in the neighbouring city. The second effect is the underestimation of the demand from people from other neighbouring cities who can seek admission to hospitals in the 20 cities analysed. To minimize this second problem, we applied an adjustment factor for hospital admissions by non-residents

(Brasil, 2005) according to the size of the population living in each hexagon, as suggested by Paez et al. (2019). A factor of 1.5, for example, would simulate that the size of the demand for admission to each hospital is 50% higher due to patients living in other cities. In a recent study, Servo, Andrade and Amaral (2019) demonstrated that in 2015 on average 30% of the hospitalizations for medium complexity treatments in cities was from patients living in other cities. Based on data from the SUS Hospital Information System for 2019, we calculated the value of the correction factors for each city (Table 1). Note that the correction factor is less than 1 in Guarulhos and São Gonçalo. This means that these cities export more people looking for healthcare in other cities than they receive from other cities.

Table 1. Inpatient care for resident and non-resident in the 20 largest Brazilian cities, 2019

City	Total residents inpatient care (A)	Total of inpatient care (B) *	Adjustment Factor B/A
Rio de Janeiro	226,630	283,946	1.3
São Paulo	608,351	694,008	1.1
Belo Horizonte	154,761	272,452	1.8
Curitiba	126,034	166,789	1.3
Brasília	181,564	229,614	1.3
Fortaleza	142,076	214,470	1.5
São Gonçalo	38,692	27,362	0.7
Porto Alegre	104,203	183,193	1.8
Duque de Caxias	42,280	44,204	1.0
Goiânia	77,235	151,762	2.0
Campinas	56,122	79,007	1.4
Guarulhos	64,252	55,369	0.9
Salvador	154,404	237,961	1.5
Recife	107,144	298,498	2.8
Campo Grande	52,322	68,952	1.3
Maceió	48,439	88,008	1.8
Belém	68,667	106,579	1.6
Manaus	113,926	124,372	1.1
São Luís	60,137	105,002	1.7
Natal	45,359	93,285	2.1

Source: Authors own elaboration. Obs. Hospitalizations by place of residence (A), and hospitalizations by hospital location (B). * Accounts for hospitalizations of patients who live inside the municipality and patients from outer areas.

5. RESULTS

5.1 Access to health services

In the 20 largest Brazilian cities nearly 228 thousand low-income people older than 50 years live more than 30 minutes by walking from a health unit that provides triage and referral services to patients with suspected infection (Table 2). The primary health care units and emergency care units, in particular, play a fundamental role as entry points to the system, to avoid hazardous agglomeration of patients with suspected coronavirus infection, so the spatial capillarity and longitudinality of this service are very important. The highest proportion of people in this situation were found in the cities of Rio de Janeiro, São Paulo, Brasília, Duque de Caxias, Campinas and Goiânia. These six cities concentrate more than 60% of the vulnerable population who live more than 30 minutes on foot from a health service point. However, analysis of the proportion in each city reveals that Duque de Caxias, São Luís, Brasília, Maceió and Campinas stand out with more than 10% of their vulnerable population living more than 30 minutes from an establishment qualified for this triage.

Furthermore, Table 2 also shows there are some 1.6 million vulnerable people who live farther than 5 Km from a health unit able to admit patients in serious condition due to COVID-19. This total represents 41% of the vulnerable population in the 20 cities. These numbers vary widely across cities due to the different patterns of urban occupation and the spatial distribution of healthcare facilities in each area. Cities like Rio de Janeiro, São Paulo, Brasília and Curitiba stand out for having more than 100 thousand inhabitants in potentially vulnerable conditions and with poor access to hospitals with ICU beds and mechanical ventilators. It is also noteworthy that half of the 20 cities have more than 50% of their vulnerable population living farther than 5 Km from inpatient facilities.

Table 2 - Low-income population above 50 years old with access to healthcare in Brazil's 20 largest cities, 2020

City	Total population	Vulnerable population**	(A) Vulnerable Pop. with poor access to basic health services	(B) Vulnerable Pop. with poor access to ICU hospitalization	(B) / Vulnerable Pop. (%)
Rio de Janeiro	6592.2	692.5	51.9	384.3	55.5
São Paulo	12142.6	1053.6	33.2	263.1	25
Brasília	3052.5	180.3	21.1	121	67.1
Curitiba	1927	172.9	5.1	116.4	67.3
Belo Horizonte	2469.9	244	7.2	92.3	37.8
Fortaleza	2651.8	193.5	6.5	77.7	40.2
São Gonçalo	1075.4	112.9	8.8	72.6	64.3
Duque deCaxias	905.1	81.3	13.5	67	82.4
Porto Alegre	1480.5	159.6	8.6	60.3	37.8
Goiânia	1509.4	118.3	11.4	59.4	50.2
Campinas	1208.9	115.1	12.2	58.1	50.5
Guarulhos	1389.9	98.7	4.3	48	48.6
Recife	1607	147.1	0.6	42.9	29.2
Campo Grande	895.6	69.7	5	42.9	61.5
Maceió	1042	74.2	8.4	38.2	51.5
Salvador	2831.6	217.4	7.8	35.3	16.2
Belém	1360.1	97.2	8.7	32.9	33.8
Manaus	2216.1	111.6	2.3	24.8	22.2
São Luís	1080.4	69.3	10.2	18.6	26.8
Natal	867.9	63	1.6	10.2	16.2
Total	48305.9	4072.2	228.4	1666	40.9

Source: authors own elaboration using data from Pereira et al. (2019), healthcare facilities data from CNES on February 2020, and population projections for 2020 from Freire et al (2020).Obs.

- Population in thousands.
- ** Population above 50 years old and in the bottom half of the income distribution.
- (A) Low-income people above 50 years old who cannot access a healthcare facility in less tan 30 minutes walking.
- (B) Low-income people above 50 years old who live more than 15 Km away from the nearest hospital with an ICU bed and mechanical ventilator.
-

As important as estimating how many vulnerable people have poor access to healthcare is mapping where this population lives. Figures 1 to 4 present for four selected cities the size and living place of the low-income population older than 50 years who (A) cannot access any primary healthcare establishment in less than 30 minutes by walking; and (B) live more than 5 Km from the nearest hospital with at least one ICU bed and one ventilator. For the sake of brevity, we only present the maps for Sao Paulo, Rio de Janeiro, Fortaleza and Manaus, the 4 cities most affected by COVID-19 in Brazil. As of the end of June, these four cities alone concentrated 18% of COVID19 confirmed cases and 32% of deaths in the country. These maps show that vulnerable populations with poor access to health services are mostly located in urban peripheries, indicating those areas which would be good candidates for local policy interventions, such as setting up field hospitals or engaging pre-hospital mobile units (such as the Urgent Mobile Response Service - SAMU) or community health agents.

Figure 1. Access to COVID-19 healthcare. Fortaleza, 2020. **(A)** Vulnerable population who cannot access a basic healthcare facility in less than 30 minutes walking. **(B)** Vulnerable population who lives farther than 5 Km to the nearest hospital with ICU bed and mechanical ventilator.

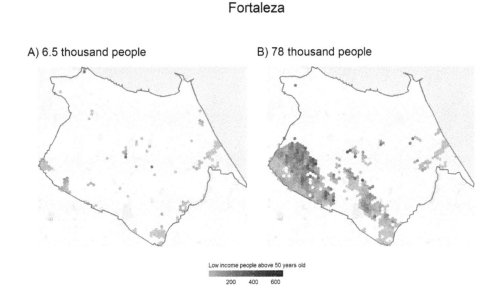

Figure 2. Access to COVID 19 healthcare. Manaus, 2020. **(A)** Vulnerable population who cannot access a basic healthcare facility in less than 30 minutes walking. **(B)** Vulnerable population who lives farther than 5 Km to the nearest hospital with ICU bed and mechanical ventilator.

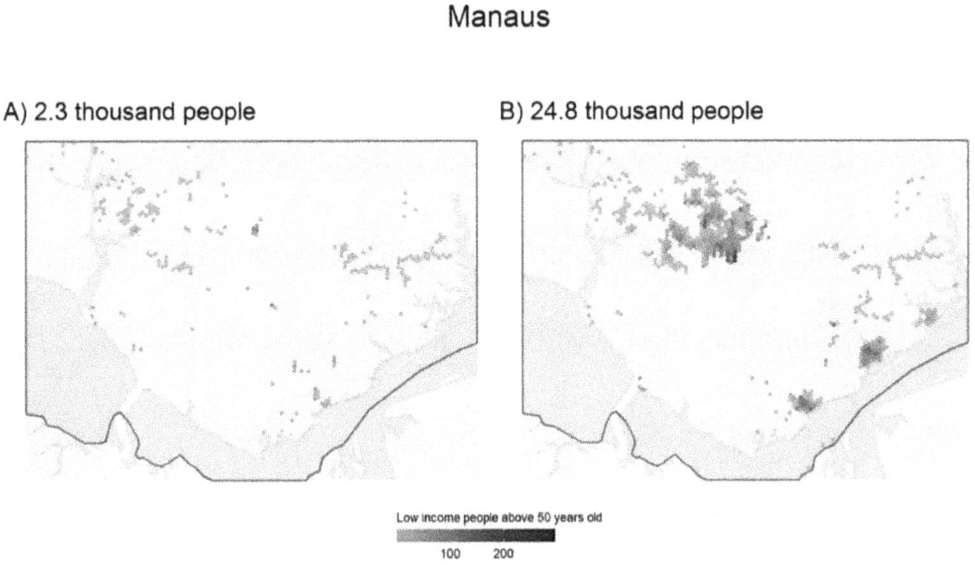

Figure 3. Access to COVID 19 healthcare. Rio de Janeiro, 2020. **(A)** Vulnerable population who cannot access a basic healthcare facility in less than 30 minutes walking. **(B)** Vulnerable population who lives farther than 5 Km to the nearest hospital with ICU bed and mechanical ventilator.

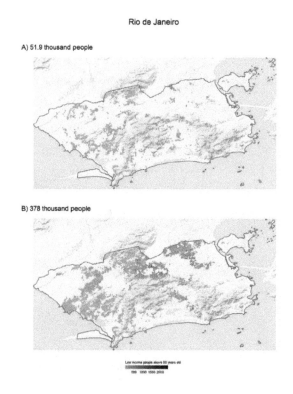

Figure 4. Access to COVID 19 healthcare. São Paulo, 2020. **(A)** Vulnerable population who cannot access a basic healthcare facility in less than 30 minutes walking. **(B)** Vulnerable population who lives farther than 5 Km to the nearest hospital with ICU bed and mechanical ventilator.

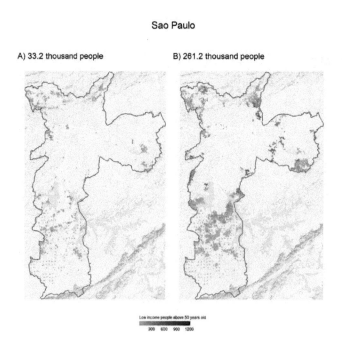

5.2. Health System Capacity

A basic indicator to measure the capacity of a health system is the number of hospital beds per inhabitant in a given area. According to the parameters defined by the Brazilian Ministry of Health (Brasil, 2015) the minimum standard provision should be 1 adult ICU bed for each 10 thousand people[1]. The average number of adult ICU beds with ventilators in hospitals in the public health system in the 20 largest Brazilian cities is 1.06 per 10 thousand people (Table 3). This value is only slightly higher than the minimum recommended by the Ministry of Health under normal circumstances. The value of 1.06 can be considered insufficient in an epidemic situation, posing a risk of overload in scenarios for COVID-19 contagion indicated in previous studies (Castro et al., 2020; Noronha et al., 2020). The ratio of beds per population also varies greatly across cities (Table 3). Thirteen out of the 20 cities analyzed are below the recommended level of service and by July 1st most of these cities had bed ICU bed occupancy rates above 80% (Folha de S.Paulo, 2020).

---

[1] Edict 1,101 of June 12, 2002, and Resolution 7 of February 24, 2010.

Table 3. Number of adult UCI beds and mechanical ventilators in SUS per 10 thousand people in Brazil's 20 greatest municipalities, 2020.

Municipality	ICU beds*	Population (in thousands)**	ICU beds per 10 thousand people
São Gonçalo	149	760.5	2
Goiânia	596	2965.9	2
Belo Horizonte	792	4348.2	1.8
Rio de Janeiro	1419	8259.4	1.7
Porto Alegre	327	2602.8	1.3
Salvador	565	4363.9	1.3
São Paulo	1211	13852.3	0.9
Campo Grande	102	1180.3	0.9
Curitiba	211	2550.1	0.8
Campinas	141	1701.9	0.8
Guarulhos	93	1197.7	0.8
Recife	373	4477	0.8
São Luís	159	1886.4	0.8
Belém	139	2111	0.7
Manaus	170	2419.3	0.7
Natal	123	1784.9	0.7
Fortaleza	241	4003	0.6
Brasília	181	3860.3	0.5
Maceió	82	1893.2	0.4
Duque de Caxias	30	946.3	0.3
Total	7,104	67,164.4	1.06

Source: authors own elaboration using data from Pereira et al. (2019), healthcare facilities data from CNES on February 2020, and population projections for 2020 from Freire et al (2020). obs.: * Number of ICU beds with mechanical ventilators in the public healthcare system. ** City population corrected by the adjustment factor from Table 1.

The greatest variations in the availability of health services, however, occur within cities. In Figures 5 to 8 below we present a set of maps that together give a detailed view of the spatial distribution of hospitals with adult ICU beds and ventilators and the level of access to these services considering competition effects.

The maps on **Panel A** show the spatial distribution of hospitals, where each hospital is represented by a circle whose size reflects the ratio between the number of beds/ventilators of that hospital and the population of its catchment area. Although the situations vary across cities, as a rule, downtown areas generally concentrate the greatest number of hospitals, especially the ones with more beds per inhabitant. This is the case for example in Fortaleza, Manaus and Rio de Janeiro. The availability of ICU beds and ventilators to serve patients with severe COVID-19 tends to be considerably lower in the peripheral regions of these cities.

In these regions, it is common to observe ratios of ICU beds per 10 thousand inhabitants between 0.5 and 1.0. These ratios can be considered critical against a backdrop of an epidemic with growing numbers of patients needing hospitalization for respiratory complications. The example of cities like Rio de Janeiro also illustrate how setting up field hospitals in farther areas can increase the capillarity of health services in epidemic situations like the COVID-19 outbreak.

Meanwhile, the maps on **Panel B** show the number of ICU beds and ventilators accessible from each location considering at the same time the level of service availability and the potential overlap of demand and supply competition effects estimated with the balanced float catchment area (BFCA). Compared to the results in Panel A, these maps present in more detail how the geographic access to COVID-19 healthcare is particularly higher in central urban areas.

This is perhaps more clearly seen in the city of São Paulo, where accessibility to equipped beds steadily declines from the central parts of the city to the periphery. Considering the average population per tile of the hexagonal grid in São Paulo, this indicates that in the regions with the highest accessibility, there are approximately 0.000012 beds per 10,000 people serving on average 1,240 persons. This translates into 9.76e-6 beds per person, compared to 8.74e-5 beds per person average for São Paulo. This shows how the regional PPR can be misleading, by assuming that every person in the region has equal access to medical facilities. Analysis using the BFCA indicator also illustrates how living close to a hospital does not necessarily translate into high levels of accessibility, once congestion effects are taken into account. This is the case in cities like Fortaleza, Rio de Janeiro, and São Paulo, where some peripheral neighbourhoods, despite being close to a hospital, face poor access to health services due to the limited capacity of the healthcare system to support the expected demand of much larger areas.

Finally, the maps on **Panel C** present bivariate choropleth maps with the combined spatial distribution of population densities and accessibility levels by automobile using city-specific thresholds so that every person could reach at least one hospital. This panel complements previous figures by highlighting those areas with large populations underserved by healthcare services (bright pink = larger population and lower accessibility) and those areas which face higher service levels for a comparable lower demand (bright green = smaller population but high accessibility). It is possible to see that even in those places with low accessibility, there are pockets where the situation is made worse by afflicting larger populations. The figures in Panel C are useful to differentiate low-accessibility areas with large and small population numbers, which can provide actionable information for policy makers to choose which low-accessibility areas should be prioritized in emergency situations.

Figure 5. Spatial distribution of hospitals with adult ICU beds and ventilators and the level of access to these services considering competition effects. Fortaleza, 2020.

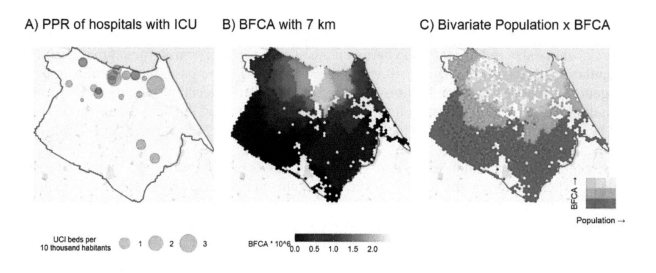

Figure 6. Spatial distribution of hospitals with adult ICU beds and ventilators and the level of access to these services considering competition effects. Manaus, 2020.

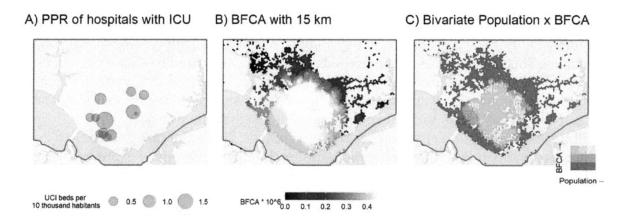

Figure 7. Spatial distribution of hospitals with adult ICU beds and ventilators and the lvel of access to these services considering competition effects. Rio de Janeiro, 2020.

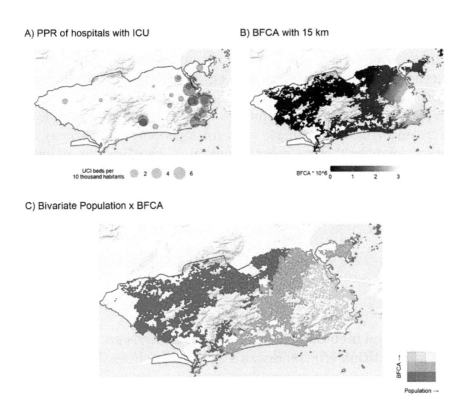

Obs. Grey circles represent field hospitals or temporarily reactivated facilities.

Figure 8. Spatial distribution of hospitals with adult ICU beds and ventilators and the level of access to these services considering competition effects. São Paulo, 2020.

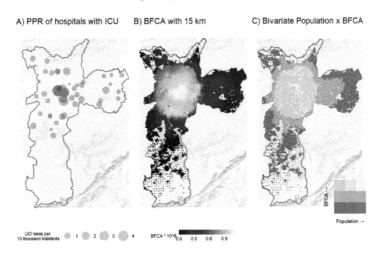

Obs. Grey circles represent field hospitals or temporarily reactivated facilities.

The geographic access to COVID-19 healthcare in Brazil presents not only spatial but also marked social inequalities. Figure 9 shows the magnitude of the racial and income inequalities in access to ICU beds and ventilators considering competition effects. One of the most extreme cases is the capital of the country Brasília, where the number of ICU beds with ventilators accessible by the wealthiest population is more than 6 times larger than for the poor. While racial inequalities are relatively lower compared to inequalities by income, they are still present in most cities.

This is particularly true in Brasília, São Paulo and Belo Horizonte, where black communities can only access half as many health resources as the white population. In summary, our findings point to a worrying pattern. Across Brazil's 20 largest cities, we find substantially lower healthcare system capacity in urban peripheral areas and among low income and black communities.

In particular, urban peripheries with high population density coupled with low incomes and poor sanitation services create a worrying scenario with strong potential for propagation of the COVID-19 precisely among communities that are most vulnerable to the disease and with lowest access to healthcare. Combined, the analyses presented provide valuable information that can help local authorities map the areas which should receive more immediate response from local healthcare community agents and perhaps the construction of new field hospitals to address short term needs induced by the COVID-19 pandemic.

Figure 9. Income and racial inequalities in access to ICU beds and ventilators considering competition effects. Brazil's 20 largest cities, 2020.4

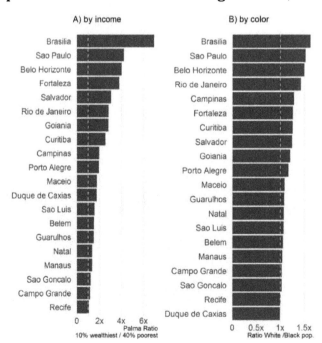

7. FINAL REMARKS

This paper examined the geographical access to COVID-19 healthcare in the 20 largest Brazilian cities, looking at both healthcare facilities with capacity for triage and referral of patients with suspected COVID-19 infections to hospitals, as well as those able to treat patients in serious condition through the support of ICU beds and mechanical ventilators. We mapped approximately 230 thousand vulnerable people (low-income above 50 years old) living more than 30 minutes walking from a public healthcare facility able to test for COVID-19 or refer suspected cases to hospitals. Our results also indicate that some 1.6 million vulnerable people live farther than 5 Km from a hospital with capacity for ICU admission.

Because patients suspected with COVID-19 might face mobility constraints due to grave conditions, it becomes crucial to develop strategies for provision of transport and health services to these people. This is particularly true of low-income people living on the outskirts of cities, where there are fewer mobility options and where health services are scarcer. The study also analysed the support capacity of the public health systems in the largest Brazilian cities, looking at the number of ICU beds/ventilators per person in the catchment area of each hospital and accessible by the population. We find that thirteen out of the 20 cities analysed have fewer ICU beds with ventilators than the minimum level recommended by the Health Ministry, which could be insufficient to deal with large growth of demand for hospital admissions in the most optimistic scenarios of COVID-19 propagation in Brazil. Accessibility analysis using the new balanced float catchment area (BFCA) shows this scenario is particularly worrisome when we account for competition effects on both supply and demand for health services. The BFCA estimates show substantially lower access to health services in low-income and black communities in urban peripheries, which generally face scarcer supply of health equipment and could more easily be overwhelmed by the near-future hospitalization demands.

As a whole, the study illustrates how transport accessibility analyses can provide actionable information to help local governments improve access to healthcare services during pandemic outbreaks. Combined, the analyses in the paper put disadvantaged communities with poor access to health services on the map, indicating in which neighbourhoods' local authorities could prioritize to build makeshift hospitals or engage mobile units or health community agents. These analyses also help local authorities identify which hospitals that might face the greatest admission overload due to competition effects, and hence would need supplementary funding to expand capacity. The application of the novel BFCA in this paper illustrates how considering competition effects in access to healthcare can have important but often overlooked implications for policy planning.

Future research could potentially combine the results of this paper with scenarios for COVID-19 infection and hospitalization rates to generate estimates of demand for beds and ventilators on an intra-urban scale. Further analysis could also indicate the areas where the construction of new makeshift hospitals would be more effective to improve healthcare accessibility at the city level and for vulnerable groups in particular. More studies however are still needed to investigate how the availability of healthcare professionals could hinder the population access to healthcare services and about the potential role of community health agents in serving people in more remote areas. Finally, although the reduction of public transportation services can potentially reduce urban mobility levels and limit the dissemination of the virus, it can also restrict access to healthcare facilities by healthcare professionals along with low-income patients and their families, who have few mobility options. The reduction of transportation services without a coordinated restriction of other activities causes longer waiting periods and can consequently increase the agglomeration of people at transport stations and crowding aboard vehicles, aggravating dissemination of the virus. In this respect, it is important for local managers to reorganize the public transit service to assure better access to healthcare facilities. This could include provision of exclusive services to healthcare professionals and providers of other essential services, without impairing the supply of services of regular lines.

REFERENCES

Amaral, P. V., Rocha, T. A. H., Barbosa, A. C. Q., ... Vissoci, J. R. N. (2017). Spatially balanced provision of health equipment: A cross-sectional study oriented to the identification of challenges to access promotion. *International Journal for Equity in Health*, *16*(1), 209. doi:10.1186/s12939-017-0704x

Arenas, A., Cota, W., Gomez-Gardenes, J., ... Steinegger, B. (2020). A mathematical model for the spatiotemporal epidemic spreading of COVID19. *MedRxiv*, 2020.03.21.20040022. doi:10.1101/2020.03.21.20040022

Brasil. (2015). *Critérios e parâmetros para o planejamento e programação de ações e serviços de saúde no âmbito do Sistema Único de Saúde*. Brasília: MS: Ministério da Saúde. Secretaria de Atenção à Saúde. Departamento de Regulação, Avaliação e Controle de Sistemas.

Brasil. (2020a). *Protocolo de Manejo Clínico do Coronavírus (Covid-19) na Atenção Primária à Saúde*.

Brasília: MS: Ministério da Saúde. Secretaria de Atenção Primária à Saúde.

Brasil. (2020b). *Protocolo de Manejo Clínico para o Novo Coronavírus (2019-nCoV)*. Brasília: MS: Ministério da Saúde. Secretaria de Atenção Primária à Saúde.

Castro, M. C., Carvalho, L. R. de, Chin, T., ... Oliveira, W. K. de. (2020). Demand for hospitalization services for COVID-19 patients in Brazil. *MedRxiv*, 2020.03.30.20047662. doi:10.1101/2020.03.30.20047662

Coelho, F. C., Lana, R. M., Cruz, O. G., ... Gomes, M. F. C. (2020). Assessing the potential impact of COVID-19 in Brazil: Mobility, Morbidity and the burden on the Health Care System. *MedRxiv*, 2020.03.19.20039131. doi:10.1101/2020.03.19.20039131

Dai, D. (2010). Black residential segregation, disparities in spatial access to health care facilities, and latestage breast cancer diagnosis in metropolitan Detroit. *Health & Place*, *16*(5), 1038–1052. doi:10.1016/j.healthplace.2010.06.012

Delamater, P. L. (2013). Spatial accessibility in sub optimally configured health care systems: A modified two-step floating catchment area (M2SFCA) metric. *Health & Place*, *24*, 30–43. doi:10.1016/j.healthplace.2013.07.012

Folha de S.Paulo. (2020, July 1). Ocupação de UTI volta a subir e supera 80% em 13 capitais. *Folha de S.Paulo*. Retrieved from https://www1.folha.uol.com.br/cotidiano/2020/07/ocupacao-de-uti-voltaa-subir-e-supera-80-em-13-capitais.shtml

Franssen, K., Neutens, T., De Maeyer, P., & Deruyter, G. (2015). A commuter-based two-step floating catchment area method for measuring spatial accessibility of daycare centres. *Health & Place*, *32*, 65–73. doi:10.1016/j.healthplace.2015.01.002

Freire, F. H. M. de A., Gonzaga, M. R., & Gomes, M. M. F. (2020). Projeções populacionais por sexo e idade para pequenas áreas no Brasil. *Revista Latinoamericana de Población*, *14*(26), 124–149. doi:10.31406/relap2020.v14.i1.n26.6

Geurs, K., & van Wee, B. (2004). Accessibility evaluation of land-use and transport strategies: Review and research directions. *Journal of Transport Geography*, *12*(2), 127–140. doi:10.1016/j.jtrangeo.2003.10.005

Grasselli, G., Pesenti, A., & Cecconi, M. (2020). Critical Care Utilization for the COVID-19 Outbreak in Lombardy, Italy: Early Experience and Forecast During an Emergency Response. *JAMA*. doi:10.1001/jama.2020.4031

Guan, W., Liang, W., Zhao, Y., ... He, J. (2020). Comorbidity and its impact on 1590 patients with Covid-

19 in   China: A Nationwide Analysis. *European Respiratory Journal*. doi:10.1183/13993003.00547-2020

InfoGripe. (2020, March 4). Monitoramento de casos reportados de síndrome respiratória aguda grave (SRAG) hospitalizados. Retrieved April 4, 2020, from http://info.gripe.fiocruz.br/

JAXA. (2011). ALOS PALSAR digital elevation model data. Japan Aerospace Exploration Agency (JAXA). Retrieved from ASF DAAC https://search.asf.alaska.edu

Ji, Y., Ma, Z., Peppelenbosch, M. P., & Pan, Q. (2020). Potential association between COVID-19 mortality and health-care resource availability. *The Lancet Global Health*, *8*(4), e480. doi:10.1016/S2214109X(20)30068-1

Lancet, T. (2020). COVID-19: Learning from experience. *The Lancet*, *395*(10229), 1011. doi:10.1016/S0140-6736(20)30686-3

Legido-Quigley, H., Mateos-García, J. T., Campos, V. R., ... McKee, M. (2020). The resilience of the Spanish health system against the COVID-19 pandemic. *The Lancet Public Health*, *0*(0). doi:10.1016/S2468-2667(20)30060-8

Luo, W., & Qi, Y. (2009). An enhanced two-step floating catchment area (E2SFCA) method for measuring spatial accessibility to primary care physicians. *Health & Place*, *15*(4), 1100–1107. doi:10.1016/j.healthplace.2009.06.002

Luo, W., & Wang, F. (2003). Measures of Spatial Accessibility to Health Care in a GIS Environment:

Synthesis and a Case Study in the Chicago Region. *Environment and Planning B: Planning and Design*, *30*(6), 865–884. doi:10.1068/b29120

Matthews, K. A., Gaglioti, A. H., Holt, J. B., ... Croft, J. B. (2019). Using spatially adaptive floating catchments to measure the geographic availability of a health care service: Pulmonary rehabilitation in the southeastern United States. *Health & Place*, *56*, 165–173. doi:10.1016/j.healthplace.2019.01.017

McGrail, Matthew R., & Humphreys, J. S. (2009). Measuring spatial accessibility to primary care in rural areas: Improving the effectiveness of the two-step floating catchment area method. *Applied Geography*, *29*(4), 533–541. doi:10.1016/j.apgeog.2008.12.003

McGrail, Matthew Richard, Humphreys, J. S., & Ward, B. (2015). Accessing doctors at times of need– measuring the distance tolerance of rural residents for health-related travel. *BMC Health Services Research*, *15*(1), 212. doi:10.1186/s12913-015-0880-6

Moghadas, S. M., Shoukat, A., Fitzpatrick, M. C., ... Galvani, A. P. (2020). Projecting hospital utilization during the COVID-19 outbreaks in the United States. *Proceedings of the National Academy of Sciences*, *117*(16), 9122–9126. doi:10.1073/pnas.2004064117

Neutens, T. (2015). Accessibility, equity and health care: Review and research directions for transport geographers. *Journal of Transport Geography*, *43*, 14–27. doi:10.1016/j.jtrangeo.2014.12.006

Noronha, K., & et al. (2020). *Análise de demanda e oferta de leitos hospitalares gerais, UTI e equipamentos de ventilação assistida no Brasil em função da pandemia do COVID-19: Impactos microrregionais ponderados pelos diferenciais de estrutura etária, perfil etário de infecção e risco etário de internação* (Nota Técnica). Belo Horizonte: Cedepar-Face-UFMG.

NTU. (2020). *COVID-19 e o transporte público por ônibus: Impactos no setor e ações realizadas*. Brasilia: Associação Nacional das Empresas de Transportes Urbanos - NTU.

Paez, A. (2020). Using Google Community Mobility Reports to investigate the incidence of COVID-19 in the United States. *Transport Findings*, 12976. doi:10.32866/001c.12976

Paez, A., Higgins, C. D., & Vivona, S. F. (2019). Demand and level of service inflation in Floating

Catchment Area (FCA) methods. *PLOS ONE*, *14*(6), e0218773. doi:10.1371/journal.pone.0218773

Paez, A., Lopez, F. A., Menezes, T., ... Pitta, M. G. da R. (n.d.). A Spatio-Temporal Analysis of the Environmental Correlates of COVID-19 Incidence in Spain. *Geographical Analysis*, *n/a*(n/a). doi:10.1111/gean.12241

Páez, A., Scott, D. M., & Morency, C. (2012). Measuring accessibility: Positive and normative implementations of various accessibility indicators. *Journal of Transport Geography*, *25*, 141–153. doi:10.1016/j.jtrangeo.2012.03.016

Pereira, R. H. M., Braga, C. K. V., Serra, Bernardo, & Nadalin, V. (2019). Desigualdades socioespaciais de acesso a oportunidades nas cidades brasileiras, 2019. *Texto para Discussão IPEA*, *2535*. Retrieved from http://www.ipea.gov.br/portal/images/stories/PDFs/TDs/td_2535.pdf

Petropoulos, F., & Makridakis, S. (2020). Forecasting the novel coronavirus COVID-19. *PLOS ONE*, *15*(3), e0231236. doi:10.1371/journal.pone.0231236

Rader, B., Astley, C. M., Sy, K. T. L., ... Kraemer, M. U. G. (2020). Geographic access to United States SARS-CoV-2 testing sites highlights healthcare disparities and may bias transmission estimates. *Journal of Travel Medicine*. doi:10.1093/jtm/taaa076

Radke, J., & Mu, L. (2000). Spatial Decompositions, Modeling and Mapping Service Regions to Predict Access to Social Programs. *Geographic Information Sciences*, *6*(2), 105–112. doi:10.1080/10824000009480538

Rocha, T. A. H., da Silva, N. C., Amaral, P. V., ... Facchini, L. A. (2017). Access to emergency care services: A transversal ecological study about Brazilian emergency health care network. *Public Health*, *153*, 9–15. doi:10.1016/j.puhe.2017.07.013

Servo, L., Andrade, M., & do Amaral, P. (2019). Análise das regiões de saúde no Brasil a partir do Pacto pela Saúde: Adequação da regionalização e acesso geográfico. In *Anais do XXI Encontro da Encontro da Associação Brasileira de Estudos Populacionais (ABEP)*.

Souza, W. M. de, Buss, L. F., Candido, D. da S., ... Faria, N. R. (2020). Epidemiological and clinical characteristics of the early phase of the COVID-19 epidemic in Brazil. *MedRxiv*, 2020.04.25.20077396. doi:10.1101/2020.04.25.20077396

Walter, P. G., & et al. (2020). *Report 12: The Global Impact of COVID-19 and Strategies forMitigation and Suppression | CRUB*. London: Imperial College London. Retrieved from http://www.crub.org.br/blog/covid-19-reports-faculty-of-medicine-imperial-college-london/

Wan, N., Zou, B., & Sternberg, T. (2012). A three-step floating catchment area method for analyzing spatial access to health services. *International Journal of Geographical Information Science*, *26*(6), 1073– 1089. doi:10.1080/13658816.2011.624987

WHO. (2020). *Addressing Human Rights as Key to the COVID-19 Response* (No. WHO/2019nCoV/SRH/Rights/2020.1). World Health Organization. Retrieved from https://www.who.int/publications-detail/addressing-human-rights-as-key-to-the-covid-19response

Wu, J. T., Leung, K., & Leung, G. M. (2020). Nowcasting and forecasting the potential domestic and international spread of the 2019-nCoV outbreak originating in Wuhan, China: A modelling study. *The Lancet*, *395*(10225), 689–697. doi:10.1016/S0140-6736(20)30260-9

Yang, J., Zheng, Y., Gou, X., ... Zhou, Y. (2020). Prevalence of comorbidities and its effects in patients infected with SARS-CoV-2: A systematic review and meta-analysis. *International Journal of Infectious Diseases*, *94*, 91–95. doi:10.1016/j.ijid.2020.03.017

Zaman, S. M. A., Cox, J., Enwere, G. C., ... Cutts, F. T. (2014). The effect of distance on observed mortality, childhood pneumonia and vaccine efficacy in rural Gambia. *Epidemiology & Infection*, *142*(12), 2491–2500. doi:10.1017/S0950268814000314

CHAPTER 8

RACIALIZED HEALTH CARE IN COVID-19 BRAZIL

1. Racism in Health Services in Brazil[1]

Cristina Gomes

Facultad Latinoamericana de Ciencias Sociales, FLACSO, Sede, México

ABSTRACT

This article discusses racial prejudices and discrimination in perceptions, attitudes and practices among health personnel in the municipality of Camaçari. The survey's methodology included racist statements in questionnaires distributed to 634 health workers and socio-determinants of health, family and work characteristics. Results indicate how masked racism is reproduced through ambiguous attitudes and practices; the feeling that speaking about race/colour would create a racist conflict, supposing that it does not exist, and resistance against accepting the need to correct injustices and promoting affirmative policies.

INTRODUCTION

With the return of democracy, Brazil has implemented various social policies covering more than 30 million people with income transference (BolsaFamilia), the reduction of poverty and elimination of hunger, the creation of more than 2 million units of affordable housing and providing more than 2 million people over 65 or people disabled with a minimum wage income.

Despite these efforts, there are still families and people with health problems and vulnerabilities, such as violence, drug abuse, disability, natural disasters and victims of discrimination. One of the barriers to full citizen inclusion is the racial disparity that has characterized Brazilian society, institutions and micro- relationships throughout its 516 years of history.

Until beginning the 20th Century, the Brazilian population was predominantly black (slave or descendant of the enslaved[1]) (Klein, H.S.; III, Ben Vinson, 2007), illiterate and defined in newspapers and by Brazilian intellectuals as "bestializada" (made beasts), a reason for national shame (Carvalho, 2004).Racism has become an intrinsic part of the formation and development of Brazilian society and has been reproduced in the present day through a false myth of "racial democracy" and the ideal of the "whitening" of society (Fernandes, 1965; Bento, 2002). A sui generis racism, masked and widespread, persists in all power structures and national, state, municipal institutions, and micro social, both individual and familial (Guimarães, 1999; Alencar, 2013; Amaral, 2011; Brasil, 2013; Brasil, 2016). As a result, blacks in Brazil have the worst rates of morbidity, mortality, and illiteracy, and have lower educational levels and higher poverty rates within the population (Brasil, 2013). There are incidents of racism witnessed on a daily basis in the media, social networks, public spaces and institutions and even among members of the same family, but prejudices and discriminatory attitudes are denied and hidden, masked by a belief that in Brazil there is a peaceful miscegenation process and an alleged racial democracy (Brasil, 2013; Brasil 2016; Alencar, 2013; Amaral, 2011).

---

[1] How to cite this paper: Gomes, C. (2016).
Racism in Health Services in Brazil. Advances in Applied Sociology, 6, 363-374.
http://dx.doi.org/10.4236/aasoci.2016.611027

According to Santos (2007), "prejudice plays its daily aggression against black people alternating silences, whispers, speeches and shouts." The first two forms are the most used, because they allow racism to hide whilst acting to keep the facade of people as "morally intact, mentally healthy" ("good"), which would have "authority" to discriminate and have power over the "other", since blacks are considered to be in an inferior social position. It is a very common and socially acceptable treatment to transmit the idea of "knowing your place"—that is, an inferior place for blacks. The referred inferior place means that "there are others who deserve more than you, there are others who have priority, you are less important". Even subconsciously, silence, looks, and attitudes can portray to black people this message of their supposed inferiority, something Brazilians learn from childhood (Brasil, 2007).

These daily witnessed incidents of racism are present in the media, social networks, public spaces and institutions and even among members of the same family. And the general opinion is that it happens by mainly denying and hiding prejudices and discriminatory attitudes, masking them in jokes, comments, views and suspicious attitudes, often without being aware of them, these characteristics having been learned from an early age. Besides this subtle and unconscious type of racial discrimination, there is also "the practice of prejudice such as irony, sarcasm and exasperation, the jokes and the nervous smile, when, for a few seconds, we realized that we would be contradictory or racist" (Ribeiro, 2012).

In Brazil, the "negro" population is composed of people who define themselves as black or mulatto/brown. In 2013, these groups represented 52.9% of the population, around one hundred million people. In the public health system (SUS), 70% of users are self-defined as black (black and brown). Brazil is the country with the second largest number of black people the first is Nigeria and Bahia is the State with the highest proportion of black inhabitants, as is the Metropolitan Region of Salvador, the capital, in which Camacari is included (Brasil, 2016).The classification of "colour or race" used in censuses and surveys is obtained using induced self-definition, i.e. the respondent is free to indicate their "colour or race" between the five categories (black, white, brown, Asiatic, indigenous) which are already well accepted as virtually the entire population responds to censuses and surveys and is able to define their colour themselves (Osório, 2003).

Civil servants of the federal agencies have more difficulties when asked about race or colour. Only 40% of the 584,000 active employees completed the question of "colour or race" in their record of personal data in 2003; in some institutions only 3% of employees responded to this question (Osório, 2003). Therefore, it is expected that public employees have a greater tendency to deny the existence of racism, and to whiten their skin colour and the colour of service users.

Available data on colour/race show that the black population (both black and brown) in Brazil has the highest rates of morbidity and mortality, the highest illiteracy rates and the lowest educational levels, the highest rates of poverty, infant and maternal mortality, mortality from diabetes, hypertension and violent deaths, and accumulate all these social disadvantages, as compared to the white population. Diseases are more prevalent in the black population; sickle cell disease, hypertensive disorders of pregnancy, arterial hypertension, and diabetes mellitus amongst others (Brasil, 2016; Batista et al., 2013; Dias et al., 2009; Araújo et al., 2010; Goes & Nascimento, 2013).

In the last two decades, Brazil has adopted actions to compensate and correct race inequalities and discrimination. Affirmative or positive policies are special and temporary measures imposed to support those who are black, disabled and those who are the poorest-the most in need of assistance to achieve equality.

These policies would be temporary and work for a limited period, until the attainment of equal opportunities for all (Silva Filho, 2008). Despite all these efforts to increase income, to equalize access to services and to diminish inequalities and disadvantages of the most vulnerable groups, it is very common in Brazil in the communications media that some population groups criticize social measures, arguing that all have the same opportunities, and that results are based upon individual merit. Controversies and conflicts in society raise the argument that race inequality is an imported issue that could create or promote a problem that "does not exist" in Brazilian society.

Another reason for conflicts is the interpretation that the inclusion of blacks with affirmative policies could generate discrimination against white people. In order to understand how these policies would work in health services, this article has the objective of analysing statements of prejudices in perceptions, attitudes and practices of workers at health services in Camaçari, Brazil, and to discuss correlations and principal components of these prejudicial statements, classified in grades from clear to masked racism. Considering the Brazilian academic consensus on the myth of racial democracy as the main characteristic of racism in Brazil, some categories were built into a scale: explicit racism, no-adherence to affirmative measures and racism denegation (based upon the denial of racial inequalities).

METHODOLOGY

A representative survey was distributed to 634 workers of the public and private health services, with a questionnaire concerning socio-demographic characteristics, family, work conditions and perceptions, and attitudes and practices in racial relationships. The vast majority of the workers are women (76%) and their mean age is 40 years old; 83% declare they are Negros (31% black and 52.2% brown or mixed race) and only 14% are white; 42% are Catholics, 21% Evangelical, 17% have no religion, 15% are spiritualists or have Afro-religions. Half of them are married, 38% single, 9% separated, 2% widowers and 2% live in other marital status. The majority have children (63%): 33% have one child and 23% have 2 or more children. Most of them (69%) are head of their households, the average size of households is 2.9 members, and they earn on average a salary of three thousand Realis per month (approximately one thousand US dollars), and 70% have a formal labour relationship as public workers.

Variables were created by adopting statements about race relationships obtained from personnel of health service in different cities of the country. These statements were accessed by previous authors using qualitative methods and published in scientific articles (Santos & Santos, 2013; Tavares et al., 2013; Grandi et al., 2013). These statements are listed in the questionnaire, applied to personnel working in different functions, from the front-of-house security and reception personnel to community agents, technical personnel, nurses, physicians and the health service managers.

Some examples of these statements are:

a) If you ask about race or colour, what is or would be the reaction of the users? Naturalness, Surprise, Distrusting, Questioning/do not understand, Uncomfortable, Refusal to answer, Irritation, Refusal to take his race: I see they are black, they say white.
b) How would you feel to ask the race-colour to users?

c) Normal, it is no big deal, Uncomfortable, Constrained, feel you are discriminating patients, Fear of offending the patient, Fear of being questioned, Fear of being misunderstood, it's unnecessary, it delays the service.
d) There is racism in Brazil? (level)
e) Have you experienced or observed of racism?
f) What is your opinion on the following statements: (totally agree, partially agree, disagree?).

- It is not necessary to differentiate people by skin colour in health services. The country is inter-bred it has no way to frame the person in a single race.
- It is important to fill this item to know the profile of people who have diseases associated with race/colour, support the treatment and identify prejudices.
- It's hard to ask the patient what his colour. We created unnecessary controversy, as there are different races in Brazil and people are in doubt about that.
- It's embarrassing to ask colour, people may take offense, create problems. They do not want to answer.
- Needless to ask the user colour. The community is not used.
- It should not be asked the user colour. It is not necessary. That's not part of my job.
- It is natural to consider the colour-race of the population, as the age or sex. I cannot take a white or black person, a teenager or a senior citizen, a man or woman in the same way.
- The black population has the worst rates of illness and death, so we have to have a focused look at the colour, differentiate the service to reduce inequalities.
- Recognize the specific health problems of the black population do not imply prejudice or discrimination against whites.
- To have true equality we have to recognize racial differences and treat them differently, so we fight against racial inequality.
- Differential treatment by colour or race is a type of discrimination it is racism, because everyone is equal according to law.
- Racial quotas discriminate against whites, it's not fair, because we have to meet all the same all have the same rights.
- Jokes about blacks and the use of the term "bad hair" or "the situation is black" are part of the culture of the population, are not racist expressions.
- Blacks tend to be more aggressive than whites.
- Brazilian law defines the crimes of racism, discrimination or race-colour prejudice like refusing access in public places, with imprisonment from 1 to 3 years as punishment.

Proportions and correlations between socio-demographic variables and discrimination statements, such as Pearson coefficients were estimated. Principal Component Analysis was used when a large number of categorical variables would be classified and grouped, as in this study, to reduce the number of variables to a few, interpretable linear combinations of the data. Each linear combination corresponds to a principal component (PCA). The First Principal Component is the linear combination of x-variables that has maximum variance (among all linear combinations), so it accounts for as much variation in the data as possible. The Second Principal Component is the linear combination of x-variables that accounts for as much of the remaining variation as possible, with the constraint that the correlation between the first and second component is 0 (zero).

All subsequent principal components have this same property—they are linear combinations that account for as much of the remaining variation as possible and they are not correlated with the other principal components. To interpret each component, we must compute the correlations between the original data for each variable and each principal component. Because of standardization, all principal components will have a mean of 0 (zero). The standard deviation is also given for each of the components and these will be the square root of the eigenvalue. More important for our current purposes are the correlations between the principal components and the original variables. Principal Component Analysis is applied for each personnel group, according to different levels of education and for the entire population. The statistical program used was SPSS version 22.

RESULTS AND DISCUSSION

Descriptive data shows that nearly 60% of the health personnel with the highest levels of education expect that patients will naturally answer their race/colour, and that it is important to include this question in health registers, to know the disease profile of the black population in order to support treatment and to identify prejudices. However, less than half of personnel in the lowest levels of education (fundamental, with 8 years of education, such as receptionists) agree with this statement. Only 40% of the personnel have positive expectations about the reaction of patients when asked about their colour. Negative expectations and personnel's fears about patients reactions are more common among personnel with low level education; around 30% of them expect that patients would feel bothered by or would not understand the question, or do not accept their own colour, or feel embarrassed, that this question would create unnecessary controversy, that people are in doubt about their colour/race, or that they may take offense, feel bad, create problems, or even that they don't want to answer about their colour. These would be interpretations of some health personnel who are transferring their own prejudices or feelings of superiority regarding patients. Half of them resent asking the colour of patients, using different excuses such as; it is not necessary, it is not part of their job; the community is not used to this; and they do not consider asking colour as natural as asking sex or age. Almost all these ambiguous answers against asking the colour of patients have higher proportions among personnel with lower levels of education, compared to doctors and other professionals with a university degree, who are more accepting of the existence of racial inequalities and its relevance to the development of health policies and actions. However, to accept the existence of inequalities does not imply accepting policies to reduce it with affirmative policies.

On the contrary, 46.8% of the personnel are against racial quotas, and 61.6% consider that giving special treatment to reduce inequalities would discriminate against whites and be reverse racism. Again, these resistances to accept actions to reduce inequalities are higher amongst less educated personnel, who are 65.6% against quotas and 78.9% against giving special treatment to black people in health services. This resistance against recognizing the need to correct inequalities with special policies is also in contrast to 80% of personnel who agree that racism exists and is very common, whilst only four people (out of 364 surveyed) directly assume that racism does not exist in the country. This contradiction could be interpreted as, in spite of almost everybody recognizing that racism exists, that the wide majority believes in racial democracy, and ambiguously believes that there is no need to differentiate people by skin colour in health care, because the country would be interbred, and that "it is not possible to fit a person into a single race category".

As inequalities are accepted as "natural", special actions to reduce it are considered "unnecessary". Some qualitative statements in this research are "it has always been so", and "it's not my problem, but a problem of my predecessors".

Principal Components Analysis

The interpretation of the principal components analysis is based upon which variables are most strongly correlated with each component. From a large number of variables, the farthest from zero in either positive or negative direction are more correlated. In this case a correlation value above 0.55 was established. For the entire population, the first principal component (PCA1) is strongly correlated with five of the original variables. The first principal component increases with the following statements scores: Recognition of black problems whilst not meaning discrimination against whites; humanizing SUS is enough to prevent racism; asking patients colour is unnecessary and it is not my job; differences exist and race inequalities are relevant; it is hard to ask colour/race and it generates unnecessary controversy; it is not necessary to ask colour/race as the country is interbred; it is unnecessary and the community is not used to such a question. This suggests that these criteria vary together. If one of them increases, then the remaining ones tend to increase as well. This component can be viewed as a measure of typical masked and defensive sentences representing the myth of racial democracy. For example, the belief that differences exist, that race inequalities should be known and are relevant.

However, these statements are immediately followed with many conditions or pretexts to immediately deny any affirmative attitudes to correct them and to promote equality (Table 1).

The second principal component (PCA2) increases with only three types of expectancies on patient's negative reactions when asked about their race/colour, justified by different reasons; people may question, misunderstand, take offense, and create problems and controversies. However, these expected conflicts, according to the myth of racial democracy, wouldn't exist in Brazilian society. So, again, prejudices are transferred to "the other". This component can be viewed as a measure of how important it is to deconstruct these expectations in training courses for health providers. In the third principal component (PCA3) any variable achieves the level established as a coefficient higher than 0.55. The highest coefficient (0.503) corresponds to the expectation that patients would deny their own race, and say they are white but the interviewer believes they are black. Explicit demonstrations of racism are only included at PCA 4: Does racism exist in Brazil? However, the coefficient is lower than the established level (0.469).

At PCA5 the statement "black people are more aggressive than whites" has the second highest coefficient (0.605). Therefore, explicit racism is uncorrelated to all the other variables in previous group. These are isolated cases. Considering that different patterns of discriminatory statements are shown according to the positions assumed by health personnel, the Principal Component Analysis is estimated to consist of four groups: doctors, other professionals with a university degree, technical staff and non-technical staff. The First Principal Component (PCA1) for doctors includes several correlated variables. This is the unique case in which PCA1 includes explicit racist statements: "Jokes on blacks is Brazilian culture, is not racism" and "Blacks are more aggressive than whites"

1. Principal components for different groups of personnel in health services, Camacari, Bahia.

Variables-Statements to agree	Total		Doctor		Other university degree		Technical		Basic school	
	1	2	1	2	1	2	1	2	1	2
Opinion on including race-colour in health records	-0.192	-0.321	-0.221	-0.337	-0.373	-0.107	-0.231	-0.204	-0.025	-0.431
Surprise	-0.093	0.313	-0.073	0.571	-0.172	0.389	0.353	-0.007	0.025	0.218
Untruth/falsehood	-0.004	0.474	0.01	0.742	-0.085	0.495	0.576	0.012	0.101	0.364
Question not understood	-0.103	0.323	-0.105	0.279	-0.052	0.544	0.399	0.065	-0.126	0.155
Bothered by	0.046	0.505	0.345	0.577	-0.186	0.461	0.548	0.216	0.083	0.443
Refusal to answer	-0.017	0.366	-0.026	0.203	-0.111	0.136	0.467	0.015	0.1	0.344
Irritation	-0.021	0.488	-0.008	0.324	-0.084	0.489	0.492	0.132	-0.02	0.412
Denial of own race, choosing white	-0.142	0.235	0.026	0.213	-0.239	0.345	0.166	-0.004	-0.126	0.223
Bothered by	0.106	0.547	0.122	0.493	0.017	0.177	0.583	0.056	0.19	0.648
Constrained	0.01	0.52	-0.072	0.057	-0.038	0.483	0.49	0.057	-0.005	0.626
Feeling that they are discriminating	0.106	0.515	0.004	0.227	0.021	0.234	0.579	0.096	0.127	0.515
Fear of offending	0.057	0.569	0.082	0.283	-0.11	0.385	0.683	0.067	0.133	0.587
Fear of being questioned	-0.011	0.637	-0.035	0.22	-0.028	0.452	0.654	0.058	-0.007	0.75
Fear of being misunderstood	0.068	0.618	0.256	0.326	-0.129	0.59	0.607	0.059	0.2	0.694
Think it is unnecessary	0.207	0.482	0.117	0.134	0.275	0.275	0.526	0.322	0.188	0.537
Delay the service	-0.018	0.494	-0.044	-0.04	-0.039	0.255	0.475	0.129	-0.049	0.577
Opinion of racism in Brazil	0.275	-0.056	-0.083	-0.015	0.457	0.177	-0.152	0.598	0.217	-0.089
Suffered, observed racism	-0.153	0.039	-0.131	0.016	-0.131	0.073	0.089	-0.006	-0.199	0.002
Not needed, country interbred	0.572	-0.033	0.616	-0.078	0.369	-0.014	-0.044	0.087	0.697	-0.096
Important racial diseases prejudice	0.522	0.003	0.743	-0.212	0.32	-0.056	0.032	-0.132	0.692	-0.083
Harsh, unnecessary controversy	0.583	-0.001	0.733	0.294	0.443	0.279	-0.046	0.484	0.654	-0.177
Embarassed, they do not want to ask	0.512	-0.029	0.713	0.01	0.378	-0.033	-0.077	0.482	0.586	-0.086
Unnecessary, community not used to it	0.555	0.008	0.109	-0.033	0.686	0.008	-0.041	0.48	0.659	-0.002
Unnecessary, it is not my job	0.587	-0.021	0.661	0.067	0.612	-0.026	-0.099	0.549	0.601	-0.096
Natural as asking age/sex, different treatment	0.488	-0.018	0.421	0.337	0.352	-0.055	-0.069	0.443	0.589	-0.06
Worst rates for blacks, focus inequalities	0.518	-0.094	0.63	0.218	0.413	-0.065	-0.13	0.17	0.605	-0.218
Black problem does not discriminate against whites	0.623	-0.003	0.762	-0.085	0.743	0.061	-0.202	0.471	0.615	0.051
Differences exist, race inequalities are relevant	0.583	-0.108	0.461	0.319	0.548	-0.088	-0.202	0.278	0.733	-0.16
Different treatment is discriminatory	0.45	0.028	0.647	0.223	0.23	0.155	-0.108	0.301	0.628	0.023
Quotas discriminate against whites	0.407	-0.001	0.447	-0.092	0.347	0.212	-0.1	0.407	0.527	0.124
Differential access for 1st/2nd class citizens	0.47	-0.054	0.619	0.059	0.573	0.127	-0.021	0.116	0.491	-0.149
Different treatment would crash the system	0.502	-0.02	0.624	-0.058	0.476	0.001	-0.134	0.362	0.569	-0.048
Black more difficulties is an imposition to differentiate	0.478	0.003	0.48	-0.273	0.214	0.069	-0.139	0.39	0.625	0.073
Humanize SUS is enough to prevent racism	0.588	-0.017	0.709	-0.38	0.546	-0.037	-0.096	0.484	0.667	0.006
Jokes on blacks is part of Brazilian culture	0.378	-0.032	0.747	-0.346	0.475	0.184	-0.098	0.051	0.57	0.077
Blacks are more aggressive than whites	0.314	-0.04	0.641	-0.33	0.252	0.071	-0.16	0.097	0.243	0.015
The Law defines racist crimes	0.372	-0.016	0.515	-0.062	0.199	0.077	-0.136	0.378	0.452	0.012

These harsh statements are as strongly correlated as the recognition of the importance and relevance of racial differences in health. Doctors combine explicit racism and ambiguity concerning the myth of racial democracy and excuses about "other" feelings; it's hard to ask because it cause unnecessary controversy; it is embarrassing because they do not want not to answer, it is not necessary because the country is interbred, and black problems do not discriminate against whites. Other statements recognizing racial differences are also correlated in doctor's opinions, such as the recognition that there exists differential access for citizens of first and second classes. The second component (PCA2) for doctors includes only negative expectations from patients when asked about their colour: surprise and falsehoods.

The group of other personnel with university degrees includes a low discrimination profile and ambiguities in their statements. Their first component (PCA1) includes only utilitarian statements like how questioning patient colour is unnecessary because the community not used to this question, it is not my job, and the program Humanize SUS is not enough to reduce racial differences. They also recognize that black problems do not discriminate against whites. It is important to note that, in opposition to doctors, this group is mainly composed of young black women. Most of them probably benefited from affirmative policies, such as racial quotas, enabling them to enter to university and public employment. In qualitative interviews at least three of them relate they have suffered racial discrimination from patients. One dentist relates that patients prefer to be treated by the other colleague who is white, and they refuse to be treated by her, just because of her colour. A nursery attendant says that patients ask her to correct and verify medications and procedures recommended by a black nurse, who is her boss; but patients do not trust her opinion, despite her university degree, just because she is black. Another nurse experiences racism daily at work, since patients never answer her public "good morning", as they answer her colleague, who is white. Technical personnel refer to few statements in their first principal component, mainly their own expectations about a patient's reaction when asking their colour, such as they feel bothered, discriminated against, offended, questioned, or misunderstood.

Personnel with the lowest level of education are mainly receptionists, security staff, ambulance drivers, telephone operators, etc. The PCA1 of this group is the largest group of discriminatory statements, including: it is important to know racial inequalities in diseases; it is as natural to ask colour, just as asking age and sex; blacks have the worst rates in health; focusing upon black problems does not discriminate against whites; race inequalities are relevant. These positive statements recognizing inequalities are also correlated to other ambiguous statements that reaffirm the myth of racial democracy, such as: it is not necessary to ask colour because the country is interbred; it causes unnecessary controversy; it is embarrassing because they do not want to answer; the community is not used to it. However, this group also has pragmatic arguments like "it is not my job" and "different treatment for blacks would crash the system"; as well as resistance to accepting affirmative policies: different treatment for blacks means to discriminate against whites; and that is because blacks have more difficulties we would not accept this imposition to differentiate between health services access.

This suggests that recognition of race inequalities, ambiguous racism of the myth of racial democracy, supposed pragmatic arguments against correcting race injustices and to be clearly against inclusive policies are correlated, and vary together. If one increases, then the remaining ones tend to do so as well. This component can be viewed as a measure of typical masked and defensive sentences representing the myth of racial democracy, but also concluding that affirmative policies are unnecessary, or even "an imposition" which can discriminate against whites.

The PCA2 of this group also includes statements that transfer to patients a feeling of being bothered, constrained, discriminated, offended, questioned, misunderstood, when asked their colour. PCA2 also includes warnings about delaying services to justify not asking the colour of the patient. The limits of this research include the tendency of respondents to answer in accordance with the expectations of the interviewers, opting for socially acceptable responses. To control partially this effect in the questionnaire including diverse types of responses. For example: according to previous studies, it was expected that almost all respondents assume that there is racism in Brazil. Therefore, in the following questions were included some common ambiguous statements related to racism, for example, the idea of reverse racism (offering affirmative policies for blacks may create discrimination against whites). Another limitation is that patients were not interviewed. It was necessary in this first approaching, to avoid the refusal of officials to answer the questionnaire in front of patients, and the embarrassment of the patient to give their opinion in front of the public servants. In participant observation it was found that indeed the majority of employees do not question the colour of patients, what reconcile whit their own answers.

CONCLUSIONS

Brazilian academic papers put an emphasis upon the sui generis Brazilian racism, masked by ambiguity and based upon the myth of racial democracy. This ambiguity would be used to deny or to hide it beneath speech and respectable attitudes. The results of this research show that race discrimination is not so ambiguous; it is firstly introduced by a formal recognition of race inequalities, but immediately denied with excuses which transfer prejudices to black people. In the case of doctors, ambiguous statements are also correlated to explicit racism.

In another extreme, health personnel with a low level of education use much more ambiguous statements to justify race inequalities and injustices. And the group of the younger, black females who recently were massively included at universities and as health personnel through inclusive policies such as racial quotas, uses much less ambiguity and pretexts to divert from common sense to deny racism and to escape from the responsibility of correcting injustices.

However, they frequently suffer race discrimination from patients, and are perceived as less qualified personnel. Explicit racism is evident in the case of patients refusing to be treated by black professionals, particularly by the group which less frequently reinforces ambiguous and explicit racist statements, compared to others. Results lead one to think a term "revived ambiguity cycle", related to the feeling that speaking about race/colour, would create a racist conflict, supposing firstly its non-existence. The mask of Brazilian racism is based upon the recognition of inequalities and injustices, but immediately followed by a resistance to asking about it and refusing to correct it through affirmative policies. This circularity allows Brazilian society to use the egalitarian discourse, to accept inequalities as something that is unjust, but natural. Universal and egalitarian statements also deny any equalitarian action to correct injustices. Results of quantitative study confirm how institutional racism is being reproduced in speech, attitudes and practices of the health personnel-from receptionists to nurses and physicians, in different levels and patterns. Racism is also present in-patient attitudes and practices when they interact with black workers at health services, as demonstrated in our qualitative approach.

The results indicate a kind of "revived ambiguity cycle", related to the recognition that race inequalities exist and are unfair, but should never be talked about, in order to avoid racist conflict and white discrimination, and therefore society can continue to conjecture that it does not exist, and to use it to deny the need of affirmative policies and a commitment to reduce racial inequalities and to correct injustices.

REFERENCES

Alencar, J. A. (2013). Stay Where You Belong: Review of Machado de Assis-Multiracial Identity and the Brazilian Novelist, by G. Reginald Daniel. Machado de Assis on line, v. 6, n. 11, pp. 134-139, June 2013. Rio de Janeiro: Foundation Casa de Rui Barbosa.

Amaral, S. P. (2011). The History of the Negro in Brazil. Training Course for the Teaching of History and Afro-Brazilian. Brasilia: Ministry of Education. Secretary of Continuing Education, Literacy and Diversity; Salvador: East Africa Studies Centre.

Araújo, C. L. F., et al. (2010). The Question of Colour/Race in Health Forms: The Vision of Health Professionals. Revista Enfermagem UERJ, 18, 241-246.http://www.facenf.uerj.br/v18n2/v18n2a13.pdf

Batista, L. E., Monteiro, R. B., & Medeiros, A. R. (2013). Racial and Health Inequities: The Cycle of Health Policy of the Black Population. Health Debate, Rio de Janeiro, 37, 571-579.

Bento, M. A. S. (2002). Bleaching and Whiteness in Brazil. In Social Psychology of Racism— Studies of Whiteness and Whitening in Brazil. Iray Carone, Maria Aparecida Silva Bento (Organizing) Petrópolis, RJ: Vozes.

Brasil (2016). SEPPIR. Promoting Racial Equality. For a Brazil without Racism. 1st Edition. Brasilia, 2016. Special Secretariat for the Promotion of Racial Equality (SEPPIR). Ministry of Women, Racial Equality, Youth and Human Rights. Organizing Katia Regina da Costa Santos & Edileuza Penha de Souza.

Brazil. Ministry of Health (2013). National Comprehensive Health of the Black Population Policy on Health Unique System (SUS) Policy (2nd ed.). Brasília: Ministry of Health.

Carvalho, J. M. (2004). The Bestialized—Rio de Janeiro and the Republic It Was Not. São Paulo: Compania Das Letras.

Dias, J., Giovanetti, M. R., & Santos, N. J. S. (2009). Asking Offends: What Is Your Colour or Race/ Ethnicity?: Answering Helps Prevention. In: Prevention of STD/AIDS. CRT-DST/AIDS.

Fernandes, F. (1965). The Integration of Black in Class Society. São Paulo: Dominus S.A

Goes, E. F., & Nascimento, E. R. (2013). Black and White Women and Levels of Access to Preventive Health Services: An Analysis of Inequalities. Saúde em Debate, 37, 571-579.http://dx.doi.org/10.1590/S0103-11042013000400004

Grandi, J., Days, M. T. G., & Glimm, S. (2013). Perceptions of Those Who Ask—What's Your Colour? Rio de Janeiro, 37, 588-596.

Guimarães, A. S. A. (1999). Racism and Anti-Racism in Brazil (Ed. 34). Sao Paulo: Foundation to support the University of São Paulo.

Klein, H. S.; III, Ben Vinson (2007). African Slavery in Latin America and the Caribbean (2nd ed.). New York: Columbia University.

OHCHR and UNESCO (2001). The World Conference against Racism, Racial Discrimination, Xenophobia and Related Intolerance. Durban.

Osório, R. G. (2003). The Classification System of "Colour or Race" at IBGE. Discussion Paper 996, Brasilia: IPEA.

Ribeiro, D. A. (2012). Ubuntu: Human Rights and the Health of the Black Population. In: L. E. Batista, J. Werneck, & F. Lopes (Org.), Health of the Black Population (2nd ed., pp. 122-145). Rio de Janeiro: Brazilian Association of Black Researchers. (Black and Black Collection: Research and Debates)

Roediger, D. (2000). Towards the Abolition of Whiteness. London: Verso.

Santos, J. E., & Santos, G. C. S. (2013). Narratives of Primary Care Professionals on the National Comprehensive Health Policy for the Black Population. Health Care Debate, 37, 571-579.

Santos, M. A. (2007). Moreninho, Neguinho, Pretinho (Little Brown, Little Negro, Little Black). Brasilia: Ministry of Education.

Silva Filho, P. (2008). Affirmative Action Policies in Brazilian Education: A Case Study of Vacancies Reserve Program for Entry into the Federal University of Bahia. Doctoral Thesis, Salvador: UFBA.

Tavares, N. O., Oliveira, L. V., & Lages, S. R. C. (2013). The Perception of Psychologists about Institutional Racism in Public Health. Health Care Debate, 37, 571-579.

2. Association Between Expansion of Primary Healthcare and Racial Inequalities in Mortality Amenable to Primary Care in Brazil: A National Longitudinal Analysis[1]

Thomas Hone[1]*, Davide Rasella[2,3], Mauricio L. Barreto[2,3], Azeem Majeed[1],Christopher Millett[1,4,5]

ABSTRACT

Background: Universal health coverage (UHC) can play an important role in achieving Sustainable Development Goal (SDG) 10, which addresses reducing inequalities, but little supporting evidence is available from low- and middle-income countries. Brazil's Estrate´gia de Sau´de da Famı´lia (ESF) (family health strategy) is a community-based primary healthcare (PHC) programme that has been expanding since the 1990s and is the main platform for delivering UHC in the country. We evaluated whether expansion of the ESF was associated with differential reductions in mortality amenable to PHC between racial groups. **Methods and findings:** Municipality-level longitudinal fixed-effects panel regressions were used to examine associations between ESF coverage and mortality from ambulatory-care-sensitive conditions (ACSCs) in black/*pardo* (mixed race) and white individuals over the period 2000–2013.Models were adjusted for socio-economic development and wider health system variables. Over the period 2000–2013, there were 281,877 and 318,030 ACSC deaths (after age standardisation) in the black/*pardo* and white groups, respectively, in the 1,622 municipalities studied. Age-standardised ACSC mortality fell from 93.3 to 57.9 per 100,000 population in the black/*pardo* group and from 75.7 to 49.2 per 100,000 population in the white group. ESF expansion (from 0% to 100%) was associated with a 15.4% (rate ratio [RR]:0.846; 95% CI: 0.796–0.899) reduction in ACSC mortality in the black/*pardo* group compared with a 6.8% (RR: 0.932; 95% CI: 0.892–0.974) reduction in the white group (coefficients significantly different, p = 0.012). These differential benefits were driven by greater reductions in mortality from infectious diseases, nutritional deficiencies and anaemia, diabetes, and cardiovascular disease in the black/*pardo* group. Although the analysis is ecological, sensitivity analyses suggest that over 30% of black/*pardo* deaths would have to be incorrectly coded for the results to be invalid. This study is limited by the use of municipal-aggregate data, which precludes individual-level inference. Omitted variable bias, where factors associated with ESF expansion are also associated with changes in mortality rates, may have influenced our findings, although sensitivity analyses show the robustness of the findings to pre-ESF trends and the inclusion of other municipal-level factors that could be associated with coverage. **Conclusions:** PHC expansion is associated with reductions in racial group inequalities in mortality in Brazil. These findings highlight the importance of investment in PHC to achieve the SDGs aimed at improving health and reducing inequalities.

---

[1] thomas.hone12@imperial.ac.uk

INTRODUCTION

Reducing inequalities within and among countries is the tenth goal of the Sustainable Development Goals (SDGs). This goal includes the target to "adopt policies, especially fiscal, wage and social protection policies" that "progressively achieve greater equality"[1]. Health systems are essential for social protection and, in addition to their contributions to other SDGs for health, may play a vital role in reducing inequalities [1]. Additionally, promoting equality in access to healthcare is a core principle of universal health coverage (UHC) [2]. Investment in primary healthcare (PHC), as part of efforts to achieve UHC, may be especially important in reducing health inequalities [3–5], but evidence is largely derived from North America and Europe. Brazil is an important setting for evaluating the relationship of PHC with health inequalities. It is a middle-income country with one of the highest levels of income inequality globally (a Gini coefficient of 52.9 in 2013 [6]) and stark health inequalities across income, education, racial, and socio-economic groups [7–13]. Brazil's considerable investments in social protection policies over the last two decades include the rollout of conditional cash transfers under the Bolsa Família programme and a commitment to UHC with the expansion of PHC through the Estratégia de Saúde da Família (ESF) (family health strategy) [14,15]. The ESF has rapidly expanded since the mid-1990s to become the largest community-based PHC program in the world [16]. In 2014, it covered ~121.2 million individuals (~62.5% of the population) [17].

Family health teams composed of a family doctor, nurses, and community health workers deliver a broad range of comprehensive and preventive healthcare services to defined local populations (approximately 3,400 individuals) [15]. Municipal governments are responsible for the provision of local ESF services, and financial incentives provided by the federal government encourage municipalities to adopt the ESF [18]. In general, municipalities with smaller populations, higher levels of poverty, and a higher proportion of residents from black/*pardo* (mixed race) racial groups exhibited greater uptake of the ESF (S1 Appendix, Figs. A–C) [19]. Expansion of the ESF has been associated with reductions in infant mortality [20–22], deaths from cardiovascular disease [4], and hospitalisations from ambulatory-care-sensitive conditions (ACSCs) [5], but there is little understanding of the associations between ESF expansion and changes in health inequalities. Recent financial and political crises in Brazil are threatening funding for social protection policies, including UHC [23]. Evidence of an association between the ESF and a reduction of inequalities in health outcomes would provide a strong argument for continued investment and political support. Assessing racial inequalities is important for evaluating the ESF, given the complex historical, sociological, and political dimensions of race in Brazil [24,25]. In contrast to ancestral and ethnic classifications of race in the US and the UK [13], institutions in Brazil use skin colour. Official classifications are *branco* (white), *preto* (black), *pardo* (brown/mixed), *amarello* (Asian), and indigenous, with white, black, and *pardo* accounting for over 98% of the population. Self-reported classification, whilst reflecting ancestral and cultural roots, also reflects an individual's perceived social identity [11,13,25]. Three main ancestral roots established the Brazilian population today—indigenous individuals, European colonisers, and African slaves [25]. Today, there is considerable admixture (evidenced by a sizeable *pardo* population), but sharp inequalities between racial groups persist [9–13]. Black and *pardo* populations have higher illiteracy, have lower average incomes, and use healthcare services less [9]. In health outcomes, they have lower life expectancy, are affected

---

[1] (http://www.un.org/ sustainabledevelopment/inequality/)

more by infectious diseases (including tuberculosis, leprosy, leishmaniasis, and schistosomiasis), and have higher mortality rates from external causes, drug overdoses, and homicides [9]. Few studies have examined the potential role of PHC in reducing health inequalities in low and middle-income countries. This study seeks to address this important gap by examining associations between ESF coverage and mortality from ACSCs in white and black/*pardo* populations in Brazil. We test the hypothesis that expansion of PHC coverage through the ESF in Brazil is associated with reduced inequalities in mortality between racial groups [26].

METHODS

Longitudinal panel data regression models were employed using routinely collected municipal-level data, which have been widely applied to evaluate the ESF previously [4,20,22,27–30]. These models estimated associations between ESF coverage and mortality from ACSCs among black/*pardo* and white populations over time, whilst controlling for other confounding factors. The main analysis was restricted to 1,622 municipalities based on previously assessed quality of vital statistics reporting to reduce bias from under-reporting of deaths [31]. Differences in our analytic approach from previous ESF evaluations were necessary to examine associations of ESF expansion and inequalities in mortality between racial groups. These were agreed before compilation and analysis of the data (which commenced in February 2016), and are set out in detail below. In response to reviewers' suggestions after initial submission, we explored factors associated with ESF uptake, tested for pre-existing trends, tested for biases from ill-defined death adjustments, explored interactions with Bolsa Família, and conducted sensitivity analyses with alternative model specifications and, for comparison with ACSC mortality, on mortality from accidents.

Data Sources

Data from individual death certificates for the years 2000–2013 were obtained from the Brazilian Ministry of Health DATASUS website [32]. Annual municipal population estimates by race and age group based on census data were obtained from the Instituto Brasileiro de Geografia e Estatística (IBGE) website [33]. Municipal-level covariate data, including illiteracy rate, poverty rate, urbanisation rate, and municipal gross domestic product (GDP), were obtained from the IBGE website [33]. Municipal ESF coverage, Bolsa Família coverage, public healthcare spending, the number of public hospital beds, the number of private hospital beds, and private health insurance coverage were obtained from the DATASUS website [32].

Variables

The mortality rate from ACSCs was the main outcome variable. ACSC deaths were encoded based on a list published by the Brazilian Ministry of Health (and restricted to those aged under 70 y) and ICD-10 codes reported on death certificates (Table 1) [34]. ACSCs were grouped by cause of death into infectious diseases, nutritional deficiencies and anaemia, chronic obstructive pulmonary disease (COPD) and asthma, cardiovascular disease, diabetes, epilepsy, and gastric ulcers. Redistribution of ill-defined deaths was performed using a published and previously utilised methodology to control for confounding trends from reductions in ill-defined deaths over time (S1 Text) [35].

Table 1. Ambulatory-care-sensitive conditions with International Classification of Diseases (ICD-10) codes.

Group	Condition	ICD-10 codes
Infectious diseases	Vaccine-preventable diseases	
	Tetanus	A33–A35
	Diphtheria	A36
	Whooping cough	A37
	Yellow fever	A95
	Acute hepatitis B	B16
	Measles	B05
	Rubella	B06
	Mumps	B26
	Haemophilus meningitis	G00.0
	Tuberculous meningitis	A17.0
	Miliary tuberculosis	A19
	Preventable conditions	
	Tuberculosis	A15–A16, A17.1–A17.9, A18
	Acute rheumatic fever	I00–I02
	Syphilis (early and late)	A51–A53
	Malaria	B50–B54
	Ascariasis	B77
	Gastrointestinal infections and complications	
	Intestinal infectious diseases	A00–A09
	Dehydration	E86
	Infections of the ear, nose, and throat	
	Otitis media	H66
	Acute upper respiratory infections	J00–J03, J06, J31
	Bacterial pneumonias	J13–J14, J15.3–J15.4, J15.8–J15.9, J18.1
	Infections of the kidney and urinary tract	
	Nephritis	N10–N12
	Cystitis	N30
	Urethritis and urethral syndrome	N34
	Urinary tract infection	N39.0
	Diseases of the prenatal period and childbirth	
	Urinary tract infection during pregnancy	O23
	Congenital syphilis	A50
	Congenital rubella	P35.0
	Infections of the skin and subcutaneous tissue	A46, L01–L04, L08
	Pelvic inflammatory disease	N70–N73, N75–N76
Nutritional deficiencies and anaemia	Anaemia	D50
	Nutritional deficiencies	
	Malnutrition	E40–E46
	Other nutritional deficiencies	E50–E64
COPD and asthma	Asthma	J45–J46
	Diseases of the lower respiratory tract	
	Bronchitis	J20, J21, J40–J42
	Emphysema	J43
	COPD	J44
	Bronchiectasis	J47
Cardiovascular disease	Hypertension	I10–I11
	Angina	I10
	Heart failure	I50, J81
	Cerebrovascular disease	I63–I67, I69, G45–G46
Diabetes	Diabetes mellitus	E10–E14
Epilepsy	Epilepsy	G40–G41
Gastric ulcers	Gastric ulcers	K25–K28, K92.0, K92.1, K92.2

Source: A list published by Alfradique et al. [34] and developed with the Brazilian Ministry of Health.
COPD, chronic obstructive pulmonary disease.

https://doi.org/10.1371/journal.pmed.1002306.t001

Race is recorded on death certificates and as part of the decennial census in Brazil. Census recording of race is self-reported. Individuals select *branco* (white), *preto* (black), *pardo* (brown/mixed), *amarello* (Asian), or indigenous. Recording of race on death certificates (using the same categories) is usually completed by the physician certifying the death and should be based on input from the family [13]. *Amarello* and indigenous deaths were very few and not examined. Black and *pardo* deaths were merged into one group, despite issues regarding differences between these populations [13]. This was to overcome potential differences in racial classification of individuals occurring either between censuses and death certificates, or over time as individuals and/or society changed reporting behaviour. Whilst evidence indicates overlap between black and *pardo* classifications in reporting of race, there are significantly clearer divisions between white and *pardo* classifications [36].

Reporting of race is near complete in censuses (99.29% in 2000 and 99.98% in 2010) and high on death certificates (total missing for 2000–2013 was 5.8%). For completeness, values were imputed for certificates with race missing using other death certificate variables (sex, age, education level, marital status, and location of death) and municipal population estimates of racial groups (S2 Text). For the period 2000–2013, race was imputed for 39,198 of the total 588,872 ACSC deaths (of those white or black/*pardo* and aged under 70 y) in the municipalities included in the analysis.

Using municipal census population data, population distributions by race (white and black/ *pardo*) and age group (0–4, 5–9, 10–14, 15–19, 20–24, 25–29, 30–39, 40–49, 50–59, and 60–69 y) were calculated for each municipality for the census years (2000 and 2010), and were linearly interpolated and extrapolated for non-census years (2001–2009 and 2011–2013). Annual total municipal population estimates were used to calculate annual age and race group population estimates for each municipality. Direct age standardisation of cause of death by race was performed, producing annual age-adjusted mortality rates for total ACSCs and ACSC groups by race. The dependent variables (for each municipality and for each year) in the regression models were the expected (from age standardisation) number of deaths from ACSCs (in total and by ACSC group) for the black/*pardo* and white populations and the standardised rate ratio (SRR) between total black/*pardo* and white ACSC mortality rates. Rate ratios (RRs) are commonly used metrics for comparing rates between groups (e.g., between males and females) [37].

In this study, the ACSC mortality rate for the black/*pardo* population was divided by the ACSC mortality rate for white population. The main variable of interest was municipal ESF coverage (percent) of the population, with official calculations based on one ESF team per 3,450 individuals [17].

A 2-y average (within the year and the year prior) of ESF coverage was employed, even though comparable results were obtained with just within-year coverage or including 2- and 3-y lags.

This approach was used to account for varying lagged and duration effects of the ESF that may differ between conditions and populations, to account for the time for ESF services to become fully operational and effective, and to permit simple comparison between the two racial groups.

Annual municipality-level covariate data were selected to include variables relating to socio-economic development, income, and the health system, which have been shown to affect mortality [38,39]. The covariates were scaled as percentages, in hundreds of Brazilian reais (R$100s) per person (adjusted for inflation), or per 1,000 inhabitants. Variables expressed as percentages were scaled between 0 and 1 so a one-unit increase would represent a 100% increase. Where necessary, logarithms were used to improve model fit. Covariates employed in all models were: Bolsa Famı́lia coverage (percent), illiteracy rate in those over 25 y (percent) (log-transformed), poverty rate (percent), population living in urban areas (percent), public healthcare spending (R$100s per person), public hospital beds per 1,000 population, private hospital beds per 1,000 population, private healthcare insurance (percent) (log-transformed), and GDP per person (R$100s per person) (log-transformed). An interaction between private healthcare insurance (percent) (log-transformed) and GDP per person (R$100s per person) (log-transformed) was included for model fit.

Statistical Analysis

Descriptive analyses were undertaken, including national trends of ACSC mortality rates for black/*pardo* and white populations and the national SRR of the two rates.

Fixed-effects longitudinal regression was employed as an appropriate method for analysing annual observations of municipalities [40]. Fixed-effects models control for time-invariant unobserved factors that may affect mortality and could bias the results [40]. Consequently, only changes *within* municipalities over time are estimated rather than differences *between* municipalities. We tested for pre-intervention trends (i.e., mortality rates prior to ESF adoption and expansion) to determine whether time-varying unobserved factors could bias the results. Examining trends in the years 2000–2003 (when many municipalities still had relatively low coverage) and employing dummy variables for the years prior to ESF adoption revealed no evidence of pre-intervention trends.

In the models with dependent count variables (ACSC deaths), a Poisson model with a population offset term was employed, allowing the dependent variable (ACSC deaths) to be modelled as a rate (deaths per population). To aid interpretability, the coefficients were exponentiated and reported as RRs. These are interpreted as a ratio of the mortality rates for a one unit increase in the independent variable (e.g., a 100% increase in ESF coverage or an additional year during the study period) (see S3 Text for more details). In other words, the difference between 1 and the RR can be interpreted as the percentage change in the rate given a one unit increase in the independent variable. For the SRR, linear longitudinal regression was employed, and β coefficients reported. These are interpreted as the change in the SRR given a one-unit increase (i.e., from 0% to 100% coverage). Two multiple regression models were undertaken examining the association between ESF expansion and ACSC mortality in the black/*pardo* and white populations separately. Differences in the effect sizes were tested for statistical significance (S4 Text). The *p*-values for the differences between the coefficients from the two models are reported in the text. The association between ESF coverage and the SRR was examined with a multiple regression model. Several regression models for the groups of ACSCs (infectious diseases, nutritional deficiencies and anaemia, COPD and asthma, cardiovascular disease, diabetes, epilepsy, and gastric ulcers) were employed in the black/*pardo* and white populations separately. Small numbers prohibited the use of SRR for groups of ACSCs. In all models, municipality-clustered robust standard errors were employed to account for possible auto-correlation and heteroscedasticity [40]. Stata 12 was used for statistical analysis.

Sensitivity Analyses

Multiple sensitivity analyses were undertaken to check the robustness of the findings. First, alternative model specifications with sequential addition of covariates, random-effect models, and negative-binomial models were employed (S2 Appendix, Tables A and B). Second, varying classifications of ESF coverage were tested (S2 Table). Third, mortality from accidents (ICD10 V01–X59) was tested, as an outcome that should have no association with ESF expansion (S3 Table). Fourth, the validity of imputing race on death certificates with race missing was assessed by excluding deaths where race was not recorded (S3 Appendix, Tables A and B). Fifth, the validity of redistributing ill-defined causes of death was tested (S4 Appendix, Tables A and B). Sixth, the analyses were repeated using data from all 5,565 municipalities in Brazil, not just those with adequate recording of vital statistics (S5 Appendix, Tables A and B). Seventh, because the potential for misclassification of race on death certificates exists (between the white and black/*pardo* populations), the effect of reclassifying black/*pardo* deaths (which are higher) as white was examined (S6 Appendix, Tables A–H). Eighth, an interaction between Bolsa Famı´lia and ESF coverage was examined (S7 Appendix).

RESULTS

Between 2000 and 2013, there were 281,877 and 318,030 deaths from ACSC causes in the black/*pardo* and white populations, respectively (after age standardisation). Age-standardised ACSC mortality rates fell 37.9%, from 93.3 to 57.9 per 100,000, in the black/*pardo* population and by 34.9%, from 75.7 to 49.2 per 100,000, in the white population (Fig 1; S7 Appendix). Mortality from ACSC causes in the black/*pardo* population was between 17% and 23% higher than in the white population during the study period. There was a sizeable expansion of the ESF over the period, both in terms of the number of municipalities adopting the ESF and the average municipal ESF coverage (Fig 2). In longitudinal Poisson regression models, ACSC mortality decreased annually by 3.4% (RR: 0.966; 95% CI: 0.954–0.976) in the black/*pardo* population and by 2.9% (RR: 0.971; 95% CI: 0.963–0.979) in the white population in adjusted models (Table 2). ESF expansion (from 0% to 100% coverage) was associated with a 15.4% (RR: 0.846; 95% CI: 0.796–0.899) reduction in ACSC mortality in the black/*pardo* population and a 6.8% (RR: 0.932; 95% CI: 0.892–0.974) reduction in the white population. These coefficients were significantly different (*p* = 0.012). ESF expansion (from 0% to 100% coverage) was associated with a 0.179 reduction (95% CI: 0.022–0.336) in the SRR (Table 3). Predicted SRRs from the model demonstrate that if ESF coverage were 0% in all municipalities, mortality amenable to PHC in the black/*pardo* population would be 29.6% higher than that in the white population (an estimated SRR of 1.296). With 100% ESF coverage in all municipalities, mortality amenable to PHC in the black/*pardo* population would be 11.7% higher than that in the white population (an estimated SRR of 1.117). Thus, expansion of the ESF (from 0% to 100%) yields a 60.5% reduction in the excess mortality that the black/*pardo* population experiences over the white population.

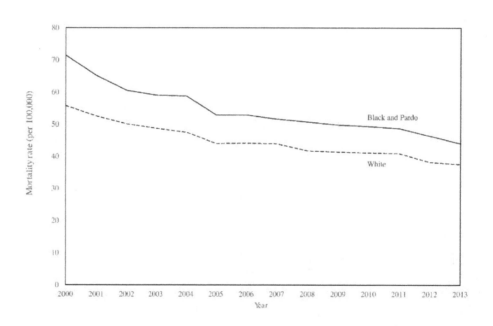

Fig 1. Age-standardised mortality rates for ambulatory-care-sensitive conditions in black/*pardo* and white populations in Brazil (2000–2013). Data only from 1,622 municipalities with adequate reporting of vital statistics. Mortality rates are age standardised to the 2010 national population estimates.

Associations With Cause-Specific Mortality

Over the study period, mortality from COPD and asthma decreased annually by 4.1% (RR: 0.959; 95% CI: 0.933–0.985) in the black/*pardo* population and by 4.5% (RR: 0.955; 95% CI: 0.939–0.971) in the white population (Table 4). Mortality from cardiovascular disease decreased annually by

3.7% (RR: 0.963; 95% CI: 0.948–0.979) in the black/*pardo* population and by 2.7% (RR: 0.973; 95% CI: 0.962–0.984) in the white population. For the black/*pardo* population, mortality from diabetes decreased 2.7% per year (RR: 0.973; 95% CI: 0.952–0.994), whilst there were non-significant trends in infectious diseases, nutritional deficiencies and anaemia, epilepsy, and gastric ulcers. For the white population, mortality from infectious diseases decreased 2.8% annually (RR: 0.972; 95% CI: 0.948–0.997), mortality from nutritional deficiencies and anaemia decreased 4.9% annually (RR: 0.951; 95% CI: 0.909–0.994), and mortality from gastric ulcers decreased 4.9% annually (RR: 0.951; 95% CI: 0.922–0.981), but there were no significant trends in diabetes and epilepsy mortality. ESF expansion (from 0% to 100%) was associated with a decrease in mortality from cardiovascular disease of 12.9% (RR: 0.871; 95% CI: 0.801–0.947) and 7.1% (RR: 0.929; 95% CI:0.876–0.985) in the black/*pardo* and white populations, respectively. In the black/*pardo* population, ESF expansion was associated with 27.5% lower mortality from infectious diseases (RR:0.725; 95% CI: 0.620–0.848) and 19.3% lower mortality from diabetes (RR: 0.807; 95% CI: 0.713–0.912), but there was no significant association with mortality for these ACSC groups in the white population.

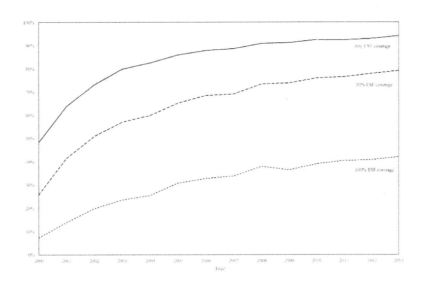

Fig 2. **Percentage of municipalities achieving any, 50%, and 100% Estrate´gia de Sau´de da Fami´lia coverage (2000–2013).** Only data from the 1,622 municipalities with adequate vital statistics reporting are included in this analysis. ESF, Estrate´gia de Sau´de da Fami´lia.

ESF expansion was associated with 17.9% lower mortality from nutritional deficiencies and anaemia (RR: 0.721; 95% CI: 0.478–0.899) in the black/*pardo* population, but in the white population, it was associated with 25.1% higher mortality (RR: 1.251; 95% CI: 1.011–1.548). For both the black/*pardo* and white populations, there was no significant association between ESF and mortality from COPD and asthma, epilepsy, or gastric ulcers.

Sensitivity Analyses

Sensitivity analyses demonstrate the robustness of our findings. Alternative model specifications (S2 Appendix, Tables A and B) demonstrate the stability and robustness of the findings. We found that controlling for additional factors (fixed effects, covariates, and state-year fixed effects) did not change our findings; in fact, the differential associations of the ESF with black/ *pardo* and white mortality became more apparent when these factors were taken into account. Alternative classifications of ESF coverage did not change the overall differences in the associations between ESF expansion and black/*pardo* and white mortality, although the results of the sensitivity analysis did suggest that greater reductions in mortality in the black/*pardo* population accrued over a longer period (S2 Table). Examining mortality from accidents as a control outcome revealed no significant association of accident deaths with ESF coverage in either racial group, adding to the robustness of our findings (S3 Table). Excluding deaths with race not recorded yielded highly comparable results, demonstrating that imputation of missing race data was not a source of bias

Table 2. Results from longitudinal fixed-effects Poisson regression of mortality from ambulatory-care-sensitive conditions in black/*pardo* and white populations.

Variable	Black/*pardo* group		White group	
	RR or *N*	95% CI	RR or *N*	95% CI
ESF coverage	0.846***	0.796, 0.899	0.932**	0.892, 0.974
Year	0.966***	0.954, 0.979	0.971***	0.963, 0.979
Bolsa Família coverage	0.873*	0.784, 0.973	0.895	0.799, 1.002
Illiteracy rate	0.940	0.757, 1.168	0.905	0.796, 1.029
Poverty rate	1.592*	1.053, 2.407	1.149	0.849, 1.555
Urbanisation rate	1.135	0.697, 1.848	0.839	0.585, 1.204
Public healthcare spending	1.009	1.000, 1.019	1.002	0.991, 1.013
Public hospital beds	1.001	0.941, 1.065	1.013	0.960, 1.069
Private hospital beds	1.193	0.913, 1.561	1.088	0.922, 1.284
Private healthcare insurance	0.831**	0.744, 0.928	0.900*	0.827, 0.979
GDP	0.846**	0.759, 0.944	0.853***	0.781, 0.932
Private healthcare insurance × GDP	0.953***	0.934, 0.972	0.974**	0.959, 0.990
N observations	22,384		22,694	
N municipalities	1,599		1,621	

Exponentiated coefficients: * $p < 0.05$, ** $p < 0.01$, *** $p < 0.001$.

The study period was from 2000 to 2013. Robust standard errors were employed. ESF coverage is a 2-y average of within-year municipal ESF coverage and coverage in the year before. Year is a continuous variable and is interpreted as the underlying annual change in mortality rate during the study period. ESF coverage, Bolsa Famı́lia coverage, poverty rate, and urbanisation rate are all expressed as percentages and are scaled so a one-unit increase represents a 100% increase. Private healthcare insurance is also expressed as a percentage, but is log-transformed. Illiteracy rate is the illiteracy rate of those aged 25 y and over and is log-transformed. Public healthcare spending is expressed as hundreds of Brazilian reais per person, as is GDP, although GDP is log-transformed. Public and private hospital beds are expressed per 1,000 municipal inhabitants. Some municipalities and/or year observations are not included for a racial group due to there being no deaths from ambulatory-care-sensitive conditions for that racial group.95% CI, 95% confidence interval; ESF, Estrate´gia de Sau´de da Famı́lia; GDP, gross domestic product; RR, rate ratio. **care-sensitive conditions in black/*pardo* and white populations.**

Table 3. Results from the longitudinal fixed-effects linear regression of standardised rate ratios for mortality from ambulatory-care-sensitive conditions in black/pardo and white populations

Variable	Coefficient or *N*	95% CI
ESF coverage	−0.179*	−0.336, −0.022
Year	0.010	−0.021, 0.041
Bolsa Famı́lia coverage	−0.170	−0.549, 0.209
Illiteracy rate	0.066	−0.476, 0.609
Poverty rate	1.226*	0.167, 2.284
Urbanisation rate	0.847	−0.361, 2.056
Public healthcare spending	0.012	−0.014, 0.039
Public hospital beds	−0.082	−0.217, 0.054
Private hospital beds	0.088	−0.207, 0.382
Private healthcare insurance	−0.114	−0.405, 0.177
GDP	−0.132	−0.450, 0.185
Private healthcare insurance × GDP	−0.038	−0.095, 0.019
N observations	21,336	
N municipalities	1,622	

The study period was from 2000 to 2013. Robust standard errors were employed. ESF coverage is a 2-y average of within-year municipal ESF coverage and coverage in the year before. Year is a continuous variable and is interpreted as the change in mortality rate for each additional year. ESF coverage, Bolsa Famı́lia coverage, poverty rate, and urbanisation rate are all expressed as percentages and scaled so a oneunit increase represents a 100% increase. Private healthcare insurance is also expressed as a percentage, but is log-transformed. Illiteracy rate is the illiteracy rate of those aged 25 y and over and is log-transformed.Public healthcare spending is expressed as hundreds of Brazilian reais per person, as is GDP, although GDP is log-transformed. Public and private hospital beds are expressed per 1,000 municipal inhabitants. Some municipalities and/or year observations are not included for a racial group due to there being no deaths from ambulatory-care-sensitive conditions for that racial group.95% CI, 95% confidence interval; ESF, Estrate´gia de Sau´de da Famı́lia; GDP, gross domestic product.

DISCUSSION

Expansion of the ESF between 2000 and 2013 in Brazil was associated with a 2-fold greater reduction in ACSC mortality in the black/*pardo* compared to the white population. This differential benefit reduced racial inequalities in mortality and was driven by greater reductions in deaths from infectious diseases, nutritional deficiencies and anaemia, diabetes, and cardiovascular disease in the black/*pardo* population.

This paper provides further evidence of the importance of expanding UHC in low- and middle-income countries. Previous literature indicates that ESF expansion is associated with reduced child mortality, mortality from cardiovascular disease, and ACSC hospitalisations [4,5,20–22]. These changes are likely due to improved access to healthcare and a focus on prevention, health promotion, proactive outreach, and early management of conditions within the ESF [3].

Whilst there is local variation in how the ESF is implemented, federal guidelines specify minimum mandatory strategic areas ESF teams must cover, including the management of hypertension, diabetes, tuberculosis, and women's and children's health [42]. In this study, ESF expansion was associated with reductions in mortality in the ACSC groups that mirror these mandatory strategic areas.

Group	Variable	Black/*pardo* group		White group	
		RR or *N*	95% CI	RR or *N*	95% CI
Infectious diseases	ESF coverage	0.725***	0.620, 0.848	0.956	0.854, 1.070
	Year	0.989	0.953, 1.026	0.972*	0.948, 0.997
	N observations	18,046		21,476	
	Total deaths	35,353		31,716	
Nutritional deficiencies and anaemia	ESF coverage	0.721**	0.578, 0.899	1.251*	1.011, 1.548
	Year	0.982	0.937, 1.031	0.951*	0.909, 0.994
	N observations	11,662		15,932	
	Total deaths	5,968		5,313	
COPD and asthma	ESF coverage	1.072	0.939, 1.223	0.988	0.914, 1.068
	Year	0.959**	0.933, 0.985	0.955***	0.939, 0.971
	N observations	19,880		22,120	
	Total deaths	27,174		48,055	
Cardiovascular	ESF coverage	0.871**	0.801, 0.947	0.929*	0.876, 0.985
	Year	0.963***	0.948, 0.979	0.973***	0.962, 0.984
	N observations	21,853		22,652	
	Total deaths	137,061		147,682	
Diabetes	ESF coverage	0.807***	0.713, 0.912	0.932	0.849, 1.023
	Year	0.973*	0.952, 0.994	0.987	0.971, 1.004
	N observations	20,244		22,526	
	Total deaths	54,873		65,003	
Epilepsy	ESF coverage	0.961	0.745, 1.240	1.017	0.806, 1.284
	Year	1.000	0.949, 1.054	0.962	0.921, 1.005
	N observations	11,578		15,848	
	Total deaths	4,045		4,908	
Gastric ulcers	ESF coverage	0.962	0.915, 1.012	0.951**	0.922, 0.981
	Year	0.864	0.697, 1.122	0.939	0.800, 1.103
	N observations	13,230		18,788	
	Total deaths	8,542		10,798	

Exponentiated coefficients:
* $p < 0.05$,
** $p < 0.01$,
*** $p < 0.001$.

The table shows select results from longitudinal Poisson regressions for groups of ambulatory-care-sensitive conditions for both the black/*pardo* population and the white population, in addition to the number of deaths for each group of conditions and racial group. The study period was from 2000 to 2013. Robust standard errors were employed. ESF coverage is a 2-y average of within-year municipal ESF coverage and coverage in the year before, and is expressed as percentages and scaled so a one-unit increase represents a 100% increase. Year is a continuous variable and is interpreted as the change in mortality rate for each additional year. Although not reported, all regressions control for Bolsa Família coverage (percent), illiteracy rate of those over 25 y (log-transformed), poverty rate (percent), urbanisation rate (percent), public healthcare spending (R$100s per person), public hospital beds per 1,000 population, private hospital beds per 1,000 population, private healthcare insurance (percent) (log-transformed), GDP per person (R$100s per person) (log-transformed), and the interaction of private healthcare insurance (percent) (log-transformed) and GDP per person (R$100s per person) (log-transformed). Some municipalities and/or year observations are not included for a racial group due to there being no deaths from ambulatory-care-sensitive conditions for that racial group.

95% CI, 95% confidence interval; COPD, chronic obstructive pulmonary disease; ESF, Estratégia de Saúde da Família; GDP, gross domestic product; R$100s, hundreds of Brazilian reais per person; RR, rate ratio.

https://dx.org/10.1371/journal.pmed.1002306.t004

Table 4. Results from longitudinal fixed-effects Poisson regressions for mortality by groups of ambulatory-care-sensitive conditions in black/ *pardo* and white populations.

We found that ESF expansion was associated with reductions in cardiovascular mortality of 12.9% and 7.1% in the black/*pardo* and white groups, respectively. We found a 27.5% reduction in mortality from infectious diseases with ESF expansion in the black/*pardo* population. ESF expansion was also associated with a 17.9% reduction in mortality from nutritional deficiencies and anaemia in the black/*pardo* population, with children under 5 y accounting for over 25% of these deaths (compared to roughly 3% of all deaths from ACSCs). Additionally, ESF-associated reductions in mortality from respiratory diseases (COPD and asthma), epilepsy, and gastric ulcers are consistent with their inclusion within ACSC definitions and the fact that these conditions are considered amenable to PHC.

We found no association between ESF expansion and mortality from accidents, which is not considered sensitive to primary care, providing reassurance that the associations of ESF expansion with ACSCs reported are not due to confounding. The differential associations between ESF expansion and mortality in black/*pardo* and white populations may be explained by numerous factors, with socio-economic differences a key explanatory factor. Black/*pardo* populations are disproportionately affected by diseases of poverty, including infectious diseases, malnutrition, and anaemia [9,43], but these conditions may be more responsive to ESF services as they are generally easier to treat in PHC settings than complex non-communicable diseases. Additionally, black/*pardo* populations in Brazil have lower utilisation of healthcare and higher rates of forgone healthcare [9], suggesting ESF expansion may have facilitated access to healthcare and reduced unmet need. Lastly, the finding that ESF has benefitted black/*pardo* populations more than white populations may not be surprising given that ESF expansion had been prioritised within poorer areas and municipalities. Surveys indicate that black/*pardo* populations now have greater ESF coverage (at 57.3% in 2008) than white populations (44.6% in 2008), but lower coverage of private health insurance, suggesting they are more reliant on publicly funded and provided services, including the ESF [9].

Our findings are consistent with evidence derived largely from studies conducted in North America and Europe that show "equity-enhancing" associations from PHC expansion [3]. However, these studies mostly examine associations of PHC with health inequalities across income groups. There are fewer studies examining the association of PHC with health inequalities between racial groups. In a study in the US, increasing the supply of primary care physicians was associated with larger reductions in African-American mortality than white mortality [38]. Inequalities in low birth weight between African-American and white infants are lower among those using PHC [44]. No evidence exists on the association between PHC and race in Brazil, although a few studies have examined inequalities between municipalities. Previous Brazilian studies have shown that ESF expansion was associated with greater reductions in infant mortality in municipalities with higher infant mortality at baseline [20,45].

Another study demonstrated greater reductions in infant mortality in municipalities with lower human development, also implying improvements in equity [20]. There are important limitations to this study pertinent to the interpretation. First, these analyses were conducted on municipal-level aggregated data, and more complete, individual data with ESF enrolment, consultation rates, and associated health outcomes are required to elucidate the mechanisms determining the greater benefits experienced by the black/*pardo* population. Second, there could be biases from the methods employed and data manipulation.

However, we conducted extensive sensitivity analyses that showed that our findings are robust to ill-defined death reclassification, varying classifications of ESF coverage, and alternative model specifications. We also found no evidence of pre-intervention trends that would bias the findings.

Third, there are important caveats regarding the use of race in this study. There is potential for misclassification bias of race (with race in censuses self-reported and race in death certificates reported by either the family or physician), although sensitivity analyses indicate the robustness of the findings. Black/*pardo* would have to be incorrectly recorded for over 30% of black/*pardo* deaths for the differences found to be non-significant. Additionally, by grouping together black and *pardo* deaths, we do not account for the large amount of heterogeneity in health outcomes between these groups [13]. Fourth, lack of statistical power due to small numbers is apparent in our analysis of associations between ESF expansion and cause specific deaths. This precluded any potential analysis with SRRs for ACSC groups. Fifth, we used mortality from ACSCs as our outcome measure rather than the more broadly defined concept of healthcare-amenable mortality [30,46]). This was principally to focus on conditions that have been defined as amenable to PHC within the Brazilian context and to exclude those that may be strongly influenced by hospital-based care. While previous research has generally examined hospital admissions for ACSCs, this was not feasible here due to low recording of race in hospital admission data in Brazil. We present a comparison of conditions included in the Brazilian Ministry of Health's definition of ACSCs and healthcare-amenable mortality as defined by Nolte and McKee [46] in S4 Table.

Policy-makers should note that in Brazil, where sharp inequalities persist and an ambition to achieve UHC has been boldly pursued over the last 20 years, the equity-promoting associations of PHC are evident [30]. The strong positive relationship between PHC and reduced racial inequalities in mortality provides impetus for a renewed government commitment to the ESF.

Current proposals that could limit public spending in Brazil and cause disinvestment from social protection programmes, including the ESF [23], may reverse the valuable progress made towards reducing health inequalities in the country. he health inequality impacts of policy changes influencing the ESF, which is the primary vehicle for UHC in Brazil, should be carefully monitored and evaluated.

Beyond the equity-enhancing nature of PHC itself, the impressive reductions in inequality in ACSC deaths between racial groups seen in Brazil may have been facilitated by numerous factors.

These include the more rapid expansion of the ESF in poorer and more deprived areas, and the proactive outreach healthcare delivered by community health workers. Whilst challenges exist, including retaining health professionals in rural areas [15] and a lack of coverage for the urban poor [47], there are valuable lessons for other countries from Brazil's efforts to achieve UHC. The pro-equity health gains demonstrated here reflect the country's adoption of a pro-poor pathway to UHC. Universal access was embraced from the start, services are publicly financed, there is a focus on expanding access through community-based models of care, and strong political commitment has enabled rapid and sizeable expansion [48].

Valuable lessons may be derived from other settings including Costa Rica, which similarly expanded PHC in poorer areas preferentially [49], and countries such as Tanzania, Uganda, and Chile, which have accelerated coverage in underserved areas through flexible budget allocations [50]. In conclusion, expansion of the ESF in Brazil was associated with improved health outcomes and reductions in health inequalities between racial groups. As countries aim to "progressively achieve greater equality" as part of the SDGs, these findings reinforce the importance of strong PHC-focused health systems for improving health and reducing health inequities.

Supporting Information

S1 Alternative Language Abstract. Portuguese translation of the abstract by Leandro Garcia.

S1 Appendix. Expansion of the Estrate´gia de Sau´de da Famı´lia by municipal population, poverty rate, and black/*pardo* population.

S2 Appendix. Sensitivity analysis: Sequential addition of covariates and alternative model specifications.

S3 Appendix. Sensitivity analysis: Excluding deaths with missing race.

S4 Appendix. Sensitivity analysis: No adjustment for ill-defined deaths.

S5 Appendix. Sensitivity analysis: Analysing all municipalities (including those with inadequate vital statistics reporting).

S6 Appendix. Sensitivity analysis: Testing potential misclassification bias.

S7 Appendix. Sensitivity analysis: Interaction between Bolsa Famı´lia and Estrate´gia de Sau´de da Famı´lia coverage. (DOCX)

S1 STROBE Checklist. STROBE checklist. (DOC)

S1 Table. National age-standardised mortality rates (deaths per 100,000) from ambulatory-care-sensitive conditions in black/*pardo* and white groups, absolute difference in rates, and standardised rate ratio in 1,622 municipalities with adequate reporting of vital statistics (2000–2013).

S2 Table. Sensitivity analysis: Different classifications of Estrate´gia de Sau´de da Famı´lia coverage.

S3 Table. Sensitivity analysis: Mortality from accidents. (DOCX)

S4 Table. Comparison of ambulatory-care-sensitive conditions and mortality amenable to primary care. (DOCX)

S1 Text. Methods for redistribution of ill-defined deaths. (DOCX)

S2 Text. Methods for imputing missing race. (DOCX)

S3 Text. Fixed-effects longitudinal Poisson regression model specification. (DOCX)

S4 Text. Calculating statistical difference in coefficients between two different models. (DOCX)

AFFILIATIONS

1 Public Health Policy Evaluation Unit, Department of Primary Care and Public Health, School of Public Health, Imperial College London, London, United Kingdom, 2 Centre for Data and Knowledge Integration for Health (CIDACS), Instituto Fonc¸alo Muniz, Fundac¸ão Oswaldo Cruz, Salvador, Brazil, 3 Instituto de Sau´de Coletiva, Universidade Federal da Bahia, Salvador, Brazil, 4 Centre for Epidemiological Studies in Health and Nutrition, University of São Paulo, São Paulo, Brazil, 5 Department of Epidemiology, Institute of Social aMedicine, Rio de Janeiro State University, Rio de Janeiro, Brazil

REFERENCES

1. Tangcharoensathien, V,, Mills, A., Palu, T.(2015).Accelerating health equity: the key role of universal health coverage in the Sustainable Development Goals. BMC Med. 2015; 13(1):101.

2. World Health Organization. The world health report (2010): health system financing—the path to universal coverage. Geneva: World Health Organization; 2010.

3. Starfield, B., Shi, L, Macinko, J. (2005).Contribution of primary care to health systems and health. Milbank Q. 2005; 83(3):457–502. https://doi.org/10.1111/j.1468-0009.2005.00409.x PMID: 16202000

4. Rasella, D., Harhay, M.O, Pamponet, M.L, Aquino, R, Barreto M.L (2014). Impact of primary health care on mortality from heart and cerebrovascular diseases in Brazil: a nationwide analysis of longitudinal data. BMJ.2014; 349:g4014. https://doi.org/10.1136/bmj.g4014 PMID: 24994807

5. Macinko, J., Dourado, I., Aquino, R., Bonolo Pde F, Lima-Costa, M.F, Medina, M.G, et al. (2020). Major expansion of primary care in Brazil linked to decline in unnecessary hospitalization. Health Aff (Millwood). 2010; 29 (12):2149–60.

6. World Bank. Brazil: country at a glance. Washington (District of Columbia): World Bank; 2016 [cited 2016 Sep 8]. http://www.worldbank.org/en/country/brazil.

7. Szwarcwald, C,L, Souza-Ju´nior PR, Damacena, G.N.(2010).Socioeconomic inequalities in the use of outpatient services in Brazil according to health care need: evidence from the World Health Survey. BMC Health Serv Res. 2010; 10:217. https://doi.org/10.1186/1472-6963-10-217 PMID: 20653970

8. Szwarcwald, C.L, Corrêa da Mota J, Damacena, G/N., Sardinha Pereira, T.G. (2011)Health inequalities in Rio de Janeiro, Brazil: lower healthy life expectancy in socioeconomically disadvantaged areas. Am J Public Health. 2011; 101(3):517–23. https://doi.org/10.2105/AJPH.2010.195453 PMID: 21233437

9. Paixão, M.J., Rossetto, I,, Montovanele, F., Carvano, L.M.(2010)Relato´rio anual das desigualdades raciais no Brasil, 2009–10. Rio de Janeiro: Editora Garamond.

10. Cardoso, A.M., Santos, R.V., Coimbra, C.E.A Jr. (2005). Mortalidade infantil segundo rac¸a/cor no Brasil: o que dizem os sistemas nacionais de informac¸ão? Cad Saude Publica. 2005; 21:1602–8.

11. Nyarko, K.A, Lopez-Camelo. J., Castilla, E.E, Wehby, G.L. (2013). Explaining racial disparities in infant health in Brazil. Am J Public Health. 2013; 103(9):1675–84. https://doi.org/10.2105/AJPH.2012.301021 PMID: 23409894

12. Rasella, D., Machado, D., Castellanos, M.E.P. Paim. J., Szwarcwald. C.L, Lima. D,et al (2016).Assessing the relevance of indicators in tracking social determinants and progress toward equitable population health in Brazil. Glob Health Action. 2016; 9:29042.

13. Travassos, C, Williams, D.R. (2004).The concept and measurement of race and their relationship to public health: a review focused on Brazil and the United States. Cad Saude Publica. 2004; 20(3):660–78. https://doi.org//S0102-311X2004000300003 PMID: 15263977

14. Rasella D, Aquino R, Santos CAT, Paes-Sousa, R., Barreto, M.L. (2013).Effect of a conditional cash transfer programme on childhood mortality: a nationwide analysis of Brazilian municipalities. Lancet. 2013; 382 (9886):57–64. https://doi.org/10.1016/S0140-6736(13)60715-1 PMID: 23683599

15. Harris, M., Haines, A. (2010).Brazil's Family Health Programme. BMJ. 2010; 341:c4945. https://doi.org/10.1136/bmj.c4945 PMID: 21115587

16. Macinko, J., Harris, MJ. (2015). Brazil's Family Health Strategy—delivering community-based primary care in a universal health system. N Engl J Med. 2015; 372(23):2177–81. https://doi.org/10.1056/ NEJMp1501140 PMID: 26039598

17. Ministe´rio da Sau´de Departamento de Atenc¸ão Ba´sica. Histo´rico de cobertura da sau´de da famı´lia. Brasilia: Ministe´rio da Sau´de; 2015 [cited 2015 Apr 11]. http://dab.saude.gov.br/portaldab/historico_ cobertura_sf.php.

18. Ministe´rio da Sau´de. Polı´tica Nacional de Atenc¸ão Ba´sica. Brasilia: Ministe´rio da Sau´de; 2011.

19. Henrique, F., Calvo, M.C (2009).. [The degree of implementation of the Family Health Program and social indicators.] Cien Saude Colet. 2009; 14(Suppl 1):1359–65.

20. Aquino R, de Oliveira, N.F., Barreto, M.L (2009). Impact of the family health program on infant mortality in Brazilian municipalities. Am J Public Health. 2009; 99(1):87–93. https://doi.org/10.2105/AJPH.2007.127480 PMID: 19008516

21. Guanais, F.C (20014). The combined effects of the expansion of primary health care and conditional cash transfers on infant mortality in Brazil, 1998–2010. Rev Panam Salud Publica. 2014; 36(1):65–9. PMID: 25211681

22. Macinko J, Marinho de Souza MdF, Guanais F.C, da Silva Simoes CC. (2007). Going to scale with communitybased primary care: an analysis of the family health program and infant mortality in Brazil, 1999–2004. Soc Sci Med. 2007; 65(10):2070–80. https://doi.org/10.1016/j.socscimed.2007.06.028 PMID: 17689847

23. Watts, J. (2016).Brazil's health system woes worsen in economic crisis. Lancet. 2016; 387(10028):1603–4. https://doi.org/10.1016/S0140-6736(16)30249-5 PMID: 27116057

24. Telles, E.E. (2004). Race in another America: the significance of skin color in Brazil. Princeton (New Jersey): Princeton University Press.

25. Lima-Costa, M.F., Rodrigues, L.C., Barreto, M.L, Gouveia, M., Horta, B.L, Mambrini, J., et al.(2015). Genomic ancestry and ethnoracial self-classification based on 5,871 community-dwelling Brazilians (the Epigen Initiative). Sci Rep. 2015; 5:9812. https://doi.org/10.1038/srep09812 PMID: 25913126

26. Purdy S, Griffin T, Salisbury C, Sharp D.(2009). Ambulatory care sensitive conditions: terminology and disease coding need to be more specific to aid policy makers and clinicians. Public Health. 2009; 123(2):169–73. https://doi.org/10.1016/j.puhe.2008.11.001 PMID: 19144363

27. Macinko J, Guanais FC, de Fatima M, de Souza M. (2006).Evaluation of the impact of the Family Health Program on infant mortality in Brazil, 1990–2002. J Epidemiol Community Health. 2006; 60(1):13–9. https://doi.org/10.1136/jech.2005.038323 PMID: 16361449

28. Guanais F, Macinko J. (2009).Primary care and avoidable hospitalizations: evidence from Brazil. J Ambul Care Manage. 2009; 32(2):115–22. https://doi.org/10.1097/JAC.0b013e31819942e51 PMID: 19305223

29. Rocha, R., Soares, R.R. (2010).Evaluating the impact of community-based health interventions: evidence from Brazil's Family Health Program. Health Econ. 2010; 19(Suppl):126–58.

30. Hone, T., Rasella, D., Barreto, M., Atun, R., Majeed, A., Millett, C. (2017). Large reductions in amenable mortality associated with Brazil's primary care expansion and strong health governance. Health Aff (Millwood). 2017; 36(1):149–58.

31. de Andrade, C.L.T., Szwarcwald, C. (2007). Socio-spatial inequalities in the adequacy of Ministry of Health data on births and deaths at the municipal level in Brazil, 2000–2002. Cad Saude Publica. 2007; 23(5):1207–16. PMID: 17486242

32. Ministe´rio da Sau´de. DATASUS. Brasilia: Ministe´rio da Sau´de; 2015 [cited 2015 Apr 4]. http://tabnet. datasus.gov.br/.

33. Instituto Brasileiro de Geografia e Estatı´stica. Banco de dados. Rio de Janeiro: Instituto Brasileiro de Geografia e Estatı´stica; 2016 [cited 2016 Dec 4]. http://www.ibge.gov.br/.

34. Alfradique, M.E, Bonolo, P.d.F, Dourado, I, Lima-Costa, M.F., Macinko, J., Mendonca, C.S., et al. (2009). Ambulatory care sensitive hospitalizations: elabouration of Brazilian list as a tool for measuring health system performance (Project ICSAP–Brazil). Cad Saude Publica. 2009; 25(6):1337–49. PMID: 19503964

35. Franc,,a E, Teixeira, R., Ishitani, L, Duncan, B.B., Cortez-Escalante, J.J., de Morais Neto, O.L, et al. (2014). Ill-defined causes of death in Brazil: a redistribution method based on the investigation of such causes. Rev Saude Publica. 2014; 48(4):671–81. https://doi.org/10.1590/S0034-8910.2014048005146 PMID: 25210826

36. Travassos, C, Laguardia, J., Marques, P.M., Mota, J.C., Szwarcwald, C.L (2011). Comparison between two race/skin color classifications in relation to health-related outcomes in Brazil. Int J Equity Health. 2011; 10:35. https://doi.org/10.1186/1475-9276-10-35 PMID: 21867522

37. Mackenbach, J.P., Kunst, A.E, Cavelaars, A.E.J.M., Groenhof, F., Geurts, J.JM. (1997). Socioeconomic inequalities in morbidity and mortality in western Europe. Lancet. 1997; 349(9066):1655–9. PMID: 9186383

38. Shi, L, Macinko, J., Starfield, B., Politzer, R, Xu, J.(2005). Primary care, race, and mortality in US states. Soc Sci Med. 2005; 61(1):65–75. https://doi.org/10.1016/j.socscimed.2004.11.056 PMID: 15847962

39. Marmot, M. (2005). Social determinants of health inequalities. Lancet. 2005; 365(9464):1099–104. https://doi.org/10.1016/S0140-6736(05)71146-6 PMID: 15781105

40. Wooldridge, J. (2013).Introductory econometrics: a modern approach. 5th ed. Boston: Cengage Learning; 2013. 878 p.

41. Rasella, D., Aquino, R., Barreto, M.L. (2010). Impact of the Family Health Program on the quality of vital information and reduction of child unattended deaths in Brazil: an ecological longitudinal study. BMC Public Health.2010; 10:380. https://doi.org/10.1186/1471-2458-10-380 PMID: 20587036

42. Ministe´rio da Sau´de. Programa Sau´de da Famı´lia: ampliando a cobertura para consolidar a mudanc,a do modelo de Atenc,ão Ba´sica. Rev Bras Saude Mater Infant. 2003; 3:113–25.

43. Stevens, P. (2004). Diseases of poverty and the 10/90 gap. London: International Policy Network; 2004.

44. Shi L, Stevens, G.D., Wulu, J.T. Jr, Politzer, R.M, Xu, J. (2004). America's health centres: reducing racial and ethnic disparities in perinatal care and birth outcomes. Health Serv Res. 2004; 39(6 Pt 1):1881–901. https://doi.org/10.1111/j.1475-6773.2004.00323.x PMID: 15533192

45. Shei, A. (2013). Brazil's conditional cash transfer program associated with declines in infant mortality rates. Health Aff (Millwood). 2013; 32(7):1274–81.

46. Nolte, E., McKee, CM. (2018). Measuring the health of nations: updating an earlier analysis. Health Aff (Millwood). 2008; 27(1):58–71.

47. Costa, N.d.R.(2016).The Family Health Strategy: primary health care and the challenge of Brazilian metropolises. Cien Saude Colet. 2016; 21(5):1389–98. https://doi.org/10.1590/1413-81232015215.24842015 PMID: 27166889

48. Bump, J., Cashin, C., Chalkidou, K., Evans, D., Gonza´lez-Pier, E., Guo, Y., et al. (2015) Implementing pro-poor universal health coverage. Lancet Glob Health. 2015; 4(1):e14–6. https://doi.org/10.1016/S2214-109X(15) 00274-0 PMID: 26700794

49. Rosero-Bixby L.(2004). Spatial access to health care in Costa Rica and its equity: a GIS-based study. Soc Sci Med. 2004; 58(7):1271–84. https://doi.org/10.1016/S0277-9536(03)00322-8 PMID: 14759675

50. World Health Organization. The world health report 2008: primary health care—now more than ever. Geneva: World Health Organization; 2008.

http://siops-asp.datasus.gov.br/CGI/deftohtm. exe?SIOPS/serhist/municipio/mIndicadores.def. Data on private health insurance were obtained from http://www.ans.gov.br/anstabnet/.

Data on primary care coverage were obtained from http:// dab.saude.gov.br/portaldab/historico_cobertura_ sf.php and are also available from http://www2. datasus.gov.br/DATASUS/index.php?area=0202.

Bolsa familia coverage can be obtained from http://aplicacoes.mds.gov.br/sagi-data/misocial/ tabelas/mi_social.php.

Population estimates were obtained from http://www.ibge.gov.br/home/ estatistica/populacao/estimativa2015/estimativa_ dou.shtm and also http://www2.datasus.gov.br/ DATASUS/index.php?area=0206&id=6942.

GDP was obtained from http://www2.datasus.gov.br/ DATASUS/index.php?area=0206&id=29610442.

Data on illiteracy, poverty, and urbanisation were obtained from http://www.atlasbrasil.org.br/ 2013/en/download/.

Funding: This work was funded by Imperial CollegeLondon through TH's PhD. CM is funded by an

NIHR Research Professorship. Imperial College London is grateful for support from the NWLondon NIHR Collabouration for Leadership in

Applied Health Research & Care (CLAHRC) and the Imperial NIHR Biomedical Research Centre. The funders had no role in study design, data collection and analysis, decision to publish, or preparation of the manuscript.

Abbreviations: ACSC, ambulatory-care-sensitive condition; COPD, chronic obstructive pulmonary disease; ESF, Estrate´gia de Sau´de da Fam´ilia; GDP, gross domestic product; PHC, primary healthcare; R$100s, hundreds of Brazilian reais; RR, rate ratio; SDG, Sustainable Development Goal; SRR, standardised rate ratio; UHC, universal health coverage.

3. COVID-19 Is Deadlier For Black Brazilians, A Legacy Of Structural Racism That Dates Back To Slavery

Kia Lilly Caldwell

Professor, African, African American, and Diaspora Studies, University of North Carolina at Chapel Hill

Edna Maria de Araújo

Professor of Public Health and Epidemiology, State University of Feira de Santana (Brazil)

The United States and Brazil have much in common when it comes to the coronavirus. Both are among the world's hardest-hit countries,[1] where hundreds die daily. Their like-minded presidents, Donald Trump and Jair Bolsonaro, have both been widely criticized for their poor handling[2] of the pandemic. And in both countries the virus is disproportionately affecting black people,[3] the result of structural racism that dates back to slavery.

Legacy of Slavery

Brazil forcibly brought some 4 million enslaved Africans into the country over three centuries, more than anywhere else in the Americas[4]. About half its 209 million people are black[5] – the world's second largest African-descendant population after Nigeria. Modern Brazil never had legalized racial discrimination like Jim Crow, but race-based inequalities are deeply entrenched. Despite a persistent myth[6] of Brazil as an integrated "racial democracy," employment discrimination and residential segregation[7] limit opportunity for black people.

These and other factors translate into lower life expectancy, education and standards of living[8] for Afro-Brazilians[9]. Black Brazilians live, on average, 73 years – three years less than white Brazilians, according to the 2017 National Household Survey[10]. The U.S. has a nearly identical life expectancy gap between races.

Because government data in Brazil is not automatically collected by race or ethnicity, though, the health impacts of racism can be hard to measure. Bolsonaro's administration did not require the collection of COVID-19 racial data[11] until late April, well into the pandemic, after much pressure. It

---

[1] https://www.nytimes.com/interactive/2020/world/americas/brazil-coronavirus-cases.html

[2] https://theconversation.com/brazil-jair-bolsonaros-strategy-of-chaos-hinders-coronavirus-response-136590

[3] https://www.americanprogress.org/issues/race/news/2020/03/27/482337/coronavirus-compounds-inequality-endangers-communities-color/

[4] https://www.bbc.com/news/world-latin-america-30413525

[5] https://www.bbc.com/news/world-latin-america-15766840

[6] https://theconversation.com/assassination-in-brazil-unmasks-the-deadly-racism-of-a-country-that-would-rather-ignore-it-94389

[7] https://www.ncbi.nlm.nih.gov/pmc/articles/PMC3863696/

[8] https://www.amazon.com.br/Solid%C3%A3o-Ensaios-Desigualdades-Raciais-Brasil/dp/8581922481

[9] https://journals.sagepub.com/doi/10.1177/0021934704264003

[10] https://www.nexojornal.com.br/grafico/2019/06/10/A-expectativa-de-vida-no-Brasil-por-g%C3%AAnero-ra%C3%A7a-ou-cor-e-estado

[11] https://noticias.uol.com.br/saude/ultimas-noticias/redacao/2020/05/04/justica-determina-coleta-de-registros-de-raca-e-etnia-em-casos-de-covid.htm

has yet to release that information. Regardless, by April the Brazilian Health Ministry[1] had already flagged high COVID-19 death rates among Afro-Brazilians, a category that includes people who identify as "black" or "brown" in the census. Officials in hard-hit São Paulo[2] had also announced that mortality rates among COVID-19 patients were higher among black residents. Now, data collected in May[3] by outside researchers for over 5,500 municipalities shows that 55% of Afro-Brazilian patients hospitalized with severe COVID-19 died, compared to 34% of white COVID-19 patients.

Health and Racism

We are health researchers – one American, one Brazilian – who for many years have studied[4] how racial disparities[5] in Brazil affect black people, looking at everything from sickle cell anemia to reproductive health. Our research over the past two months finds structural racism[6] – in the form of high-risk working conditions, unequal access to health and worse housing conditions – is a major factor shaping Brazil's COVID-19 pandemic. For over a decade, black activists and public health researchers have been pointing out that institutional racism[7] creates worse health outcomes for Brazil's black population[8]. Black Brazilians experience higher rates of chronic illnesses[9] like diabetes, high blood pressure, and respiratory and kidney problems due to food insecurity, inadequate access to medicine and unaffordable prescriptions[10]. Racism itself also takes a severe physical toll on black people. Studies in the United States demonstrate that daily experiences of racism and discrimination can lead to dangerously high stress hormones and diminish the body's ability to fight disease[11]. Racial bias from medical professionals[12] then compounds poor outcomes for black patients. Unlike the U.S., Brazil has free, universal health care. But its public hospitals have been woefully underfunded since a deep recession that began in 2015[13]. Intensive care beds are now in short supply[14] at public hospitals in several cities fighting coronavirus outbreaks. This is especially detrimental to black COVID-19 patients, since Afro-Brazilians rely more heavily on the public health system[15] than white Brazilians, who often have private health insurance through their jobs.

---

[1] https://g1.globo.com/bemestar/coronavirus/noticia/2020/04/11/coronavirus-e-mais-letal-entre-negros-no-brasil-apontam-dados-do-ministerio-da-saude.ghtml

[2] https://www.prefeitura.sp.gov.br/cidade/secretarias/upload/saude/PMSP_SMS_COVID19_Boletim Quinzenal_20200430.pdf?fbclid=IwAR0mNVdNtmO7ODqPCAqH0QfkzsX1hpMKNkvmgySqi1k2XD42E3F8vjz2OjU

[3] https://drive.google.com/file/d/1tSU7mV4OPnLRFMMY47JIXZgzkklvkydO/view

[4] https://www.ethndis.org/edonline/index.php/ethndis/article/view/878

[5] https://www.scopus.com/scopus/inward/record.url?partnerID=10&rel=3.0.0&view=basic&eid=2-s2.0-85035756709&md5=329eac49bd35f8a77849586b7daae38b

[6] https://www.sciencedirect.com/science/article/abs/pii/S0277953617304410

[7] https://www.scielo.br/pdf/sausoc/v25n3/1984-0470-sausoc-25-03-00535.pdf

[8] https://www.sciencedirect.com/science/article/abs/pii/S0277953617304410

[9] http://portalarquivos2.saude.gov.br/images/pdf/2019/julho/25/vigitel-brasil-2018.pdf

[10] https://ethndis.org/edonline/index.php/ethndis/article/view/878/1199

[11] https://theconversation.com/coronavirus-deaths-and-those-of-george-floyd-and-ahmaud-arbery-have-something-in-common-racism-139264

[12] https://www.nationalgeographic.com/history/2020/04/coronavirus-disproportionately-impacts-african-americans/

[13] https://www.theguardian.com/world/2016/dec/13/brazil-approves-social-spending-freeze-austerity-package

[14] https://www.scielo.br/scielo.php?script=sci_arttext&pid=S0102-311X2020000500101

[15] https://nacoesunidas.org/quase-80-da-populacao-brasileira-que-depende-do-sus-se-autodeclara-negra/

Poverty and Exposure

Extreme economic inequality is another critical factor shaping the general health of Afro-Brazilians[1]. With the top 10% of the population earning 55% of domestic income, Brazil trails only Qatar in concentration of wealth, according to a 2019 United Nations report[2].

Few, if any, Afro-Brazilians rank among Brazil's super-rich. National household survey data[3] shows that black and brown Brazilians make far less money than white Brazilians, even with equivalent educational background. The racial wage gap in Brazil actually outweighs the gender wage gap[4]: White women earn up to 74% more than black men. The higher the salary, the less likely Afro-Brazilians[5] are to have a job. Many work in the informal and service sectors, as house cleaners[5] or street vendors. Others are self-employed or unemployed. During the pandemic, this economic insecurity severely lessens Afro-Brazilians' ability to socially distance[6] and makes them highly dependent on staying in their jobs despite the health threat. Maids, for example – most of whom are black women – are proving to be a high-risk group[7]. Domestic workers were among Brazil's first COVID-19 deaths[8].

Neighbourhood Risks

Brazil's coronavirus outbreak originated in wealthy neighborhoods whose residents had traveled to Europe, but the disease is now spreading fastest[9] in its poor, dense, long-neglected urban neighborhoods. Just over 12 million Brazilians, most of them black, live in such informal urban settlements, from Rio de Janeiro's favelas to the "peripheries" of São Paulo. These areas have inadequate access to water and sanitation[10], making it difficult to follow basic hygiene recommendations like washing one's hands with soap.

So while the disparate impact of COVID-19[11] on black Brazilians was not inevitable, our research explains why it's unsurprising. The racism that pervades nearly every facet of Brazilian society increases black people's exposure to the virus – then reduces their ability to get to quality care.

---

[1] https://temas.folha.uol.com.br/global-inequality/brazil/brazils-super-rich-lead-global-income-concentration.shtml

[2] https://nacoesunidas.org/relatorio-de-desenvolvimento-humano-do-pnud-destaca-altos-indices-de-desigualdade-no-brasil/

[3] https://biblioteca.ibge.gov.br/visualizacao/livros/liv101681_informativo.pdf

[4] https://biblioteca.ibge.gov.br/visualizacao/livros/liv101681_informativo.pdf

[5] https://theconversation.com/in-brazils-raging-pandemic-domestic-workers-fear-for-their-lives-and-their-jobs-138163

[6] https://www.hypeness.com.br/2020/03/coronavirus-e-a-inabilidade-social-do-governo-ameacam-negros-e-pobres/

[7] https://theconversation.com/in-brazils-raging-pandemic-domestic-workers-fear-for-their-lives-and-their-jobs-138163

[8] https://g1.globo.com/rj/sul-do-rio-costa-verde/noticia/2020/03/17/idosa-de-63-anos-morre-por-suspeita-coronavirus-em-miguel-pereira-diz-secretaria-municipal.ghtml

[9] https://nacla.org/news/2020/03/31/brazil-favelas-covid19

[10] https://theconversation.com/megacity-slums-are-incubators-of-disease-but-coronavirus-response-isnt-helping-the-billion-people-who-live-in-them-138092

[11] https://www.theguardian.com/world/2020/jun/09/enormous-disparities-coronavirus-death-rates-expose-brazils-deep-racial-inequalities?emci=94d478d2-52aa-ea11-9b05-00155d039e74&emdi=45829873-54aa-ea11-9b05-00155d039e74&ceid=4606001

4. Decolonising Stereotypes: A Brief Reflection On Racial Violence And Cultural Relations During The COVID-19 Crisis

Bruna Alves Gonçalves Affiliations[1]

ABSTRACT

During these first moments of the current coronavirus crisis, world powers have been pointing the finger at each other and finding unilateral solutions, rather than creating an international cooperative movement. Their actions have included, among others, the demonization of Asian countries, peoples and their descendants, creating a wave of violence and persecution; and the suggestion that African territory should be used as a vaccine trials labouratory. As both these actions repeat a historical treatment of these communities as socially inferior on the international stage, this paper investigates the influence of the *coloniality of power* as described by Anibal Quijano and decolonial studies in the current international discourse. It considers racial and ethnic elements as the basis of analysis for understanding the social and cultural relations in the crisis context. The findings reveal how international and Western attitudes are still embedded in colonially established stereotypes and epistemologies, regardless of a supposedly neutral discourse from politics, the media or academia.

INTRODUCTION

According to the Cambridge Dictionary, the adjective *embedded* holds two basic meanings: [1] "fixed into the surface of something"; or [2] "If an emotion, opinion, etc. is embedded in someone or something, it is a very strong or important part of him, her, or it". Following the second definition, it seems the colonial mindset of the past has remained *embedded* in the imaginary of the contemporary global society, supported by both the media, academia and politics.

The colonial worldview remains structurally intact even to current times and our thoughts and expressions are still shaped by it. Even though colonialism as a political form of direct domination ended a few decades ago, its analytical concepts and epistemology were perpetrated and remain valid, a phenomenon named by Anibal Quijano as the *coloniality of power* [1,2,3], which refers to the continued subordination of other societies, their citizens and cultures to Western standards (European-American axis). During the current international crisis and the resulting need to reach out internationally to find solutions, these colonial organizations and divisions have been responsible for intensifying the situation of vulnerability of certain ethnic groups and national populations in the global context. Since Covid19 emerged, the exclusion and objectification of racial groups has become been vivified by political discourses, both when trying to find a responsible

---

[1] Largo São Francisco, 95, São Paulo – Brazil: Faculdade de Direito da Universidade de São Paulo;
Largo São Francisco 26, São Paulo – Brazil: Instituto Almeida Mantelli.
E-mail: Bruna.alves.goncalves@usp.br
Current Address: Rua Sargento Jair Baptista de Olibeira, 193 – Chácaras Reunidas São Jorge, Sorocaba, São Paulo - Brasil

subject and when searching for a solution. These solutions have sought to articulate political interests, instead of the common interests and needs of the entire international population.

It is in this context that people phenotypically associated with Asian countries and the African continent as a whole, as it is treated by the Western discourse, have become the main victims of the effect. Recently, Asian immigrants and descendants who reside in European countries started facing several racist and xenophobic attacks as a result of the public blaming the People's Republic of China [4]. At the same time, respected medical institutions suggested using Africa as potential labouratory for vaccine and treatment trials, not only treating the continent as a unitary rather than a plural environment, in a complete objectification of its citizens [5].

As both of these expressions against these groups are prime examples of colonial constructions towards the populations, the article will focus on discussing the relation between racial colonial stereotypes and the current exercise of power on the international system amidst the COVID-19 pandemic crisis. The paper will analyse in order the historical construction of the "Asian" and "African" ethnic categories, its application nowadays, and its role in the international crisis.

MATERIALS AND METHODS

The situation of prejudice, exclusion and persecution of phenotypically Asian people became acknowledged through the broad repercussion of physical attacks and the social media campaign "#IamNotaVirus", organized by victims all around the world aiming to raise awareness about the commonly neglected racism against Asians in Western countries. The violent situation emerged after several media and political discourses from Western countries' leaders attributing the virus to what they say to be cultural Chinese practices, or even calling it the China Virus [4, 6].

The situation of Africa was also stressed by virtual means: between March and April 2020, when the coronavirus crisis spread rapidly around the world, social media comments from the footballers Didier Drogba and Samuel Eto'o [7,8] drove the world's attention to Jean-Paul Mira's, head of intensive care unit at Cochin hospital in Paris, insinuating the use of Africa as the place for vaccine trials [9,5]. The doctor has, since then, justified himself by indicating his true intention was to point the continent as more vulnerable and therefore in desperate need for medication. Nonetheless, his first affirmation was followed, as the videos show, by the statement "[a] bit like as it is done elsewhere for some studies on Aids. In prostitutes, we try things because we know that they are highly exposed and that they do not protect themselves" [5], which shows (i) a paternalistic view that remits to the generalist white saviour syndrome; and (ii) an indication that the "help" would come in the shape of trials. As it is known, trials present a great risk for the subjects, since the cure's efficacy is obviously not yet proven and they may come with negative side effects. Even taking into account later comments, he still referred to a hypothesis of trials, objectifying the African population, and suggesting the continent should be used as the world's labouratory, which is historically problematic. While the first situation demonstrates a political and societal response to the COVID-19 crisis, the second outlines the role of academia in reinforcing racial and geographical colonial organizations. Racial and geographical classifications, according to Aníbal Quijano and the decolonial studies' academics that follow him, were the structures that allowed Western domination between the 15th and 20th century [1, 10]. As explained by the author, the concept and classification of "races" and the attribution of biological and intrinsic characteristics to each one of the groups contemplated by it, created during colonialism, created a hierarchy of social groups with European primacy and the justification of control of non-European populations [1].

Therefore, according to one's origin and phenotype, people from the Global South were forcibly attributed characteristics said to be natural and biological that supposedly attested their inferiority through different stereotypes [11]. The characteristics were attributed according to the role each one of the societies could play in the West's plans of development and according to its needs. It seemed useful or even egocentrically logical for the global powers to establish an objectification of certain human beings, presenting non-European cultures as barbaric, retrograde and anti-modern and therefore subservient to *superior peoples'* goals. It is in that context that Latin America emerges as the scenario for the creation of ethnic and racial categories during 15th and 16th centuries, as the starting point of colonialism [10]. The notion of race became the means for determining who were the dominators and who were the dominated, in a society of racial states.

We need to mention, that the period was marked by the exploitation of non-European populations, indigenous genocide and the subsequent African diaspora, where the racial hierarchy was born. Post-colonial and decolonial studies were created within academia in the latter half of the 20th century, as a questioning of how knowledge was created. It questioned the Western vision of modernity and how it used its own culture as the objective standard of comparison from which it analysed other cultures, norms and societies, and how, per definition, they lack neutrality and objectivity [12]. It questions exactly how gender, racial, ethnic and geographical categories were created as referenced to the White Western class, how the Global South became the political "Other", the subaltern, and how current universal and modern categories still retain concepts of colonial differentiation [12]. Considering the aforementioned events and this historical background, and using decolonial and post-colonial theoretical frameworks and specifically the categories proposed by Aníbal Quijano, this research aims to evaluate the pertinence of "race" and "ethnicity" as relevant categories of analysis to the COVID-19 crisis' effects on social inequality and violence. One must also consider that the presented point of view comes from a Brazilian background, where the author is inserted. This is important to mention, since Brazil experienced the construction of the colonial order, sharing the experience of the Global South, but is still deeply embedded in these structures of White and Western superiority, with strong racial division. Thus, this is subject for an article of its own...

Africa And the Black Question in the World Order

The first colonial processes sought to exploit *natural resources* and the individuals that resided in close to these natural resources, mostly Latin-American indigenous groups and individuals from the African civilizations [11]. The contact between the societies and the domination processes motivated, in that context, a multiracial society organized through racial estates subservient to European (Portuguese and Spanish) interests. Black African individuals represented the main work force of colonial American countries from their beginning, once the indigenous communities were wiped out and achieved their *supply* limit [13]. Even though African societies had entire functioning empires, integrated communities and individual lives, the entire process of slavery and human exploitation was based on a process of dehumanization. As the citizens were not considered humane when confronted by Europeans - taken as the referential of modernity and led by anthropocentric views - their exploitation was made morally accepted and slavery was justified. Removed from their original lands and taken to the American continent, the black African became the lowest in the racial hierarchy of the European colonies [13]. Despite the formal abolition acts, mostly during the 19th century, the estates remained almost intact. This is due to the fact that the abolitionist movements worldwide were not mainly motivated by the recognition of black and indigenous men and women's humanity, but to the ascension of liberalism as the new economic system and its organization not being compatible with the structures of the old regime, along with the economic weight of slavery structures by the end of the century [14]. It is with that motivation that on the beginning of the 20th century the approach taken by land owners in Brazil was importing work force from European countries – mainly white workers, to whom it was socially accepted to exchange their labour and in an attempt to "lighten the population" [15]. The racial hierarchy had been established in Brazil as it was in former Hispanic colonies, spreading for the entire Western world while being defended by academia biologically and sociologically. Beyond the topic of African diaspora and slavery exploitation related to Latin America's colonialism process, African countries suffered a second wave of occupation dubbed as neo-colonialism [16]. The African continent was divided and conquered in the so-called "scramble for Africa", and its position in the ethnic and racial hierarchy of the world was consolidated.

In terms of academic and medical subjugation of Africa, not only *Scientific racism* persisted for years in an attempt of medicine and biology academia to prove the biological differences between races as determined by Western powers, but the literal use of African countries and its nationals for experimental trials remained a common practice of Western countries until less than a century ago. In *Africa as a Living Labouratory: Empire, Development, and the Problem of Scientific Knowledge, 1870-1950*, Hellen Tilley (2011) describes the use of African goods and individuals for scientific experiments of all kinds - medical, sociological, anthropological, amongst others – by the British and other European colonizers. As described by the author, during the entire neo-colonial period African subjects were experimented on.

Medicine and biology exploited and dehumanized racially and geographically excluded people. It was only in 1947 after the Nuremberg trials on the Nazi regime's actions that medical ethics started seeking consent from the subjects prior to testing, in a revealing decision on scientific atrocities and dehumanization of racialized bodies [17]. An example of this is the iconic Tuskegee case, in which *The Times* reported on the four decades of medical experimentation on syphilis effects done by the United States on black male individuals for trials. Even though the case does not directly concern Africans, this case is still relevant through its use of the racial category colonially attributed to the continent, as can be seen in the name given to this group as *African-Americans* [18]. This mirrors the contemporary claims of Dr. Jean-Paul Mira. It leaves clear how the contemporary situation was rooted in colonial structures: medical experiments and the characterization of African citizens as trials subjects are a historical practice proposed by colonial ideologies.

Even when justified by him through his supposedly humanitarian motivation, it suggests an appropriation and objectification of the subjects and their narratives. It downplays the humanity of African citizens and submits its interests to Western attitudes and goals through(i) reinforcing the notion of Africa as a homogenous society, with no internal differences, conflict and specific demands through the image of a constantly in-need continent subjected to the permanent need of foreign help; (ii) disregarding the autonomy, wills and narratives of the people; and (iii) perpetuating the colonial culture of using Africa as the "world's lab": an area with limited social responsibility. Any intervention would mean an attempt to implement *modernity standards*, as explained by decolonial scholars. The strengthening of the image of Africa as the starving black baby is both racist and ethnocentric. The African continent is formed by fifty-four countries, each one a collection of different cultural identities, ethnicities, and economic situations. Reaffirming the disadvantaged geographical and racial position of African individuals in the international order and homogenizing all of their interests in order for them to benefit from Western benevolence brings back the Lacanian concept of infantilization. Lélia Gonzales summarizes the concept in reference to black women as the appropriation of a subject's authority over their own narrative, as is often done with children when adults address them in the third person: the individual is "excluded, ignored, and considered absent despite its presence"[1] [19].Basically, Western speakers appropriate voices and transform them as if it was a homogenous truth without effective dialogue with the nations.

It is also in that context that Escobar argues that the "Third World (sic.) reality is inscribed with precision and persistence by the discourses and practices of economists, planners, nutritionists, demographers and the like, making it difficult for people to define their own interests in their own terms—in many cases actually disabling them to do so" [20]. The relativizing process of internal wills and narratives reveals misleading conductions of humanitarian actions, that either on purpose or through embedded concepts enhance colonial attitudes. As providing medicine trials could supposedly help the solution arrive in African countries more easily (which is internationally seen as positive), the greater advantage for Western countries would be to not put their own citizens at risk and reduce liability while looking generous themselves [21]. Another aspect of this conflict is the exact risk of an immediate interpretation of the action as positive.

As trials, there is neither guaranteed safety of the medication or knowledge of the side effects. Hydroxychloroquine, for example, endorsed by the media and presidents such as Donald Trump and Jair Bolsonaro during its trials, led to several incidents of death by heart attack during the medical trials, costing human lives in spite of political and academic confidence [22].

Still, besides physical and medical risks, any form of international intervention must be taken with precaution. One must not forget the events that led to the current positioning of Africa in the international order or the destruction of its civilizations as direct consequences to Western intervention. The designation of a restricted geographical and ethnic region to put uncertain trials in practice endorses the sociological and cultural view of African individuals as inhumane and at the will of the Western population's needs, regardless of a dialogue with them.

Like everywhere else, there is a current demand for medication and scientific solutions in African countries. Similarly, to other regions, racially and economically oppressed groups happen to be more vulnerable to lack of health care and prevention measures, therefore contracting the virus and not healing. Nonetheless, the access to medicine must not be derived from missionary intentions or through imposed experiments that use citizens for its own interests. The discourse perpetuated reinforces these social international categories created by colonialism and should be revised while paying attention to history.

China and the Virus

Different from the Latin American sense of colonialism, the Asian exploitation and stereotype formation follows an intellectual and neo-colonial process, especially when it comes to China. The "far East" portrayal emerged in the 17th and 18th centuries, when the European academics evaluated Chinese society as immutable and stuck in the past. Described as "inferior and barbarous, narrow-minded and xenophobic", the Chinese became subjects of intellectual subordination and Western fear [23, 24]. Amidst the Western/Eastern dichotomy which aligned with the Modern/Barbarous one, Western thinkers established the notion of the *Yellow Peril*. Once again conceiving the continent as homogenous according to the concept of race, the Asian individual was biologically determined

---

[1] Translated from Portuguese

to be cruel, and therefore a threat to the West [25]. The negative attributions of the Asian stereotype not only remained but worsened through the 20th century. Especially during the 1929 financial crisis, Japanese and Chinese groups were portrayed by European and American politicians and media as oppressors to the low and medium-income White classes. The deplorable situation of common workers in Europe and the USA was blamed on Asian immigrants, which served as a scapegoat, accused of taking the *true American*'s job.

This was considered even more unacceptable as their race was considered to be biologically inferior. Following the political trends, the media started to openly defend racial politics, while phenotypically Asian individuals were then harassed within Western countries [25].

Due to exclusion based on race and ethnicity, Asian groups became geographically excluded from the society, forced to create and live in ghettos, so-called *Chinatowns*. Due to the lack of social integration and poor sanitary conditions, they became known as *dirty*, a stereotype that prevails until nowadays [26], and has been reinforced with the COVID-19 crisis. Besides dirtiness, they included the consumption of animals considered *exotic* and *weird* [26]: rats, mice, cats, puppies, or even bats – which were the result of living in extreme poverty and cultural habits limited to certain classes and regions of Asian countries which were than generalized to represent the entire continent's culture. While highly criticised by post-colonial academia, sinologism[1], stereotypes, and xenophobic and racist expressions continue to be widely spread in the West. The COVID-19 crisis has only worsened this cultural violence and narrative denial. As for past epidemics, the origin of COVID-19 was internationally attributed to elements of "dirtiness" and "exoticism" of the artificially homogenized Chinese culture, in specific reference to the existence of the *wet markets* in the region. The wet markets are central elements of food commercialization and consumption in Asia, spread in several countries around the continent and specialized in fresh products. They do not differ much from the European or Brazilian open markets both in their aspects and social function [27], a comparison that may cause some discomfort to Western citizens confronted by the *coloniality of power* context.

Besides the theoretical distancing of the cultures, nonetheless, it is important to question what would be the difference between the criticized commercialization of porcupine and deer meat in Chinese wet markets and the alligator and armadillo meat consumption in Latin America? If we take Europe as the comparative element, what is the difference between the European open market commercialization of game meat such as rabbit, quail, horse, venison or even frogs and the Chinese consumption of parallel species? When confronted by these questions, the conventional Western answer defends that Chinese commercialization of living organisms is the issue, even for meat eaters. However, a first response is to point to the commercialization of living animals in any French, American, Brazilian or Luxembourgish countryside cows, hens, goats, either for consumption or procreation and fish market. This does not make "Chinese/Asian culture" peculiar, as similar practices exist around the world, with their associated sanitary problems, consistent all around the world [26]. In addition, a second response questions European standards of normal and exotic.

The commercialization and consumption of *exotic* species is rare not only in China but in throughout Asia, especially in big cities [27]. Their commerce is limited to certain regions and have been addressed by the Chinese government since the SARS epidemics of the early 2000s, similarly to other countries [27]. For example, the consumption of snakes, bear paws, tiger and pangolin meat,

---

[1] Ming Dong Du defines sinologism as the "Sinologism is primarily an implicit system of ideas, notions, theories, approaches, and paradigms, first conceived and employed by the West in the encounter with China to deal with all things Chinese and to make sense of the bewildering complexity of Chinese civilization" [24].

is already extremely restricted, and when not forbidden, strongly discouraged in the country [28 Despite the several problematic political statements made by China during the current international crisis, there is no justification for the attribution of individual responsibility or strengthening of violent historical stereotypes towards Asian and Chinese peoples. The idea of 'contaminated culture' in China simply is not the case, and such broad stereotypes mistake Asia for a homogenous continent. The national stereotype, as seen, was socially built in a context of racial conflict and subjugation of racialized individuals to white western citizens and its interests. The image of homogeneity emerges way earlier, along with the geographical and ethnical organization proposed by the colonial powers, as described earlier in this paper, outlining Quijano's work.

RESULTS, DISCUSSION AND CONCLUSION

The complexity of the current international situation and the damaging effects of the subordination culture to the already vulnerable minorities amidst the crisis demonstrate the need for questioning the practices of marginalization of the current global order. The context of despair in international relations outlines the existent colonial stratification in terms of race, ethnicity and geography. When it comes to the situation regarding the status of African citizens and Black people inside the international community, the COVID-19 crisis reveals the impunity Western powers have in objectifying individuals and reducing their conditions to its own wills and interests. The fact that a respected figure in the medical community can speak on TV of prostitutes or African citizens as second-class humans demonstrates the structure of power that is prevailing since colonial times. This has only been possible or even tolerable because of deeply embedded gendered, ethnic, racial and geographical divisions in the social structure.

Additionally, this structure seems to have been exposed and strengthened rather than reduced with this crisis: any behaviour is legitimized under the disguise of international help, rather than finding joint solutions. The circumstances of the Asian and Chinese communities were more evidenced by the media through racist attacks. Nonetheless, it is important to recall the origins and the structure shaping the motivations for such attacks in order to stop the perpetuation of damaging stereotypes and social exclusion. In addition, political discourses that blame specific peoples and countries for the international spreading of the virus enhance the social division produced by race and perpetuates White and Western dominance as the moral and cultural standard that the global South must accept. The roles and stereotypes enforced by the measures taken during the crisis reveal the current unsustainability of the Western epistemological perspective. The analysis categories by decolonial scholars has proved effective in revealing its effects on the current situation. As a worldwide phenomenon, COVID-19 reinforces the international structure of power not only in economic terms, but also socially, culturally and within academia.

Acknowledgements

First and foremost, I would like to express my deep gratitude to Professor Gabriel Mantelli, my academic mentor at Espaço Almeida Mantelli, my current research institution, for giving me guidance and motivation to write this article. Secondly, I am extremely grateful for Oscar Brisset, my partner and editor, for helping with English spelling and grammar corrections and for his constant support of my researches.

REFERENCES

1. Quijano, A. (2000). Coloniality of Power and Eurocentrism in Latin America, International Sociology 15 (2), 2000:215 – 232.

2. Quijano, A. (2007).Coloniality and Modernity/Rationality, Cultural Studies, 21: 2-3 2007: 168-178, DOI: 10.1080/09502380601164353

3. Gosfoguel, R. (2008). Para descolonizar os estudos de economia política e os estudos pós-coloniais: transmodernidade, pensamento de fronteira e colonialidade global, Revista Crítica de Ciências Sociais, n. 80 (2008): 115-147.

4. de Lima, Juliana Domingos (2020). Como o racismo aflora diante do medo do coronavírus. Nexo Jornal (February 3rd), available at https://www.nexojornal.com.br/expresso/2020/02/03/Como-o-racismo-aflora-diante-domedo-do-coronav%C3%ADrus.

5. BBC. Coronavirus: France racism row over doctors' Africa testing comments (April 3rd), available at https://www.bbc.com/news/world-europe-52151722.

6. Chiu, A. (2020). Trump has no qualms about calling coronavirus the 'Chinese Virus'. That's a dangerous attitude, experts say. The Washington Post (March 20), available at https://www.washingtonpost.com/nation/2020/03/20/coronavirus-trumpchinese-virus/.

7. Drogba, Didier [@didierdrogba] (2020, April 2nd). "Let us save ourselves from this crazy virus that is plummeting the world economy and ravaging populations health worldwide.Do not take African people as human guinnea pigs! It's absolutely disgusting..." [Tweet]. Retrieved from https://twitter.com/didierdrogba/status/1245798251720314880

8. Eto'o, Samuel [setoo9] (2020, April 2nd). "Fils de P...Vous n'êtes que de la MERDE, N'est-ce pas l'Afrique est vôtre terrain de jeu...adrénaline". Retrieved from https://www.instagram.com/p/B-d6SUMCid6/?utm_source=ig_web_copy_link.

9. Rossman, R. (2020). Racism row as French doctors suggest virus vaccine test in Africa. Al Jazeera (4 de abril), available https://www.aljazeera.com/news/2020/04/racism-row-french-doctors-suggest-virusvaccine-test-africa-200404054304466.html.

10. Mignolo, W; Walsh, C. (2018). On Decoloniality. London, Duke University Press.

11. Young, S. (2016). Race and the Global South in Early Modern Studies. Shakespeare Quarterly 67(1): 125-135.

12. Adelia Miglievich-Ribeiro (2014). Por uma razão decolonial: Desafios éticopolítico-epistemológicos à cosmovisão moderna. Dossiê Diálogos do Sul. Civitas, Porto Alegre 14(1): 66-80.

13. Ortegal, L. (2018). Relações Raciais no Brasil: colonialidade, dependência e diáspora.Serv. Soc. Soc., São Paulo, n. 133: 413-431.

14. Fernandes, F. (2008). A integração do negro na sociedade de classes, Volume 1. Editora Globo: São Paulo, 5th edition.

15. Santos, Ricardo Augusto dos. (2008). 'Branqueamento' do Brasil. História, Ciências, Saúde-Manguinhos, 15(1): 221-224. https://doi.org/10.1590/S0104-59702008000100014

16. Zeleza, P.T. (2006). The Troubled Encounter between Postcolonialism and African History. Journal of the Canadian Historical Association, New Series, 17(2): 89-129.

17. Tilley, H.(2011). Africa as a Living Labouratory: Empire, Development, and the Problem of Scientific Knowledge, 1870-1950. University of Chicago Press, DOI: 10.7208/chicago/9780226803487.001.0001

18. Rothman, L. (2017). The Disturbing History of African-Americans and Medical Research Goes Beyond Henrietta Lacks. The Times (21 de abril), available at https://time.com/4746297/henrietta-lacks-movie-history-research-oprah/ .

19. Gonzáles, L. (2020). Por um Feminismo Afro-Latino-Americano, in *Pensamento Feminista Hoje: perspectivas decoloniais* (org. Heloisa Buarque de Holanda). Bazar do Tempo: 38-51.

20. Escobar, A. (1992). Imagining a post-development era: Critical thought, development and social movements. Social Text, 31/32: 20–56.

21. Pogge, T. (2010). Politics as Usual: What Lies Behind the Pro-Poor Rhetoric. Cambridge, UK: Polity.

22. Wong, J.C. (2020). Hydroxychloroquine: how an unproven drug became Trump's coronavirus 'miracle cure', The Guardian (April 7), available at https://www.theguardian.com/world/2020/apr/06/hydroxychloroquine-trumpcoronavirus-drug.

23. Martínez-Robles, D. (2007). The Western Representation of Modern China: Orientalism, Culturalism and Historiographical Criticism. Digithum, issue 10.

24. Gu, Ming Dong (2012). Sinologism: An Alternative to Orientalism and Postcolonialism, Taylor & Francis Group. ProQuest Ebook Central, http://ebookcentral.proquest.com/lib/oxford/detail.action?docID=1097826.

25. Lovell, J. (2014). The Yellow Perril: Dr. Fu Manchu & the Rise of Chinophobia by Christopher Frayling – review. The Guardian (October 30), available at https://www.theguardian.com/books/2014/oct/30/yellow-peril-dr-fu-manchu-rise-ofchinaphobia-christopher-frayling-review

26. Shim, D.(1998). From Yellow Peril through Model Minority to Renewed Yellow Peril. Journal of Communication Inquiry 22 (4): 385-409.

27. Westcott, B; Wang, S. (2020). China's wet markets are not what some people think they are. CNN (April 16): disponível em
https://edition.cnn.com/2020/04/14/asia/china-wet-market-coronavirus-intlhnk/index.html

28. J. Li, Peter; Sun, Jian; Yu, Dezhi (2017). Dog "Meat" Consumption in China: A Survey of the Controversial Eating Habit in Two Cities. Society and Animals 25: 513-532; 515

5. Anti-Blackness of The Pandemic In The US And Brazil

João Costa Vargas and Ana Flauzina[1]

Antiblackness of the Pandemic in the US and Brazil

At the heart of health disparities is antiblackness, a social code that

renders Black people disposable.

"In Brazil the virus is far more lethal to Blacks than it is for whites."

In spite of COVID-19's destructive capacity, in the U.S. and in Brazil antiblackness is the ultimate facilitator of preventable death. The pandemic only exacerbates social and institutional patterns that consistently devalue the lives of Black people. Such patterns are not incidental or temporary, but rather are the very foundation of modern empire-states. Because antiblackness establishes the value of life – who lives and who dies – it sets up the conditions within which the pandemic advances and breaks havoc. While it is known that underlying medical conditions increase the chances of one's death once the virus infects a person, such conditions are a function of social codes and institutional practices. Antiblackness is certainly not the only social code related to underlying medical conditions, but it is a central one. We often hear the term "health disparities" as an explanation for vulnerable social groups' greater susceptibility to disease, lack of available health care, and preventable death. Yet at the heart of such disparities is antiblackness: a social code that, because it is based on a scale of humanity that renders Black people disposable, impacts them singularly and disproportionately. Antiblackness causes and naturalizes Black death.

On April 8, 2020, the Centres for Disease Control and Prevention (C.D.C.) released a study on people who were hospitalized from the coronavirus during the month of March. Considering a subset of 178 adult patients, the study found that 89.3 percent of them had one or more underlying conditions. The most frequent were the following: hypertension (49.7 percent), obesity (48.3 percent), chronic lung disease (34.6 percent), diabetes mellitus (28.3 percent), and cardiovascular disease (27.8 percent). What is evident in the C.D.C. report is that COVID-19 is the most devastating among Black people. In hospitalizations due to the coronavirus among those on whom there were race/ethnicity data, Blacks were by far the most disproportionately represented, and thus the most impacted: they comprised 33.1 percent, whereas Whites were 45 percent, Hispanics 8.1 percent, Asians 5.5 percent, and 0.3 percent were American Indian/Alaskan Native.[1]

---

[1] https://blackagendareport.com/antiblackness-pandemic-us-and-brazil

"COVID-19 Is the Most Devastating Among Black People."

It can be surmised from this data that in the U.S., Black people are most likely to experience underlying conditions, and thus most likely to suffer the worst consequences of the pandemic. (We hesitate to state that Black people are the most likely to be hospitalized, as the C.D.C. data suggest, because for them treatment and access to health care are historically deficient. Accordingly, it would be more accurate to affirm that hospitalization and death rates for Black people, due to patterns of social exclusion, are consistently underestimated.)The problem is amplified in cities where Blacks are either a majority or a large minority. For example, in Milwaukee, Chicago, and New Orleans, Black people experience 70 to 80 percent of all COVID-19-related deaths. To put this in another way: the greater the proportion of Black people in a city, the worst the outcome of the pandemic will be; conversely, the smaller the proportion of Black people in a city, the greater will be the chances of controlling the pandemic. Thus, it is not only the presence of Black people that is correlated with the most devastating traits of the pandemic; the absence of Black people seems to be a predictor of how well a city or region will do. The states of Washington, Oregon, and California, without majority Black cities, are doing relatively well in terms of hospitalizations and deaths caused by the virus.[2]

Similar patterns are already evident in Brazil, where the pandemic is only now beginning to show signs of its spread. Even though the first official cases of infection were of relatively affluent White people who had access to health care and tests, it is now apparent that Blacks, which in Brazil correspond to pretos and pardos, constituting 54 percent of the population, are the most severely affected. In other words, the pandemic is quickly spreading, from the privileged neighbourhoods to disadvantaged areas where people are segregated away from the country's infrastructure, including quality health care. Currently, whereas Black people are 23.1 percent of all hospitalizations due to COVID-19-related symptoms, they are 32.8 percent of deaths caused by the virus. The contrast to Whites is clear: whereas they are 73.9 percent of those hospitalized due to the coronavirus, they are 64.5 percent of those who die from it. The virus is far more lethal to Blacks than it is for whites.

"The absence of Black people seems to be a predictor of how well a city or region will do in the epidemic."

These data bring to the surface mutually reinforcing aspects of antiblackness. Black people have less access to hospitals and effective care. As in the U.S., Brazil is highly segregated, and Black people consistently live in areas that are more violent, bereft of urban infrastructure such as sewage, piped water, trash, and transportation services, where quality public services and access to healthy food are absent, closer to environmental toxins, with high concentration of unemployment, and disproportionately dependent on the informal economy. Housing in those areas is scares and expensive; households are markedly denser, with several family members sharing small spaces. Social distancing in these conditions is not only difficult, but it also cripples the income of households that overwhelmingly rely economically on being in public spaces, often crowded ones, selling goods and performing services. So, the hospitalization numbers are reflections of the constitutive antiblack patterns of residential hyper segregation, which in turn determines access to health care. Black people in Brazil are 67 percent of all those who depend exclusively on the public health care system, which has been severely defunded by the current federal administration.

Like the U.S., Black people in Brazil are the majority among those with diabetes, tuberculosis, hypertension, and chronic kidney disease, all underlying conditions that increase the likelihood of COVID-19's lethality. As the pandemic advances, it is expected that the proportion of Black people's hospitalizations and deaths will only increase. [3] The 1951 Civil Rights Congress denunciation of genocide in the U.S. provides a useful diasporic framework to reflect on this current moment, marked by COVID-19 and how it intersects and actualizes a myriad of processes of antiblack social exclusion.[4]

Encompassing residential segregation and blocked access to health care, but also discriminatory policing, punitive schooling, industrial incarceration, and widespread unemployment all of which reveal Black people's unique condition of social death that often leads to physical death – the concept of antiblack genocide forces us to recognize the ways in which Black lives continue to not matter. When the presidents of Brazil and the U.S. signal recommendations that go against the advice of epidemiologists, they only reinforce long-term patters of antiblack genocide that far exceed their most ludicrous and murderous impulses.

"Black people in Brazil are 67 percent of all those who depend exclusively on the public health care system." To oppose antiblack genocide is a must, and urgent. At the forefront of the fight against antiblack genocide, autonomous organizations such as React or Die! in Salvador know exactly what to do. Drawing on long term work in prisons and Black neighbourhoods, when the country's authorities were pathetically vacillating on the appropriate measures, they provide basic cleaning supplies, food, and assistance to incarcerated women and men, and the elderly.[5] The Network of Communities and Movements Against State Violence instantly mobilized to provide basic foods to vulnerable Black women in favelas.[6] Cooperative Jackson in Mississippi immediately started using their arduously-acquired production capacity to manufacture masks for those most affected by the pandemic.[7] In their unflinching and immediate actions, these and many other Black autonomous collectives are informed by a long tradition of diasporic interventions that recognizes the uniqueness of Black people's multiple vulnerabilities.

To fight against the devastating effects of COVID-19 is to relearn, adapt, and apply the lessons from the diasporic Black campaigns focusing on police abuse and state terror, nutrition and food security, schooling, the elimination of domestic pests, sickle-cell anaemia, Aids/HIV, domestic and sexual violence, LGBTQ phobia, incarceration, assistance and transportation for the elderly, exposure to environmental toxins, residential hyper segregation, and many other facets of antiblack genocide.

To come to terms with antiblackness is to recognize that the pandemic intensifies social patterns of exclusion and death that fundamentally impact Black people disproportionately.

We stress fundamentally because such patterns, rooted in a social unconscious that constantly reinforces the correspondence between being and not being Black, structure empire-states with a high presence of Black people and a past in slavery. In the U.S. and in Brazil, antiblackness is at the core of the country's social and ontological makeup. COVID-19's lethality is as much about the virus's craftiness as it is about antiblackness as a social encryption that determines who lives and who dies. Antiblackness is an underlying condition that makes the pandemic all the more devastating.

Notes and Links

[1] https://www.cdc.gov/mmwr/volumes/69/wr/mm6915e3.htm#F2_down

[2]https://www.nytimes.com/2020/04/08/opinion/coronavirus-black-cities.html?action=click&module=RelatedLinks&pgtype=Article

[3]https://www1.folha.uol.com.br/cotidiano/2020/04/coronavirus-e-mais-letal-entre-negros-no-brasil-apontam-dados-da-saude.shtml

[4]Patterson, William. *We Charge Genocide: The Historic Petition to the United Nations for Relief for a Crime of the United States government against the Negro People.* New York: Civil Rights Congress, 1951.

[5] https://g1.globo.com/ba/bahia/noticia/2020/04/10/organizacao-distribui-itens-de-higiene-e-promove-trabalho-educativo-sobre-o-coronavirus-em-unidades-prisionais-de-salvador.ghtml

[6] https://www.vakinha.com.br/vaquinha/doando-esperanca-ajuda-nas-atividades-da-rede-contra-violencia-2019

[7] https://cooperationjackson.org/

João Costa Vargas works at the University of California - Riverside.Ana Flauzina works at Universidade Federal da Bahia (Federal University of Bahia). In 2017 they co-edited a book in Brazil called, Motim: Horizontes do genocidio antinegro na diaspora (Uprising: Horizons of antiblack genocide in the Diaspora).

6. In Brazil, COVID-19 Death Rate For Black Community Is Higher Than For Other Populations

Written by **Agencia Pública**
Translated by **Liam Anderson**

This article was first published in Portuguese on May 6, 2020, and translated into Spanish by our Brazilian partner Agência Publica. It was then republished and edited by Global Voices with their permission.

The number of black people who have died from COVID-19 in Brazil increased fivefold over a period of two weeks. From 11 to 26 April, the number of federally confirmed deaths rose from just over 180 to more than 930 among black Brazilians infected with the coronavirus. The number of black patients hospitalized for severe acute respiratory syndrome (SARS) caused by the coronavirus increased 5.5 times. For the white Brazilian population, the rise in deaths during these same two weeks was significantly smaller: deaths increased three times and the number of hospitalizations increased by a similar proportion.

By 18 June, the total number of deaths from the coronavirus in Brazil had risen[1] to 46,842. Since the beginning of the pandemic, President Jair Bolsonaro has minimized[2] the seriousness of COVID-19 and argued for keeping the economy open. Quarantine rules have been decided by regional governors. Today the country has the second-highest number of cases in the world.

The large increase in the number of black people who have been hospitalized or have died due to COVID-19 has highlighted issues of racial inequality in Brazil. Among the black population, one in three patients has died from complications due to the virus compared to one in 4.4 deaths among white Brazilian patients.

[Translators' note: Below, the graphs include "branco", referring to white people and "preto" and "pardo", referring to black and mixed-black people. For the English translation, we will refer to the latter group as black people.]

---

[1] https://www.coronatracker.com/country/brazil/
[2] https://www.bbc.com/news/world-latin-america-52868854

Deaths From COVID-19 In Brazil Increase More Among Black People. Graph Used With Permission.

Mortes por Covid-19 no Brasil crescem mais entre negros

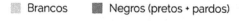

Brancos   Negros (pretos + pardos)

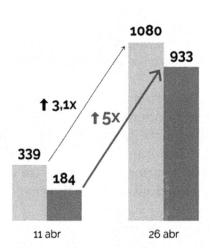

A % de mortes por Covid-19 entre brancos tem caído, a de negros tem aumentado

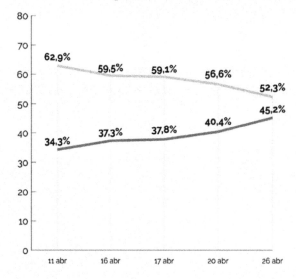

°Os dados de % do Ministério da Saúde não incluem fichas de notificação com informação de raça/cor ignorada

The percentage of deaths among white people has decreased, while among black people it has increased. Graph used with permission.

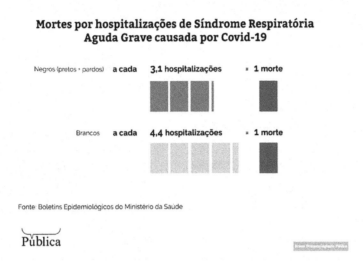

Deaths caused by Severe Acute Respiratory Syndrome among hospitalized COVID-19 patients. Graph used with permission.

These data is taken from an analysis carried out by Agência Pública based on epidemiological reports from the Ministry of Health which contain information on race in hospitalisations and deaths from coronavirus. The federal government published these updated figures on 26 April. São Paulo, the country's biggest city and the one with the highest number of deaths from COVID-19, has registered increased death rates in neighbourhoods where the black population is larger. According to Agência Pública, of the ten neighbourhoods with the highest death rate from coronavirus, eight have a larger percentage of black residents than the São Paulo average.

The neighbourhood with the highest number of deaths is Brasilândia[1], where 103 coronavirus patients have died. Nearly 50 percent of the residents in this area identify as black (the average in São Paulo is 37 percent). In contrast, Moema, the neighbourhood with the lowest percentage of black residents (less than 6 percent), registered 26 deaths.

When adjusting the figures proportionally, the two neighbourhoods still have different realities: compared to the number of residents in Moema, Brasilândia has approximately 25 percent more deaths. Agência Pública used data from the last census (2010) to analize the population size and residents' race.

.

---

[1] https://apublica.us8.list-manage.com/track/click?u=47bdda836f3b890e13c9f416d&id=7b0d394abd&e=dda8916e3f

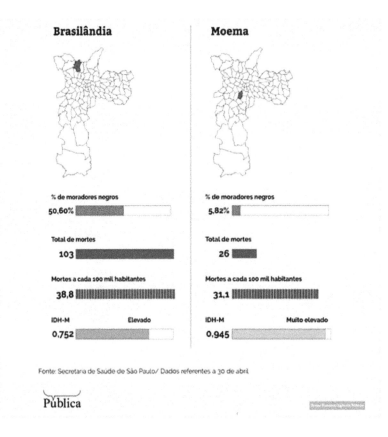

COVID-19 data for black residents in Brasilândia and Moema.
Graph used with permission.

In Jardim Ângela, the neighbourhood with the highest percentage of black people in the whole city, deaths from coronavirus almost tripled in about two weeks. In other neighbourhoods with a majority black population, such as Grajaú, Parelheiros, Itaim Paulista, Jardim Helena, Capão Redondo and Pedreira, deaths from COVID-19 more than doubled during the same period.

The spread of the coronavirus in São Paulo's suburbs has slowed down in wealthier neighbourhoods where the first cases of COVID-19 appeared. On 17 April, neighbourhoods with fewer black people than the city average had 13 percent more deaths than areas where more black people live. Two weeks later, that difference fell to 3 percent. If the trend continues, deaths from COVID-19 in neighbourhoods with a majority black population will exceed those in neighbourhoods where fewer black people live. The areas with denser populations of black people are the areas where the Municipal Human Development Index (MHDI) — which calculates longevity, education and income — is at its lowest. The ten neighbourhoods with the worst MHDI in São Paulo are where more black people live than the city average. The ten neighbourhoods with the best MHDI are where fewer black people live. In the ten neighbourhoods with the highest number of deaths, eight have an average MHDI below 0.8. The percentage of black people in these eight neighbourhoods is higher than the city average. In Rio, neighbourhoods with more black people than the city average already have already seem more deaths in absolute numbers than neighbourhoods with fewer black people. Currently, Campo Grande, which has more than 50% black inhabitants, is the neighbourhood with the most deaths. The neighbourhood overtook Copacabana, which previously had the highest number of deaths from COVID-19. After Copacabana, Bangu and Realengo, two neighbourhoods with a majority black population are the third and fourth most affected in the city.

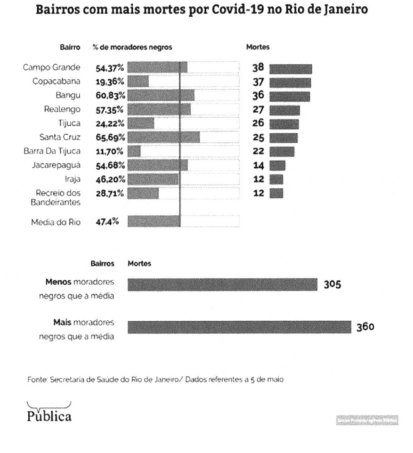

Bairros com mais mortes por Covid-19 no Rio de Janeiro

Bairro	% de moradores negros		Mortes	
Campo Grande	54.37%		38	
Copacabana	19.36%		37	
Bangu	60.83%		36	
Realengo	57.35%		27	
Tijuca	24.22%		26	
Santa Cruz	65.69%		25	
Barra Da Tijuca	11.70%		22	
Jacarepaguá	54.68%		14	
Irajá	46.20%		12	
Recreio dos Bandeirantes	28.71%		12	
Média do Rio	47.4%			

Bairros	Mortes
Menos moradores negros que a média	305
Mais moradores negros que a média	360

Fonte: Secretaria de Saúde do Rio de Janeiro/ Dados referentes a 5 de maio

Pública

Neighbourhoods With Most COVID-19 Deaths In Rio De Janeiro. Graph Used With Permission.

In Rocinha, the city's largest poor neighbourhood, there were nine deaths according to official data at the time of the investigation. Doctors[1] working in that community questioned the number and pointed out that there were already 22 deaths in the favela.

The relationship between the number of confirmed cases and deaths is also quite different between the rich and poor neighbourhoods of Rio de Janeiro, which may indicate difficulties to get tested for residents of favelas and suburbs.

In Amazonas, white people survive more than black people In Amazonas state, where the public health system has collapsed[2], black people are dying in higher numbers than white people who are severely

---

[1] https://apublica.us8.list-manage.com/track/click?u=47bdda836f3b890e13c9f416d&id=66cd74f145&e=dda8916e3f

[2] https://www.nexojornal.com.br/expresso/2020/04/13/Por-que-o-Amazonas-%C3%A9-o-1%C2%BA-estado-a-ter-um-colapso-na-sa%C3%BAde

affected COVID-19 patients. According to Agência Pública, one black person dies for every 2.4 patients in serious condition, while among white people there is one death for every 3.2 seriously ill patients.

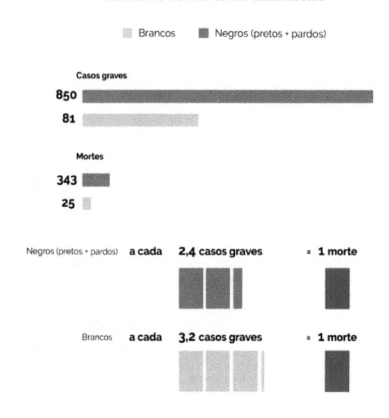

Dados de Covid-19 no Amazonas

Brancos   Negros (pretos + pardos)

Casos graves

850

81

Mortes

343

25

Negros (pretos + pardos) **a cada** **2,4 casos graves**   = **1 morte**

Brancos **a cada** **3,2 casos graves**   = **1 morte**

Fonte: Secretaria de Saúde do Estado do Amazonas/ Dados referentes a 29 de abril

Pública

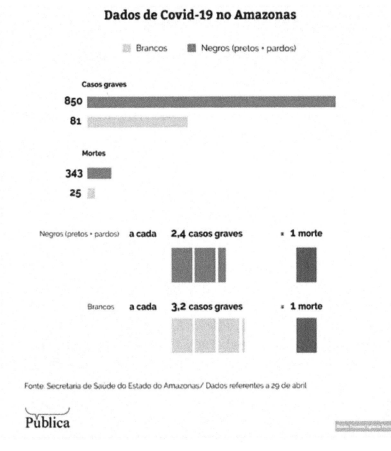

Dados de Covid-19 no Amazonas

Brancos   Negros (pretos + pardos)

Casos graves
850
81

Mortes
343
25

Negros (pretos + pardos) a cada **2,4 casos graves** = **1 morte**

Brancos a cada **3,2 casos graves** = **1 morte**

Fonte: Secretaria de Saúde do Estado do Amazonas/ Dados referentes a 29 de abril

Pública

The state of Amazonas, which was the first to reach its maximum capacity of intensive care units for patients with COVID-19, has recorded a more significant increase among black people severely affected by COVID-19 than among white people. At the end of April, the number of seriously ill black patients doubled. In Amazonas,13 black people died for every white person who died.

The health department had registered about 850 black patients with severe coronavirus infections and over 340 deaths. Among white people, there were 81 serious cases and 25 deaths. The data on race was updated[1] on 29 April. Despite data that shows a greater increase in deaths in the black population and more deaths among hospitalized patients, the Federal Government does not release details about this information. For example, there is no information available about how many cases were confirmed by race, nor the number of tests done on black people, white people, and other populations. The lack of official data on race has a long history in the country, says lawyer Daniel Teixeira, director of the Centre for the Study of Labour Relations and Inequalities (Ceert). According to Teixeira: There are several factors that may explain the high lethality [of COVID-19 among the black population]. Indeed, having more information means that we can even confirm or exclude the importance or relevance of each of these factors, as the case may be. That's where the importance of the data lies. Teixeira believes that the gap is not only in the area of health and that it is widespread in the country. The lack of this type of data could prevent people from having public policies that take into account this situation which, historically, ignores the factors of structural inequalities in Brazil.

---

[1] https://apublica.us8.list-anage.com/track/click?u=47bdda836f3b890e13c9f416d&id=5be4460ef4&e=dda8916e3f

7.COVID-19 Pandemic In Brazil:
Do Brown Lives Matter?

[1]Helena Ribeiro,[a] Viviana Mendes Lima,[c] and
Eliseu Alves Waldman [b]

In *The Lancet Global Health*, a pioneering study by Pedro Baqui and colleagues[1] confirms in Brazil findings observed in other countries hit hard by COVID-19: that mortality rates from the pandemic differ by geographical region and ethnicity, with disproportionate impact for Black populations and other ethnic minorities.[2,3] We can discuss these findings in the context of the social protests occurring in the past few months against structural racism and to the slogan "Black lives matter".

However, in this Comment, we go beyond ethnicity, focusing on social and environmental determinants of health for about 50% of Brazilians. Using COVID-19 hospital mortality data from SIVEP-Gripe (*Sistema de Informação de Vigilância Epidemiológica da Gripe*) dataset, Baqui and colleagues did a cross-sectional observational study to assess regional variations in patients with COVID-19 admitted to hospital by state and by two socioeconomically grouped regions (north and central-south).

The ethnicity of patients was categorised according to the five categories used by the Brazilian Institute of Geography and Statistics: *Branco* (White), *Preto* (Black), *Amarelo* (East Asian), *Indígeno* (Indigenous), or *Pardo* (mixed ethnicity). The authors used mixed-effects Cox regression survival analysis to estimate the effects of ethnicity and comorbidity at an individual level in the context of regional variation. Baqui and colleagues found that, compared with White Brazilians, *Pardo* and Black Brazilians who were hospitalised had significantly higher mortality risk (hazard ratio 1·45, 95% CI 1·33–1·58 for *Pardo* Brazilians; 1·32, 1·15–1·52 for Black Brazilians). *Pardo* ethnicity was the second most important risk factor after age for death.

The authors also showed that, in the north region, hospitalised patients had higher risk of death from COVID-19 than those in the central-south region. Rio de Janeiro was an outlier, with mortality rates similar to those of northern states. We add to their findings that incidence rates were also higher in northern regions.[4] Speculation that severe acute respiratory syndrome coronavirus 2 would have milder transmission in low latitudes has delayed actions in northern regions. However, historically, these areas face several challenges that directly affect their capacity to respond to the COVID-19 pandemic: shortages of doctors and intensivists; fragile epidemiological surveillance; poorer network of health services than in other regions; and fewer family health teams, hospital beds, and number of intensive care units (ICUs) per inhabitant than in other regions. Therefore, discussions regarding ethnicity and regional variations must be integrated, not only because northern states and Rio de Janeiro have higher proportions of *Pardo* and Black populations, but also because the root causes of higher mortality are overlapping.

The percentage of low-income families living in subnormal housing, with higher average numbers of individuals per room, is more elevated in northern areas than in the central south region and higher among *Pardo* and Black families than in White families.

---

[1] *Helena Ribeiro, Viviana Mendes Lima, Eliseu Alves Waldman lena@usp.br

These conditions favour intense circulation of respiratory pathogens. Low-income neighbourhoods also have higher population density and low adherence to social distance measures. In these often hot and crowded neighbourhoods, the streets and sidewalks have cultural importance and become part of the living space.

Additionally, lower schooling in northern regions and among *Pardo* and Black populations might jeopardise the comprehension of risks and measures proposed by sanitary authorities, as well as judgment of the right time to seek medical assistance. Additionally, in the north region, lower percentages of the urban population are served by piped water compared with those of other regions (69·5% in the north, 88·7% in the northeast, and 96% in southern regions).[5] This situation means that a substantial proportion of the northern urban population has difficulty in adhering to the simplest prevention recommendation of hygiene, such as washing hands.

The prevalence of comorbidities among *Pardo* and Black populations in Brazil is higher than among other ethnicities, including overweight and obesity,[6] risk factors for severity of symptoms of COVID-19.[2-4] Hypovitaminosis D is also more prevalent among *Pardo* and Black people in Brazil than among other ethnicities.[7] The lower the level of schooling, the higher the chances of obesity in Brazilian women.[6] With soaring numbers of cases, cities in the northern region faced collapse of their health system, with worst cases occurring in Manaus, Fortaleza, and Natal.

However, we note that phases of the epidemic vary within the country, and the northern region has probably reached the peak of the first wave of transmissions, whereas this might not be the case for other regions. The situation is dynamic, and Baqui and colleagues' research portrays a snapshot in a timeline. Additionally, substantial under-reporting of deaths and cases of COVID-19 is occurring, related to low testing. This under-reporting is more intense in the northern region, which might reinforce health inequities.

We draw attention to issues of mobility and historical shortages of doctors in villages and poverty areas, which are not discussed in Baqui and colleagues' study. In the Amazon, most people move around by boat through *igarapés* and rivers, and trips to cities with health equipment and medical doctors might take hours or even days. In Rio de Janeiro, mobility plays a role too.

The poor, mostly *Pardo* and Black, live in shantytowns on steep slopes with no streets or health services, where ambulance access is difficult; or in suburbs with precarious and very crowded public transportation, facilitating transmission. In those cases, the delay to hospital admission might be fatal. Additionally, this population works mainly in unstable jobs with no payment for sick days, and thus are likely to postpone going to health services until disease symptoms are acute. Most doctors are White and might show less empathy for *Pardo* and Black patients. By contrast, the majority of non-medical health staff is composed of *Pardo* and Black people, who are more exposed to COVID-19 risks, as pointed out by Baqui and colleagues, sometimes without adequate protection equipment and tests to identify early contagion. In Rio de Janeiro, but not exclusively, hospital equipment, beds, and ICUs were poorly managed, which left many people to die in inadequate places or at home. Irresponsibility and corruption have also played a role in this context. Therefore, there are people for whom and places where vulnerability and susceptibility[8] act together to exacerbate the risks of COVID-19, and this is compounded by a resistance of the Ministry of Health to account for ethnicity in its approach to the pandemic.

Shedding light on these issues is a merit of Baqui and colleagues' study. We declare no competing interests. We thank the Brazilian National Council for Scientific and Technological Development for a productivity grant for HR and postdoc scholarship for VML.

AFFILIATIONS

Departamento de Saúde Ambiental, Faculdade de Saúde Pública, Universidade de Sao Paulo, São Paulo 01246-904, Brazil
b Departamento de Epidemiologia, Faculdade de Saúde Pública, Universidade de Sao Paulo, São Paulo 01246-904, Brazil
c Laboratório de Estudos das Cidades, Departamento de Planejamento Urbano e Regional, Universidade do Vale do Paraíba, São José dos Campos, Brazil
Helena Ribeiro: rb.psu@anel

REFERENCES

1   Baqui P, Bica I, Marra V, Ercole A, van der Schaar M. Ethnic and regional variations in hospital mortality from COVID-19 in Brazil: a cross-sectional observational study. *Lancet Glob Health* 2020; published online July 2. https://doi.org/10.1016/S2214-109X(20)30285-0.
2   Ravi K. Ethnic disparities in COVID-19 mortality: are co-morbidities to blame? *Lancet* 2020; published online June 19. https://doi.org/10.1016/ S0140-6736(20)31423-9.
3   Haywood EGP, Burton J, Fort D, Seone L. Hospitalization and mortality among Black patients and White patients with COVID-19. *N Engl J Med* 2020; **382:** 2534–43.
4   Ministério da Saúde, Secretaria de Vigilância em Saúde. Boletim epidemiológico especial. Doença pelo Coronavírus COVID19. 2020. http://saude.gov.br/images/pdf/2020/June/18/Boletim-epidemiologicoCOVID-2.pdf (accessed June 26, 2020).
5   Sistema Nacional de Informações sobre Saneamento. Diagnóstico dos serviços de água e esgotos—2018. 2019. https//snis.gov.br/diagnosticoanual-agua-e-esgotos/diagnostico-dos-servicos-de-agua-e-esgotos-2018 (accessed June 20, 2020).
6   Ferreira APS, Szwarcwald CL, Damacena GN. Prevalence of obesity and associated factors in the Brazilian population: a study of data from the 2013 National Health Survey. *Rev Bras Epidemiol* 2019; **22:** e190024.
7   Ribeiro H, de Santana KVdS, Oliver SL, et al. Does vitamin D play a role in the management of COVID-19 pandemic in Brazil? *Rev Saúde Púb* 2020; **54:** 53.
8   Diderichsen F, Hallqvist J, Whitehead M. Differential vulnerability and susceptibility: how to make use of recent development in our understanding of mediation and interaction to tackle health inequalities. *Int J Epidemiol* 2019; **48:** 268–274.

CHAPTER 9

THE RELATIONSHIP BETWEEN ETHNICITY NEIGHBOURHOOD AND COVID-19

1. The Risk Of COVID-19 Transmission In Favelas And Slums In Brazil

R.J. Pereira*,

G.N.L.do Nascimento Curso de Nutriçao, Universidade Federal Do Tocantins, Quadra 109 ~ Norte, Avenida NS-15, ALCNO-14 Plano Diretor Norte, Palmas Tocantins, CEP 77001-090, Brazil

L.H.A. Gratao

~ Faculdade de Medicina, Departamento de Pediatria,
Universidade Federal de Minas Gerais, Avenida

Professor Alfredo Balena,

190, Santa Efig^enia, Belo Horizonte, Minas Gerais, CEP 30130-100, Brazil

R.S. Pimenta

Curso de Medicina, Universidade Federal Do Tocantins, Quadra 109 Norte, Avenida NS-15,
ALCNO-14 Plano Diretor Norte, Palmas Tocantins, CEP 77001-090, Brazil

At a time when the coronavirus disease-2019 (COVID-19) pandemic affects a large part of the continents, populations who live in subnormal clusters, especially in developing countries, appear as an additional concern. Subnormal clusters is a group of at least 51 housing units, arranged in a disorderly and dense manner, lacking essential public services, occupying land owned by others; commonly called favelas, invasions, caves, lowlands, communities, villages, undertow, irregular subdivisions, huts, and stilts.[1] In Brazil, these areas were home to 11,425,644 people, or 6% of the Brazilian population, in accordance with the 2010 population census, the last conducted in the country. It is known that 5.6% (3,224,529) of the total Brazilian households are located in these areas. In the country, 6329 subnormal clusters were identified, in 323 municipalities.[1]

The Southeast region, the most populous in the country, concentrated in 2010 the largest number of homes in these types of agglomerates (49.8% of the total in Brazil), with greater concentrations in the States of Sao Paulo (23.2%) and Rio de Janeiro (19.1%). Then, the Northeast region concentrated 28.7% of the Brazilian subnormal agglomerates, the North region, 14.4%; the South region, 5.3%; and the Midwest, 1.8%.[2] Geometric estimate of the growth of slum dwellings in Brazil shows an average growth trend of 6.93% in these numbers, between 2010 and 2020, reaching up to 11.7% in the Northeast region.[3]

The average demographic density in Brazilian settlements is 67.5 inhabitants/hectare (inhab./ha); reaching up to 99.1 inhab./ ha, as observed in the Southeast region. About 72.6% (2.3 million) of the households in these agglomerations coexist without spacing between them.[3] The profile of people living in these settlements shows that the average age in these areas was 27.9 years in 2010. The range from 0- to 14-years-old corresponded to 28.3% and the range of 60-years-old or older was 6.1%.[2] Subnormal agglomerations have a high demographic density, so it is inevitable the agglomeration of socio-economically vulnerable people, with low education, in precarious conditions of basic sanitation and with less access to health goods and services, which predisposes its inhabitants to a greater risk of contracting the new coronavirus and to perpetuate the spread of the disease.[4] COVID-19 cases have spread throughout the country, with a tendency to exponentially increase the number of infected people in all Brazilian regions. In times when isolation of cases, quarantine of contacts and social detachment are the most effective strategies to contain the pandemic, Brazil faces a challenge that is unknown to European countries: the living conditions in the subnormal agglomerations. In these types of houses, social distance becomes almost impossible because residents must coexist, in quarantine, within a space that does not hold all residents together at the same time. Isolating sick individuals within multigenerational households, in which five or more individuals share the same room and bathroom, becomes impractical. The precarious conditions of basic sanitation in the houses mean that there is even a lack of drinking water and minimal hygiene. The poor socio-economic conditions do not allow adequate availability of sanitizers and disinfectants, not even soap.[4]

Although the impact of the spread of COVID-19 on these clusters is not noticed, little is discussed between government and the population about these communities. There are few proposals for coping with COVID-19 in these communities, which lack differentiated strategies, considering their particularities and their spatial distribution.[4] Health authorities have not considered the inevitable agglomeration in conditions of economic fragility and in unequal territory, which hinder the dissemination and understanding of the minimum information on hygiene and protection against the virus, and which often also make the acquisition and use of disinfectant agents unfeasible. In this way, the peculiarities of populations living in subnormal agglomerations emerge as a major public health challenge, especially in the face of a pandemic, which can spread to these communities, with irreversible consequences for an entire country, including the inhabitants of urbanized regions.

REFERENCES

1. Brasil. Ministerio do Planejamento, Orçamento e Gestao. Instituto Brasileiro de Geo~ grafia e Estatística. Censo Demografico de 2010. Aglomerados Subnormais: informaço~es territoriais. Rio de Janeiro: MPOG; 2010.
2. Meirelles R. (2014). Um país chamado favelas: a maior pesquisa ja feita sobre a favela brasileira. Sa~
3. Pasternak S, D' Ottaviano C. (2016). Favelas no Brasil e em Sa~o Paulo: avanços nas analises a partir da Leitura Territorial do Censo de 2010. Cad Metrop 2016;18: 75e99.
4. Central Única das Favelas. Propostas de medidas para reduzir os impactos dapandemia de Covid19 nos territorios das favelas brasileiras. Available at: https://www.cufa.org.br/noticia.php?n¼MjYx.

*
Corresponding author. E-mail address: renatajunqueira@uft.edu.br (R.J. Pereira).

2. Neighbourhood Effects and Urban Inequalities: The Impact of COVID-19 on the Periphery of Salvador, Brazil

Lucas Amaral de Oliveira

Department of Sociology, Federal University of Bahia, Brazil

Rafael de Aguiar Arantes,

Department of Sociology, Federal University of Bahia, Brazil

On March 29, two weeks after the first COVID-19 case was confirmed and on the same day of the first pandemic-related death in the city, Salvador turned 471 years old. However, the streets did not showcase the celebrations that distinguish one of the most culturally active cities in Brazil. From the confinement of our homes, we witnessed an empty, suspended city. The isolation measures taken by local authorities, essential to reduce the virus' transmission, have shaken the dynamics of sociability as well as disrupted the use of public spaces in Salvador, recognized by UNESCO as the "city of music" and "national capital of Afro-Brazilian culture".

Besides changing socio-cultural patterns, isolation has economic implications in a city that essentially depends on commerce, tourism and services. Commercial sector organizations estimate daily losses in the millions in a scenario in which only key services remain open. Tourist activities are paralyzed, beaches are closed, and cinemas, theatres, museums and nightclubs are suspended. At the same time, the number of flights that usually reach the city during this season has decreased dramatically. According to the Brazilian Hotel Industry Association of Bahia, in the last week of March the hotel occupancy rate was 4%. Such a slowdown has a more severe impact on the lives of informal workers, who constitute 1/3 of the employed population. Much of this population lives in the urban peripheries. In view of the pandemic context that threatens a city with high rates of urban and socioracial inequalities, we aim to offer a brief diagnosis about the potential impacts of Covid19 on the peripheries of Salvador in terms of *neighbourhood effects*. We address the following question: to what extent does urban location determine health and socioeconomic risks in the current pandemic?

A Poor, Uneven and Peripheral City

Salvador is one of the oldest cities in Brazil. Its foundation in 1549 consolidated the project of the Portuguese crown to create a "fortress-city" that could host the new General Government in the Brazilian territory. As the country's first capital, Salvador became the main pillar of the colonial agro-mercantile economy, profoundly based on sugar and tobacco plantations, as well as on the intense slave trade. The city prospered over the next two centuries as a commercial, religious and administrative centre, until it lost its political influence when Portugal transferred the capital to Rio de Janeiro in 1763. The city experienced solid modernization processes only in the 1950s, when it received investments in infrastructure, oil exploration, and petrochemical industrial sectors, with the development of its metropolitan region in 1973 (Gordilho-Souza, 2008). Despite the impact of investments on the city economy and the social structure, the industrialization process was tightly linked to the flows of the south-southeast regions, with a robust supply of unskilled labour and precarious occupations. This condition worsened in the 1990s, when the city suffered a disruption of its labour market.

Currently, the third sector constitutes the most important activity of the economy in Salvador. About 20% of the population is unemployed, whereas informality represents 35%, and the average income is US$430 per month[1]. According to Census data, 37% of citizens have a per capita income of up to ½ minimum wage (U$100), an empirical condition of poverty. Precariousness is even more perverse when we consider race: unemployment and informality are higher among the black population, which is 83% of the city (Carvalho, 2018).In the 1970s, Salvador underwent rapid changes that culminated in the development of three vectors of territorial expansion: "Orla Marítima Norte", "Miolo" and "Subúrbio Ferroviário" – which added to the old central region close to the port.

The first is a "noble" area, where wealth, investments, facilities, opportunities, and services are concentrated. The second, in the city geographic epicentre, was initially composed of housing estates for the working classes, expanded through popular allotment programs (*loteamentos populares*), and presents today an area with limited availability of goods and services. The latter, which emerged along with the construction of the railway line, in 1860, grew in the 20th century, and became the most deprived region of Salvador, with irregular occupations, precarious housing, high levels of violence, and deficiencies in infrastructure, transportation and services (Carvalho & Pereira, 2014). Nowadays, Salvador maintains a pattern of urban segregation so uneven that 1/3 of its citizens live in "subnormal agglomerates", such as slums or *favelas*. In these areas, population density may exceed 27,000 inhab/km², whereas the municipal average is 3,859 inhab/km² (Carvalho & Pereira, 2014).

Pandemic's Impacts on The Peripheries

Initial reports show that COVID-19 arrived in Brazil via wealthy people who were in Europe during the epidemiological outbreak.

If we consider the residential patterns of the infected so far, we notice a concentration in middle- and upper-class neighbourhoods, including in Salvador. Notwithstanding, the current concern turns to the peripheries, as projections indicate that in the coming weeks there will be an alarming spike in cases and deaths in poorer neighbourhoods. According to a report published by the Oswaldo Cruz Foundation[1], Brazilian regions will face the peaks of the disease at different points: first, major urban centres such as São Paulo and Rio de Janeiro; then, other decentralized cities like Recife and Salvador. Freitas, Napimoga and Donalisio (2020) sustain that it is necessary to consider the heterogeneity of the current indicators among different Brazilian regions, as they depend on political actions, availability of supplies and equipment, structure of health services, and inequality indices. Since the first confirmed cases, Salvador City Hall and the Bahia State Government decided to ignore President Jair Bolsonaro, who has insisted that social isolation should not be a measure in the fight against coronavirus. Local authorities quickly implemented mitigation protocols indicated

---

[1] See report by *Observatório Covid-19 Fiocruz*: <cutt.ly/jtDXHhH>. Access: 8 April 2020.

3 See report by the Group *GeoCombate Covid-19*: <cutt.ly/OtDXNZZ>. Access:8 April 2020.

by WHO, seeking to "flatten the curve" and help the health system to avoid collapse during the most intense phase of the pandemic. However, even with the adoption of these health procedures, COVID-19's impacts on the peripheries might be horrific.

A study led by the Federal University of Bahia[3] analysed the potential risks faced by different districts of Salvador during the pandemic. The analysis considered the flow of people in the city and the distribution of official reported cases, crossing the variables "potential danger" (where people are more likely to get the virus) and "health vulnerability" (where vulnerable groups live) from each neighbourhood. One of the conclusions is that the population that live in the regions of "Miolo" and "Subúrbio Ferroviário" would be exposed to a greater danger due to the rates of poverty and precarious housing. Many of these peripheral neighbourhoods have a high population density, deficiencies in health services and a lack of basic sanitation. Recently, there have been complaints of water rationing in some neighbourhoods, just now when the recommendation is for everyone to stay at home and increase hygiene measures.

These complaints led us to the idea of "neighbourhoods effects", which constitutes the benefits or losses that potentially may affect socio-racial groups based on location. We argue that "territory" is a central variable to analyse the production and reproduction of inequalities, insofar as it would impact both the available structure of goods and services, and the social capital, networks and resources of each group (Andrade & Silveira, 2013; Farber & Sharkey, 2015). Therefore, the agglomeration of vulnerable groups in relatively homogeneous and segregated spaces can contribute to dispossession (Carvalho, 2018; Sampson, 2008).

These "potential" effects, which vary from neighbourhood to neighbourhood, are a real challenge in Salvador, which is one of the most unequal cities in the country (Serpa, 2001). On the one hand, poorer neighbourhoods tend to suffer from poor health services; on the other, there are inequalities associated to the place of residence in relation to those who have access to private health plans and those who depend on the Unified Health System (SUS). Accordingly, urban infrastructure implies unequal conditions in the efficient fight against the coronavirus. For instance, in many cases, inhabitants of peripheral areas find it difficult to acquire basic hygiene items, such as soap, hand sanitizer, and masks. In others, they feel obliged to refuse social isolation under threat of not having minimum conditions to survive and pursue informal employment.

The question then becomes: how to adopt strict mitigation protocols, special care for risk groups and their relatives, and quarantine in the most symptomatic cases when we are dealing with an urban reality in which, usually, a large family lives in a single-room house in a slum? President Bolsonaro has insisted on underestimating the ramifications of inequality, not only in Salvador but also throughout Brazil. Moreover, he denies that we are facing an unprecedented crisis and accuses governors, media and scientists of inciting "hysteria" by adopting "horizontal isolation" (restriction on movement and commerce). Disregarding the president's denial, several local self-organizing actions have emerged across the peripheries of Salvador, in order to mitigate the impacts of COVID-19 on unassisted populations[1]. These actions include money, food and sanitary materials donation, crowdfunding, the construction of databases to facilitate the assistance of risk groups, cleaning efforts and disseminating information about the disease. The Salvador City Hall also created a project called "Salvador For All", which will transfer US$52 over three months to 20,000 informal workers. The State Government, in turn, will exempt low-income citizens from water and electricity bills for the same period. Nevertheless, these measures may be insufficient to reduce the effects of the crisis on the population most at risk.

---

[1] See the article written by Luciene Santana e Monique Evelle: <cutt.ly/EtD0uL1>. Access: 8 April 2020.

In addition to these important solidarity initiatives among residents of peripheral neighbourhoods, as well as the health precautions and financial assistance protocols adopted by local government, we urge that specific actions must be taken, at the state and federal levels, so that the urban peripheral populations can survive the pandemic. To avoid a catastrophe that is already on the horizon, the public authorities must work with peripheral communities to offer the conditions for a "safe isolation". These procedures involve the increase of the number of Intensive Care Unit beds and a more feasible management and distribution of detection tests. In addition, we must have well-designed minimum-income policies in areas whose indicators reveal greater inequalities and vulnerabilities. COVID-19, although global, is not an "egalitarian" or "democratic" disease. On the contrary, it tends to have an uneven impact on different territories and socio-racial groups that constitute the urban space, which can further deepen the already overwhelming inequalities in a city like Salvador.

REFERENCES

Andrade, L., Silveira, L (2013). Efeito Território: explorações em torno de um conceito sociológico. *Civitas*, 13(2): 2013.

Carvalho, I. Desigualdade raciais no espaço urbano. Seminário *A Cidade e a Sujeição Racial.* São Paulo: Laboratório de Estudos sobre Raça e Espaço Urbano da USP, 2018.

Carvalho, I.; Pereira, G. (eds.)(2014). *Salvador: transformações na ordem urbana*. Rio de Janeiro: Letra Capital.

Faber, J.; Sharkey, P.(2015) Neighborhood Effects. *International Encyclopedia of the Social & Behavioural Sciences*, 2: 443-449.

Freitas, A.; Napimoga, M.; Donalisio, M.R. (2020).Análise da gravidade da pandemia de Covid19. *Epidemiologia e Serviço de Saúde*, 29(2), e2020119, 8 April 2020.

Gordilho-Souza, A. (2008) *Limites do habitar*. Salvador: EDUFBA.

Sampson, R. J., (2008) Moving to inequality: neighborhood effects and experiments meet social structure. *American Journal of Sociology,* 114, 189–231.

Serpa, A. (2001) *Fala, periferia: uma reflexão sobre a produção do espaço periférico metropolitano*. Salvador: EDUFBA.

	Brazilian population*	Hospital admission	ICU admission	Death	Death/ hospitalisation	Death (not ICU)	Death (ICU)
North (n=2043)							
White	27·8 %	342 (16·7%)	127 (19·4%)	136 (15·6%)	39·8 %	69 (14·9%)	67 (16·5%)
Pardo	61·5 %	1567 (76·7%)	481 (73·8%)	683 (78·4%)	43·6 %	368 (79·3%)	315 (77·4%)
Black	8·8 %	85 (4·2%)	26 (4·0%)	35 (4·0%)	41·2 %	20 (4·3 %)	15 (3·7%)
Fast Asian	1·2 %	36 (1·8%)	13 (2·0%)	12 (1·4%)	33·3 %	5 (1·1 %)	7 (1·7%)
Indigenous	0·7 %	13 (0·6%)	5 (0·8%)	5 (0·6%)	38·5 %	2 (0·4%)	3 (0·7%)
Central-south (n=9278)							
White	58·7 %	6291 (67·8%)	2344 (69·4%)	1560 (63·5%)	24·8 %	616 (60·3%)	944 (65·8%)
Pardo	33·2 %	2112 (22·8%)	731 (21·6%)	627 (25·5%)	29·7 %	278 (27·2%)	349 (24·3%)
Black	6·8 %	667 (7·2%)	220 (6·5%)	210 (8·6%)	31·5 %	108 (10·6%)	102 (7·1%)
Fast Asian	1·1 %	195 (2·1%)	82 (2·4%)	57 (2·3%)	29·2 %	19 (1·9%)	38 (2·7%)
Indigenous	0·3 %	13 (0·1%)	2 (0·1%)	3 (0·1%)	23·1 %	1 (0·1%)	2 (0·1%)

Data are % or n (%). ICU=intensive care unit. *Census values of the Brazilian population.

Table 2: Ethnic composition of patients at each stage of the COVID-19 trajectory

3. Ethnic and Regional Variation In Hospital Mortality From COVID-19 In Brazil

Pedro Baqui,[1, 1] Ioana Bica,[2,3, *] Valerio Marra,[1,4, †] Ari Ercole,[5] and Mihaela van der Schaar[3,6,7]

1 Núcleo de Astrofísica e Cosmologia (Cosmo-ufes),
Universidade Federal do Espírito Santo, 29075-910, Vitória, ES, Brazil
2 Department of Engineering Science, University of Oxford, Parks Road, Oxford OX1 3PJ, UK
3 The Alan Turing Institute, 96 Euston Rd, London NW1 2DB, UK
4 PPGCosmo & Departamento de Física, Universidade Federal do Espírito Santo, 29075-910, Vitória, ES, Brazil
5 University of Cambridge Department of Medicine,
Addenbrooke's Hospital, Hills Road, Cambridge CB2 0QQ, UK
6 Centre for Mathematical Sciences, University of Cambridge, Wilberforce Rd, Cambridge CB3 0WA, UK
7 Department of Electrical Engineering, University of California, Los Angeles, Los Angeles, CA 90095 USA

ABSTRACT

Background The COVID-19 pandemic is quickly spreading throughout Brazil, which is rapidly ascending the ranking of countries with the highest number of cases and deaths.
A particularly unstable federal regime and fragile socioeconomic situation is likely to have contributed to the impact of the disease. Amid this crisis there is substantial concern in the possible socioeconomic, geopolitical and ethnic inequity of the impact of COVID-19 on the country's particularly diverse population.
Methods We performed a cross-sectional observational study of COVID-19 hospital mortality using observational data from the SIVEP-Gripe dataset. We present descriptive statistics to quantify the COVID-19 pandemic in Brazil. We assess the importance of regional factors such as education, income and health either on a state-by-state basis or by splitting Brazil into a North and a Central South region. Mixed-effects survival analysis was used to estimate the effects of ethnicity and comorbidity at an individual level in the context of regional variation.
Findings Our results show that, compared to *branco* comparators, hospitalised *pardo* and *preto* Brazilians have significantly higher risk of mortality, with hazard ratios and 95% CI of 1.47 (1.331.58) and 1.32 (1.15-1.52), respectively. In particular, *pardo* ethnicity was the second most important risk factor (after age). We also found that hospitalised Brazilians in North regions tend to have more comorbidities than in the Central-South, with similar proportions between the various ethnic groups. Finally, we found that states in the North have a higher hazard ratio as compared to the Central-South, and that Rio de Janeiro obtained one of the highest hazard ratios, similar to the ones of the more underdeveloped Pernambuco and Amazonas.
Interpretation Our results can be interpreted according to the interplay of two independent, but correlated, effects: i) mortality by COVID-19 increases going North (vertical effect), ii) mortality increases for the *pardo* and *preto* population (horizontal effect). We speculate that the vertical effect is driven by increasing levels of comorbidity in Northern regions where levels

---

[1] These authors contributed equally to this work. [†] Corresponding author: marra@cosmo-ufes.org

of socioeconomic development are lower, whereas the horizontal effect may be related to lower levels of healthcare access or availability (including intensive care) for *pardo* and *preto* Brazilians. For most states the vertical and horizontal effects are correlated giving a larger cumulative mortality. However, Rio de Janeiro was found to be an outlier to this trend: It has an ethnicity composition (horizontal effect) similar to the states in the North region, despite high levels of socioeconomic development (vertical effect). Our analysis motivates an urgent effort on the part of Brazilian authorities to consider how the national response to COVID-19 can better protect *pardo* and *preto* Brazilians as well as the population of poorer states from their higher death risk from SARS-CoV-2 infection.

INTRODUCTION

The COVID-19 pandemic has created an unprecedented worldwide strain on healthcare. Whilst early reports from East Asia and Europe meant that Brazil was well positioned to implement non-pharmaceutical interventions, Brazilians, like those in many developing countries, have limited access to testing and social security. The former makes it difficult to assess the growth of the pandemic, while the latter prevents a sizable fraction of society from engaging in physical distancing. This has been further complicated by an unstable federal government[1] that has failed to support measures such as social distancing and attempted to downplay the gravity of the pandemic. Worryingly, as of May 19th, Brazil ranks fourth worldwide for total COVID-19 cases and sixth for deaths, with the highest estimated rate of transmission in the world ($R_0 = 2.81$),[2] second only to USA for the daily increase of confirmed cases and deaths. Worldwide there is substantial interest in the emerging societal inequity of the impact of COVID-19, and there is emerging evidence to suggest variability in the impact of the disease across ethnicities in a variety of settings in- Informação da Vigilância Epidemiológica da Gripe") respiratory infection registry data, which is maintained by the Ministry of Health for the purposes of recording cases of Severe Acute Respiratory Syndrome (SARS) across both public and private hospitals. Using this rich dataset, we characterize the COVID19 pandemic in Brazil, particularly with regard to risk factors related to comorbidities, symptoms and ethnicity, similarly to previous analyses in countries such as the UK.5, [11-13]

RESEARCH IN CONTEXT

Evidence Before This Study

Brazil is a highly ethnically and socioeconomically diverse country. The severe impact of COVID-19, coupled with an unstable federal regime, may make it particularly susceptible to outcome inequities. Although the issue of the disproportionate effect of COVID-19 on ethnic groups has been debated in the Brazilian media, quantitative / systematic studies assessing the ethnic and regional variation in mortality from SARS-CoV-2 in Brazil are lacking. Added value of this study. We found that hospitalised pardo and preto Brazilians have statistically significant higher mortality compared to a branco comparator group. In particular, pardo ethnicity was the second most important risk factor after age. We also found that mortality by COVID-19 increases in socioeconomically comparable Northern regions, and that Rio de Janeiro has an exceptionally high risk as compared to its neighbouring states.

Implications of All The Available Evidence

Our results have serious social implications: pardo and preto Brazilians have, on average, less economic security, are less likely to be able to stay at home and work remotely and comprise a significant proportion of health and care workers. We hope that this analysis assists the authorities in better directing and aligning their response to COVID-19 in order to protect pardo and preto Brazilians from their higher death risk from SARS-CoV-2. Our results also indicate that the states in the North and Northeast macroregions are more vulnerable to the COVID-19 pandemic, an issue that merits further urgent attention by the federal government.

including in the UK,[3-5] USA[6-8] and Norway.[9] Brazil's population is particularly diverse, comprising many races and ethnic groups. The Brazilian Institute of Geography and Statistics (IBGE) racially classifies the Brazilian population in five categories (percentages as of 2010): *branca* (47.7%), *parda* (43.1%), *preta* (7.6%), *amarela* (1.1%) and *indígena* (0.4%). We will use the Portuguese terms throughout this work. This IBGE classification is based on colour and, as in international practice, individuals are asked to self identify as either: *Branco* ('white'), *preto* ('black'), *amarelo* ('yellow'), *indígeno* ('Amerindians') or *pardo*. The term *pardo* is particularly complex one and is used in Brazil to refer to people of mixed ethnic ancestries: *pardo* Brazilians represent a diverse range of ethnic backgrounds. While *branco* and *pardo* Brazilians together comprise the majority of the population, with approximately equal proportions, their distribution varies considerably regionally. For example, the population in the South macro-region is 78% *branca* and 17% *parda*, while the North macro-region's population is 23% *branca* and 67% *parda*.[10]The combination of the severity of the outbreak, governmental failure to implement non-pharmaceutical interventions and complex social and ethnic societal composition makes Brazil a particularly important as well as interesting country in which to study the impact of COVID-19. In this work, we analyze COVID-19 hospital mortality from the prospectively collected SIVEPGripe ("Sistema de Informação da Vigilância Epidemiológica da Gripe") respiratory infection registry data, which is maintained by the Ministry of Health for the purposes of recording cases of Severe Acute Respiratory Syndrome (SARS) across both public and private hospitals. Using this rich dataset, we characterize the COVID19 pandemic in Brazil, particularly with regard to risk factors related to comorbidities, symptoms and ethnicity, similarly to previous analyses in countries such as the UK.[5,11-13]

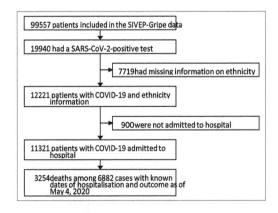

Figure 1: Flowchart of SIVEP-Gripe data used in this study SARS-CoV-2=severe acute respiratory syndrome coronavirus 2. SIVEPGripe=Sistema de Informação de Vigilância Epidemiológica da Gripe

METHODS

Our analysis is based on the SIVEP-Gripe public dataset.[14] As of the time of access, this contains epidemiological data for 99,557 patients from different states. Each entry has 139 features, including symptoms, age, sex, ethnicity and comorbidities. Applying the condition of having tested positive for COVID-19 leaves data for 19,940 patients. As we are interested in the relation between ethnicity and health risk, we then consider only data with ethnicity recorded, leaving data for 12,221 patients. Furthermore, we consider only the subset that was hospitalized: this is our base dataset of 11,321 patients, see **Fig. 1**. The date of diagnosis spans the time interval from 27th February 2020 to 4th May 2020. Our analysis employs descriptive statistics to quantify the COVID-19 pandemic in Brazil, and Cox regression to estimate hazard ratios. Cox regression needs a reliable date of outcome, and, therefore, we further restrict the dataset as depicted in **Fig. 1**. Brazil is a very heterogeneous country, a federation composed of the union of 26 states and a federal district. In the Cox analysis we assess the importance of factors such as education and income of each Brazilian state, as also health indexes such as the number of ICU beds, ventilators, doctors and nurses in the public and private health care system.[15]

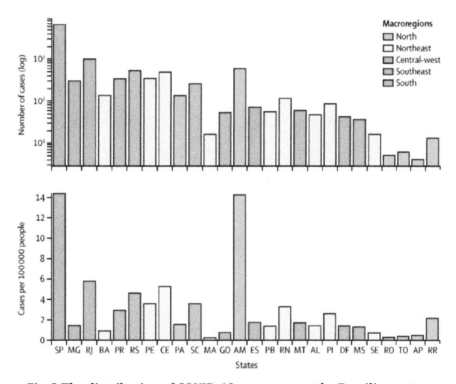

Fig. 2 The distribution of COVID-19 cases among the Brazilian states.

Brazil Is Divided Geopolitically Into 5 Macroregions:

North: Acre (AC), Amapá (AP), Amazonas (AM), Pará (PA), Rondônia (RO), Roraima (RR), Tocantins (TO); Northeast: Alagoas (AL), Bahia (BA), Ceará (CE), Maranhão (MA), Paraíba (PB), Pernambuco (PE),Piauí (PI), Rio Grande do Norte (RN), Sergipe (SE);Central-West: Distrito Federal (DF), Goiás (GO), Mato Grosso (MT), Mato Grosso do Sul (MS);Southeast: Espírito Santo (ES), Minas Gerais (MG), Rio de Janeiro (RJ), São Paulo (SP);South: Paraná (PR), Rio Grande do Sul (RS), Santa Catarina (SC).

For descriptive purposes we chose to dichotomise the data into two maximally contrasting regions based on similar education (literacy, higher education and school drop-out rates), income (per-capita gross domestic product, salary and poverty level) and health (life expectancy, child mortality and food security). Ethnicity was not considered at this point. We do not consider a finer subdivision in order to maximize statistical significance. The two regions that we consider are:

- "Central-South" which comprises the Central West, Southeast and South macroregions for a total of 9278 patients (81%)

- "North" which comprises the North and Northeast macroregions for a total of 2043 patients (19%).

As shown in the supplementary materials, this division appears quite naturally once the socioeconomic factors are combined and is also the customary one when one splits Brazil into a Northern and a Southern region. The SIVEP-Gripe file that is used at the hospitals includes information on comorbidities and symptoms.

Fig 1a Hospitalized Patients with COVID-19 for Brazilian States

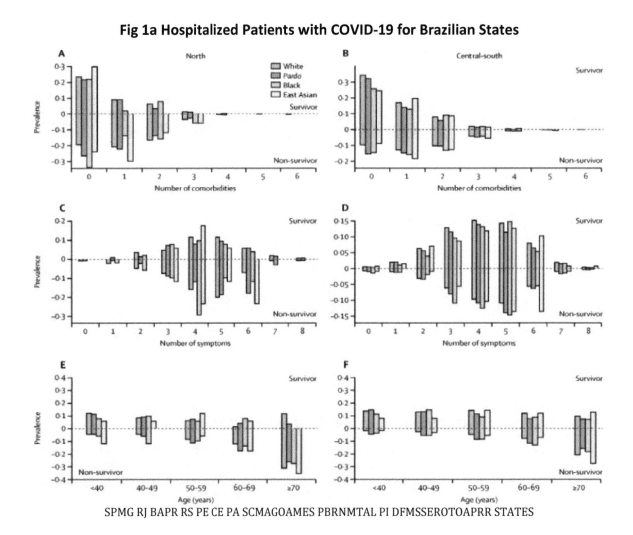

SPMG RJ BAPR RS PE CE PA SCMAGOAMES PBRNMTAL PI DFMSSEROTOAPRR STATES

We interpret missing values as absence of comorbidities or symptoms as we assume that doctors mainly filled in the information for the present comorbidities. Missing values are also present for ICU admissions. In this case we consider missing values as non-admissions to ICU. The number of patients with missing data for symptoms and comorbidities can be found in the supplementary materials, as per STROBE requirement. To investigate the effects of record-level risk factors, we fitted a multivariate mixed-effects Cox regression model to estimate hazard ratios for in-hospital mortality. We used patient-level clinical features, namely age group, sex, ethnic group and comorbidities as fixed effects, with geographical location (i.e. state of Brazil) as the random effect, similarly to previous analyses in the context of UK NHS hospitals.[16] For the categorical variables age group and ethnic group, we used Age < 40 and *branco* as reference categories, respectively. Statistical testing was used to evaluate the proportional hazards assumption[17] and we did not find any statistically significant evidence that it was violated (p=0.11).

RESULTS

Descriptive Statistics

Fig. 2 shows the distribution of COVID-19 cases among the Brazilian states. One sees that SP, RJ and AM have the highest number of cases, both absolute and per capita. Table I shows the distribution of demographic characteristics and comorbidities among survivors and non survivors of COVID-19, while Table II shows the ethnic composition of patients at each stage of the COVID-19 trajectory.

	Survivors (n=4043)	Non-survivors (n=3328)
North (n=1350)	479 (35·5%)	871 (64·5%)
Age (years)	46·9 (19·3)	65·3 (16·0)
Sex		
Men (n=795)	261 (32·8%)	534 (67·2%)
Women (n=555)	218 (39·3%)	337 (60·7%)
Ethnic group		
White (n=225)	89 (39·6%)	136 (60·4%)
Pardo (n=1049)	366 (34·9%)	683 (65·1%)
Black (n=51)	16 (31·4%)	35 (68·6%)
East Asian (n=17)	5 (29·4%)	12 (70·6%)
Indigenous (n=8)	3 (37·5%)	5 (62·5%)
Comorbidities		
Cardiovascular disease	95 (22·6%)	325 (77·4%) (n=420)
Asthma (n=35)	22 (62·9%)	13 (37·1%)
Diabetes (n=371)	74 (19·9%)	297 (80·1%)
Pulmonary disease (n=51)	15 (29·4%)	36 (70·6%)
Obesity (n=58)	13 (22·4%)	45 (77·6%)
Immunosuppression (n=49)	28 (57·1%)	21 (42·9%)
Renal disease (n=69)	13 (18·8%)	56 (81·2%)
Liver disease (n=17)	4 (23·5%)	13 (76·5%)
Neurological disease (n=33)	7 (21·2%)	26 (78·8%)
Central-south (n=6021)	3564 (59·2%)	2457 (40·8%)
Age (years)	52·2 (16·6)	67·0 (15·8)
Sex		
Men (n=3495)	2039 (58·3%)	1456 (41·7%)
Women (n=2526)	1525 (60·4%)	1001 (39·6%)
Ethnic group		
White (n=4108)	2548 (62·0%)	1560 (38·0%)
Pardo (n=1355)	728 (53·7%)	627 (46·3%)
Black (n=425)	215 (50·6%)	210 (49·4%)
East Asian (n=126)	69 (54·8%)	57 (45·2%)
Indigenous (n=7)	4 (57·1%)	3 (42·9%)
Comorbidities		
Cardiovascular disease	936 (44·9%)	1147 (55·1%) (n=2083)
Asthma (n=244)	158 (64·8%)	86 (35·2%)
Diabetes (n=1521)	641 (42·1%)	880 (57·9%)
Pulmonary disease (n=336)	115 (34·2%)	221 (65·8%)
Obesity (n=266)	130 (48·9%)	136 (51·1%)
Immunosuppression (n=260)	104 (40·0%)	156 (60·0%)
Renal disease (n=320)	87 (27·2%)	233 (72·8%) Liver
disease (n=66)	25 (37·9%)	41 (62·1%)
Neurological disease (n=283)	84 (29·7%)	199 (70·3%)

Data are n (%) or mean (SD). For this table, we considered patients for which the outcome was known but not the corresponding dates. Therefore, the total number of survivors and non-survivors (n=7371) is larger than that reported in figure 1 (6882).

Table 1: Demographic characteristics and coexisting conditions among survivors and non-survivors of COVID-19

From **Table** I one sees that, in both the North and Central-South regions, survivors are younger and more likely to be white and female, while non-survivors are more likely to be *preto* and *pardo*, respectively (results regarding the other ethnicities are more difficult to interpret due to the lower numbers). In the North region, non-survivors display a great prevalence of almost all comorbidities. This suggests that the overall health condition in the North region is worse compared to the Central-South region.

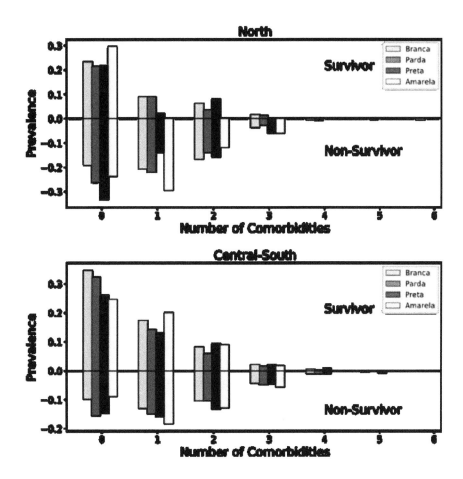

Figure 3. Distributions according to number of comorbidities and ethnicity. The normalization is such that all the fractions of a given ethnicity add to unity. We exclude *indígeno* patients for clarity due to their small numbers.

This Is Confirmed By The Significantly Larger Percentage Of Non-Survivors In The North.

The same trend is observed by comparing the total number of hospitalized patients to the number of deaths (fifth column of Table II). Again we see that mortality is significantly higher in the North as compared to the Central-South and that *preto* and *pardo* Brazilians are less likely to survive the virus. In other words, we are observing two independent effects: i) mortality by COVID19 increases going North (vertical effect), ii) mortality increases for the *preto* and *pardo* population (horizontal effect). To better assess the prevalence of comorbidities, Fig. 3 shows the distributions by ethnicity and number of comorbidities, for survivors and non-survivors, excluding *indígeno* patients because of the small numbers. There is a notable North/Central-South asymmetry with more non-survivors in the former. Fig. 4 shows the distributions according to number of symptoms and ethnicity, split according to mortality. We consider the following symptoms: fever, cough, sore throat, shortness of breath, respiratory discomfort, SpO2 < 95%, diarrhoea, and vomiting. Most patients present between 3 and 6 symptoms, suggesting again that in this dataset, it is the more severe presentations that were tested for COVID-19. Fig. 5 presents the distributions according to age and ethnicity for survivors and non-survivors.

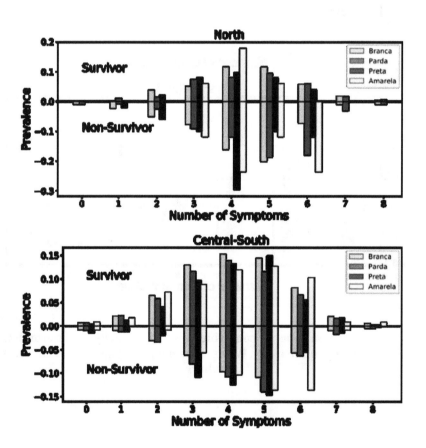

Figure 4. Distributions according to number of symptoms and ethnicity. The normalization is such that all the fractions of a given ethnicity add to unity. We exclude *indígeno* patients for clarity due to their small numbers.

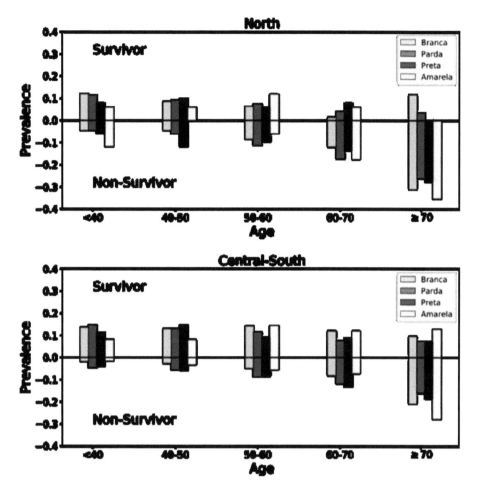

Figure 5. Distributions according to age and ethnicity. The normalization is such that all the fractions of a given ethnicity add to unity. We exclude *indígeno* patients for clarity due to their small numbers.

The expected trend that younger patients are more likely to survive is much more pronounced in the North. Also, younger *pardo* and *preto* Brazilians seem to be less likely to survive the virus compared to *branco* Brazilians, with the difference being more pronounced in the Central-South region.

Risk Factors

Fig. 6 shows hazard ratios with 95% confidence intervals for all clinical features (fixed effects) considered in the fitted multivariate mixed-effects Cox model for in hospital mortality. Compared to *branco* comparators, hospitalised *pardo* and *preto* Brazilians have significantly higher risk of mortality. In particular, *pardo* ethnicity was the second most important risk factor (after age).

Fig. 7 shows hazard ratios with 95% confidence intervals for all different states in Brazil (random effects) considered in the fitted multivariate mixed-effects Cox model for in-hospital mortality. A substantial between-states variation is apparent. The states in the North region tend to have higher hazard ratios than the ones belonging to the Central-South region, further justifying our approach of splitting Brazil into two sets. This also agrees with the significantly larger percentage of non-survivors in the North as shown in Tables I and II (vertical effect discussed earlier).

DISCUSSION

We present, to our knowledge, the largest study of COVID-19 hospital survival in Brazil. We show that survivors are younger[18] with female preponderance[19] and tend to have fewer comorbidities,[20] replicating worldwide findings. However, we also reported other important sociodemographic trends which are specific to Brazil. There is significant regional variation in both case-mix and outcome. The high number of cases (both in absolute and per-capita terms) seen in SP, RJ and AM (Fig. 2) are interesting. Of note, these regions are important ports of entrance to Brazil: AM hosts the Free Economic Zone of Manaus and most of the international flights route through SP and RJ: in 2019 7.7 million international passengers landed in SP and 2.2 million in RJ[21] (further details in the supplementary materials).

Therefore, these states are characterized by a higher international circulation of people. Furthermore, both SP and RJ are characterized by a particularly high population density and the COVID-19 outbreak coincided with the rainy season in AM, which is usually associated with a peak in respiratory infections. In order to explore regional differences, we split the Brazilian states into socioeconomically comparable North and Central-South regions.

The finding of a higher comorbidity burden in hospitalised patients in the North region is concordant with a lower life expectancy[22] and is also borne out by differences in the average age of survivors/non-survivors between the North and Central South regions, as well as the significantly larger percentage of non-survivors in the North. In addition, we found that, in both regions, survivors are more likely to be *branco* and that *branco* Brazilians are more likely to be admitted to ICU than *pardo* Brazilians. In other words, the increased death rate of *pardo* Brazilians seems to be due in part to non-ICU admission, raising concerns regarding the organization of public and private medical resources.

It is also noteworthy that the distribution of hospitalized COVID-19 patients between the Central-South (81%) and North (19%) regions in our data is discordant with the actual population sizes of these two regions (64% and 36% respectively).[10]

This highlights the diversity in the country and may, at least in part, be due to either intrinsically lower hospitalization rates in the North region and/or disproportionate impact of COVID-19 in populous areas such as São Paulo and Rio de Janeiro (both in the Central-South region), the populations of which total about 20 million people. The disparity in comorbidity among hospitalized patients between the North and Central-South regions is also striking (Table I), with non-survivors displaying a greater prevalence of almost all comorbidities in the North: Only asthma and immunosuppression are below hospital prevalence 70%. By contrast, for the Central South region, the only comorbidities affecting more than 70% of non-survivors are renal and neurological diseases. Whilst a number of structural explanations are of course possible, this is likely to reflect poorer health status overall in the North region which, again, has a substantially larger percentage of non-survivors.

The disproportionately large percentage of comorbidity-free survivors in the Central-South region (Fig. 3) is remarkable. We may speculate that this may be due to differences in comorbidity ascertainment either due to structural differences in the way data is collected – perhaps comorbidity data was less available from patients who were sicker at the time of presentation – or because less severe patients, perhaps with concerns regarding their comorbid health, presented to hospital preferentially in the Central-South region. It is interesting to observe that *branco* and *pardo* Brazilians have a similar number of comorbidities in these populations.

Therefore, it seems that comorbidities are not associated with ethnicity in the group studied, but are correlated with regional socioeconomic development (education, income and health).However, an interplay between ethnic and regional socioeconomic factors is apparent in Fig. 5 with younger *pardo* and *preto* Brazilians seemingly less likely to survive the disease compared to the *branco* population; the difference being more pronounced in the Central-South region. It is worth placing this in the context of the typical life-expectancy in Brazil of 76 years (as of 2017).[23] By way of comparison the life expectancy in the European Union is 80.9 years.[24] Note also that the average life expectancy varies significantly by region, being higher in the Central-South than in the North: Santa Catarina has a life expectancy of 79.4 years while that of Maranhão is 70.9. This provides a baseline for the trend shown in Fig. 5. From the ethnic distribution of patients admitted to ICU shown in Table II it appears that *branco* Brazilians are more likely than *pardo* Brazilians to be admitted to ICU once hospitalised. Also, by comparing percentages of hospitalization with deaths, one sees that *branco* Brazilians are more likely to survive than *pardo* Brazilians. However, by comparing total hospitalization with deaths after ICU admission, one sees more similar proportions between both ethnicities.

Table II. Ethnic composition of patients at each stage of the COVID-19 trajectory

	Brazilian population*	Hospital admission	ICU admission	Death	Death/ hospitalisation	Death (not ICU)	Death (ICU)
North (n=2043)							
White	27·8%	342 (16·7%)	127 (19·4%)	136 (15·6%)	39·8%	69 (14·9%)	67 (16·5%)
Pardo	61·5%	1567 (76·7%)	481 (73·8%)	683 (78·4%)	43·6%	368 (79·3%)	315 (77·4%)
Black	8·8%	85 (4·2%)	26 (4·0%)	35 (4·0%)	41·2%	20 (4·3 %)	15 (3·7%)
East Asian	1·2%	36 (1·8%)	13 (2·0%)	12 (1·4%)	33·3%	5 (1·1%)	7 (1·7%)
Indigenous	0·7%	13 (0·6%)	5 (0·8%)	5 (0·6%)	38·5%	2 (0·4%)	3 (0·7%)
Central-south (n=9278)							
White	58·7%	6291 (67·8%)	2344 (69·4%)	1560 (63·5%)	24·8%	616 (60·3%)	944 (65·8%)
Pardo	33·2%	2112 (22·8%)	731 (21·6%)	627 (25·5%)	29·7%	278 (27·2%)	349 (24·3%)
Black	6·8%	667 (7·2%)	220 (6·5%)	210 (8·6%)	31·5%	108 (10·6%)	102 (7·1%)
East Asian	1·1%	195 (2·1%)	82 (2·4%)	57 (2·3%)	29·2%	19 (1·9%)	38 (2·7%)
Indigenous	0·3%	13 (0·1%)	2 (0·1%)	3 (0·1%)	23·1%	1 (0·1%)	2 (0·1%)

Data are % or n (%). ICU=intensive care unit. *Census values of the Brazilian population.

Table 2: Ethnic composition of patients at each stage of the COVID-19 trajectory

It appears that there are substantial ethnic differences in the proportion of patients admitted to ICU, and this also varies between North and Central-South regions. The greater proportion of deaths without admission to ICU for *pardo* is noteworthy. This is likely to reflect higher levels of access to private healthcare for *branco* as compared to *pardo* Brazilians as ICU admission policies are known to differ between public and private hospital settings.[25] This may suggest that the lower rate of admission to ICU may be a factor for the increased proportion of deaths among *pardo* Brazilians. Note that the distribution of comorbidities, symptoms and age does not show strong ethnic variations, especially between *pardo* and *branco*.

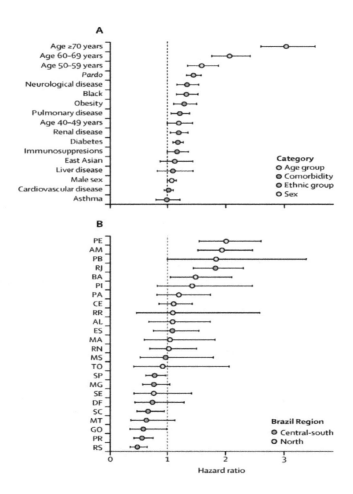

Fig 6 (a) and Fig 7 (b)[1]

That the proportions of the different ethnicities admitted to ICU with COVID-19 are similar to those in the full 2019 SIVEP-Gripe dataset[14] The data suggests that this is not a specific feature of COVID-19. At an individual level survival analysis showed that, after age, the most important factor for hospital mortality was being of *pardo* or, to a lesser extent, *preto* ethnicity with hazard ratios of 1.47(1.33-1.58) and 1.32(1.15-1.52) (95% CI) compared to the *branco* baseline.

The other risk factors largely replicate worldwide findings although we see that male sex is perhaps slightly less of a risk factor compared to what has been found in other series.[19] This ethnic inequity has important social roots and implications: *pardo* and *preto* Brazilians have, on average, less economic security, are less likely to be able to stay at home and work remotely, and comprise a significant proportion of health and care workers, making them disproportionately the most vulnerable to COVID-19.[26] We also performed the Cox regression separately on the patients in the North and South regions, on patients in São Paulo and also excluding the São Paulo and Amazonas states (the ones with the highest number of cases per capita, see Fig. 2) to test robustness of our

---

[1]

Figure 6. Fixed effects (hazard ratio) estimates with their 95% confidence intervals for in-hospital mortality.
Figure 7. Random effects (hazard ratio) showing between-Brazilian-state variation with their 95% confidence intervals.

findings to outliers: The results were qualitatively consistent and did not change our conclusions that ethnicity is a key risk factor (details in the supplementary materials).

Examining the magnitude of the random effect estimates, we see substantial variation in hazard by region. The states that belong to the North region tend to have higher hazard ratios than the ones belonging to the Central-South region, which provides additional justification for splitting Brazil into two socioeconomically similar sets.

It is also in agreement with the significantly larger percentage of non-survivors in the North as shown in Table I. Incorporating number of ICU beds/ventilators and nurses per 100 million inhabitants for each region as proxies for physical availability of healthcare resources did not qualitatively change our result (supplementary materials) suggesting a more fundamental difference in healthcare access and trajectory. Rio de Janeiro, despite high standards of education, income and health, has one of the highest hazard ratios, very similar to those seen for the less developed Pernambuco and Amazonas regions. It is possible that this represents the effect of a highly populous area on viral spread.

At the same time, Table IV shows the ethnic distribution for the seven states with highest number of cases, together with their hazard ratios. States in the North region have a hazard ratio greater than unity and a high proportion of *pardo* Brazilians, while states in the Central-South region have a hazard ratio less than one and a higher proportion of *branco* Brazilians. The notable exception is Rio de Janeiro, which exhibits a much higher hazard ratio than the neighbouring state of São Paulo and an ethnicity similar to the states in the North region.

Many *preto* Brazilians may identify themselves as *pardo* Brazilians.[27] For this reason, it is reasonable to consider the *preto* and *pardo* populations together. Indeed, as seen from our analysis, both ethnic groups share higher percentages of non-survivors and higher hazard ratios. The results of our analysis can then be interpreted according to the interplay of two independent, but correlated, effects:

i) mortality by COVID-19 increases going North: 'vertical' effect,

ii) mortality increases for the *pardo* and *preto* population: 'horizontal' effect.

We may speculate that the vertical effect is due to expected increasing levels of comorbidities (or poorly controlled comorbidities) and general healthcare access, which we might expect in regions such as the North where socioeconomic levels are lower. We similarly postulate that the horizontal effect is likely driven by the greater reliance on publicly-funded healthcare in *pardo* and *preto* communities whereas *branco* Brazilians on average have greater access to private healthcare.

This may explain the lower ICU admission for *pardo* as compared to *branco* Brazilians as ICU admission policy and availability vary substantially between public and private hospitals.[25]

For most states the vertical and horizontal effects are correlated, giving a larger cumulative akin to those of Central-South states. In other words mortality. Indeed, lower socioeconomic development correlates with a larger *pardo* and *preto* population. Again, Rio de Janeiro is an outlier with an ethnic composition (horizontal effect) that is similar to the states in the North region, but high levels of development (vertical effect) more, Rio de Janeiro violates the typical correlation between vertical and horizontal effects seen elsewhere.

Whilst we believe our work is the most comprehensive of its kind to date in Brazil, there are a number of limitations which are worthy of discussion. Limitations and possible biases in case ascertainment cannot be ruled out, in common with all observational / database research. Ethnicity is missing in 39% of our data. This is not specific to COVID-19 (32% for the full SIVEP-Gripe dataset) but we cannot be sure that this is not subject to bias. We have limited our analysis to patients who were hospitalised since testing in the community is more likely to be biased according to local factors. However, again here, we cannot be sure that the availability of testing practice is homogeneous even in this population. Indeed, the fact that a large fraction of patients that have tested positive are admitted to the hospital clearly shows that testing, at least as far as this dataset is concerned, is performed only when symptoms are severe, indicating in turn that the number of COVID-19 cases in Brazil is likely to be much higher than suggested by available data.[28,29]

It is possible that health-seeking behaviour varies with both ethnicity and region and late presentation may be an important determinant of ultimate hospital outcome. We are not able to consider this in our analysis as physiological severity at hospital presentation / admission data is not available in the SIVEP-Gripe dataset. However, a recent UK study did not demonstrate an important effect of physiological severity[16] at least for ICU mortality, suggesting a high degree of homogeneity at admission, at least for this group. We cannot comment on whether this applies to Brazil or for the hospital population as a whole, and this would be an interesting area for future research. We conducted our study during the Brazilian outbreak in the hope of generating actionable results. However, the analysis of early data introduces the possibility of lead time and outcome ascertainment bias, although since our data encompasses a period substantially longer than the typical hospital stay, we hope that this does not affect our results qualitatively in any substantial way. Whilst we have focused on hospital mortality, it is important to appreciate that we do not have data on out-of hospital mortality (which may be appreciable) and neither can we robustly address the question of access to hospital services both by region or ethnicity / socioeconomic status. As such, a consideration of hospital mortality is likely to substantially underestimate the true effects of COVID-19 and it is plausible to assume that healthcare availability inequities would be further amplified in patients who are not hospitalized.

In conclusion, we present evidence suggesting a higher risk of death among *pardo* and *preto* Brazilians and in the North region. We hope that this analysis assists the authorities in better directing and aligning their response to COVID-19 in order to protect *pardo* and *preto* Brazilians from their higher death risk from SARSCoV-2. Our results also indicate that the states in the North and Northeast macroregions are more vulnerable to the COVID-19 pandemic, an issue that merits further urgent attention by the federal government.

CONTRIBUTORS

MvdS conceived the research question. All authors designed the study and analysis plan. VM obtained the epidemiological and socioeconomic data. PB carried out the analysis with descriptive statistics. IB carried out the analysis with Cox regression. VM drafted the initial version of the manuscript. AE oversaw the clinical review of the methods and manuscript. All authors critically reviewed early and final versions of the manuscript.

DATA SHARING

SIVEP-Gripe data ispublicly available from

http://plataforma.saude.gov.br/coronavirus/dadosabertos/sivep-gripe. Our analysis code is made available in the supplementary material.

ACKNOWLEDGMENTS

We would like to thank Roberto Andre Kraenkel for help with the SIVEP-Gripe catalog, and the CCE/UFES COVID-19 group and Fabiana V. Campos for useful comments and discussions.

REFERENCES

1. The Lancet. COVID-19 in Brazil: "So what?". *Lancet* 2020; **395**: 1461.

2. Imperial College COVID-19 response team. Shortterm forecasts of COVID-19 deaths in multiple countries, 2020.

3. Kirby T. (2020) Evidence mounts on the disproportionate effect of COVID-19 on ethnic minorities. *Lancet Respir Med* 2020; published online May 8. doi:10.1016/S2213-2600(20)302289

4. Pareek, M., Bangash M.N, Pareek, N., et al. (2020) Ethnicity and COVID-19: an urgent public health research priority. *Lancet* 2020; **395**: 1421–2.

5. Williamson, E., Walker, A,J., Bhaskaran, K.J., et al. (2020). OpenSAFELY: factors associated with COVID-19-related hospital death in the linked electronic health records of 17 million adult NHS patients. medRxiv 2020; published online May 7. doi:10.1101/2020.05.06.20092999.

6. Centres for Disease Control and Prevention. COVID19 in Racial and Ethnic Minority Groups, 2020.
7. https://www.cdc.gov/coronavirus/2019-ncov/html (accessed May 10, 2020).

8. Centres for Disease Control and Prevention. Hospitalization Rates and Characteristics of Patients Hospitalized with Labouratory-Confirmed Coronavirus Disease 2019 – COVID-NET, 14 States, March 1-30,2020, 2020. https://www.cdc.gov/mmwr/volumes/69/ wr/mm6915e3.htm?s_cid=mm6915e3_w (accessed May 10, 2020).

9. APM research lab staff. The colour of coronavirus: COVID19 deaths by race and ethnicity in the U.S., 2020. https://www.apmresearchlab.org/covid/deaths-by-race (accessed May 10, 2020).

10. Cookson, C. and Milne R. (2020) Nations look into why coronavirus hits ethnic minorities so hard, 2020.

11. Brazilian Institute of Geography and Statistics. Tabela 2094 - População residente por cor ou raça e religião,2010. https://sidra.ibge.gov.br/tabela/2094#/n1/all/n2/all/n3/all/v/1000093/p/last%201/c86/allxt/ c133/0/d/v1000093%201/l/v,p+c86,t+c133/resultado (accessed May 10, 2020).

12. Mehra, M.R., Desai. S.S., Kuy, S., Henry, T.D., and Patel, A.N. (2020) Cardiovascular Disease, Drug Therapy, and Mortality in COVID-19. *New England Journal of Medicine* 2020; published online May 1. doi:10.1056/NEJMoa2007621.
13. Brat, G.A., Weber, G.M,, Gehlenborg, N., et al. (2020) International Electronic Health Record-Derived COVID19 Clinical Course Profiles: The 4CE Consortium. medRxiv 2020; published online April 30.

14. Ministry of Health. SIVEP-Gripe public dataset,2020. http://plataforma.saude.gov.br/coronavirus/ dados-abertos/ (accessed May 10, 2020).

15. Brazilian Institute of Geography and Statistics. Informações de Saúde, 2020. https://mapasinterativos. ibge.gov.br/covid/saude/ (accessed May 10, 2020).

16. Qian, Z, Alaa, A.M., van der Schaar M, and Ercole A. (2020) Between-centre differences for COVID-19 ICU mortality from early data in England. medRxiv 2020; published online May 15. doi:10.1101/2020.04.19.20070722.

17. Grambsch, P.M. and Therneau, T.M. (1994) Proportional hazards tests and diagnostics based on weighted residuals. *Biometrika* 1994; **81**: 515–26.

18. The Epidemiological Characteristics of an Outbreak of 2019 Novel Coronavirus Diseases (COVID-19) – China, 2020. *China CDC Weekly* 2020; **2**: 113–22.

19. Wenham, C. Smith, J. and Morgan, R.(2020) COVID-19: the gendered impacts of the outbreak. *Lancet* 2020; **395**: 846–8.

20. Halpin, D.M.G, Faner, R., Sibila, O., Badia, J.R., and Agusti, A. (2020) Do chronic respiratory diseases or their treatment affect the risk of SARS-CoV-2 infection? *Lancet Respir Med* 2020; **8**: 436–8.

21. Agência Nacional de Aviação Civil. Dados Estatísticos, 2020. https://www.anac.gov.br/assuntos/ dados-e-estatisticas/dados-estatisticos/ dados-estatisticos (accessed May 10, 2020).

22. Wikipedia. Lista de unidades federativas do Brasil por expectativa de vida, 2017. https://pt.wikipedia.org/wiki/Lista_de_unidades_ federativas_do_Brasil_por_expectativa_de_vida (accessed May 10, 2020).

23. Brazilian Institute of Geography and Statistics. Tábua completa de mortalidade para o Brasil – 2017,2018. ftp://ftp.ibge.gov.br/Tabuas_Completas_de_ Mortalidade/Tabuas_Completas_de_Mortalidade_2017/ tabua_de_mortalidade_2017_analise.pdf (accessed May 10, 2020).

24. Eurostat. Life expectancy at birth in the EU: men vs. women, 2017. https://ec.europa.eu/eurostat/web/ products-eurostat-news/-/DDN-20190725-1 (accessed May 10, 2020).

25. Costa, N.d.R. (2020) A Disponibilidade de Leitos em Unidade de Tratamento Intensivo no SUS e nos Planos de Saúde Diante da Epidemia da COVID-19 no Brasil, 2020. http://www.ensp.fiocruz.br/portal-ensp/informe/ site/arquivos/ckeditor/files/DISPONIBILIDADE% 20DE%20UTI%20NO%20BRASIL_27_03_2020(1).pdf (accessed May 10, 2020).

26. Tavares, F. and Betti, G.,(2020)Vulnerability, Poverty and COVID-19: Risk Factors and Deprivations in Brazil,2020. https://www.researchgate.net/publication/ 340660228_Vulnerability_Poverty_and_COVID-19_ Risk_Factors_and_Deprivations_in_Brazil (accessed May 10, 2020).

27. Bailey, S.R. and Telles, E.E. (2016) Multiracial versus Collective Black Categories: Examining Census Classification Debates in Brazil. *Ethnicities* 2006; **6**: 74–101.

28. Cintra, P.H.P., and Fontinele Nunes, F. (2020) Estimative of real number of infections by COVID-19 on brazil and possible scenarios. medRxiv 2020; published online May 12. doi:10.1101/2020.05.03.20052779.

29. Alves, D., Gaete R, Miyoshi, N,, Carciofi, B,, Olveira, L, and Sanchez, T.(2020) Estimativa de Casos de COVID-19, 2020. https://ciis.fmrp.usp.br/covid19-subnotificacao/ (accessed May 10, 2020).

4. A Population-Based Study of The Prevalence Of COVID-19 Infection In Espírito Santo, Brazil: Methodology and Results of The First Stage

[1]Cristiana Costa Gomes[1] Crispim Cerutti Junior[2] Eliana Zandonade[2] Ethel Leonor Noia Maciel[2] Filomena Euridice Carvalho de Alencar[2] Gilton Luiz Almada[1] Orlei Amaral Cardoso[1] Pablo Medeiros Jabor[3] Raphael Lubiana Zanotti[1] Tania Queiroz Reuter[2,4] Vera Lucia Gomes de Andrade[5] Whisllay Maciel Bastos[1] Nésio Fernandes de Medeiros Junior [1].

ABSTRACT

BACKGROUND:COVID-19 is affecting almost the entire world, causing more than four hundred thousand deaths and undermining the health care systems, as much as the economy, of the afflicted countries. The strategies for prevention depend on largely lacking information, as infection prevalence and virus pathogenicity. This study aimed to determine the prevalence, the pathogenicity, and the speed of infection spreading in a large population in Brazil.

MATERIALS AND METHODS: This is a serial cross-sectional study designed on a population basis and structured over houses as the sampling units. The sampling consisted of four visits at 15 days intervals in randomly selected census-designated sectors of the State major municipalities (reference municipalities) and two visits at 30 days intervals in smaller municipalities of the same regions of those of reference. At each visit, the investigators sampled houses and sampled one individual in each house for data collection. After the informed consent, the investigators performed a rapid antibody detection test (Celer Technology, Inc) and applied a questionnaire containing clinical and demographic questions.

RESULTS: From May 13th—May 15th the investigators performed 6,393 rapid tests in 4,612 individuals of the reference municipalities, 1,163 individuals of the smaller municipalities, and 166 contacts of the positive individuals. Ninety-seven dwellers were positive in the reference municipalities, giving a prevalence of 2.1% (CI 95%:1.67-2.52%). In the smaller municipalities, the figure was 0.26% (CI 95%: 0.05%-0.75%) (three positives).There was an association of the positive result with female sex (p = 0.013) and houses with five dwellers or more (p = 0.003). Seventy-eight positive individuals reported symptoms in the previous 15 days (80.4%), being anosmia (45.4%), cough (40.2%), and myalgia (38.1%) the more frequent. About one-third of them reported fever (28.9%).

CONCLUSIONS: The results reveal a still small prevalence of infection in the study area, despite the significant number of sick people overloading the health system. The figures indicate an important underreporting in the area and a frequency that still can grow, making necessary public health actions for the containment of the transmission.

---

[1] 1Secretaria de Estado da Saúde do Espírito Santo, SESA
2   Universidade Federal do Espírito Santo, UFES
3   Instituto Jones dos Santos Neves, IJSN
4   Hospital Universitário Cassiano Antônio Moraes, HUCAM 5 Epidemiologist. Independent consultant.

INTRODUCTION.

In December 2019, Chinese health authorities detected a novel coronavirus transmitted in the city of Wuhan, province of Hubei, China, which was called SARS-CoV-2.It belongs to the betacoronavirus group, with SARS-CoV and MERS-CoV [1, 2, 3]. The coronavirus respiratory disease (COVID-19) has clinical manifestations ranging from asymptomatic infection to severe forms, and its case-fatality ratio is expressive. The clinical picture is pleomorphic because the virus is capable of infecting several different types of cells, as respiratory, neural, muscle, and endothelial [4].

Therefore, life-threatening conditions, including severe pneumonia, thromboembolic phenomena, myocardial injury, and multiple forms of neurological damage, frequently impose the need for intensive care [4]. Some unusual manifestations are also present in the less severe presentations, as anosmia [5].Approximately 15% to 20% of the symptomatic cases need hospitalisation, which represents an enormous burden over the national health systems [6].In a scenario of broad dissemination and absence of prophylactic or therapeutic choices, social distancing became the only alternative to prevent the health systems from collapsing.

The COVID-19 had a fast dissemination to all the continents [7].The World Health Organisation classified the disease as a public health emergency of international concern on January 30th, changing its status progressively until the final classification as a pandemic on April 11th [8]. When considering the several moments in the history of this pandemic, it is possible to verify that the infections were occurring, at first, because of the contact with travellers arriving from China, returning from business or tourism travels. Soon later, there was the inclusion of other countries to the list of those from where the infection was coming. The disease progression to countries like Italy and Spain [9, 10], disclosed the disease contagiousness and the epicentre moved from China to Italy and the United States of America, with increasing reported cases and deaths [11].The epidemiological scenario in Brazil is not different, with a sharp increase in the number of reported cases, challenging the health system, and resulting in a high mortality [12].

The source of COVID-19 case reporting in Brazil is the hospital admissions, but the real extension of the disease in the population is unknown. It is imperative to know the disease extension, including the status of the asymptomatic people, which are known to be fit for transmitting to other people [13]. Additionally, in Brazil, given the speed of the disease propagation, people with flu symptoms without severity received the instruction to remain home for fourteen days, reserving the attendance to a health facility to the situation of the appearance of severe symptoms. In this sense, there is an impairment in the calculation of the incidence, prevalence, and case-fatality, underestimating the first two and overestimating the last one, as it depends on the real number of affected individuals and not on only those admitted to a hospital. Consequently, surveys conducted on a population-basis are of utmost importance for the understanding of the real dimension of the pandemic in the different scenarios of its occurrence.

They are likewise critical to foster actions to prevent the spread of the disease and to assist in the organisation of a healthcare network fit for offering enough health assistance as indicated by the requirements of the affected population. Another potential benefit of population-based surveys is the tuning of the restrictive measures. Such measures generally apply to a community as a whole in geographic terms, mainly departing from a policy determined by local authorities. However, health authorities do not know if the spread of the infection takes place in the same way in small communities as it does in big cities. The understanding of this epidemiologic aspect would provide better reasoning in the establishment of policies, adapting them to the several different realities. The design of the present study comprises two concomitant steps with four phases, each one. The main step, called study of prevalence, plans to ascertain the percent of residents in Espírito Santo infected with SARS-CoV-2, to establish the frequency of asymptomatic or subclinical episodes and to establish the disease spreading during 45 days every two weeks, as an approach to measure its speed. The second step, designated extension study, aims to establish the extension of the disease to the several cities of the State.

MATERIALS AND METHODS.

Study area:

Espírito Santo is a coastal Brazilian State, located in the south eastern region. It has 46,095.5 Km^2 encompassing 78 municipalities distributed in eight census regions. Each region except one has the most populous municipality as a reference, in which populations vary from 16,000 to 400,000 inhabitants each. The capital, Vitória, is a harbour city, being part of a large metropolitan area that encompasses seven other municipalities. The State has an exuberant agricultural production, comprising coffee, fruits, and vegetables, as much as a developed industrial park and a marked trade activity.

Study Design:

This is a serial cross-sectional study designed on a population basis and structured over houses as the sampling units. The approach involves two concomitant steps, the prevalence study and the extension study. The 'prevalence study' comprises the sampling of each reference municipality, added by the four most populous in the metropolitan region and one elected municipality in the region lacking a reference. Therefore, there are 11 municipalities allocated to the prevalence study. The step called 'extension study' comprises the sampling on 16 lesser populous municipalities, being two in each one of the eight regions. The urban population of these municipalities varies from approximately 14,000 to about 100,000 inhabitants each, but only three of them have more than 30,000 inhabitants. The sampling plan includes four visits to the 'prevalence study', one every 15 days. The visits in the 'extension study' are two, with 30 days interval, being, in each region, one of the municipalities visited at the same time of the first and the third visits of the 'prevalence study', and the other at the same time of the second and the fourth visits of the 'prevalence study'. Each visit constituted a stage of the study. This paper presents the complete planning, the methods, and the results of the study first stage.

Sample Size Calculation:

The calculation for each one of the stages considered the estimation of the prevalence in a simple random sampling. The estimative was a priori prevalence of 3% in the first stage, progressing to 20% in the fourth stage (table 1).For ethical reasons, the study teams are performing additional tests for dwellers in houses with a positive individual. Thirty-two thousand tests should be performed along the entire study to include up to four members of the family of the selected subject plus the team members.

Table 1. Parameters and estimates used for sample size and total number of tests calculation. A Population-based study of the prevalence and extension of COVID-19 in Espírito Santo, Brazil.

Survey stages	Estimated prevalence	N	Total precision (%)	N	Total precision (%)	Additional tests		
		Prevalence study		Extension study		Cont. Prev*	Cont.Exten*	Team
1	3%	4,500	0.5	1,160	1.0	540	35	400
2	5%	4,500	0.6	1,040	1.3	900	52	400
3	10%	4,500	1.0	1,160	1.7	1,800	116	400
4	20%	4,500	1.2	1,040	2.4	3,600	208	400
Total		18,000		4,400		6,840	411	1,200

* Contacts of the prevalence study and contacts of the extension study: values obtained from the estimated prevalence multiplied by four (mean number of dwellers by house, not including the selected subject).

Sampling Procedures:

The house is the sampling unit of the study. The total number of houses included in each municipality is proportional to the total population of the given municipality. The study applies to census-designated sectors defined by Instituto Brasileiro de Geografia e Estatística (IBGE) [14] as the random selection primary level. A census-designated sector is a territorial unit delimited by IBGE to organise data collection in the household surveys.

It is a continuous area located in a defined rural or urban region and having a dimension and number of houses that allow the work accomplishment by an enumerator individual alone. After the sectors randomised selection, the secondary level encompasses the houses. The third level is the random selection of one individual in the house. The sectors included for selection were those located in urban areas, with more than 100 hectares in extension and comprising more than 200 houses. The sampling included 80 to 120 houses for cities with less than 50,000 urban residents, 200 for 51,000 to 99,000 residents, and 240 for 100,000 to 120,000 inhabitants. From this population size on, the houses number was approximately 1 for every 450 inhabitants, with a limit at 1,360 houses.

The samples were multiples of 40 because it was the number established for sampling in each one of the sectors, in 171 random selected sectors. A waypoint in the central area guided the entrance of the team in each sector, supported by Google maps™. The investigators always moved from the right to the left, starting on the first house. They followed the same direction inside a block of flats if this was the first kind of habitation encountered, taking a photograph of each sampled house or each building, after permission of the dwellers for participation. The strategy consisted of including one house at each five or one flat on each four floors. In case of refusal, they included the next house or flat on the left. If the building was a business establishment, they selected the next one. When the sampling started on a building earth floor, it started on the last of the other.

At each stage, the team will collect in the same sector, but in different houses. Each team received a map of their sector. The production of the maps was the responsibility of Instituto Jones dos

Santos Neves, a local government institution dedicated to technical advising to support logistic decisions. Google maps™ was the basis for the maps manufacturing.

Before starting data collections, the study coordinators trained adequately all the fieldwork teams involved, and a coordinator of each region kept permanent contact with the coordination board during the entire period of fieldwork, to solve on time any unexpected trouble. All the investigators performed the sampling using personal protective equipment (PPE) according to the guidelines of the National Sanitary Surveillance Agency (ANVISA) [15].They also received meals and all the necessary materials to accomplish their task. The study coordination board performed anti-SARS-CoV-2 tests in each one of the investigators on the day before sampling, with the replacement of any positive investigator and those with respiratory symptoms independently of the test result. Testing will occur at each one of the stages.

Inclusion Criteria:

The included individuals were older than two years. The legal guardian answered the questions for those younger than 16.

Data Collection:

After the informed consent, the volunteers participated in an interview that provided information regarding the following variables: sex, age, education level of the person with the highest level of education in the house, and self-referred skin colour. The interview also included questions about COVID-19 symptoms in the previous 15 days (cough, fever, tiredness, pain in the body, shortness of breath, changes in taste and smell or any other symptom) and chronic morbid conditions (respiratory, renal, cardiac, endocrine and others). Apart from the interview, the investigators performed a rapid serological immunochromatographic test for the detection of IgM and IgG antibodies against SARSCoV-2 in every volunteer (Celer Technologies Inc; sensitivity86.4% and specificity 97.63%) (ANVISA registration number:80537410048).The test processes blood collected from the fingertip.

Data Analysis:

The procedures for data collection include the use of the e-SUS Atenção Primária platform [16], a standard electronic form of the Brazilian Unique Health System. Tablets with internet access received the platform download, being possible the data recording in the device if the internet had a failure. Data analysis included the organisation of tables of frequencies and the estimation of the point prevalence and its 95% confidence interval. Statistical methods used to verify the association between the study variables and the test results were Chi-squared and Fisher Exact. The statistical package used for data analysis was SPSS version 20.0 (IBM).The limit for statistical significance was 5%.

Ethical issues:

All the selected individuals received information regarding the objectives of the study, the risks and the benefits involved. The procedures took place only after each volunteer provided the signed informed consent form, and all the selected volunteers had access to the result of their tests. The investigators reported the positive cases to the local health service for the application of the necessary measures. There was strictly adoption of all biologic safety measures during all the collections, to guarantee the health integrity of all the field investigators and volunteers. This study had the approval of the Committee on Ethics of Research on Human Beings of the University Hospital Cassiano Antonio de Moraes of the Federal University of Espírito Santo, under the insertion number CCAE 31417020.3.0000.5064 and the approval number 4.009.337.

RESULTS

The fieldwork teams performed 6,393 rapid tests, being 4,612 in individuals selected for the prevalence study, 1,163 in participants of the extension study, 140 in contacts of the positive individuals of the prevalence study, 26 in contacts of those of the extension study and 452 in the fieldwork investigators. The results presented here refer to the prevalence study, excluding four individuals with inconclusive tests. Ninety-seven individuals had positive results in the prevalence study, giving a frequency of 2.1% (CI 95%:1.67% to 2.52%).On the other hand, three had positive results in the extension study, giving a prevalence of 0.26% (CI95%:0.05% to 0.75%).

This result indicates 84,391 (CI 95%:64,299 to 100,485) individuals infected by SARSCoV2 in Espírito Santo.Among 140 additional tests carried out on the contacts of the positive individuals, there were 50 positives (35.7%), one for every two positive individuals.

Regarding sociodemographic variables, female sex was predominant (p = 0.013), with age ranging from 21 to 40 years (p = 0.09), living in dwells with five or more residents (p = 0.003) and with the resident with the higher level of schooling being in middle year (equivalent to high school) (p = 0.074) (table 2). The symptoms occurrence was statistically associated with the positive rate for the test (p < 0.001) (Figure 1), but 19.6% of the positive individuals were asymptomatic. The questionnaire included 12 different symptoms, including others. The most prevalent symptoms were anosmia (45.4%), cough (40.2%), myalgia (38.1%), fatigue (34%), dyspnoea (28.9%) and fever (28.9%).Other symptoms included headache (7.4%), sore throat (9.3%), diarrhoea (6.4%), abdominal pain (5.3%), tachycardia (5.3%), and vomiting (2.2%) (Figure 2).

The positive result for the test was also statistically associated with the presence of a symptomatic individual at home. Among the positive selected individuals, 40.2% had attended a health care facility (table 3). Comorbidities like diabetes (18.6%), asthma (16.5%), and obesity (22.7%) were more frequent among the individuals with a positive test (p < 0.05).Positive individuals more frequently had three, four or more comorbidities when compared to negative individuals, indicating their greater susceptibility to infection (table 3).

DISCUSSION

The first step of this cross-sectional study conducted in Espírito Santo disclosed an infection prevalence of 2.1%, corresponding to 84,391 infected individuals in the whole State. It is a high frequency when compared to 0.05%, 0.13%, 0.22%, and 0.18% prevalence observed in the first, second, third, and fourth steps of a Southern State survey [17, 18].However, the one-month difference between the two studies can explain the discrepancy between the frequencies, as this period is long enough for a significant expansion of this rapidly spreading disease [17, 18].Furthermore, there are differences between both the control strategies adopted in each region and the frequency of social distancing observed in these populations [17].Results of prevalence studies are not always directly comparable, as they depend on the moment of their performance regarding the evolution of the epidemics and the type of the tests used. Therefore, whilst Brazil uses rapid antibody-detection tests, the basis of surveys performed in Italy, Spain, United States, and other countries was antibody detection blood tests or molecular tests [19, 20, 21]

The performance of additional tests in cohabitants of the positive individuals (contacts) revealed 35.7% percent of positive results (50 of 140).Hence, there was one positive contact for every two selected individuals found positive. The presence of positive contacts is an expected finding in a fast-evolving epidemic like COVID-19 [17, 22, 23], and it will be possible to better ascertain its frequency after the future steps of this serial cross-sectional study. However, at this point, it is possible to observe a higher probability of positive contacts when the number of dwellers was five or more. Whilst it points to a clustering behaviour of the transmission, the study did not evaluate other contributing factors, like house dimensions and the amount of rooms. The confinement in agglomeration opposes the policy of social distancing because it is useless to stay at home, the place where the possibility of infection is higher.

The finding of 19.4% of asymptomatic among positive individuals is in contrast with data from other studies, which reveal frequencies as high as 81% [24]. However, the percentage of asymptomatic may also depend on the type of test performed and the testing time related to the moment of infection. If the test has a high sensitivity, the possibility of detecting asymptomatic individuals is also higher.

Table 2:Sociodemographic profile of the individuals included in the population-based study of COVID-19 in Espírito Santo, Brazil – first stage (prevalence study), according to the test result.

Variable	Category	Total		Test result N = 4608				p-value
				Positive		Negative		
		N	%	N	%	N	%	
	Female	2809	61.0	**71**	**73.2**	2738	60.7	**0.013**
Sex	Male	1799	39.0	26	26.8	1773	39.3	
	Untill 20 years	434	9.4	12	12.4	422	9.4	**0.090**
	21 to 40 years	1367	29.7	**36**	**37.1**	1331	29.5	
	41 to 60 years	1583	34.4	25	25.8	1558	34.5	
	61 to 80 years	1081	23.5	24	24.7	1057	23.4	
Age range	81 years and more	143	3.1	0	0.0	143	3.2	
	Mixed	2026	44.0	45	46.4	1981	43.9	0.199
	White	1795	39.0	28	28.9	1767	39.2	
	Black	710	15.4	22	22.7	688	15.3	
	Yellow	46	1.0	1	1.0	45	1.0	
Race/color	Indian	12	0.3	0	0.0	12	0.3	
	Illiterate	174	3.8	5	5.2	169	3.7	0.499
	1 to 8 years	1723	37.4	34	35.1	1689	37.4	
Years of education	9 years or more	2678	58.1	57	58.8	2621	58.1	
	1	496	10.8	8	8.2	488	10.8	**0.003**
	2	1243	27.0	21	21.6	1222	27.1	
	3	1217	26.4	19	19.6	1198	26.6	
	4	925	20.1	20	20.6	905	20.1	
Total of residents in the house	**5 or more**	727	15.8	**29**	**29.9**	698	15.5	
	Illiterate	74	1.6	1	1.0	73	1.6	0.074
	Basic grade	1116	24.2	24	24.7	1092	24.2	
	Middle grade	1887	41.0	**46**	**47.4**	1841	40.8	
	College	1170	25.4	14	14.4	1156	25.6	
Higher level of education in the dwell	Incomplete College level	361	7.8	12	12.4	349	7.7	
	Selected individual	4317	93.7	93	95.9	4224	93.6	0.614
	Mother	167	3.6	2	2.1	165	3.7	
	Other guardian or caretaker Father	100	2.2	1	1.0	99	2.2	
Questionnaire respondent		24	0.5	1	1.0	23	0.5	

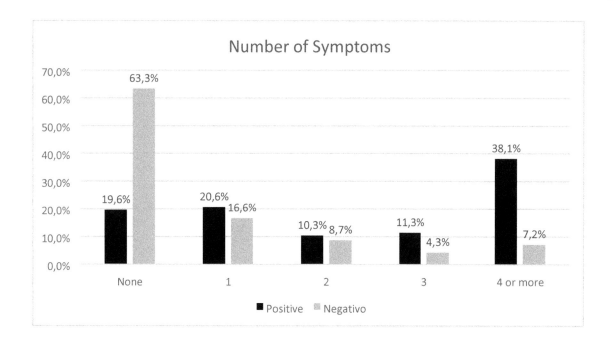

Figure 1:Number of symptoms informed by the individuals selected for the population based study of COVID-19 in Espírito Santo, Brazil – first stage (prevalence study), according to the test result.

The symptoms more frequent were anosmia and cough, also frequently reported in other surveys [23, 25].Anosmia is a distinctive feature of SARS-CoV-2 infection, being complete in 86.4% of the participants of a population-based study [25].Animal models suggest a neural propagation of the virus from the nasal cavity first to the olfactory bulb, and then to the pyriform cortex and the brainstem [26].

Symptoms were more frequent in positive individuals, indicating validity for the test and agreeing with similar results from other studies[27, 28].The information about symptoms was referent to their occurrence in the last 15 days in this study, as it was for the study conducted in south of Brazil[18], whilst other studies reported symptoms occurring in the previous thirty days[29].A longer lag time between symptoms occurrence and reporting could increase their frequencies, but, on the other hand, increases the possibility of memory bias.

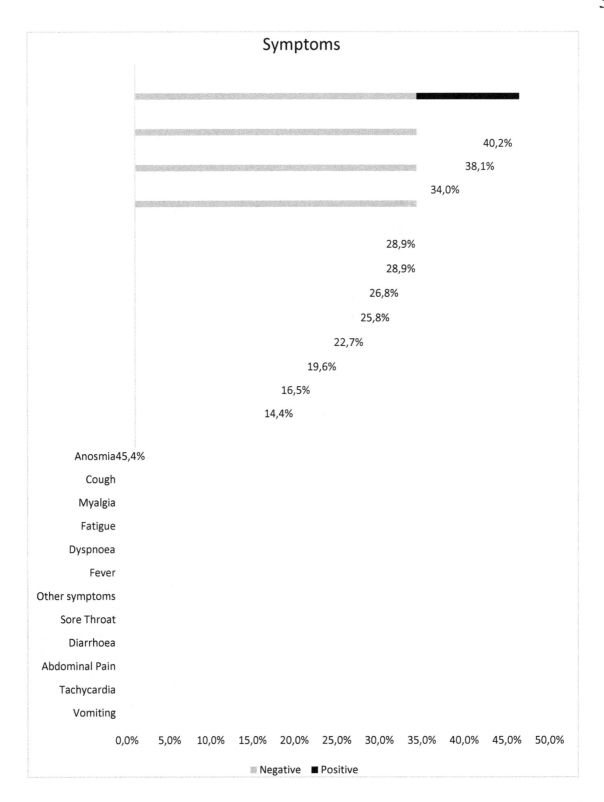

Figure 2: Frequency of symptoms informed by the individuals selected for the population-based study of COVID-19 in Espírito Santo, Brazil – first stage (prevalence study), according to the test result.

This study has several limitations. As any cross-sectional study, it is not possible to determine causality, as investigators did not measure events occurrence along time. Interviews served as the bases for data collection, giving room to information bias, particularly interviewer and memory biases. Selective survival, a type of selection bias, was possibly a consequence of the sampling procedure, as the selection included only individuals in the disease mild spectrum because of the hospital admission or death of those with the severe form of the clinical presentation. Furthermore, a sensitivity of the test lower than 90% may have enabled false-negative results, but, even in these cases, the low prevalence probably kept a high negative predictive value.

Table 3:Presence of symptomatic persons at home, search for health care services, and frequency of comorbidities among the individuals included in the population-based study of COVID-19 in Espírito Santo, Brazil – first stage (prevalence study), according to the test result.

Variable	Category	Total		Test result N = 4608				p-value
				Positive		Negative		
		N	%	N	%	N	%	
Is there a symptomatic person at home?	Yes	129	2.8	**15**	**15.5**	114	2.5	**0.001**
	No	4479	97.2	82	84.5	4397	97.5	
Search for health care unit		800	17.4	**39**	**40.2**	761	16.9	**0.001**
Systemic arterial hyperthension		1399	30.4	32	33.0	1367	30.3	0.569
Diabetes		549	11.9	**18**	**18.6**	531	11.8	**0.041**
Asthma		391	8.5	**16**	**16.5**	375	8.3	**0.004**
Neoplasia		115	2.5	2	2.1	113	2.5	0.782
Renal disease		85	1.8	3	3.1	82	1.8	0.356
Heart disease		323	7.0	5	5.2	318	7.0	0.470
Obesity		565	12.3	**22**	**22.7**	543	12.0	**0.002**
Other chronic disease		476	10.3	13	13.4	463	10.3	0.315
	none	2275	49.4	41	42.3	2234	49.5	**0.016**
	1	1282	27.8	26	26.8	1256	27.8	
	2	670	14.5	13	13.4	657	14.6	
	3	272	5.9	**11**	**11.3**	261	5.8	
	4 or more	109	2.4	**6**	**6.2**	103	2.3	
Number of comorbidities								

The detection of a 2.1% prevalence of infected individuals in the first stage of this cross-sectional study is probably a consequence of the very early application of the mitigation measures by the State Health Department. Such measures included partial social isolation and closure of schools, malls, and gyms since the detection of the first few cases by the health care system in March, as well as sanitary barriers in the motorway highways. On the other hand, this low prevalence indicates an epidemic still in its beginning capable of spreading to a huge contingent of susceptible individuals and overload the health care facilities, at the cost of many human lives. In this sense, this is vital information for the health administrators, giving them the basis for planning the correct strategies for coping with this disease. The future stages can add more help for this planning, indicating through the speed of growth of the prevalence, the need for adjustments in the mitigation strategies. An adequate analysis of the extension study will be possible only after the next stages, as the intervals are longer for this study component. Nevertheless, such analysis will be able to clarify the necessity for other measures targeted to the smaller municipalities like sanitary blockades, for example.

CONCLUSIONS

The first stage of this serial cross-sectional study disclosed a prevalence of 2.1% for infection by SARS-CoV-2 in Espírito Santo, indicating a potentially growing epidemic and the necessity of adequate strategies for its containment. Furthermore, the marked frequency of asymptomatic infected individuals and the association of the positive status with indoor clustering reinforce the need for health education and social distancing as interventions for control.

Conflicts of interest

Nésio Fernandes de Medeiros Junior is the head of the Espírito Santo Department of Health, which funded this study. The other authors declare that they have no conflicts of interest.

REFERENCES:

1. Roujian Lu, Xiang Zhao, Juan Li, Peihua Niu, Bo Yang, Honglong Wu *et al.*Genomic characterization and epidemiology of 2019 novel coronavirus:implications for virus origins and receptor binding. Lancet 2020; 395:565-74.
2. Hussin A, Rothan HA, Byrareddy SN.The epidemiology and pathogenesis of coronavirus disease (COVID-19) outbreak.J Autoimmun 2020; 109:102433.
3. Hui DS, Ia E, Madani TA, Ntoumi F, Kock R, Dar O *et al.*The continuing 2019-nCoV epidemic threat of novel coronaviruses to global health – the latest 2019 novel coronavirus outbreak in Wuhan, China.Int J Infect Dis 2020; 91:264-6.
4. Zaim S, Chong J H , Sankaranarayanan V, Harky A. COVID-19 and Multiorgan Response. Curr Probl Cardiol. 2020:100618. doi: 10.1016/j.cpcardiol.2020.100618.
5. Hopkins C, Surda P, Whitehead, E and Kumar, BN. Early recovery following new onset anosmia during the COVID-19 pandemic – an observational cohort study. J Otolaryngol Head Neck Surg. 2020;4;49(1):26. doi: 10.1186/s40463020-00423-8.
Lippi G, Sanchis-Gomar F, Henry BM.Coronavirus disease 2019 (COVID19): the portrait of a perfect storm. Ann Transl Med. 2020;8(7):497. doi: 10.21037/atm.2020.03.157.
6. Lai C-C, Li T-P, Ko W-C, Tang H-J, Hsue P-R.Respiratory syndrome coronavirus 2 (SARS-CoV-2) and coronavirus disease-2019 (COVID-19): The epidemic and the challenges.Int J Antimicrob Agents 2020; 55(3): 105924.

7. Abduljalil JM, Abduljalil BM.Mini-review epidemiology, genome, and clinical features of the pandemic SARS-CoV 2: a recent view.New Microbes New Infect 2020; 35:100672.
8. Piva S, Filippini M, Turla F, Cattaneo S, Margola A, De Fulviis S, *et al.*Clinical presentation and initial management critically ill patients with severe acute respiratory syndrome coronavirus 2 (SARS-CoV-2) infection in Brecia, Italy.J Crit Care 2020; 58:29-33.
9. Saez M, Tobias A, Varga D, Barceló MA.Effectiveness of the measures to flatten the epidemic curve of COVID-19.The case of Spain.Sci Total Environ 2020; 727:138761.
10. Wells CR, Fitzpatrick MC, Sah P, Shoukat A, Pandey A, El-Sayed AM, *et al.*Projecting the demand for ventilators at the peak of the COVID-19 outbreak in the USA.Lancet Infect Dis 2020;pii:S1473-3099(20)30315-7.
11. BOLETIM EPIDEMIOLÓGICO ESPECIAL - 16 | SE 21 - 18 de maio de 2020. Available from:https://coronavirus.saude.gov.br/index.php/boletinsepidemiologicos. Accessed 25th May 2020.
12. Gandhi M, Yokoe DS, Havlir DV.Asymptomatic transmission, the Achilles' heel of current strategies to control COVID-19.N Eng J Med 2020.doi: 10.1056/NEJMe2009758 [Epub ahead of print].
13. Instituto Brasileiro de Geografia e Estatística. Available from: https://www.ibge.gov.br/ Accessed 12th jun 2020.
14. Agência Nacional de Vigilância Sanitária – ANVISA. NOTA TÉCNICA GVIMS/GGTES/ANVISA N° 04/2020. Orientações para serviços de saúde: medidas de prevenção e controle que devem ser adotadas durante a assistência aos casos suspeitos ou confirmados de infecção pelo novo coronavírus (SARS-CoV-2). Atualizada em 08.05.2020.Available from http://portal.anvisa.gov.br/documents/33852/271858/Nota+T%C3%A9cnica +n+04-2020+GVIMS-GGTES-ANVISA/ab598660-3de4-4f14-8e6fb9341c196b28 Accessed 12th June 2020.
15. e-SUS Atenção Primária. Available from https://aps.saude.gov.br/ape/esus Accessed 12th June 2020.
16. Silveira M, Barros A, Horta B, Pellanda L, Victora G, Dellagostin O *et al.* Repeated population-based surveys of antibodies against SARS-CoV-2 in Southern Brazil.medRxiv 2020.05.01.20087205 doi: https://doi.org/10.1101/2020.05.01.20087205
17. Epidemiologia da COVID-19 no Rio Grande do Sul. Estudo de base populacional. Available from https://estado.rs.gov.br/quarta-etapa-depesquisa-aponta-estabilidade-no-total-de-infectados-por-coronavirus-no-rs Accessed 12th June 2020.
18. Study shows Spain far from having 'herd immunity' to virus. ABC News. Available from https://abcnews.go.com/Health/wireStory/study-shows-spainherd-immunity-virus-71072709 Accessed 12th June 2020.
19. Bendavid E, Mulaney B, Sood N, Shah S, Ling E, Bromley-Dulfano R *et al.* COVID-19 Antibody Seroprevalence in Santa Clara County, California. medRxiv 2020.04.14.20062463; doi: https://doi.org/10.1101/2020.04.14.200 62463
20. Gudbjartsson DF,Helgason A, Jonsson H,Magnusson OT, Melsted P, Norddahl GL *et al.* Spread of SARS-CoV-2 in the Icelandic population . N Engl J Med . 2020;382(24):2302-2315.
21. Leung GM, Lim WW, Ho LM, Lam T-H, Ghan AC, Donelly CA *et al.* Seroprevalence of IgG antibodies to SARS-coronavirus in asymptomatic or subclinical population groups. Epidemiol Infect. 2006;134, 211–221.
22. Wang Z, Ma W, Zheng X, Wu G, Zhang R. Household transmission of SARSCoV-2. J Infect 2020;81:179-182
23. Ing AJ, Cocks C, Green JP. COVID-19: in the footsteps of Ernest Shackleton. Thorax Epub ahead of print: May-12-2020;0:1–2. doi:10.1136/thoraxjnl2020-215091.
24. Hopkins C, Surda P, Whitehead E, Kumarb, BN. Early recovery following new onset anosmia during the COVID-19 pandemic –an observational cohort study. J Otolaryngol Head Neck Surg 2020; 49:26 https://doi.org/10.1186/s40463-020-00423-8
25. Dubé M, Le Coupanec A, Wong AHM, Rini JM, Desforges M, Talbot PJ.Axonal Transport Enables Neuron-to-Neuron Propagation of Human Coronavirus OC43. J Virol 2018;92 (17) e00404-18; doi: 10.1128/JVI.00404-18.
26. Xiang F, Wang X, He X, Peng Z, Yang B, Zhang J *et al.* Antibody Detection and Dynamic Characteristics in Patients with COVID19. Clin Infect Dis, ciaa461, https://doi.org/10.1093/cid/ciaa461
27. Wang Y, Tong J, Qin Y, Xie T, Li J, Li J *et al.* Characterization of an asymptomatic cohort of SARS-COV-2 infected individuals outside of Wuhan, China. Clin Infect Dis, ciaa629, https://doi.org/10.1093/cid/ciaa629
28. Garcia-Basteiro AL, Tortajada M, Vidal M, Guinovart C, Jimenez A, Santano R *et al.* Seroprevalence of antibodies against SARS-CoV-2 among health care workers in a large Spanish reference hospital. doi: https://doi.org/10.1101/2020.04.27.20082289

5. Perceptions and Experiences Regarding the Impact of Race on The Quality of Healthcare in Southeast Brazil: A Qualitative Study

Aneela Chauhan[a], Gilles de Wildt[b],
Marcos da Cunha Lopes Virmond[c,d],
Derek Kyte[e],Noemi Garcia de Almeida Galan[f],
Renata Bilion Ruiz Prado[g]
Vidya Shyam-Sundar[h]

[a] Population Sciences and Humanities, University of Birmingham, Birmingham, UK;[b]Primary Care Clinical Sciences, Institute of Clinical Sciences, University of Birmingham, Birmingham, UK; [c]Former President of the International Leprosy Association, Director at Instituto Lauro de Souza Lima, Bauru, Brazil; [d]Professor of Public Health, University of the Sacred Heart, Bauru, Brazil; [e]Centre for Patient-Reported Outcomes Research, Institute of Applied Health Research, University of Birmingham, Birmingham, UK; [f]Scientific Researcher, Therapeutic Clinical Techniques Team, Instituto Lauro de Souza Lima, Bauru, Brazil; [g]Scientific Researcher, Rehabilitation Techniques Team, Instituto Lauro de Souza Lima, Bauru, Brazil; [h]University of Birmingham, UK

ABSTRACT

Objective: To explore the impact of race on the quality of healthcare received by patients attending a primary care centre in Brazil. **Design**: This was a qualitative study consisting of 19 semi-structured interviews conducted on patients from six racial groups (as defined in Brazil as white, yellow, brown, black and indigenous and one self-identified 'other' group). The interviews were analysed using thematic analysis. **Results**: Four main themes were identified during analysis; factors affecting the access to healthcare, experiences regarding quality of healthcare, discrimination in healthcare and deep-rooted societal discrimination, which were categorised into a number of sub-themes. Within these themes, interviewees reported (1) experiences of racism in society towards the black racial group, (2) one personal perception and two observations of racial discrimination in healthcare, (3) perceived racial discrimination due to healthcare professional behaviour and (4) other factors, such as delays in appointments and long waiting times in health facilities were felt to impact access to care. **Conclusion:** The findings suggest that racial discrimination exists in Brazilian society but its direct impact on healthcare access was felt to be less obvious. Instead, organisational level factors were felt to contribute to difficulty accessing care. Interviewees perceived that racial discrimination may affect the quality of care, particularly for those designated as 'black'. Socio-economic factors were felt to influence discrimination in healthcare. The findings can help inform further studies and educational initiatives to help address discrimination and access to healthcare in Brazil.

INTRODUCTION

The population of Brazil is diverse, a product of the native indigenous population, the immigration of people from Europe, Asia, the Middle East and the importation of African slaves (Telles 2004; The Economist 2013). Alongside its North American counterparts, Brazil has a long-standing history of involvement in the slave trade. During the 16th to 19th centuries, 4.9 million black Africans were imported into Brazil (Telles 2004; The Economist 2012). This contributed to the socio-cultural views of white superiority over other racial groups (The Economist 2012). Such historically embedded views are difficult to change and, although less obvious in the twenty-first century, may still exist.

According to Bhopal (2007), race can be defined as a social construct that categorises humankind based on their physical characteristics. Racism can be subcategorised into internalised, personally mediated and institutionalised (Jones, 2000). Personally, mediated racism is prejudice and discrimination on a person to person level whereas institutionalised racism is differential treatment at an organisation level (Jones, 2000). Internalised racism is when members of the affected group accept the negative comments and undermine their own self-worth (Jones, 2000). Currently there is no universal classification of race.As a result, categorisation varies from country to country making the collection of data on an individual's race a complex, multidimensional process.

In Brazil, the official classification of race is based solely around the colour of a person's skin resulting in the formation of 5 main racial groups: brancos (white), amarelos (yellow), pardos (brown), pretos (black) and indigenous (Bhopal, 2007; Censo Demográfico 2011).

Taking Brazil's history into consideration, it is interesting that non-white citizens make up the majority of its population (52.3%) (Censo Demográfico 2011). In contrast to this, the United Kingdom categorises race based on both skin colour and ethnic descent through self-identification (Bhopal, 2007). These differences in the classification of race may affect the perceptions of race and the extent of racism in different countries. Brazil prides itself on being a racially integrated society that promotes racial equality. The Sistema Único de Saúde (SUS) established in 1988 follows this principle by providing 'universal and equal access to health services' (Telles, 2004; WHO 2008). Even with the promotion of racial equality, huge economic and health disparities have persisted between different racial groups (The Economist 2012; Drumond et al. 2013). While socio-economic status is strongly associated with health, there may be further health disparities due to unequal access to healthcare (Adler et al. 1994).

Internationally, numerous studies have identified inequalities in health and access to healthcare secondary to race, with some showing the black racial group, in particular, to be disadvantaged (Murrell et al. 1996; Boyer-Chammard, Taylor, and Anton-Culver 1999; Janevic et al. 2011; MacDorman and Mathews, 2011; Souza de Bairros et al, 2011; Quach et al, 2012; Trad, Castellanos, and Guimaraes 2012; Emmanuelli et al. 2015). However, many of these studies were conducted in the United States of America therefore the findings may lack generalisability to the Brazilian population. Literature searches have revealed conflicting results in relation to the impact of race and discrimination in healthcare in Brazil. Whilst Macinko et al. (2012) and Blay et al. (2008) found that racial discrimination was not perceived by patients when accessing healthcare services; several other studies found that accessibility to healthcare services varied depending on race (Vieira and Souza 2009; Souza de Bairros et al. 2011). Trad, Castellanos, and Guimaraes (2012) investigated the accessibility of primary healthcare by black families in Salvador and found that many factors were perceived to affect access, two of which were: belonging to the black race and being poor.

Poor socio-economic status was more strongly associated with discrimination than skin colour. The limitations of this study are that only black families were interviewed therefore no comparisons with other racial groups were made. Additionally, this paper only concentrated on primary care access. Further research needs to be conducted involving a variety of racial groups and healthcare services in order to gain a fuller overview and allow comparisons to be made. This study therefore aimed to investigate the experiences and perceptions regarding the accessibility and quality of healthcare in patients from different racial groups, attending a Primary Care Centre in Brazil. The two primary aims of this study were: 1) to explore peoples' experiences when accessing a range of healthcare facilities in Southeast Brazil and 2) to explore peoples' perceptions and beliefs about the impact of race on the quality of healthcare. A secondary aim in this study was to investigate patients' beliefs and perceptions about racism and discrimination in Brazilian society to provide appropriate cultural context and explore whether societal discrimination bears any influence on patients' experiences of healthcare.

METHODS

Research Design and Sampling

This was a qualitative study that took place in a Primary Care Centre in the city of Bauru, Southeast Brazil over a period of 6 weeks in 2016. Data was gathered using face-to-face, semi-structured interviews, which explored participants' experiences and beliefs regarding healthcare access, quality of care and discrimination. Given the potentially sensitive nature of the discussion topic, individual interviews were chosen to allow participants to feel more comfortable to speak honestly. At the time of the study there were 38 healthcare professionals (HCPs) interacting with users in the Primary Care Centre (11 doctors, 3 nurses, 2 dentists, 2 dental assistants, 13 health assistants, 1 physical therapist, 1 nutritionist, 1 phonologist and 4 administrative assistants), 81.5% of which were female and 92.1% white. Most of them (65%) were only working in this health care centre, with an average load of 34 h a week. Inclusion criteria were patients: i) registered and attending the Primary Care centre through the government-run SUS, ii) over the age of 18, iii) able and willing to give informed consent and iv) able to speak Portuguese or English fluently. Purposive sampling was used to identify participants from all five racial groups in Brazil and with a range of demographics. This was done to increase the breadth of experiences and investigate the impact of racism on a wider scale resulting in a richer data set.

Recruitment and Interviewing Procedure

Potential participants were recruited by NG or RB, who were researchers from the Instituto Lauro de Souza Lima (ILSL). Suitable participants were identified in the waiting room at the health centre by HCPs at the centre alongside NG or RB, using an eligibility sheet as an aid. Eligible patients were approached, and the study was explained to them using a script provided by AC, the primary researcher. If interest was expressed, full information was given to the participant and informed consent was obtained. The interviews were conducted by NG/RB, using an iterative topic guide (Table 1). AC was present to take field notes. A verbal summary of the interview was relayed to AC at the close, to allow reflection and alteration of the interview style and questions.

A piloting phase was undertaken during the first week of interviewing. Minor modifications were made to the topic guide based on discussions with the interviewer after the pilot interviews. For example, it became clear that the word 'race' was not understood by all participants therefore the term 'skin colour' was used instead. All interviews were conducted in Brazilian Portuguese and were audio-recorded.

ANALYSIS

The audio-recordings were transcribed verbatim and translated into English directly from the Portuguese recording, by an independent qualified translator. AC conducted the primary analysis, after data collection was complete, using Braun and Clarke's (2006) six step process to thematic analysis. This analytical approach was used due to its flexibility in the analysis of the data allowing unexpected themes to be included. Data collection and analysis was conducted taking into consideration a constructivist epistemological stance held by the primary researcher. Repeated readings of the transcripts were undertaken to achieve familiarisation with the overall nature of the data. The early coding process drew upon Jones (2000) Theoretical Framework on the levels of racism. However, this framework could only be used to code racism related responses hence inductive coding was applied to the rest of the data (Saldana, 2013).

As shown by the themes, there were numerous factors, not just racial discrimination, found to affect accessibility and quality of healthcare therefore, Jones' framework[5] did not have a significant influence on theme identification.

Initially, in vivo and descriptive coding were used. This progressed to applying process codes in the second cycle of coding (Saldana, 2013). Therefore, initially a theoretical approach to analysis was taken which developed into a predominately data-led, inductive approach making thematic analysis an appropriate methodology due to its flexibility. The data analysis and management process was aided by the use of NVivo qualitative data analysis software (version 10). Once coding was complete, a list of 478 codes was compiled. Related codes were grouped together using lists and mind maps to examine the relationships between them to formulate sub-themes and overarching themes. Subsequently, the entire data set was re-read ensuring that the themes were appropriate.

Extracts were chosen by reading through the quotes complied under each sub-theme and picking the most appropriate quotes to illustrate the finding. The appropriateness of the quote was based on AC's judgement after immersion in the data. Minor errors in translation were corrected by re-reading the relevant transcript and listening to the audio-recording with GdW, who is a Portuguese speaker. It was crucial to maintain reflexive practice throughout the data collection and analysis process in order to be aware and interrogate researcher preconceptions and ensure that when analysing the results they had minimal conscious influence on theme formation. It was important to consider the potential impact that the researchers may have had on the data.

Table 1. Interview Topic Guide

Area to be discussed	Questions
Introduction/explanation to patient Introductory questions	Please could you tell me a little bit about your health? . Why have you come to the health centre today? . Why do you normally attend this centre? . Do you have any health conditions that you seek medical attention for?
Experience/ quality of care	If they have any health conditions: How did you come to be diagnosed with this condition? . Probe: which health services did you come into contact with? . Probe: What was your experience of these? How do you feel about your care at these healthcare facilities? . If not good: why? Reasons? . Have you ever felt discriminated against when you were receiving care? . Why do you think this is? If they do not have any medical conditions: Have you attended any healthcare facilities in the past? . Probe: What are your feelings about the care you received at this facility? . Probe: Can you tell me about your experience at this health centre? . Have you ever felt discriminated against when you were receiving care? . Why do you think this is?
Accessibility	How accessible have you found the health services that you have needed? . In what ways/ why or why not accessible? . Any challenges/ barriers?
Discrimination (if not brought up in other questions)	Have you ever been made to feel uncomfortable or discriminated against in a healthcare setting? . Probe: Can you tell me about this experience . Probe: Why did you feel uncomfortable/ discriminated against? Have you ever been made to feel uncomfortable or discriminated against in any other places? . General life, education, work etc. How did you feel when you experienced this? . Why do you think people would discriminate against you?
Race	What racial group would you identify yourself as? . What do you understand by the term racism? . What is your opinion about racism in Brazil? Do you feel that your skin colour has affected your access to healthcare? . How? Do you feel that your skin colour has affected the quality of healthcare? . How? Do you think other people from your racial group may have similar thought about this? Do you think people from other races would have been treated in the same way as you have been treated? Have you ever experienced racism when accessing or receiving care? . Can you tell me more about this? In Brazilian society there are many different racial groups. Do you think that the colour of a person's skin affects their access to healthcare? . How do you think it affects this? . In your opinion, are there any groups in general that are affected more than others?
Closing	Do you have any other things that you would like to tell me?

The fact that the interviewers are white, native Brazilians and that AC is a British person of Indian parentage may have influenced the questioning or participant responses during data collection. Analyst triangulation was conducted by VS to increase the credibility of the results (Patton 2002). This comprised reading 20% of the original transcripts and examining the derived codes and themes. This method also ensured that analysis was not unduly influenced by the primary researcher's preconceptions and allowed the identification of alternative interpretations of the data thus facilitating reflexivity. This project was approved by the BMedSc Population Sciences and Humanities Internal Ethics Review Committee at the University of Birmingham and the Research Ethics Committee at Instituto Lauro de Souza Lima (Reference numbers: 2015–2016/ C2/SF and 53623916.7.0000.5475 respectively). Data will be archived according to the University's code of practice, for 10 years.

Participant Characteristics

Data saturation was reached at 19 interviews. The interviews were on average 32 minutes in duration. The characteristics of the interviewees are summarised in Table 2. Interviewees belonging to all five racial groups were sampled in this study; white (n = 6, 31.6%), yellow (n = 2, 10.5%), brown (n = 4, 21.0%), black (n = 5, 26.3%), indigenous (n = 1, 5.3%) and other (n = 1, 5.3%). There appeared to be a disparity regarding self-identified and observed race in 15.8% of the participants; similar to Telles' (2002) study. This racial ambiguity is due to the fact that race in Brazil is measured on a colour spectrum (Telles 2004; Bhopal 2007). For the purposes of this study, self-identified race will be used because the interviewees' beliefs and experiences will be based on their perceived race. There were twelve females and seven males interviewed; representative of the population visiting primary care centres as females tend to use healthcare services more than males (Travassos et al. 2002). The age of the participants ranged from 22–70 years. A large proportion (n = 16, 84.2%) of the participants were above the age of 41. This appears consistent with the use of healthcare services in Brazil as underutilisation of healthcare is more prevalent in younger age groups, particularly below the age of 30 (Boccolini and de Souza Junior 2016). In terms of education, majority of participants (n = 12, 63.2%) had completed up to Primary school 1 or 2. One participant did not complete primary school and six participants had completed secondary school or above.

Table 2. Participant Demographic Table

Demographic	Proportion (n, %)
Gender Male	
	7, 36.8
Female	12, 63.2
Age 18–25	
	2, 10.5
26–40	1, 5.3
41–60	10, 52.6
>60	6, 31.6
Race (self-identified) White	
	6, 31.6
Yellow	2, 10.5
Brown	4, 21.1
Black	5, 26.3
Indigenous	1, 5.3
Other	1, 5.3
Race (observed) White	
	7, 36.8
Yellow	2, 10.5
Brown	3, 15.8
Black	6, 31.6
Indigenous	1, 5.3
Religion Catholic	
	8, 42.1
Protestant	8, 42.1
Christian (not specified)	3, 15.8
Education	
Read and write	1, 5.3
Primary school 1 (First 5 years of school)	6, 31.6
Primary school 2 (Next 9 years of education)	6, 31.6
Secondary school	5, 26.3
College or University	1, 5.3

FINDINGS

Four main themes were identified from the data; 1) Factors affecting the access to healthcare, 2) Experiences regarding quality of healthcare, 3) Discrimination in healthcare and 4) Deep-rooted societal discrimination. The themes were then split into various subthemes as illustrated by Figure 1. Major themes and their sub-themes are summarised below.

Factors Affecting The Access To Healthcare

Interviewees reported mixed experiences regarding the accessibility of health services, identifying both barriers to accessing the health system as a whole; and specific factors that facilitated access.

Delays In The Health System

A majority of the participants (n = 18, 94.7%) identified barriers to accessing the health system. The negative experiences reported by participants were centred around delays and difficulties accessing services in a variety of healthcare settings. This included delays in receiving appointments, long waiting times in health facilities, and delays in receiving test results and treatment. Such issues were attributed to a supply and demand problem. It was believed that there were not enough appointments and HCPs available to manage the high demand for health services, particularly in the public health setting.

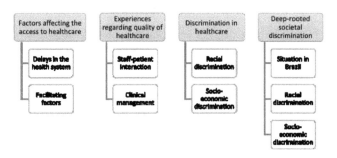

Figure 1. Flow Chart of Themes and Subthemes

The time it takes to get an appointment is the biggest problem. It is too long ... . At 7 they distribute the numbers so I need to arrive at 5 to be among the first 20 [patients] otherwise I don't get it. There are many people here ... they would not be here if they didn't need it [Participant 2, Black] D There were too many people and only two doctors for everybody [Participant 58, Brown]

Delays In Receiving Appointment

However, delays in other aspects of the service such as scheduling investigations and receiving test results, were evident in both primary and hospital care in the public health system. Interviewees stated that the main difference between the public and private sector was that the private service was faster. These problems were experienced by participants from all racial groups.

It was very difficult for me and I know it was not because of my colour or race or anything like that, it's a problem with the whole of Brazil. It's been difficult for the health system [Participant 98, Yellow]The only difference is the private service is faster [Participant 11, White]

Facilitating Factors

Interviewees recounted some positive experiences regarding access to healthcare services. In terms of appointment scheduling, accessibility was facilitated if the participant tended to book routine appointments for monitoring of chronic conditions. For example, participant 15 was having regular monitoring for hypertension in the primary care centre.

My appointments are always with Dr. [Anonymised], after the appointment we immediately schedule the next one.[Participant 15, White]

Personal connections within the health centres was also identified as a facilitating factor as this was shown to increase the availability of appointments. Some participants expressed having personal experience of this whilst others expressed a belief that this eased access to health services.

I only gained access because I had a friend who started working here who got it for me because I came here and I couldn't get [an appointment] [Participant 98, Yellow]The ones who have easy access are the ones who know somebody in the system [Participant 86, White]

Experiences regarding quality of healthcare

Interviewees reported mixed experiences regarding the quality of care. These experiences revolved around staff attitude and communication as well as the clinical management of their condition. The majority of interviewees expressed positive experiences.

> I was very well treated ... I've never been disrespected [Participant 35, Yellow]

Staff-Patient Interaction

With regards to attitude and communication of staff members, the majority of experiences appeared to be positive. This involved interactions between the patient and a variety of HCPs such as doctors and nurses. Some interviewees reported feelings of appreciation towards the HCPs and believed that the HCPs felt genuine concern and empathy towards them. This led to a positive patient experience in the healthcare setting resulting in patient satisfaction about the quality of care received.

> *The nurses used to treat me and the other patients with affection; whenever I got back to the hospital they would talk to us and ask how the treatment was going. They used to be sad because of our situation [Participant 15, White]*

> *The doctor was wonderful. I think she gave me a lot of attention and was very dedicated when she spoke to me so I wasn't uncomfortable to talk to her about my problems [Participant 98, Yellow]*

Some negative experiences regarding staff interaction and communication were identified. Participants discussed experiences during consultations with HCPs and other observations in healthcare settings including poor attitude from reception staff. They felt that the HCP's behaviour affected the quality of care and amount of attention received.

> *There was a doctor ... He was so rude to me. I told my husband I would never come back to see this doctor again. He told me: 'you are a mess!' screaming at me, 'You're going to lose your leg! I said to him 'hey this is not the way you should talk to me' but he kept going on [Participant 2, Black]*

> *The nurses keep talking and looking at their phones looking at photos instead of assisting us. It's terrible! [Participant 58, Brown]*

The participants interpreted these negative experiences in two ways. A few participants perceived their experience to be due to racial prejudice by staff; however, the majority believed their experience was due to the general attitude and communication of that individual. In addition, for interviewees' experiences, no obvious trend was found in relation to racial groups.

Clinical Management

Interviewees expressed both positive and negative beliefs regarding the quality of care received throughout their diagnosis and treatment. Positive views conveyed the efficiency of the diagnostic process and the high quality of treatment received.

> *I was well treated in my opinion because I was pregnant. When I got to the doctor's office, the doctor already knew what has happened to me. [Participant 72, Black]*

It was excellent. My surgery was a success and the Doctor was very careful with me and gave me all the attention, I didn't have any problems after the surgery. I felt very safe because the doctor gave me all the support ... The Doctor who did my surgery was excellent. [Participant 98, Yellow]

A number of interviewees reported negative experiences and beliefs concerning their clinical management. Some expressed feelings of frustration due to medication errors whilst others felt that lack of adequate monitoring and attention by HCPs had impacted on their healthcare. These negative experiences were reported in both the public and private sector.

She [the Doctor] said to my granddaughter that it was an allergic cough and gave her a prescription ... My granddaughter got worse. Then I started reading the prescribing information leaflet but after reading it I didn't give it to my granddaughter, I bought it and didn't give her because it said for those who need chemotherapy, tuberculosis ... Next day I was at [hospital] to see another doctor ... showed the medication and told him that I hadn't given it to my granddaughter ... He said that it was not the correct medication and that I was lucky because I hadn't given it to her. [Participant 35, Yellow]

Positive and negative experiences were identified across a range of racial groups and therefore did not exhibit any obvious trends in relation to race.

Discrimination In Healthcare

Participants discussed their experiences and beliefs about discrimination in the healthcare setting. In addition, to racial discrimination, beliefs and perceptions regarding socio-economic discrimination emerged as an additional discriminatory factor.

Racial Discrimination

The majority of participants (n = 16, 84.2%) reported no personal experiences or observations of discrimination in healthcare. This perception appeared to be present in a variety of racial groups. Several participants that reported negative experiences in healthcare did not believe that these were associated with racial discrimination.

At all places I went, three health centres like here, I felt like a common citizen without any discrimination [Participant 4, White]
No. Discriminated no. [Participant 54, Brown]

There were few first-hand experiences of racial discrimination in healthcare (n = 3, 15.8%). There was one personal perception, and two observations; one of reception staff and the other of a doctor. However, these experiences were not of active racial discrimination, defined as 'blatant, intentional acts of racial discrimination' (Tatum 2003), by HCPs but perceived by the patient to be due to race. The personal account of racial discrimination was towards a black participant who perceived that the negative behaviour of the HCP was due to her skin colour and that a white person would get more attention.

Once I asked to change my gynaecologist in the private clinic because she didn't even care when I entered the room, she stayed sitting on the other side of the table, didn't even look at me, only asked some questions and order the investigations.

-And do you think it is racial discrimination?
-Yes.
-Do you think that if it were a white person she would give more attention?
-Yes, I do. [Participant 2, Black]

The observations were from participants who did not belong to the black racial group. Both participants perceived differential treatment of black or dark-skinned patients; one resulting in problems accessing healthcare due to discrimination by a receptionist and the other resulting in poor quality of care by a HCP.

> *I compare the way they treated my grand daughters, the brunette was not treated the same as the yellow ones. Even in the way they talk to them. I've seen that in the private clinic too. I've seen it happen and with the same doctor she talked to one of my granddaughters in one way and to the other one in a very different way. I always paid much attention to them and I didn't like this way of treating my granddaughters so I said to myself I will change this doctor. [Participant 35, Yellow (Japanese Ancestry)]*

Although few experiences of racial discrimination were identified, over half of the participants (n = 10, 53%) believed that racial discrimination exists in the healthcare setting, towards the black racial group. Even participants who had not personally experienced or observed any racial discrimination believed that racism could exist in healthcare. Some participants felt that their skin colour affected their healthcare experience. They perceived a negative attitude or less attention from HCPs. Other participants felt that racism had not affected their healthcare but acknowledged the possibility of it affecting other races, particularly the black racial group. Several of these beliefs and perceptions were based on hearsay of racial discrimination in healthcare. The type of discrimination appeared to be subtle, mainly revolving around the HCPs' attitude and communication.

> *Many times you see people giving more attention to the other [racial groups] ... you can see it only in the way they look at you [Participant 2, Black]*
>
> *I think if I were white, people would treat me better. They would be nicer and talk to me longer [Participant 58, Brown]*
>
> *They talk to me more. They give me more attention [Participant 67, White]*

When discussing racial discrimination, participants highlighted that in their opinion, black patients are more likely to be discriminated against because their racial group is associated with stereotypes of crime and being poor.

> *They think that because they are black that they are poor or a criminal, unfortunately. And it's not only the health services it's everywhere. [Participant 98, Yellow]*
>
> *Many people associate your behaviour with your colour. People think that because you're black you are not a good person, that you cannot be trusted. This is ridiculous. [Participant 72, Black]*

Alternatively, some interviewees felt that racism does not exist in the healthcare setting and believed that all racial groups are treated equally. Several participants based this on their own experiences of accessing healthcare. This belief did not appear to be associated with the participant's racial group.

> *I don't believe that they would pass a white person before a black person, there is no need for that. [Participant 93, White]*
>
> *I don't believe so. I've seen other people having the same treatment as me. If I had seen it I would be the first to complain [Participant 37, Brown]*

Socio-Economic Discrimination

During discussions it became clear that a number of participants felt that socio-economic status impacted on the access to and quality of healthcare. Similar to racial discrimination, there were few first-hand experiences and three observations of socio-economic discrimination.

It was terrible! I asked the nurse why it was taking so long and she said: "why don't you pay a private one?" [Participant 58, Brown]I've seen a lot of people being treated badly. The poor people, mainly because they are dirty. [Participant 25, Black]

In contrast, some participants did not report any experiences of socio-economic discrimination in healthcare. Despite this, a number of interviewees expressed beliefs of socioeconomic discrimination (n = 9, 47%) where people of a lower socio-economic status are disadvantaged in terms of accessibility and treatment by HCPs, revolving around assistance and communication. Again, participants that had not observed socio-economic discrimination still believed that it could exist in healthcare.

We see here even the simplest person not being treated badly but out there I am sure it happens, because we see on the news that it has happened [Participant 17, Black]Once in the emergency room, I saw a very well dressed child and many people believed he would be treated better [Participant 67, White]

Deep-Rooted Societal Discrimination

Throughout the interviews, participants discussed a number of situations relating to discrimination in general life. These can be separated into: 1) racial discrimination and 2) socio-economic discrimination.

Situation in Brazil

There was a common belief that racism and discrimination in Brazil is a widespread problem in all aspects of life. It was felt that discrimination exists: between racial groups and within racial groups. Discrimination between racial groups was thought to be racially motivated, mainly directed at the black race whereas discrimination within racial groups was based on perceived socio-economic status.

Black people have problems everywhere, not only the health services. I think that people when they see a black person, the Brazilian people normally look differently to the black people. [Participant 98, Yellow]
I also know black people who discriminated black people [Participant 72, Black]

All participants emphasised their beliefs that society should be equal and expressed feelings of hopelessness towards the resolution of discrimination. In addition, interviewees reported that racism is a man-made phenomenon and its existence is due to lack of progression from deeply, embedded historical views.

I think it is cultural because of the time the black people were slaves [Participant 2, Black]
No matter the colour you have, everybody is equal. What defines the person is your character and your morals. [Participant 67, White]

Racial Discrimination

Within society, interviewees reported many experiences of racial discrimination. Personal experiences affected the black racial group and participants from other races spoke about their observations of such discrimination.

I worked at a bus station and I was attending a customer, another one arrived and interrupted me. I asked her to wait a little to finish with the customer that I was already attending. She called me a nigger and stupid [Participant 25, Black]

You see this with the police, if they see a car coming with four white people inside that is no problem but if they see a car with four black men inside, it's a robbery [Participant 93, White]

Socio-Economic Discrimination

Socio-economic discrimination in society was experienced across a range of racial groups. Some interviewees felt that people with a lower socio-economic status were given less attention and experienced negative behaviour.

The worst is in the shops. The people discriminate the poor because of the way we dress. For example the people who come from the rural areas and they need to buy something then they see the dirty clothes and they think we don't have money to pay. [Participant 90, Indigenous]

In the healthcare setting, a participant who was perceived to be from a higher social group felt discrimination from patients, rather than HCPs, for using the public health system, SUS.

From people who are next to you who think ... "there are people who shouldn't be using the SUS", maybe because of our race they think I am rich [Participant 35, Yellow]

DISCUSSION AND PRINCIPAL FINDINGS

In this study, there were no experiences of direct racial discrimination in the healthcare setting. However, few participants (n = 3,15.8%) perceived negative behaviour of HCPs and staff to be due to racial prejudice. This perceived racial discrimination appears to be the personally mediated type (Jones, 2000).These experiences and observations suggest, that if present, racism may affect the way patients are communicated with by HCPs, rather than necessarily directly affecting the clinical management of the patient and outcomes.

It appears to be more subtle than experiences demonstrated in society. In addition, there were mixed beliefs regarding the impact of racism on healthcare services, with majority of participants believing that racial discrimination influences healthcare. It was believed that the impact of race in healthcare appeared to be subtle mainly affecting the amount of assistance that patients would receive and staff behaviour. Interviewees reported a perception that discrimination was often directed towards the black racial group; consistent with Murrell et al. (1996) where beliefs regarding differential treatment of the black patients were reported in the United States of America. In Bahia state, Trad, Castellanos, and Guimaraes (2012) reported few perceptions of subtle discrimination in healthcare. The findings of our study conducted in São Paulo state which is mainly white, are consistent with those in Bahia where the racial composition is predominately black or brown (Censo Demográfico 2011). This suggests that the perceptions and beliefs regarding black discrimination are not confined to one part of Brazil. However, further research in other parts of Brazil is needed to substantiate these findings.

Responses regarding racial discrimination in society suggested the existence of widespread, obvious racism towards the black racial group, not only personal discrimination but observations from participants belonging to other races. These findings are consistent with related research, where racism was perceived by people who identify themselves as black in a variety of social situations including employment and education (Murrell 1996; Macinko 2012). Participants' beliefs regarding racial discrimination in healthcare may have been influenced by their experiences of societal racism.

Socio-economic discrimination was identified as a potential factor for affecting healthcare. The few experiences and observations discussed, suggest that this may affect quality of care through HCP behaviour and access to services for people with a lower socio-economic status. Some participants expressed a belief that black people are discriminated against due to negative stereotypes linked with their racial group. For example, blacks are associated with poverty, crime and slavery. This suggests that racial and socio-economic discrimination sit hand-in-hand resulting in a double disadvantage for people belonging to the black race, both in healthcare and society. This is emphasised by research showing that a disproportionate number of black and brown citizens are socially disadvantaged in terms of income, poverty and education further suggesting the intertwining nature of socio-economic and racial discrimination (Telles and Lim 1998; Telles 2004; The Economist 2012). Since majority of people living in poverty are non-white (Skidmore 1995; Telles and Lim 1998), this may indicate that race indirectly affects healthcare and that socio-economic status is actually the primary discriminatory factor.

Melo et al. (2016) found that socioeconomic status and race were found to affect access to mammography in Brazil, although the significance of these factors varied depending on the region investigated. Other issues identified in the interviews were the delays in the health system and factors facilitating accessibility. Institutional racism did not appear to play a role. Instead, it seemed that these factors were due to a widespread, organisation level problem. Furthermore, similar barriers to accessibility, such as long waiting times and referral to specialist services were identified in Dilelio et al.'s (2015) and Borghi et al. (2015) studies. Although the study participants in Borghi et al.'s (2015) study were indigenous people, the authors observed that delays in treatment occurred in the entire population.

Strengths and Limitations

A strength of this study is the semi-structured interview format which allowed exploration of novel issues affecting access and quality of healthcare raised by the participant themselves. In addition, the use of purposive sampling led to the inclusion of members from each racial group, allowing informative comparisons of experiences. Analyst triangulation was conducted in order to increase the credibility of the data and address any potential analyst bias.

Finally, during the pilot interviews, two additional researchers were present, observing non-verbal communication. This allowed modification of the interview questions and style based on a consensus between three researchers. A limitation was that the interviews were conducted in Portuguese, meaning the lead researcher could not guide probing of participant responses. However, this method was deemed necessary to maximise participant acceptability and allow them to feel more comfortable throughout the interview. Although the interviews explored participants' experiences in all healthcare facilities they had accessed, a potential shortcoming is that the findings may predominantly relate to the health centre where recruitment took place. The sample only included participants who were present at the health centre for an appointment and not the general public therefore the results may not be transferrable to other patient groups. Concurrent data collection and analysis was not possible due to delays in the transcription and translation process. To address this, modifications were implemented based on discussions with the interviewers. Finally, all of the translations could not be double-checked for accuracy however some quotations from 16 interviews were checked and improved with GdW.

Implications of The Research

Based on the findings of this study, there is scope for further qualitative studies in other parts of Brazil on this topic. In addition, the results have highlighted the need for further investigation into the organisation of healthcare in Brazil as this was a notable finding in this study. These qualitative studies can inform large-scale, quantitative studies in order to investigate the magnitude of the problem and generalisability of the findings. This study adds to the evidence base regarding the impact of discrimination in healthcare and society. The findings can help to inform educational initiatives in health services and society to address discrimination in all its forms including racism. For example, training programmes can be implemented at a primary care level in order to educate HCPs and staff regarding the effects of racial and social discrimination. In addition, the findings can also inform initiatives at an organisational level to improve accessibility.

CONCLUSION

Interviewees suggested few Brazilians may have direct experience of impaired healthcare access secondary to racial discrimination. Rather, participants felt other non-racially driven factors, such as delays in the health system affected healthcare access for participants belonging to all racial groups. Instead, interviewees gave examples regarding their perceptions showing that those designated as 'black', were more likely to affect the quality of care received through negative HCP behaviour. Socio-economic factors, including income and educational level, were also felt to influence discrimination in the healthcare setting.

Acknowledgements

I wish to thank the staff and participants at the Health centre for their support and participation. I would like to acknowledge the University of Birmingham for providing the opportunity to carry out this research and for their continuing support. I wish to acknowledge and thank the Yorke Williams Bequest for their support. I would also like to thank the translator for the transcription and translation of the transcripts.

Funding:

This study was supported by the University of Birmingham.

REFERENCES

Adler, N. E., T. Boyce, M. A. Chesney, S. Cohen, S. Folkman, R. L. Kahn, and S. L. Syme. (1994). "Socioeconomic Status and Health: The Challenge of the Gradient." American Psychologist 49 (1): 15–24.

Bhopal, R. S. (2007). Ethnicity, Race and Health in Multicultural Societies. 1st ed.New York: Oxford University Press Inc.

Blay, S. L., G. G. Fillenbaum, S. B. Andreoli, and F. L. Gastal. (2008). "Equity of Access to Outpatient Care and Hospitalization among Older Community Residents in Brazil." Medical Care 46 (9): 930–937. doi:10.1097/MLR.0b013e318179254c.

Boccolini, C. S., and P. R. B. de Souza Junior. (2016). "Inequalities in Healthcare Utilization: Results of the Brazilian National Health Survey, 2013." International Journal for Equity in Health 15: 1778. doi:10.1186/s12939-016-0444-3.

Borghi, A. C., A. M. Alvarez, S. S. Marcon, and L. Carreira. (2015). "Cultural Singularities: Indigenous Elderly Access to Public Health Service." Revista da Escola de Enfermagem da USP 49 (4): 0589– 0595. doi:10.1590/S0080-623420150000400008.

Boyer-Chammard, A., T. H. Taylor, and H. Anton-Culver. (1999). "Survival Differences in Breast Cancer among Racial/Ethnic Groups: A Population-Based Study." Cancer Detection and Prevention 23 (6): 463–473.

Braun, V., and V. Clarke. (2006). "Using Thematic Analysis in Psychology." Qualitative Research in Psychology 3 (2): 77–101.

Censo Demográfico (Instituto Brasileiro de Geografia e Estatística. Censo Demográfico 2010). 2011. http://biblioteca.ibge.gov.br/visualizacao/periodicos/93/cd_2010_caracteristicas_populacao_ domicilios.pdf.

Dilélio, A. S., E. Tomasi, E. Thumé, D. S. Silveira, F. C. V. Siqueira, R. X. Piccini, S. M. Silva, B. P. Nunes, and L. A. Facchini. (2015). "Lack of Access and Continuity of Adult Health Care: a National Population-Based Survey." Revista de Saúde Pública 49: 384.

Drumond, E., D. M. Abreu, C. Machado, F. Gomes, and E. Franca. (2013). "Racial Disparities and Avoidable Infant Mortality in a City of Southeastern Brazil, 2001–09." Journal of Tropical Pediatrics 59 (1): 23–28. doi:10.1093/tropej/fms039.

The Economist. (2012). Race in Brazil: Affirming the divide. Accessed December 7, 2015. http://www. economist.com/node/21543494.

The Economist. (2013). Affirmative action in Brazil: Slavery's legacy.

Emmanuelli, B., A. A. Kucner, M. Ostapiuck, F. Tomazoni, B. A. Agostini, and T. M. Ardenghi. (2015). "Racial Differences in Oral Health-Related Quality of Life: A Multilevel Analysis in Brazilian Children." Brazilian Dental Journal 26 (6): 689–694. doi:10.1590/0103-6440201300478.

Janevic, T., P. Sripad, E. Bradley, and V. Dimitrievska. (2011). "'There's no Kind of Respect Here': A Qualitative Study of Racism and Access to Maternal Health Care among Romani Women in the Balkans." International Journal for Equity in Health 10 (53), doi:10.1186/14759276-10-53.

Jones, C. (2000). "Levels of Racism: A Theoretic Framework and a Gardener's Tale." American Journal of Public Health 90 (8): 1212–1215.

MacDorman, M. F., and T. J. Mathews. (2011). "Understanding Racial and Ethnic Disparities in U.S. Infant Mortality Rates." National Centre for Health Statistics Data Briefing(s) (74): 1–8.

Macinko, J., P. Mullachery, F. A. Proietti, and M. F. Lima-Costa. (2012). "Who Experiences Discrimination in Brazil? Evidence from a Large Metropolitan Region." International Journal for Equity in Health 11: 80. doi:10.1186/1475-9276-11-80.

Melo, E. C. P., E. X. G. de Oliveira, D. Chor, M. S. Cavalho, and R. S. Pinheiro. (2016). "Inequalities in Socioeconomic Status and Race and the Odds of Undergoing a Mammogram in Brazil." International Journal for Equity in Health 15: 986. doi:10.1186/s12939-016-0435-4.

Murrell, N., R. Smith, G. Gill, and G. Oxley. (1996). "Racism and Health Care Access: A Dialogue with Childbearing Women." Health Care for Women International 17: 149–159. doi:10.1080/ 07399339609516229.

Patton, M. Q. (2002). Qualitative Research and Evaluation Methods. 3rd ed.Thousand Oaks, CA: SAGE Publication, Inc.

Quach, T., A. Nuru-Jeter, P. Morris, L. Allen, S. J. Shema, J. K. Winters, G. M. Le, and S. L. Gomez. (2012). "Experiences and Perceptions of Medical Discrimination among a Multiethnic Sample of Breast Cancer Patients in the Greater San Francisco Bay Area, California." American Journal of Public Health 102 (5): 1027–1034.

Saldana, J. (2013). The Coding Manual for Qualitative Researchers. 2nd ed.Los Angeles: SAGE Publications.

Skidmore, T. (1995). "Fact and Myth: Discovering a Racial Problem in Brazil." In Population, Ethnicity, and Nation-Building, edited by C. Goldscheider, 91–117. Boulder: Westview Press.

Souza de Bairros, F., S. N. Meneghel, J. Dias da Costa, D. Bassani, A. M. B. Menezes, D. Gigante, and M. T. Olinto. (2011). "Racial Inequalities in Access to Women's Health Care in Southern Brazil." Cadernos de Saúde Pública 27 (12): 2364–2372.

Tatum, B. D. (2003). "Why are All the Black Kids Sitting Together in the Cafeteria?" and Other Conversations About Race. New York: Basic Books.

Telles, E. E. (2002). "Racial Ambiguity Among the Brazilian Population." Ethnic and Racial Studies 25 (3): 415–441.

Telles, E. E. (2004). Race in Another America: The Significance of Colour in Brazil. 1st ed.United Kingdom: Princeton University Press.

Telles, E. E., and N. Lim. (1998). "Does it Matter who Answers the Race Question? Racial Classification and Income Inequality in Brazil." Demography 35 (4): 465–474.

Trad, L., M. Castellanos, and M. Guimaraes. (2012). "Accessibility to Primary Health Care by Black Families in a Poor Neighbourhood of Salvador, Northeastern Brazil." Revista de Saúde Pública 46 (6): 1007–1013.

Travassos, C., F. Viacava, R. Pinheiro, and A. Brito. (2002). "Utilization of Health Care Services in Brazil: Gender, Family Characteristics, and Social Status." Revista Panamericana de Salud Pública 11 (5-6): 365–373.

Vieira, E., and L. Souza. (2009). "Access to Surgical Sterilization Through the National Health System, Ribierao Preto, Southeastern Brazil." Revista de Saúde Pública 43 (3): 398–404.

WHO (World Health Organization). 2008. Flawed but Fair: Brazil's health system reaches out to the poor. Accessed April 26, 2016. http://www.who.int/bulletin/volumes/86/4/08-030408/en/.

6. Differences In The Prevalence Of Risk Factors For Severe COVID-19 Across São Paulo City Regions

Beatriz Thomé[1], Leandro F. M. Rezende[1],
Mariana Cabral Schveitzer[1],
Camila Nascimento Monteiro[2],
Moises Goldbaum[3]

INTRODUCTION

São Paulo city stands as the epicentre of the outbreak sparked by SARS-Cov-2 in Latin America. On July 2nd there were 134,984 confirmed COVID-19 cases and 7,370 deaths, roughly 10% of confirmed cases and deaths in Brazil[1]. São Paulo city is composed of 5 regions
(North, East, South, Midwest and Southeast), each with unique socioeconomic and epidemiological characteristics. São Paulo health systems are currently being challenged in the attempt to control transmission of SARS-CoV-2 while providing adequate care in particular to a subset of infected patients with severe disease.

In Brazil it has been observed that among deaths due to COVID-19, 69% were 60 years or older, and 63% had at least one of the identified clinical risk factors for severe disease, amongst which the most prevalent were cardiovascular disease and diabetes[2].As part of response planning it becomes of utmost importance to identify segments of the population who may be at risk for severe COVID-19 and describe their sociodemographic characteristics and how they are geographically distributed.

The scientific community has been calling attention to the disproportionate impact of the pandemic among the population subgroups of lower socioeconomic status[3]. In this study we estimated the prevalence of risk factors for severe COVID-19 living in São Paulo city by sociodemographic characteristics based on routinely collected public health data.

METHODS

We retrieved data from the most recent household-based survey conducted in São Paulo, ISA Capital 2015, which collected information from a representative sample of non-institutionalized residents. ISA-Capital 2015 collected respondents' self-reported health conditions, weight and height, smoking habit, among other information. The survey was based on probabilistic sample.

Two-stage sampling was done within census tracts (primary sampling unit) and households (second stage). A total of 4,043 respondents were interviewed. Data were collected through a structured questionnaire with mostly closed questions.

The design, characteristics, and questionnaires of ISA-Capital 2015   have been described in detail[1] In our analysis we included risk factors for severe disease described in the literature and

---

[1] https://www.prefeitura.sp.gov.br/cidade/secretarias/saude/epidemiologia_e_informacao/ isacapitalsp/.

other reliable public health resources[4] which were available in ISA-Capital survey. From the total of people interviewed we included data from 3,223 adults (≥18 years) for whom information on chronic diseases and lifestyle risk factors was available. Criteria for risk for severe disease included people aged ≥65 years or with a diagnosis of cardiovascular disease, diabetes, chronic respiratory disease, hypertension, (current) cancer, history of stroke, obesity (BMI ≥30 kg/m2), current smoking, or moderate to severe asthma (defined as asthma that moderately/severely limits daily activities as per respondents). We estimated the prevalence of one or more risk factors for severe COVID-19 by sex, age, education, income, race/ethnicity and São Paulo city region. All statistical analyses considered ISA complex multistage sampling design and were carried out using Stata 15.0 software (StataCorp, TX, USA).

RESULTS

Participants included in our study were 47% were men, 66% had at least secondary education, 51% were white, and 54% lived on less than a minimal wage per capita. Prevalence of single risk factors for severe COVID-19 among older adults ≥65 years were as high as 58% (hypertension), while for younger adults (<65 years) obesity was the most prevalent risk factor (21%). In general, risk factors were more prevalent among older adults with two exceptions: obesity and smoking were more prevalent in younger adults (data not shown).The prevalence of one or more risk factors for severe COVID-19 was 56.4% (4.7 million) in the city of São Paulo (Table 1). The proportion was higher in adults <65 years old (51%) vs. in the older adults (80%). Among less educated adults, that is, those who had no formal education reported, 86% had at least 1 risk factor for severe COVID-19, as compared to 49% among those with university education initiated. Distribution of risk factors was similar according to income or race (Figure 1). Southeast (59.8%), North (58.7%) and South (56%) had higher prevalence of one or more risk factors, while in the Midwest it was relatively lower (53.8%) (Table 1), despite the high proportion of adults ≥65 years (data not shown).

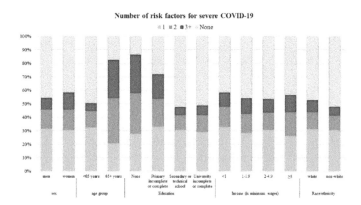

Figure1. Distribution of risk factors for severe COVID-19 by sociodemographic characteristics.

Table 1.Prevalence and 95% confidence intervals (CI) of one or more risk factors for severe COVID-19 by region of São Paulo city, ISA-Capital 2015.

Characteristics	Regions of São Paulo city					
	North	Mid-west	Southeast	South	East	Total
	(n=624)	(n=499)	(n=690)	(n=746)	(n=664)	(n=3223)
Risk factors for Severe COVID-19						
Cardiovascular disease	8.0	9.1	11.9	5.6	8.0	8.6
	(6.2, 10.3)	(5.8, 13.9)	(8.9, 15.7)	(4.1, 7.6)	(6.5, 9.9)	(7.5, 9.9)
Diabetes	7.1	6.6	7.3	8.2	7.8	7.5
	(5.2, 9.8)	(4.6, 9.4)	(5.9, 9.0)	(6.4, 10.6)	(6.0, 10.0)	(6.6, 8.4)
Chronic respiratory disease	2.9	2.5	2.4	2.5	3.9	2.8
	(1.6, 5.3)	(1.4, 4.3)	(1.4, 4.3)	(1.5, 4.1)	(2.7, 5.4)	(2.2, 3.5)
Hypertension	23.1	22.8	24.8	19.7	21.9	22.5
	(19.1, 27.7)	(17.5, 29.1)	(21.7, 28.3)	(16.3, 23.7)	(18.4, 25.8)	(20.7, 24.4)
Cancer (currently)	1.8	0.4	1.1	0.2	0.3	0.8
	(0.8, 3.9)	(0.1, 1.4)	(0.5, 2.3)	(0.1, 0.6)	(0.1, 1.1)	(0.5, 1.2)
Stroke	1.0	1.9	1.4	1.1	1.3	1.3
	(0.6, 1.9)	(0.9, 3.9)	(0.7, 2.8)	(0.6, 2.0)	(0.6, 2.7)	(1.0, 1.8)
Obesity (BMI ≥30 kg/m2)	23.0	17.5	23.1	19.7	18.8	20.7
	(19.6, 26.8)	(13.9, 21.9)	(19.3, 27.5)	(17.0, 22.8)	(15.9, 22.3)	(19.2, 22.4)
Smoking	18.3	16.7	17.8	20.4	14.8	17.8
	(15.7, 21.2)	(13.2, 20.8)	(14.2, 22.2)	(17.3, 23.9)	(12.2, 17.8)	(16.3, 19.4)
Moderate to severe asthma	2.4	1.4	2.4	3.2	2.2	2.4
	(1.5, 3.8)	(0.8, 2.7)	(1.5, 3.8)	(2.1, 4.9)	(1.3, 3.7)	(1.9, 3.0)
Number of risk factors for severe COVID-19[a]						
None	41.3	46.2	40.2	44.0	48.2	43.6
	(37.2, 45.6)	(39.7, 52.9)	(35.6, 45.1)	(40.0, 48.2)	(45.0, 51.4)	(41.6, 45.7)
1	33.0	28.2	31.0	33.1	29.1	31.1
	(29.2, 37.1)	(23.3, 33.6)	(27.2, 35.1)	(29.8, 36.5)	(26.0, 32.3)	(29.3, 32.9)
2	15.8	13.3	15.1	15.0	13.4	14.6
	(12.9, 19.1)	(10.3, 17.2)	(12.0, 18.8)	(12.5, 17.9)	(11.0, 16.2)	(13.3, 16.1)

	9.9	12.3	13.7	7.9	9.4	10.6
3+	(7.4, 13.0)	(8.8, 16.9)	(11.0, 16.8)	(6.1, 10.1)	(7.3, 11.9)	(9.4, 12.0)
Adult population living in São Paulo city[b]	1.787.806	1.253.318	2.180.543	2.120.010	1.894.605	8.411.089
Number of adults with risk factors for severe COVID-19[c]	1.049.442	674.285	1.303.965	1.187.206	981.405	4.743.854

[a]Criteria: age ≥65 years or diagnosis of cardiovascular disease, diabetes, chronic respiratory disease, hypertension, cancer (currently), stroke, obesity (body mass index - BMI ≥30 kg/m2), current smoking, moderate to severe asthma (limit moderate/severe daily activities). [b]Adult population (≥18 years) living in São Paulo city in 2020.
[c]Adult population (≥18 years) presenting with one or more risk factors for severe COVID-19 (age ≥65 years, cardiovascular disease, diabetes, chronic respiratory disease, hypertension, cancer (currently), stroke, obesity (BMI ≥30 kg/m2), smoking, moderate to severe asthma, in São Paulo city, 2020.

DISCUSSION

We found that more than half of the population, and hence a large number of adults, presented with at least one risk factor for severe COVID-19 in the city of São Paulo, including under the age of 65 years. A similar estimate for worldwide risk for severe disease pointed out to a fifth of the population, but is likely to be underestimated, since the calculation did not include obesity, a highly prevalent risk factor globally[5].We also described how the prevalence of risk factors is unequally distributed across São Paulo city: in the North and Southeast these risk factors were more prevalent, which may partially explain the higher deaths rates, alongside with inequalities in resources for care, particularly in the North. Subgroups of the population with lower education rates, a robust indicator of lower socioeconomic status, had higher prevalence of risk factors for severe disease. Data analysis of the first weeks of the pandemic in the city of São Paulo pointed out to a concentration of COVID-19 cases in the Midwest and Southeast regions, while COVID-19 deaths concentrate in the North, Southeast and East regions[6]. probably also reflecting disparities in accessing the necessary health services. As part of an effective COVID-19 response it is important to describe the distribution of risk factors for severe disease in the population in order to identify vulnerabilities and tailor prevention and care strategies. The present study has limitations. Risk factors were self-reported and therefore prone to misclassification bias. In addition, ISA-Capital dates from 2015, and other risk factors (known and unknown) were not captured. Nevertheless, our findings contribute to a better understanding of the greater impact of COVID-19 in lower-resource settings and population subgroups. Response strategies will need to be tailored to address such vulnerabilities.

AFFILIATIONS

[1]Universidade Federal de São Paulo, Escola Paulista de Medicina, Departamento de Medicina Preventiva
[2]Hospital Israelita Albert Einstein
[3] Faculdade de Medicina da Universidade de São Paulo
Corresponding author: Beatriz Thomé; biathome@gmail.com, https://orcid.org/00000002-3941-3756; Universidade Federal de São Paulo, Escola Paulista de Medicina,
Departamento de Medicina Preventiva. Rua Botucatu, 740 - São Paulo, São Paulo, Brazil. +55 11 55754848 VoIP 2197

Leandro F.M. Rezende; leandro.rezende@unifesp.br; https://orcid.org/0000-0002-74691399; Universidade Federal de São Paulo, Escola Paulista de Medicina, Departamento de Medicina Preventiva. São Paulo, São Paulo, Brazil.

Mariana Cabral Schveitzer; mariana.cabral@unifesp.br; https://orcid.org/0000-00019833-2932; Universidade Federal de São Paulo, Escola Paulista de Medicina,
Departamento de Medicina Preventiva. São Paulo, São Paulo, Brazil.
Camila Nascimento Monteiro; c.nascimentomonteiro@gmail.com;
https://orcid.org/0000-0002-0121-0398; Hospital Israelita Albert Einstein, São Paulo, São Paulo, Brazil.

Moisés   Goldbaum;   mgoldbau@usp.br; https://orcid.org/0000-0002-8049-7824;
Faculdade de Medicina da Universidade de São Paulo, São Paulo, São Paulo, Brazil.
Author contribution:
Study design: BT, LR. Data analysis: BT, LR, MCS, CN, MG. ISA conceptualization and analysis: MG, CN. Manuscript write up and review: BT, LR, MCS, CN, MG.

REFERENCES

Fundação SEADE. https://www.seade.gov.br/ . Accessed June 21, 2020.
Ministério da   Saúde   - Boletim Epidemiológico Especial.
https://www.saude.gov.br/images/pdf/2020/May/29/2020-05-25---BEE17--Boletim-do-COE.pdf. Accessed June 21, 2020.
Chiriboga D, Garay J, Buss P, Madrigal RS, Rispel LC. Health inequity during the COVID-19 pandemic: a cry for ethical global leadership. Lancet.
2020;395(10238):1690-1691. doi:10.1016/S0140-6736(20)31145-4
CDC. People Who Are at Increased Risk for Severe Illness. https://www.cdc.gov/coronavirus/2019-ncov/need-extra-precautions/people-atincreasedrisk.html?CDC_AA_refVal=https%3A%2F%2Fwww.cdc.gov%2Fcoronavirus%2F2019-ncov%2Fneed-extra-precautions%2Fpeople-at-higher-risk.html. Accessed June 29, 2020.
Clark A, Jit M, Warren-Gash C, Guthrie B, Wang HHX, Mercer SW, et al. Global, regional, and national estimates of the population at increased risk of severe COVID-19 due to underlying health conditions in 2020: a modelling study. Lancet Glob Health. 2020 Jun 15:S2214-109X(20)30264-3. doi: 10.1016/S2214-109X(20)30264-3. Epub ahead of print. PMID: 32553130; PMCID: PMC7295519.
Boletins - Secretaria Municipal da Saúde - Prefeitura da Cidade de São Paulo.
https://www.prefeitura.sp.gov.br/cidade/secretarias/saude/vigilancia_em_saude/
doencas_e_agravos/coronavirus/index.php?p=295572. Accessed June 21, 2020.

7. Underreporting of Death by COVID-19 In Brazil's Second Most Populous State

[1]Thiago Henrique Evangelista Alves[1†], Tafarel Andrade de Souza[1†],
Samyla de Almeida Silva[1], Nayani Alves Ramos[1],
Stefan Vilges de Oliveira[1*]

[1] Federal University of Uberlândia, Uberlândia, Minas Gerais, Brazil

ABSTRACT

The COVID-19 pandemic brings to light the reality of the Brazilian health system. The underreporting of COVID-19 deaths in the state of Minas Gerais (MG), where is concentrated the second largest population of the country, reveals government unpreparedness, as there is a low capacity of testing in the population, which prevents the real understanding of the general panorama of Sars-Cov-2 dissemination. The goals of this research are to analyze the causes of deaths in the different Brazilian government databases (ARPEN and SINAN) and to assess whether there are sub-records shown by the unexpected increase in the frequency of deaths from causes clinically similar to COVID-19. A descriptive and quantitative analysis of the number of COVID-19 deaths and similar causes was made in different databases. Ours results demonstrate that the different official sources had a discrepancy of 209.23% between these data referring to the same period. There was also a 648.61% increase in SARS deaths in 2020, when compared to the average of previous years. Finally, it was shown that there was an increase in the rate of pneumonia and respiratory insufficiency (RI) by 5.36% and 5.72%, respectively. In conclusion, there is an underreporting of COVID-19 deaths in MG due to the unexplained excess of SARS deaths, Respiratory insufficiency and pneumonia compared to previous years.

INTRODUCTION

Coronavirus 2 (COV-2) is a new betacoronavirus related to Severe Acute Respiratory Syndrome (SARS) that emerged in December 2019 in China and became a pandemic in March 2020 due to its high infection and mortality rates[1] [2] [3].COVID-19 was the official name given by the World Health Organization (WHO) to the disease caused by the new coronavirus of 2019(SARS-CoV-2) [1]. The first epicentre of COVID-19 was observed in Wuhan, the capital of Hubei, China, in December 2019 based on the several pneumonia cases notifications [4]. Since then, COVID-19 has rapidly

---

[1] * Mailing address
Department of Collective Health, Faculty of Medicine, Federal University of Uberlândia. Uberlândia (MG), Brazil. Avenue Pará 1720, Block 2U, Campus Umuarama, ZIP Code: 38.405-320. E-mail: stefan@ufu.br

spread around the world and, as of May 12th 2020, more than 4.4 million cases of the disease have been confirmed, causing over 299,000 deaths worldwide. [5]. Of this total, Brazil has reported more than 188,000 cases and over 13,000 deaths, according of Coronavírus Brasil database [6]. COVID-19 is classified according to the symptoms' severity. Patients with the mild form (80% of the cases) present fever, dry cough, chills, malaise, muscle pain, and sore throat. Patients with moderate form present fever, respiratory symptoms, and radiographic characteristics. Severe patients (5% of the cases) manifest dyspnoea (> 30 bpm), low oxygen saturation (<93%) and low PaO2/FiO2 ratio (< 300 mmHg), and may evolve to a respiratory failure, septic shock, and multiple organ failure [7] [8] [9].

Furthermore, increased age and the presence of comorbidities, such as hypertension, diabetes, and coronary disease, are associated with mortality in COVID-19 patients [10] [11].

The accurate diagnosis of COVID-19 is carried out by searching the genetic material of the virus and, in a complementary way, by imaging methods. Computed tomography and radiographs can identify lesions in the lungs due to viral multiplication [12] [13].Laboratory confirmation is essential for the timely management of cases to avoid the spread of transmission. However, Brazil is far below the ideal number of tests for COVID-19, as there are not enough laboratory inputs to understand the overall panorama of the virus' spread. Furthermore, confirmatory molecular tests depend on the availability of imported reagents, which are globally scarce, and on government investments that prioritize this strategy.

This scenario leads Brazil to a delay in the number of COVID-19 cases and deaths confirmations. These aspects become more aggravated when the patient evolves to death, because the effectiveness of tests, for these cases, is even more difficult. In addition, the recommendation is to collect blood and sputum to perform the culture, since these samples have a higher viral load – considering the studies done to date [14]. The difficulty regarding death registration have been also presented in the state of Minas Gerais, which, by the end of April 2020, had 584 suspected deaths notifications, of which 81 (13%) had not yet been confirmed or discarded [15]. Thus, it is possible to state that there is a disparity between the real number of COVID-19 deaths and the numbers that are reported in different Brazilian sources of information, since not all deaths have been tested for confirmation or exclusion and are potentially being confirmed by others causes than COVID-19. The present study aims to analyse the death causes in the notary records and in the Brazilian National disease notification system records, and thus evaluate the sub registries and the possible increase in the frequency of deaths with clinically compatible causes to COVID-19 in the Minas Gerais territory.

METHOD

This study is a descriptive and quantitative analysis of the deaths records clinically compatible with COVID-19, registered in the notary offices records and in the Brazilian National Disease Notification System Records (SINAN) of the state of Minas Gerais (MG), Brazil. The state of MG has an estimated population of 21,168,791 people in a territory of 586,521.121 km^2, having the second largest population and being the fourth largest state in the country [16]. Its Human Development Index (HDI) is 0.731, with a population composed of approximately 22.25% from 0 to 15 years old, 69.31% from 15 to 64 years old, and 8.12% over 65 years old [17]. For this study, the notary offices records were analysed from January to April of 2020 in the state of MG. Additionally, to assess the deaths excess in this period according to their causes, information from the SINAN was accessed referring to the range of years 2017 to 2019. The notary data were obtained from the Civil Registry

Transparency Portal, which is a free access platform developed to provide information about births, marriages, and deaths. Due to the COVID-19 pandemic, these data are being grouped in the Special sections COVID-19 and the COVID Registral Panel made available on ARPEN database [18]. The information presented here (accessed on 05/05/2020) is based on Death Certificates (DD), presenting only one cause for each death certificate [19].To evaluate sub-registrations in the different Information Systems in Brazil, SINAN data were collected through the InfoGripe platform of the Oswaldo Cruz Foundation (Fiocruz) InfoGripe database [20] is an initiative that aims to monitor and present alert levels for reported cases of Severe Acute Respiratory Syndrome (SARS) in SINAN [20]. The data in this system were compared with the notary data.

On this platform, the records of SARS and COVID-19 were selected on 05/07/2020 according to the Epidemiological Week (EPI Week) from 1 to 18 of the years 2017 to 2020 for the state of Minas Gerais. We also evaluated the death excess from causes that present clinical compatibility with COVID-19, according to the following aetiology:

Severe Acute Respiratory Syndrome (SARS), Pneumonia, Respiratory insufficiency (RI), Sepsis (sepsis/septic shock), Indeterminate Causes (deaths related to respiratory diseases, but not conclusive), and Other deaths (all other types of deaths that are not listed above) [19].

The data were collected and analysed in spreadsheet by descriptive statistics and presented in raw numbers, relative frequency, and central tendency measures. To assess the death excess per EPI week, the average, minimum and maximum values of deaths from the years 2017 to 2019 were calculated and confronted with diseases that presented changes in the pattern of distribution in the fourth quarter of 2020. All graphs were prepared using GraphPadPrism 7 software (GraphPad Software, Inc. San Diego, CA).

RESULTS

A total of 201 COVID-19 deaths were identified in the notary records and this number differs in 209.23% of the deaths registered in the SINAN at the same period (Table 1).

Table 1: Number of COVID-19 deaths according to the information in the notary offices records and the Brazilian National Disease Notification System Records (SINAN).

COVID-19	January		February		March	April
	N	%	N	%	N%	N%
Notary offices records	0	0	0	0	23 11.44	17 88.56
SINAN records	0	0	0	0	23 35.38	42 64.62

The evaluation of the death causes on the notaries' offices showed an increase in the frequency of SARS deaths in 2020 in relation to the number of deaths from the same disease in 2019. There was also a slight increase in the number of pneumonia and respiratory failure deaths in 2020 between January and March (SARS), Pneumonia, Respiratory insufficiency (RI), Sepsis (sepsis/septic shock), Indeterminate Causes (deaths related to respiratory diseases, but not conclusive), Other Deaths (all other types of deaths that are not listed above), according to the notary offices records from January to April 2019 and 2020, in the state of Minas Gerais, Brazil. The increase of SARS case sin 2020 was in the order of 152.7% compared to 2019. Regarding to the elevation in the rates of pneumonia and respiratory insufficiency from January to March compared to the same period in 2019, it was around 5.36% and 5.72%, respectively. When analysing the excess of deaths in 2020 according to epidemiological weeks 1st to 18th, there was an increase of 648.61% in SARS deaths compared to the average of previous years (2017/2019). Such ascendancy of SARS deaths was observed from epidemiological week number 10 and the records of COVID-19 deaths in the state of MG are reported from epidemiological week number 12.

DISCUSSION

The study points out divergences of information between different death registrations systems.
The important increase in SARS deaths that started earlier than those from COVID-19, in epidemiological week 10, is also highlighted, suggesting the underreporting of COVID-19 deaths in the state of Minas Gerais. The COVID-19 situation is particularly challenging because, besides being a new and unprecedented disease,
it is also capable of triggering other conditions, such as pneumonia and SARS, which can be characterized as the main cause of death. In other words, the COVID-19 may be the underlying cause, that is, it may not be the direct cause of death that has been registered. In this perspective, there is a subjectivity bias, since the physician can attest or not the death from COVID-19 according to his clinical knowledge without the need of laboratory tests [21].
This finding corroborates with data from Hubei, China and Northern Italy, where mortality calculations were adjusted for the biases of preferential verification, symptomatic and severe cases, and delay in death records.
An increase in the mortality rate was found, which confirms the existence of underreporting COVID-19 deaths in those regions [22].In relation to underreporting in Brazil, the Ministry of Health (MH) reports that the number of under-reported deaths is low according to the Mortality Information System (MIS), because states and municipalities are advised to include deaths from COVID-19, either confirmed cases or only suspects, in the system as a priority, in order to advance analysis of these cases [23]. However, our results show that there is a significant underreporting of the occurrences by COVID-19, given the excess of SARS deaths. Another issue that should be analysed is that although the Civil Registry Information Centre takes into consideration both confirmed deaths and suspects, the MH discloses in its reports only the laboratory proven COVID-19 deaths [23].However, suspect deaths need to be considered in the count, even though it is noted that they have not been confirmed. This is stated because it is known that many of these deaths will not be able to be analysed, given the difficulties in collecting, transporting, and wrapping the *post-mortem* samples. Thus, if they are not mentioned, there will be a relaxation of the real situation in Brazil and, consequently, in the state of MG.
The Brazilian MH also points out that in the same death certificate more than one cause of death can be described, so that the record of COVID-19 can be associated with other diseases.

However, the Civil Registry Transparency Portal presents these causes separately, even those included or registered in the same death certificate. Thus, one cannot only add up the deaths made available on the portal by the different diseases, because they would generate false over-notification. A thorough investigation must be made when considering each death and the causes that were cited in the death certificate [23]. However, according to the hierarchical criteria exposed in the Civil Registry Transparency Portal, only one cause of death is selected to make the count, and not all the causes present in the same death certificate [24], which validates the data exposed in this platform and the information presented here.

It is worth noting that the different systems of deaths registration of the government, such as the municipalities and states, are not fully connected and that several of them depend on manual labour to be registered. This is capable of causing discrepancies and delays in data traffic and, consequently, in the production of timely and reliable information. WHO has been advising countries on the need to expand laboratory testing capacity as a strategy to overcome the pandemic [25]. This action will enable the real knowledge of a population's immunity, providing reliable statistics for a better understanding of the circulation of the disease. Consequently, strategies to control the pandemic and even the relaxation of non-pharmacological measures, such as social isolation and quarantines, may be proposed. In Brazil, a network formed by referenced laboratories was established to help fight COVID-19 [14]. However, the country is far below the optimal number of tests for COVID-19, as there are not enough tests to have a reliable panorama of the real number of cases and deaths. This scenario leads Brazil to have a delay in accounting the records of COVID-19. In conclusion, our results reveal that COVID-19 deaths in the state of Minas Gerais are higher than the official statistics presented. In view of these aspects, it is necessary to expand Brazil's diagnostic capacity, which will allow us to recognize the real number of COVID-19 deaths and cases in Minas Gerais.

ACKNOWLEDGEMENT

Thanks to Gabriela Geraldo Mendes and Adélio Tiago da Mota for the collaborations.
Thanks to the Department of Collective Health of the Faculty of Medicine of the Federal University of Uberlândia for the encouragement.

REFERENCES

1   World Health Organization (WHO) database (https://www.who.int/dg/speeches/detail/who-director-general-s-opening-remarks-atthe-media-briefing-on-COVID-19---11-march-2020). WHO Director-General's opening remarks at the media briefing on COVID-19. Accessed 22 March 2020.

2   Guan, W.J, et al. (2020). Clinical characteristics of coronavirus disease 2019 in China. *New England Journal of Medicine*. Published online: 30 April 2020. doi:10.1056/NEJMoa2002032.

3   Cobb, J.S,, Seale, M.A. (2020). Examining the effect of social distancing on the compound growth rate of SARS-CoV-2 at the county level (United States) using statistical analyses and a random forest machine learning model. *Public Health*. Published online: 28 April 2020. doi: https://doi.org/10.1016/j.puhe.2020.04.016 (in press).

4   Velavan, T.P., Meyer, C.G. (2020). The COVID-19 epidemic. *Tropical Medicine & International Health*. Published online: 16 February 2020. doi: 10.1111/tmi.13383.

5   Worldometers database (https://www.worldometers.info/coronavirus). COVID-19 coronavirus pandemic. Accessed: 12 May 2020.

6   Coronavírus Brasil database (https://covid.saude.gov.br). Painel de casos de doença pelo coronavírus 2019 (COVID-19) no Brasil pelo Ministério da Saúde. Accessed: 12 May 2020.

7   Wang, Y., et al. (2020). Unique epidemiological and clinical features of the emerging 2019 novel coronavirus pneumonia (COVID- 19) implicate special control measures. *Journal of medical virology* 2020; 92: 568-576.

8   Rodriguez-Morales, A.J, et al.(2020).Clinical, laboratory and imaging features of COVID19: A systematic review and meta-analysis. *Travel medicine and infectious disease.* Published online: 13 March 2020. doi: 10.1016/j.tmaid.2020.101623.

9   Ministério da Saúde (MS) do Brasil database (https://coronavirus.saude.gov.br/sobre-a-doenca#transmissao). Sobre a doença. Accessed: 7 May 2020.

10 Huang, C, et al. (2020). Clinical features of patients infected with 2019 novel coronavirus in Wuhan, China. *The Lancet.* Published online: 24 January 2020. doi: 10.1016/S0140-6736(20)30183-5

11 Zhou, F., et al. (2020). Clinical course and risk factors for mortality of adult inpatients with COVID-19 in Wuhan, China: a retrospective cohort study. *The Lancet.* Published online: 9 March 2020. doi: 10.1016/S0140-6736(20)30566-3

12 Colégio Brasileiro de Radiologia e Diagnóstico por Imagem (CBRDI) database (https://cbr.org.br/recomendacoes-de-uso-de-metodos-de-imagem-para-pacientessuspeitos-de-infeccao-pelo-COVID-19/). Recomendações de uso de métodos de imagem para pacientes suspeitos de infecção pelo COVID-19. Accessed: 7 May 2020.

13 Kanne, J.P. et al (2020)..Essentials for radiologists on COVID-19: An update radiology scientific expert panel. *Radiology.* Published online: 27 February 2020. doi: https://doi.org/10.1148/radiol.2020200527

14 Ministério da Saúde (MS) do Brasil database (https://portalarquivos.saude.gov.br/images/pdf/2020/April/07/ddt-COVID-19.pdf) Diretrizes para diagnóstico e tratamento da COVID-19. Accessed: 6 May 2020.

15 Secretaria De Estado De Saúde De Minas Gerais (SESMG) database (https://www.saude.mg.gov.br/component/gmg/story/12594-informe-epidemiologicocoronavirus-30-04-2020). Informe Epidemiológico Coronavírus 30/04/2020. Accessed: 6 May 2020.

16 Instituto Brasileiro de Geografia e Estatística (IBGE) database (http://www.atlasbrasil.org.br/2013/pt/perfil_uf/minas-gerais#demografia) Perfil de Minas Gerais. Accessed: 29 April 2020.

17 Instituto Brasileiro de Geografia e Estatística (IBGE) database (https://cidades.ibge.gov.br/brasil/mg/panorama). Panorama de Minas Gerais. Accessed: 29 April 2020

18 Associação dos Registradores de Pessoas Naturais (ARPEN) do Brasil database (https://transparencia.registrocivil.org.br/registros). Portal da Transparência: Registro Civil do Brasil em 2020. Accessed: 7 May 2020.

19 Associação dos Registradores de Pessoas Naturais (ARPEN) do Brasil database (https://transparencia.registrocivil.org.br/registral-covid). Painel COVID Registral. Accessed: 29 April 2020.

20 InfoGripe database (http://info.gripe.fiocruz.br/). Monitoramento de casos reportados de síndrome respiratória aguda grave (SRAG) hospitalizados. Accessed: 5 April 2020.

21 Our World in Data (OWD) database (https://ourworldindata.org/coronavirus). Statistics and research coronavirus pandemic (COVID-19). Accessed: 2 May 2020.

22 Hauser, A. et al. (2020). Estimation of sars-cov-2 mortality during the early stages of an epidemic: a modelling study in Hubei, China and northern Italy. *MedRxi.* Published online: 30 March 2020. doi: https://doi.org/10.1101/2020.03.04.20031104

23 Ministério da Saúde (MS) do Brasil database (https://portalarquivos.saude.gov.br/images/pdf/2020/April/27/2020-04-27-18-05hBEE14-Boletim-do-COE.pdf). Boletim epidemiológico especial 14. Accessed: 26 April 2020.

24 Associação dos Registradores de Pessoas Naturais (ARPEN) do Brasil database (https://transparencia.registrocivil.org.br/especial-covid). Especial COVID-19. Accessed: 29 April 2020.

25 Pan American Health Organization (PAHO) database (https://www.paho.org/bra/index.php?option=com_content&view=article&id=6101:cov id19&Itemid=875). Folha informativa – COVID-19 (doença causada pelo novo coronavírus). Accessed: 12 May 2020.

CHAPTER 10

CONVERGING AND CONTRASTING AGE RELATED RISKS

1. Regional COVID-19 Mortality in Brazil by Age

Emerson A. Baptista
Asian Demographic Research Institute emersonaug@gmail.com

Bernardo Lanza Queiroz
Universidade Federal de Minas Gerais lanza@cedeplar.ufmg.br

ABSTRACT

In this study, we introduce a ternary colour coding to visualize and compare the age structure of deaths by COVID-19 (until 06/30/2020) in Brazilian small-areas using the tricolore package in R. The analysis of age profile is important to better understand the dynamics of the pandemic and how it affects the population according to age groups (0-19, 20-59, and >60 years) and regions of the country. The results highlight the importance of looking at the small-areas and show that there are many pandemics going on in Brazil at the same time, instead of a single one. The pandemic is increasing in the interior of the country, but we still observed several cases and deaths in the major cities and, as of today, very few signs of reduction in the spread of the disease. We also show that the number of cases is more concentrated in females, but deaths are prevalent among men. The CFR for males is greater than the ones for females, but also mortality for young adult males is greater when compared with other countries.

INTRODUCTION

The COVID-19 pandemic has negatively impacted public health worldwide. Recently, Latin America and Brazil have become the new epicentre of the disease (Anderson et al. 2020; Barreto et al. 2020; Rodriguez-Morales et al. 2020; The Lancet 2020). By not following WHO recommendations and ignoring effective measures that were implemented in most countries that successfully control the pandemic, Brazil is following a very bad path. Currently, the country is the second in number of confirmed cases and deaths, behind only the United States(Dong, Du and Gardner 2020). However, there are important regional disparities in the progress of the pandemic, which leads us to investigate and evaluate the spatial distribution of mortality by COVID-19, as well as to understand how the pandemic spread across regions in a less developed and younger population (Codeço et al. 2020; Souza et al. 2020).COVID-19 deaths show a considerable gradient by age, very similar to that observed in the general mortality rates of a population (Goldstein and Lee 2020). Mortality rates are much higher for the elderly than for adults and the young, and in most countries, higher for males than for females.

Therefore, population age structure is a risk factor for higher mortality, so that in locations with an older population a relatively higher overall number of deaths is expected (Dowd et al. 2020; Goldstein and Lee 2020). However, COVID-19 also appears to be more dangerous for people with previous health problems. Evidence shows that cardiovascular diseases, diabetes and obesity increase the risk of complications and deaths for infected people (Jordan et al. 2020; Nepomuceno et al. 2020; Shuchman 2020). In developing countries, therefore, the level of morbidity of the younger population may act as an additional risk for COVID-19. If, on the one hand, a younger age structure is a protective factor, general levels of morbidity may have the opposite effect (Nepomuceno et al. 2020; Shuchman 2020). These studies are important for understanding the different aspects of the spread of the pandemic at the national level. However, sub-national variations and differences should also be considered in the analysis to provide support for public health interventions.

In the first moments of the epidemic in Brazil, most deaths were concentrated in places where the first infections were registered (Souza et al. 2020). However, throughout the process of spreading and internalizing the pandemic, understanding the spatial pattern of mortality (Schmertmann and Gonzaga 2018; Baptista and Queiroz 2019) and of the age structure of the population (Dowd et al. 2020; Kashnitsky 2020) before the pandemic can help policymakers to respond to potential regional differentials of mortality due to diseases, as well as contribute to the understanding of possible differences in the age structure of mortality by COVID-19 (Barreto et al. 2020). In short, the risks of death in Brazil are largely related to the age structure of the population, general health conditions and socioeconomic situation to which the population is exposed (Borges 2017; França et al. 2017).

Therefore, in a country marked by major regional and socioeconomic differences (Ribeiro and Leist 2020), which occur regardless of geographic level (Queiroz et al. 2017; Schmertmann and Gonzaga 2018; Baptista and Queiroz 2019), this analysis is essential. Additionally, there is an hypothesis that mortality by COVID-19 in Brazil has a younger age structure than observed in other countries (Guilmoto 2020) and this regional analysis might shed some light on this discussion.

In this study, we introduce a ternary colour coding to visualize and compare the age structure of deaths by COVID-19 (until 06/30/2020) in Brazilian small-areas using the tricolore package (Kashnitsky and Schöley 2018) in R. In addition, we calculate COVID-19 case fatality rates and mortality ratios. The analysis of age profile is important for better understanding the dynamics of the pandemic (Dudel n.d.; Guilmoto 2020) and how it affects the population according to age groups (0-19, 20-59, and >60 years) and regions of the country. In most countries, mortality is higher for older individuals (Goldstein and Lee 2020; Jin et al. 2020; Kang, undefined/ed), but recent research highlights the possibility of high mortality rates for younger ages in less developed economies. In the case of Brazil, one can add the large regional differences that may also play an important role in mortality risks (Nepomuceno et al. 2020; Rezende et al. 2020).

DATA AND METHODS

Data source and level of analysis

We use the database of the Ministry of Health of Brazil, DATASUS, which is publicly available online[1]. The Ministry of Health, through the Health Surveillance Secretariat (SVS), has been developing surveillance for Serious Acute Respiratory Syndrome (SARI) in Brazil since 2009, due to the Influenza A (H1N1) pandemic. Thereafter, SARS was incorporated into the surveillance network for Influenza and other respiratory viruses and, recently (2020), COVID-19, the human infection caused by the new Coronavirus that generated a global pandemic, also became part of the

---

[1] (https://opendatasus.saude.gov.br/dataset/casos-nacionais)

network. We collected the information on June 30th, when Brazil had registered 54.470 deaths and 1.113.682 cases. The original data are available at the individual level (case by case) and by municipality. The main limitation in using city level data in Brazil is that the population sizes, as well as the number of cases and deaths, are very small in some localities, which can cause many random fluctuations. To avoid problems but maintaining the importance of analysing and understanding regional variations, we aggregated municipalities in 137 comparable small areas, using the IBGE definition of geographic meso-regions. These geographical areas are statistical constructions aggregated using regional and socioeconomic similarities and have not changed their boundaries over time. In addition, they have been used elsewhere (Lima and Queiroz 2014; Baptista and Queiroz 2020). We also produce estimates using standardized rates so that we can compare COVID-19 mortality levels, thereby eliminating effects of population age structure (Dowd et al2020).

Ternary colour coding

We used the approach proposed by Kashnitsky and Schöley (2018) to investigate the spatio-temporal variation of deaths by COVID-19 in Brazilian meso-regions. We map the age profile (0-19, 20-59, and >60 years) of COVID-19 deaths using ternary colour coding. This technique maximises the amount of information conveyed by colours. Each element of a three-dimensional array of compositional data, in our case, three age groups, is represented with a unique colour. In other words, ternary colour coding is designed to visualize proportions of a whole, that is, anything that splits in three non-negative parts that add up to unity. This is perhaps its biggest limitation, and a second one occurs when there is unbalanced data. In this study, COVID-19 deaths are concentrated in adults and the elderly; that is, there is little variation with regards to the visual reference point, which is the grey point that marks perfectly balanced proportions (Kashnitsky and Aburto 2019; Schöley 2019). Therefore, and to see the internal variation of the data, we have changed the point of reference to the location of the average Brazilian mortality structure of COVID-19, thereby visualizing direction and magnitude of the deviations from that average.

RESULTS

Figure 1 shows Case Fatality Rates (CFR) for males and females. CFR is the proportion of COVID-19 deaths by the total number of people diagnosed with the disease, by age, sex and in a specific period of time. It is important to stress that CFR for COVID-19 changes constantly and it is different over time and regions. Specifically, here, our goal is just to show the differences by age and sex in Brazil. CFR is not an appropriate measure of mortality risk by COVID-19, as it is affected by the number of people who receive the proper diagnostic. That is, in countries with very few tests we might observe very high CFR because only those in hospitals or severe symptoms are being tested. In addition, we are counting deaths at a specific point of time, but some people with the disease might have a positive or negative outcome. In the case of Brazil, we observed that CFRs for males are higher than for females in all age groups – as observed in other countries. However, CFRs for younger adults are greater than observed in other countries.

Figure 1. COVID-19 Case Fatality Rates (CFR), by age groups and sex, Brazil, 2020 (June, 30th)

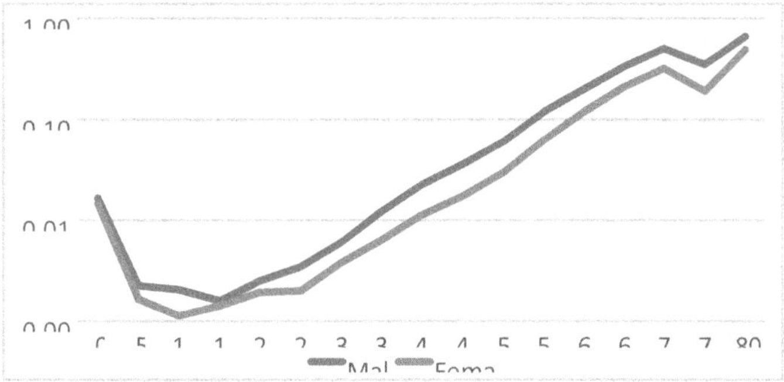

Table 1 shows summary results for the country and the main regions. The distribution of COVID-19 deaths by age in Brazil follows a very similar pattern than observed in other countries. For males, we find that 0.60 % of deaths are for individuals younger than 19 years of age, 28.20% for those aged 20 to 59, and 71.20% for those aged 60 and above. For females, the values are 0.77%, 24.70% and 74.02%, respectively. In addition, there is some variation across regions of the country that we will highlight later. The observed CFR for males is higher than for females for all age groups, and the difference increases for young adults and extends to older ages (Natale et al. 2020; Rezende et al. 2020).There is also an interesting gender pattern. In the country, we observe the ratio male to female for deaths in around 1.44, that is, there are 144 male deaths to 100 female deaths. The ratio ranges from 1.52 in the North to 1.29 in the Centre-West. For confirmed cases in the country, we calculate a ratio of 0.88, that is, 88 male cases for every 100 female cases.

Table 1. Summary Statistics, COVID-19, Brazil And Regions, 2020

Region	M/F deaths	M/F cases	CFR - Females	CFR - Males	% deaths 20-59	% deaths 60+
North	1.52	0.76	0.0225	0.0435	24.40	74.74
Northeast	1.44	0.86	0.0195	0.0327	27.07	71.49
Centre-West	1.29	0.98	0.0167	0.0219	31.02	67.34
Southeast	1.33	0.98	0.0331	0.0446	31.28	68.06
South	1.46	0.92	0.0145	0.0232	32.46	66.48
Brazil	1.44	0.88	0.0218	0.0368	27.04	71.89

Figure 2 shows, for males and females, the proportional distribution of COVID-19 deaths by age groups across Brazilian meso-regions. The overall results show that, for both sexes, the percentage of deaths in the older age group (above 60) is higher in 9 out of 10 meso-regions. When comparing men and women, in approximately 73%, 85% and 82% of meso-regions, the number of deaths of men is higher than that of women in the 0-19, 20-59, and 60 and above age groups, respectively.

The figure also shows the Brazilian mortality by COVID-19 with the colour scale altered so that the visual point of reference (point of intersection of the three lines within the triangle) is positioned at the Brazilian average. The colours present direction and magnitude of the deviation from the Brazilian average distribution of COVID-19 mortality by age groups. *Yellow, green and pink* show a higher than average share of COVID-19 deaths in the 0-19, 20-59 and 60+ age groups.

The saturation of the colours exhibits the amplitude of that deviation with perfect grey indicating a region that has age distribution of mortality composition equal to the Brazilian average (Kashnitsky and Schöley 2018). The results show that the spatial distribution is quite heterogeneous. Some meso-regions, for both males and females, in the South and Southeast, as well as in the state of Mato Grosso do Sul, have higher levels of mortality when compared to the Brazilian average in the age groups of 20-59 and 60+. On the other hand, in the central region of the country there are meso-regions with a higher mortality percentage in the 0-19 age group. Finally, we can also observe that many meso-regions in the North and Northeast (especially on the coast) have levels of mortality close to the Brazilian average. The results depicted in the maps highlight the importance of looking at small areas. We can observe that results for meso-regions and states do not represent the differences observed within each area. For instance, in the state of Minas Gerais, the results indicate different patterns of mortality by age. The northern part of the state has a higher prevalence in adults (20-59) compared to the southern part, which has an older than the reference point. A similar pattern is observed in other areas, for males and females.

Figure 2. Spatial Distribution Of Deaths By COVID-19, Age Groups And Sex In Brazilian Mesoregions, 2020

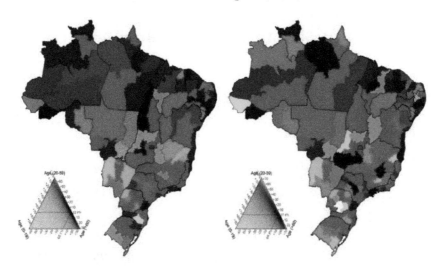

Males   **Females**

Source: Datasus (2020)

CONCLUSION

The results presented in this paper show that there are many pandemics going on in Brazil at the same time, instead of a single one. The pandemic is increasing in the interior of the country, but we still observed several cases and deaths in the major cities and, as of today, very few signs of reduction in the spread of the disease. We also show that the number of cases is more concentrated in females, but deaths are prevalent among men. The CFR for males is greater than the one for females, and mortality for young adult males is greater than it is in other countries (Natale et al. 2020).

REFERENCES

Anderson, R. M., Heesterbeek, H., Klinkenberg, D., & Hollingsworth, T. D. (2020). How will country-based mitigation measures influence the course of the COVID-19 epidemic? *Lancet (London, England)*, *395*(10228), 931–934.

Baptista, E. A., & Queiroz, B. L. (2020). Age Patterns of COVID-19 and Severe Acute Respiratory Illness in Brazil. unpublished manuscript.

Baptista, E. A., & Queiroz, B. L. (2019). The relation between cardiovascular mortality and development: Study for small areas in Brazil, 2001–2015. *Demographic Research*, *41*(51), 1437–1452.

Barreto, M. L., Barros, A. J. D. de, Carvalho, M. S., Codeço, C. T., Hallal, P. R. C., Medronho, R. de A., Struchiner, C. J., Victora, C. G., Werneck, G. L., Barreto, M. L., Barros, A. J. D. de, Carvalho, M. S., Codeço, C. T., Hallal, P. R. C., Medronho, R. de A., Struchiner, C. J., Victora, C. G., & Werneck, G. L. (2020). O que é urgente e necessário para subsidiar as políticas de enfrentamento da pandemia de COVID-19 no Brasil? *Revista Brasileira de Epidemiologia*, *23*.

Borges, G. M. (2017). Health transition in Brazil: Regional variations and divergence/convergence in mortality. *Cadernos de Saúde Pública*, *33*(8). https://doi.org/10.1590/0102311x00080316

Codeço, C. T., Villela, D., Coelho, F., Bastos, L. S., Gomes, M. F. C., Cruz, O. G., Lana, R. M., Piontti, A. P. y, Vespignani, A., & Davis, J. T. (2020). *Estimativa de risco de espalhamento da COVID-19 no Brasil e o impacto no sistema de saúde e população por microrregião*. https://www.arca.fiocruz.br/handle/icict/40509

Dong, E., Du, H., & Gardner, L. (2020). An interactive web-based dashboard to track COVID-19 in real time. *The Lancet. Infectious Diseases*, *20*(5), 533–534. https://doi.org/10.1016/S1473-3099(20)30120-1

Dowd, J. B., Andriano, L., Brazel, D. M., Rotondi, V., Block, P., Ding, X., Liu, Y., & Mills, M. C. (2020). Demographic science aids in understanding the spread and fatality rates of COVID-19. *Proceedings of the National Academy of Sciences*, *117*(18), 9696–9698. https://doi.org/10.1073/pnas.2004911117

Dudel, C. (n.d.). *Monitoring trends and differences in COVID-19 case fatality rates using decomposition methods: Contributions of age structure and age-specific fatality*. 17.

França, E. B., Passos, V. M. de A., Malta, D. C., Duncan, B. B., Ribeiro, A. L. P., Guimarães, M. D. C., Abreu, D. M. X., Vasconcelos, A. M. N., Carneiro, M., Teixeira, R., Camargos, P., Melo, A. P. S., Queiroz, B. L., Schmidt, M. I., Ishitani, L., Ladeira, R. M., Morais-Neto, O. L., Bustamante-Teixeira, M. T., Guerra, M. R., … Naghavi, M. (2017). Cause-specific mortality for 249 causes in Brazil and states during 1990–2015: A systematic analysis for the global burden of disease study 2015. *Population Health Metrics*, *15*(1), 39. https://doi.org/10.1186/s12963-017-0156-y

Goldstein, J., & Lee, R. (2020). *Demographic Perspectives on Mortality of COVID-19 and Other Epidemics* (No. w27043; p. w27043). National Bureau of Economic Research. https://doi.org/10.3386/w27043

Guilmoto, C. Z. Z. (2020). COVID-19 death rates by age and sex and the resulting mortality vulnerability of countries and regions in the world. *MedRxiv*, 2020.05.17.20097410. https://doi.org/10.1101/2020.05.17.20097410

Jin, J.-M., Bai, P., He, W., Wu, F., Liu, X.-F., Han, D.-M., Liu, S., & Yang, J.-K. (2020). Gender Differences in Patients With COVID-19: Focus on Severity and Mortality. *Frontiers in Public Health*, *8*. https://doi.org/10.3389/fpubh.2020.00152

Jordan, R. E., Adab, P., & Cheng, K. K. (2020). COVID-19: Risk factors for severe disease and death. *BMJ*, *368*. https://doi.org/10.1136/bmj.m1198

Kang, Y.-J. (undefined/ed). Mortality Rate of Infection With COVID-19 in Korea From the Perspective of Underlying Disease. *Disaster Medicine and Public Health Preparedness*, 1–3. https://doi.org/10.1017/dmp.2020.60

Kashnitsky, I. (2020).*COVID-19 in unequally ageing European regions.*

Kashnitsky, I., & Aburto, J. M. (2019). Geofaceting: Aligning small multiples for regions in a spatially meaningful way. *Demographic Research*, *41*, 477–490. JSTOR. https://doi.org/10.2307/26850657

Kashnitsky, I., & Schöley, J. (2018). Regional population structures at a glance. *The Lancet, 392*(10143), 209–210.

Lima, E. E. C. de, & Queiroz, B. L. (2014). Evolution of the deaths registry system in Brazil: Associations with changes in the mortality profile, under-registration of death counts, and ill-defined causes of death. *Cadernos de Saúde Pública, 30*(8), 1721–1730. https://doi.org/10.1590/0102-311X00131113

Natale, A., Ghio, D., Tarchi, D., Goujon, A., & Conte, A. (2020). *COVID-19 Cases and Case Fatality Rate by age.* (Knowledge for Policy,).

Nepomuceno, M. R., Acosta, E., Alburez-Gutierrez, D., Aburto, J. M., Gagnon, A., & Turra, C. M. (2020). Besides population age structure, health and other demographic factors can contribute to understanding the COVID-19 burden. *Proceedings of the National Academy of Sciences, 117*(25), 13881–13883.

Queiroz, B. L., Freire, F. H. M. de A., Gonzaga, M. R., & Lima, E. E. C. de. (2017). Completeness of death-count coverage and adult mortality (45q15) for Brazilian states from 1980 to 2010.
Revista Brasileira de   Epidemiologia, 20, 21–33.https://doi.org/10.1590/19805497201700050003

Rezende, L. F. M., Thome, B., Schveitzer, M. C., Souza-Júnior, P. R. B. de, Szwarcwald, C. L., Rezende, L. F. M., Thome, B., Schveitzer, M. C., Souza-Júnior, P. R. B. de, & Szwarcwald, C. L. (2020). Adults at high-risk of severe coronavirus disease-2019 (COVID-19) in Brazil. *Revista de Saúde Pública, 54*. https://doi.org/10.11606/s1518-8787.2020054002596

Ribeiro, F., & Leist, A. (2020). Who is going to pay the price of COVID-19? Reflections about an unequal Brazil. *International Journal for Equity in Health, 19*(1), 91. https://doi.org/10.1186/s12939-020-01207-2

Rodriguez-Morales, A. J., Gallego, V., Escalera-Antezana, J. P., Méndez, C. A., Zambrano, L. I., Franco-Paredes, C., Suárez, J. A., Rodriguez-Enciso, H. D., Balbin-Ramon, G. J., SavioLarriera, E., Risquez, A., & Cimerman, S. (2020). COVID-19 in Latin America: The implications of the first confirmed case in Brazil. *Travel Medicine and Infectious Disease.*

Schmertmann, C. P., & Gonzaga, M. R. (2018). Bayesian Estimation of Age-Specific Mortality and Life Expectancy for Small Areas With Defective Vital Records. *Demography, 55*(4), 1363–1388. https://doi.org/10.1007/s13524-018-0695-2

Schöley, J. (2019). *The centreed ternary balance scheme: A technique to visualize surfaces of unbalanced three-part compositions.* PAA Anual Conference.
https://portal.findresearcher.sdu.dk/en/publications/the-centreed-ternary-balance-schemea-technique-to-visualize-surf

Shuchman, M. (2020). Low- and middle-income countries face up to COVID-19. *Nature Medicine.*

Souza, C. D. F. de, Paiva, J. P. S. de, Leal, T. C., Silva, L. F. da, Santos, L. G., Souza, C. D. F. de, Paiva, J. P. S. de, Leal, T. C., Silva, L. F. da, & Santos, L. G. (2020). Spatiotemporal evolution of case fatality rates of COVID-19 in Brazil, 2020. *Jornal Brasileiro de Pneumologia, 46*(4). https://doi.org/10.36416/1806-3756/e20200208

The Lancet. (2020). COVID-19 in Brazil: "So what?" *The Lancet, 395*(10235), 1461.

2. The Changing Age-Structure Of Coronavirus SARS-Cov-2 Deaths And Cases: A Case Study Of Paraná, Brazil

Raquel Guimaraes[1]

Marília Nepomuceno[2]

Acácia Nasr[3]

Junior R. Garcia[4]

Maria Goretti David Lopes[5]

Nestor Werner Junior[6]

Carlos Alberto Gebrim Preto[7]

ABSTRACT

The goal of this paper is to explore the demographic evolution of the Coronavirus SARS-CoV-2 deaths and cases in the state of Paraná, Brazil. We focus on changes in the age-pattern of cases and deaths attributed to the COVID-19. Paraná is an interesting case of study in Brazil due to several aspects. First, it is one of the most developed states of the country. Second, the population growth rate is rapidly approaching zero growth, with an observed average growth rate of 0.78 percent per year in the decade 2010/2020, and of 0.28 percent per year in the period 2030/2040. Third, Parana has an older population age-structure than that of the whole country. Finally, although the state government pushed for earlier Non-Pharmaceutical Interventions to control the pandemic, data shows that they only took effect in the very late stages. Taken together, we claim that these aspects created a very particular setting, in which changes over time in the age-structure of the deaths attributed to COVID-19 could be observed: in the beginning of the pandemic, the age-structure of the deaths was concentrated among the elderly. As the pandemic unfolds, deaths were spreading over younger ages. Finally, we speculate on mechanisms behind the changes in the age structure of the COVID-19 deaths in Paraná.

[1] Federal University of Parana (Brazil) and International Institute for Applied System Analysis (Austria). Corresponding author: raquel.guimaraes@ufpr.br.

[2] Max Planck Institute for Demographic Research (Germany).

[3] Coordination of Epidemiological Surveillance, Health Secretariat, State of Parana (Brazil).

[4] Federal University of Parana (Brazil).

[5] Director of Health Care and Surveillance, Health Secretariat, State of Parana (Brazil).

[6] General Director, Health Secretariat, State of Parana (Brazil). [7] Secretary of Health, State of Parana (Brazil).

INTRODUCTION

The state of Parana is located in the southern region of Brazil. Historically populated by European migrants fleeing from the first world war, Parana is a state based on highly innovative agriculture and industry. The Human Development Index (HDI) for Parana in 2010 was 0.749, similar to Costa Rica and higher than the observed for Brazil (0.726). According to the 2018 Population Projection Revision from the Brazilian Institute of Geography and Statistics (IBGE, 2020), the state of Parana represented 5.4 percent of the total Brazilian population in 2020. As per the demographic profile of the State, Parana has an older population age-structure and a higher life expectancy than that of the whole country. The state had a life expectancy (both sexes) of 74.8 years in 2010, approximately one year higher than the observed for Brazil: 73.9. In other words, the age structure of Parana is slightly aged than observed in Brazil, as illustrated by Figure 1.Therefore, by its population characteristics, the state of Parana brings an interesting case study for the assessment of the evolution of COVID-19 pandemics. Instituto Paranaense de Desenvolvimento Econômico e Social, a state-level unit that develop social studies to subsidize policymaking, produced population projection estimates at the municipality level and showed that, from the 399 municipalities in the state, 83 had more than 20 percent of elderly among the total population (IPARDES 2020).

Figure 1: Population age-structure of Brazil and Parana, 2020

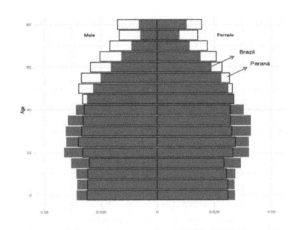

Source: Authors' own elaboration based on IBGE (2020) and Ipardes (2020).

Given these unique features of Parana state, and the availability of administrative microdata by gender, age and sex for the confirmed COVID-19 cases and deaths, the goal of this paper is to explore the demographic evolution of the Coronavirus SARS-CoV-2 deaths and cases in the state. We hypothesize that, although the mortality and fatality rates are found to be, around the word, more concentrated among the elderly, the development of the pandemics in an environment of loose restrictions of social isolation leads to a younger age-structure of the deaths and cases.

BACKGROUND

The first case of COVID-19 in the state of Parana was documented on March 12, 2020. As of July 27, 2020, the state registered 68,000 cases and 1,703 deaths, and, in standardized rates, a COVID-19 death coefficient of 0.05 per 100,000 inhabitants (Brazil: 42 per 100,000 inhabitants) and a fatality rate of 2.5 percent (Brazil: 3.6 percent). An important issue regarding COVID-19 investigations is the underreporting of cases due to limited testing (Mills, 2020; Paixão et al., 2020). Using the ISO calendar as reference, the number of tests, starting from the ISO week 11 (when the first case was documented), 116 tests were performed with a positivity rate of 6 percent. In the week 30, 17,290 were conducted, with a positivity rate of 7.31 percent. Overall, during the full evolution of the pandemic, 217,558 tests were carried out with a positivity rate of 19.25 percent (State of Parana, Health Secretariat, 2020).In Brazil, one important characteristic of the policies aimed to tackle the COVID-19 pandemic was the decentralization of the actions to the state and local levels. In April 2019, the Supreme Court of the country ruled that states and municipalities had autonomy to carry out sanitary, epidemiological and administrative measures related to combating COVID-19. Henceforth, governors and mayors were in charge of establishing rules for isolating, quarantining and restricting transport and transit on highways and ports (BRASIL, 2020).

Even before the documentation of the first COVID-19 case in the state of Parana (a woman, on March 12), the state government had released in February orientations regarding the prevention of COVID-19. Afterwards, in late March, the government announced its first decree (Estado do Paraná, 2020a) suspended public events consisting of more than 50 people; reduced the workload in public offices as well as the possibility of adhering to teleworking; suspended face-to-face classes in public and private state schools and public universities; suspended visits to theatres, cinemas, libraries, museums; obliged the availability of alcohol gel in public offices; suspended the activities of shopping malls, gyms and physical activity centres. A few days later, other decrees from the state government suspended non-essential activities indefinitely (Estado do Paraná, 2020b); prohibited the sale and consumption of alcoholic beverages in public places from 10 pm to 6 am(Estado do Paraná, 2020c) As anticipated by several scholars for the impacts of COVID-19 for Latin America (Enrique Acosta et al., 2020), families across the state of Parana are struggling financially because of the severe impact that COVID-19 has had on the economy. Although the state is amongst the most developed of the country, it was not the case that families andfirms had difficult choices to make during the pandemic. There was a stark reduction in sales, job losses and decreases in tax revenues by the state (Marcelino et al., 2020).

DATA AND METHODS

Our study draws on administrative records from the Parana Health Secretariat shared according to the approved research project UFPR/202038043 (Guimaraes, Raquel et al., 2020). We monitor COVID-19 cases and confirmed COVID-19 deaths by single age, sex and municipality of residence. The Health Secretariat follows a rigid protocol for notification: deaths of residents in the state are included in the statistics if COVID-19 was given as cause following clinical-epidemiological criteria. Also, COVID-19 cases are included in the notification system if only reported when using tests approved by the National Institute for Quality Control in Health/Fiocruz.

It should be noted that the state of Parana uses as sources of information data obtained via information systems or via direct notification from the local health departments.

RESULTS

Indeed, results of COVID-19 cases and deaths in the state of Parana endorse the rejuvenation of the age-structure when the pandemic unfolds in the State. Figure 2 presents the relative age-distribution by sex of COVID-19 cases and deaths according to the temporal evolution of the disease: (a) ISO weeks 11-15; (b) ISO weeks 11-25; and the cumulative scenario (c) ISO weeks 11-30. Comparing the figures, we can infer two patterns: first, that the cases are more concentrated among individuals in the economic active age groups (prime ages). However, this was not the case in the very beginning of the pandemic. Also, for COVID-19 deaths, the initial age-sex distribution was more concentrated among the 50-60s and above. However, with the increase in the number of cases over the weeks (more exposure), there was a clear rejuvenation of the age structure of deaths.

We also explore the heterogeneity in space on the demographic ageing process at the local level and the relationship with the age-distribution of cases and deaths in the 399 municipalities of the state. Figure 3 displays the regional distribution of the confirmed COVID-19 cases according to the percentage of elderly in the municipality and temporal evolution of the pandemic, as in the previous exercise a) ISO weeks 11-15; (b) ISO weeks 11-25; and the cumulative scenario (c) ISO weeks 11-30.Each map display two dimensions, obtained by three quartiles of the variables: percentage of individuals aged 65 years or more, and number of cases. The first variable is fixed over the epidemiological weeks because the information is drawn from annual estimates. Therefore, municipalities are classified in low, medium, high as per the percentage of elderly in the population, and low, medium, high as per the number of confirmed COVID-19 cases (cumulative) in the period of reference. We can see that, with the evolution of the pandemic, the number of low-low municipalities decreases (blue).Out of 109 municipalities with this condition in Figure 3a, only45 persist until the week 30. The rejuvenation process can be seen as from the medium-low municipalities in week 11-15 (green), 112 localities, 77 migrate to the state medium-medium on weeks 11-25 and 22 municipalities to the medium-high state in the weeks 11-30.

A quite similar pattern can be show for the temporal evolution of the deaths on the space (Figures 4a, 4b and 4c). But the changes are quite remarkable: for the municipalities with more percentage of elderly (high), the number of municipalities that turn out to have higher number of deaths (red) increases systematically over the weeks (from 5, to 47, and then to 59 localities). Besides, 1the number of municipalities with the lower percentage of elderly and lower number of registered deaths (low-low, blue) decreases from 126 on week 11-15 to92 on weeks 11-25 and67 on weeks 11-30. On the other hand, from the initial number of medium-low municipalities in week 11-15 (green), 129 localities, 32 migrate to the state medium-high on weeks 11-25 and 20 municipalities continue in this state in the weeks 11-30.

Figure 2: Relative age-distribution by sex of COVID-19 cases and deaths in Parana State by ISO weeks.

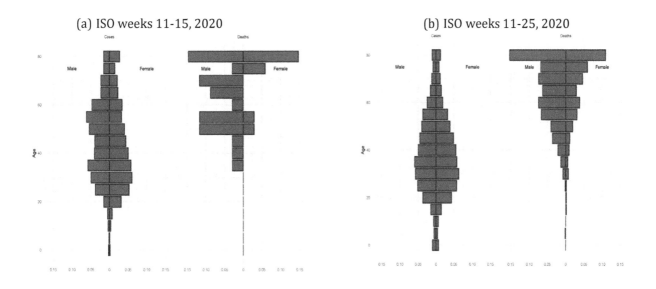

(a) ISO weeks 11-15, 2020

(b) ISO weeks 11-25, 2020

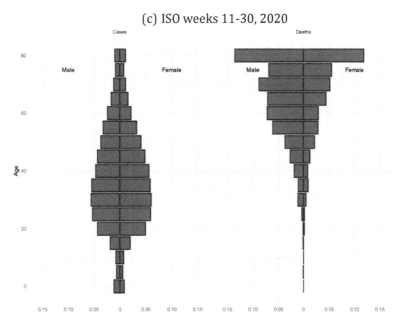

(c) ISO weeks 11-30, 2020

Source: Source: Authors' own elaboration based on IBGE (2020) and Ipardes (2020).

Figure 3: Regional distribution of the confirmed COVID-19 cases, according to the percentage of elderly in the municipality and temporal evolution of the pandemic.

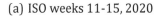

(a) ISO weeks 11-15, 2020   (b) ISO weeks 11-25, 2020

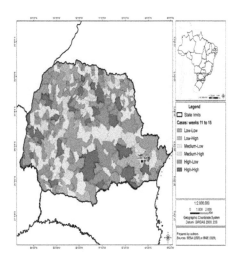
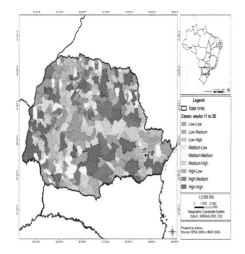

(c) ISO weeks 11-30, 2020

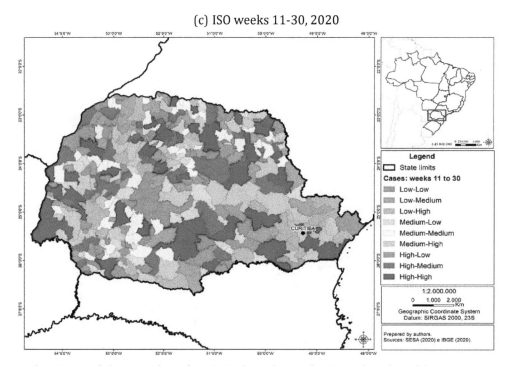

Source: Authors' own elaboration based on IBGE (2020), Ipardes (2020) and Health Secretariat (2020)

Figure 4: Regional distribution of the number of COVID-19 deaths, according to the percentage of elderly in the municipality and temporal evolution of the pandemic.

(a) ISO weeks 11-15, 2020 (b) ISO weeks 11-25, 2020

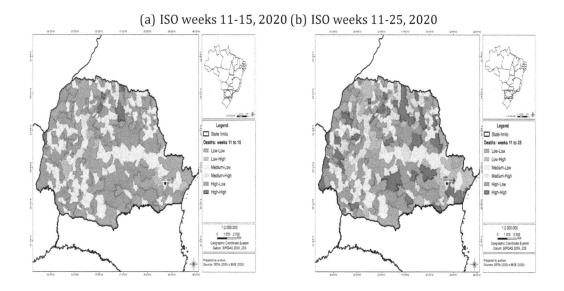

(c) ISO weeks 11-30, 2020

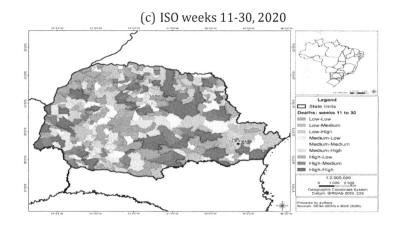

Source: Authors' own elaboration based on IBGE (2020), Ipardes (2020) and Health Secretariat (2020)

CONCLUSION

The demography of COVID-19 cases and deaths has started to gain attention from the academic and policy community. Not only sex and age help in the design of interventions and in understanding the mechanisms behind the disease, but also the heterogeneity in the territory has to be explored. In this article we explore unique administrative records from the Health Secretariat of the Parana State to understand the changes in the demographic age structure of the deaths and cases. As a result of loose incentives from the population to stay in social isolation (which is explained by the huge inequality in the country), cases and deaths are increasing. In a particular old state, Parana, our results demonstrate that, with the evolution of the pandemic and small take up to the measures of social isolation by the population, the age distribution of deaths and cases has rejuvenated over time. As a future research agenda, besides the age-structure, we will incorporate the structure of morbidity in the state, as claimed by several researchers as being an important feature for comparisons (Nepomuceno et al., 2020).

REFERENCES

BRASIL, 2020. MEDIDA PROVISÓRIA Nº 926, DE 20 DE MARÇO DE 2020 [WWW Document]. URL http://www.planalto.gov.br/ccivil_03/_ato2019-2022/2020/Mpv/mpv926.htm (accessed 7.27.20).

Enrique Acosta, Aburto, J.M., Alburez-Gutierrez, D., Guimaraes, R., Nepomuceno, M., 2020. Latin American and Caribbean governments must increase the COVID-19 test coverage drastically to mitigate the humanitarian impact of the pandemic, OSF Preprint. https://doi.org/10.17605/OSF.IO/WG3B2

Estado do Paraná, 2020a. Decreto 4230 - 16 de Março de 2020 [WWW Document]. URL https://www.legislacao.pr.gov.br/legislacao/listarAtosAno.do?action=exibirImpressao&codAto=232854 (accessed 7.27.20).

Estado do Paraná, 2020b. Decreto 4317 - 21 de Março de 2020 [WWW Document]. URL https://www.legislacao.pr.gov.br/legislacao/listarAtosAno.do?action=exibirImpressao&codAto=232854 (accessed 7.27.20).

Estado do Paraná, 2020c. Decreto 4886 - 19 de Junho de 2020 [WWW Document]. URL https://www.legislacao.pr.gov.br/legislacao/listarAtosAno.do?action=exibirImpressao&codAto=232854 (accessed 7.27.20).

Guimaraes, Raquel, Junior Garcia, Welters, Angela, Maia, Denise, Nasr, Acácia, Maranho, Eron, Ciminelli, Rossana, Paganotto, Luís, 2020. A Demografia Econômica do COVID-19 no Paraná: diagnóstico e perspectivas. https://doi.org/10.17605/OSF.IO/YTU3C

IBGE, 2020. Projeções da População do Brasil e Unidades da Federação por sexo e idade: 2010-2060: Indicadores implícitos na projeção [WWW Document]. URL https://www.ibge.gov.br/estatisticas/sociais/populacao/9109-projecao-da-populacao.html?=&t=resultados (accessed 7.27.20).

Marcelino, J.A., Rezende, A., Miyaji, M., 2020. Impactos iniciais da COVID-19 nas micro e pequenas empresas do estado do Paraná - Brasil. Bol. Conjunt. BOCA 2, 101–112. https://doi.org/10.5281/zenodo.3779308

Mills, M., 2020. Demographic Science COVID-19. https://doi.org/10.17605/OSF.IO/SE6WY

Nepomuceno, M.R., Acosta, E., Alburez-Gutierrez, D., Aburto, J.M., Gagnon, A., Turra, C.M., 2020. Besides population age structure, health and other demographic factors can contribute to understanding the COVID-19 burden. Proc. Natl. Acad. Sci. 117, 13881–13883. https://doi.org/10.1073/pnas.2008760117

Paixão, B., Baroni, L., Salles, R., Escobar, L., de Sousa, C., Pedroso, M., Saldanha, R., Coutinho, R., Porto, F., Ogasawara, E., 2020. Estimation of COVID-19 under-reporting in Brazilian States through SARI. ArXiv200612759 Cs Stat.

State of Parana, Health Secretariat, 2020. Notifica COVID-19/SESA, July 27, 2020.

3. COVID-19 Diagnostic and Management Protocol for Paediatric Patients

Ana Paula de Carvalho¹ Panzeri Carlotti,ᴵ Werther Brunow de Carvalho,ᴵᴵ,*
Cı´ntia Johnston,ᴵᴵIsadora Souza Rodriguez,ᴵᴵ
Artur Figueiredo Delgadoᴵᴵ

ᴵ Departamento de Pediatria, Hospital das Clinicas, Faculdade de Medicina de Ribeirao Preto, Universidade de Sao Paulo, Ribeirao Preto, SP, BR. ᴵᴵ Instituto da Crianca e do Adolescente (Icr), Hospital das Clinicas HCFMUSP, Faculdade de Medicina, Universidade de Sao Paulo, Sao Paulo, SP, BR.

Carlotti APCP, Carvalho WB, Johnston C, Rodriguez IS, Delgado AF. COVID-19 Diagnostic and Management Protocol for Pediatric Patients. Clinics. 2020;75:e1894 *

ABSTRACT

This review aims to verify the main epidemiologic, clinical, laboratory-related, and therapeutic aspects of coronavirus disease 2019 (COVID-19) in critically ill paediatric patients. An extensive review of the medical literature on COVID-19 was performed, mainly focusing on the critical care of paediatric patients, considering expert opinions and recent reports related to this new disease. Experts from a large Brazilian public university analysed all recently published material to produce a report aiming to standardize the care of critically ill children and adolescents. The report emphasizes on the clinical presentations of the disease and ventilatory support in paediatric patients with COVID-19. It establishes a flowchart to guide health practitioners on triaging critical cases. COVID-19 is essentially an unknown clinical condition for the majority of paediatric intensive care professionals. Guidelines developed by experts can help all practitioners standardize their attitudes and improve the treatment of COVID-19.

INTRODUCTION

Coronavirus disease 2019 (COVID-19) is a viral respiratory illness caused by severe acute respiratory syndrome coronavirus 2 (SARS-CoV-2), a single-stranded RNA virus that most likely originated in bats. The virus is thought to spread mainly from person-to-person via close contact (the virus can be transferred from the hands to the eyes, nose, or mouth) and respiratory droplets (produced when an infected person coughs or sneezes). There is no evidence of vertical transmission or transmission via breastfeeding. Transmission from asymptomatic or mildly symptomatic carriers or during the incubation period, estimated to be between 1 and 14 days (mean, 5 days), can also occur; 95% of patients develop symptoms up to 12.5 days after exposure. This gave rise to the established quarantine period of 14 days after exposure (1,2).Clinical presentation The clinical spectrum of COVID-19 ranges from being asymptomatic to being in severe

---

¹ Corresponding author. E-mail: werther.brunow@hc.fm.usp.br

acute respiratory distress (Figure 1) (3). According to a case series of 2143 paediatric patients (3) registered in the China Centre for Disease Control and Prevention (CDC) database, 731 cases were confirmed using laboratory testing, 94 (4.4%) patients were asymptomatic, 1091 (50.9%) patients presented with mild symptoms, and 831 (38.8%) patients presented with moderate symptoms. Only 125 (5.8%) patients developed severe or critical disease. Younger children were more susceptible to severe or critical symptoms (10.6% o1 year old vs. 3% X16 years old); there were 13 critical cases, and in seven (53.8%) of them the patient was less than 1 year old. Only one death was reported, that is, of a 14-year-old boy. According to another series of 171 paediatric cases (4) (1 day to 15 years old; median, 6.7 years) admitted to a hospital in Wuhan, China, all patients tested positive for COVID-19, 27 (15.8%) were asymptomatic, 33 (19.3%) had upper airway symptoms, and 111 (64.9%) had pneumonia. Seventy-one paediatric patients presented with fever (41.5%) which lasted 1 to 16 days (median, 3 days).

Clinical Presentation of Covid-19

Asyntomatic Infection	Absence of clinical signs and symptoms of the disease and normal chest X-ray or CT scan associated with a positive test for SARS-CoV-2
Mild Infection	Upper airway symptoms such as fever, fatigue, myalgia, cough, sore throat, runny nose and sneezing. Pulmonary clinical exam is normal. Some cases may not have fever and others may experience gastrintestinal symptoms such as nauseas, vomiting, abdominal pain, and diarrhea.
Moderate Infection	Clinical signs of pneumonia. Persistent fever, initially dry cough, which becomes productive, may have wheezing or crackles on pulmonary auscultation but shows no respiratory distress. Some individuals may not have symptoms or clinical signs, but chest CT scan reveals typical pulmonary lesions.
Severe Infection	Initial respiratory symptoms may be associated with gastrointestinal symptoms such as diarrhea. The clinical deterioration usually occurs in a week with the development of dyspnea and hypoxemia (blood oxygen saturation [SaO$_2$] <94%)
Critical Infection	Patients can quickly deteriorate to acute respiratory distress syndrome or respiratory failure and may present shock, encephalopathy, myocardial injury or heart failure, coagulopathy, acute kidney injury, and multiple organ dysfunction.

Figure 1 - Clinical Presentation of COVID-19.

Three patients were admitted to the intensive care unit; all of them had comorbidities such as hydronephrosis, leukaemia (during chemotherapy), and intussusception. The patient presenting with intussusception was 10 months old; the patient's condition deteriorated, leading to multiple organ dysfunction and death. Various cutaneous rashes have been recently observed in some paediatric cases with variable clinical presentations (5,6).

Laboratory Findings

The white blood *cell* count can be normal or reduced. A series of 171 paediatric cases of COVID-19 reported leukopenia in 26.3% of patients; only 3.5% developed lymphocytopenia. C-reactive protein levels can be normal or elevated. Severe or critical cases may be accompanied by an elevation in hepatic and muscular enzyme levels and high D-dimer levels (2,4).

Imaging Findings

During the initial phase of illness, chest radiography findings can show signs of pneumonia, such as small irregular lung opacities and interstitial alterations, usually affecting peripheral areas. Ground glass opacities (GGO) and consolidation may be observed in severe cases. Pleural effusion is uncommon. Chest computed tomography also exhibits GGO and segmental consolidation in both lungs. Children presenting with severe infection may show lobar consolidation bilaterally (2). Lung ultrasonography (US) exhibits single or grouped, usually bilateral, pneumogenictype vertical artefacts and/or small areas of white lung. Advanced COVID-19 pneumonia is characterized by evident consolidation, particularly in the poster basal regions, and widespread patched artefactual changes, similar to those in acute respiratory distress syndrome (ARDS) (7). Thoracic electrical impedance tomography can be used to monitor the distribution of regional ventilation in patients with ARDS and to identify refractory hypoxemia that requires alveolar recruitment manoeuvres.

Detection of etiological agent

The detection of SARS-CoV-2 nucleic acid using real-time reverse transcriptase-polymerase chain reaction (RT-PCR) is the reference standard for COVID-19 diagnosis. The virus can be detected in upper airway or inferior airway secretions (nasopharynx swab or tracheal aspirates [if intubated], sputum, and bronchoalveolar lavage), blood, urine, and stool (1,8). In a case series of 10 paediatric patients from Shanghai (9), viral RNA was detected in the nasopharynx of all patients from 4 to 48h after the beginning of symptoms up to 6 to 22 days (mean, 12 days) after the first day of illness. In five patients, SARS-CoV-2 RNA was detected in the stool until 18 to 30 days after the initial symptoms. According to the 22-38 SS Resolution, 3-17-2020, from São Paulo's State Health Secretary (10), RT-PCR for SARS-CoV-2 should be performed only for patients in a severe or critical condition, those in sentinel units, and health care professionals with symptoms typical of COVID-19. The test should not be performed in asymptomatic individuals.

Diagnostic Criteria

A diagnosis is made considering clinical findings, epidemiology, and laboratory testing to confirm SARS-CoV-2infection (2). Figure 2 shows the flowchart for patients with flu-like symptoms as proposed by the São Paulo State Health Secretary (10,11).Differential diagnosis. Other viral respiratory illnesses. Respiratory syncytial virus, influenza, parainfluenza, adenovirus, and metapneumovirus are frequent causes of lower airway infection in children and have similar clinical presentation to COVID-19. The diagnosis can be made by identifying the etiological agent in respiratory secretions using polymerase chain reaction. Bacterial pneumonia. The main clinical manifestations of bacterial pneumonia are high fever and taxemic state.

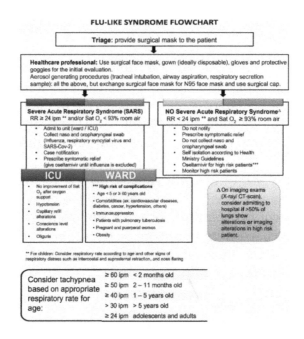

Figure 2- Flu-like syndrome flowchart.

Frequently, there is leucocytosis with neutrophilia and increased numbers of younger cells. Blood and aspirate tracheal cultures are very important. Bronchoalveolar lavage (BAL) in intubated patients can be very useful in making a diagnosis. **Atypical pneumonia. Mycoplasma pneumoniae** and **Chlamydia pneumoniae** are important causative agents of community-acquired pneumonia in children, and serologic tests can be used to confirm the diagnosis (2).

Therapeutic Management

The four main principles for adequate therapeutic management are early identification, early isolation, early diagnosis, and early treatment. When dealing with a case of suspected COVID-19, the patient should be kept in a single room with all precautions to prevent and control infections before laboratorial confirmation. Mild cases should be treated with symptomatic relief medication, preferably paracetamol or dipyrone, to control fever. Antiviral agents, including Oseltamivir, Ribavirin, Ganciclovir, Remdesivir, Lopinavir, And Ritonavir, have been used to reduce the viral load to prevent potential respiratory complications but with no apparent benefits thus far (1,2,12). A Chinese study (13) of more than 100 patients reported that chloroquine was secure and effective in treating COVID-19-associated pneumonia, inhibiting exacerbation of pneumonia, reducing radiographic alterations, promoting virus elimination, and decreasing the period of time of the disease. Another French study (14) enrolled 20 patients with COVID-19 and showed that treatment with hydroxychloroquine was associated with cure of the viral infection, with the utilization of azithromycin leading to increased benefit.

There are other current studies analysing the drug's efficiency in critically ill patients with a higher risk of death and considering the use of hydroxychloroquine/chloroquine (5–10 mg/kg/day of basic chloroquine for 10 days) and azithromycin (10 mg/kg on the first day, followed by 5 mg/kg/day for 4 days with a maximum dose of 30 mg/kg or 1,500 mg) (14-16). Severe cases with respiratory distress and/or hypoxia (SaO^2 o94%) (Severe Acute Respiratory Syndrome) should be admitted to the hospital. Indications for ICU admission are: respiratory failure requiring mechanical ventilation, shock or other organ dysfunction requiring treatment (9,17). The main characteristic of the critical cases is the occurrence of ARDS with hypoxemic acute respiratory distress and bilateral pulmonary infiltrates that are not explained by cardiac dysfunction or fluid overload.

The main treatment principles of ARDS are as follows (17-20):arly tracheal intubation rapid sequence intubation is the best practice in this situation. Preoxygenation should be performed using a flexible nasal cannula (up to flows of 4 L/min) or a reservoir mask with a lower flux to maintain an SaO$_2$ 493%. Positive pressure ventilation with a bag-valve-mask or other similar apparatus should be avoided to not generate aerosols. Sedation can be performed using fentanyl (1–2 mg/ kg) or ketamine (1–2 mg/kg, if there is no contraindication such as pulmonary hypertension) and neuromuscular blocking with rocuronium (0.6–1.2 mg/kg), preferably. Video laryngoscopy should be utilized if available. Non-invasive ventilation (NIV) should be avoided because of the high risk of aerosol dispersion and contamination among health practitioners.

Protective mechanical ventilation using a pressure controlled or volume cycled, with a low tidal volume (around 6 mL/kg) and plateau pressure p30 cmH$_2$O. The positive end-expiratory pressure (PEEP) should be titrated such that FiO$_2$ is reduced (p50%), with PaO$_2$ 460 mmHg and SaO$_2$ 490–93%. The general recommendation is to start with PEEP at 5–6 cmH$_2$O and increase progressively to 12–14 cmH$_2$O if necessary. It's very important to maintain a driving pressure (plateau pressure PEEP) o15 cmH$_2$O and tolerate hypercapnia with pH 47.2 (permissive hypercapnia), except for patients with pulmonary hypertension. Prone positioning, especially if PaO$_2$/FiO$_2$ o150 mmHg. The patient should be maintained in this position for at least 18 hours per day with oximetry and capnography monitoring. Closed tracheal aspiration systems should be used.

Treatment with nitric oxide and/or sildenafil (0.5–2 mg/ kg/dose each 4–6 hours with a maximum of 20 mg/dose each 8 hours) for patients with persistent hypoxemia.

Venovenous extracorporeal membrane oxygenation (ECMO) can be used in patients with PaO$_2$/FiO$_2$ o70–80 mmHg in whom conventional treatment (protective mechanical ventilation, prone positioning, nitric oxide/sildenafil) was not successful, according to its availability in the hospital. Conservative fluid therapy, including volume restriction in patients with hemodynamic stability, starting with 50% of the normal recommendation based on the Holliday-Segar rule, and adjustments according to the fluid balance and hemodynamic clinical conditions. Patients with wheezing and lower airway obstruction should be treated with the aim of reducing respiratory droplet dispersion inside the environment. Aerosol bronchodilators should be avoided and spray or dosimetric inhalers should be used. It is possible to utilize NIV in some cases but it should use a mechanical ventilator with a double circuit, with filters in both parts (to warm and humidify in the inspiratory circuit and a high-efficiency particle separator in the expiratory circuit).

It is necessary to emphasize that NIV support has been used in isolation hospital rooms with negative pressure only. After 1 to 2 hours of non-invasive mechanical ventilation without adequate evolution, tracheal intubation is recommended. Mechanical ventilation support should avoid pulmonary hyper insufflation, auto-PEEP, and barotrauma. Pressure-controlled ventilation is preferred in synchronized intermittent mandatory ventilation with support pressure, low breathing rate, inspiration/expiration time rate of 1:3–1:4 and PEEP=5 cmH$_2$O.

Antibiotics should be used only in patients with secondary bacterial infections on the basis of the culture and antibiogram results. Corticosteroids can suppress lung inflammation but also inhibit immune responses and pathogen clearance and should be avoided except for those with a specific indication (e.g., bronchospasm or some cases of septic shock) (1,2).

There is a report that intravenous immunoglobulin treatment in a 3-year-old critically ill child was effective (21). Patients with cardiocirculatory dysfunction and shock should be treated with fluid therapy or vasoactive/inotropic drugs. Milrinone (0.1–1.0 mg/kg/min) or dobutamine (5–15 mg/kg/min) can be useful in patients with a low cardiac index as a consequence of pulmonary hypertension and normal arterial pressure. Epinephrine at an inotropic dose (p0.3 mg/kg/min) can be used in patients with hypotension. In children and adolescents with other organic dysfunctions, continuous renal replacement therapy may be necessary because renal dysfunction is an indicator of a poor prognosis (1,2,7). Microthrombosis and associated ischemic events are very common (e.g., strokes), mainly in adolescents and adults. D-dimer levels should be monitored frequently. Appropriate medical transport for the patient (and their parent/caregiver) to the hospital should be provided by medical transport teams. Community paediatricians should advise parents to wait for this service and to not seek secondary care themselves, for example, by going to the hospital via car or public transport (22).

REFERENCES

1. He F, Deng Y, Li W. Coronavirus disease 2019: What we know? J Med Virol. 2020 doi: 10.1002/jmv.25766. [PMC free article] [PubMed] [CrossRef] [Google Scholar]
2. Chen ZM, Fu JF, Shu Q, Chen YH, Hua CZ, Li FB, et al. Diagnosis and treatment recommendations for pediatric respiratory infection caused by the 2019 novel coronavirus. World J Pediatr. 2020 doi: 10.1007/s12519-020-00345-5. [PMC free article] [PubMed] [CrossRef] [Google Scholar]
3. Dong Y, Mo X, Hu Y, Qi X, Jiang F, Jiang Z, et al. Epidemiological Characteristics of 2143 Pediatric Patients With 2019 Coronavirus Disease in China. Pediatrics. 2020:pii e20200702. doi: 10.1542/peds.2020-0702. [CrossRef] [Google Scholar]
4. Lu X, Zhang L, Du H, Zhang J, Li YY, Qu J, et al. SARS-CoV-2 Infection in Children. N Engl J Med. 2020 doi: 10.1056/NEJMc2005073. [PMC free article] [PubMed] [CrossRef] [Google Scholar]
5. Recalcati S. Cutaneous manifestations in COVID-19: a first perspective. J Eur Acad Dermatol Venereol. 2020 doi: 10.1111/jdv.16387. [PubMed] [CrossRef] [Google Scholar]
6. Joob B, Wiwanitkit V. COVID-19 can present with a rash and be mistaken for Dengue. J Am Acad Dermatol. 2020:pii: S0190-9622(20)30454-0. doi: 10.1016/j.jaad.2020.03.036. [PMC free article] [PubMed] [CrossRef] [Google Scholar]
7. Soldati G, Smargiassi A, Inchingolo R, Buonsenso D, Perrone T, Briganti DF, et al. Is there a role for lung ultrasound during the COVID-19 pandemic? J Ultrasound Med. 2020 doi: 10.1002/jum.15284. [PMC free article] [PubMed] [CrossRef] [Google Scholar]
8. Bouadma L, Lescure FX, Lucet JC, Yazdanpanah Y, Timsit JF. Severe SARS-CoV-2 infections: practical considerations and management strategy for intensivists. Intensive Care Med. 2020;46((4)):579–82. doi: 10.1007/s00134-020-05967-x. [PMC free article] [PubMed] [CrossRef] [Google Scholar]
9. Cai J, Xu J, Lin D, Yang Z, Xu L, Qu Z, et al. A Case Series of children with 2019 novel coronavirus infection: clinical and epidemiological features. Clin Infect Dis. 2020:pii: ciaa198. doi: 10.1093/cid/ciaa198. [PMC free article] [PubMed] [CrossRef] [Google Scholar]
10. Resolução SS-28, 17-03-2020 . Diário Oficial do Estado de São Paulo, 130 (54), pages 24-25. [Google Scholar]
11. Protocolo de Tratamento do Novo Coronavírus (2019-nCoV) Ministério da Saúde; Brasil: 2020. [Google Scholar]
12. Cao B, Wang Y, Wen D, Liu W, Wang J, Fan G, et al. A Trial of Lopinavir-Ritonavir in Adults Hospitalized with Severe COVID-19. N Engl J Med. 2020 doi: 10.1056/NEJMoa2001282. [PMC free article] [PubMed] [CrossRef] [Google Scholar]
13. Gao J, Tian Z, Yang X. Breakthrough: Chloroquine phosphate has shown apparent efficacy in treatment of COVID-19 associated pneumonia in clinical studies. Biosci Trends. 2020;14((1)):72–3. doi: 10.5582/bst.2020.01047. [PubMed] [CrossRef] [Google Scholar]
14. Gautret P, Lagier JC, Parola P, Hoang VT, Meddeb L, Mailhe M, et al. Hydroxychloroquine and azithromycin as a treatment of COVID-19: results of an open-label non-randomized clinical trial. Int J Antimicrob

Agents. 2020:105949. doi: 10.1016/j.ijantimicag.2020.105949. [PMC free article] [PubMed] [Cross-Ref] [Google Scholar]

15. Cortegiani A, Ingoglia G, Ippolito M, Giarratano A, Einav S. A systematic review on the efficacy and safety of chloroquine for the treatment of COVID-19. J Crit Care. 2020:pii: S0883-9441(20)30390-7. doi: 10.1016/j.jcrc.2020.03.005. [PMC free article] [PubMed] [CrossRef] [Google Scholar]

16. Smith ER, Klein-Schwartz W. Are 1-2 dangerous? Chloroquine and hydroxychloroquine exposure in toddlers. J Emerg Med. 2005;28((4)):437–43. doi: 10.1016/j.jemermed.2004.12.011. [PubMed] [CrossRef] [Google Scholar]

17. Wang H, Wang S, Yu K. COVID-19 infection epidemic: the medical management strategies in Heilongjiang Province, China. Crit Care. 2020;24((1)):107. doi: 10.1186/s13054-020-2832-8. [PMC free article] [PubMed] [CrossRef] [Google Scholar]

18. Murthy S, Gomersall CD, Fowler RA. Care for Critically Ill Patients With COVID-19. JAMA. 2020 doi: 10.1001/jama.2020.3633. [PubMed] [CrossRef] [Google Scholar]

19. Ferguson ND, Guérin C. Adjunct and rescue therapies for refractory hypoxemia: prone position, inhaled nitric oxide, high frequency oscillation, extra corporeal life support. Intensive Care Med. 2018;44((9)):1528–31. doi: 10.1007/s00134-017-5040-5. [PubMed] [CrossRef] [Google Scholar]

20. Associação de Medicina Intensiva Brasileira . Manuseio do paciente com infecção pelo Coronavírus COVID-19, pneumonia e insuficiência respiratória. 2020. Pelo Comitê de Ventilação Mecânica da AMIB. [Google Scholar]

21. Liu W, Zhang Q, Chen J, Xiang R, Song H, Shu S, et al. Detection of COVID-19 in Children in Early January 2020 in Wuhan, China. N Engl J Med. 2020 doi: 10.1056/NEJMc2003717. [PMC free article] [PubMed] [Cross-Ref] [Google Scholar]

22. European Centre for Disease Prevention and Control (2020, March 4) Situation update worldwide, March 4th 2020 . 2020. Available from: https://www.ecdc.europa.eu/en/geographical-distribution-2019-ncov-cases. [Google Scholar]

4. The Challenging And Unpredictable Spectrum Of COVID-19 In Children And Adolescents

Marco Aurelio Palazzi Safadi[a] , Clovis Artur Almeida da Silva[b,*]

A novel coronavirus, named severe acute respiratory syndrome coronavirus 2 (SARS-CoV-2), emerged in China in the end of 2019 and after less than 6 months its related disease (COVID-19) has already affected more than 6 million individuals in almost all countries worldwide. COVID-19 was declared a pandemic by the World Health Organization on March 11, 2020, becoming one of the most challenging and concerning public health crisis faced by this generation.[1-4]

A striking feature of COVID-19 pandemic is that children and adolescents seem to be less frequently infected by SARS-CoV-2 comparing to adults. Preliminary evidence also shows that, unlike influenza or respiratory syncytial virus, children do not play a critical role in SARS-CoV-2 transmission in the community.[5] Furthermore, although most infected children and adolescents are asymptomatic or present mild symptoms, recent unexpected data showing the emergence of a late-onset severe inflammatory syndrome temporally associated with SARS-CoV-2 highlights the importance of continued surveillance around the world.[6]

Data from laboratory-confirmed COVID-19 cases in Asia, Europe and North America, by age groups, showed that the prevalence of children and adolescents in these case series ranged from 1.0 to 1.7%. The clinical spectrum of paediatric COVID-19 is wide, ranging from asymptomatic to critically ill cases. Fever and cough were consistently the most common reported symptoms in these case series, although less frequently than in adults, followed by pharyngeal erythema, shortness of breath, rhinorrhoea, nausea, abdominal pain, vomiting and diarrhoea.

Additional symptoms reported included myalgia, tiredness, headache, anosmia and ageusia. More recently, variable cutaneous manifestations have been described in paediatric populations with COVID-19, including erythematous rashes, urticaria, vesicular and chilblain-like lesions.[7]

Leukopenia, lymphopenia and increased inflammatory markers (erythrocyte sedimentation rate, C-reactive protein or procalcitonin) were the most frequently reported laboratorial findings in children and adolescents with COVID-19.

Although data is limited comparing to adults, lymphopenia, high levels of C-reactive protein, procalcitonin, D-dimer and creatine kinase muscle and brain (MB) biomarkers were laboratorial findings associated with more severe disease.[1-7] Clinical course of COVID-19 in children and adolescents uncommonly resulted in life-threatening illness with severe outcomes. In the largest reported case series from USA, with information on hospitalization status, approximately 20% of the children and adolescents were hospitalized and 2% of them were admitted in Paediatric Intensive Care Units (PICU). Importantly, infants aged <1 year represented the age group with the highest percentage of hospitalization among COVID-19 paediatric patients. Less than 1% of children and adolescents had severe COVID-19 with acute respiratory distress syndrome or multiorgan failure.[8] A recent study reporting the outcomes of children and adolescents with COVID-19 admitted to USA and Canadian PICU showed severe disease is less frequent, and early outcomes in children hospitalized are far better comparing to adults. Interestingly, among 46 children and adolescents (median age 13 years) admitted to the PICU, 40 (83%) were found to have chronic underlying health conditions, 18 (38%) of them required invasive ventilatory support and only 2 (4.2%) died.[9] In the end of Abril, cases of a severe rare syndrome, temporally associated with COVID-19, have been reported in children and adolescents, initially in Europe and then in North and Latin America.

This syndrome, named multisystem inflammatory syndrome in children (MIS-C), occurs days to weeks after acute SARS-CoV-2 infection. The clinical characteristics of MIS-C share similar features with Kawasaki disease (KD), KD shock syndrome, macrophage activation syndrome (MAS) and toxic shock syndrome. Although many patients with MIS-C meet criteria for complete or incomplete KD, affected children were older, presented more intense inflammation and higher levels of markers of cardiac injury.

A broad spectrum of presenting signs and symptoms and disease severity were observed among reported MIS-C cases, including persistent fever, gastrointestinal symptoms (abdominal pain, vomiting, diarrhoea), rash, conjunctivitis, progressing in some cases to shock, myocarditis, acute heart failure and development of coronary artery aneurysms. Patients who have presented with this syndrome were, in general, previously healthy, and most of them have tested negative for SARS-CoV-2 RNA but positive for antibodies, suggesting an unbalanced immune response following SARS-CoV-2 infection. Laboratory findings include lymphocytopenia, increased inflammatory (C-reactive protein, erythrocyte sedimentation rate, D-dimer, ferritin) and cardiac biomarkers (troponin, brain natriuretic peptide [BNP]).[6]

Based on current evidence, older adults and people of all ages with underlying medical conditions, including severe obesity, chronic lung disease, cardiovascular disease, diabetes mellitus, chronic kidney disease, liver disease, active cancer, transplantation and immunocompromised have been associated with poor clinical outcomes and higher fatality rates from COVID-19.[1,3] There are limited data on which underlying conditions in children and adolescents are associated with increased risk of infection or severe illness. Infants <1 year of age and children with chronic pulmonary diseases (including moderate to severe asthma), cardiovascular illnesses (including congenital heart disease), malignancy, immunosuppression and obesity appear to be at increased risk of severe disease.[8-10]

Data of immunocompromised patients with autoimmune diseases and COVID-19 are scarce. Although the true risk of life-threatening complications of this emerging infectious disease for these chronic illnesses is not yet known, there are particular concerns regarding SARS-CoV-2 infection for patients treated with immunosuppressive, biological agents and disease-modifying antirheumatic drugs.[11] One of the most important Latin American reference centres for paediatric liver diseases and paediatric liver transplantation in Brazil described their experience with 169 non-transplant children and adolescents suspected and tested for SARS-CoV-2. Of note, 13/169 (8%) of them had laboratory-confirmed COVID-19. All of them had mild COVID-19, except one that died due to a serious genetic syndrome. Furthermore, during the study period, none of 190 paediatric liver transplant patients had COVID-19.[12]

Overall morbidity and mortality of COVID-19 in paediatric patients with cancer seem to be low. One of the largest paediatric cancer programs in the USA, in New York city, reported that 20/178 (11%) children and adolescents with cancer had positive test for SARS-CoV-2. Only one patient with COVID-19 required noncritical hospitalization.[13] Malignancy in paediatric populations are generally aggressive, needing multiple chemotherapy or stem cell transplantation. Therefore, postponing these therapies are not recommended during COVID-19 pandemic. Importantly, the long-term effects of this pandemic, with school closure and social isolation during quarantine/lockdown for children and adolescents, may influence sedentary behaviour and consumption of calories-dense comfort foods, increasing the risk of weight gain and contributing for metabolic and cardiovascular diseases, particularly among those living in urban districts.[11]

Challenges related to this pandemic in children/ adolescents. Non-pharmacological interventions have been an essential preventive measure, recommended by national and international public health authorities. Besides the risk of limited or even no education for children and adolescents during COVID-19 crisis, home confinements may induce longer screen time, physical inactivity, sleep abnormalities, increase alcohol intake risk and domestic violence, particularly in adolescents. Drug adherence should also be reinforced for patients with pre-existing chronic disease and their families due to risk of disease flare or disease damage.

Patients with suspected or confirmed COVID-19 must be strictly monitored for the possible risk of disease reactivation after the resolution of this viral infection.[11]

The overwhelmed public health systems by the COVID19 pandemic represents a serious risk for paediatric general health, limiting access of children and adolescents to basic health care, compromising immunization coverages and postponing consultations for patients with underlying conditions. Moreover, mental health burden and socio-economic issues may contribute for short and long-term negative outcomes in children and adolescents and their families. Acute stress, anxiety, mild to severe depression, post-traumatic stress disorder, and emotional exhaustion may be first diagnosed during or after COVID-19 pandemic.

Thus, online mental health care delivery, using teleconsultation or telephone support lines, may be required for paediatric populations.[14]

Identification of a safe and effective antiviral therapy, that could improve disease outcomes, has been object of extensive research worldwide. However, there is no convincing data showing that any of the several antivirals inhibitor such as Lopinavir/Ritonavir, Remdesivir Or Favipiravir) that are being tested proved to be safe and efficacious against SARS-CoV-2. Moreover, it must be acknowledged that the majority of these trials have been performed in adults, with very limited data, if any, for most of the different candidate antiviral therapies in children.[15]It is also of paramount importance to have in mind that the overwhelming majority of children and adolescents with COVID-19, once infected, will develop a mild, self-limited form of disease. It means that a large number of patients would have to be treated in order to demonstrate the benefits of an antiviral, raising concerns of the potential adverse events associated with this intervention.

This way, it is our opinion that, given the lack of evidence supporting safety and efficacy of the current available drugs for the treatment of COVID-19 in children and adolescents, only supportive care should be routinely recommended for the majority of cases. In selected cases, of severe disease presentations or potential risk for disease progression due to the presence of strong risk factors, the use of antiviral therapy might be considered on a case-by-case individualized decision, assuming that the benefits outweigh risks of potential adverse events of the drug used. It is recommended that, ideally, these off-label antiviral therapies for COVID-19 should occur as part of a clinical trial. Post-exposure prophylaxis is another potential strategy for using antiviral therapies. In this context, a recent double-blind randomized trial tested the use of hydroxychloroquine within four days after the reported exposure. However, results did not show any effect of this drug on the prevention of illness compatible with COVID-19 or confirmed SARS-CoV-2 infection when used as post-exposure prophylaxis.[16] The most exciting and fascinating chapter of the battle against COVID-19 is undoubtedly the development of a safe and effective vaccine. We currently have more than 130 candidate vaccines being developed, at least 10 of them already being tested in humans, using different vaccine platforms, including nucleic acid-based (mRNA and DNA), vector-based, and inactivated or recombinant protein vaccines. Studies performed with several vaccine strategies against the other zoonotic coronavirus, SARS-CoV and MERS-CoV, focused on the S protein target, paved the way to facilitate a more rapid development of the current SARS-CoV-2 vaccine.[17]

Although significant progress has been made in a very short period of time, we still have several unanswered questions and challenges to the development of a vaccine against SARS-CoV-2, including the theoretical risk of Antibody Dependent-Enhancement, the lack of clear correlates of protection, the long-term persistence of the immune responses induced by vaccination, the number of vaccine doses required for different age groups, the probable need of adjuvants to trigger TH1 response, and high neutralizing antibodies to spare antigen dosing. It is also difficult to anticipate whether these vaccines will provide protection against infection (which would also have the possibility to decrease transmission in the community once high coverage is achieved) or only prevent disease severity and/or death.[17]

The role of a recent Bacille-Calmette-Guerin (BCG) immunization in the prevention of COVID-19 is also being investigated in clinical trials. Previous studies have shown that BCG immunization, besides its specific effect against severe forms of tuberculosis, induces a nonspecific protective immune response against other infections.[17] In conclusion, almost six months into the COVID-19 pandemic, its epicentre has displaced from China, Europe and USA to Brazil, exposing our vulnerable population to devastating consequences. Despite the fact that children and adolescents appear to have lower prevalence, milder clinical manifestations and lower fatality rates, compared to other age groups, COVID-19 global crisis has a potentially profound, long-term negative impact on paediatric populations. The recent identification of rare and severe inflammatory syndrome cases of COVID-19 in older children and adolescents highlights its unpredictable pathogenesis spectrum and outcomes. Mental health burden, social impact and financial loss are important challenges for children and adolescents of this and future generations. Further multicentre and longitudinal paediatrics studies with large populations will be necessary to clarify these findings and to evaluate specific healthy and pre-existing chronic diseases in children and adolescents.

Funding

This study was supported by grants from Conselho Nacional de Desenvolvimento Científico e Tecnológico (CNPq 303422/2015-7 to CAS), Fundação de Amparo à Pesquisa do Estado de São Paulo (FAPESP 2015/03756-4 to CAS), and by Núcleo de Apoio à Pesquisa "Saúde da Criança e do Adolescente" da USP (NAP-CriAd) to CAS.

REFERENCES

1. World Health Organization (WHO) [homepage on the Internet]. Coronavirus disease (COVID-19) pandemic. Geneva: WHO; 2020 [cited 2020 Jun 05]. Available from: https://www.who.int/emergencies/diseases/novel-coronavirus-2019

2. Safadi MA. The intriguing features of COVID-19 in children and its impact on the pandemic. J Pediatr (Rio J). 2020;96:265-8. https://doi.org/10.1016/j.jped.2020.04.001

3. Palmeira P, Barbuto JA, Silva CA, Carneiro-Sampaio M. Why is SARS-CoV-2 infection milder among children? Clinics. 2020;75:e1947. https://doi.org/10.6061/clinics/2020/e1947

4. Almeida FJ, Olmos RD, Oliveira DB, Monteiro CO, Thomazelli LM, Durigon EL, et al. Hematuria associated with SARS-CoV-2 infection in a child. Pediatr Infect Dis J. 2020;39:e161. https://doi.org/10.1097/inf.0000000000002737

5. Lee B, Raszka Jr WV. COVID-19 transmission and children: the child is not to blame. Pediatrics. 2020;e2020004879. https://doi.org/10.1542/peds.2020-004879

6. Whittaker E, Bamford A, Kenny J, Kaforou M, Jones CE, Shah P, et al. Clinical characteristics of 58 children with a pediatric inflammatory multisystem syndrome temporally associated with SARS-CoV-2. JAMA. 2020. Epub 2020 Jun 08. https://doi.org/10.1001/jama.2020.10369

7. Parri N, Lenge M, Buonsenso D, Coronavirus Infection in Pediatric Emergency Departments (CONFIDENCE) Research Group. Children with COVID-19 in pediatric emergency departments in Italy. New Engl J Med. 2020. Epub 2020 May 01. https://doi.org/10.1056/NEJMc2007617

8. Centres for Disease Control and Prevention (CDC) COVID-19 Response Team. Coronavirus disease 2019 in children - United States, February 12-April 2, 2020. MMWR Morb Mortal Wkly Rep. 2020;69:422-6. https://doi.org/10.15585/mmwr.mm6914e4

9. Shekerdemian LS, Mahmood NR, Wolfe KK, Riggs BJ, Ross CE, McKiernan CA, et al. Characteristics and outcomes of children with coronavirus disease 2019 (COVID-19) infection admitted to US and Canadian pediatric intensive care units. JAMA Pediatr. 2020. Epub 2020 May 11. https://doi.org/10.1001/jamapediatrics.2020.1948

10. Chao JY, Derespina KR, Herold BC, Goldman DL, Aldrich M, Weingarten J, et al. Clinical characteristics and outcomes of hospitalized and critically Ill children and adolescents with coronavirus disease 2019 (COVID-19) at a tertiary care medical centre in New York City. J Pediatr. 2020;S0022-3476;30580-1. https://doi.org/10.1016/j.jpeds.2020.05.006

11. Silva CA, Queiroz LB, Fonseca CB, Silva LE, Lourenço B, Marques HH. Spotlight for healthy and preexisting chronic diseases adolescents during COVID-19 pandemic. Clinics. 2020;75:e1931. https://doi.org/10.6061/clinics/2020/e1931

12. Tannuri U, Tannuri AC, Cordon MN, Miyatani HT. Low incidence of COVID-19 in children and adolescent post-liver transplant at a Latin American reference centre. Clinics. 2020;75:e1986. https://doi.org/10.6061/clinics/2020/e1986

13. Boulad F, Kamboj M, Bouvier N, Mauguen A, Kung AL. COVID-19 in children with cancer in New York city. JAMA Oncol. 2020. Epub 2020 May 13. https://doi.org/10.1001/jamaoncol.2020.2028

14. Brooks SK, Webster RK, Smith LE, Woodland L, Wessely S, Greenberg N, et al. The psychological impact of quarantine and how to reduce it: rapid review of the evidence. Lancet. 2020;395:912-20. https://doi.org/10.1016/S0140-6736(20)30460-8

15. Chiotos K, Hayes M, Kimberlin DW, Jones SB, James SH, Pinninti SG, et al. Multicentre initial guidance on use of antivirals for children with COVID-19/SARS-CoV-2. J Pediatric Infect Dis Soc. 2020;piaa045. https://doi.org/10.1093/jpids/piaa045

16. Boulware DR, Pullen MF, Bangdiwala AS, Pastick KA, Lofgren SM, Okafor EC, et al. A randomized trial of hydroxychloroquine as postexposure prophylaxis for COVID-19. N Engl J Med. 2020. Epub 2020 Jun 03. https://doi.org/10.1056/NEJMoa2016638

17. Diamond M, Pierson T. The challenges of vaccine development against a new virus during a pandemic. Cell Host Microbe. 2020;27:699-703. https://doi.org/10.1016/j.chom.2020.04.021

5. Adults At High-Risk Of Severe Coronavirus Disease-2019 (COVID-19) In Brazil[1]

Leandro F. M. Rezende[I], Beatriz Thome[I], Mariana Cabral Schveitzer[I],
Paulo Roberto Borges de Souza-Júnior,
Célia Landmann Szwarcwald[II]

[I] Universidade Federal de São Paulo. Escola Paulista de Medicina. Departamento de Medicina Preventiva. São Paulo, SP, Brasil
[II] Fundação Instituto Oswaldo Cruz. Instituto de Comunicação e Informação Científica e Tecnológica em Saúde. Rio de Janeiro, RJ, Brasil

ABSTRACT

OBJECTIVE: To estimate the proportion and total number of the general adult population who may be at higher risk of severe COVID-19 in Brazil. **METHODS:** We included 51,770 participants from a nationally representative, household-based health survey (PNS) conducted in Brazil. We estimated the proportion and number of adults ($\geq$ 18 years) at risk of severe COVID-19 by sex, educational level, race/ethnicity, and state based on the presence of one or more of the following risk factors: age $\geq$ 65 years or medical diagnosis of cardiovascular disease, diabetes, hypertension, chronic respiratory disease, cancer, stroke, chronic kidney disease and moderate to severe asthma, smoking status, and obesity. **RESULTS:** Adults at risk of severe COVID-19 in Brazil varied from 34.0% (53 million) to 54.5% (86 million) nationwide. Less-educated adults present a 2-fold higher prevalence of risk factors compared to university graduated. We found no differences by sex and race/ethnicity. São Paulo, Rio de Janeiro, Minas Gerais, and Rio Grande do Sul were the most vulnerable states in absolute and relative terms of adults at risk. **CONCLUSIONS:** Proportion and total number of adults at risk of severe COVID-19 are high in Brazil, with wide variation across states and adult subgroups. These findings should be considered while designing and implementing prevention measures in Brazil. We argue that these results support broad social isolation measures, particularly when testing capacity for SARS-CoV-2 is limited.

INTRODUCTION

The World Health Organization (WHO) suggests that most people infected with the virus may develop mild or uncomplicated (80%) coronavirus disease 2019 (COVID-19), while the remaining 20% may develop its severe variation, requiring hospitalization (14%) or intensive care unit (6%)[1]. Established risk factors for severe disease among inpatients with COVID-19 in China included older age[2,3] and serious medical conditions such as cardiovascular disease[2-4], diabetes[2-4], chronic respiratory disease (in particular chronic obstructive pulmonary disease COPD)[2], hypertension[2,4], cancer[2,5], and cerebrovascular disease[3,4]. Recent findings from United States (US) and Europe

[1] https://doi.org/10.11606/s1518-8787.2020054002596

confirmed these risk factors and proposed new ones, such as chronic kidney disease, obesity, asthma and smoking[6-9]. The emergence of a highly transmissible pathogen[10] in a completely susceptible population has resulted in an exponential growth of new cases worldwide and a wide dissemination across the globe. As of April 12, 2020, the number of SARS-CoV-2 infections was above 1.8 million, reported in 185 countries/regions of the world[11]. High- and low-income regions are already facing overload of health facilities and facing scarcity of resources to fight the pandemic. In lower resource settings, countries have a short time to prepare prevention and management strategies, including the identification of high-risk populations and regions within countries. Herein, we propose a calculation of the proportion and total number of the general adult population who may be at higher risk for severe COVID-19, based on routinely collected data from a nationwide, household-based survey in Brazil. We argue that this method could be easily and rapidly applied within and across countries in order to craft tailored prevention strategies such as social isolation.

METHODS

We obtained data from the most recent representative, household-based survey conducted in Brazil, the National Health Survey (PNS, 2013 – *Pesquisa Nacional de Saúde*), carried out by the Ministry of Health in partnership with the Brazilian Institute of Geography and Statistics (IBGE). The PNS enrolled 62,202 adults who responded to a comprehensive questionnaire about several health-related issues. In this study, we included 51,770 participants who responded to the questionnaire about medical diagnosis and lifestyle risk factors, and had their weight and height measured. Further details about PNS have been described elsewhere[12].

Risk Factors for Severe COVID-19

We included risk factors for severe COVID-19 based on currently available information from clinical studies and expertise[2-9], and for which exposure data were available in the PNS[12]. Age and medical diagnosis of cardiovascular disease, diabetes, hypertension, chronic respiratory disease, cancer, stroke, chronic kidney disease and asthma were assessed. We also obtained time (in years) since cancer diagnosis and treatment/medication use for chronic kidney disease (e.g. dialysis) and asthma to match definitions from the literature (e.g. moderate to severe asthma). Information about age, smoking status and measured body mass index (BMI) were also obtained/estimated.

Prevalence of one or more risk factors for severe COVID-19 was estimated using two criteria Criterion 1 included first identified and established risk factors for severe COVID-19 such as age ≥ 65 years or medical diagnosis of cardiovascular disease, diabetes, hypertension, chronic respiratory disease, cancer or stroke. Although ≥ 60 years have been used to define older adults in Brazil, herein we considered ≥ 65 years to match the definition of risk factors for COVID-19 obtained from the literature and allow comparisons with other publications[2-9]. Criterion 2 additionally included diagnosis of chronic kidney disease and moderate to severe asthma, smoking status (current smokers) and obesity (BMI ≥ 30 kg/m^2). Criterion 2 was used to provide a higher sensitivity for the proportion of adults at risk of severe illness. Denominator for both criteria 1 (n = 52,511) and 2 (n = 51,770) included all participants with complete questionnaires. We also estimated the sum of all risk factors for severe illness (0, 1, 2, 3 + risk factors).

Table 1 Definition of risk factors for severe COVID-19 according to two different proposed criteria.

Risk factors	Definition	Presence of risk factor for severe COVID-19	
		Criterion 1	Criterion 2
Age	in years	≥ 65 years	≥ 65 years
Cardiovascular disease	Has a doctor ever diagnosed you with a heart disease such as infarction, angina, heart failure or other?	Yes	Yes
Diabetes	Has a doctor ever diagnosed you with diabetes?	Yes	Yes
Hypertension	Has a doctor ever diagnosed you with hypertension (high blood pressure)?	Yes	Yes
Chronic respiratory disease	Has a doctor already diagnosed you with any lung disease such as pulmonary emphysema, chronic bronchitis, or COPD (Obstructive Pulmonary Disease Chronic)?	Yes	Yes
Cancer	Has any doctor ever diagnosed you with cancer (excluding skin cancer)?	Yes	Yes
	How many years ago since your cancer diagnosis?	< 5 years	< 5 years
Stroke	Has any doctor ever diagnosed you with stroke?	Yes	Yes
Obesity	Measured body mass index	No	≥ 30 kg/m²
Smoking	Current smoker	No	Yes (daily or less than daily)
Chronic kidney disease	Has any doctor ever diagnosed you with chronic kidney disease?	No	Yes
	What do you currently do or have done because of the chronic kidney disease?	No	Hemodialysis, peritoneal dialysis, took medication, underwent a kidney transplant
Moderate to severe asthma	Has any doctor ever diagnosed you with asthma (or asthmatic bronchitis)?	No	Yes
	What do you currently do because of asthma?	No	Use of inhalers, aerosol or tablets

Sociodemographic Covariates

Information on covariates including sex, race/ethnicity, educational level, and Brazilian state (26 states and the Federative District) were obtained to describe the proportion of adults at risk of severe COVID-19 by population strata. We also retrieved the total projected number of the Brazilian adult population (≥ 18 years) in 2020 by sex and state from the IBGE[13].

Statistical Analysis

We estimated the prevalence and 95% confidence intervals of adults at risk for severe COVID-19 (Criterion 1 and Criterion 2) by sex, education, race/ethnicity and Brazilian state. We performed sensitivity analyses for prevalence by considering two other definitions for older adults (≥ 60 years and ≥ 70 years). In order to obtain the total number of adults at risk of severe illness, we applied the prevalence to the number of adult's population (≥ 18 years) by sex and state.

The sample design was considered for all analyses using the survey prefix command (svy) in Stata version 15.0. Participants characteristics and risk factors for severe illness are presented by age group (Table 2). Compared with younger participants, older adults (≥ 65 years) were less educated, more likely women, white and presented higher prevalence of risk factors for severe COVID-19, except for smoking. Prevalence of one or more risk factors for severe illness was 47.3% in younger vs 75.9% in older adults.

RESULTS

Table 2 Characteristics and risk factors for severe COVID-19 by age group in Brazil, PNS 2013

Characteristics	Age groups		Total
	< 65 years	≥ 65 years	
Number of participants	23.838	27.932	51.770
Mean age, years (se)	39.7 (11.4)	73.5 (14.1)	44.3 (15.0)
Sex (%)			
Men	45.4	42.9	45.0
Education (%)			
None or incomplete primary education	15.1	67.0	22.2
Complete primary or incomplete secondary education	27.2	14.0	25.4
Complete secondary education or incomplete undergraduate course	42.7	10.3	38.3
University Graduate	15.0	8.7	14.1
Race/ethnicity (%)			
White	48.3	55.9	49.4
Non-white	51.7	44.1	50.6
Risk factors for Severe COVID-19 (%)			
Cardiovascular disease	3.4	13.0	4.7
Diabetes	5.1	20.7	7.2
Chronic respiratory disease	1.5	4.4	1.9
Hypertension	18.8	55.3	23.7
Cancer	0.6	2.2	0.8
Stroke	1.0	6.1	1.7
Obesity (BMI ≥30 kg/m^2)	22.0	22.7	22.1
Smoking	14.6	9.6	13.9
Chronic kidney disease	0.7	2.0	0.9
Moderate to severe asthma	1.5	1.7	1.5
Number of risk factors for severe COVID-19* (%)			
None	52.7	24.1	48.8
1	30.9	35.1	31.5
2	12.0	25.2	13.8
3+	4.4	15.6	5.9

SE: standard error

* Diagnosis of cardiovascular disease, diabetes, chronic respiratory disease, hypertension, cancer (< 5 years of diagnosis), stroke, obesity (BMI ≥ 30 kg/m^2), current smoking, chronic kidney disease (diagnosis and under haemodialysis, peritoneal dialysis, taking medication or did a kidney transplant), moderate to severe asthma (diagnosis and taking inhalers, aerosol or tablets)Proportion and total number of adults at risk for severe COVID-19 in Brazil varied from 34.0% (53 million adults) to 54.5% (86 million adults) (Table 3). Overall, 46% of the sample presented no risk factor, 30.0% with one, 15.0% with two, and 9% with 3 or more risk factors for severe illness. Sensitivity analyses considering older adults ≥ 60 years and ≥ 70 years suggested that prevalence could vary from 36.7%–56.2% to 32.3%–53.3%, respectively (Table 4).

Table 3 Prevalence of one or more risk factor for severe COVID-19 among the Brazilian general adult population by risk criteria and sociodemographic characteristics, PNS 2013.

Characteristics	Prevalence of one or more risk factors for severe COVID-19			
	Criterion 1 (n = 52,511)		Criterion 2 (n = 51,770)	
	Prevalence (%)	95%CI	Prevalence (%)	95%CI
Total	34.0	33.2–34.7	54.4	53.6–55.2
Sex				
Men	31.6	30.5–32.8	53.3	52.1–54.5
Women	35.9	34.9–36.8	55.4	54.3–56.4
Education				
None or incomplete primary education	66.3	64.7–67.9	80.2	78.9–81.4
Complete primary or incomplete secondary education	30.5	29.2–31.9	55.0	53.5–56.5
Complete secondary education or incomplete undergraduate course	20.4	19.4–21.4	42.2	40.9–43.6
University Graduate	27.0	25.1–29.1	46.1	44.1–48.3
Race/ethnicity				
White	34.9	33.8–36.0	55.0	53.9–56.2
Non-white	33.1	21.1–34.0	53.9	52.8–54.9

Criterion 1: age $\geq$ 65 years or diagnosis of cardiovascular disease, diabetes, chronic respiratory disease, hypertension, cancer (< 5 years of diagnosis), or stroke

Criterion 2: additionally, obesity (BMI $\geq$ 30 kg/m^2), current smoking, chronic kidney disease (diagnosis and under Hemodialysis, peritoneal dialysis, taking medication or did a kidney transplant), moderate to severe asthma (diagnosis and taking inhalers, aerosol or tablets)

Table 4 Sensitivity analysis: prevalence of one or more risk factors for severe COVID-19 among the Brazilian general adult population by risk criteria, definitions of older age and sociodemographic characteristics in Brazil, PNS 2013.

Characteristics	Risk factors for severe COVID-19							
	Criterion 1 (n = 52,511)				Criterion 2 (n = 51,770)			
	Older age defined as ≥ 60 years		Older age defined as ≥ 70 years		Older age defined as ≥ 60 years		Older age defined as ≥ 70 years	
	Prevalence (%)	95%CI	Prevalence (%)	95%CI	Prevalence (%)	95%CI	Prevalence (%)	95%CI
Total	36.7	36.0–37.5	32.3	31.6–33.0	56.2	55.3–57.0	53.3	52.5–54.0
Sex								
Men	34.5	33.3–35.6	30.0	28.9–31.1	54.9	53.7–56.1	52.2	51.0–53.4
Women	38.6	37.6–39.5	34.2	33.3–35.1	57.2	56.1–58.2	54.2	53.2–55.2
Education								
None or incomplete Primary	72.0	70.4–73.4	62.2	60.5–63.8	83.4	82.3–84.6	77.5	76.2–78.8
Complete primary or incomplete secondary	32.2	30.9–33.6	29.3	28.0–30.6	56.2	54.6–57.7	54.1	52.5–55.6
Complete secondary or incomplete university	22.1	21.1–23.2	19.8	18.8–20.8	43.4	42.0–44.7	41.8	40.4–43.2
University Graduate	30.0	28.0–32.1	25.6	23.7–27.5	48.1	45.9–50.2	45.1	43.0–47.2
Race/Ethnicity								
White	38.0	36.9–39.2	33.1	32.0–34.2	57.0	55.8–58.2	53.8	52.6–54.9
Non-white	35.5	34.5–36.5	31.6	30.6–32.5	55.3	54.3–56.3	52.8	51.8–53.9

Criterion 1: age group or diagnosis of cardiovascular disease, diabetes, chronic respiratory disease, hypertension, cancer (< 5 years of diagnosis), or stroke; Criterion 2: additionally obesity (BMI ≥ 30 kg/m^2), current smoking, chronic kidney disease (diagnosis and under haemodialysis, peritoneal dialysis, taking medication or did a kidney transplant), moderate to severe asthma (diagnosis and taking inhalers, aerosol or tablets). Proportion of adults at risk for severe COVID-19 was 2-fold higher in less educated participants compared with university graduated.

We found no differences in prevalence estimates by sex and race/ethnicity (Table 3). Estimates varied widely across states, with higher prevalence in the South and Southeast regions of the country (Figure). The highest prevalence was 39.5%–58.4% in Rio Grande do Sul, followed by 36.0–55.8% in Rio de Janeiro and 35.6%–58.2% in São Paulo. The lowest prevalence was found in Amapá (23.4%–45.9%), followed by Roraima (25.0%–48.6%) and Amazonas (25.1%–48.7%). The highest number of adults at risk of severe illness was found in São Paulo (17-21 million), Minas Gerais (6–9 million) and Rio de Janeiro (5–7 million) (Table 5).

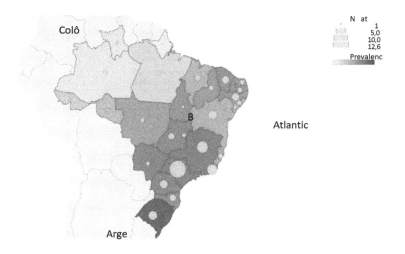

Criterion 1

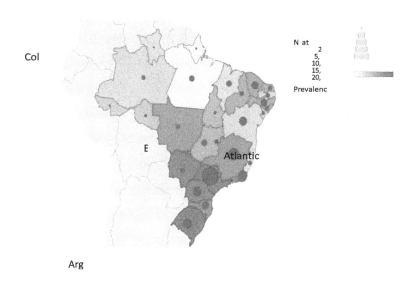

Criterion 2

Figure. 1 Adults at high-risk of severe COVID-19 in Brazil by state and risk criteria. a Criterion 1 (C1): age ≥ 65 years or diagnosis of cardiovascular disease, diabetes, chronic respiratory disease, hypertension, cancer (<5 years of diagnosis), or stroke;b Criterion 2 (C2): additionally, obesity (BMI ≥ 30 kg/m2), current smoking, chronic kidney disease (diagnosis and under hemodialysis, peritoneal dialysis, taking medication or did a kidney transplant), moderate to severe asthma (diagnosis and taking inhalers, aerosol or tablets).

Table 5 Prevalence of one or more risk factors for severe COVID-19 among the Brazilian general adult population by risk criteria and Brazilian states, PNS 2013.

Brazilian States	Adult population (≥ 18 years)	Prevalence of one or more risk factors for severe COVID-19, %					
		Criterion 1 (n = 52,511)			Criterion 2 (n = 51,770)		
		Prevalence (%)	95%CI	N at risk	Prevalence (%)	95%CI	N at risk
Brazil	158,255,554	34.0	33.2–34.7	53,806,888	54.4	53.6–55.2	86,091,021
Brazilian States							
Rondônia	1,296,218	29.6	26.7–32.7	383,681	50.3	47.3–53.2	651,998
Acre	581,754	28.1	25.3–31.0	163,473	50.0	46.8–53.2	290,877
Amazonas	2,769,201	25.1	22.6–27.8	695,069	48.7	45.7–51.7	1,348,601
Roraima	430,939	25.0	22.3–27.9	107,735	48.6	45.0–52.2	209,436
Pará	5,971,477	26.2	23.2–29.3	1,564,527	45.2	41.8–48.7	2,699,108
Amapá	570,298	23.4	20.2–26.9	133,450	45.9	41.6–50.3	261,767
Tocantins	1,125,023	33.1	29.0–37.6	372,383	52.2	48.7–55.7	587,262
Maranhão	4,873,279	30.0	26.3–34.0	1,461,984	48.5	43.9–53.0	2,363,540
Piauí	2,383,425	32.7	29.4–36.1	779,380	53.0	49.6–56.3	1,263,215
Ceará	6,788,403	33.8	31.0–36.7	2,294,480	53.7	50.8–56.6	3,645,372
Rio Grande do Norte	2,632,403	33.2	30.2–36.3	873,958	52.9	49.7–56.1	1,392,541
Paraiba	2,984,647	33.4	30.6–36.3	996,872	49.0	46.0–51.9	1,462,477
Pernambuco	7,035,040	33.2	30.7–35.8	2,335,633	53.4	50.8–55.9	3,756,711
Alagoas	2,377,983	31.7	28.6–35.0	753,821	53.5	49.7–57.3	1,272,221
Sergipe	1,688,955	30.8	28.0–33.8	520,198	50.0	46.7–53.2	844,478
Bahia	11,044,986	30.3	26.8–34.1	3,346,631	48.9	44.8–53.0	5,400,998
Minas Gerais	16,425,183	35.6	33.1–38.2	5,847,365	55.1	52.0–58.2	9,050,276
Espírito Santo	3,047,439	31.5	27.6–35.6	959,943	48.1	43.6–52.7	1,465,818
Rio de Janeiro	13,419,464	36.0	33.8–38.1	4,831,007	55.8	53.6–58.0	7,488,061
São Paulo	35,414,776	35.6	33.7–37.4	12,607,660	58.2	56.2–60.2	20,611,400
Paraná	8,736,014	34.9	31.7–38.2	3,048,869	57.1	53.3–60.9	4,988,264
Santa Catarina	5,578,842	34.1	30.2–38.2	1,902,385	55.9	51.6–60.1	3,118,573
Rio Grande do Sul	8,902,263	39.5	36.8–42.3	3,516,394	58.4	55.6–61.1	5,198,922
Mato Grosso do Sul	2,045,881	34.7	31.6–37.8	709,921	57.6	54.5–60.7	1,178,427
Mato Grosso	2,543,642	31.9	28.9–35.1	811,422	54.8	51.9–57.6	1,393,916
Goiás	5,277,383	34.4	31.5–37.4	1,815,420	52.0	49.1–54.9	2,744,239
Distrito Federal	2,310,636	29.9	27.3–32.5	690,880	49.2	46.3–52.1	1,136,833

N at risk: number of adults (≥18 years) at risk of severe COVID-19

Criterion 1: age ≥ 65 years or diagnosis of cardiovascular disease, diabetes, chronic respiratory disease, hypertension, cancer (< 5 years of diagnosis), or stroke; Criterion 2: additionally obesity (BMI ≥ 30 kg/m^2), current smoking, chronic kidney disease (diagnosis and under Hemodialysis, peritoneal dialysis, taking medication or did a kidney transplant), moderate to severe asthma (diagnosis and taking inhalers, aerosol or tablets)

DISCUSSION

In this study, we estimated that a third (53 million) to over a half (86 million) of Brazilian adults present at least one risk factor for severe COVID-19. Our findings point to high prevalence of serious medical conditions in younger, but mostly, among older adults. Less educated adults present 2-fold higher prevalence of risk factors compared with university graduated. São Paulo, Rio de Janeiro,

Minas Gerais and Rio Grande do Sul were the most vulnerable states in absolute and relative terms of adults at high-risk. Contrasts between South and Southeast vs North and Northeast regions might be due to different age structure, prevalence of health condition and/or access to medical diagnosis and care. Estimating the proportion of the population at risk for severe COVID-19 within and across countries is key to improve prevention measures. However, to our knowledge, these estimates are still sparse worldwide. In the US, it was estimated that four in ten (37.6%) adults ≥ 18 years may be at high-risk of severe COVID-19[14]. During the pandemic, time is limited and hence the use of existing health information to support countries' response is imperative. These findings and methods to identify high-risk settings may be useful to plan and manage prevention strategies in Brazil and other low- to middle-income settings with routinely collected data from population-based surveys, but limited testing capacity for SARS-CoV-2. The understanding of risk factors for severe COVID-19 has so far supported the implementation of prevention strategies.

It is interesting to note that non-communicable diseases such as cardiovascular disease, cancer, respiratory diseases, and diabetes, which accounts for most of deaths globally[15], play a role on worsening the impact of the COVID-19 pandemic. Since isolation of infected cases and contact tracing alone will not likely suffice to control the pandemic[16], countries have largely implemented social isolation measures. The combination of different interventions such as case isolation, social distancing of the entire population, household quarantine, school closure and, ultimately, complete lockdown is predicted to have significant impact on transmission[17]. Protecting the groups that are most at risk[18], such as older adults and people with comorbidities, by widely and temporarily refraining from engaging in social contact, remains imperative. As knowledge on the clinical course of COVID-19 advances, the understanding of risk factors for severe disease will be improved, and so will the estimates of most-at-risk populations.

Our results have some limitations. Prevalence of risk factors for severe COVID-19 is likely underestimated due to self-reported medical diagnosis of comorbidities and smoking status. Underlying diseases have been associated with poorer prognosis among inpatients with COVID-19, but some people may have lower risk due to well-controlled blood pressure and serum glucose, for instance, which may have overestimated the proportion and number of adults at risk. Undiagnosed, asymptomatic diseases such as diabetes and hypertension are concerns, especially in low-income settings. This may partially explain differences of adults at risk between Brazilian states. Estimates considered the same weight for all risk factors assessed, which may not be applicable. Furthermore, other known risk factors for severe COVID-19 such as living in a nursing home or long-term care facility, and immunosuppression could not be captured in our study. Lastly, risk factors information date from 2013, the most recent representative, household-based health survey of Brazilian adults. The proportion of older adults has increased in Brazil in the past seven years, as well as the prevalence of obesity and other non-communicable diseases[19], which may have underestimated our estimates. On the other hand, the prevalence of tobacco smoking has decreased, which may have overestimated the adults at risk of severe COVID-19. In conclusion, proportion and total number of adults at risk of severe COVID-19 is high in Brazil, with wide variation across states and adult subgroups. These findings should be considered while designing and implementing prevention measures. We argue that these results support broad social isolation measures, particularly while testing capacity for SARS-CoV-2 is limited.

REFERENCES

1. Novel Coronavirus Pneumonia Emergency Response Epidemiology Team. [The epidemiological characteristics of an outbreak of 2019 novel coronavirus diseases (COVID-19) – China]. Zhonghua Liu Xing Bing Xue Za Zhi. 2020;41(2):145-51. Chinese. https://doi.org/10.3760/cma.j.issn.0254-6450.2020.02.003

2. Wu Z, McGoogan J.M. (2020). Characteristics of and important lessons from the coronavirus disease 2019 (COVID-19) outbreak in China: summary of a report of 72314 cases from the Chinese Centre for Disease Control and Prevention [published online ahead of print, 2020 Feb 24]. JAMA. 2020. https://doi.org/doi:10.1001/jama.2020.2648

3. Du RH, Liang. L.R, Yang, C.Q., Wang, W., Cao, T.Z, Li M, et al. (2020).Predictors of mortality forpatients with COVID-19 Pneumonia caused by SARS-CoV-2: a prospective cohort study [published online ahead of print, 2020 Apr 9]. Eur Respir J. 2020. https://doi.org/10.1183/13993003.00524-2020

4. Wang. D., Hu B, Hu C, Zu, F., Liu, X, Zhang J, et al. (2020). Clinical characteristics of 138 hospitalized patients with2019 novel coronavirus-infected pneumonia in Wuhan, China [published online ahead of print, Feb 7]]. JAMA. 2020;323(11):1061-9. https://doi.org/10.1001/jama.2020.1585

5. Liang, W., Guan, W., Chen, R., Wang, W., Li J, Xu K, et al. (2020). Cancer patients in SARS-CoV-2 infection: a nationwide analysis in China. Lancet Oncol. 2020.21(3):335-7. https://doi.org/10.1016/S1470-2045(20)30096-6

6. Grasselli, G., Zangrillo, A., Zanella, A., Antonelli, M., Cabrini, L, Castelli, A,, et al. (2020). Baseline characteristics and outcomes of 1591 patients infected with SARS-CoV-2 admitted to ICUS of the Lombardy Region, Italy [published online ahead of print]. JAMA. 2020;323(16):1574-1581. https://doi.org/10.1001/jama.2020.5394

7. Centres for Disease Control and Prevention - CDC COVID-19 Response Team. Preliminary estimates of the prevalence of selected underlying health conditions among patients with Coronavirus Disease 2019 - United States, February 12-March 28, 2020. MMWR Morb Mortal Wkly Rep. 2020;69(13):382-6. https://doi.org/10.15585/mmwr.mm6913e2

8. COVID-19 Surveillance Group. Characteristics of COVID-19 patients dying in Italy: report based on available data on March 20th, 2020. Rome (ITA): Istituto Superiore di Sanità; 2020 [cited 2020 Apr 28

9. Leung, J.M, Yang, C.X., Tam, A., Shaipanichi, T., Hackett, T.L, Singhera, G.K, et al. (2020). ACE-2 expression in the small airway epithelia of smokers and COPD patients: implications for COVID-19 [published online ahead of print, 2020 Apr 8]. Eur Respir J. 2020. https://doi.org/10.1183/13993003.00688-2020

10. World Health Organization. Report of the WHO-China Joint Mission on Coronavirus Disease 2019 (COVID-19). Geneva: WHO; 2020 [cited 2020 Apr 28].

11. Sanche, S., Lin, Y.T., Xu, C., Romero-Severson, E., Hengartner, N., Ke R. (2020).The Novel Coronavirus, 2019nCoV, is highly contagious and more infectious than initially estimated [preprint]. medRxiv.

12. Szwarcwald, C.L, Malta, D.C., Pereira, C.A., Vieira MLFP, Conde. W.L,Souza Júnior, P.R/B, et al. [National Health Survey in Brazil: design and methodology of application]. Cienc Saude Coletiva. (2014) 19(2):333-42. Portuguese. https://doi.org/10.1590/1413-81232014192.14072012 Instituto Brasileiro de Geografia e Estatística. Projeções da população: Brasil e unidades da federação: revisão 2018. Rio de Janeiro: IBGE; 2018.

13. Koma. W, Neuman, T, Claxton, G, Rae, M., Kates J, Michaud J. (2020).How many adults are at risk of serious illness if infected with Coronavirus? updated data. San Francisco (USA): Kaiser Family Foundation- KFF; 2020.

14. GBD 2017 Causes of Death Collaborators. Global, regional, and national age-sex-specific mortality for 282 causes of death in 195 countries and territories, 1980-2017: a systematic analysis for the Global Burden of Disease Study 2017. Lancet. 2018;392(10159):1736-88. https://doi.org/10.1016/S0140-6736(18)32203-7 Imai, N., Cori. A., Dorigatti, I., Baghelin, M., Donnelly, C.A., Riley, S., et al. (2020). Report 3: transmissibility of 2019-nCoV. London: Imperial College London; 2020. https://doi.org/10.25561/77148

15. Ferguson, N.M., Laydon, D., Nedjati-Gilani, G., Imai, N., Ainslie, K., Baguelin, M., M, et al. (2020). Report 9: impact of non-pharmaceutical interventions (NPIs) to reduce COVID-19 mortality and healthcare demand. London: Imperial College London; 2020. https://doi.org/10.25561/77482

16. Centres for Disease Contol and Preventiion. Implementation of mitigation strategies for communities with local COVID-19 transmission. Atlanta, GA: CDC; 2020 [cited 2020 Apr 28].

17. Ministério da Saúde (BR), Secretaria de Vigilância em Saúde, Departamento de Análise em Saúde e Vigilância de Doenças Não Transmissíveis. VIGITEL Brasil 2018: vigilância de fatores de risco e proteção para doenças crônicas por inquérito telefônico: estimativas sobre frequência e distribuição sociodemográfica de fatores de risco e proteção para doenças crônicas nas capitais dos 26 estados brasileiros e no Distrito Federal em 2018. Brasília, DF; 2019.

6. COVID-19 and Long-Term Care in Brazil: Impact, Measures and Lessons Learned[1]

Fabiana Da Mata and Déborah Oliveira[2]

KEY POINTS

- The COVID-19 pandemic is on its ascending period in Brazil and mortality rates have risen exponentially;
- Several initiatives have been implemented and recommendations have been published by the public sector to support unpaid carers, older and disable people, and Long-Term Care (LTC) professionals with regards to ways to protect from the infection;
- There is a paucity of specific population data in relation to the pandemic (e.g. infection and mortality rates in people living in care homes vs. living at home) and most actions so far have been taken by the public health sector;
- It is unclear the extent to which the private care sector (e.g. private care homes, health insurances) have been following national and international guidance;
- Unpaid carers, vulnerable populations, and LTC workers have been mostly unassisted financially and with the necessary equipment to face the pandemic;
- There is a lack of evidence on COVID-19 is affecting older people and those with disabilities living together with several other family members in vulnerable communities (such as "favelas");
- It appears that most of the actions so far have been carried out remotely or digitally, and there is a lack of information with regards to the extent to which such actions have reached those who do not have access to online information;
- Brazil has a large proportion of the population who is illiterate or semi-illiterate and it is unclear the extent to which the preventative measures and recommendations implemented/published so far have taken into account individual literacy and health literacy levels.

Impact of COVID19 On Long-Term Care Users and Staff So Far

Number of positive cases in population and deaths

[1] Da Mata FAF & Oliveira D. COVID-19 and Long-Term Care in Brazil: Impact, Measures and Lessons Learned. Available at LTCcovid.org, International Long-Term Care Policy Network, CPEC-LSE, 6 Mayl 2020.

[2] Da Mata FAF, PT MSc PhD (Department of Psychiatry, School of Medicine, Universidade Federal de São Paulo - UNIFESP - https://orcid.org/0000-0003-3762-9091). Email: fagfigueiredo@hotmail.com

Oliveira D, RN MSc PhD (Department of Psychiatry, School of Medicine, Universidade Federal de São Paulo - UNIFESP - http://orcid.org/0000-0002-6616-533X). Email: oliveiradc.phd@gmail.com

ltccovid.org

On January 10, a federal committee was created by the Ministry of Health to monitor the spread of COVID-19 in Brazil. On January 16, the Ministry of Health published the first report in Brazilian Portuguese about what was known about the disease worldwide up to that point. On 20 January the Ministry of Health met with PAHO to align the public health strategies to be used to control the pandemic in the Americas. On 27 January Brazil had its first suspected case and the country status was changed from "alert level 1" to "imminent danger". On 3 February, it was declared National Public Health Emergency and on 7 February the Quarantine Law was sanctioned by the President. On 26 February, the first COVID-19 case was confirmed in Sao Paulo, Brazil. Every suspected and confirmed case is registered by the health services in a national electronic surveillance system (e-SUS VE)[1] controlled by the Ministry of Health. In Brazil, up to 27 April 2020, there were 61,888 confirmed cases of COVID-19 and 4,205 deaths nationally. The numbers of cases and deaths continue to grow in the country with all the states having confirmed cases (Brazilian Ministry of Health, 2020)[2]. Detailed national reports on the epidemiology of the COVID-19 pandemic situation in Brazil is published periodically here.[3] Figure 1 shows the geographical distribution of cases (A) and deaths (B) per city across the country (Brazilian Ministry of Health, 2020)[4]. Table 1 shows the basic epidemiology of the COVID-19 pandemic in Brazil compared to other European countries (Brazilian Ministry of Health, 2020)[5]. Worldwide, Brazil is in the 11th position in the number of confirmed cases and in the 11th position in the number of deaths. However, if the mortality rate per 1 million people is considered, Brazil is in 37th in the world's ranking.

Figure 1. Geographical distribution of the number of cases (A) and deaths (B) per city across the country.

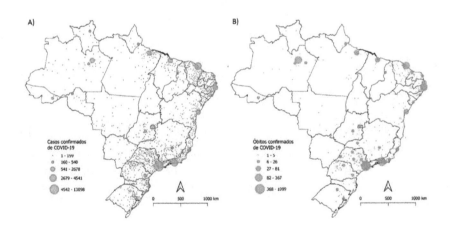

Source: Brazilian Ministry of Health, 2020

---

[1] https://notifica.saude.gov.br/onboard

[2] https://covid.saude.gov.br/

[3] https://www.saude.gov.br/boletins-epidemiologicos

[4] https://portalarquivos.saude.gov.br/images/pdf/2020/April/27/2020-04-27-18-05h-BEE14-Boletim-do-COE.pdf

[5] https://portalarquivos.saude.gov.br/images/pdf/2020/April/27/2020-04-27-18-05h-BEE14-Boletim-do-COE.pdf

Table 1. Comparison of the COVID-19 pandemic situation between Brazil, Italy, Germany and Spain* (based on the National Epidemiological Report)[1]

Country	Date when the 100th case was registered	Number of days after the 100th confirmed case	Date of the 1st confirmed death	Days after mortality reaches 0.1 million	Mortality rate for 1 million people
Brazil	15 March	42	17/03	34	20
Italy	24 February	62	23/03	60	436
Germany	1 March	56	10/03	41	67
Spain	3 March	53	05/03	49	482

*26 April 2020

Up to 26 April, approximately 60% of the people who had died from SARS-CoV2 were men, 70% were aged 60 and over and 67% had at least one comorbidity. Cardiomyopathy has been the most common condition associated with higher mortality rates (present in 1,566 deaths), followed by diabetes (n=1,223), renal diseases (n=296), pneumopathy (n=279) and neurological conditions (n=265). In all vulnerable groups, the majority were aged 60 and over, except for those with obesity (Brazilian Ministry of Health - SVS)[2]. The mortality rate by COVID-19 in the Brazilian population is 6.8% and the infection rate in the population is 4.3 cases per 100,000 people. However, as only a small percentage of people are tested for COVID-19, it is likely that these infection rates are higher. Even though mortality rate statistics in Brazil are considered relatively robust because the sub notification number is considered generally low (Brazilian Ministry of Health - SVS, 2020)[3].

Rates of Infection and Mortality Among Long-Term Care Users and Staff

Official information about rates in LTC facilities is not yet available in Brazil. On 28 April 2020, a magazine[4] published a report of a LTC home in Piracicaba (a town in the state of Sao Paulo) where, out of 82 residents, there had been 28 cases of infection and 6 deaths that were confirmed to be from COVID-19.

---

[1] https://portalarquivos.saude.gov.br/images/pdf/2020/April/27/2020-04-27-18-05h-BEE14-Boletim-do-COE.pdf
[2] https://portalarquivos.saude.gov.br/images/pdf/2020/April/27/2020-04-27-18-05h-BEE14-Boletim-do-COE.pdf
[3] https://portalarquivos.saude.gov.br/images/pdf/2020/April/27/2020-04-27-18-05h-BEE14-Boletim-do-COE.pdf
[4] https://revistaforum.com.br/coronavirus/asilo-tem-28-casos-e-6-mortos-por-coronavirus-no-interior-de-sao-paulo/

Population Level Measures to Contain Spread Of COVID-19

The measures to contain the spread of COVID-19 have been established and implemented at federal, state and municipal levels. On 6 February 2020 law nº 13.979 was sanctioned, which established national measures to deal with the public health emergency of international importance – the COVID-19 pandemic.

At the federal level[1], lay and specialist information about the disease, forms of transmission, as well as individual and population measures to control the virus spread are available online[2] and via public health services, including accessible information for deaf and blind people. An online chat for questions from the general public and health professionals has been implemented in the same webpage. Clinical guidelines and the number of COVID-19 treatment beds and equipment per region/state, legislations, reports, are all published online regularly and in a transparent manner (Brazilian Ministry of Health, 2020)[3].Locally, the measures include social distancing for the general public, social isolation for those who had tested positive for COVID-19.

However, no strict lockdown measures have been in place yet. All public and private services such as shopping malls, pet shops, stores, offices, schools were gradually closed from 11 March 2020, with the exception of shops providing basic supplies (supermarkets, pharmacies and bakeries) and health units. Restaurants were allowed to continue to sell food through delivery or self-collection. In some country regions, especially large urban areas, the police were allowed to arrest those who were found 'conglomerating' in groups of eight people or more. Stores or services which were found working can be fined by the councils. The first state to adopt social distancing measures was the Federal District, it closed schools and service providers establishments on 11 March 2020. It was followed by the states of São Paulo and Rio de Janeiro that adopted social distancing measures on 16 and 17 March 2020, respectively (Brazilian newspaper, 2020)[4]. All the federal regulations and laws with regards to the national response to the COVID-19 pandemic are published and regularly updated here[5].

Brief Background To The Long-Term Care System

In Brazil, long-term care is available through public and private systems. The Unified Social Assistance System (SUAS) provides some public long-term care services to the population, such as long-term care institutions, day centres, palliative care, advance care directives and others. The system's coverage is means tested, provided to people without means to pay for their care or without family support (Ministry of Citizenship, 2020)[6]. Long term care may also be accessed privately. Very often family members are the main providers of care (unpaid care). However, private options such as paid carers, Day Care Centres (Getting Quite Popular In The Last Years) And Long-Stay Institutions (The Most Traditional Model Of Long-Term Care In Brazil, After The Provision Of Care By Family Members) Are Available In The country (Camarano and Barbosa, 2016)[7].

---

[1] https://coronavirus.saude.gov.br/

[2] https://coronavirus.saude.gov.br/sobre-a-doenca#como-se-proteger

[3] https://covid-insumos.saude.gov.br/paineis/insumos/painel_leitos.php

[4] https://g1.globo.com/bemestar/coronavirus/noticia/2020/04/06/coronavirus-veja-a-cronologia-da-doenca-no-brasil.ghtml

[5] https://portalarquivos.saude.gov.br/images/pdf/2020/April/23/23042020-Portarias-publicadas-sobre-COVID-com-edilcao.pdf

[6] https://www.gov.br/cidadania/pt-br/desenvolvimento-social

[7] http://repositorio.ipea.gov.br/bitstream/11058/9146/1/Institui%C3%A7%C3%B5es de longa perman%C3%AAncia.pdf

Long-Term Care Policy And Practice Measures : Whole Sector Measures

Measures created by the Government and by expert commissions are being carried out to address the pandemic with regards to LTC. The Brazilian Ministry of Health has recently published a national contingency plan[1]. This plan includes Federal Technical guidance documents (e.g., 7/2020,8/2020 and 9/2020)[2] about the prevention and control of COVID-19 in LTC institutions for older people. Recommendations regarding the assessment and monitoring of residents, hygiene strategies, education, strategies for group activities, management of suspect cases etc. are expressed in the documents to orientate LTC managers, workers, residents, family and visitors. There is also a website called "ILPI.me" which was voluntarily produced by institutions such as UFMG, FMUSP, residential homes etc. that informs LTC institutions regarding an action plan for fighting against COVID-19. This website makes protocols of care available, so LTC institutions may follow them. These protocols contain information about measures of care during the pandemic aiming at healthcare professionals, administrative, and auxiliary personnel from LTC institutions.

Care Coordination Issues: Hospital Discharges To The Community

Hospital discharges are recommended to take place only after the diagnosed person has been isolated for 14 days counting from the beginning of the symptoms. In cases of hospital discharges before the recommended period of isolation, the person should be kept isolated at home until the 14 days have been completed (Brazilian Ministry of Health, 2020)[3].

Hospital Discharges To Residential And Nursing Homes

Persons who have recovered from COVID-19, should return from hospitals to the institution where they came from if they have been tested positive by the immunity cure test (IgG) 14 days after being hospitalized and if they do not present symptoms of any other disease for 72 hours. If it is not possible to do the test, the person should be isolated for 14 days in the institution where they used to live (FN-ILPI, 2020).

Care Homes (Including Supported Living, Residential And Nursing Homes, Skilled Nursing Facilities)

Prevention of COVID19 Infections

A thorough technical guideline was created by a national commission to strengthen the long term care responses to the COVID-19 pandemic in Brazil (FN-ILPI, 2020)[4].

This guidance was published at the end of April 2020 aiming to inform the Government of the current situation in LTC institutions as well as of the management of COVID-19 outbreaks in these institutions. The document firstly provides a situational analysis about LTC institutions, including recommendations regarding general health care, family contact, preventive measures and good

---

[1] National Contingency Plan for the Care of Institutionalized Older People in Situation of Extreme Social Vulnerability.

[2] https://aps.saude.gov.br/noticia/8196

[3] https://www.conasems.org.br/wp-content/uploads/2020/03/guia_de_vigilancia_2020.pdf

[4] https://sbgg.org.br/wp-content/uploads/2020/04/Relato%CC%81rio-final-vCAU-2.pdf

habits to follow in LTC institutions. The document also details recommendations on specific steps of care to be followed in LTC institutions during COVID-19 pandemic (FN-ILPI, 2020)[1].

Apart from that document, Federal Technical Guidelines were developed as part of the National Contingency Plan, to prevent and controlCOVID-19 infections in LTC institutions (Federal Technical Guidelines -numbers 7/2020,[2]8/2020[3] and 9/2020)[4]. Regarding prevention of COVID-19 infections, many recommendations have been proposed for care homes since the pandemic reached Brazil. These include, for instance, that all products received from third parties should be delivered outside the institution, that external packaging should be discarded, and the internal packages should be cleaned with alcohol (liquid, 70%).

All workers are advised not go to work if they feel symptoms of cold. Before entering the care home, workers should measure their body temperature and use a face mask on their way to the care home. They should enter the care home through another entrance door than of that used by the care home residents, wash their hands with water and soap, change their clothes and shoes, take a shower (when possible), use a face mask and surgical cap. The workers are advised to wash their hands before and after caring for an older person, use alcohol gel 70% after touching any furniture, use N95 masks when exposed to aerosols, use gloves when in contact with urine, faeces or any other secretion. Before leaving the LTC institution, the workers are advised to remove their masks, gloves, surgical caps, change their clothes, measure their body temperature, and put on another mask. After arriving home, they should wash their hands, take a shower and put on clean clothes (FN-ILPI, 2020[5] and Federal Technical Guideline 09/2020)[6].

All residents should have their body temperature measured daily and should be monitored for respiratory symptoms and symptoms of a cold (Federal Technical Guideline 09/2020)[7]. They should be encouraged to wash their hands every two hours as well as before and after having meals. The LTC institutions' workers should be trained to wash hands and apply alcohol gel.

All the entrances of the institutions should have carpets with a solution of sodium hypochlorite (30%); all the door handles, handrail, wheelchair holders should be cleaned twice a day with alcohol 70% (FN-ILPI, 2020)[8].In terms of general prevention, the institutions are advised to stimulate the ingestion of fruit and water among residents, reorganise the number of older people per meals in the dining hall (to keep a distance of 1 to 2 meters between residents) and arrange both Influenza and Pneumococcal vaccines for their residents in the nearest basic health unit (Federal Technical Guideline 09/2020[9] and FN-ILPI, 2020).

---

[1] https://sbgg.org.br/wp-content/uploads/2020/04/Relato%CC%81rio-final-vCAU-2.pdf
[2] https://drive.google.com/file/d/1hzfRUBJW3F2DG5ajSgzGN8vd0XMyDuaO/view
[3] http://189.28.128.100/dab/docs/portaldab/documentos/notatecnica82020COSAPICGCIVIDAPESSAPSMS02abr2020COVID-19.pdf
[4] https://aps.saude.gov.br/noticia/8196
[5] https://sbgg.org.br/wp-content/uploads/2020/04/Relato%CC%81rio-final-vCAU-2.pdf
[6] Federal Technical Guideline 09/2020).
[7] http://189.28.128.100/dab/docs/portaldab/documentos/NT_N_9_2020_COSAPI_CGCIVI_DAPES_SAPS_MS.pdf
[8] https://sbgg.org.br/wp-content/uploads/2020/04/Relato%CC%81rio-final-vCAU-2.pdf
[9] (Federal Technical Guideline 09/2020

Controlling Spread Once Infection Is Suspected
Or Has Entered A Facility

Once a resident has been infected, this person should be isolated, use a mask for 14 days and be moved to a bedroom with proper ventilation and with a bathroom to avoid contact with others in the institution. It is important to note, however, that many of the institutions only have shared rooms and lack important supplies. This makes it difficult for them to comply with some of these recommendations (FN-ILPI, 2020)[1]. In such cases, a regional manager from SUS should be contacted by the institution to arrange the transfer of the infected resident to a reference hospital (Federal Technical Guideline 09/2020)[2]. Workers from the LTC institution who present with fever or/and acute respiratory symptoms must be immediately removed from their functions in the institution and should ideally be tested for COVID-19 (Federal Technical Guideline 09/2020)[3]. Besides, social distancing measures should be reinforced among the whole institution (FN-ILPI, 2020)[4]. The Ministry of Health has published a flowchart for the management of suspect cases (Brazilian Ministry of Health, 2020)[5].

Managing Staff Availability And Wellbeing

The importance of managing carers' physical and mental aspects during the pandemic has been recognised. Apart from the day to day burden already experienced by many LTC workers in institutions, dealing with the responsibility of LTC activities during COVID-19 pandemic brings fear, uncertainty and the need for greater hygienic rigour. In this context, it is important to promote physical and psychological wellbeing to those persons, to avoid bringing new responsibilities (e.g.; buying individual protection equipment) during the period of pandemic, to take care of mourning in case of death from an older person in the institution, and to promote interventions to support care worker's mental health (FN-ILPI, 2020)[6].

Community-Based Care: Measures To Prevent Spread Of COVID19 Infection

The measures to prevent the spread of COVID-19 in community-based care are the same recommended for the rest of the population.

Managing Staff Availability And Wellbeing

The federal, state and municipal governments have opened emergency calls to contract healthcare staff to replace those who have been infected or who are part of vulnerable groups (such as older workers) in hospitals and community health services. However, there is no specific information available with regards to expected long-term contracts for professionals to work on LTC institutions or community health services. Up to 28 April 2020, almost 400,000 healthcare professionals have

[1] https://sbgg.org.br/wp-content/uploads/2020/04/Relato%CC%81rio-final-vCAU-2.pdf
[2] http://189.28.128.100/dab/docs/portaldab/documentos/NT_N_9_2020_COSAPI_CGCIVI_DAPES_SAPS_MS.pdf
[3] http://189.28.128.100/dab/docs/portaldab/documentos/NT_N_9_2020_COSAPI_CGCIVI_DAPES_SAPS_MS.pdf
[4] https://sbgg.org.br/wp-content/uploads/2020/04/Relato%CC%81rio-final-vCAU-2.pdf
[5] http://189.28.128.100/dab/docs/portaldab/documentos/Fluxograma_nt9_COSAPI-ILPI.pdf
[6] https://sbgg.org.br/wp-content/uploads/2020/04/Relato%CC%81rio-final-vCAU-2.pdf

registered to voluntarily work on the front line responding to the COVID-19 pandemic (Brazilian Ministry of Health, 2020)[1]

Impact On Unpaid Carers And Measures To Support Them

Up to the end of April, no data has been published regarding the impact of the pandemic on unpaid carers in Brazil. The media and the Brazilian Alzheimer Associations have published several articles highlighting the concerns from experts and authorities about the high risk for social isolation and abuse which this population is potentially subjected to (see for example here[2] and here)[3]. Older people's and disease-specific associations (such as the Brazilian Society of Geriatrics and Gerontology and the Brazilian Alzheimer Associations) have published specific guidance for carers, with particular issues being addressed in each situation. However, only technical and educational advice has been published, with no specific social or financial support measure implemented to aid this specific group. The National Institute for Health Care Research FioCruz has produced, in collaboration with academic and clinical experts, a booklet with clear and objective guidance to inform family carers of older people about how they can control the spread of respiratory viruses and protect themselves and the people they care for from COVID-19. This manual can be accessed here.[4] The Ministry of Health, in collaboration with PAHO, have released a campaign to help Brazilians to cope with the impact of the pandemic on their mental health. A series of videos have been produced and can be accessed online here.[5] This could potentially be used and/or implemented with unpaid carers to help tackle feelings of loneliness, distress and isolation. Several online surveys and studies are ongoing, and it is hoped that data will be published soon with regards to the impact of the COVID-19 pandemic on this population.

Impact On People With Intellectual Disabilities And Measures To Support Them

Approximately 22% of the entire country's population (45 million people) have at least one disability. About 60% of this population are aged 50 and over and 70% are socio-economically deprived (Brazilian newspaper, 2020)[6]. This population group is considered to be highly vulnerable to COVID-19, however, no formal data has been published about this by the end of April 2020. The Ministry of Women, Family and Human Rights has created a dedicated webpage to help people with rare conditions and disabilities (including people who are blind, deaf, and/or live with physical and intellectual disabilities) and their families to find relevant information about how to cope with the pandemic. This webpage can be accessed here[7].

Impact On People Living With Dementia And Measures To Support Them

Brazil has approximately 1.5 million people with dementia, and it has been estimated that 77% of these people are undiagnosed (Nakamura et al, 2015)[8]. We do not have official data on the number

---

[1] https://www.saude.gov.br/noticias/agencia-saude/46805-500-mil-profissionais-dispostos-a-atuarem-no-combate-ao-coronavirus

[2] https://www.cartacapital.com.br/saude/cuidadoras-de-idosos-enfrentam-abusos-e-riscos-na-pandemia-de-coronavirus/

[3] http://abraz.org.br/web/2020/04/17/o-impacto-da-pandemia-do-coronavirus-nos-cuidadores-de-pacientes-com-doenca-de-alzheimer/

[4] http://www.rets.epsjv.fiocruz.br/biblioteca/orientacoes-para-cuidadores-domiciliares-de-pessoa-idosa-na-epidemia-do-coronavirus-covid

[5] https://www.saude.gov.br/noticias/agencia-saude/46750-ministerio-da-saude-e-opas-lancam-campanha-para-cuidados-em-saude-mental

[6] https://g1.globo.com/bemestar/coronavirus/noticia/2020/03/24/quais-os-cuidados-as-pessoas-com-deficiencia-devem-tomar-para-nao-serem-infectadas-com-o-novo-coronavirus.ghtml

[7] https://sway.office.com/tDuFxzFRhn1s8GGi?ref=Link

[8] https://www.thelancet.com/journals/lancet/article/PIIS0140-6736(15)60153-2/fulltext

of people with dementia who have been affected by the COVID-19 pandemic. However, given the high vulnerability of this population group, we expect this number to be high. As mentioned previously, educational and technical information has been published to inform carers and health professionals with regards to infection prevention and management of social isolation in long-term care more generally. The Alzheimer's Associations and other NGOs have created helplines, as well as online forums, blogs and videos with educational materials to help address key potential unmet needs of carers and people with dementia. See an example here.[1]

Lessons Learnt So Far

The COVID-19 pandemic in Brazil brought together a great deal of fake news that affect society. This misinformation might have contributed to increased levels of uncertainty and anxiety among people. Besides, fake news might have delayed people's early compliance with preventive measures regarding COVID-19. Until April 2020, the Ministry of Health clarified on its website around 80 COVID-related fake news that were disseminated throughout the internet (Brazilian Ministry of Health, 2020)[2]. Another important point is the current political context in Brazil.

The president has been making speeches against the importance of physical distancing and comments underestimating the severity of the COVID-19 infection. Besides, the Health Minister and Minister of Justice were replaced in April 2020 because their views differed from those of the president. The political situation, combined with the pandemic, has led to constant dissatisfaction of the population. Even though the state governors have the independence to place their states under quarantine and lockdown measures (as Brazil is a federation with autonomous subnational governments), the political situation created by the national government adds more anxiety to the population on the steps Brazil will take to control the spread of COVID-19. On the other hand, a number of citizens have grouped together in an attempt to promote psychosocial activities whilst maintaining social isolation, such as, for example, the Brigades (Brincada de Apoio and Brincada da Educação)[3] and the Age Knitting (Tecer Idades)[4] – this last one aims to supporting older people. In many cities, the public sector also managed to develop a network where information and support can be found (Londrina City Council, 2020[5] and Sao Paulo City Council, 2020)[6].

Short-Term Calls For Action

Several actions have been implemented and/or recommended to protect vulnerable people who are receiving LTC and their unpaid carers, living either at home or in care homes.
However, there is still the need for further actions, such as the following:

We need to establish specific population data in relation to the pandemic (e.g. infection and mortality rates in people living in care homes vs. living at home);

---

[1] http://abraz.org.br/web/2020/03/13/covid-19-o-novo-coronavirus-e-a-doenca-de-alzheimer/
[2] https://www.saude.gov.br/component/tags/tag/novo-coronavirus-fake-news?limitstart=0
[3] https://www.facebook.com/brincadadaeducacao/
[4] https://www.facebook.com/Programa-Tecer-Idades-438961066536319/
[5] https://www.londrina.pr.gov.br/coronavirus-londrina
[6] https://www.prefeitura.sp.gov.br/cidade/secretarias/saude/vigilancia_em_saude/doencas_e_agravos/coronavirus/index.php?p=291766

Most actions have been taken by the public health sectors and it is unclear the extent to which private care sectors (e.g. private care homes, health insurances) have been following national and international guidance;

There needs to be effective and continuous financial and health support actions for paid and unpaid caregivers and vulnerable groups living alone;

It appears that most of the actions so far have been done remotely or digitally, and there is a lack of information with regards to the extent to which such actions have reached out to those who do not have access to online information. More efforts should be made to reach out to vulnerable / disabled groups;

Brazil has a large proportion of the population who is illiterate or semi-illiterate and it is unclear the extent to which the preventative measures and recommendations implemented/published so far have taken into account individual literacy and health literacy levels;

There is a lack of evidence on how older people living together with several other family members in vulnerable communities (such as "favelas") are doing to prevent and treat respiratory infections.

Relevant information sources

https://portalarquivos.saude.gov.br/images/pdf/2020/April/23/23042020-Portariaspublicadas-sobre-COVID-com-edilcao.pdf
 https://www.ilpi.me/
https://drive.google.com/file/d/1FRf1xTY6XNQ7KrcyGPsorjSNB7ohyCwQ/view
https://drive.google.com/file/d/1bfkLTZsfqzOZYFukNTaVQ0CfIMHczruL/view

CHAPTER 11

OBESITY, DIABETIS AND SUSCEPTIBILITY TO COVID-19

1. COVID-19, Sedentary Behaviour And Dynapenic[1] Abdominal Obesity In Brazilian Older People

André Bonadias Gadelha

Department of Physical Education and Sports, Federal Institute of Education, Science and Technology Goiano. Rodovia Geraldo Silva Nascimento Km 2.5, Urutaí - GO, 75790-000, Brazil, Phone +55 64 993404092.E-mail: andrebonadias@gmail.com

The novel coronavirus (COVID-19) epidemic has been caused by respiratory tract infectious disease which is motivated by a Severe Acute Respiratory Syndrome 2 (SARS-2), and has been recognized as a public health emergency by the World Health Organization, 2020). In this scenario, COVID-19 was recently declared a global pandemic by the World Health Organization on 11th March 2020, being associated with substantial morbidity and mortality (Eurosurveillance Editorial Team, 2020). Currently, medical records indicate that the pandemic has affected more than 200 countries around the world, with approximately 260,000 deaths until May 6th 2020. In Brazil, rate of deaths by COVID-19 has increased close to eight thousand people until the aforementioned date. Based on what is known, a group in imminent danger of contagion and even death by COVID-19 are the aged people ($\geq$ 65 years old). Noteworthy, eight out of ten deaths caused by COVID-19 reported in the US have been related to older adults.

In Italy, aged people ($\geq$85 years old) infected by COVID-19 present case-fatality rate ranging from 15 to 20% (Onder, Rezza, & Brusaferro, 2020); additionally, in Brazil, according to Ministry of Health, approximately 80% of deaths by COVID-19 has been related to aged people. Therefore, policies that aimed to contain this pandemic have been adopted, especially for older adults, who are at imminent risk for SARS-2.

In general, the main preventive procedure to avoid contamination by COVID-19 include frequent and adequate hand sanitizing, covering the nose and mouth with a mask and social distancing (Lynch, Mahida, Oppenheim, & Gray, 2020), being the latter highly recommended for aged people. However, social distancing imposes more time at home, which might negatively influence the sedentary behaviour. For example, spending more sitting time.

Briefly, this kind of sedentary behaviour has been linked to increased risks of chronic conditions and even mortality, especially for older adults (Ekelund et al., 2016). Paradoxically, it has been recommended to aged people to keep physically active (Fragala et al., 2019) to avoid excess of fat accumulation, while losing both strength and functionality, which are phenotypes of obesity and dynapenia, respectively. Obesity is consistently recognized as a relevant public health problem and can be easily monitored by waist circumference (abdominal obesity measure).

The term dynapenia has been used to define the age-related loss of strength and functionality (Gadelha, Neri, Vainshelboim, Ferreira, & Lima, 2019). Thus, the coexistence of abdominal obesity and dynapenia has introduced as dynapenic abdominal obesity (DAO) (Gadelha et al., 2019), and have been linked to falls (Gadelha et al., 2019), frailty, disability and even mortality (da Silva Alexandre, Scholes, Santos, de Oliveira Duarte, & de Oliveira, 2018).

---

[1] DOI: http://dx.doi.org/10.33837/msj.v3i1.1224

It is known that inactivity (i.e., sedentary behaviour) can favour traits of DAO. Therefore, attention in older adults during this worldwide pandemic must be given. Home stay has been linked to both lower energy expenditure and muscle unloading, which provide excess of fat mass accumulation (Church & Martin, 2018) and decline in muscle strength (Onder et al., 2020), respectively. Also, in this critical moment, inaccurate and often harmful "old person" stereotypes in combination with the social distancing have hinder actions to maintain physical and functional capacity of those people by honest valuing and care.

In Brazil, appropriate places for physical activity remain closed due to the pandemic. Thus, while fearing the pandemic growth, sedentary behaviour has been favoured. Regarding the sedentary behaviour of aged people, honestly, I am afraid to believe that the panic displayed by part of society right now may be causing more harm than good. It is paradoxical like the "old saying of short blanket". Although there is no treatment for COVID-19, physical activity cannot be limited to the aforementioned places. Therefore, important questions should be considered in this regard: a) "how to stimulate waist circumference monitoring among older Brazilians during home stay?" and b) "how to promote strength training during this social distancing period?"

By this time, strategies and stand positions from geriatric entities and government are extremely necessary to meet the current need of physical activities. We cannot ignore the fact that sedentary behaviour related to quarantine might be harmful to aged people. Therefore, this discussion should be considered for health promotion in Brazil.

REFERENCES

Church, T., & Martin, C. K. (2018). The obesity epidemic: a consequence of reduced energy expenditure and the uncoupling of energy intake? *Obesity, 26*(1), 14-16.

da Silva Alexandre, T., Scholes, S., Santos, J. F., de Oliveira Duarte, Y. A., & de Oliveira, C. (2018). Dynapenic abdominal obesity increases mortality risk among English and Brazilian older adults: a 10-year follow-up of the ELSA and SABE studies. *The journal of nutrition, health & aging, 22*(1), 138-144.

Ekelund, U., Steene-Johannessen, J., Brown, W. J., Fagerland, M. W., Owen, N., Powell, K. E., ... Group, L. S. B. W. (2016). Does physical activity attenuate, or even eliminate, the detrimental association of sitting time with mortality? A harmonised metaanalysis of data from more than 1 million men and women. *The Lancet, 388*(10051), 1302-1310.

Eurosurveillance Editorial Team. (2020). Updated rapid risk assessment from ECDC on the novel coronavirus disease 2019 (COVID-19) pandemic: increased transmission in the EU/EEA and the UK. *Eurosurveillance, 25*(10).

Fragala, M. S., Cadore, E. L., Dorgo, S., Izquierdo, M., Kraemer, W. J., Peterson, M. D., & Ryan, E. D. (2019). Resistance training for older adults: position statement from the National strength and conditioning association. *The Journal of Strength & Conditioning Research, 33*(8).

Gadelha, A. B., Neri, S. G., Vainshelboim, B., Ferreira, A. P., & Lima, R. M. (2019). Dynapenic abdominal obesity and the incidence of falls in older women: a prospective study. *Aging Clin Exp Res*, 1-8.

Lynch, C., Mahida, N., Oppenheim, B., & Gray, J. (2020). Washing our hands of the problem. *Journal of Hospital Infection*.

Onder, G., Rezza, G., & Brusaferro, S. (2020). Case-fatality rate and characteristics of patients dying in relation to COVID-19 in Italy. *Jama*.

World Health Organization. (2020). Report of the WHO-China Joint Mission on coronavirus disease 2019 (COVID-19). 2020. *World Health Organization: Geneva, Switzerland. Available at https://www. who. int/docs/default-source/coronaviruse/who-chinajointmission-on-COVID-19-final-report. pdf. Accessed, 6.* _____

2. The Impact Of COVID-19 On People With Diabetes In Brazil[1]

Mark Thomaz Ugliara Barone,[a,b,c,d,*] Simone Bega Harnik,[e] Patrícia Vieira de Luca,[c,f] Bruna Letícia de Souza Lima,[b,c] Ronaldo José Pineda Wieselberg,[a,b,c,d] Belinda Ngongo,[g] Hermelinda Cordeiro Pedrosa,[d,h] Augusto Pimazoni-Netto,[d,i] Denise Reis Franco,[b,d] Maria de Fatima Marinho de Souza,[c,j] Deborah Carvalho Malta,[k] and Viviana Giampaoli[e]

ABSTRACT

The present study aims at identifying main barriers faced by people living with diabetes in Brazil during the COVID-19 pandemic.

INTRODUCTION

The COVID-19 outbreak has led to an unprecedented global health crisis, testing health systems' preparedness and ability to cope with a pandemic response [1], [2], [3], [4]. Brazil experienced a similar challenge. The first SARS-CoV-2 case was officially reported in December 2019 in Wuhan, China, and rapidly spread in the entire country and beyond within 30 days [5], [6], [7]. The first suspected case in Latin America was reported on January 27th in Brazil and the first case was confirmed in the same country on February 26th of 2020 [2], [3], [7]. A series of measures were put in place to prepare Brazil for the anticipated health crisis prior to the declaration of COVID-19 as a Public Health Emergency of International Concern, on January 30th [2], and then a pandemic, on March 11th [8]. Following these international alerts, less than a month after the first confirmed case, on March 20th, the Brazilian Ministry of Health recognized that community transmission was already happening in Brazil [2].

Infection by SARS-CoV-2 causes major disruptions and threats, in addition to the loss of human lives, with case fatality rate ranging from 0.2% in Germany, to 7.7% in Italy [9], the impact of COVID-19 is beyond imagination and is sparkling a global mourning, booming a feeling of unsafety and uncertainty. On July 5th, according to the World Health Organization (WHO), 11,301,850 cases and 531,806 deaths due to COVID-19 were confirmed in 216 countries areas or territories with cases [10]. On this same day, the number of cases and mortality in Brazil had reached 1,603,055 and 64,867 respectively, with a case fatality rate of 4.0% [11]. While this is the highest number of cases and one of the highest case fatality rate in Latin America [12], scientists argue that cases and

[1] Diabetes Res Clin Pract. 2020 Aug; 166: 108304.
Published online 2020 Jul 3. doi: 10.1016/j.diabres.2020.108304

mortality are extremely underscored due to the low number of tests performed among other reasons [1], [4], [12], [13] by possible 14–20 times the official reported figures [14].Authors of the first Chinese and Italian reports alerted for the worse prognosis of individuals with diabetes and other noncommunicable disease (NCDs), in comparison with populations of the same age group without chronic health conditions [5], [15], [16], [17], [18]. Further retrospective studies have revealed that, within this group of individuals, hyperglycaemia was associated with higher severity and mortality rates[15], [19], [20], [21], for reasons under investigation [22], [23]. Additionally, usual comorbidities such as hypertension, cardiovascular disease, older age, and gender (male) also complement increased severity and mortality risks of individuals with diabetes hospitalized due to COVID-19 [24].

With a prevalence as high as 16.8 million people or 11.4% of the population between 20 and 79 years old, Brazil is among the top 5 countries regarding diabetes prevalence [25]. Moreover, its observes more than 135,000 deaths caused by this condition and its complications yearly [25]. Brazil struggles with the continuous treatment routine of impacted populations; only 28.8% are considered to be in target, having a glycated haemoglobin A1C below 7.0% (53 mmol/mol) [26]. Consequently, 71.2% of Brazilians with diabetes belong to a subgroup more exposed to hyperglycaemia, which makes them vulnerable to even higher risk of poor outcomes when infected by the SARS-CoV-2 virus. This situation calls for deep commitments from the public health in all its forms and a concrete alignment with the WHO. Unfortunately, in the midst of the fight against this novel virus, Brazil experienced a troublesome atmosphere of political disputes, blinding authorities to making decisions aligned with the global technical recommendations [1], [4], [12]. This also harmed adjustments to continue the proper follow-up and management of other diseases, including both communicable and NCDs. For these reasons, the present study aims to investigate challenges encountered by people living with diabetes in Brazil during the COVID-19 pandemic.

METHOD

In a convenience sampling study, data were collected from 1701 individuals, aged 18 or above; 75.54% female participants; 60.73% T1D and 30.75% T2D, between April 22nd and May 4th, using an anonymous and untraceable survey containing 20 multiple choice questions Relationship between variables was established using the multiple correspondence analysis technique. Data from individuals with diabetes were collected through an anonymous and untraceable survey containing 20 multiple choice questions in Portuguese. The authors shared this survey on websites and social media including Facebook and WhatsApp, through their affiliated institutions, co-ligated or partner entities, and diabetes social media groups. Hence, the convenience sampling nature of this study. In addition to being a person living with diabetes, individuals needed to be legally adults (above 18 years old) and accept the terms to share anonymous and untraceable answers. Survey responses were collected from April 22nd through May 4th. The first question provided a complete overview of the questionnaire and required confirmation of the health condition (diabetes) by the respondent. This was followed by socio-demographic questions related to age, gender, state of residence, capital/inland/coast, education level, number of people living in the household, and nature of the health system which could be public, private or both. Subsequent questions served to identify the health status of the participants, asking about diabetes type, and presence and type of comorbidity. All remaining questions covered aspects attributed to the COVID-19 pandemic: frequency of going outside, strategies to protect from infection when outside, noted changes in the glycaemic levels, access to medical care, changes in eating habits and physical activity, changes in smoking and drinking habits, and suspected or confirmed COVID-19 infection by the respondent or cohabitant family member. At the end of the survey, the respondent could leave a comment. Several questions and their answers were regarding subjective perceptions, such as "my blood glucose increased", "I am eating more" or "I am exercising much less" than before the pandemic. Therefore, answers should not be interpreted as objective measurements, but as subjective comparisons with the pre-pandemic states. A multivariate analysis of dimensions of COVID-19 and types of diabetes (type 1 diabetes - T1D; type 2 diabetes - T2D; others: LADA, MODY, gestational; and unknown) was performed with multiple correspondence analysis (MCA) in R (version 3.6.1) and RStudio (version 1.1.453) [27].

RESULTS

The survey was answered by 1701 individuals, 75.54% were female respondents, 70.78% between 18 and 50 years old, 64.96% of respondents were from Southeast of Brazil, and the main diabetes types were type 1 (60.73%) and type 2 (30.75%)[1] (full socio-demographic profile in table 1). Among the main reported consequences of the COVID-19 pandemic were: 95.1% reduced frequency of going outside home (26.9% never went outside since the beginning of the pandemic); among the ones who monitored their blood glucose at home (91.5%), the majority (59.4%) experienced a deterioration, which included: 31.2% reported greater variability than before the pandemic, 20% higher glycemia and 8.2% lower glycaemic levels. Moreover, 38.4% postponed medical appointments and/or routine exams, and 40.2% did not schedule a medical appointment since the onset of the pandemic. Among recommended habits, slated for diabetes treatment, physical activity was the most impacted, with a reduction reported by 59.5% of the respondents (14.7% with a slight reduction and 44.8% with a great reduction). [2]

Regarding comorbidities, for the current study and analysis, we opted to group them into the following: 1) "Mental Health" which includes the following conditions: depression, anxiety, bulimia, anorexia and diabulimia; and 2) "Cardiovascular Diseases" comprising: stroke, infarction, hypertension and dyslipidaemia. Two other groups were already established in the survey as single answers, which had a parenthesis to facilitate comprehension, the "Diabetes Related Complications" with: retinopathy, neuropathy and diabetic renal disease; and the "Respiratory Diseases": asthma and COPD,[3].The analysis revealed the association between age and the occurrence of symptoms of COVID-19, type of diabetes and some of the comorbidities evaluated.[4]. People with T1D were among the youngest and appeared in proximity to mental health diseases category, but also close to the no-cardiovascular conditions, no-obesity and no-respiratory disease categories.

They were alarmingly close to the category that, despite having symptoms of COVID-19, had no testing for SARS-CoV-2. Not measuring the blood glucose is close to T2D and unknown diabetes type. T2D, not surprisingly, was more associated than other types with older age, cardiovascular diseases and obesity. It is also worth noting that T2D and older group were the closest to test positive for SARS-CoV-2. In opposition, individuals who had symptoms of COVID-19 and were not tested (125 people or 7.35%) presented higher proximity to increased blood glucose.[5]Measuring

[1] Suplementary Tables and Figures and data Diabetes Res Clin Pract. 2020 Aug; 166: 108304.
[2] See Suplementary Tables and Figures and data Diabetes Res Clin Pract. 2020 Aug; 166: 108304.
[3] Suplementary Tables and Figures and data Diabetes Res Clin Pract. 2020 Aug; 166: 108304.
[4] Suplementary Tables and Figures and data Diabetes Res Clin Pract. 2020 Aug; 166: 108304.
[5] Suplementary Tables and Figures and data Diabetes Res Clin Pract. 2020 Aug; 166: 108304.

blood glucose was related with food consumption and working out[1] Individuals that experienced decrease in blood glucose levels, increased physical activity and decreased food consumption. Meanwhile, higher food consumption and reduced physical activity were associated with higher blood glucose levels. While it seems that the pandemic had a higher impact on habits and glycaemic levels of T1D individuals.[2], with significant perceived changes, T2D respondents seem to have maintained most of their habits during this period.

Individuals who exclusively use the Brazilian public health system (Unified Health System - SUS), which serves more than 70% of the Brazilian population [28] (in our case, 28.16% of the respondents), were who kept venturing out during the pandemic and experienced an increase of blood glucose levels,[3] . T1D individuals were the closest to the use of both health systems (SUS and private) and experienced higher glycaemic variability (ups and downs). They had the ability to have friends or relatives to buy or collect their medicines and medical supplies. Users of the private health system were closer to experience no glycaemic changes during the pandemic (the same), and used their own stocks of medicine and medical supplies or ordered for home delivery from private pharmacies.[4]MCA for glycaemic measures, method for buying/receiving medicine, health system, and type of diabetes[5]

4. DISCUSSION

The results above unveil short, mid and long-term risks for individuals with diabetes in Brazil. While the federal government and some states made initial commitments and plans [2], knowing the risks for poor prognosis among individuals living with diabetes and/or other NCDs if infected by SARS-CoV-2, our data revealed that implemented measures did not cover most of this population. The strategy to distribute medicines and medical supplies for 90 days, as recommended by different organizations in order to avoid monthly trips [29], [30], were effective for only 21% of the 64.5% who received their medication and supplies from SUS (or 13.5% of the total respondents). This provision of medicines and supplies for 3 months, avoiding the monthly rounds to public primary healthcare facilities or pharmacies, seemed to be one of the only specific policies to protect individuals with diabetes and others NCDs in Brazil [31], [32]. Although limited, if working well, this would at least protect them from encountering infected people seeking care. Meanwhile, at municipality level, certain locations successfully implemented alternative strategies, as hailed by one participant from an inland town: "my town adopted a delivery of medicine method for people with chronic diseases".

According to our data, especially individuals who exclusively depended on SUS were at higher risk, venturing out of home more often and experiencing an increase in blood glucose levels.[6]. Differences would not be expected, since Brazil prides itself for its Universal Health Coverage, and most people, including the ones with private insurance, rely on SUS to receive part or all their medicines and supplies. We hypothesise that this finding highlights the socioeconomic inequalities in the country, which exposes the less privileged more often to unsafe environments by forcing them to continue going out to work during the pandemic and/or to access affordable food. Even though 44.3% of the individuals reported having a family member or friend going monthly to public pharmacies on their

---

[1] Supplementary Tables and Figures and data Diabetes Res Clin Pract. 2020 Aug; 166: 108304.
[2] Supplementary Tables and Figures and data Diabetes Res Clin Pract. 2020 Aug; 166: 108304.
[3] Supplementary Tables and Figures and data Diabetes Res Clin Pract. 2020 Aug; 166: 108304.
[4] Supplementary Tables and Figures and data Diabetes Res Clin Pract. 2020 Aug; 166: 108304.
[5] Supplementary Tables and Figures and data Diabetes Res Clin Pract. 2020 Aug; 166: 108304.
[6] Supplementary Tables and Figures and data Diabetes Res Clin Pract. 2020 Aug; 166: 108304.

behalf to collect medicines and supplies, 49.9% went themselves, perhaps due to lack of direct support. It is important to highlight that family member's or friend's support may reduce but not eliminate the risk of infection, especially if residing in the same location, acting as a potential vehicle of indirect transmission. Another uncomfortable answer came from 5.8% of the individuals who reported halting collection of their medicines and medical supplies and relying on personal stocks, which might not last the entire pandemic period.

This situation may place those who avoided leaving their homes during the pandemic in a risky untreated situation, a globally shared concern [15], [17], [33], [34], [35]. While it is hard to predict social, economic and health impacts of a pandemic, specialists alert to the consequences of implementing only light measures [4], [12], [13], [36], [37], [38], but, at the same time, also the harmful consequences of lockdowns, mobility restrictions and social distancing on the prevention and control of diabetes and other NCDs [17], [34], [39]. Barone et al. [39] reported an association between stricter measures against the pandemic and perceived challenges and fear in the diabetes community in South and Central America, which, when disconnected from information and educational strategies, would increase the pressure on the health systems [37], [39]. Although decentralized (defined by states and municipalities) and delayed [1], [4], [12], [13], [40], the measures to contain the SARS-CoV-2 spread in Brazil, and reflected on mobility reduction, was experienced by 95.1% of this study's respondents in different degrees (with 26.9% never going outside their homes).

Differently from Kluge et al.'s prediction [17], in our case it was not associated with increased consumption of alcohol, tobacco and unhealthy foods. Notwithstanding, physical activity was affected, being reduced for 59.5% of the respondents. Other researchers have also reported physical activity reductions during the pandemic, and alerted for the potential negative consequences on metabolic, cardiovascular and musculoskeletal health [41], [42].

They alert that these effects are observed even after short periods of inactivity, are hard to recover and, not only increase premature mortality, but also favour the development of diabetes chronic complications [41], [42]. A strategy to minimize those consequences would be developing good channels and partnerships for informing these populations through the internet, TV broadcasting and messaging through mobile phone applications in a structured manner, focusing on preventive measures and maintenance or improvement of habits and behaviours, such as regular physical activity [17], [34], [41], [42], [43].

This recommendation is compatible with the present findings where 87.4% of the individuals maintained or increased their time watching TV and 90.7% maintained or increased their time on the internet. Regarding treatment, the COVID-19 pandemic, as predicted and observed by different authors, is impacting availability and access to healthcare professionals (HCPs) for the routine care of people with diabetes, since many of them relocated to emergency rooms, testing sites, ICUs and other services to attend infected individuals [15], [17], [33], [34], [39]. We found that 38.4% postponed their medical appointments and/or examinations. We attributed these results to shortage of HCPs, as expressed by 3 individuals in the comments space of the survey, reporting appointment cancelation or absence of physician; or personal decision because of the fear of getting infected at a hospital or clinic, as identified in other studies [39], [35].

The potential consequence of this phenomenon of fear during the pandemic was reported in a paediatric emergency department, in Italy, with reduction and delay in children's arrival, which included cases of severe diabetes ketoacidosis and hypoglycaemia [35]. Although online consultation and other telemedicine strategies were not investigated profoundly in the present study, one of the respondents commented that he/she was having online medical appointments.

Brazilian laws and regulations became more flexible allowing this type of approach during the COVID-19 pandemic [44]. In alignment with other authors and international organizations, we highly recommend it [15], [33], [36], [45], [46], [47], [48], reinforcing Primary Healthcare's role during the pandemic through ensuring close and timely monitoring of people with diabetes and other NCDs [37], [44], [49]. The results show that all types of diabetes were close to additional risk factors for poor prognosis of individuals infected by SARS-CoV-2. While T2D and unknown diabetes type (Fig. 1) appear near other NCDs (especially cardiovascular and obesity) [18], [24], [47], [50], [51], T1D and other types (LADA, MODY and gestational grouped) presented close proximity to glycaemic variability[1][5], [15], [52]. Therefore, we suggest that none of the types should feel safe.

Although, not surprising, T2D was associated with the category "50 years and older"[2]reason to be vigilant, since the COVID-19 mortality and severity increase with age [5], [24], [53]. An unfortunate result was the proximity of individuals reporting increased blood glucose levels and the presence of COVID-19 symptoms without testing.[3]The global shortage of tests for SARS-CoV-2 poses a grand challenge [2], [3], [4], however, cognizant that high blood glucose increases the risk for infection severity and death [15], [19], [20], [21], [22], [23], early testing efforts must be prioritized in this group. In addition, supporting the intensification of diabetes self-care practices to quickly bring individuals' glycemia back on track must be prioritized [45], [51], [54]. [4] depicts the importance of balancing food and exercise, since individuals who increased or decreased any of them experienced changes in their blood glucose levels, whereas those able to maintain exercise and food consumption avoided glycaemic changes.

While the present study focused only on diabetes, WHO's data show that other NCDs serviced in similar health systems and pandemic environment are facing comparable challenges [55]. In terms of unattended needs of individuals with diabetes during this COVID-19 crisis, Brazil is not the only country with unaddressed demands. In a collection of testimonials from people with diabetes in different countries, the International Diabetes Federation exposed some similar issues whilst others different from the Brazilian context [56]. While the absence of specific measures to protect those with diabetes was reported in Greece and Spain, access to medicines was a challenge in Zimbabwe, Iran and India [56]. However, countries like Argentina, Italy, Portugal, and South Korea seemed to have adopted measures that made people with diabetes feel safer [48], [56].

It is urgent for Brazil to follow international best practices and recommendations, since, as stated by the WHO Regional Office for Europe, "the prevention and control of NCDs have a crucial role in the COVID-19 response and an adaptive response is required to account for the needs of people with NCDs" [17].The limitations of the present study include the fact that, although efforts were made to disseminate the survey as much as possible, its sample neither reflects the proportion of Brazilian population nor its fraction with diabetes.

Thus, it is a convenience sample, without post-stratification weights. Questions about behaviours, habits and glycaemic changes were subjective comparisons with the pre-pandemic state, therefore, we did not have access to objective data to validate the subjective responses. As an online survey, it is biased by individuals who have internet access. While 17% of the Brazilian population have a college degree [57] and 27.9% have private health insurance [28], among the respondents of the present survey, 51.8% had at least one college degree and only 28.2% exclusively access care services through SUS.

---

[1] Supplementary Tables and Figures and data Diabetes Res Clin Pract. 2020 Aug; 166: 108304.
[2] Supplementary Tables and Figures and data Diabetes Res Clin Pract. 2020 Aug; 166: 108304.
[3] Supplementary Tables and Figures and data Diabetes Res Clin Pract. 2020 Aug; 166: 108304.
[4] Suplementary Tables and Figures and data Diabetes Res Clin Pract. 2020 Aug; 166: 108304.

Other demographic limitations are related to the age groups distribution, younger than the general population with the great majority of the respondents from Sao Paulo state, which would be about 20% of the country, not 42.6% as in our group of respondents. We understand that one of the main factors leading to this bias is the network in which the authors are engaged, the geographic location of diabetes associations and the profile of their active members; tendency to have more individuals with T1D than T2D, mostly young and highly educated. An additional limitation is the number of choices for each question and the aggregation made for analysis purposes. This includes the fact that if separated, diseases aggregated in the Cardiovascular Disease group, for example, could behave differently in terms of proximity to other factors. Moreover, increase or decrease of the blood glucose, interpreted as distancing from the target, would in fact have led the glycemia to target, while the ones who successfully maintained the blood glucose in pre-pandemic levels, may have kept it out of target.

5. CONCLUSION

As revealed for the first time in the current study, individuals with diabetes were not spared by the COVID-19 pandemic in Brazil. Measures and adjustments lacked or were insufficient, paving the way to unhealthy and unsafe behaviours such as postponing medical appointments, reducing physical activity and refraining from collecting medicines and supplies, which led to a high percentage of glycaemic worsen reports. Additionally, announced measures for prevention and mitigation of COVID-19 consequences on this population, such as supply of medicines for 3 months, worked just for a minority. In conclusion, we see a pressing need from the Brazilian federal, states and municipal authorities to broaden the implemented measures in order to reach more people, and partner with civil society, private sector and media channels to quickly improve the response and, this way, prevent a surge of individuals with diabetes infected by SARS-CoV-2 and of acute and chronic diabetes complications.

Measures to keep individuals healthy, ensuring their glycemia is on target and allowing them to stay at home as much as possible must be prioritized. We recommend that the public and the private health systems maintain, adapt and strengthen programs for the continuity of care of individuals with diabetes and other NCDs, and develop information and educational campaigns on how to access these programs. In addition to focusing on reducing the risk of infection and continuity of their healthcare, these measures should facilitate access to healthcare professionals' counselling for therapeutic adjustment.

Finally, as key measures we foresee are a) active monitoring, informing, educating and responding to communities' needs at primary healthcare level; b) high quality telehealth for consultations, monitoring and examining; c) distribution of medications and supplies for three or more months, ideally with home delivery; and d) home sampling for scheduled lab exams, using mobile point-of-care strategies or appointment in specific facilities with well-established disinfection protocols. Consequently, we believe that the pandemic's challenges can be lessened if appropriate measures protecting individuals with diabetes and other chronic conditions are adopted, and investments are not solely directed to purchasing mechanical ventilators and equipping tertiary care.

ACKNOWLEDGEMENTS

The authors acknowledge Vanessa Pirolo's support and assistance sharing the survey through her network and the non-governmental organizations ADJ Diabetes Brasil (ADJ), Institute for Children with Diabetes (ICD), Brazilian Diabetes Society (SBD), Brazilian Hypercholesterolemia Association (AHF), Fórum DCNTs and their member and partner entities for assisting in sharing the survey and providing general support.

REFERENCE

1. Rafael R., Neto M., Carvalho M. Epidemiology, public policies and COVID-19 pandemics in Brazil: what can we expect? Revista de Enfermagem Uerj. 2020;28 [Google Scholar]
2. Croda J., Oliveira W., Frutuoso R. COVID-19 in Brazil: advantages of a socialized unified health system and preparation to contain cases. Sociedade Brasileira de Medicina Tropical. 2020;53 doi: 10.1590/0037-8682-0167-2020. [PMC free article] [PubMed] [CrossRef] [Google Scholar]
3. Rodriguez-Morales A.J., Gallego V., Escalera-Antezana J.P., Méndez C.A., Zambrano L.I., Franco-Paredes C., Suárez J.A., Rodriguez-Enciso H.D., Balbin-Ramon G.J., Savio-Larriera E., Risquez A., Cimerman S. COVID-19 in Latin America: the implications of the first confirmed case in Brazil. Travel Med Infect Dis. 2020;35:101613. doi: 10.1016/j.tmaid.2020.101613. [PMC free article] [PubMed] [CrossRef] [Google Scholar]
4. Kirby T. South America prepares for the impact of COVID-19. Lancet. 2020 doi: 10.1016/S2213-2600(20)30218-6. [PMC free article] [PubMed] [CrossRef] [Google Scholar]
5. Wu Z., McGoogan J. Characteristics of and important lessons from the coronavirus disease 2019 (COVID-19) outbreak in China. JAMA Network. 2020;323(13):1239–1242. doi: 10.1001/jama.2020.2648. [PubMed] [CrossRef] [Google Scholar]
6. Yang X., Yu Y., Xu J. Clinical course and outcomes of critically ill patients with SARS-CoV-2 pneumonia in Wuhan, China: a single-centreed, retrospective, observational study. Lancet. 2020 doi: 10.1016/S2213-2600(20)30079-5. [PMC free article] [PubMed] [CrossRef] [Google Scholar]
7. Rodriguez-Morales AJ, Sánchez-Duque JA, Hernández Botero S et al. Preparación y control de la enfermedad por coronavirus 2019 (COVID-19) en América Latina. Acta Med Peru 2020;37(1):3 10.35663/amp.2020.371.909. [CrossRef]
8. Bedford J., Enria D., Heymann D. COVID-19: towards controlling of a pandemic. Lancet. 2020;395(10229):P1015–P1018. [PMC free article] [PubMed] [Google Scholar]
9. Lazzerini M., Putoto G. COVID-19 in Italy: momentous decisions and many uncertainties. Lancet. 2020;8(5):E641–E642. doi: 10.1016/S2214-109X(20)30110-8.
10. WHO. Coronavirus Disease (COVID-19) Pandemic, https://www.who.int/emergencies/diseases/novel-coronavirus-2019?gclid=Cj0KCQjwhtT1BRCiARIsAGlY51IENPlv2UGpmxXy8AuUGkFbDKbMq5inFN5BVmJuo2O6n34GouGgdwAaAvEZEALw_wcB; 2020 [accessed 6 July 2020].
11. Coronavírus Brasil. Painel Coronavírus, https://covid.saude.gov.br/; 2020 [accessed 6 July 2020].
12. Lancet T. COVID-19 in Brazil: "So what?" Lancet. 2020;395:1461. doi: 10.1016/S0140-6736(20)31095-3. [PMC free article] [PubMed] [CrossRef] [Google Scholar]
13. Mellan T, Hoeltgebaum H, Mishra S, et al. Report 21: Estimating COVID-19 cases and reproduction number in Brazil. Imperial College London. 2020; 10.25561/78872. [CrossRef]
14. Ziegler MF. Pesquisadores estimam haver mais de 1,6 milhão de casos de COVID-19 no Brasil. Agência Fapesp. 2020; http://agencia.fapesp.br/pesquisadores-estimam-haver-mais-de-16-milhao-de-casos-de-COVID-19-no-brasil/33116/ [accessed 17 May 2020].
15. Gentile S., Strollo F., Ceriello A. Ceriello, COVID-19 Infection in italian people with diabetes:lessons learned for our future (an experience to be used) Diabetes Res Clin Pract. 2020 doi: 10.1016/j.diabres.2020.108137. [PMC free article] [PubMed] [CrossRef] [Google Scholar]
16. Wang W., Lu J., Gu W., Zhang Y., Liu J., Ning G. Care for diabetes with COVID-19: advice from China. J Diabetes. 2020;12(5):417–419. doi: 10.1111/jdb.v12.510.1111/1753-0407.13036. [PubMed

17. Kluge H., Wickramasinghe K., Rippin H. Prevention and control of non-communicable diseases in the COVID-19 response. Lancet. 2020 doi: 10.1016/S0140-6736(20)31067-9. [CrossRef] [Google Scholar]

18. Zhou F., Yu T., Du R. Clinical course and risk factors for mortality of adult inpatients with COVID-19 in Wuhan, China: a retrospective cohort study. Lancet. 2020 doi: 10.1016/S0140-6736(20)30566-3. [PMC free article] [PubMed] [CrossRef] [Google Scholar]

19. Zhu L., She Z., Cheng X. Association of blood glucose control and outcomes in patients with COVID-19 and pre-existing type 2 diabetes. Cell Metab. 2020 doi: 10.1016/j.cmet.2020.04.021. [PMC free article] [PubMed] [CrossRef] [Google Scholar]

20. Iacobellis G., Penaherrera C.A., Bermudez L.E. Admission hyperglycemia and radiological findings of SARS-CoV2 in patients with and without diabetes. Diabetes Res Clin Pract. 2020;164 doi: 10.1016/j.diabres.2020.108185. [PMC free article] [PubMed] [CrossRef] [Google Scholar]

21. Bode B., Garrett V., Messler J. Glycemic characteristics and clinical outcomes of COVID-19 patients hospitalized in the United States. J Diabetes Sci Technol. 2020:1–9. doi: 10.1177/1932296820924469. [PubMed]

22. Codo A.C., Davanzo G.G., Monteiro L.B. Elevated glucose levels favor Sars-Cov-2 infection and monocyte response through a Hif-1α/glycolysis dependent axis. Cell Metab. 2020 doi: 10.2139/ssrn.3606770.

23. Ceriello A. Hyperglycemia and the worse prognosis of COVID-19. why a fast blood glucose control should be mandatory. Diabetes Res Clin Pract. 2020;163:108186. doi: 10.1016/j.diabres.2020.108186. [

24. Shi Q., Zhang X., Jiang F. Clinical characteristics and risk factors for mortality of COVID-19 patients with diabetes in Wuhan, China: a two-centre retrospective study. Diabetes Care. 2020;43(5):1–10. doi: 10.2337/dc20-0598. [PubMed] [CrossRef] [Google Scholar]

25. International Diabetes Federation (IDF). IDF Diabetes Atlas. 9th ed. Brussels, Belgium: International Diabetes Federation; 2019.

26. Malta DC, Duncan BB, Schmidt MI et al. Prevalence of diabetes mellitus as determined by glycated hemoglobin in the Brazilian adult population, National Health Survey. Rev. Bras. Epidemiol. 2019;22(S2). 10.1590/1980-549720190006.supl.2. [PubMed] [CrossRef]

27. Tenenhaus M., Young F. An analysis and synthesis of multiple correspondence analysis, optimal scaling, dual scaling, homogeneity analysis and other methods for quantifying categorical multivariate data. Psychometrika. 1985;50:91–119. doi: 10.1007/BF02294151. [CrossRef] [Google Scholar]

28. Malta D., Stopa S., Pereira C. Private health care coverage in the Brazilian population, according to the 2013 Brazilian National Health Survey. Ciência & Saúde Coletiva. 2017;22(1):179–190. doi: 10.1590/1413-81232017221.16782015. [PubMed] [CrossRef] [Google Scholar]

29. PAHO. If I have diabetes, what do I need to know about COVID-19?, https://iris.paho.org/bitstream/handle/10665.2/52213/PAHONMHNVCOVID-19200014_eng.pdf?sequence=5&isAllowed=y; 2020 [accessed 10 June 2020].

30. Bachireddy C., Chen C., Dar M. Securing the safety net and protecting health during a pandemic: medicaid's response to COVID-19. JAMA. 2020;323(20):2009–2010. doi: 10.1001/jama.2020.4272. [PubMed] [CrossRef] [Google Scholar]

31. Ministerio da Saude. Alterações no Programa Farmácia Popular devido à situação de emergência de saúde pública decorrente do coronavírus (COVID19), https://www.saude.gov.br/noticias/farmacia-popular/46566; 2020 [accessed 10 June 2020].

32. Governo do Estado de Sao Paulo. Saúde amplia entrega de remédios nas farmácias de alto custo para prevenção do coronavírus, http://www.portaldenoticias.saude.sp.gov.br/saude-amplia-entrega-de-remedios-nas-farmacias-de-alto-custo-para-prevencao-do-coronavirus/; 2020 [accessed 10 June 2020].

33. Ma R.C.W., Holt R.I.G. COVID-19 and diabetes. Diabet Med. 2020;37:723–725. doi: 10.1111/dme.14300. [PMC free article] [PubMed] [CrossRef] [Google Scholar]

34. Katulanda P., Dissanayake H., Ranathunga I. Prevention and management of COVID-19 among patients with diabetes: an appraisal of the literature. Diabetologia. 2020 doi: 10.1007/s00125-020-05164-x

35. Lazzerini M., Barbi E., Apicella A., Marchetti F., Cardinale F., Trobia G. Delayed access or provision of care in Italy resulting from fear of COVID-19. Lancet Child Adolesc Health. 2020;4(5):e10–e11. doi: 10.1016/S2352-4642(20)30108-5. [PMC free article] [PubMed] [CrossRef] [Google Scholar]

36. Puig-Domingo M., Marazuela M., Giustina A. COVID-19 and endocrine diseases. A statement from the European Society of Endocrinology. Endocrine. 2020;68:2–5. doi: 10.1007/s12020-020-02294-5.

37. Sánchez-Duque J.A., Arce-Villalobos L.R., Rodríguez-Morales A.J. Enfermedad por coronavirus 2019 (COVID-19) en América Latina: papel de la atención primaria en la preparación y respuesta. Aten Primaria. 2020 doi: 10.1016/j.aprim.2020.04.001. [PMC free article] [PubMed] [CrossRef] [Google Scholar]

38. Inglesby T.V. Public health measures and the reproduction number of SARS-CoV-2. JAMA. 2020 doi: 10.1001/jama.2020.7878. [PubMed] [CrossRef] [Google Scholar]

39. Barone M, Villarroel D, de Luca P, et al. COVID-19 Impact on People with Diabetes in the South and Central America. Diabetes Res Clin Pract 2020 (submitted). 10.1016/j.diabres.2020.108301 [PMC free article] [PubMed] [CrossRef]

40. Cimerman S., Chebabo A., da Cunha C.A. Deep impact of COVID-19 in the healthcare of Latin America: the case of Brazil. Braz J Infect Dis. 2020 doi: 10.1016/j.bjid.2020.04.005. [PMC free article] [PubMed] [CrossRef] [

41. Peçanha T., Goessler K.F., Roschel H. Social isolation during the COVID-19 pandemic can increase physical inactivity and the global burden of cardiovascular disease. Am J Physiol Heart Circ Physiol. 2020;318(6):H1441–H1446. doi: 10.1152/ajpheart.00268.2020. [PMC free article] [PubMed] [CrossRef] [Google Scholar]

42. Roschel H., Artioli G.G., Gualano B. Risk of increased physical inactivity during COVID-19 outbreak in older people: a call for actions. J Am Geriatr Soc. 2020 doi: 10.1111/jgs.16550. [PubMed] [CrossRef] [Google Scholar]

43. Hopman J., Allegranzi B., Mehtar S. Managing COVID-19 in low- and middle-income countries. JAMA. 2020;323(16):1549–1550. doi: 10.1001/jama.2020.4169. [PubMed] [CrossRef] [Google Scholar]

44. Sarti T., Lazarini W., Fontenelle L. What is the role of primary health care in the COVID-19 pandemic? Epidemiol Serv Saude. 2020;29(2) doi: 10.5123/S1679-49742020000200024. [PubMed] [CrossRef] [Google Scholar]

45. Bornstein S., Rubino F., Khunti K. Practical recommendations for the management of diabetes in patients with COVID-19. Lancet. 2020 doi: 10.1016/S2213-8587(20)30152-2. [PMC free article] [PubMed]

46. Peters A., Garg S. The silver lining to COVID-19: avoiding diabetic ketoacidosis admissions with telehealth. Diabetes Technol Ther. 2020;22(6):1–

47. Drucker D. Coronavirus infections and type 2 diabetes - shared pathways with therapeutic implications. Endocr Rev. 2020;41(3):1–13. doi: 10.1210/endrev/bnaa011. [PMC free article] [PubMed] [CrossRef] [Google Scholar]

48. World Health Organization, Regional Office for Europe. Ensuring people-centred diabetes care during the COVID-19 pandemic Experiences from Portugal (2020),

49. Beran D., Perone S.A., Perolini M.C. Beyond the virus: Ensuring continuity of care for people with diabetes during COVID-19. Primary Care Diabetes. 2020 doi: 10.1016/j.pcd.2020.05.014. [PMC free article] [PubMed]

50. ai Q., Chen F., Wang T. Obesity and COVID-19 severity in a designated hospital in Shenzhen, China. Diabetes Care. 2020 doi: 10.2337/dc20-0576. [PubMed] [CrossRef] [Google Scholar]

51. Hussain A., Bhowmik B., Vale Moreira N.C. COVID-19 and diabetes: knowledge in progress. Diabetes Res Clin Pract. 2020;162. doi: 10.1016/j.diabres.2020.108142. [PMC free article] [PubMed] [CrossRef] [Google Scholar]

52. Ebekozien OA, Noor N, Gallagher MP et al. Type 1 Diabetes and COVID-19: preliminary findings from a multicentre surveillance study in the U.S. Diabetes Care. 2020:dc201088. doi: 10.2337/dc20-1088. [PubMed]

53. Grasselli G., Pesenti A., Cecconi M. Critical care utilization for the COVID-19 outbreak in Lombardy, Italy. JAMA Network. 2020;323(16):1545–1546. doi: 10.1001/jama.2020.4031. [PubMed] [CrossRef] [Google Scholar]

54. Gupta R., Ghosh A., Singh A.K. Clinical considerations for patients with diabetes in times of COVID-19 epidemic. Diabetes Metabolic Syndrome: Clin Res Rev. 2020;14(3):211–212. doi: 10.1016/j.dsx.2020.03.002. [PMC free article] [PubMed] [CrossRef] [Google Scholar]

55. World Health Organization, Rapid assessment of service delivery for NCDs during the COVID-19 pandemic, https://www.who.int/docs/default-source/ncds/ncd-COVID-19/for-web---rapid-assessment---29-may-2020-(cleared).pdf?sfvrsn=6296324c_8&download=true; 2020 [accessed 10 June 2020].

56. International Diabetes Federation. COVID-19: Perspectives from people with diabetes. Diabetes Res Clin Pract. 2020 May;163:108201. doi: 10.1016/j.diabres.2020.108201. [PubMed]

57. OECD. Education at a Glance 2019. Country Note Brazil; https://www.oecd.org/education/education-at-a-glance/EAG2019_CN_BRA.pdf; 2019 [accessed 10 June 2020].

3. Chronic Heart Diseases As The Most Prevalent Comorbidities Among Deaths By COVID-19 In Brazil[1]

Julianne Pachiega[1] Alexandre José dos Santos Afonso[1]
Géssica Thaís Sinhorin[1] Bianca Teshima de Alencar[2]
Marta dos Santos Mirandade Araújo[3] Fabiana Gulin Longhi[4] Andernice dos Santos Zanetti[3] Omar Ariel Espinosa[5]

ABSTRACT

Age, sex and the presence of comorbidities are risk factors associated with COVID-19. Hypertension, diabetes and heart disease are the most common comorbidities in patients with COVID-19. The objective of this study was to estimate the prevalence of patients with comorbidities who died of COVID-19 in Brazil. Searches of data were carried out on the official pages of the 26 State health departments and the federal district. The random-effect method was used to calculate the prevalence of patients with comorbidities who died. From the beginning of the pandemic in Brazil until May 20, 2020, 276,703 cases of COVID-19 were notified in Brazil, 6.4% died, 58.6% of whom were male. The prevalence of comorbidities among deaths was 83% (95% CI: 79 - 87), with heart disease and diabetes being the most prevalent. To our knowledge, this study represents the first large analysis of cases of patients with confirmed COVID-19 in Brazil. There is a high prevalence of comorbidities (83%) among patients who died from COVID-19 in Brazil, with heart disease being the most prevalent. This is important considering the possible secondary effects produced by drugs such as hydroxychloroquine.

INTRODUCTION

The coronavirus disease 2019 (COVID-19) pandemic has infected more than seven million people worldwide in 216 countries, and, until Jun 16, 2020, it had caused over four hundred thousand deaths[1]. Its etiological agent is the severe acute respiratory syndrome coronavirus 2 (SARS-CoV-2), transmitted by contact with an infected person or contaminated fluids[2,3]. A multicentre cohort study showed that gender and advanced age are significantly correlated with COVID-19 and these findings are consistent with the higher incidence among older people and men[4]. Another study observed that the presence of any comorbidity increases the patient's risk of developing respiratory distress, possibly leading to an intensive care unit (ICU) hospitalization and/or death[5,6]. Cardiovascular diseases, diabetes, hypertension, and chronic obstructive pulmonary disease are among the most prevalent comorbidities in COVID-19 cases[7].

[1] Rev. Inst. Med. trop. S. Paulo vol.62 São Paulo 2020 Epub June 29, 2020

In Brazil, the first confirmed case of COVID-19 was reported on February 26, 2020[8], and the first known death was reported 20 days later, on March 17. Until June 21, the country had confirmed 1,073,376 cases and 50,182 deaths, with an incidence of 5.08 cases per million inhabitants.

This study aimed to estimate the prevalence of patients with comorbidities that died of COVID-19 in the Brazilian Federative Units.

METHODS

Data were extracted from the bulletin on the epidemiological situation of COVID-19, made available by each of the 26 Brazilian States and the Federal District, on their official websites. The obtained data were evaluated according to the following variables: confirmed cases, ICU hospitalizations and deaths. The epidemiological and clinical profiles of the death's cases were also described, considering sex, age, and the presence and type of comorbidities, respectively. Because not all States reported the presence of comorbidities in fatal cases, the random-effects model to estimate the pooled prevalence of comorbidities in deaths and their respective confidence intervals (CI) of 95%, was used. The heterogeneity of prevalence was analysed by State using the Higgins test (I^2), which presents the percentage of variation across them. These analyses were performed using the Stata statistical software, version 12 (Stata Corp LLC, Texas, USA).

RESULTS

Data collection from the official websites of each State Health Department took place from the beginning of the pandemic in Brazil to May 20, 2020. During this period, we found 276,703 reported cases of COVID-19, among which 11,278 (4.8%) were admitted to ICU, and 17,752 (6.4%) cases resulted in deaths. When analysing ICU hospitalization percentage by State, Rio de Janeiro (23.3%) and Minas Gerais (19.6%) were the States with the highest prevalence's. [1]The States with the highest death percentages were Rio de Janeiro (10.7%), Para (9.4%), Sao Paulo (7.8%), Pernambuco (8.1%), Amazonas (6.9%) and Parana (5.2%)[2]

The epidemiological and clinical profiles of confirmed and deaths cases of COVID-19 were obtained through the bulletin information on the epidemiological situation of COVID-19, which each Brazilian State makes available on its official websites. ICUs = Patients admitted to intensive care units; 95% CI = 95% confidence interval; N.S. = Not specified. AC (Acre); AL (Alagoas); AP (Amapa); AM (Amazonas); BA (Bahia); CE (Ceara); DF (Distrito Federal); ES (Espirito Santo); GO (Goias); MA (Maranhao); MT (Mato Grosso); MS (Mato Grosso do Sul); MG (Minas Gerais); PA (Para); PB (Paraiba); PR (Parana); PE (Pernambuco); PI (Piaui); RJ (Rio de Janeiro); RN (Rio Grande do Norte); RS (Rio Grande do Sul); RO (Rondonia); RR (Roraima); SC (Santa Catarina); SP (Sao Paulo). SE (Sergipe); TO (Tocantins).

Regarding the epidemiological profile of fatal cases, 22 States segregated a total of 7,531 cases by sex, of which 58.6% were male and 41.4% female. The age of the death cases was reported only in epidemiological bulletins of 25 States. From 17,752 cases of death, only in 14,728 (83%) the age was reported, the population over 60 years old was the most affected (71.4%)[3].

---

[1] https://www.scielo.br/scielo.php?pid=S0036-46652020000100605&script=sci_arttext#t1
[2] https://www.scielo.br/scielo.php?pid=S0036-46652020000100605&script=sci_arttext#t1
[3] https://www.scielo.br/scielo.php?pid=S0036-46652020000100605&script=sci_arttext#t1

Conversely, the clinical profile was only reported in 2,116 deaths (12%) from 15 States, 1,768 of which presented comorbidities, resulting in an 83% prevalence (95% CI: 79 – 87).[1]The clinical descriptions of the comorbidities in the death cases were extracted from the epidemiological bulletins of each State, which reported diseases grouped according to: Chronic Heart Diseases, Diabetes, Chronic Lung Diseases including Chronic Obstructive Pulmonary Disease, asthma, Chronic Kidney Diseases, Stroke, Hypertension, Obesity,

Immunosuppressive Diseases, Chronic Liver Diseases, Cancer, Digestive System Diseases, Pneumonia, Haematological diseases, Tuberculosis, Metabolic Diseases, different than diabetes., Smoking habit, Others . Among the cases of death, that showed one or more previous diseases, a total of 14,737 comorbidities were recorded. The most prevalent comorbidities found were: 35% chronic heart diseases, 28.7% diabetes, 8.2% chronic lung diseases, including asthma and Chronic Obstructive Pulmonary Disease, 5.9% kidney diseases, 5.3% stroke, 5.1% hypertension, 4.4% obesity, and 3.8% immunosuppressive diseases.[2]

DISCUSSION

To our knowledge, this study represents the first large analysis of cases of sequentially patients with confirmed COVID-19 in Brazil. By June 21, 2020, Brazil was the second country in number of confirmed cases of COVID-19, reporting over a million cases of confirmed COVID-19 and our analysis included approximately a quarter of these cases. As in different parts of the world, a higher prevalence in men and people aged 60 years or in elderly people were found among deaths by COVID-19[9-11]. We found that 4.8% of COVID-19 patients were admitted to ICU, a percentage comparable with a previous study conducted in the United States of America (USA) that analysed 74,439 COVID-19 patients, among whom 1.4% required ICU[12]. Data collected from 138 patients in China showed that 26% were admitted to ICUs[13]. Thus, States such as Rio de Janeiro and Minas Gerais, with the highest hospitalization percentages in the country (23.3% and 19.6%, respectively), should strengthen measures to avoid the collapse of their hospital's intensive care units.

By June 21, 2020, Brazil has exceeded 50,000 deaths, a mark, so far, reached by only two countries worldwide. Considering that, Rio de Janeiro, Para, Sao Paulo, Pernambuco, and Amazonas, which present higher percentages than that calculated for the overall country, represent a great national concern. When dealing with the COVID-19 pandemic, mortality, as well as establishing priorities for controlling it, is the most important concern.

The capacity of the healthcare system thus becomes a major issue, especially considering that the number of confirmed cases in communities is rapidly increasing, as is the case in Brazil. The pooled prevalence of comorbidities in deaths by COVID-19 in Brazil was 83% (95% CI: 79 – 87). Previous studies conducted in Korea (90.7%) and China (68.2%) warned about a higher prevalence of severe acute respiratory syndrome caused by SARS-CoV-2 among patients with comorbidities[11,14].

They also point hypertension, cardiovascular diseases, and diabetes as the main comorbidities among deaths by the disease. Several studies suggest that hypertension is the most common comorbidity in COVID-19 patients[15]. Likewise, a meta-analysis carried out recently by our team showed that hypertension is the most prevalent comorbidity among deaths from COVID-

---

[1] https://www.scielo.br/scielo.php?pid=S0036-46652020000100605&script=sci_arttext#t1
[2] https://www.scielo.br/scielo.php?pid=S0036-46652020000100605&script=sci_arttext#t2

19,followed by diabetes and chronic heart diseases ranking third[16]. Now, in Brazil we found that the main comorbidities among deaths are chronic heart diseases and diabetes.

The third most common comorbidity were the chronic lung diseases, followed by chronic kidney diseases, stroke, hypertension, obesity and immunosuppressive diseases which may include HIV infection and organ transplant patients. The epidemiological bulletins of each State do not specify what were the chronic heart diseases of patients who died from COVID-19, although this group may include patients with coronary heart disease, arrhythmias, infarction, patients with pacemakers and others. Our results showed that this group of comorbidities was the most important in the population studied, and this is an important finding, because the Ministry of Health defends the use of hydroxychloroquine for treating COVID-19.

A recent study claims that some cardiac manifestations, such as cardiac arrhythmias, and even conduction disorders without repercussion, may represent the initial manifestations of toxicity related to chloroquine or hydroxychloroquine[17]. Therefore, the use of these drugs can lead to serious complications and even death in patients with previous heart disease. On the other hand, the use of these drugs as post exposure prophylaxis (PEP), has also proved unsuccessful[18].

Some difficulties to develop this study were found. Firstly, not every Health Department updates their epidemiological bulletins daily, so the daily updating of data unfeasible. Secondly, the epidemiological bulletins were not standardized, not all of them provide epidemiological data such as age, nor clinical data such as the presence of comorbidities, which impaired the collection of complete data. Thirdly, many epidemiological bulletins provide information only as graphics and the absolute numbers were lacking, hampering data replication. Finally, each Secretariat reported different age groups, which impaired the comparisons among them.

We concluded that there is a high prevalence of comorbidities among deaths by COVID-19, affecting mainly men aged over 60 years. The group of chronic heart diseases and diabetes were the main comorbidities among these patients, and this is relevant considering the possible adverse effects produced by drugs such as hydroxychloroquine. On the other hand, we recommend conducting studies based on medical records analyses, with the purpose of knowing specifically the proportion of each heart disease in patients affected by COVID-19. Acknowledging such factors may help to better defining the risks of death among these COVID-19 patients, enabling a more targeted and specific approach to avoid probable deaths. In a scenario without effective antivirals or vaccines available, governments should apply continuous countermeasures for different pandemic situations to reduce mortality, especially in States with high percentages of ICU hospitalization and deaths.

REFERENCES

1. World Health Organization. Coronavirus disease 2019 (COVID-19): situation report – 124. [cited 2020 Jun 22]. Available from: https://www.who.int/docs/default-source/coronaviruse/situation-reports/20200523-COVID-19-sitrep-124.pdf?sfvrsn=9626d639_2 [Links]
2. Gorbalenya AE, Baker SC, Baric RS, de Groot RJ, Drosten C, Gulyaeva AA, et al. The species severe acute respiratory syndrome-related coronavirus: classifying 2019-nCoV and naming it SARS-CoV-2. Nat Microbiol. 2020;5:536-44. [Links]
3. Chan JF, Yuan S, Kok KH, To KK, Chu H, Yang J, et al. A familial cluster of pneumonia associated with the 2019 novel coronavirus indicatingperson-to-person transmission: a study of a family cluster. Lancet. 2020;395:514-23. [Links]
4. Cai H. Sex difference and smoking predisposition in patients with COVID-19. Lancet Respir Med. 2020;8:e20. [Links]
5. Chen N, Zhou M, Dong X, Qu J, Gong F, Han Y, et al. Epidemiological and clinical characteristics of 99 cases of 2019 novel coronavirus pneumonia in Wuhan, China: a descriptive study. Lancet. 2020;395:507-13. [Links]

6. Wang D, Hu B, Hu C, Zhu F, Liu X, Zhang J, et al. Clinical characteristics of 138 hospitalized patients with 2019 novel coronavirus-infected pneumonia in Wuhan, China. JAMA. 2020;323:1061-9. [Links]

7. Yang J, Zheng Y, Gou X, Pu K, Chen Z, Guo Q, et al. Prevalence of comorbidities and its effects in coronavirus disease 2019 patients: a systematic review and meta-analysis. Int J Infect Dis. 2020;94:91-5. [Links]

8. Brasil. Ministério da Saúde. Secretaria de Vigilância em Saúde. Boletim Epidemiológico Especial COE-COVID19. Brasília: Ministério da Saúde; 2020. [cited 2020 Jun 22]. Available from: https://portalarquivos.saude.gov.br/images/pdf/2020/April/27/2020-04-27-18-05h-BEE14-Boletim-do-COE.pdf [Links]

9. Du RH, Liu LM, Yin W, Wang W, Guan LL, Yuan ML, et al. Hospitalization and critical care of 109 decedents with COVID-19 pneumonia in Wuhan, China. Ann Am Thorac Soc. 2020 In Press. [Links]

10. Chen T, Dai Z, Mo P, Li X, Ma Z, Song S, et al. Clinical characteristics and outcomes of older patients with coronavirus disease 2019 (COVID-19) in Wuhan, China (2019): a single-centreed, retrospective study. J Gerontol A Biol Sci Med Sci. 2020:glaa089 In Press. [Links]

11. Korean Society of Infectious Diseases, Korea Centres for Disease Control and Prevention. Analysis on 54 mortality cases of coronavirus disease 2019 in the Republic of Korea from January 19 to March 10, 2020. J Korean Med Sci. 2020;35:e132. [Links]

12. CDC COVID-19 Response Team. Preliminary estimates of the prevalence of selected underlying health conditions among patients with coronavirus disease 2019 - United States, February 12-March 28, 2020. MMWR Morb Mortal Wkly Rep. 2020;69:382-6. [Links]

13. Wang D, Hu B, Hu C, Zhu F, Liu X, Zhang J, et al. Clinical characteristics of 138 hospitalized patients with 2019 novel coronavirus-infected pneumonia in Wuhan, China. JAMA. 2020;323:1061-9. [Links]

14. Du Y, Tu L, Zhu P, Mu M, Wang R, Yang P, et al. Clinical features of 85 fatal cases of COVID-19 from Wuhan: a retrospective observational study. Am J Respir Crit Care Med. 2020;201:1372-9. [Links]

15. Wang B, Li R, Lu Z, Huang Y. Does comorbidity increase the risk of patients with COVID-19: evidence from meta-analysis. Aging (Albany NY). 2020;12:6049-57. [Links]

16. Espinosa OA, Zanetti AS, Antunes EF, Longhi FG, Matos TA, Battaglini PF. Prevalence of comorbidities in patients and mortality cases affected by SARS-CoV2: a systematic review and metaanalysis. Rev Inst Med Trop Sao Paulo. 2020;62:e43. [Links]

17. Chatre C, Roubille F, Vernhet H, Jorgensen C, Pers YM. Cardiac complications attributed to chloroquine and hydroxychloroquine: a systematic review of the literature. Drug Saf. 2018;41:919-31. [Links]

18. Boulware DR, Pullen MF, Bangdiwala AS, Pastick KA, Lofgren SM, Okafor EC, et al. A randomized trial of hydroxychloroquine as postexposure prophylaxis for COVID-19. N Engl J Med. 2020 In Press. [Links]

Correspondence to: Omar Ariel Espinosa Faculdade do Pantanal, Av. São Luiz, 2522, CEP 78200-000, Cáceres, MT, Brazil Tel: +55 65 99999-5940 E-mail: omar.espinosa@fapan.edu.br

AFFILIATION

[1]Universidade do Estado de Mato Grosso, Faculdade de Ciências da Saúde, Departamento de Medicina, Cáceres, Mato Grosso, Brazil

[2]Universidade do Estado de Mato Grosso, Faculdade de Ciências da Saúde, Departamento de Enfermagem, Cáceres, Mato Grosso, Brazil

[3]Universidade do Estado de Mato Grosso, Faculdade de Ciências Agrárias e Biológicas, Programa de Pós-Graduação em Ciências Ambientais, Cáceres, Mato Grosso, Brazil

[4]Centro de Excelência do Instituto Joanna Briggs, Centro Brasileiro para o Cuidado à Saúde Informado por Evidências, São Paulo, São Paulo, Brazil

[5]Faculdade do Pantanal, Cáceres, Mato Grosso, Brazil

CHAPTER 12

SEXUAL BEHAVIOUR IN THE MIDST OF THE COVID-19

1. The Prostitute, the City, and the Virus

Dr. Soraya Simões
Associate Professor of Anthropology at IPPUR, UFRJ;

Dr. Thaddeus Blanchette
Associate Professor of Anthropology at PPGCiaC, UFRJ-Macaé;

Dr. Ana Paula da Silva
Adjunct Professor of Social Sciences at PCH at UFF- Santo Antônio de Pádua;

Dr. Laura Murray
Public Health specialist

ABSTRACT

The present article has two goals. First, it seeks to establish, for non-specialized readers, the history of what we label "hygenization" in Brazilian urban and health policies and their intersections with the sale of sex and the prevention of pandemic disease. Secondly, we want inform readers as to how the challenges of the COVID-19 pandemic are being met within the context of this history, particularly by Brazil's organized sex workers. By necessity and location, in this time of quarantine, our focus is on the city of Rio de Janeiro, which has historically provided an example for what has been called "the Brazilian model of urbanization". We begin our article with a brief overview of this model and then proceed to a historical look at two prior pandemics, how they were dealt with and, in particular, their intersections with sex work. We finish by analyzing what the COVID-19 pandemic may mean for sex workers in Brazil in light of the country's ambiguous public health traditions.

Introduction: Prostitution and Pandemics in Belindia

Brazil has been an odd case in global history since at least the beginning of the 20th Century. Simultaneously understood to be "western" and "non-western", it is a "puzzle" that exists on (or perhaps constitutes part of) the "borderland of the Western World" (DaMatta & Hess, 1985). Its Cold War nickname – Belindia (Belgium in the middle of India) – expresses this ambiguity well (O Estado de São Paulo, 2017), which hasn't been much altered by its recent identification as one of the BRIC nations. As political scientist Oliver Stuenkel points out, the country is, at most, a "partly Western" emerging power that continues to strongly identify with its "non-western, under developed side" (Stuenkel, 2011: 194).Stuenkel's qualification is particularly apt because it puts the finger upon the essential characteristic that makes a "Western" nation: more than cultural affinities, it is a question of wealth, power, and relative economic development. This is well reflected in the field work of one of the authors of the present article, who has interviewed many foreigners on this very topic (Blanchette: 2001).

"Gringos" often point to economics when defining Brazil as "the most Western of non-Western nations and the most non-Western of Western nations"[1].Whether or not Europe, Japan, China, and the U.S. consider Brazil to be "Western", however, the country has historically oriented itself, as best it can, towards the U.S. and Western Europe. However, "oriented" does not mean "blindly copy" or even "able to copy". Nowhere are the contradictions of "Belindia" more apparent than in the intersections between urban policy, public health, and prostitution[2], particularly in the city of Rio de Janeiro, historically the country's first metropolis and still Brazil's "post card to the world". The on-going COVID-19 pandemic has cast these contradictions into sharp relief. As a group of scholars and activists, centred in an Urban Policy Studies Institute in Rio de Janeiro and dedicated to ethnographic and historical research on sex work and public policy and collaborating with the organized sex worker movement in Brazil over the past 15 years, we are charting how these contradictions develop while helping sex workers to organize for survival and political power.

The present article is being written almost in "real time" as events unfold in Brazil. Every day, new information comes in or new policies are announced that supersede what was the state of affairs a few days earlier. As such, it is a necessarily preliminary look at the intersection between sex work, public health, urban policy in Brazil in syn- and diachronic terms.

The present article has two goals. First, we want to briefly establish for non-specialized readers the history of what we label "hygenization" in Brazilian urban and health policies and their intersections with the sale of sex; secondly, we want inform readers as to how the challenges of the COVID-19 pandemic are being met within the context of this history, particularly by Brazil's organized sex workers. By necessity and location, in this time of quarantine, our focus is on the city of Rio de Janeiro. However, it should be noted that Rio, Brazil's capital until 1960, has for most of the country's history been synonymous with its urban and public health policies and has thus formed the basis for what Brazilian urbanist Maurício de Abreu has described as a Brazilian model of urbanization (Abreu, 1987). We start our article with a brief overview of this model and then proceed to a historical look at two prior "plagues", how they were dealt with and, in particular, their intersections with sex work. We then analyse what the pandemic may mean for sex workers in Brazil in light of the country's ambiguous public health traditions. We conclude by looking at Brazilian sex worker mobilizations on-going in the face of COVID-19.

We want to remind readers that there is a history of struggle against stigma in the Brazilian prostitutes' movement (Lenz 2008) and a good part of this struggle was welcomed, supported and empowered by and through the field of public health, particularly in the late 20th century (Murray et al 2018). The very concept of *health* can expand during times of crisis, contemplating positive recognition as the essence of health, be it emotional, physical, or social. The *care of the self*, extensively historicized by Foucault (2005, 2006), returns as a debate under the demand that *care for oneself* implies *care for the other*. Under these conditions, one can think of both comfort (of a social position, of a house, or of the streets of a neighbourhood) and of social valourization expressed through the treatments experienced in the most diverse everyday situations.

---

[1] Quote taken from ethnographic fieldwork among Anglophone sex tourists in the Copacabana region of Rio de Janeiro.

[2] The terms "sex work" and "prostitution" will be used interchangeably in this article to refer to the commercial sale of physical sexual/affective acts. We do not include sex work such as phone sex, pornography, or camming in the definition used in the present article, but such things as erotic massage or being a "paid companion" (with a sexual relationship implied) are included.

However, Brazil's history also holds a darker lesson regarding public health and prostitution, one in which those who sell sex (particularly women) are understood to be especially contagious, potentially dangerous and needing to be controlled and contained (Carrara 1996). On this side of Belinida, prostitutes are lumped together with a (poor, black and brown) Brazilian majority understood to be an agency less mass, affectable, but not effective, which needs to be tutored and even occasionally violently pruned if the country is to reach its long-dreamt of goal of being an unqualified part of the West (Ferreira da Silva, 2007). Which Brazil will become dominant in the current pandemic is still an open question at the moment this article goes to the editor (April 29th, 2020)? Organized sex workers, however, a politically active and particularly stigmatized population that have historically occupied a strategic position in public health reactions to pandemic disease, are a group that should be carefully watched as the COVID-19 drama unfolds if we want an answer to this question.

Hygenization: Public Health and Social Distancing in Rio De Janeiro

Rio de Janeiro began its existence as a "European" city in the16th century, in a context of Great Power conflicts for control over the trade routes of the South Atlantic and, in particular, the African slave trade (Alencastro, 2000). During the colonial period, Rio's political economy revolved around two principal focuses: international trade and national/colonial administration. Historian Manolo Florentino emphasizes the city's relative lack of direct economic production, pointing out that, to keep the city supplied, Portuguese sugar merchants had to be ordered by the Portuguese king to stop off in Rio on their way to the more lucrative sugar colonies of the Brazilian northeast (Ibid).

Possessing one of the best natural harbours of the South Atlantic, however, Rio became increasingly important to international trade following the Brazilian gold rush of the 18th century. In 1763, it became the capital of the Portuguese Empire's "State of Brazil" and, finally, the capital of the Empire itself in 1808, as the Portuguese Court fled to the city to escape Napoleon Bonaparte's armies. Historians generally understand this moment as the foundational mark for modern Brazil (Malerba, 2000; Morel, 2016; Souza, 2000), emphasizing the simultaneous opening of the colony's ports to international trade, which transformed Rio into one of the principal cities of theSouth Atlantic and an almost obligatory stop-over for shipping heading around the Capes of Good Hope and Horn. As gold poured out of Rio (helping to finance the British industrial revolution, African slaves poured in and were distributed throughout the hinterlands of South America (Alencastro, 2000). The profits accumulated in this trade were partially spent on the importation of European luxury goods (whose traces were widely encountered by archaeologists during the urban renewal projects leading up to the 2014 World Cup and 2016 Olympic Games (Veja, 2013)). Rio became *the* "European" city of Brazil, a showcase for the nation and the world. This status only intensified with Brazil's transition to independence in 1822, when Rio became the capital of the new nation.

But at the base of this "Europeanization" lay slavery. And – unlike the case of Bristol in the U.K. or Boston in the U.S. – Rio could not hold this fact at a comfortable distance. Africans passed through its port daily. They were employed in every aspect of the city's economy. Their cultural and even political influence (at least in the realm of street politics) was enormous and at times appeared almost overwhelming. And what Gilberto Freyre would later label their "biological influence" could be seen in almost every Carioca[1] face. Black women – slave and free -- were particularly important

---

[1] "Carioca" is the adjective form for people and things from Rio de Janeiro.

in this context, given that the slave trade was overwhelmingly skewed to the importation of men and there were relatively few white women of any class (Freyre, 1933).

Slave brothels were an ubiquitous feature of 19th century Rio de Janeiro (Graham, 1991).

With the arrival of Abolition in Brazil in 1888 and the consequent overthrow of the Brazilian Empire a year later, the capital of the new Republic of the United States of Brazil began a prolonged period of urban crisis and renewal. (Abreu, 1987). To simplify a complex and nuanced situation, the problem was that Rio retained all the architectural and social baggage of a semi feudal slaveocratic metropolis when it wanted to be seen as a Paris of the tropics, a rival to Buenos Aires and Montevideo.. With the collapse of Brazilian agriculture brought on by the end of slavery, a wave of free black migration hit Rio, which did not possess an infrastructure capable of adequately housing, feeding, employing, or policing its new masses. At the same time, the Republic began to open Brazil to mass migration from Europe, believing that "whitening" the country's population would pave the way to establishing Brazil as a modern nation state along Western European line. Poor European immigrants also began to flood into the city (Schwarcz, 1993).Rio's impoverished masses were agglomerated in tenement slums, generally dilapidated buildings from the colonial period stitched together with ad hoc constructions into giant complexes known as *cortiços*.. These housed almost 25% of Rio's population in the last decade of the 19th century (Santucci, 1997). One *cortiço*, the infamous "Pig's Head" located in the port zone, reputably had over 4000 residents (Benchimol, 1990; Carvalho, 1990; Valladares, 2000).Prostitution was rife in the city, possibly due to the imbalance in the male-to-female ratio of the population and the general lack of work for the poorer strata of the population.

In fact, the sale of sex was understood to be so common among the female lower classes that the doctors and lawyers who investigated the city's "plague" of prostitution at the time qualified any independent female worker – flower saleswomen, washerwomen, actresses, kiosk clerks, etc. – as belonging to the ranks of "clandestine prostitutes"(Blanchette & Schettini, 2017; Engel, 1990).While much has been written about the relatively upper-class sex working women of this period, known as *francesas* (French women), relatively little is known about the vast majority of poor women and men who sold sex.The *cortiços*, however, were seen at the time as their universe, where they mixed in with *capoeiristas[1]*, dock workers, itinerant laborers, washing women, and other "disorderly bums" (Gazeta de Notícias, 5/21/1893, APUD Santucci, 2008). The *cortiços* were a world unto themselves, often directly opposed to State authority of any sort. As historian Jane Santucci describes them, they were:

to urban health. With the advent of the Republic, Brazil's first generation of urban planners began a protracted campaign to demolish them (and a significant portion of the old A territory that was closed to the police, who were prevented from entering even to resolve internal conflicts, such as fights between residents. On these occasions, as soon as they saw the police, the people immediately forgot their quarrels in order to unite and push out the authorities. These were fights in which everyone participated – men, women, and children – furiously attacking in defence of local autonomy. (Santucci, 2008: 58).As such, the *cortiços* were seen as both a physical and moral threat Rio) under the banner of urban sanitation and the struggle against the city's perennial smallpox and yellow fever epidemics (Cukierman,2007).

As many authors have pointed out (Santucci, 2008; Abreu, 1987; Chalhoub, 1996 Lowy, 2005) , this campaign cannot be understood simply in terms of physical improvements to the city, although it

---

[1] Practitioners of the Afro-Brazilian martial art of *capoeira*, criminalized during the period and long understood to be the reigning kings of the carioca streets and slave hierarchies (Santucci, 2008).

was always carefully wrapped in the rhetoric of defeating Rio's many epidemics. Using the term employed by its authors, this "hygenization" of Rio de Janeiro was as much social as physical and depended upon separating the "dangerous classes" (particularly the poor brown and black cariocas) from "proper citizens",envisioned as white and bourgeois. Thus, while the city's port district, Downtown and the neighbourhood of Lapa were lavishly made over according to Hausmannian models, little attention was paid tothe perennial urban housing crisis. *Cortiço* residents were pushed into the streets and, finally, up into the hills of Rio de Janeiro, founding the first of the *favela* slums that today garnish the city. In fact, the first hillside slum which would give the *favelas* their name[1], established on the Morro da Providência, literally sprang up in what was the back yard of the "Pigs Head", one of the first great *cortiços* to be demolished.

As Santucci documents, in the period stretching from 1890 to 1905, Rio was rocked by periodic revolts in the face of this "top down" urban renewal conducted in the name of physical and social health, culminating in the most famous rebellion of them all: the "Vaccine Revolt" of October November 1904. The spark which ignited 5 days of street fighting in the city and an abortive coup d'etat was the Republic's Mandatory Vaccination Law, which authorized the use of the police in order to forcibly vaccinate the population against smallpox. The revolt was swiftly crushed, and its results were ambiguous.

Mandatory vaccination was repealed, only to be reinstated five years later after a smallpox epidemic killed 9,000 cariocas (Meade, 1986; Needel, 1987). More importantly, following the revolt, hygenization picked up steam, culminating in the establishment of what urbanist Maurício de Abreu describes as the Brazilian model of urbanization. This can be characterized as a city divided into three parts: a wealthy centre and south zone; a suburbanized working class; with *favelas* and other "areas of exception" sprinkled throughout (Abreu, 1987). In truth, this model can be even further simplified – as Cariocas are wont to do – into the two antagonistic, socially distanced, and yet complimentary emic categories: *morro* (hill) and *asfalto* (asphalt). On the "asphalt", the municipal laws regarding planning, hygiene, fire control, and sanitation more-or-less apply, or at least are applicable. The "hill" (an allusion to favelas' traditional hilltop locations), however, is a world unto itself. Much like the old *cortiços*, police can only enter in well-armed bands and local authority overrules municipal law.

And although favelas are traditionally understood to be "hill", there are many other places and people in Rio de Janeiro which also occupy a similar position, most notoriously the demi-monde of sex work.In the decades following the Vaccine Revolt, prostitution became increasingly subject to police control in a model of non-regulated regulation. The earlier urban model in which sex work was more-or-less evenly distributed throughout the city was replaced by one in which prostitutes would have an official place; a quarantine zone. Dubbed "The Mangue", this was situated on the outskirts of town in a section of recently drained marshland. Most sex workers – particularly black, brown and poor white – were forcibly removed by police to the new district, which became synonymous with prostitution and was provided with its own venereal disease hospital (Simões,

---

[1] There are many conflicting stories about how this settlement came to be named "favela", but most trace it back to soldiers returning from the Canudos campaign, where the Republic brutally put down a messianic rebellion in the Brazilian northeast (Cunha, 1902). Supposedly, the veterans of this war were detained in Rio de Janeiro while awaiting the government to pay out their war bonuses (Santucci, 2008). Joining refugees from the urban hygenization campaign and dock workers, they founded the Morro da Providência colony, naming it after the hill upon which the Brazilian Army Headquarters and principal artillery batteries stood. It must be understood, in this context, that the Morro da Providência stands in relation to the then Ministry of War as the Morro da Favela stood in relation to the city of Canudos. "Favela" can thus be understood to imply a threat. This was not lost on reporters of the time, one of whom claimed that "following the Canudos War, the most daring delinquents began to inhabit the top of the hill, calling it Favela, because in that redoubt no police could enter without being defeated" (Gazeta de Notícias, 5/21/1903, APUD Santucci, 2008: 58).

2010; Caulfield, 2000; Leite, 2005; Moraes, 2006). Meanwhile, brothels catering to the elite were allowed to continue to operate in the now Bohemian districts of Lapa and Glória.

In both cases, however, prostitution was subject to an official, unwritten set of laws, codified in judicial decisions and in police power. Legally, houses of prostitution were prohibited under Brazilian law. "Women's boarding houses", however, were allowed if their owners were female, they paid a licensing fee to the city, and registered all boarders with the police and public health authorities (with obligatory gynaecological exams).

Thus, in both the Mangue and elsewhere, Rio de Janeiro created a form of French-style regulated prostitution without ever formally legalizing brothels. Police were ultimately the "pimps" in this scheme as they were the authorities who had the real power to say where, when, and how the sale of sex could take place. Licensing fees – as well as numerous bribes and "tips" for extra service – went directly into the force's pocket, culminating in the establishment of a police precinct specialized in overseeing "Popular Parties and Entertainments" which, in effect, administered sex work in Rio de Janeiro (Blanchette & Schettini, 2017; Blanchette, Mitchell & Murray, 2015; Chaumont, et al, 2017; Engel. 1990; Leite, 2005). This model of sex work organization would, mutandis mutatis, continue in operation for most of the 20th century and is arguably functioning even today. While the days of "boarding houses" being officially overseen by the police are long gone, the authors' fieldwork, carried out over the last two decades, has made it clear that police and other carioca authorities are still "silent partners" in almost all of our city's commercial sex venues. The overriding objective of this model has been one of both physical and moral quarantine and "social distancing", with sex work portrayed as an integral part of the urban landscape (Saint Augustine and Aquinas'proverbial "necessary sewer under the palace" (Richards, 1991: 118)), but also a "zone of exception" in terms of laws and morality, which needed to be kept under firm police control and set apart from the bourgeois world of family and propriety.

Sueann Caulfield points out (Caulfield, 2000) and our present day ethnographic work confirms that this "corralling" of prostitution has never been wholly successful. In fact, as Blanchette & Schettini remark (2017), no region in which prostitution has ever established itself in Carioca history has ever been made "family safe" again. Even in the 21st century, one of the main downtown "strolls" is located precisely where early 19th century Rio had its principal slave brothels, right between two of the city's most famous parks and its largest popular commercial district. Anthropologist Soraya Simões has described how the Mangue never fulfilled its role as Rio's only red light district and how later attempts to shut it down only resulted in its migration and transformation into today's Vila Mimosa, Rio's largest concentration of commercial sex venues (Simões, 2010).But for most of the past century, sex work in Rio de Janeiro has continued operating under the control of the police, either directly or indirectly (Blanchette, Mitchell , & Murray, 2015), being largely restricted to certain areas. This paradigm began to change, however, with two simultaneous events in the 1980s: the end of the Brazilian military dictatorship and the explosion of the AIDS/HIV crisis, as part of processes that Jeffery Weeks has referred to as a balancing between "reform and control" or "reform as a means of control" (Weeks 2012:2010).

AIDS and the Brazilian Prostitutes' Movement

The beginning of the AIDS epidemic was characterized by widespread fear and blame constructed and spread by scientific and media discourses that in turn shaped the ways in which government and civil society responses to the epidemic took shape (Triechler 1987). As a virus transmitted by blood, semen and vaginal secretions, it quickly became associated with certain subjects, who, alongside with their practices, were classified as "dangerous" and "risk groups"; that is, those who were members of populations considered to be the most exposed to the risk of HIV infection. The criterion most employed to define "at risk groups" was that these fell outside of a certain norm (heteronormativity, to be precise).

As was the case around the world, in Brazil the government responded slowly to the urgency of the epidemic. The country's first case of AIDS was reported in 1982 and rapidly transformed the country's political, sexual and public health landscapes. Civil society mobilization around the HIV epidemic began alongside a much larger and powerful sanitary reform movement that was key in push to establish health as a universal right in the country's 1988 democratic constitution (Daniel and Parker 1991;Parker, 2003). At first, the federal government's lack of response to the first cases of AIDS contrasted with civil society mobilizations, particularly in São Paulo, not only the site of the most reported AIDS cases as compared to any other city, but also the centre of Brazil's recent gay liberation movement and opposition to the dictatorship (Teixeira, 1997;Parker, 2003) and the first documented sex worker mobilization against police violence in 1979.

When the epidemic first emerged, it was primarily concentrated among men who have sex with men (MSM) and intravenous drug users (IDUs) (Barbosa Jr., 2009), yet by 1987, sex workers were also fighting the stigma of having been identified as one of the primary "risk groups". They would come to occupy a critical political and cultural position at the beginning of the Brazilian epidemic. On the one had, they were still understood to be subjects of sanitary control and intervention.

On the other, however, sex workers became fierce public critics of the deadly consequences of epidemic research and prevention models cantered upon stigmatizing and shaming populations (de Zalduondo, 1991).

One sex worker in particular, Gabriela Leite, who had led protests against police violence in São Paulo in 1979 and had worked in Vila Mimosa (the successor of Rio's Mangue), would come to occupy a central role in the defining the country's response to the epidemic.In the late 1980s, Gabriela was working at the Institute for Religious Studies (ISER), leading a project called, "Prostitution and Civil Rights."She was invited to Brazil's capital, Brasilia to discuss a national HIV prevention project – PREVINA – with sex workers, prisoners and drug users.

Many people from the sanitary reform movement had taken jobs within the Ministry of Health during the redemocratization process, and as such, despite initial missteps and silences in the mid-1980s, by 1988 were directly engaging with civil society.

The previous, "traditional" model of public health promulgated under hygenization, saw the "unfavoured" masses as agency less human objects upon which unilateral action could be taken, eroded as part of the broader process of constructing Brazil's Universal Health Care System (SUS). Despite a climate of broad civil society mobilization and the emerging sex worker movement, however, the original project design of PREVINA presented a conservative and morally charged vision of prostitution (typical of the broad Brazilian political Left at the time), associating it with exploitation and suffering (Murray et al 2018). In this way it was remarkably similar to the discourses surrounding prostitution at the turn of the twentieth century, employed by earlier generations of urban hygenizers in that it linked prostitution to poverty and the sexual exploitation of minors.

The direction of the project drastically changed , however, with the involvement of Gabriela Leite and Lourdes Barreto, a leader of the sex worker movement from the North-eastern state of Pará. These women co-organized a national meeting of sex workers in 1987. Though not the focus of the event, AIDS prominently figured in its discussions, focusing in particular on sex workers' resistance to the "risk group" category. As Enir Gonçalvez, one of the sex workers at the 1987 meeting was quoted as saying, "Enough of talking about us as a risk group!

We use condoms. I am a woman of the life [referring to prostitution] and a human being like any other. I deserve respect" (Jornal do Brasil 1987).

Sex worker criticisms contemplated not only their occupation as part of a larger universe of jobs (looking at what working conditions were capable of promoting preventive practices and prevent various types of abuse) but, above all, a necessary recognition that prostitution, as a stigmatized behaviour, should be interpreted as *work* and, therefore, be *respected*.

Two years later, at another national meeting focused on "AIDS and Prostitution", sex workers rebelled against the exclusivity of medical specialists discourse. In the *Beijo da Rua* (a sex worker newspaper) article about the event, Gabriela Leite stated that she "felt that people were distant from everything and that the doctors were, of course, involved in a debate with themselves. So the next morning, I came back in a low cut black dress, high heels, exaggerated make-up and I talked about my life" (Lenz, 1990:4). Gabriela's intervention reversed more than the meeting's dynamic: it set the tone for a partnership with the Ministry of Health that respected the protagonist role of sex workers, crafting a public policy response that placed sexuality, pleasure, and respect for sex work at the centre of the sanitationist discourse cast in Caroica emic terms, the *morro* and the *asfalto* had met and the "doctors" of the asphalt had conceded that, not only could they learn from the "whores" of the hill, an equal partnership needed to be established between the two groups in order to effectively combat HIV.

As part of this process, adapting to both national and international pressures from a variety of social movements and AIDS researchers, the Brazilian Ministry of Health adopted the concept of *vulnerability,* eschewing the concept of *risk groups*, which became less and less relevant in the plans to contain the epidemic. First developed in the context of HIV research by Jonathan Mann, and expanded upon by Brazilian researchers (Mann et al. 1993; Paiva et al. 2012) vulnerability provided a framework for politicizing the epidemic and including citizenship as a core component of HIV prevention. *Vulnerability* made it possible to better see, and therefore intervene, in the social and cultural contexts in which vulnerable subjects were inserted. Foundational concepts of the early organizing of around the epidemic (Daniel and Parker 1991; de Souza 1994), "solidarity" and "mobilization" came to be understood as central parts of the government response. Individual, collective, programmatic, structural, and institutional vulnerabilities were highlighted in State interventions and research, and all forms of discrimination that "vulnerable" groups were subjected to started to be treated as an integral part of the response (Parker, 2003; Paiva et al 2012). Many new frameworks for addressing the epidemic were forged and new "worldviews" created a process that seems to occur on extreme occasions (such as our present COVID 19 crisis) when the unknown manifests itself as a *trickster* or a *ghost in the machine* .

Over the following two decades, social movements would continue to make decisive contributions to the struggle against HIV. The virus itself forced a reorientation of politics, moving away from being a "gay disease" as the international media first called it, and becoming increasingly seen as something that also affected children, mothers, and fathers. The Brazilian family's sexuality was exposed to public scrutiny and it was found that, in practice,

it necessarily so different from that of the so-called *vulnerable groups*. Apparently, the *asfalto* wasn't so far removed from the *morro* in its sexual and moral habits, a finding that overturned the hygenizationist presumptions of the previous century's public health policies.

City, work, gender, sexuality, and stigma were thus brought together in one package, re-situating the debate on HIV/AIDS prevention in Brazil, a country which came to be seen as a global example of best practices in its combat and treatment of HIV/AIDS, thanks to its mobilization of society and, in particular, the members of so-called "risk groups."

The sex worker movement continued to be a foundational component of the country's HIV/AIDS response, strategically leveraging aspects of "puta subjectivity" in Brazil to mobilize allies, media attention and State power in favour of prostitute rights. Referred to as "puta politics" by Murray (2015), this is a form of politics invested in the transformative potential of what is often perceived of as immorality. Constantly disrupting and blurring divisions between "asphalt" institutional structures and the realities of the populations occupying the streets and hills, puta politics did, on a national level, what Gabriela Leite had done at the first AIDS and Prostitution meeting when she showed up in her low cut dress and demanded to be heard. Important gains were made such as the inclusion of "sex professional" in the Brazilian Ministry of Labour and Employment's Classification of Occupations in 2002 (Simões, 2010b). Brazil also achieved widespread international attention when it refused more than $40 million in US funds because USAID, the US's development arm, demanded that organizations receiving said funds condemn prostitution as a precondition.

Reaction and Retrenchment

Over the past 10 years however, Brazil's leadership in the AIDS response and, in particular, its solidarity and community mobilization based approaches to health have slowly begun to fade. This has been due to many complex and overlapping factors, yet two in particular stand out and have been highlighted by activists and scholars (Seffner and Parker 2016; Correa 2016; Malta 2013). .First, the aggressive neoliberalization of Brazil's economy that began in the 1990s has continued with increasing force while the country is confronting one of its worst economic crisis in decades. This has resulted in a decrease of federal investment in public health overall and changes in the ways in which the HIV/AIDS program was funded, which subsequently meant less funding for the program and for the NGOs that were at the forefront of the Brazil's social response to the epidemic (Seffner and Parker 2016). A second factor has been the increased moralization of all aspects of politics, as conservative and evangelical religious forces in Brazil have gained power, pressuring the leftist Workers' Party government to censor HIV prevention campaigns for gays in 2012 and sex workers in 2013 (ABIA and Davida 2013; Murray et al 2018).Without projects, many sex worker organizations also drastically reduced their actions and, consequently, reach. These processes culminated in the election of far-right president Jair Bolsonaro in 2018, but sex workers were some of the first groups to feel the pressure of both gentrification and police repression even under the previous Workers' Party government (Amar 2013, Blanchette et al, 2014).

Aside from an increase in police violence directed at sex workers, there have been numerous small, but symbolic changes such as removing the word *puta* from the CBO (ABIA & Davida, 2013). As Paul Amar (2013) notes, however, the conservative moralities now flexing their political muscle in Brazil are deeply ingrained in both police and paramilitary forces, which have also been intimately tied to the gentrification efforts we have been investigating in prostitution areas in Rio since 2005. In many ways, what we see here is a re-emergence of the racialist, sexist, and classist values and structures that drove urban hygenization and social distancing in the years of the early Republic – not surprising, given that President Jair Bolsonaro much admires the second President of the Republic, authoritarian Marshal Floriano Peixoto, a man who inaugurated the period of late 19th century violent repression described above (Topik, 1996).

Amar draws many parallels between post-liberal urbanization and development in Brazil and Egypt, which should also be read in the light of human rights analyst Scott Long's extensive discussions of the engendered and ethnic/racial dimensions of Egypt's authoritarian turn .

In essence, what Bolsonarismo represents is a return to the "social distancing" of top-down driven development and sanitation that sees the majority of Brazilians not as citizens partners, but as a problem to be managed violently, if necessary.

Nowhere has this been more clearly demonstrated than in Bolsonaro's March 26th speech to the nation, where he claimed that Brazilians have an in-built resistance to COVID-19 because "they play in sewers" (Gomes, 2020). Obviously, Bolsonaro does not see himself as "playing in sewers" and yet he speaks of this as a defining characteristic of "Brazilians", who are simultaneously cast as unclean, perversely immune to the new coronavirus, and consequently not needing any special treatment or policies in the face of the epidemic. One needs to ask: which Brazilians is the President imagining here? In Rio de Janeiro, one of Bolsonaro's principal allies, Congressman Rodrigo Amorim, is demonstrating who is being contemplated and how they should be dealt with. Brought into power on the same conservative wave that elected Bolsonaro, Amorim made a name for himself during the election by publicly destroying a street sign that paid homage to black and LGBT city councilwoman, Marielle Franco. (Fig. 4) Franco had been politically assassinated in early 2018 and the probable murderers are reported as having intimate ties to the Bolsonaro family and to Amorim himself (Lourenço, 2020).

The sign had taken the place of an earlier sign giving homage to Marshal Floriano Peixoto and (Dimenstien, 2019) and the remains of the sign paying tribute to Marielle have been mounted on Congressman Amorim's office wall as a trophy. Amorim has taken a particular interest in the São Cristovão neighbourhood of Rio de Janeiro, which has long been marked for urban renewal (Costa, 2013; Extra, 2011). Shortly following his inauguration, the state congressman launched an unauthorized invasion of the Maracanã Indian Village, an urban occupation conducted by Native Brazilians in the neighbourhood. After calling the Village "urban trash" and saying that "those who like Indians should go to Bolivia" (in a clear allusion to the on-going racist coup against Bolivia's Native President Evo Morales), Amorim invaded the Village in a surprise "inspection" (Capelli, 1/2019; 3/2019). A few months later, Amorim conducted an unauthorized invasion of Pedro II high school, one of Brazil's oldest and most prestigious learning institutions and a cornerstone of São Cristovão, alleging that the school was a factory for "leftist militants" (Werneck, Leal, & Rodrigues, 2019).

Amorim's greatest impact on Rio's new frontier of urban cleansing, however, has come through his leadership of the State Parliamentary Inquiry Commission into fires and firefighting. Following a disastrous series of blazes (one of which, coincidentally, razed Brazil's national Museum, located in São Cristovão, and another a downtown brothel), this commission was detailed to "clean up" Rio de Janeiro. Echoing the forced sanitation campaigns of the early 20th century, Amorim's Commission has emphasized actions against racialized and engendered "areas of exception", and his largest target to date is Vila Mimosa, the red light district descended from the old Mangue, which lies in the heart of São Cristovão. In December 2019, when COVID-19 was still a distant threat for most Cariocas, firemen under the direction of Amorim's Commission, shut down the Vila, putting some 4000 sex workers out of work. The alleged reasons for VM's closing were that it was both a fire and health threat (although the city had ignored the conditions in the Vila for three decades). For weeks on end, many prostitutes had to suspend their activities, feeling the same economic fragility that today afflicts billions of people around the world. Leadership from the Vila Mimosa's community association were able to pressure Amorim to hold a public hearing about the situation with representation from the state legislature, fire fighters and interested parties from the Vila on March 13th, 2020. The hearing opened with Amorim showing a series of photographs from his report, including everything from the precarious and illegal electrical wiring systems to the cubicles where sex workers attend to clients (which he narrated as, "I know it isn't the focus of this investigation, but look at the level of human degradation of this place"). Images of condoms on the floor, narrow hallways and food left out at one of the kilo restaurants were used as further evidence of what he referred to as the "inhuman" and "grotesque" nature of the Vila Mimosa. Despite the stigmatizing nature of the presentation (and his insistence that his goal was to dignify, not denigrate, when later questioned), the hearing ended with a decision that pending approval of their superiors, the fire department would sign a temporary order to reopen the Vila the following Friday while they resolved the more expensive electrical wiring renovations. The mood was thus hopeful as the hot pink coloured bus that had taken dozens of women to the State Assembly to witness the hearing returned to Vila Mimosa with everyone eager to get back to work. On that same day, however, much of Rio de Janeiro was already starting to close down due to of the new coronavirus and the on the day that the Vila had planned to re-open, it too shut down many of its houses as part of the state-wide lockdown that is still in place as we write this piece.

CONCLUSIONS

As sex workers have arguably been targets of the moral and economic forces currently overtaking Brazil longer than many other groups, they find themselves today, confronting the COVID-19 epidemic from an especially precarious place, both from the perspective of the institutional fragilities of the organized movement and the ambiguous nature of sex work as an occupation in Brazil. In this sense, the COVID-19 pandemic sheds new light on this distressing collective experience through a nostalgia for the times of formulation of public health policies with integrated the effective participation of social movements. It also calls up fears of what can happen when critical populations are left out of State responses or indeed are they themselves targeted as groups which must be eliminated for the greater good.

The coronavirus epidemic helps us to review past Brazilian political responses to epidemic and endemic disease and to think about the collective sentiments regarding the importance of a public health system and the end of health inequalities. Critical moments such as the present favour the recognition of what can and should be fundamental and universal. We are again immersed in a distressing collective experience, on a global scale, and the procedures for identifying a disease, its forms of contagion and its origins open a wide field for *subjects* to also be identified and recognized as a *major* part of the transmission chain. In the case of COVID-19, some examples of this process of subjectification have already occurred, all of them containing racist and xenophobic aspects, as often happens when human collectivises search of the origin of "evil". As we've shown above, even before the new virus hit, sex workers, Native Brazilians, and "communist" youth were already being recast by the governing party in Rio de Janeiro as "trash" and threats to both moral and physical health in terms that frankly (and apparently consciously) recover the ideological content of the city's early 20th century hygenization campaigns. The new coronavirus, with its so far unbeatable capacity for propagation, outlined an overwhelming social imaginary. The "risk group" the elderly are our grandfathers and grandmothers, fathers, mothers, uncles and aunts. The virus necessarily reminds one of the family -a type of family that in no way refers to those affinities that are constituted by those who have been cast out by or on the run from their birth families. In all of this, there is an oppression that sustains a certain organization of the city as well, marked by mores that, although very contested, remain in force, operating various forms of oppression. Red light districts, hotels, motels, bars, clubs, spas, roadside gas stations, beaches... Prostitution presents itself where the people are and where the people go. It even creates *deviations,* drawing people away from the "normal".

The COVID-19 pandemic and the controversies surrounding the resulting lockdown have diluted cities, emptying their streets and eliminating or greatly reducing the activities that take place in them. Those who depend on the living, populated street have had to resort to local ties more than ever before while waiting for action from the same State that, in recent years has been dismantling of social safety nets, labour rights, and the SUS. As at the beginning of the HIV / AIDS epidemic, COVID-19 shows the weaknesses and prejudices of state structures, especially with regards for the care of the elderly and informal workers including sex workers. And as during the sanitation battles of the early 20th century, sex workers have used their political savvy cultivated through decades of responding to the HIV epidemic to mobilize local networks of power and influence, bridging once again the *morro* e *asfalto* together .Social Assistance Secretariats are on duty to register homeless people, the LGBT population, sex workers and refugees.

In Paraíba and Rio Grande do Norte, APROS-PB, APROS-RN, APRO CE (Association of Prostitutes of Paraíba, Rio Grande do Norte and Ceará), APPS (the Pernambucan Association of Sex Professionals) are encouraging women to register as "sex workers" so that, with this, a number of workers are "officially" produced in the records. Currently, the profession is quite invisible in statistical terms. While there are many organizations doing admirable work to read out to and aid Brazilian sex workers in the current pandemic, exemplary of this dynamic is CasaNem in Rio de Janeiro. In Copacabana, CasaNem, a squat organized by trans sex workers that now occupies a seven-storey building on Rua Dias da Rocha, continued to welcome residents and collaborators. Affiliated with the Internationalist Front of the Homeless (FIST), CasaNem collectively organized a series of measures to guarantee the functioning of the building in times of coronavirus.

One floor of the building has been set aside for those who need to be quarantined. The others inhabited by everyone else, conducting social isolation in the building. The collective kitchen works on a rotating basis and, according to Indian are Siqueira, creator of CasaNem, everyone must clean their hands with alcohol gel (distributed by volunteers) in order to enter the building. CasaNem serves 147 people with 65 are residing in the building, in Copacabana, in social isolation. A number of online collaborations have earmarked resources for the inhabitants. Among these, FIST has organized a WhatsApp list releasing information regarding the distribution of supplies to LGBTQI+ host houses and to supply prostitutes who work in rooms in commercial buildings, bars, hotels, brothels, nightclubs, cabarets, squares, and streets across the country. Ironically, CasaNem's squat currently occupies a building that was built by and housed one of the few "old money" families that actively resisted the forced vaccination campaigns that lead to the Vaccine Revolt of 1904.

Meanwhile, in the Centre, the region of Rio de Janeiro with the highest concentration of sexual commerce in the city of, all the dozens of spas, *fast fodas*, *relaxs*, nightclubs and massage parlours in the region have been closed since March 23rd. There is also no street commerce in places like the Praça da República. However, there is still a small amount of movement around the Central do Brasil rail station, where prostitutes – particularly older ones, who do not have other resources -- look for clients among the already reduced flow of workers that come and go via the suburban trains. The vast majority of these sex workers are not politically organized and have been largely abandoned by the Ministry of Health in the last years of the Workers' Party government. Any health-related outreach among them directed at COVID-19 will thus have to begin from zero.

The Brazilian Network of Prostitutes, which brings together sex worker associations based in cities in all regions of the country, is attempting to create a campaign to analyse Brazil's precarious occupations and the gender of those who perform this sort of work. Manicurists, depilators and other workers who deal with body care services have been able to get help directly from some of their clients. In the case of prostitutes, the same sort of solidarity is rare. Lourdes Barreto of GEMPAC (in the northern Brazilian state of Pará), one of the founders of the Brazilian Network of Prostitutes interprets this as a change in prostitution itself. The migration from street corners to the digital environment has affected various forms of sociability in the cities and, with this, has hindered the establishment of more or less durable bonds marked by relationships of trust. According to Lourdes, a part of the women receive help from their clients to pay bills or buy domestic supplies, but these days, this is an exception in the relations established in prostitution.

Currently, the COVID-19 pandemic has thrown Brazil into a unique balancing act that is highlighted by its past history of dealing with pandemics, particularly among urban and marginalized populations such as men and women who sell sex.

The division between the "asphalt" and the "hill" in Rio de Janeiro – which can also be glossed as rich versus poor and white versus black – is the Carioca representation of Brazil's more global ambiguous positioning on the "frontier of the West". But as anthropologist Gilberto Freyre once pointed out in his classic work *The Masters and the Slaves*, Brazil really only exists where these two polarities must deal with each other and work out some form of modus vivendi. The past has shown us that the "asphalt" is fully capable of treating large sections of their fellow citizenry –particularly those who are most heavily stigmatized, such as poor black sex workers – as, essentially, expendable – less than animals, really. Sacrifices to be made in the name of a national "whitening" process that is both simultaneously physical and moral.

At the same time, however, the past shows us what can be done when the "asphalt" listens to the "hills" and sits down at the same table with them, as partners, to forge creative responses to pandemic disease. The current political moment in Brazil is very dark and many of the actors who were responsible for the HIV/AIDS policies of the late 20th century are now dead, retired, it side-lined by a government that is frank in its portrayal of certain Brazilian populations as unnecessary and even eliminable *en masse*. Sex worker organizations across Rio and, particularly in Rio de Janeiro, have begun a flurry of local organization in the face of the existential threat posed by the combination of COVID-19 and quasi-fascist authoritarian government. These actors, however, have been greatly weakened by the past decade's retrenchment in human rights, public health, and social responsibility – of which sex workers were one of the first groups to be thrown under the bus.

What will happen in the upcoming months is not clear. The pandemic has weakened the Bolsonaro government even as it has thrown Brazilian sex workers to the brink of physical extinction. Nonetheless, we take comfort (however small) in Brazil's rich past of subaltern insurrection, often protaganized and even led by sex workers. Whether we are on the brink of another hopeless revolt against genocidal hygenization, or the dawn of a new era of rapprochement between the "asphalt" and the "hills", we can be sure that Brazilian sex workers will be leading change from the front.

Emails:
Soraya Silveira Simões sosimoes01@gmail.com

REFERENCES

Abia & Davida. (2013) Analysis of Prostitution Contexts In Terms Of Human Rights, Work, Culture, And Health In Brazilian Cities.. Rio De Janeiro: Abiu. .

Abreu, Maurício De. A Evolução(1987) Urbana Do Rio De Janeiro. Rio De Janeiro: Iplanrio; Zahar,

Alencastro, Luiz Felipe De. O Trato Dos Viventes. A Formação Do Brasil No Atlântico Sul. São Paulo, Companhia Das Letras, 2000.

Amar, P. (2013).The Security Archipelago: Human-Security States, Sexuality Politics, And The End Of Neoliberalism. Durham: Duke University Press.

Bachelard, G. (1996). A Formação Do Espírito Científico: Contribuição Para Uma Psicanálise Do Conhecimento. Rio De Janeiro: Contraponto, 1996.

Barbosa Jr., Aristides, et al. (2009)."Trends In The Aids Epidemic In Groups At Highest Risk In Brazil, 1980-2004". Cadernos De Saúde Pública 25(4). 2009. Pp.727-737.

Benchimol, Jaime L. Pereira Passos; Um Haussmann (1990). Tropical. A Renovação Urbana Do Rio De Janeiro No Início Do Século Xx. Rio De Janeiro: Biblioteca Carioca V. 11, 1990.

Blanchette, Thaddeus. Gringos. Masters Thesis In Social Anthropology, Defended In 2001 At Ppgas, Mn, Ufrj, Rio De Janeiro.

Blanchette, T.G; Mitchell, G.; Murray, L. (2015)"Discretionary Policing, Or The Lesser Part Of Valor: Prostitution, Law Enforcement, And Unregulated Regulation In Rio De Janeiro's Sexual Economy". Criminal Justice And Law Enforcement Annual: Global Perspectives. V.7. 2015.

Blanchette, T.G.; Schettini, C. (2017) "Sex Work In Rio De Janeiro: Police Management Without Regulation". In: Garcia, M.R., Van Voss L.H, Van Nederveen Meerkerk, E. Orgs. Sex Sold In World Cities: 1600s-2000s. Leiden, The Netherlands: Brill. 2017.

Blanchette, T.G.; Silva, A.P.; Ruvolo, J.; Murray, Laura Rebecca. "A Orgia Que Não Aconteceu: A Copa Do Mundo Fifa (2014) E O Comércio Do Sexo No Rio De Janeiro". In: Conrado, M.P.; Bernardo, C .C.; Santos, R.M.P.; Silva, M.P.. (Org.). Prostituição, Tráfico E Exploração Sexual De Crianças: Diálogo Multidisciplinar.Lisboa: Editora Vewstnik. 2104. P. 98-130.

Capelli, Paulo. "'Aldeia Maracanã É Lixo Urbano. Quem Gosta De Índio, Vá Para A Bolívia', Diz Rodrigo Amorim", O Globo, 01/04/2019. Accessed On 04/26/2020 At Https://Oglobo.Globo.Com/Rio/Visita-Surpresa-De-Deputado-Rodrigo-Amorim-Aldeiamaracana-Acaba-Em-Confusao-23545971

Capelli, Paulo. "'Visita Surpresa De Deputado Rodrigo Amorim À Aldeia Maracanã Acaba Em Confusão", O Globo, 03/23/2019. Accessed On 04/26/2020 At Https://Oglobo.Globo.Com/Rio/Visita-Surpresa-De-Deputado-Rodrigo-Amorim-Aldeiamaracana-Acaba-Em-Confusao-23545971

Carrara, Sérgio. Tributo A Vênus: (1996) A Luta Contra A Sífilis No Brasil, Da Passagem Do Século Aos Anos 40. Rio De Janeiro: Fiocruz,

Carvalho, José Murilo. Os Bestializados (1987) – O Rio De Janeiro E A República Que Não Foi. Rj: Companhia Das Letras.

____. A Formação Das Almas: O Imaginário Da República No Brasil. Rj: Companhia Das Letras, 1990.

Caulfield, Sueann. "O Nascimento Do Mangue: Raça, Nação E Controle Da Prostituição No Rio De Janeiro, 1850-1942", Tempo, 9. 2000.

Chalhoub, Sidney. Cidade Febril: Cortiços E Epidemias Na Corte Imperial. Rio De Janeiro: Companhia Das Letras, 1996.

Chaumont, J.M.; García, M.R.; Servais, P. Trafficking In Women 1924-1926 - The Paul Mckinsie Reports For The League Of Nations. Vienna: United Nations.

Corrêa, S. O."The Brazilian Response To Hiv And Aids In Troubled And Uncertain Times". In: A. Basthi, R. Parker & V. Terto Júnior (Eds.), Myth V Reality: Evaluating The Brazilian Response To Hiv In 2016. Rio De Janeiro: Brazilian Interdisciplinary Aids Association - Abia - Global Aids Policy Watch. 2016.

Costa, Célia. "Bairro Imperial, São Cristovão Espera Novos Tempos". O Globo, 11/20/2013. Accessed On 26/04/2020 At Https://Oglobo.Globo.Com/Rio/Bairro-Imperial-Sao-Cristovaoespera-Novos-Tempos-De-Gloria-10741355.

Cunha, Euclides. Cunha, (2007) Rebellion In The Backlands. University Of Chicago Press, 1957 (1902).

Cukierman, Henrique. Yes, Nós Temos Pasteur. Rio De Janeiro: Editora Relume Dumará /
Faperj.

Daniel, Herbert, And Parker, Richard. (1991) Aids: A Terceira Epidemia (Ensaios E Tentativas).
São Paulo: Iglu.

Da Matta & Hess, Eds. The Brazilian Puzzle: (1995) Culture On The Borderlands Of The Western World. New York:
Columbia University Press.

Dimenstein, Gilberto. "Instagram Mostra Suspeita Amizade Do Destruidor Da Placa Marielle". Catraca Livre,
02/08/2019. Accessed On 04/26/2020 At
Https://Catracalivre.Com.Br/Dimenstein/Instagram-Mostra-Suspeita-Amizade-Dodestruidor-Da-Placa-Marielle/.

Engel, Magalí. Meretrizes E Doutores: O Saber Médico E A Prostituição (1990) Na Cidade Do Rio De Janeiro, 1845-
1890. São Paulo.

Extra. "Vila Mimosa Pode Estar Com Os Dias Contados Para Construção Do Trem-Bala, Ligando O Rio A São Paulo".
Extra, 06/01/2011. Acessed On 04/26/2020 At
Https://Extra.Globo.Com/Noticias/Rio/Vila-Mimosa-Pode-Estar-Com-Os-Dias-Contados-Paraconstrucao-Do-Trem-
Bala-Ligando-Rio-Sao-Paulo-1933760.Html

Ferreira Da Silva, Denise. Towards(2007)A Global Idea Of Race. Minneapolis: University Of Minnesota Press..

Foucault, Michel (2005). História Da Sexualidade Iii. São Paulo: Graal.

_____. A Hermenêutica Do Sujeito. São Paulo: Martins Fontes, 2006

Freyre, Gilberto. Casa Grande E Senzala. Rdj: Record. 1994 (1933)

Gomes, Pedro Henrique. "Brasileiro Pula Em Esgoto E Acontece Nada, Diz Bolsonaro Em Alusão A Infecção Pelo
Coronavírus". T.V. Globo, 03/26/2020. Accessed On 04/26/2020 At
Https://G1.Globo.Com/Politica/Noticia/2020/03/26/Brasileiro-Pula-Em-Esgoto-E-Naoacontece-Nada-Diz-
Bolsonaro-Em-Alusao-A-Infeccao-Pelo-Coronavirus.Ghtml.

Graham, S.L. (1991) "Slavery's Impasse: Slave Prostitutes, Small-Time Mistresses, And The Brazilian Law Of 1871".
Comparative Studies In Society And History,Vol. 33, No. 4. Pp.
669-694

Leite, Juçara Luzia. República Do Mangue: Controle Policial E Prostituição No Rio De Janeiro (1954-1974). São Paulo:
Yendis, 2005.

Lenz, Flavio. Daspu: (2008) A Moda Sem Vergonha. Rio De Janeiro: Aeroplano.

Lenz, Flavio. Beijo (1990) Da Rua. Rio De Janeiro.

Lourenço, Cleber. "Revelação Do Intercept Coloca Família Bolsonaro No Caso Marielle
(Novamente)." Revista Fórum, 04/25/2020. Accessed On 04/26/2020 At
Https://Revistaforum.Com.Br/Blogs/Ocolunista/Revelacao-Do-Intercept-Coloca-Familiabolsonaro-No-Caso-Marielle-
Novamente/.

Lowy, Ilana.(2005) Vírus, Mosquitos E Modernidade: A Febre Amarela No Brasil – Entre Ciência E
Política. Rio De Janeiro: Fiocruz.

Malta, M And Breyner, C. (2013) The Hiv Epidemic And Human Rights Violations In Brazil. Jias. 16(1).

Mann, Jonathan; Tarantola, Daniel; And Netter, T.W., Eds. Aids No Mundo. Rio De
Janeiro: Relume Dumará. 1993

Meade, Teresa. (1986) "'Civilizing Rio De Janeiro': The Public Health Campaign And The Riot Of 1904". Journal Of
Social History. 20 (2).

Malerba, Jurandir. (2000) A Corte No Exílio – Civilização E Poder No Brasil Às Vésperas Da Independência (1808-
1821). Rio De Janeiro: Companhia Das Letras.

Moraes, Aparecida Fonseca. Mulheres Da Vila. Petrópolis: Vozes, 2006.

Morel, Marco. As Transformações Dos Espaços Públicos: Imprensa, Atores Políticos E
Sociabilidades Na Cidade Imperial. Jundiaí: Paco Editorial, 2016.

Murray, L. (2005)Not Fooling Around: The Politics Of Sex Worker Activism In Brazil. (Phd Thesis), Columbia
University, New York. 2015.

Murray, L., Kerrigan, D., Paiva, V. (2019) "Rights Of Resistance: Sex Workers Fight To Maintain Pleasure And Sex At
The Centre Of The Hiv Response In Brazil". Global Public Health. 14 (6-7). 2019. Pp. 939-953.

Museu Da Manha. Porto Do Rio E A Construção Da Alma Carioca Exhibition. Museu Da Amanha, Accessed At
Https://Museudoamanha.Org.Br/Portodorio/?Share=Timelinehistoria/11/O-Inderrubavel-Cabeca-De-Porco On
04/22/2020.

Needell, Jeffrey D. (1987) "The Revolta Contra Vacina Of 1904: The Revolt Against
"Modernization" In Belle-Époque Rio De Janeiro". The Hispanic American Historical Review. 67 (2). 1987. 266–8.

O Estado De São Paulo, "O Homem Que Cunhou O Termo 'Belíndia". Estado De São Paulo, 4/14/2017. Accessed On 4/22/2020 At Https://Economia.Estadao.Com.Br/Noticias/Geral,Ohomem-Que-Cunhou-O-Termo-Belindia,70001738802

Paiva, Vera; Ayres, Jose Ricardo And Buchalla, Cassia (2012) Eds. Vulnerbilidade E Direitos Humanos, Prevenção E Promoção Da Saúde. Livro I: Da Doença À Cidadania. Curitiba: Juruá Editora.

Parker. Building The Foundations For The Response To Hiv/Aids In Brazil: The Development Of Hiv/Aids Policy, 1982-1996. Divulgação Em Saúde Para Debate 27. 2003. Pp143-183

Ramos, Diana Helène. Preta, Pobre E Puta: A Segregação Urbana Da Prostituição Em Campinhas. Tese De Doutorado Defendida Em 2015, No Ppgpur/Ippur-Ufrj.

Richards, J. (1991). Sex, Dissidence And Damnation: Minority Groups In The Middle Ages. New York: Routledge. 1991.

Schwarcz, Lilia Moritz (1993)Espectâculo Das Raças. Cientistas, Instituições E Questão Racial No Brasil Do Século Xix. São Paulo: Cia. Das Letras.

Seffner, F., & Parker, R (2016). "The Neoliberalization Of Hiv Prevention In Brazil". In: A.

Basthi, R. Parker & V. Terto Júnior (Eds.), Myth Vs. Reality: Evaluating The Brazilian Response To Hiv In 2016 (Pp. 22-30). Rio De Janeiro: Brazilian Interdisciplinary Aids Association (Abia) - Global Aids Policy Watch. 2016.

Simões, Soraya Silveira. Vila Mimosa: Etnografia Da Cidade Cenográfica Do Rio De Janeiro. Niterói: Eduff, 2010.

_____. "Identidade E Política: A Prostituição E O Reconhecimento De Um Métier No Brasil". Revista R@U,Ppgas-Ufscar, V.2, N.1, Jan.-Jun., P.24-46, 2010b.

Souza, Herbert. (1994) Cura Da Aids. Rio De Janeiro: Relumé Dumará.

Souza, Iara Lis Carvalho. (2000) A Independência Do Brasil. Rio De Janeiro: Jorge Zahar Editor, 2000

Stuenkel, Oliver. "Identity And The Concept Of The West: The Case Of Brazil And India". In: Re.

Bras. De Polit. Int. 54.1, 2011. Pp. 178-195.

Topik, Steven C. (1996) Trade And Gunboats: The United States And Brazil In The Age Of Empire. Stanford: Stanford University Press.

Teixeira, Paulo Roberto. (2003) "Políticas Públicas Em Aids". In: R. Parker, Ed Políticas, Instituições E Aids: Enfrentando A Epidemia No Brasil. Rio De Janeiro: Jorge Zahar/Abia. Pp. 43-68.

Toussaint, Eric. "A Pandemia Do Capitalismo, O Coronavírus E A Crise Econômica". Accessed On 28/04/2020 At Https://Www.Cadtm.Org/A-Pandemia-Do-Capitalismo-Ocoronavirus-E-A-Crise-Economica. 2020.

Treichler, Paula. (1987). "Aids, Homophobia, And Biomedical Discourse: An Epidemic Of Signification." October. 43: 31-70.

Valladares, Lícia. A Gênese Da Favela Carioca (2000): A Produção Anterior Às Ciências Sociais. Rbcs, Vol.15, N.44,

Vieira Da Cunha, Neiva ; Mello, Marco Antonio Da Silva (2006). "Rito E Símbolo Na Cosmologia Do Sanitarismo : Considerações Sobre A História E A Memória Urbana Do Rio De Janeiro". Revista Candelária, Nº3, Rio De Janeiro, 2006.

Viveiros De Castro, Eduardo. "O Capitalismo Sustentável É Uma Contradição Em Seus Termos". Accessed On 04/28/2020 At Http://Www.Ihu.Unisinos.Br/Noticias/526606-Ocapitalismo-Sustentavel-E-Uma-Contradicao-Em-Seus-Termos-Diz-Eduardo-Viveiros-Decastro

Veja. "No Rio, Lixo Do Século Xix Vira Tesouro Arqueológico." Veja, 9/24/2013. Accessed On 4/22/2020 At Https://Veja.Abril.Com.Br/Entretenimento/No-Rio-Lixo-Do-Seculo-Xix-Viratesouro-Arqueologico/

Werneck, A., Leal, A, & Rodrigues, R. "Deputados Do Psl Entram No Colégio Pedro Ii Sem Autorização Para 'Vistoria' E Provocam Confusão", O Globo, 10/11/2019. Accessed On 04/26/2020 At Https://Oglobo.Globo.Com/Rio/Deputados-Do-Psl-Entram-No-Colegiopedro-Ii-Sem-Autorizacao-Para-vistoria-provocam-confusao-24012387

2. Casual Sex Among MSM During the Period of Sheltering in Place to Prevent the Spread of COVID-19: Results of National, Online Surveys in Brazil and Portugal

[1]Alvaro Francisco Lopes Sousa[1,2], Layze Braz de Oliveira[1], Artur Acelino Francisco Luz Nunes Queiroz[1], Hérica Emilia Felix de Carvalho[1], Guilherme Schneider[1], Emerson Lucas Silva Camargo[1]; Telma Evangelista de Araujo[3], Sandra Brignol[4], Isabel Amélia Costa Mendes[1], Willi McFarland[5], Inês Fronteira[2].

ABSTRACT

Background: Sheltering in place to reduce the spread of COVID-19 may have adverse effects on mental and sexual health, particularly for LGBT populations whose social support may be fragile. In this study, we investigated the extent to which Brazilian and Portuguese MSM had casual sex partners outside their homes during the period of sheltering in place for the COVID19 pandemic. **Methods:** An online survey was implemented nationally in Brazil and Portugal in April 2020, during the period of social isolation for COVID-19, with a sample of 2,361 MSM (1,651 in Brazil, 710 in Portugal). Recruitment was done through meeting apps and Facebook groups catering to MSM. Data collection was online via CASI. **Results:** Over 95% of MSM were sheltering at least partially at the time of the survey. Nearly 50% said sheltering had a high impact on their lives. A majority (53.0%) had casual sex partners during sheltering. Factors that increased the odds of engaging in casual sex in Brazil were having group sex (adjusted odds ratio [aOR] 2.1, 95% CI 1.3-3.4), living in a urban area (aOR 1.6, 95% CI 1.1-2.2), feeling that sheltering had high impact on daily life (aOR 3.0, 95% CI 1.1-8.3), having casual vs steady partners (aOR 2.5, 95% CI 1.8-3.5), and not decreasing the number of partners during the COVID-19 epidemic (aOR 6.5, 95% CI 4.2-10.0). In Portugal, the odds of engaging in casual sex increased with using Facebook to find partners (aOR 4.6, 95% CI 3.0-7.2), not decreasing the number of partners during the COVID-19 epidemic (aOR 3.8, 95% CI 2.9-5.9), usually (pre-COVID-19) finding partners in physical venues (aOR5.4, 95% CI 3.2–8.9), feeling that the isolation had high impact on daily life (aOR 3.0, 95% CI 1.3-6.7), and HIV positive serostatus (aOR 11.7, 95% CI 4.7-29.2). Surprisingly, taking PrEP/Truvada to prevent COVID-19 was reported by 12.7% of MSM. **Conclusions:** The COVID-19 epidemic has not stopped the majority of Brazilian and Portuguese MSM from finding sexual partners outside their home, with high risk sexual behaviours continuing. Public health messages for the prevention of COVID-19 need to be crafted to explicitly link sexual behaviour to reduce pandemics in the current moment.

[1] Affiliations:
1. Human Exposome and Infectious Diseases Network, Escola de Enfermagem de Ribeirão Preto, Universidade de São Paulo, Brazil.
2. Global Health and Tropical Medicine, Instituto de Higiene e Medicina Tropical, Universidade Nova de Lisboa, Portugal.
3. Universidade Federal do Piaui, Brazil.
4. Departamento de Saúde Coletiva, Universidade Federal Fluminense, Brazil.
5. Department of Epidemiology and Biostatistics, University of California at San Francisco, USA.
Funding: Conselho Nacional de Pesquisa – CNPq, Brazil.

BACKGROUND

By June 01, 2020, Brazil became one of the most severely affected countries by the COVID-19 pandemic. With 35,000 deaths and 690,000 cases of COVID-19 officially confirmed [1], Brazil ranked in the second position in the world [2]. Portugal, where the spread the infection began nearly one month before Brazil, had 34,000 confirmed cases and 1,400 deaths by COVID19 by the same date [3]. Without a vaccine or effective treatment, general preventive measures for respiratory infections remain the main means of containing the spread of the virus. Minimizing the gathering and movement of people, that is, "sheltering in place" to varying degrees of strictness have been adopted by many countries, including Brazil and Portugal [4,5].

There appear to be positive effects of sheltering on reducing the speed of COVID-19 infection. However, mental and other aspects of health, including sexual health, may be suffering [6].Social support is a known protective factor for general health [7] and social withdrawal can potentiate, or trigger, harmful consequences for mental and physical health. In populations where this support is more fragile, as in the case of LGBT populations, interruptions in social support can have severe negative consequences, including greater risk of exposure to COVID-19, which is still not fully understood [6].To measure the potential consequences of COVID-19 on the mental health and sexual behaviour of MSM, the In_PrEP Group in Brazil and Portugal implemented an online questionnaire. In particular, the questionnaire sought to measure whether MSM were seeking casual partners outside their homes during the period when shelter in place directives were in effect and measures they were undertaking to reduce the risk of COVID-19, HIV, and STI. Brazil and Portugal were selected as they share language and a large flow of people between these countries each year (28,210 thousand) [8], through immigration, professional and student activities, and tourism [9].

METHODS

Study Design, Population, Sampling, And Recruitment

This project entitled "40tena" is derived from the In_PrEP cohort study, a multicentre survey implemented in all 26 Brazilian states and the Federal District, and in 15 districts of Portugal. A rapid and dynamic data collection process took place in April 2020 at a time when the two countries were under sheltering directives. Recruitment of MSM was done using a combination of strategies for dating apps and Facebook. The design was a modified time-space sampling technique adapted to the virtual environment, following procedures used in previous studies [10, 11, 12]. Two dating applications catering to the MSM population were chosen to meet participants through direct chat with online users. The researchers registered as users with the apps, changing their selected locations to produce a diversified sample within the targeted coverage areas planned for the research. We included only individuals who identified themselves as male (cis or trans), aged 18 or over, and living in one of the two countries. Non-Portuguese speakers and tourists were excluded. For Facebook recruitment, the researchers used the boost on the social network feature to target MSM in both countries. A fixed post on the official research page[1]was accompanied by an electronic link which provided access to the informed consent form and the survey questionnaire.

---

[1] (https://www.facebook.com/taafimdeque/)

Measures

Data were collected by Computer-Assisted Technique Interview (CASI). The data collection questionnaire was hosted on a study website, only allowing answers from IP for security reasons. The questionnaire was divided into five sections including sociodemographic information, sheltering, issues of sexual health, sexual behaviour in the period of sheltering, and COVID-19 prevention measures.

Analysis

Descriptive analysis was performed for key numerical and categorical variables. Bivariate and multivariate logistic regression was used to characterize associations with having casual sex with partners outside the home during the period of sheltering. A final model was selected based on retaining those variables with $p<0.1$ while using the cut-off of $p<0.05$ for significance.

Ethical Considerations

The research project obtained ethical approval from the Universidade Nova de Lisboa and Universidade de São Paulo. Informed consent was obtained from all users online, before proceeding with the questionnaire.

RESULTS

A total of 2,361 MSM participated in the online surveys, including 1,651 (69.9%) from Brazil and 710 (30.1%) from Portugal (Table 1). The median age was 29 years (range 18-66). Majorities in both countries lived in urban areas (69.0% in Brazil, 95.4% in Portugal) and were single (69.2% in Brazil, 82.3% in Portugal). One in ten (9.9%) MSM respondents in Brazil self-reported their HIV status as positive, as did 12.1% of respondents in Portugal. In Brazil, 10.5% reported testing and 5.5% reported being diagnosed with COVID-19. In Portugal, 15.5% had tested and 1.8% were diagnosed with COVID-19.Majorities of MSM in Brazil (71.0%) and Portugal (74.6%) reported that they were sheltering at the time of the survey. Most of the remaining reported partially sheltering. Only 4.5% of MSM respondents in Brazil and 4.2% in Portugal said they were not sheltering in any form. Nearly half of MSM respondents (48.0% in Brazil, 49.0% in Portugal) felt sheltering had high impact on their lives.

Table 1 also describes how the COVID-19 epidemic changed the respondents' sexual behaviour. Respondents reported a median of 1.0 sex partners (range 0-32) during the period of sheltering. Two-thirds reported having only casual partner (66.4%), with many having both casual and steady partners (14.0%). Overall, 14.6% of respondents lived with their sex partner. Substantial majorities of MSM (75.9% in Brazil, 72.5% in Portugal) reported a decreased number of sexual partners and sexual frequency (72.0% in Brazil, 86.6%) during the sheltering period. Nonetheless, over half of respondents (53.0%) had casual sex, with paying for sex (3.0%), group sex (15.8%), sex under the influence of alcohol or drugs (39.0%), and condomless sex (30.4%) also reported.

Many MSM reported behaviours that they believed would reduce the risk of COVID-19 transmission. Apart from measures taken with respect to sex, general preventive measures (25.8%), asking if the partner was sheltering (30.7%), and asking if the partner had symptoms (27.5%) were mentioned.

Other measures to reduce the spread of COVID-19 included avoiding kissing during sex (16.2%), washing hands before and after sex (27.6%), and disinfecting the area before and after sex (14.6%). Of note, some mentioned taking PrEP/Truvada (12.7%) and using condoms (21.9%) as measures adopted to prevent COVID-19 transmission. Table 2 presents correlates of leaving the house or having someone in their house for casual sex during the sheltering period in bivariate and multivariate logistic regression models for each country.

In Brazil, the odds of engaging in casual sex increased with having group sex (adjusted odds ratio [aOR] 2.1, 95% CI 1.3-3.4), living in a urban area (aOR 1.6, 95% CI 1.12.2), feeling that sheltering had average (aOR 2.2, 95% CI 1.5-3.2) or high impact on their daily life (aOR 3.0, 95% CI 1.1-8.3) compared to low impact, having casual partners (aOR 2.5, 95%CI 1.8-3.5), and not decreasing the number of partners during the COVID-19 epidemic (aOR 6.5, 95% CI 4.2-10.0). In Portugal, the odds of engaging in casual sex increased with using Facebook to find partners (aOR 4.6, 95% CI 3.0-7.2), not decreasing the number of partners during the COVID-19 epidemic (aOR 3.8, 95% CI 2.9-5.9), usually (pre-COVID-19) finding partners in physical venues (aOR5.4, 95% CI 3.2–8.9), feeling that the isolation had high impact on their daily life (aOR 3.0, 95% CI 1.3-6.7), and reporting HIV-positive serostatus (aOR 11.7, 95% CI 4.7-29.2).

DISCUSSION

Our study showed that the COVID-19 epidemic and the period of sheltering in place did not stop the majority of Brazilian and Portuguese MSM from finding sexual partners outside their home. Nonetheless, over 95% of respondents say they adopted at least partial sheltering in place. For Brazil, this level may be higher than typically reported by local authorities for the general population (between 40% and 55%) [13] – levels which have cause for concern in overcrowding hospitals [14]. For Portugal, compliance in the general population appears to have been high enough to avert overwhelming the hospital system [15]. Although slightly over half of MSM still found casual partners outside their homes, three-fourths had fewer partners compared to before the COVID-19 epidemic. MSM reported other measures to reduce the risk for COVID-19 akin to harm reduction practices. For example, more than one in four asked if their partners were otherwise sheltering and if they had any symptoms of COVID-19.

Although close contact was inherent or implied in having casual sex, many MSM reported avoiding kissing, handwashing before and after sex, and disinfecting the area before and after sex.

A surprising and unexpected finding was the use of PrEP/Truvada for COVID-19 prophylaxis. In the absence of evidence of efficacy for COVID-19 prevention, the assumption risks causing people on PrEP to neglect effective measures. A possible explanation for the adoption of this practice might be misunderstanding the discussion of potential of prophylaxis drugs for SARS-CoV2 in the popular media [26]. Some MSM may have mistaken Truvada, promoted for HIV prophylaxis, as having a similar mechanism for SARS-CoV2.

Specific messaging may be needed to dispel this false connection through programs promoting PrEP for HIV.Our study also found continuation of behaviours that may place MSM at high risk for acquiring or transmitting HIV and STI during the COVID-19 epidemic. More than one in six MSM reported group sex, implying the meeting of several people in very close contact, thus amplifying potential COVID-9 exposure [18]. Engaging in group sex was further associated with increased odds of having casual partners outside the home among Brazilian MSM. Sexual encounters under the influence of drugs or alcohol, also common during the sheltering period, can decrease reasoning capacity and hinder the adoption of preventive measures for HIV/STI and COVID-19 [19]. Condomless sex itself was reported by over one in three Brazilian MSM and one in five Portuguese MSM during the shelter in place period, apparently high levels [12].The duration of the sheltering period, with accompanying feelings of isolation, may partly explain the high-risk sexual behaviours. The large majority of participants had been isolated for at least 30 days, and many recognized a high impact of social isolation on their lives. This in turn may have led MSM to feel a greater need for social contact, to seek a "break" in isolation to seek partners [16], with an additional break for HIV preventive measures. This hypothesis is corroborated by the findings of the multivariate analysis, in which acknowledging high impact of the sheltering period was associated with seeking outside casual sex partners in both in Brazil and in Portugal.

The effect of a prolonged isolation period is particularly worrisome as Brazil moves towards becoming a COVID-19 epicentre in Latin America and the world [17]. There are some studies in the literature implying social isolation may lead to higher utilization of virtual networks to search for sexual encounters [6, 23]. Tinder connections increased 15% in the US and 25% in Italy and Spain during the COVID-19 epidemic [23]. The duration of chat activity also increased by 30% [23]. Notably, the use of Facebook was significantly associated with an increasing odds for Portuguese MSM seeking partners through this platform. Another hypothesis is that partnering through Facebook can provide a false sense of controlling exposure by enabling sex with someone known and belonging to the same social network (friend/acquaintance). Yet another possible explanation for the association of increased casual partnering during COVID-19 and use of Facebook, not yet documented in the literature, may be fear of judgment (i.e., for breaking sheltering) by closer friends, which leads MSM to seek out like-minded strangers. On the other hand, to the extent that social media can assist with keeping to smaller social groups and the adoption of virtual sex and masturbation [20, 22], it may reduce risks for transmissible infections.

Other significant associations with seeking causal sex during COVID-19 are notable. Being HIV positive also increased the odds of engaging in casual sex in Portuguese MSM. One hypothesis may be a false sense of protection due to antiretrovirals for HIV currently being tested in COVID-19 patients [24]. This may be consistent with assumptions or misunderstandings about PrEP, as mentioned above. In both Brazil and in Portugal, living in an urban area increased the odds of casual sex, likely explained by a access to greater numbers of MSM [25] easy to locate and select partners by dating Apps or other social media [12].This study has limitations. First, we recognize the data derive from a convenience sample in both countries. Understandably, venue-based and peer referral mechanism to sample and recruit are made harder during the COVID-19 epidemic. Second, we did not measure variables recognized as important in hindsight, such as exact days sheltering, different sexual practices, and the organization of other events, such as parties where sex may have occurred. Lastly, we did not test for COVID-19 and therefore could not fully link behaviours directly to acquisition of infection.

CONCLUSIONS

We were able to identify a high frequency of casual sex among MSM, and associated factors that might increase exposure to SARS-CoV-2, HIV, and other STI during a period of high COVID19 transmission when sheltering in place was implemented. Although many strategies were adopted to minimize the exposure to SARS-CoV-2, the effectiveness of those measures is threatened by high-risk practices common to COVID-19 and HIV, including condomless sexual intercourse and group sex. By analysing two countries with different outcomes in terms of the control of the COVID-19 epidemic, our results demonstrate the vulnerability of MSM communities and if left unaddressed they may hamper the pandemic response. We suggest that governments craft messages for the prevention of COVID-19 explicitly linked to messages on sexual behaviour to reduce the impact of the current era on both pandemics.

REFERENCES

1. Ministério da Saúde (Brazil). Painel Coronavírus. 2020. Available at: https://covid.saude.gov.br/

2. WHO. Coronavirus disease (COVID-2019) situation reports. Available from: https://www.who.int/emergencies/diseases/novel-coronavirus-2019/situation-reports

3. Ministério da Saúde (Portugal). SNS-24. Temas da saúde - COVID-19. Available at: https://www.sns24.gov.pt/tema/doencas-infecciosas/COVID-19/

4. Peixoto, V.R., Vieira, A., Aguiar, P. Sousa., Abrantes, A. (2020) "Timing", Adesão e Impacto das Medidas de Contenção da COVID-19 em Portugal. NOVA National School of Public Health report 2020.

5. Albuquerque, L.P., Silva, R.B., Araújo, R.M.S. (2020) COVID-19: origin, pathogenesis, transmission, clinical aspects and current therapeutic strategies. Rev Pre Infec e Saúde. 2020; 6:10432.

6. Brennan, D.J, Card, K.G., Collict, D., Jollimore, J., Lachowsky, N.J. (2020).How Might Social Distancing Impact Gay, Bisexual, Queer, Trans and Two-Spirit Men in Canada? AIDS Behav 2020 30:1–3.

7. McDonald, K. (2018). Social Support and Mental Health in LGBTQ Adolescents: A review of the literature. Issues Ment Health Nurs 2018; 39(1):16-29.

8. Portugal. Serviço de Estrangeiros e Fronteiras, 2018. Available at:https://sefstat.sef.pt/Docs/Rifa2018.pdf

9. Barbosa, B., Santos, C.M., Santos, M., (2020) Tourists with migrants' eyes: the mediating role of tourism in international retirement migration. J Tour Cult Chang 2020.

10. Queiroz, A.A.F.L.N, Sousa, A.F.L, Matos, M.C.B, Araújo, T.M.E, Reis, R.K., Moura, M.E.B.(2018) Knowledge about HIV/AIDS and implications of establishing partnerships among Hornet® users. Rev Bras Enferm 2018; 71(4): 1949-1955.

11. Queiroz, A.A.F.L.N., Sousa, Á.F.L., Matos, M.C.B, et al. (2019).Factors associated with self-reported noncompletion of the hepatitis B vaccine series in men who have sex with men in Brazil. BMC Infect Dis 2019;19(1):335.

12. Queiroz, A.A.F.L.N. Sousa, A.FL, Brignol, S, Araújo, T.M.E, Reis, R.K. (2019) Vulnerability to HIV among older men who have sex with men users of dating apps in Brazil. Braz J Infect Dis 2019; 23(5): 298-306.

13. Lana, R.M., Coelho, F.C., Gomes, M.F.C. Cruz, O.G., Bastos, L.S., Villela, D.A,M. et al. (2020). The novel coronavirus (SARS-CoV-2) emergency and the role of timely and effective national health surveillance. Cad Saúde Pública 2020; 36 (3): e00019620.

14. Freitas, A.R.R., Napimoga, M. Donalisio, M.R. (2020) Assessing the severity of COVID-19. Epidemiol Serv Saúde 2020; e2020119.

15. Peixoto, V.R., Vieira, A., Aguiara, P., Carvalho, C., Thomas, D., Abrantes, A. (2020). Rapid assessment of the impact of "lockdown" on the COVID-19 epidemic in Portugal. MedRxiv 2020.

16. Sanchez, T.H., Zlotorzynska, M., Rai, M., Baral, S.D. (2020).Characterizing the Impact of COVID-19 on Men Who Have Sex with Men Across the United States in April, 2020. AIDS and Behav 2020; 1-9.

17. Menezes, P.L, Garner, D.M., Valenti, V.E. (2020).Brazil is projected to be the next global COVID-19 pandemic epicentre. Medrxiv 2020.

18. Yuen, K.S., Ye, Z.W., Fung, S.Y., Chan, C.P. (2020). Jin DY. SARS-CoV-2 and COVID-19: The most important research questions. Cell Biosci 2020 16;10:40.

19. Wong, N.S., Kwan, T.H., Lee, K.C.K., Lau, J.Y.C., Lee, S.S., (2020). Delineation of chemsex patterns of men who have sex with men in association with their sexual networks and linkage to HIV prevention. Int J Drug Policy. 2020 ;75:102591.

20. NYC. Sex and COVID-19 Fact Sheet. Available from: https://www1.nyc.gov/assets/doh/downloads/pdf/imm/covid-sexguidance.pdf?utm_source=morning_brew. Acess 27 May 2020.

21. Yeo, C., Sanghvi, K., Yeo, D. (2020) Enteric involvement of coronaviruses: is faecal-oral transmission of SARS-CoV-2 possible?. Lancet Gastroenterol. 2020, 5:P335-337. 10.1016/ S2468-1253(20)30048-0

22. UNAIDS. Safer sex in the time of COVID-19. Available from:

    https://www.unaids.org/en/resources/covid-blog, acess in 27 may 2020

23. Sullivan, A. (2020). Love in the time of coronavirus: COVID-19 changes the game for online dating. Deutsche Welle. 2020. https://www.dw.com/en/love-in-the-time-of-coronavirusCOVID-19changes-the-game-for-online-dating/a-52933001. Accessed 27 May 2020.

24. Cao, B. Wang, Y. Wen, D. et al. (2020)A Trial of Lopinavir-Ritonavir in Adults Hospitalized with Severe COVID-19. N Engl J Med **2020;** 382:1787-1799.

25. Whitfield, D.L, Kattari, S.K., Walls, N.E., Al-Tayyib, (2017) A. Grindr Scruff, and on the Hunt: Predictors of Condomless Anal Sex, Internet Use, and Mobile Application Use Among Men Who Have Sex With Men. Am J Mens Health. **2017**;11(3):775-784.

26. https://www.pharmacytimes.com/ajax/development-of-prep-for-COVID-19-could-allowcountry-to-open-safely-before-a-vaccine-is-available

Table 1. Characteristics and sexual practices during the COVID-19 shelter in place period, men who have sex with men, Brazil and Portugal, 2020.

Variables	Brazil (N=1,651)			Portugal (N=710)		Total (N=2,361)	
	n	%		n	%	n	%
Gender identity							
Man	1637	99.2	697	98.2	2334	98.9	
Trans man or non-binary	14	0.8	13	1.8	27	1.1	
Lives in urban area	1140	69.0	677	95.4	1817	77.0	
Relationship status							
Single	1143	69.2	584	82.3	1727	73.1	
Monogamous	480	29.1	86	12.1	566	24.0	
Polyamorous	28	1.7	40	5.6	68	2.9	
Self-reported HIV status							
HIV negative	1285	77.8	488	68.7	1773	75.1	
HIV positive	163	9.9	86	12.1	249	10.5	
I do not know	203	12.3	136	19.2	339	14.4	
Tested for COVID-19	174	10.5	110	15.5	284	12	
Diagnosed with COVID-19	90	5.5	13	1.8	103	4.4	
Are you now sheltering in place?							
No	74	4.5	26	3.7	100	4.2	
Partially	405	24.5	154	21.7	559	23.7	
Yes	1172	71.0	530	74.6	1702	72.1	
For how long have you been sheltering?							
1 to 14 days	60	3.6	54	7.6	114	4.8	
15 to 29 days	331	20.1	62	8.8	393	16.7	
30 to 45 days	1035	62.7	326	45.9	1361	57.6	
More than 45 days	225	13.6	268	37.7	493	20.9	

How would you rate the impact that

sheltering has had on your life?

Low impact	215	13.0	70	9.9	285	12.1
Average impact	643	38.9	292	41.1	935	39.6
High impact	793	48.0	348	49.0	1141	48.3
Usual type of sex partner						
Casual	1155	70.0	413	58.2	1568	66.4
Steady	291	17.6	40	5.6	331	14.0
Both casual and steady	205	12.4	257	36.2	462	19.6
Lives with sex partner	236	14.3	109	15.4	345	14.6
Usual ways respondent finds sex partners before period of sheltering						
Dating apps	1285	77.8	544	76.6	1829	77.5
Facebook, Twitter, or Instagram	560	33.9	286	40.3	846	35.8
Other sites	446	27.0	173	24.4	619	26.2
Bars, clubs, saunas, cruising areas	72	4.4	25	3.5	97	4.1
Does not search for partners	292	17.7	98	13.8	390	16.5
Decreased number of sexual partners during sheltering	1253	75.9	515	72.5	1768	74.8
In this sheltering period, would you say that…						
Your sexual frequency						
Decreased	1188	72.0	615	86.6	1803	76.4
Did not change	364	22.0	66	9.3	430	18.2
Increased	99	6.0	29	4.1	128	5.4
Your interaction with social media						
Decreased	117	7.1	248	34.9	365	15.5
Did not change	357	21.6	136	19.2	493	20.9
Increased	1177	71.3	326	45.9	1503	63.6
Your alcohol consumption						
Decreased	705	42.7	384	54.1	1089	46.1
Did not change	608	36.8	212	29.9	820	34.7

Increased	338	20.5	114	16.0	452	19.2

During sheltering, the respondent

Had casual sex	875	53.0	377	53.1	1252	53.0
Sought to pay for sex	63	3.8	9	1.3	72	3.0
Had sex with 2 or more people at the same time	259	15.7	113	15.9	372	15.8
Had sex under the influence of drugs or alcohol	777	47.1	143	20.1	920	39.0
Had condomless sex	576	34.9	142	20.0	718	30.4

To protect from COVID-19, the respondent

Took general protective measures	423	25.6	187	26.3	610	25.8
Asked if the partner was sheltering	513	31.1	212	29.9	725	30.7
Asked if the partner had symptoms	452	27.4	197	27.7	649	27.5
Avoided kissing during sex	219	13.3	164	23.1	383	16.2
Washed hands with soap and water for at least 20 seconds before and after sex	450	27.3	202	28.5	652	27.6
Disinfected area before and after sex	209	12.7	136	19.2	345	14.6
Used PrEP/Truvada	191	11.6	110	15.5	301	12.7
Used a condom with anal sex	403	24.4	114	16.1	517	21.9
Did not adopt any strategy	610	36.9	247	34.8	857	36.3

Country	Variables	Bivariate OR (95% CI)	MultivariateaOR (95% CI)
Brazil	Sought to pay for sex	2.7 (1.5-4.8)	0.4 (0.2-1.1)
	Sex with ≥2 at the same time (group sex)	10.0 (6.6-15.1)	2.1 (1.3-3.4)
	Lives in urban area	1.4 (1.1-1.7)	1.6 (1.1-2.2)
	Impact of sheltering on daily life:		
	Low	1.0	1.0
	Average	1.2 (0.9-1.5)	2.2 (1.5-3.2)
	High	1.1 (0.8-1.40	3.0 (1.1-8.3)
	Type of sex partner(s):		
	Steady	1.0	1.0
	Casual and steady	3.3 (2.2-4.8)	1.6 (0.9-2.8)
	Casual	1.5 (1.2-2.0)	2.5(1.8-3.5)
	Used condom with anal sex	0.4 (0.3-0.5)	0.6 (0.4-0.9)
	Did not decrease number of partners during sheltering	21.3 (15.0-30.4)	6.5 (4.2-10.0)

Portugal	Used Facebook to find partners	3.0 (2.2-4.2)	4.6 (3.0-7.2)
	Did not seek partners Time in isolation: 15-29 days	0.5 (0.4-0.7)	0.3 (0.1-0.5)
	30-45 days	1.0	1.0
	>45 days	0.5 (0.3-0.8)	0.2 (0.1-0.4)
	Not in isolation	0.8 (0.4-1.4)	0.4 (0.2-0.8)
	Did not decrease number of partners during sheltering	0.5 (0.3-1.1)	0.2 (0.1-0.8)
	Usually found partners at bars, clubs, saunas, etc.	1.2 (0.9-3.8)	3.8 (2.9-5.9)
	Impact of isolation on daily life: Low	2.3 (1.6-3.3)	5.4 (3.2-8.9)
		1.0	1.0
	Average	0.8 (0.5-1.4)	0.7 (0.3-1.7)
	High	3.1 (1.9-5.4)	3.0 (1.3-6.7)
	Self-reported HIV status: HIV negative	1.0	1.0
	HIV positive	10.4 (4.9-22.0)	11.7 (4.7-29.2)
	Does not know	0.9 (0.8-1.1)	1.4 (0.7-2.3)

Table 2. Factors associated with having casual sex during the COVID-19 shelter in place period, men who have sex with men, Brazil and Portugal, 2020.

3.LGBT+ Community During The COVID-19 Pandemic In Brazil

Ricardo H. D. Rohm e José Otávio A. L. Martins

At a time when the World Health Organization and other government officials say "do stay at home!", which home does the LGBTQ+ community has the option to stay in? This article illuminates the struggles lived by the LGBTQ+ community during the COVID-19 crisis, also illustrating some of the initiatives taken in response.

May 17th the International Day Against Homophobia, Transphobia, and Biphobia was celebrated, a date aiming to promote international events that raise awareness of LGBTQ+ rights violations worldwide. This date was chosen due after the World Health Organization (WHO) chose to remove the term "homosexuality" from the list of mental disorders of the International Classification of Diseases in 1990, disregarding homosexuality as a pathology.

Even though the date is now remembered as the day against LGBTQphobia, it is important to remember that the so-called "gender incongruence" was only removed by the WHO from the International Classification of Diseases and Related Health Problems (ICD 11) on June 18, 2018.

This date is a great achievement for the LGBTQ+ community, especially if we consider the context in which the decision took place the early 1990s, still reverberating the spread of AIDS. For the LGBTQ+ community, notably for those who were born in the 1950s and 1960s and fully experienced the demonization of their bodies during the 1980s, the situation in which we live today, with the COVID-19 pandemic, recalls painful memories. Still recovering from being considered as the source and proliferator of HIV/AIDS, the "gay cancer", the LGBTQ+ community seems nowadays once again being held accountable by some authorities and public personalities, without grounds other than homophobia, for the current pandemic, as we can see in examples in the United States[1],Israel[2] and Iraq[3]. Situations like these portray the constant and hostile prejudice, discrimination, and attack which the LGBTQ+ community suffers, day after day, year after year, century after century. Even if we are not at the heart of the matter, we are blamed for it.

This system of oppression constantly puts our community in a situation of social and emotional vulnerability. The vast majority only lives in the fullness of their sexual orientation and gender identity far away from the utopian coziness which family and home should symbolize. Many LGBTQ+ people, however, are only free when they are among friends, a *chosen family*, lovers, on a stage performing with a wig on or waving their flags, once a year, at the pride parades. This distance from their family and home could be by choice, when it is unbearable to cope with prejudice, or not – just like when they are rejected, abused, or thrown out of their home. We should ask again, therefore, at a time when the WHO and other government officials say "do stay at home!", which home does the LGBTQ+ community has the option to stay in?

In Marseille, France, a couple was kicked out[4] of the apartment they rented because they were "the first to be contaminated" by the COVID-19, an affirmation that has no scientific base, just

---

[1] https://theintercept.com/2020/03/24/trump-cabinet-bible-studies-coronavirus/
[2] https://www.timesofisrael.com/israeli-rabbi-blames-coronavirus-outbreak-on-gay-pride-parades/
[3] https://www.middleeasteye.net/news/coronavirus-iraq-muqtda-sadr-covid-19-same-sex-marriage
[4] https://www.metroweekly.com/2020/04/gay-couple-told-to-leave-home-because-homosexuals-are-contaminated-by-covid-19/

homophobia. Exposed to a peculiar extra vulnerability now, which increases the existing one which the LGBTQ+ population has been facing, our community is even more targeted within the coronavirus crisis, as pointed out by the High Commissioner for Human Rights of the United Nations (UN),Michelle Bachelet. The UN draws attention to those who are HIV positive in the LGBTQ+ community. In Brazil, HIV among men who have sex with men is a reality classified as an epidemic and, although they are not part of the risk group, they do have a specific health care routine and ongoing medical treatments which require, for example, going out to withdraw retroviral drugs in health units.

The UN also reinforces the importance of the local authorities to ensure the maintenance of these treatments and the continuous supply of HIV medication during the pandemic, not allowing prejudices to affect access and availability of these drugs. Other health issues raise worries when we are facing the dissemination of a virus which attacks the respiratory system. Some Studies show that the LGBTQ+ population uses tobacco at rates that are 50% higher than the general population. The community still has a significant amount of people with cancer and, consequently, with a fragile immune system. It is important to note that LGBTQ+ people are historically discriminated by both health employees and the health system itself. As a result, many are reluctant to seek medical care, even in urgent situations. That can mean a health risk in times of COVID-19.

Talking about employment issues in Brazil, a national survey[1] conducted by the group #VoteLGBT, with the participation of researchers from two major Brazilian universities, points out that, within the LGBTQ+ community, 21.6% of respondents are unemployed and 20.7% have no income. This survey was conducted through online questionnaires, therefore, there is a considerable possibility that it has not reached some of the most vulnerable people in the community and the results could be worrisome. It is also relevant to highlight the difficulty in the access to income by trans and transvestite women who are sex workers[2] (90% of Brazilian trans population uses prostitution as a source of income) who, in times of social distancing, can no longer carry out their activities, losing their source of income (unless able to resort to virtual sessions instead).

Opening a short parenthesis to talk about the trans population, as if the suffering of the most vulnerable portion of the LGBTQ+ community was not enough, transphobia does not cease during a pandemic. Some Latin American countries have determined that, among the measures of social distancing, men and women can only leave their houses on separate days. There have been cases of trans women being fined for leaving their home on the day designated for women, making the pandemic period even more difficult for the trans population, who in addition to fighting the virus, has to still fight to reaffirm who they are.

Addressing the issues associated with staying at home during the pandemic and the difficulty of finding a safe place to be protected, a global survey[3] conducted by the relationships app Hornet, with gay, bisexual, cis or transgender men points out that 1 out of 3 men feels physically and emotionally insecure in their own homes. The reasons are not only due to the intrafamilial prejudice, for those who live with their families, but also the loneliness of those living alone – data from #VoteLGBT`s survey also pointed out that 28% of the Brazilian respondents have been diagnosed with depression, which worsens the scenario presentedby Hornet`s survey. When talking about LGBTQ+ people who are unable to earn a living or who have been kicked off from their families' homes, an alternative to survival are the shelters (in Portuguese "*Casas de Acolhimento*"),

---

[1] https://docs.google.com/document/d/1FkdQib_mrApYY_PpGhE8HzOMPxvBGJkoyO3aqFRZUBE/edit
[2] https://antrabrasil.files.wordpress.com/2020/03/dicas-profissionais-do-sexo-antra.pdf
[3] https://hornet.com/about/hornet-report-coronavirus-anxiety/

present in several cities in Brazil. Although each has its administration, they support each other on joint projects to collect donations and carry out cultural actions. In addition to a shelter, they provide food and personal hygiene products for marginalized LGBTQ+ people, as well as develop academic, capacitation, and cultural activities for their residents and the external public, always relying on donations and sponsorships to maintain their activities. During the pandemic, where everything is more urgent and scarce compared to normal times, the shelters see the decrease of donations while the requests for shelter are increasing.

Initiatives To Cope With This Scenario

Amid the plight that the LGBTQ+ community faces today, some initiatives deserve not only visibility but also our support. They are the result of the mobilization of the community itself and, eventually, with the support of some LGBTQ-friendly companies and celebrities. Links to the initiative and organizations are copied herein under to bring awareness and visibility to the cause. Speaking about the shelters mentioned above, some fundraising initiatives have managed to obtain significant support to these institutions in this time of crisis.

A virtual live concert with a famous Brazilian DJ organized by NGO Casinha, produced by Tenho Orgulho[1], FestivalUniverso, andTODXS[2], raised more than 5,000 BRL for organizations such as Cas[3]a Nem,LGBT+[4] Movimento[5] and for Casainha[6] itself.

Another virtual live concert titled Festival do Orgulho was organized by Amstel Brewery and payment app AME.

The Festival was headlined by artists of great national visibility (among them singer/*drag queen* Pabllo Vittar) and raised 115,000 BRL[7] that were donated to the NGOsCasa Florescer,[8] Grupo Pela Vidda[9] andProjeto[10] Séfora's,[11]Família [12]Stronger and Arco Íris de Ribeirão Preto

Another fundraising initiative for shelters across the country – in this case, without musical performances – was the crowdfunding organized by All Out Brazil[13] movement to support these institutions in their maintenance, purchase, and distribution of cleaning and hygiene materials, as well as food. The initiative raised approximately 54,000 BRL and will benefitCasAmor LGBTQI+ [14] (Aracaju),Astra Human Rights and LGBT Citizenship[15] | Acódi LGBT[16] (Aracaju),Casa Transformar[17](Fortaleza), Casa Miga Acolhimento LGBT+[18](Manaus),Casa da Diversidade

---

[1] https://www.instagram.com/tenhoorgulho/
[2] https://www.todxs.org/
[3] https://www.instagram.com/casanem_/
[4] https://www.instagram.com/lgbtmaismovimento/
[5] https://www.instagram.com/lgbtmaismovimento/
[6] https://www.instagram.com/casinhaacolhida/
[7] https://www.cidademarketing.com.br/marketing/2020/05/01/live-festival-do-orgulho-arrecada-r115-mil-com-shows-de-pabllo-vittar-pepita-aretuza-lovi-urias-e-mateus-carrilho/
[8] https://www.instagram.com/casaflorescer_/
[9] https://www.instagram.com/pelaviddarj/
[10] https://www.instagram.com/projeto.seforas/
[11] https://www.instagram.com/projeto.seforas/
[12] https://www.instagram.com/redefamiliastronger/
[13] https://action.allout.org/
[14] https://www.instagram.com/casamorlgbtqi/
[15] https://www.instagram.com/astraglbt/
[16] https://www.instagram.com/astraglbt/
[17] https://www.instagram.com/casatransformar/
[18] https://www.instagram.com/casamigalgbt/

Niterói[1] (Niterói),Transviver[2] (Recife), CasaNem (Rio de Janeiro), Casa Aurora [3] (Salvador), Casa dos Direitos da Baixada (São João de Meriti), Casa Chama (São Paulo), Casa Florescer 1 (São Paulo) and Casa Florescer 2 (São Paulo).

Another initiative, linked to the arts, was created by #VoteLGBT, the same group which conducted the aforementioned survey. Created during quarantine, LGBTFLIX is a free-access platform, not linked to any streaming service, that compiles more than 200 LGBTQ+ themed short films! The initiative aims to bring entertainment to the LGBTQ+ community during this period of social isolation; on the platform, you can choose short films with homosexual, bisexual or transgender themes. Some nationwide initiatives are still ongoing and accepting donations. One of them is The Emergency Fund for TRANS people organized by Casa Chama, in São Paulo, which has already raised 83,000 BRL (all information about this initiative is listed in this link). Those initiatives show a path of light amid so many adversities and also the capacity of the LGBTQ+ community to once again unite efforts to face another major challenge with COVID-19. It is essential to understand the reality of the LGBTQ+ community during this pandemic, to highlight good movements that have already accomplished significant results and call on everyone to support initiatives such as those mentioned herein, not only during the pandemic. With prudence, responsibility, union, and following scientific and WHO`s guidelines the COVID-19 pandemic will be surpassed.

---

[1] https://www.instagram.com/transviver/
[2] https://www.instagram.com/transviver/
[3] https://www.instagram.com/aurora_casalgbt/

4.Impact of COVID-19 Pandemic on Sexual Minority Populations in Brazil

[1]Thiago S. Torres[1] ⓘ · Brenda Hoagland[1] · Daniel R. B. Bezerra[1] · Alex Garner[2] · Emilia M. Jalil[1] · Lara E. Coelho[1] · Marcos Benedetti[1] · Cristina Pimenta[3] · Beatriz Grinsztejn[1] · Valdilea G. Veloso[1]

ABSTRACT

We conducted a web-based survey to understand the impact of social distancing measures on Brazilian MSM and transgender/non-binary lives. A total of 3486 respondents were included in this analysis and the great majority were cismen (98%). The median age was 32 years (IQR: 27–40), 44% non-white, 36% low schooling and 38% low income.

Most of participants reported HIV negative/unknown status (77%). Participants on-PrEP reported more condomless anal sex than those off-PrEP. Conversely, 24% off-PrEP were at substantial HIV-risk. PrEP/ART continuation were reported by the majority, despite reports of impediments to medication refill.

Transgender/non-binary reported more mental health problems and challenges to access health care. Social and racial disparities were associated with unattainability of maintaining social distancing. Tailored social and economic support policies during COVID-19 pandemic should be made available to these populations. Challenges for PrEP/ART access will demand the implementation of innovative solutions to avoid the expansion of the HIV epidemic.

INTRODUCTION

On March 11, 2020 the World Health Organization (WHO) recognized the novel coronavirus (SARS-CoV-2) disease 2019, or "COVID-19", as a pandemic months after the initial reports from Wuhan, China in December, 2019 [1]. Brazil at the present has the second-highest number of confirmed SARS-CoV-2 cases in the world. From February 26, 2020 to July 30, 2020 there have been more than 2,500,000 confirmed cases and more than 90,000 deaths in the country [2]. The Southeast region account for the largest number of cases, although incidence and mortality rate per 00,000/ inhabitants is higher in the North region [2].

To avoid the spread of COVID-19 and the collapse of the health system, the Brazilian Ministry of Health, Brazilian States Governors and City Mayors have adopted social distancing and community containment measures since March 2020. These measures have been criticized by part of the Federal government, albeit the continuous rise of new cases, no availability of effective treatment nor prevention and limited availability of hospital and intensive care units [3]. Despite the

[1] Thiago S. Torres thiago.torres@ini.fiocruz.br

1Fundação Oswaldo Cruz, Instituto Nacional de Infectologia Evandro Chagas, STD/AIDS Clinical Research Lab, Av. Brasil 4365, Manguinhos, Rio de Janeiro 21040-900, Brazil

2Hornet INC, Los Angeles, CA, USA

3Brazilian Ministry of Health, Brasilia, DF, Brazil

importance of such measures, low income Brazilians may face barriers to adhere to social distancing measures, especially due to financial constraints. Almost 14 million Brazilians live in low-income communities (favelas or "slums") [4] mostly concentrated in metropolitan areas of big cities, such as Rio de Janeiro and São Paulo. These communities are highly populated and have precarious living conditions, with limited access to hygiene and sanitation, posing sanitary recommendations as a challenge, thus increasing vulnerability to COVID-19 infection.

Moreover, Brazil has a great proportion of informal jobs, especially among low-income individuals, with no possibility of doing home office, what may impact in adhering to social distancing. During the first quarter of 2020, unemployment rate was 12.2% corresponding to 12.9 million Brazilians unemployed [5], and it may increase between 50 and 100% due to the COVID-19 pandemic impact [6], especially considering the limited social support measures adopted by the Brazilian government.

Adding to economic and social challenges, sexual minorities such as cisgender gay, bisexual and other men who have sex with men (MSM) and transgender/non binary (TGNB) individuals may be facing other vulnerabilities during the COVID-19 pandemic, such as lack of access to HIV prevention, treatment and care [7]. Brazil accounts for almost half of HIV cases in Latin America [8], with a disproportional prevalence of infection among some sexual minorities, such as MSM (18%) and transgender women who have sex with men (31%) [9–12]. Brazil has long been at the forefront of HIV treatment and prevention in Latin America [13]. The Brazilian Public Health System (SUS) provides free of charge antiretroviral therapy (ART) to HIV-infected individuals since 1996 and daily oral pre-exposure prophylaxis (PrEP) with emtricitabine and tenofovir disoproxil fumarate (FTC/TDF) to those at substantial HIV risk since December, 2017 [14]. In addition, sexual minorities, especially transgender women, often present housing instability that may impact in adherence to social distancing measures [15].

In this context, we conducted a web-based survey targeting Brazilian MSM and TGNB individuals to understand how social distancing measures and the COVID-19 pandemic are impacting their personal lives, sexual behaviour, and PrEP/ART access and use. In addition, we assessed the factors associated with unattainability of maintaining social distancing.

METHODS

Study Design

This cross-sectional web-based study, conducted during social distancing period (April 16 to May 31, 2020), recruited MSM and TGNB using a geosocial networking (GSN) app for sexual encounters (Hornet), WhatsApp groups and Facebook. Individuals who met eligibility criteria (age ≥ 18 years, MSM and TGNB individuals, Brazilian resident) and acknowledged reading the informed consent were directed to the online questionnaire programmed on SurveyGizmo®. Cisgender men self-identifying heterosexual and cisgender women were excluded from this analysis. The Instituto Nacional de Infectologia Evandro Chagas (INI-Fiocruz) institutional review board (#CAAE 82021918.0.0000.5262) reviewed and approved this study. No identification of participants was collected and no incentives were provided.

Survey Instrument

The survey instrument was composed of six sections (55 questions) addressing: sociodemographic information, social distancing/COVID-19 pandemic impact in personal life, substance use, HIV testing, PrEP and ART use/access and sexual behaviour.

Variables

Socio-Demographic

Variables were as following: age at the time of the survey (categorized in 3 brackets: 18 to 24; 25 to 35 and > 35 years); gender in cisgender men, transgender men, transgender women, and non-binary/gender fluid; sexual orientation in gay, bisexual, heterosexual or other (e.g. pansexual, asexual); race/color (categorized in white, black, *pardo* or mixed-black, native or indigenous and Asian); schooling (categorized in low [≤ 12 years or completed secondary school or less] and high [> 12 years or more than secondary school]). We also collected data on family monthly income, grouped into the following strata considering Brazilian minimum wage (MW) in 2020 (R$998 or US$268): low (up to 2 MW), middle (> 2–6 MW), and high (> 6 MW). Region was defined according to the Brazilian administrative division: North (7 states), Northeast (9 states), Central-west (3 states and Federal District), South (3 states) and Southeast (4 states); individuals living in the metropolitan area of the State Capital were considered as resident of metro area.

Social Distancing/COVID-19 Pandemic Impact In Personal Life

Fear to be infected by COVID-19 had 5 categories: high, moderate, low, none or infected or previously infected by COVID-19. We asked how concerned individuals were if a close relative or friend got infected by COVID-19 (rate between 0 and 100); answers were stratified in 100, 99–75, 74–50, < 50%. Participants also answered how much social distancing measures impacted their personal life (high, medium, low/none) and which aspect was the most affected (economic, affective/sexual, family/friendship, or none).

We also assessed challenges during social distancing/COVID-19 pandemic presented in a pre-determined list: access to hand sanitizer and water, salary/job reduced or lost, transportation availability, access to food, access to health/mental care support, access to daily medication/hormones and housing. Respondents could answer yes/no to any of the challenges. The question: "Were you unable to maintain recommended social distancing due to any reason, such as work or housing challenges?" (yes/no) assessed unattainability of maintaining social distancing.

Mental Health, Binge Drinking and Substance Use

Mental health problems were assessed by the question:
"Have you felt depressed, lonely, angry, nightmares, panic attack, sleeping or concentration problems during the social distancing period?"(yes/no). Participants were also asked about suicidal thoughts and physical/sexual/emotional abuse (yes/no). Binge drinking [16] was evaluated with

the question "During the social distancing period, did you drink 5 or more drinks in a couple of hours?" (yes/no). Tobacco and any illicit drug use during social distancing period were dichotomized into yes/no. Individuals answered about the habit of using alcohol, tobacco and illicit drug during that period (increased, decreased, or the same).

HIV Testing

HIV self-reported status derived from the question "Have you ever had an HIV test?", whose potential answers were positive, negative, or never.

Pre-exposure Prophylaxis (PrEP)

Participants self-reporting HIV negative/unknown status answered if they were using oral PrEP before the issuance of social distancing recommendations. Those on PrEP prior to social distancing answered if they stopped PrEP (no FTC/ TDF refill) after such recommendations and choose the main reason to stop from a selected list of options (including an open field for other reasons). Those who continued using PrEP answered about PrEP regimen (daily, event-driven PrEP, or [ED]-PrEP and other nonstandard regimens). We assessed awareness and intention to use PrEP for those not on PrEP prior to social distancing recommendations. Awareness was defined as a positive answer to the question "Have you ever heard of PrEP?". A brief explanation about PrEP was provided after this question. Intention to use PrEP was defined as the "High interest" answer to the question "Would you be using PrEP currently available at the Brazilian Public Health System (SUS) to prevent HIV?" with a five-point Likert scale as potential answers.

Antiretroviral Therapy (ART)

Participants self-reporting HIV-positive status answered about ART use (yes/no) and the impact of social distancing recommendations on ART refill. Those reporting "yes" also had to select the main reason to stop from pre-existing options (including an open field for other reasons). They rated ART adherence from 0 (missed all ART doses during social distancing period) to 100 (no missing dose). We dichotomized self-reported ART adherence in complete (rating = 100) and poor (rating < 100).

Sexual Behaviour, PrEP Eligibility Criteria and HIV Perceived Risk

Participants self-reporting HIV-negative/unknown status answered questions on sexual behaviour during social distancing period, including sex frequency, steady partner HIV status [HIV-negative, -unknown, -positive with undetectable viral load (VL), -positive with detectable/unknown VL, no steady partner], number of casual partners, condomless receptive anal sex with steady and casual partners, and transactional sex. Sex abstinence was defined as no physical contact with partners. Participants were also asked if the number of casual partners has changed during this period and the main venue used to find them. PrEP eligibility criteria was based on Brazilian recommendations for PrEP use [17] and defined as one of the following during social distancing period: (1) condomless receptive anal sex, (2) sex with HIV-positive partner, and/or (3) transactional sex.

The question "In your opinion, what is your risk of getting HIV during social distancing period?", which had five possible options ("No risk", "Low risk", "Moderate risk/50%", "High risk", and Certain/100%"), assessed the HIV perceived risk. We categorized that variable into three groups: "No risk", "Low risk", and "High risk" (which included the categories "Moderate risk/50%", "High risk" and "Certain/100%"), as previously described [18].

Statistical Analysis

Sociodemographic characteristics and HIV self-reported status were described considering the entire sample. We used chi-square test to compare sexual behaviour, PrEP eligibility criteria and HIV perceived risk between PrEP users during social distancing period (on PrEP vs not on PrEP). We compared social distancing/COVID-19 pandemic impact in personal life, binge drinking and substance use according to gender (cisgender men vs. TGNB) using chi-square or Fisher's exact test when appropriate. Finally, we used logistic regression modelling to assess the factors associated with unattainability of maintaining social distancing. Variables were included in the adjusted model regardless of significant p-value thresholds in univariate analysis. To build the model, race was dichotomized into white/Asian vs. non-white (black/mixed-black/native), and country region was dichotomized into Southeast/South vs. other, following previous study conducted among Brazilian MSM [18]. Analyses were performed using Software R version 4.0.0 [19].

RESULTS

A total of 5490 individuals accessed the questionnaire, 715 (13.0%) did not meet inclusion criteria or did not consent, and 3486 (63.5%) completed it and were included in this analysis (Fig. 1). Median age was 32 years (interquartile range [IQR 27–40]); 505 (14.5%) participants were aged 18–24 years; 61.3% (n = 2137) were recruited on Hornet. The great majority of respondents were cisgender men (3400; 97.5%), self-identified as gay (2961; 84.9%) and lived in the Southeast Brazil (2784; 80.4%). Non-white individuals accounted 44.0% (n = 1534), about a third (1252; 35.9%) had low schooling and 38.0% (n = 1323), low family income.

Social Distancing/COVID-19 Pandemic

About one quarter of participants reported unattainability of maintaining social distancing (917/3486; 26.3%). Most of individuals had high/moderate fear to get infected by COVID-19 (2699; 77.4%), and 72.3% were very worried (scale: 75–100) about close relatives/friends getting infected (2519; 72.3%) Only 61 (1.7%) reported had being infected by COVID-19. Social distancing measures had highly impacted most of participants' lives (2195; 63.0%), and the economic aspect was the most affected (1474; 42.3%). Challenges more frequently reported during social distancing were: salary/job reduced or lost (1575; 45.2%), access to hand sanitizer (1201; 34.5%), and transportation availability (676; 19.4%). Compared to MSM, TGNB individuals had more challenges to access food, hormones, health/mental care, medication refill, and higher frequency of unsafe housing (p < 0.01).

Mental Health and Substance Use

TGNB individuals reported more mental health problems during the social distancing period, access to mental health care, and suicidal thoughts (p < 0.001). Among respondents reporting alcohol use (n = 2181), 29.7% (n = 647) reported an increased use during social distancing period. Almost half of the overall sample reported binge drinking (48.9%, n = 1705/3486), Among tobacco smokers, 49.4% (397/804) increased its use during this period.

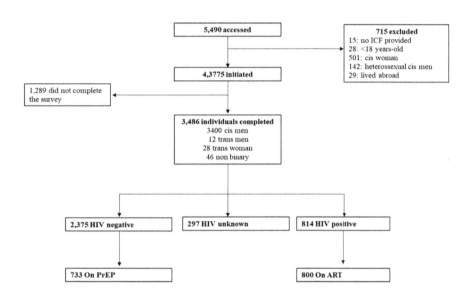

Any illicit drug use was reported by 23.1% (n = 806), and the most common were marijuana (586; 16.8%) and cocaine (233; 6.7%); 30.4% reported increased use of illicit drugs during social distancing period. Comparing to MSM, TGNB people reported more tobacco and illicit drug use (p < 0.001).

HIV Status/PrEP and ART Access During Pandemic

Most respondents reported to be HIV-negative (2375/3486; 68.1%) and 8.5% (n = 297) reported unknown HIV status. Among HIV-negative respondents, 30.9% (n = 733) were on oral PrEP before social distancing recommendations, mostly through the Public Health System (SUS) [PrEP SUS (342/733; 46.7%) and the ImPrEP study (338/733; 46.1%)]. A total of 68.5% (502/733) maintained daily oral PrEP during social distancing period, while 27.8% (204/733) stopped it completely, 1.5% (11/733) used ED-PrEP, and 2.2% (16/733), nonstandard PrEP regimens. Main reasons for stopping PrEP use were: impediments to pick up PrEP refill at the health service (95/204; 46.6%) and sexual abstinence (81/204; 39.7%). Main reasons for continuing PrEP were: fear of HIV infection (327/529; 61.8%), sex with casual partners (90/529; 17.0%), HIV-positive partner (63/529; 11.9%), and belief that PrEP protected against COVID-19 (49/529; 9.3%). The large majority of participants self-reporting HIVpositive status were on ART (800/814; 98.2%), and 18.2% (146/800) reported poor ART adherence during social distancing period.

Only 17.2% (138/800) reported impact of social distancing measures on ART refill; most frequent reasons were: fear of going out (68/138; 49.2%), non-availability of public transportation (29/138; 21.0%), and closing of health care unit (21/138; 15.2%). Considering only those with poor adherence, 37.7% (55/146) reported impact on ART refill.

Sexual Behaviour

The evidence describes sexual behaviour characteristics among HIV-negative/unknown status according to PrEP use during social distancing period. Overall, almost half of participants (1213/2672; 45.4%) reported sex abstinence during social distancing period; among these, 28.8% (349/1213) reported virtual sex. Most of participants reported decreased number of sexual partners during social distancing period. More than three quarters of respondents Brazil, 2020 reported finding casual partners mainly online (779/1012; N = 3486 76.8%). Almost half of individuals who maintained any regimen of PrEP during social distancing period reported having sex (273/529; 51.6%) and, compared to those not on PrEP, more condomless receptive anal sex, number of casual partners and transactional sex (p < 0.001). Almost a quarter of those not on PrEP (23.9%; 513/2143) were eligible for PrEP and 10.5% (n = 225) reported condomless receptive anal sex with casual partner, but only 8.5% (183/2143) reported high HIV perceived risk. Among those who stopped PrEP during the social distancing period, 33.3% (68/204) maintained PrEP eligibility and could have continued its use. Considering those not on PrEP prior to this period, 86.6% were aware of PrEP (1679/1939), and 22.9% (445/1939) had PrEP eligibility, among whom 48.1% (214/445) reported intention to use PrEP.

Factors Associated with Unattainability of Maintaining Social Distancing

Black/*Pardo*/native race (adjusted odds ratio [aOR] 1.23; 95% confidence interval [CI] 1.05–1.44), lower schooling (aOR 1.47; 95% CI 1.23–1.75), lower income (aOR 1.30; 95% CI 1.03–1.66), and binge drinking (aOR 1.28; 95% CI 1.09–1.49) were associated with unattainability of maintaining social distancing in the logistic multivariate analysis. There was no difference in the unattainability of maintaining social distancing according to self-reported HIV status nor gender/sexual orientation.

DISCUSSION

In this study, we have shown that maintaining social distancing is a challenge among MSM and TGNB surveyed. Socioeconomic (low schooling and low income) and racial disparities were associated with unattainability in maintaining social distancing among these groups. Social distancing measures had highly impacted most of participants' lives, and TGNB populations reported more mental health problems and more challenges to access health care than cisgender MSM. Non-white, low schooling, and low income MSM and TGNB had higher odds of unattainability in maintaining social distancing. Our findings reinforce that social and racial inequalities are also of utmost importance among sexual minorities. Brazil is a highly stigmatized, transphobic, and homophobic country [20, 21], and the adverse context surrounding sexual minorities populations in the country may act synergistically with the social disruption linked to the pandemic and disproportionally affect MSM and TGNB. Moreover, despite being the 9th largest economy by nominal Gross Domestic Product (GDP = US$ 1.9 trillion), Brazil is the 9th most unequal country in the world and the 1st in the Americas according to GINI index from The World Bank [22, 23]. Inequality is a major challenge regardless of the population group, and racial disparities, which have been historical since the inception of the country, have now reached one of their worst periods according to some authors [24, 25]. This unfair system forces low income people, mostly of black and *Pardo* race and of lower schooling, to maintain their professional activities, which are frequently informal or unstable, even during social distancing recommendations. For those people, home office and social distancing are not an option [26].

Besides that, Brazilian social policies have been dismantled, and the governmental support during the epidemic is very limited. Recent data has shown that 37% of favela inhabitants who requested the Federal COVID-19 emergency support (US$120 for 3 months) have not received it, although 73% of these families have lost half or the entire family income [27]. The COVID19 pandemic emphasizes the relationship between social/ racial disparities and health outcomes [28], as seen in recent studies conducted in Brazil, which identified that adults with lower schooling presented higher prevalence of risk factors for severe COVID-19 compared to university graduated [29] and that black and *Pardo* populations had higher risk of mortality compared to white Brazilians [30].Sexual behaviour, PrEP eligibility criteria and HIV perceived risk among individuals reporting negative/unknown HIV status according to PrEP use during social distancing period

Social distancing measures had highly impacted sexual minorities, and gender disparities were observed. Challenges related to access to hand sanitizer and economic issues have been equally reported regardless of gender. However, TGNB reports of challenges in accessing health care are worrisome. Transgenders usually face relevant barriers in accessing health care that may be magnified when compared to other groups [31]. In a qualitative study among Brazilian transgender women, past experiences of transgender-identity related discrimination was the most prominent barrier to seek for PrEP or health care in general [32]. Of note, Brazil is the country with the highest rate of murders against transgenders, 118.5 cases per year since 2008 [20].

Our findings on mental health problems, suicidal thoughts and tobacco/illicit drug use, although restricted to this online sample, indicate that social distancing measures may be disproportionally affecting TGNB individuals. Transphobia and stigma may lead to the high rates of mental health problems and substance use among transgender women in Brazil [9, 33], and the COVID-19 pandemic may be an additional burden for this population. In-depth assessments among transgender populations are necessary to better understand such associations. Moreover, online mental health support specific for these populations could be implemented by the Public Health System.

Another concern related to the COVID-19 pandemic relates to HIV vulnerability, access to HIV care and prevention. Although HIV high-risk behavior was more frequent among participants on PrEP compared to those not on PrEP during the social distancing period, almost a quarter of individuals not on PrEP were at substantial HIV risk. Most of respondents continued their medications (PrEP or ART), but an important percentage of people reported barriers to pick up medication refill. Among those reporting impediments to pick up PrEP refill at the health service, 40% (38/95) maintained PrEP eligibility criteria and could have continued its use.

We identified a high percentage of poor ART adherence (20%), considering the short period since social recommendations initiation, which is consistent with ART adherence data before COVID-19 pandemic [34].

People living with HIV in China also reported difficulties to access ART during the COVID-19 pandemic [7]. In Central and Eastern Europe, there have been concerns regarding a shortage of resources and an inevitable impact on HIV care. To avoid PrEP/ART shortage, the Brazilian Ministry of Health has recommended an extension of the PrEP refill dispensation from 90- to 120days and for ART from 90- to 180-days [35]. In addition, telemedicine and HIV self-testing have been used as options to maintain PrEP programs, including in Brazil [36–38]. These and other initiatives such as PrEP/ART home delivery would be essential to avoid medication shortage. Future impacts of COVID-19 pandemic on HIV epidemics are yet to be established.

Our results show that more than half of MSM and TGNB reported sexual activity during social distancing period, although the majority decreased the number of sexual partners. In a large web-based survey conducted among 11,367 MSM in Brazil before COVID pandemic, only 8% reported no sex in previous 6 months [39]. Although the recall time frames used in the surveys are different, this indicates a strong change in sexual behaviour among this population. This is corroborated by the fact that 30% had PrEP eligibility criteria in the present survey, while 70% had the same criteria in the previous survey [39]. Almost half of PrEP users engaged in higher risk behaviours, indicating that health services in Brazil should continue PrEP provision for those populations.

However, some PrEP users were not at substantial HIV risk and could have stopped PrEP. In such cases, ED-PrEP currently recommended by WHO [40] could be an option [17]. Awareness of PrEP among non-PrEP users was higher than previously reported [39, 41–43], showing that efforts of non-governmental, civil society, and projects such as ImPrEP [44] to advertise PrEP information on social media and dating apps have been effective. Conversely, only half of respondents not on PrEP showed interest in using PrEP. This could be explained by the misinformation on PrEP efficacy or side effects [43] and by the fact that daily oral pills may be a regimen not suitable for all individuals. These individuals could be benefited by other prevention technologies on the pipeline, such as long-acting injectable PrEP [45], and by continuous education programs on PrEP.

This study has limitations. First, web-based studies are not probabilistic sampling strategies, precluding the generalization of the findings to all Brazilian MSM and TGNB populations. Moreover, our findings are based on those who have access to cellphones and who use GSN apps or social media, thus they are not generalizable to all MSM and TGNB in Brazil. Nevertheless, recent data show that 85% of Brazilians have mobile phones [46] and 79% have access to internet connection [47]. Also, the cross-sectional study design precludes to infer causality and the direction of association. In addition, we do not have pre-COVID-19 period data for some of the measures. Subsequent surveys are planned to understand sexual behaviour and PrEP use during relaxing of social distancing measures and posCOVID-19 pandemic period in Brazil. Other limitation is that all collected data were self-reported by participants and may be subject to bias.

However, individuals tend to be more open and honest through web-based surveys, thereby reducing social desirability bias [48]. Lastly, other issues specific to LGBTQI + populations (e.g. discrimination, stigma or homonegativity) were not explored in this study.

CONCLUSION

Maintaining social distancing is challenging, particularly for the most vulnerable MSM and TGNB people, likely increasing their risk of acquiring COVID-19. Furthermore, these individuals may also suffer the biggest consequences of the COVID-19 pandemic on the health care system, thus impacting their HIV care and prevention and ultimately the Brazilian HIV epidemic control. Tailored social, economic and mental health support policies during the COVID-19 pandemic should be made available to those individuals. In the context of the COVID-19 pandemic, challenges for PrEP and ART access will demand the implementation of innovative solutions to fulfill the needs of prevention and treatment and avoid the expansion of the HIV epidemic in Brazil.

Acknowledgements This project was made possible, thanks to Unitaid's funding and support. Unitaid accelerates access to innovative health products and lays the foundations for their scale-up by countries and partners. Unitaid is a hosted partnership of the WHO. TST acknowledges funding from the National Council of Technological (CNPq, #28/2018). BG acknowledges funding from the National Council of Technological and Scientific Development and the Research Funding Agency of the State of Rio de Janeiro (Programa Cientista do Nosso Estado; Edital No. 03/2018). This work has been presented as late breaker in a Poster Session at the 23rd International AIDS Conference (AIDS 2020: Virtual), held on 6–10 July 2020.

REFERENCES

1. WHO. WHO Timeline - COVID-19. https ://www.who.int/newsroom/detai l/27-04-2020-who-timel ine-covid -19. Accessed 4 Jun 2020.
2. Brasil. Painel Coronavírus. 2020. https ://covid .saude .gov.br/. Accessed 30 July 2020.
3. The Lancet. COVID-19 in Brazil: "So what?". Lancet. 2020;395(10235):1461.
4. Agência Brasil. Brasil tem 13,6 milhões de pessoas morando em comunidades. https: //agenciabras il.ebc.com.br/gera l/notici a/2020 01/morad ores-de-favel as-movim entam -r-1198-bilho es-por-ano. Accessed 3 Jun 2020.
5. IBGE. Pesquisa Nacional por Amostra de Domicílios Contínua - PNAD Contínua. 2020. https ://www.ibge.gov.br/es-tat istic as/ socia is/traba lho/9173-pesqu isa-nacio nal-por-amost ra-de-domic ilios -conti nua-trime stral .html?=&t=resul tados .
6. Anadolu Agency. COVID-19 triggers massive unemployment in Latin America. 2020. https ://www.aa.com.tr/en/ameri cas/covid -19-trigg ers-massi ve-unemp loyme nt-in-latin -ameri ca/18250 29.
7. Jiang H, Zhou Y, Tang W. Maintaining HIV care during the COVID-19 pandemic. Lancet HIV. 2020;7:e308.
8. UNAIDS. UNAIDS data 2019 [Internet]. 2019. https: //www.unaid s.org/sites/ default/files/ medi a_asset/ 2019-UNAI DS-data_en.pd f. Accessed 24 Apr 2020.
9. Grinsztejn B, Jalil EM, Monteiro L, Velasque L, Moreira RI, Garcia ACF, et al. Unveiling of HIV dynamics among transgender women: a respondent-driven sampling study in Rio de Janeiro, Brazil. Lancet HIV. 2017;4(4):e169–e176176.
10. Kerr L, Kendall C, Guimarães MDC, Salani Mota R, Veras MA, Dourado I, et al. HIV prevalence among men who have sex with men in Brazil: results of the 2nd national survey using respondentdriven sampling. Medicine. 2018;97:S9–15.
11. De Boni R, Veloso VG, Grinsztejn B. Epidemiology of HIV in Latin America and the Caribbean. Curr Opin HIV AIDS. 2014;9(2):192–8.
12. Luz PM, Veloso VG, Grinsztejn B. The HIV epidemic in Latin America: accomplishments and challenges on treatment and prevention. Curr Opin HIV AIDS. 2019;14(5):366–73.
13. Galea JT, Baruch R, Brown B. ¡PrEP Ya! Latin America wants PrEP, and Brazil leads the way. Lancet HIV. 2018;5(3):e110–e11212.
14. WHO. Brazil begins PrEP roll-out on World AIDS Day [Internet]. World Health Organization. 2017. Available from: https ://www. who.int/hiv/media centr e/news/brazi l-prep/en/. Accessed 29 Oct 2018.
15. Jalil EM, Wilson EC, Luz PM, Velasque L, Moreira RI, Castro CV, et al. HIV testing and the care continuum among transgender women: population estimates from Rio de Janeiro, Brazil. J Int AIDS Soc. 2017;20(1):21873.
16. National Institute on Alcohol Abuse and Alcoholism (NIAAA), Abuse and Alcoholism (NIAAA). NIAAA approves definition of binge drinking [Internet]. 2004. https ://pubs.niaaa .nih.gov/publi catio ns/Newsl etter /winte r2004 /Newsl etter _Numbe r3.pdf
17. Brasil, Ministério da Saúde. Protocolo Clínico e Diretrizes Terapêuticas para Profilaxia Pré-Exposição (PrEP) de Risco à Infecção pelo HIV [Internet]. 2018. https ://www.aids.gov.br/ pt-br/pub/2017/proto colo-clini co-e-diret rizes -terap eutic as-paraprofi laxia -pre-expos icao-prep-de-risco

18. Torres TS, Marins LMS, Veloso VG, Grinsztejn B, Luz PM. How heterogeneous are MSM from Brazilian cities? An analysis of sexual behavior and perceived risk and a description of trends in awareness and willingness to use pre-exposure prophylaxis. BMC Infect Dis. 2019;19(1):1067.

19. The R Project for Statistical Computing. [cited 2020 May 26]. Available from: https ://www.r-proje ct.org/

20. Benevides BG, Nogueira SNB. Dossiê assassinatos contra travestis brasileiras e violência e transexuais em 2019 [Internet]. 2020. https ://antra brasi l.files .wordp ress.com/2020/01/dossi c3aa-dosassas sinat os-e-da-violc 3aanc ia-contr a-pesso as-trans -em-2019. pdf. Accessed 11 Jun 2020.

21. Grupo Gay Bahia. RELATÓRIOS ANUAIS DE MORTES LGBTI+ [Internet]. https ://grupo gayda bahia .com.br/relat orios -anuai s-de-morte -de-lgbti /. Accessed 4 May 2020.

22. The world bank. GINI index (World Bank estimate) [Internet]. https ://data.world bank.org/indic ator/SI.POV.GINI?most_recen t_value _desc=true

23. UNITED NATIONS ECONOMIC COMMISSION FOR LATIN AMERICA AND THE CARIBBEAN. SOCIAL PANORAMA OF LATIN AMERICA 2019. [Internet]. 2020. https: //www.cepal .org/en/public ations/44989- soci al-panora ma-lati n- americ a-2019. Accessed 4 Jun 2020.

24. Brasil de Fato. "We're living one of the worst moments of Brazilian racism," writer says [Internet]. https: //www.brasildefat o.com . br/2019/05/13/were-livin g-one-of-the-worst -momen ts-of-brazi lian-racis m-write r-says. Accessed 17 Jul 2020.

25. United Nations. Racial Discrimination and Miscegenation: The Experience in Brazil [Internet]. Racial Discrimination and Miscegenation: The Experience in Brazil. https: //www.un.org/en/chron icle/artic le/racia l-discr imina tion-and-misce genat ion-exper ience -brazi l. Accessed 17 Jul 2020.

26. DW Brasil. Epidemia de coronavírus expõe vulnerabilidades da "uberização" [Internet]. https: //www.dw.com/pt-br/epidemia-de-coron av%C3%ADrus -exp%C3%B5e-vulne rabil idade s-da-uberi za%C3%A7%C3%A3o/a-52830 974. Accessed 11 Jun 2020.

27. UOL. 3,9 milhões das famílias mais ricas recebem auxílio de R$ 600, diz pesquisa. [Internet]. https ://econo mia.uol.com.br/notic ias/redac ao/2020/06/03/pesqu isa-insti tuto-locom otiva -auxil ioemerg encia l.htm. Accessed 4 Jun 2020.

28. Bilal U, Alazraqui M, Caiaffa WT, Lopez-Olmedo N, Martinez-Folgar K, Miranda JJ, et al. Inequalities in life expectancy in six large Latin American cities from the SALURBAL study: an ecological analysis. Lancet Planetary Health. 2019;3(12):e503–e510510.

29. Rezende LFM, Thome B, Schveitzer MC, de Souza-Júnior PRB, Szwarcwald CL. Adults at high-risk of severe coronavirus disease-2019 (COVID-19) in Brazil. Rev Saude Publica. 2020;54:50.

30. Baqui P, Bica I, Marra V, Ercole A, van der Schaar M. Ethnic and regional variations in hospital mortality from COVID-19 in Brazil: a cross-sectional observational study. Lancet Glob Health. 2020;8:e1018.

31. Safer JD, Coleman E, Feldman J, Garofalo R, Hembree W, Radix A, et al. Barriers to healthcare for transgender individuals. Curr Opin Endocrinol Diab Obes. 2016;23(2):168–71.

32. Wilson EC, Jalil EM, Castro C, Martinez Fernandez N, Kamel L, Grinsztejn B. Barriers and facilitators to PrEP for transwomen in Brazil. Glob Public Health. 2019;14(2):300–8.

33. Garcia Ferreira AC, Esteves Coelho L, Jalil EM, Luz PM, Friedman RK, Guimarães MRC, et al. Transcendendo: a cohort study of HIV-infected and uninfected transgender women in Rio de Janeiro, Brazil. Transgender Health. 2019;4(1):107–17.

34. de Costa M, Torres TS, Coelho LE, Luz PM. Adherence to antiretroviral therapy for HIV/AIDS in Latin America and the Caribbean: Systematic review and meta-analysis. J Intern AIDS Soc. 2018;21(1):e25066.

35. Ministério da Saúde. OFÍCIO CIRCULARNº 8/2020/CGAHV/. DCCI/SVS/MS [Internet]. 2020. https ://www.aids.gov.br/pt-br/ legis lacao /ofici o-circu lar-no-82020 cgahv dccis vsms

36. Barney A, Buckelew S, Mesheriakova V, Raymond-Flesch M. The COVID-19 pandemic and rapid implementation of adolescent and young adult telemedicine: challenges and opportunities for innovation. J Adolesc Health. 2020. https: //doi.org/10.1016/j. jadoh ealth .2020.05.006.

37. Hoagland B, Torres TS, Bezerra DRB, Geraldo K, Pimenta C, Veloso VG, et al. Telemedicine as a tool for PrEP delivery during the COVID-19 pandemic in a large HIV prevention service in Rio de Janeiro-Brazil. Braz J Infect Dis. 2020. https ://doi. org/10.1016/j.bjid.2020.05.004.

38. Dourado I, Magno L, Soares F, Massa P, Nunn A, et al. Adapting to the COVID-19 pandemic: continuing HIV prevention services for adolescents through telemonitoring, Brazil. AIDS Behav. 2020;24:1994.

39. Torres TS, Luz PM, De Boni RB, de Vasconcellos MTL, Hoagland B, Garner A, et al. Factors associated with PrEP awareness according to age and willingness to use HIV prevention technologies: the 2017 online survey among MSM in Brazil. AIDS Care. 2019;31(10):1193–202.

40. WHO. What's the 2+1+1? Event-driven oral pre-exposure prophylaxis to prevent HIV for men who have sex with men: Update to WHO's recommendation on oral PrEP. https ://www.who.int/hiv/ pub/prep/211/en/. Accessed 4 Jun 2020 Jun 4.

41. Torres TS, De Boni RB, de Vasconcellos MT, Luz PM, Hoagland B, Moreira RI, et al. Awareness of prevention strategies and willingness to use preexposure prophylaxis in Brazilian men who have sex with men using apps for sexual encounters: online cross-sectional study. JMIR Public Health Surveill. 2018;4(1):e11.

42. Hoagland B, De Boni RB, Moreira RI, Madruga JV, Kallas EG, et al. Awareness and willingness to use pre-exposure prophylaxis (PrEP) among men who have sex with men and transgender women in Brazil. AIDS Behav. 2017;21(5):1278–87.

43. Torres TS, Konda KA, Vega-Ramirez EH, Elorreaga OA, DiazSosa D, Hoagland B, et al. Factors associated with willingness to use pre-exposure prophylaxis in Brazil, Mexico, and Peru: webbased survey among men who have sex with men. JMIR Public Health Surveill. 2019;5(2):e13771.

44. ImPrEP study team. ImPrEP Facebook fanpage [Internet]. 2020.

45. Coelho LE, Torres TS, Veloso VG, Landovitz RJ, Grinsztejn B. Pre-exposure prophylaxis 20: new drugs and technologies in the pipeline. Lancet HIV. 2019;6(11):e788–e799799.

46. Comitê Gestor da Internet no Brasil (CGIBR). J2 - INDIVÍDUOS QUE POSSUEM TELEFONE CELULAR 2019 [Internet]. 2020.

47. Comitê Gestor da Internet no Brasil (CGIBR). C2A - USUÁRIOS DE INTERNET - INDICADOR AMPLIADO 2019 [Internet]. 2019. https ://cetic .br/pt/tics/domic ilios /2019/indiv iduos /C2A/. Accessed 4 Jun 2020.

48. Heerwegh D. Mode differences between face-to-face and web surveys: an experimental investigation of data quality and social desirability effects. Int J Public Opin Res. 2009;21(1):111–21.

CHAPTER 13

THE BIRTH OF BRAZILIAN COVID-19 MATERNAL CRISIS

Table 2 The Thematic Analysis

Phases of the Thematic Analysis	Description	Means of stablishing trustworthiness
Phase 1: Familiarizing yourself with data	Phase in which the researchers are familiarized with the depth and breadth of the available data (interviews transcripts and field diary). The process of creating initial ideas about the data begins.	- Prolonged involvement with the data - Triangulation of different types of qualitative data - Documentation of reflective and theoretical thoughts - Documentation of potential codes and themes - Storage of raw data in organized files - Keep records of field diaries, transcripts, and scientific articles
Phase 2: Generating initial codes	Production of initial codes, a theorizing activity that requires researchers to revisit the data constantly. The codes will index important sections of the text, using software such as NVivo.	- Peer debriefing - Reflective diary on data analysis - Structuring the coding process - Review of produced codes - Documentation of all meetings with researchers
Phase 3: Searching for themes	Production of themes that will unite the codes, bringing meaning and identity to the data according to the research question.	- Discussion or triangulation with researchers - Layout to give meaning to the text (use of maps, flowcharts, etc.) - Keep detailed notes on the development of hierarchical themes and concepts
Phase 4: Reviewing themes	Refining the themes to check if there is a coherent standardization, according to the entire data. It is possible to return to the raw data and produce new codes that were not covered in the previous phases.	- Discussion or triangulation with researchers - Approval of themes and sub-themes by team researchers - Referential suitability test through the return to raw data
Phase 5: Defining and naming themes	The researchers determine which aspect of the data each theme captures and identify what is interesting about it and why.	- Discussion or triangulation with researchers - Team consensus on topics - Documentation of team meetings on the topics - Documentation of the theme naming process
Phase 6: Producing the report	When the themes are already defined, it is possible to complete the final analysis. Provide a concise, coherent, logical, non-repetitive, and interesting description of the data within and between themes	- Discussion with researchers - Describe the coding and analysis process in sufficient detail - Detailed context descriptions - Description of the audit process - Report on the reasons for the theoretical, methodological and analytical choices throughout the study

DISCUSSION

This study will shine light on the lived experience of women infected by the COVID-19 during pregnancy. We have not found other studies adopting this approach, and the results will make valuable contributions to health care services and policy, especially for understanding the personal context, the immediate social context, and the expanded social context influencing the feelings of this women. This is important due to the relevance of the COVID-19 pandemic and may offer insights for health professionals and police makers.

Abbreviations
SARS-CoV-2: Severe acute respiratory syndrome-novel coronavirus; COVID19: Coronavirus

Authors' contributions
All authors contributed to the overall study design and specific methodologies. All authors approved the final version for submission.

Funding
The authors JVFJ and LR received doctoral scholarships by the Coordenação de Aperfeiçoamento de Pessoal de Nível Superior - Brasil (CAPES). The protocol was not peer reviewed.
Availability of data and materials Not applicable.

Ethics approval and consent to participate
The Declaration of Helsinki and Resolution 466/12 of the National Health Council are being followed. Women who are 18 years old or more will be invited to the study and will be included after reading the consent form. The researcher will explain the consent form and will inform them that they can withdraw from the study without any harm or loss. The study data will be used for the sole purpose of this study, and a commitment will be made to maintain confidentiality as to the identity of the interviewees in the disclosure of the data. This study was approved by the Ethics and Research Commission of UNICAMP under the number CAAE: 30721120.8.0000.5404.

Author details
1
 Postgraduate Program in Obstetrics and Gynecology, School of Medical Sciences, University of Campinas, Campinas, Brazil. 2Department of Obstetrics and Gynecology, School of Medical Science, University of Campinas, Av. Alexander Fleming, 101, Campinas, SP, Brazil.

REFERENCES

1. Zhu N, Zhang D, Wang W, Li X, Yang B, Song J, et al.(2019)A novel coronavirus from patients with pneumonia in China, 2019. N Engl J Med. 2020;382(8): 727–33. Cited 2020 Mar 30. Available from. https://doi.org/10.1056/NEJMoa2001017.
2. Huang C, Wang Y, Li X, Ren L, Zhao J, Hu Y, et al. Clinical features of patients infected with 2019 novel coronavirus in Wuhan, China. Lancet. 2020;395(10223):497–506.
3. World Health Organization. Coronavirus disease (COVID-19) Situation Report-123. 2020. Available from: https://www.icao.int/Security/COVID-19/ EBandSL/eb027e.pdf. Cited 2020 May 23.
4. Lauer SA, Grantz KH, Bi Q, Jones FK, Zheng Q, Meredith HR, et al.(2020). The

Incubation Period of Coronavirus Disease 2019 (COVID-19) From Publicly Reported Confirmed Cases: Estimation and Application. 2020; Available from: https://zenodo.org/record/3692048. Cited 2020 Apr 18.

5. Kucharski AJ, Russell TW, Diamond C, Liu Y, Edmunds J, Funk S, et al. (2020).Early dynamics of transmission and control of COVID-19: a mathematical modelling study. Lancet Infect Dis. 2020;20(5):553–8.

6. Rothan, H.A., Byrareddy, S.N. (2020).The epidemiology and pathogenesis of coronavirus disease (COVID-19) outbreak. 2020. Available from: www. elsevier.com/locate/jautimm. Cited 2020 Apr 18.

7. Zhou F, Yu T, Du R, Fan G, Liu Y, Liu Z, et al. Articles Clinical course and risk factors for mortality of adult inpatients with COVID-19 in Wuhan, China: a retrospective cohort study. Lancet. 2020;395. Cited 2020 Apr 18. Available from. https://doi.org/10.1016/S0140-6736(20)30566-3 www.thelancet.com.

8. Fang L, Karakiulakis G, Roth M. (2020).Are patients with hypertension and diabetes mellitus at increased risk for COVID-19 infection? Lancet Respir. 2020;8:e21. Cited 2020 Apr 18. Available from. https://doi.org/10.1016/S22132600(20)30116-8.

9. Sanders, J.M., Monogue, M.L Jodlowski, .TZ, Cutrell. J.B. (2020).Pharmacologic Treatments for Coronavirus Disease 2019 (COVID-19): A Review. JAMA. 2020; Available from: http://www.ncbi.nlm.nih.gov/pubmed/32282022. Cited 2020 Apr 18.

10. Rasmussen, S.A., Smulian, J.C, Lednicky, J.A, Wen, T.S, Jamieson, D.J..(2019).Coronavirus Disease 2019 (COVID-19) and Pregnancy: What obstetricians need to know. Am J Obstet Gynecol. 2020; Cited 2020 Mar 30. Available from. https://doi. org/10.1016/j.ajog.2020.02.017.

11. Dotters-Katz SK, Hughes BL. Considerations for Obstetric Care during the COVID-19 Pandemic. Am J Perinatol. 2020; Available from: http://www.ncbi. nlm.nih.gov/pubmed/32303077.

12. Larson, H.J. (2018).The biggest pandemic risk? Viral misinformation. Nature. 2018; 562:309 Nature Publishing Group.

13. Lancet, T.. (2020). COVID-19: fighting panic with information. 2020; Available from: www.ny-times.com/2020/02/15/. Cited 2020 Apr 18.

14. Depoux A, Martin S, Karafillakis E, Preet R, Wilder-Smith A, Larson H. The pandemic of social media panic travels faster than the COVID-19 outbreak. J Travel Med. 2020;27(3):taaa031.

15. Chattu, V.K., Yaya, S.. (2020). Emerging infectious diseases and outbreaks: implications for women's reproductive health and rights in resource-poor settings. Reprod Health. 2020;17(1):1–5.

16. WHO | Maternal mental health. Available from: https://www.who.int/mental_ health/maternal-child/maternal_mental_health/en/. Cited 2020 Mar 30.

17. Tong, A., Sainsbury, P., Craig, J., (2007).Consolidated criteria for reporting qualitative research (COREQ): a 32-item checklist for interviews and focus groups. Int J Qual Heal Care. 2007;19(6):349–57 Available from: http://www.ncbi.nlm.nih. gov/pubmed/17872937. Cited 2018 Mar 25.

18. Glaser, B., Strauss, A. (199). The discovery of grounded theory: strategies for qualitative research. Aldine Transaction: New Brunswick; 1999.

19. Nowell, L.S., Norris, J.M., White, D.E., Moules, N.J. (2017).Thematic analysis : striving to meet the trustworthiness criteria. Int J Qual Methods. 2017;16:1–13.

20. Shenton, A.K. (2004). Strategies for ensuring trustworthiness in qualitative research projects. Educ Inf. 2004;22:63–75.

1. Expert Recommendations For The Care Of Newborns Of Mothers With COVID-19[1]

Werther Brunow de Carvalho,[I,*]
Maria Augusta Bento Cicaroni Gibelli,[II]
Vera Lucia Jornada Krebs,[II,III]
Valdenise Martins Laurindo Tuma Calil,[II]
Cíntia Johnston[I2]

ABSTRACT

This article presents expert recommendations for assisting new-born children of mothers with suspected or diagnosed coronavirus disease 2019 (COVID-19). The consensus was developed by five experts with an average of 20 years of experience in neonatal intensive care working at a reference university hospital in Brazil for the care of pregnant women and new-borns with suspected or confirmed COVID-19. Despite the lack of scientific evidence regarding the potential for viral transmission to their foetus in pregnant mothers diagnosed with or suspected of COVID-19, it is important to elaborate the lines of care by specialists from hospitals caring for suspected and confirmed COVID-19 cases to guide multidisciplinary teams and families diagnosed with the disease or involved in the care of pregnant women and new-borns in this context. Multidisciplinary teams must be attentive to the signs and symptoms of COVID-19 so that decision-making is oriented and assertive for the management of the mother and new-born in both the hospital setting and at hospital discharge.

INTRODUCTION

To date, the impact of coronavirus disease 2019 (COVID-19), the disease caused by infection by severe acute respiratory syndrome coronavirus 2 (SARS-CoV-2) during pregnancy is not fully known. Although there remains no evidence of transplacental transmission of the virus, this possibility may exist [1-7]. In this context, it is necessary to determine the likely mechanisms of contamination of the foetus, such as maternal fluids and intrapartum, as well as neonatal factors that may influence the perinatal transmission of the virus [8]. The clinical signs and symptoms, results of laboratory tests, and chest tomography findings of nine pregnant women with COVID-19 pneumonia in Wuhan-China were recently described [9]. These women were diagnosed based on oral swabs positive for SARS-CoV-2.

[1] Clinics (Sao Paulo). 2020; 75: e1932.
[2] Terapia Intensiva em Neonatologia/Pediatria, Departamento de Pediatria, Faculdade de Medicina (FMUSP), Universidade de Sao Paulo, Sao Paulo, SP, BR
IICentro Neonatal e Terapia Intensiva Neonatal, Instituto da Crianca e do Adolescente (ICr), Hospital das Clinicas HCFMUSP, Faculdade de Medicina, Universidade de Sao Paulo, Sao Paulo, SP, BR
IIICurso de Pos-Graduacao, Departamento de Pediatria, Faculdade de Medicina (FMUSP), Universidade de Sao Paulo, Sao Paulo, SP, BR*Corresponding author. E-mail: rb.psu.mf.ch@wonurb.rehtrew

Vertical intrauterine transmission was investigated by testing amniotic fluid, cord blood, and oral swabs from the new-borns as well as breast milk, all of which were negative for the presence of the virus in all mothers and their new-borns. Premature birth occurs in an estimated 47% of pregnant women with confirmed COVID-19. Among 19 neonates of mothers positive for COVID-19, delivery occurred up to 13 days after disease onset. In new-borns born to mothers with COVID-19, the clinical findings ranged from asymptomatic to manifestations such as respiratory distress requiring ventilatory support, disseminated intravascular coagulation, multiple organ dysfunction, and shock. Despite the presence of signs and symptoms in the mothers, these new-borns were negative for COVID-19 [4].Fan et al. [5] reported two cases of COVID-19 in the third trimester of pregnancy.

The mothers and their new-borns showed good clinical evolution. The virus was not detected in breast milk or in swabs or serological samples from the new-borns. The authors concluded that the risk of infection by vertical transmission of SARS-CoV-2 was low. Another case report [10] presented a preterm new-born (gestational age 30 weeks) whose mother was symptomatic with a positive swab for COVID-19 2 days before delivery. Oral swabs and faeces from the new-born tested negative for coronavirus on the third, seventh, and ninth days after birth. Hong et al. [10] proposed the presence of at least one of following clinical signs or symptoms as criteria for the neonatal diagnosis of COVID-2: thermal instability, hypoactivity, feeding difficulty, respiratory distress, chest X-ray with changes (including single or bilateral ground-glass patterns), COVID-19 diagnosis in family or caregiver of the new-born, intimate contact with people with suspected or confirmed COVID-19, or patients with unclear pneumonia. Based on the reports in the literature so far on the subject, as well as on the expertise of the authors, the objective of this article was to present expert recommendations for assisting the new-born children of mothers with suspected or diagnosed COVID-19.

RECOMMENDATIONS FOR NEONATAL CARE
Personal Protective Equipment (PPE) and Insulation Precautions

SARS-CoV-2 is a respiratory virus transmitted person-to-person mainly by respiratory droplets. The infection is mediated by virus present in the respiratory secretions of an infected person that meet the mucous membranes of another person. High-risk exposure is defined as a person with COVID-19 disease requiring direct physical or close contact (<1.8 meters) for an extended time. It is recommended that precautions be taken to prevent droplets and contact, during contact between new-borns and their mothers with COVID-19 through the use of PPE including aprons, gloves, surgical masks, and eye protection (goggles or face protector) [8],. Contact and droplet precautions are recommended in situations that could generate aerosols; these precautions include the use of PPE such as aprons, gloves, N95 or PFF2 masks, and eye protection (glasses or face protector). Consideration of the potential for generating aerosols is recommended, including bag-mask ventilation, tracheal intubation, airway aspiration, tracheal extubating, high-flow nasal oxygen therapy (oxygen flow greater than 2 litres per minute/kg), and non-invasive ventilation (continuous positive airway pressure [CPAP] or bilevel) [20,21].

Assistance in the Delivery Room

Following the normal routine assistance for new-born's is recommended in the delivery room according to the hospital. During new born resuscitation, multidisciplinary teams must be fitted with

PPE as a precaution against transmission by air, droplets, and contact due to the increased probability of aerosols with maternal viruses and the potential need for tracheal intubation, airway aspiration, and ventilation with positive pressure, which can also generate aerosols for the new-born.

Recommendations for the Care of Pregnant Women

a. Collect COVID-19 samples from pregnant women in lab or with suspected COVID-19 or with disease confirmation in the 14 days preceding labour.

b. Suspend skin-to-skin contact between the mother and newborn in cases of symptomatic parturient or those with home contact with a person with flu-like symptoms or positive for COVID-19.

c. After the birth, refer the puerperal woman to the inpatient sector for the suspected and confirmed patients of COVID-19.

Recommendations for Newborn Care

a. Newborns should be resuscitated under radiant heat in the delivery room.

b. The multidisciplinary team in contact with the newborn must wear PPE (N95 or PFF2 masks, glasses and face protectors, waterproof aprons, and sterile gloves and caps).

c. In cases of new borns with respiratory distress, treatment must follow the assistance routines of each service.

Newborn Transport and ICU Admission

It is recommended that all new-borns of pregnant women in labour with suspicion or confirmed COVID-19 in the 14 days preceding labour be transported in a heated incubator from the delivery room to the neonatal centre or neonatal intensive care unit (ICU) and admitted to an isolation room. The following steps are recommended for the dressing and undressing of the transport team:

a. Wear all garments until arrival at the neonatal ICU.

b. If individual rooms with negative pressure are available, the hospitalization of new-born's positive for COVID-19 should be prioritized.

c. Remove gloves and aprons in the patient's room and caps, glasses, and masks in the anteroom.

New-borns requiring intensive care should ideally be admitted to an isolation room with the potential for negative ambient pressure or other available air filtration systems. If this feature is not available, cribs or incubators should be kept at a minimum distance of 1.5 meters. For new-born's with indications for non-invasive ventilation (CPAP or bilevel), high-flow oxygen therapy, or invasive mechanical ventilation, precautions should be taken to avoid aerosols, droplets, and contact thought the use of PPEs recommended for this purpose.

Care in the Neonatal Centre and Clinical Evaluation of Newborns

The following routine care is recommended for new-born's upon arrival to the Neonatal Centre based on the infant's clinical condition and COVID-19 severity:

a) Asymptomatic new-born's and mothers negative for COVID-19

- If the puerperal woman is clinically well, she can receive the newborn in the Joint Accommodation (JA); at discharge, they should be referred to the basic health unit to receive routine guidance.

b) Asymptomatic new-born's awaiting the mother's COVID-19 test results

- The new-born must be kept in the isolation sector to prevent contact and droplets and should be bathed immediately after birth to remove viruses potentially present on the skin surface.

- The multidisciplinary team must use precautions against droplets and close contact.

- The mother will be able to receive the new-born at the JA after being instructed on cough etiquette, hand hygiene, use of a surgical mask for new-born routines and breastfeeding, maintaining a distance of at least 1.8 meters between the new-born's crib and the postpartum bed. Breastfeeding should be started as soon as possible after hygiene care and measures to prevent contamination of the newborn.

- The maintenance of a single (regular) companion is recommended, provided that he or she is asymptomatic and does not have home contact with a person with flu-like symptoms or positive for COVID-19, in places that promote distance between hospitalized patients or with private accommodation.

- Routine newborn care: 1st day: vaccination against hepatitis B and vitamin K injection; 2nd day: red reflex and otoacoustic emission, tongue; pulse oximetry, and neonatal screening tests with 48 hours of birth.

- For mothers positive for COVID-19: the indications for testing of asymptomatic new-borns are evaluated on a case-by-case analysis.

- At hospital discharge, the person responsible for the new-born should receive guidance on home isolation care and warning signs. Social services must provide a support network including a family member or guardian (wearing a surgical mask) at the time of discharge who can provide home new-born care for mothers under investigation or positive for COVID-19.

c) Symptomatic new-borns

Recommendations for the care of new-borns with acute ventilatory failure:

- Intern in an isolation room.

- COVID-19 investigation.

- Among diagnostic hypotheses, consider COVID-19 infection.

- Start treatment according to the service's protocol.

- Multidisciplinary team wearing PPE to protect against aerosols and contact.

- Departmentation: removal of gloves and apron in the patient's room and removal of caps, glasses, and mask in that order in the anteroom before entering the hall.

The risk of postnatal infection in the immediate postpartum period due to mother-new-born contact has not yet been established. Temporary separation of the mother from her newborn will minimize the risk of postnatal infection from maternal respiratory secretions. The likely benefits of this temporary separation to decrease the risk of neonatal infection should be discussed with the mother, preferably before delivery.

Breastfeeding

The presence of coronavirus in breast milk has not yet been demonstrated. Mothers can express breast milk (after hand and breast hygiene), which can be offered to the newborn by caregivers. Pumps and accessories must be thoroughly cleaned according to the standard measures of the breast milk banks, which must include cleaning the pump with disinfectant wipes and washing the accessories with hot water and soap. In addition to the known benefits of breastfeeding, mothers' milk can provide infant protection factors after maternal SARS-CoV-2 infection.

Viral Testing of the Newborn

If available, molecular tests for SARS-CoV-2 infection should also be performed in new-borns. This strategy can facilitate care planning after hospital discharge and contribute to the understanding of viral transmission. If the test is not readily available or there is a shortage, clinicians may choose to perform only clinical monitoring. New-borns requiring care in the intensive care unit should be tested to determine the potential contribution of COVID-19 to the observed clinical disease. The testing of new-born's in the intensive care unit will allow scheduling of discontinuation of contact precautions (droplets and aerosols) for negative results.

The need for testing and the ideal time for testing has not yet been established. Viral detection data are limited. The following are recommended to distinguish transient viral colonization from established infection:

- The first molecular test must be carried out within approximately 24 hours of birth.

- The test should be repeated with approximately 48 hours after birth. For new-born's in good general condition who will be discharged within 48 hours of birth, this test may not be performed. However, the possibility of new-born's with negative results within 24 hours of birth becoming positive within 48 to 72 hours of birth cannot be ruled out.

- New-borns requiring hospitalization can be transitioned to the use of precautions (contact/droplets/aerosols) following two negative test results at least 24 hours apart. For neonates with positive initial CRP test results, follow-up tests should be performed at intervals of 48 to 72 hours until two consecutive negative results are obtained.

Maternal and Family Visits to Hospitalized Newborns

Symptomatic mothers or fathers or those who have had home contact with individuals with influenza syndrome or positive for COVID-19 should not visit hospitalized new-born's until they become asymptomatic and the period of COVID-19 transmissibility has passed (approximately 14 days). Daily screening for respiratory symptoms and flu syndrome is recommended for fathers and mothers visiting new-borns. In cases in which the father or mother cannot stay, the family may designate an asymptomatic substitute without home contact with an individual with flu syndrome or positive for COVID-19.

Newborn Hospital Discharge

New-borns should be discharged according to the criteria of each hospital and avoiding the use of public transport. Social visits at home to the mother and newborn should be suspended. The following situations are recommended to be considered:

- Asymptomatic newborn with no results or no tests for COVID-19: can be discharged home with due precautions and outpatient monitoring by phone or telemedicine for up to 14 days after birth. Guidance on the use of gloves and hand hygiene should be provided to family members and caregivers. Uninfected individuals over 60 years of age and with comorbidities should not care for the newborn.

- New-borns with negative molecular tests for COVID should be discharged from the care of an uninfected caregiver. If the mother is in the same house, she should keep a distance of at least 1.8 m for as long as possible. When the mother is closest to the Newborn, she should wear a surgical or tissue mask and frequently perform hand hygiene. The distance between the mother and the Newborn must be maintained until negative COVID-19 results are obtained for at least two consecutive nasopharyngeal swab samples collected at an interval of ≥24 hours.

- Caregivers under observation for the development of COVID-19 should wear masks and perform hand hygiene until their test results are known.

- Frequent outpatient follow-up by telephone or telemedicine or face-to-face assessments up to 14 days after hospital discharge are recommended for New borns positive for COVID-19 or at risk of postnatal coronavirus infection who are unable to be tested.

At the time of hospital discharge, mothers should be educated on the warning signs of illness in her Newborn; namely:

1. Fever;
2. Poor feeding or vomiting or bloating;
3. Lethargy, drowsiness;
4. Breathing difficulty, groaning;
5. Worsening jaundice intensity;
6. Decreased diuresis;
7. Pallor;
8. Cyanosis.

In the presence of any of the above clinical signs, the following are recommended:
a. Identify the Health facility closest to the residence.
b. If positive for COVID-19: use a mask and inform the health professional who provides care to the family.
c. If the mother still does not have her COVID-19 screening results, advise her to contact the hospital by phone.

Recommendations For Home Isolation Of Mothers Positive Or Under Investigation For COVID-19

- Maintain breastfeeding as long as the mother desires and is in adequate condition;

- Educate the mother regarding precautions for the prevention of virus transmission (contact/droplets/aerosols) during contact with the infant, including breastfeeding, such as: washing hands for at least 20 seconds before touching the New born and before removing breastmilk (by hand or pump); wearing a face mask (completely covering the nose and mouth) while breastfeeding; avoiding talking or coughing while breastfeeding; and changing the mask immediately in case of coughing or sneezing or with each breastfeeding;

- Strictly follow the recommendations for cleaning breast pumps after each use.

- Consideration should be given to requesting the help of a person without evidence of viral infection to offer the Newborn breast milk in a cup, cup, or spoon (this person must learn how to do this task with help from a health professional).

CONCLUSIONS

Despite the lack of scientific evidence regarding the potential viral transmission to their foetus by pregnant women with suspected or positive for COVID-19, multidisciplinary teams must be attentive to the disease signs and symptoms for guided and assertive decision making in the management of both mothers and Newborns in the hospital environment and discharge.

REFERENCES

1. Lu Q, Shi Y. J Med Virol. (2020). Coronavirus disease (COVID-19) and neonate: What neonatologist need to know.
2. Chen, D. Yang, H., Cao, Y., Cheng, W., Duan, T., Fan, C., et al. (2020) Expert consensus for managing pregnant women and neonates born to mothers with suspected or confirmed novel coronavirus (COVID-19) infection. Int J Gynaecol Obstet. 2020;149((2)):130–6. doi: 10.1002/ijgo.13146.
3. Chen, Y. Peng, H., Wang, L., Zhao, Y., Zeng, L., Gao, H., et al. (2020) Infants Born to Mothers With a New Coronavirus (COVID-19) Front Pediatr. 2020;8:104. doi: 10.3389/fped.2020.00104.
4. Dong, L., Tian, J., He S, Zhu, C., Wang, J., Liu, C., et al. JAMA. (2020). Possible Vertical Transmission of SARS-CoV-2 From an Infected Mother to Her Newborn.
5. Fan, C., Lei, D., Fang, C, Li C, Wang, M, Liu Y, et al. Clin Infect Dis. 2020. Perinatal Transmission of COVID-19 Associated SARS-CoV-2: Should We Worry? p. ciaa226. pii.
6. Kimberlin, D.W., Stagno, S. JAMA. (2020). Can SARS-CoV-2 Infection Be Acquired in Utero?: More Definitive Evidence Is Needed.
7. Zeng, H., Xu, C., Fan, J., Tang, Y., Deng, Q.,, Zhang, W., et al. JAMA. (2020). Antibodies in Infants Born to Mothers With COVID-19 Pneumonia.

8. Puopolo, K.M., Hudak, M.L., Kimberlin, D.W., Cummings, J. (2020). INITIAL GUIDANCE: Management of Infants Born to Mothers with COVID-19 Date of Document: April 2. 2020. Available from: https://downloads.aap.org/AAP/PDF/COVID%2019%20Initial%20New born%20Guidance.pdf. [Google Scholar]

9. Chen, H., Guo, J., Wang, C,, Luo, F., Yu X, Zhang, W, et al. (2020) Clinical characteristics and intrauterine vertical transmission potential of COVID-19 infection in nine pregnant women: a retrospective review of medical records. Lancet. 2020;395((10226)):809–15. doi: 10.1016/S0140-6736(20)30360-3. [PMC free article] [

10. Wang X, Zhou Z, Zhang J, Zhu F, Tang Y, Shen X. Clin Infect Dis. (2020). A case of 2019 Novel Coronavirus in a pregnant woman with preterm delivery; p. ciaa200. pii. [PMC free article] [PubMed] [CrossRef] [Google Scholar]

11. Considerations for Inpatient Obstetric Healthcare Settings .

12. Sociedad Espanola de Neonatologia . Recomendaciones para el manejo del recién nacido en relatión con la infección por SARS-CoV-2. Available from: https://www.aeped.es/noticias/recomendaciones-manejo-recien-nacido-en-relacion-con-infeccion-por-sars-cov-2. [Google Scholar]

13. Royal College of Obstetricians and Gynaecologists . Coronavirus (COVID-19) Infection in Pregnancy. Information for healthcare professionals Version 1: Published Monday. March 9th, 2020.

14. Ministério da Saúde . Nota técnica n°10/2020-COCAM/CGCIVI/DAPES/SAPS/MS.

15. Ministério da Saúde . Agência Nacional de Vigilância Sanitária. Brasil. Resolução RDC n° 171, de 04 de setembro de 2006. 2006. Dispõe sobre o Regulamento Técnico para o funcionamento de Bancos de Leite Humano. Diário Oficial da União; Poder Executivo, de 05 de setembro de. Available from: https://bvsms.saude.gov.br/bvs/saudelegis/anvisa/2006/res0171_04_09_2006.html. [Google Scholar]

16. Schwartz, D.A. Arch Pathol Lab Med. (2020). An Analysis of 38 Pregnant Women with COVID-19, Their New born Infants, and Maternal-Fetal Transmission of SARS-CoV-2: Maternal Coronavirus Infections and Pregnancy Outcomes.]

17. van Doremalen N, Bushmaker T, Morris DH, Holbrook MG, Gamble A, Williamson BN, et al. (2020).Aerosol and Surface Stability of SARS-CoV-2 as Compared with SARS-CoV-1. N Engl J Med. 2020;382((16)):1564–7. doi: 10.1056/NEJMc2004973. [PMC free article] [PubMed] [CrossRef] [Google Scholar]

18. Hong, H,, Wang, Y., Chung, H.T., Chen. C.J. Clinical characteristics of novel coronavirus disease 2019 (COVID-19) in New borns, infants and children. Pediatr Neonatol. 2020;61((2)):131–2. doi: 10.1016/j.pedneo.2020.03.001. [PMC free article] [PubMed] [CrossRef] [Google Scholar]

19. Wang, J., Qi H, Bao L, Li F, Shi Y,(2009).National Clinical Research Centre for Child Health and Disorders and Pediatric Committee of Medical Association of Chinese People's Liberation Army A contingency plan for the management of the 2019 novel coronavirus outbreak in neonatal intensive care units. Lancet Child Adolesc Health. 2020;4((4)):258–9.

20. De Luca, D. (2020). Managing neonates with respiratory failure due to SARS-CoV-2. Lancet Child Adolesc Health. 2020;4((4)):e8. doi: 10.1016/S2352-4642(20)30073-0. [PMC free article] [PubMed] [CrossRef] [Google Scholar]

21. Niederman, M.S., Richeldi, L, Chotirmall, S.H., Bai, C., (2020) Rising to the Challenge of COVID-19: Advice for Pulmonary and Critical Care and an Agenda for Research. Am J Respir Crit Care Med. 2020;201((9)):1019–22.

2. A Review Of Initial Data On Pregnancy During The COVID-19 Outbreak: Implications For Assisted Reproductive Treatments[1]

Pedro A.A. Monteleone,[1,2] Mayra Nakano,[1,2] Victor Lazar,[1] Alecsandra P Gomes,[1] Hamilton de Martin,[1,2] and Tatiana C.S. Bonetti[1,3] [2]

[2]Disciplina de Ginecologia - Departamento de Obstetrícia e Ginecologia. Faculdade de Medicina da Universidade de São Paulo (FMUSP)
[3]Departamento de Ginecologia. Universidade Federal de São Paulo - Escola Paulista de Medicina (UNIFESP-EPM)

ABSTRACT

The current outbreak of the novel 2019 coronavirus disease (COVID-19) started in China in December 2019 and has since spread to several other countries. On March 25, 2020, a total of 375,498 cases had been confirmed globally with 2,201 cases in Brazil, showing the urgency of reacting to this international public health emergency. While in most cases, mild symptoms are observed, in some cases the infection leads to serious pulmonary disease. As a result, the possible consequences of the COVID-19 outbreak for pregnant women and its potential effects on the management of assisted reproductive treatments, demand attention. In this review, we summarize the latest research progress related to COVID-19 epidemiology and the reported data of pregnant women and discuss the current evidence of COVID-19 infections during pregnancy and its potential consequences for assisted reproductive treatments. Reported data suggest that symptoms in pregnant women are similar to those in other people, and that there is no evidence for higher maternal or fetal risks. However, considering the initial data and lack of comprehensive knowledge on the pathogenesis of SARS-CoV-2 during pregnancy, human reproduction societies have recommended postponing the embryo transfers and do not initiate new treatment cycles. New evidence must be considered carefully in order to adjust these recommendations accordingly at any time and to guide assisted reproductive treatments.

BACKGROUND

The current outbreak of the novel 2019 coronavirus disease (COVID-19) caused by severe acute respiratory syndrome coronavirus 2 (SARS-CoV-2) emerged in China in December 2019 and subsequently spread to many other countries. On January 30 2020, the Emergency Committee of

[1] JBRA Assist Reprod. 2020 Apr-Jun; 24(2): 219–225.
[2] Corresponding author: Tatiana CS Bonetti, Centro de Reprodução Humana Monteleone, São Paulo - SP. Email: rb.dem.enoeletnom@ocifitneic Laboratório de Ginecologia Molecular - Departamento de Ginecologia, Universidade Federal de São Paulo - Escola Paulista de Medicina, São Paulo - SP, Brasil. E-mail: rb.psefinu@ittenobt

the World Health Organization (WHO) declared a global health emergency, and less than one month later, almost 80,000 cases were confirmed in China and more than 7,000 cases outside of China. Numerous countries have reported increasing numbers of confirmed cases and deaths per day, and despite all efforts, spreading of COVID-19 currently continues; therefore, on March 11 2020, the WHO declared COVID-19 a pandemic (WHO, 2020a).

In numerous countries, current disease dynamics resemble those observed in China following the emergence of COVID-19. On March 5 2020, an issue of Euro Surveillance Journal reported the first confirmed COVID-19 case in Europe (Spiteri *et al*., 2020), according to the WHO case definition (WHO, 2020b). On March 15 2020, COVID-19 cases have been detected in all 30 countries of the European Union/European Economic Area and in the United Kingdom with a total of 39,768 cases and 1,727 deaths, of which 17,775 cases and 1,441 deaths occurred in Italy alone (European Centre for Disease Prevention and Control, 2020). The Brazilian Health Ministry confirmed the first COVID-19 case on February 26 2020 in São Paulo. The patient was a 65-year-old man who had recently returned from northern Italy, where a significant outbreak had occurred.

This was also the first confirmed case in South America, a continent with a population of over 640 million people who have previously experienced significant outbreaks of infections such as zika, dengue, and measles. The number of COVID-19 cases has been increasing constantly since the first reported case, and while initial cases were associated with travellers arriving from countries with ongoing COVID-19 epidemics, since March 13 2020, the stage of 'community transmission' was announced to be reached in São Paulo and Rio de Janeiro. At the time this manuscript was drafted (March 25 2020), 2,201 cases have been confirmed in Brazil, and the pandemic continues to increase worldwide, with currently 375,498 confirmed cases and 16,362 deaths in 195 countries (WHO, 2020c).

SARS-CoV-2 shows rapid community transmission, and nosocomial infections are common (Novel Coronavirus Pneumonia Emergency Response Epidemiology, 2020). Evidence suggests that when the number of initial cases reaches 40, the likelihood of losing control is high, and the number of infections should double within a week, on average, which highlights the urgency of early detection and rapid response measures (Hellewell *et al*., 2020). China enacted a program of strict social isolation to control further spreading of COVID-19, with measures including isolation of cases and limited contact, lock-down of cities, mass quarantine, social distancing mandates, school closures, and intense case identification and contact tracing executed by health care professionals (Chen *et al*., 2020a). These steps helped control local outbreaks, and Chinese authorities reported absence of community transmission cases in China as of March 19 2020. Following this strategy, numerous countries also adopted social isolation regulations to contain the pandemic (WHO, 2020b). However, it is important to emphasize that transmissibility of SARS-CoV-2 is high and infection growth rates are exponential, ranging from 2.2 to 3.6 (Li *et al*., 2020; Zhao *et al*., 2020). The rapid increase in suspected and confirmed cases of COVID-19 suggests that virus transmission may occur by droplet infection and a faecal-oral route. Moreover, transmission from people with mild or no symptoms or before symptom onset may reduce the effect of such isolation strategies (Khan *et al*., 2020; Niud & Xu, 2020; Rothe *et al*., 2020).

SARS-Cov-2 Pathogenesis

Coronaviruses are a large family of viruses known to cause symptoms ranging from a common cold to more severe diseases, such as the severe acute respiratory syndrome (SARS) and the Middle East respiratory syndrome (MERS). The severe acute respiratory syndrome coronavirus (SARS-CoV) caused a SARS outbreak in China in 2002 (Drosten *et al*., 2003; Ksiazek *et al*., 2003), and MERS coronavirus (MERS-CoV) was the pathogen responsible for severe respiratory disease outbreaks in the Middle East in 2012 (Zaki *et al*., 2012). SARS-CoV-2 is the seventh identified member of the family of coronaviruses which infect humans, and the main symptoms including fever, cough and fatigue are similar to those following SARS-CoV and MERS-CoV infection (Liu *et al*., 2020 a).

Coronaviruses are large, enveloped, positive-sense single-stranded RNA viruses that infect humans and a wide range of animals. SARS-CoV-2 belongs to the genus beta-coronavirus, and it may originate from a virus of bats, as the genome sequence of SARS-CoV-2 is to approximately 90% identical with that of a bat coronavirus. In contrast, SARS-CoV-2 sequences show only about 80% sequence identity with SARS-CoV and about 50% with MERS-CoV (Lu *et al*., 2020; Zhou *et al*., 2020). ARS-CoV-2 has four key structural proteins: the nucleocapsid protein (N), spike protein (S), small membrane protein (SM), and membrane glycoprotein (M). The angiotensin-converting enzyme 2 (ACE2), which is expressed on type-I and type-II alveolar epithelial cells, is the main SARS-CoV-2 receptor, and infection causes respiratory symptoms and eventually the acute respiratory syndrome. This receptor is also expressed in the gut, albeit at a low abundance, and infection may lead to diarrhoea and vomiting, despite it is less frequent. The S protein is required for the virus to fuse with the host cell through the receptor-binding domain. This protein includes two subunits, S1 and S2, and while S1 determines cellular tropism, S2 mediates virus-cell membrane fusion.

After membrane fusion, viral RNA is released into the cytoplasm, and viral replication is initiated. Newly formed viral particle buds then fuse with the plasma membrane through virion-containing vesicles to release the virus (Guo *et al*., 2020; Sun *et al*., 2020). It is noteworthy that SARS-Cov also uses ACE2 as a receptor for cell entry; however, receptor binding ability of SARS-CoV-2 is 10- to 20-fold higher than that of SARS-CoV, and the number of infections with SARS-CoV-2 has exceeded that of SARS infections during the outbreak in China in 2002/2003, indicating higher transmission rates. Moreover, men typically have higher ACE2 levels than women, and Asians show higher levels of ACE2 expression in alveolar cells than Caucasian and African American people, which would suggest Asian males to be most susceptible to infection (Sun *et al*., 2020).

SARS-CoV-2 is predominantly transmitted from person to person through droplets and close contact (Chan *et al*., 2020). After contact with a virus-shedding patient, the mean incubation period is about 5 days, ranging from 1 to 14 days (Li *et al*., 2020). The spectrum of clinical presentations of SARS-CoV-2 infections has been reported to range from asymptomatic infections to severe respiratory failure. However, most cases experience a similar course of disease as SARS and MERS patients, with the most common symptoms including fever and cough which frequently leads to lower respiratory tract disease with poor clinical outcomes in elderly patients and in those with pre-existing health conditions. Confirmation of infection requires nucleic acid testing of respiratory tract samples (e.g., pharyngeal swabs), whereas clinical diagnoses can be made based on symptoms, exposure to infection, and chest imaging (Wu & McGoogan, 2020).

The study describing approximately 45.000 cases of COVID-19 in China showed that in most cases (86%), the course of disease was mild (i.e., no or mild pneumonia), and it was severe in 14% (i.e., dyspnoea, respiratory frequency $\geq$ 30/min, blood oxygen saturation $\leq$ 93%, partial pressure of arterial oxygen to fraction of inspired oxygen ratio <300, and/or lung infiltrates >50% within 24-

48 hours) and critical in 5% (i.e., respiratory failure, septic shock, and/or multiple organ dysfunction or failure). The overall case fatality rate was 2.3%, but it was 8.0% in patients aged 70-79 years and 14.8% in patients aged 80 years and older; no deaths occurred in patients aged 9 years or younger and among mild and severe cases. However, case fatality rates were higher in patients with pre-existing comorbid conditions, varying from 5.6% to 10.5%, depending on comorbidity (Wu & McGoogan, 2020). SARS and MERS infections, which also showed widespread transmission, produced fatality rates of 9.6% and 35%, respectively (Hui *et al*., 2020). Despite considerably higher case-fatality rates in SARS and MERS patients, COVID-19 seems to be more transmissible and has led to a higher number of deaths due to the large number of cases. In addition, the true number of COVID-19 cases can be presumed to be higher than the number of reported cases owing to inherent difficulties in identifying mild and asymptomatic cases in addition to insufficient COVID-19 testing capacities in all affected countries (Wu & McGoogan, 2020).

COVID-19 and Pregnancy

Immunosuppression and other physiological changes during pregnancy cause high susceptibility to respiratory pathogens and severe pneumonia in pregnant women (Jamieson *et al*., 2006) which may require hospitalization in intensive care units and ventilatory support (Goodnight & Soper, 2005). Hormone levels and immune competence show considerable variation throughout pregnancy. Early pregnancy seems to be more risk-prone due to adaptive changes in response to foetal antigens, but conditions typically stabilize with gradual adjustment of the mother's immune and endocrine systems, with highest stability in the late stages of pregnancy.

Early pregnancy is a crucial period of foetal organ development, and the immune system is particularly sensitive at this stage, which likely affects the course of infections (Wong *et al*., 2004). Experience with previous respiratory virus epidemics may offer some insights regarding COVID-19 susceptibility and complication rates during pregnancy. Swine-origin influenza A (H1N1) virus is an influenza virus type A, which also causes respiratory disease that can develop into an acute respiratory syndrome. During the H1N1 epidemic in 2009, pregnant women were found to be at higher risk of complications as they were four times more likely to be hospitalized than the rest of the population (Jamieson *et al*., 2009). Regarding other coronaviruses, the SARS epidemic in 2002/2003 produced 8,442 cases and 916 deaths, and studies have shown that clinical outcomes during this epidemic were worse in pregnant women than in non-pregnant women. In addition, increasing rates of premature births and abortions have been associated with SARS-CoV infections (Schwartz and Graham, 2020). Approximately 50% of pregnant women suffering from SARS required intensive care, and approximately 33% needed mechanical ventilation.

The death rate of pregnant women suffering from SARS reached 25% (Wong *et al*., 2004). From the MERS epidemic which produced 2,500 confirmed cases and caused 858 deaths, we can affirm that MERS progresses much more quickly to respiratory failure and results in higher mortality rates than SARS. However, there was no evidence of vertical transmission of MERS or SARS. Based on this evidence, there is no doubt that SARS-CoV and MERS-CoV infections, as even the H1N1, are associated with higher rates of complications in pregnant women (Schwartz and Graham, 2020). Despite that COVID-19 epidemic is ongoing and the data are limited, recent reports indicate that clinical characteristics reported in pregnant women with confirmed SARS-CoV-2 infections are similar to those of non-pregnant women with COVID-19 pneumonia, and no evidence of vertical transmission of SARS-CoV-2 in late pregnancy has been produced so far.

Nine studies reported COVID-19 in pregnant women, with a total of 69 patients; however, some of these patients may have been included in more than one study.

The reported cases included five patients in the second trimester of pregnancy, and all other patients were in the third trimester. Most women showed mild or moderate symptoms, and three of them required intensive care. Preterm birth occurred in 8 out of 61 women who gave birth (Chen *et al.*, 2020b; Chen *et al.*, 2020c; Fan *et al.*, 2020; Liu *et al.*, 2020b; Liu *et al.*, 2020c; Wang *et al.*, 2020a; Wen *et al.*, 2020; Zhang *et al.*, 2020; Zhu *et al.*, 2020). A joint investigation carried out by the WHO and China evaluated 147 pregnant women in China (64 confirmed and 82 suspected COVID-19 cases and an asymptomatic patient), 8% showed severe symptoms, and 1% showed a critical course of disease. It was concluded that pregnant women with COVID-19 were not at a higher risk of developing severe symptoms (WHO, 2020d). Most likely, there are many other pregnant women with no or mild symptoms who were not included in these statistics.

One case of a neonate infected with SARS-CoV-2 was confirmed 36 hours after birth; however, it is unclear whether this was due to vertical transmission from mother to child (Wang *et al*., 2020b).Regardless of the small number of reported cases, the combined data suggest that susceptibility to infection and frequencies of severe courses of disease due to SARS-CoV-2 infection in pregnant women are similar to those in other young adults, and no case of vertical transmission has been reported. Moreover, according to the WHO definition of preterm delivery as birth occurring before 37 weeks of gestation and an estimated rate of preterm births of 10% (WHO, 2018), preterm birth rates in pregnant women affected by COVID-19 seems to follow the general rate. Regarding premature births, it should be considered that many pregnant patients who are hospitalized near term presenting symptoms of COVID-19, the anticipation of delivery by elective caesarean section can be a medical decision that is influenced by the patient and epidemic pressure and is not necessarily a result of current SARS-CoV-2 infection.

No studies on severe COVID-19 and obstetric complications during the first trimester of gestation are available so far; therefore, we lack information on potential effects of infection on pregnancy during the initial stages. Regarding other coronaviruses, SARS and MERS epidemics showed no correlation with frequencies of malformations. Moreover, data from the current epidemic should be considered for managing COVID-19 infections during pregnancy, as the clinical course of this disease and the response to treatments seem to differ from those of previous outbreaks of other types of coronaviruses (Chen *et al*., 2020d; Liang & Acharya, 2020). Further research is needed in order to understand pathogenesis and epidemiology of SARS-CoV-2 during pregnancy, including aspects such as the time of maternal infection, gestational age, effects of comorbidity factors, and frequencies of adverse outcomes; however, preliminary observations of pregnant women infected with SARS-CoV-2 suggest an optimistic outlook regarding the clinical course.

It is important to consider that the COVID-19 pandemic elicited psychological stress and anxiety in the general population, including pregnant women.

Several concerns regarding potential infection during pregnancy have been raised, including (i) presence of family members given quarantine constraints, (ii) potential SARS-CoV-2 exposure during visits to physicians, (iii) potential requirement of early termination of pregnancy through elective caesarean section; (iv) constant use of sodium hypochlorite and alcohol as disinfectants which may exert toxic effects, and (v) potential postpartum complications, e.g., during breastfeeding or neonatal care (Rashidi Fakari & Simbar, 2020).

COVID-19 and Assisted Reproduction Treatments

In view of the current COVID-19 pandemic and uncertainties regarding effects of SARS-CoV-2 on mothers and foetuses during pregnancy, human reproduction societies published suggestions for managing patients who currently are or will be undergoing infertility treatments through Assisted Reproductive Technologies (ART). T
he International Federation for Fertility Societies (IFFS) recommended on March 12 2020 that patients who are considering pregnancy or who are currently undergoing fertility therapies should consult with their personal physician for planning further steps (IFFS, 2020).

The same day, the American Society for Reproductive Medicine (ASRM) published a bulletin suggesting that patients who are highly likely to suffer from COVID-19 (i.e., patients who were tested SARS-CoV-2 positive or who have been exposed to confirmed COVID-19 cases within 14 days of onset of their symptoms) should consider freezing oocytes or embryos and avoid embryo transfer until they are symptom-free; however, this recommendation was emphasized to not necessarily apply to suspected COVID-19 cases as symptoms of COVID-19 closely resemble those of other more common forms of respiratory disease (ASRM, 2020a).

On March 17 2020, the ASRM published a new document named "Patient Management and Clinical Recommendations During the Coronavirus (COVID-19) Pandemic" in which the key recommendations were:

1. Suspend initiation of new treatment cycles, including ovulation induction, intrauterine inseminations (IUIs), in vitro fertilization (IVF) including retrievals and frozen embryo transfers, as well as non-urgent gamete cryopreservation.

2. Strongly consider cancellation of all embryo transfers whether fresh or frozen.

3. Continue to care for patients who are currently "in-cycle" or who require urgent stimulation and cryopreservation.

4. Suspend elective surgeries and non-urgent diagnostic procedures.

5. Minimize in-person interactions and increase utilization of telehealth (ASRM, 2020b).

The European Society of Human Reproduction and Embryology (ESHRE) issued a statement on March 14 2020 detailing that so far, only few cases of COVID-19 during pregnancy have been reported, thus the respective data must be interpreted with caution as no information is available regarding potential effects of COVID-19 infection during the initial stages of pregnancy; furthermore, medical treatment administered to severe COVID-19 cases may include drugs that are contraindicated during pregnancy (ESHRE, 2020).

The same publication advised that all patients considering or planning treatments, independently of confirmation or suspicion of COVID-19 infections, should avoid becoming pregnant at this time and consider deferring pregnancy by freezing oocytes or embryos for embryo transfer at a later point (ESHRE, 2020). The Brazilian Society for Human Reproduction (SBRH), the Brazilian Society for Assisted Reproduction (SBRA), and the Latin American Network of Assisted Reproduction (REDLARA) also published statements concerning patients undergoing assisted reproductive treatments.

The SBRH stressed that there is no cause for panic in pregnant women and urged that the ASRM recommendations for women undergoing or planning infertility treatments be followed. However, treatment plans should be individually discussed with physicians as postponing of treatments may, in some cases, reduce chances of success (SBRH, 2020).

The SBRA and the REDLARA published a joint note on March 17 2020, firstly suggesting that infertility treatments should continue as planned to avoid reducing prospects of success in infertile women but that the advice of international societies to postpone embryo transfers should be followed (SBRA & REDLARA, 2020). Then, an update launched on March 20 2020 recommended that ongoing cycles should be finalized and new procedures should not be initiated.

Embryo transfer must be assessed individually with strict controls on the patients and teams involved and the exceptions lies on oncological and others situations in which the postponement may cause loss to the patient, since the decision need to be shared (SBRA & REDLARA, 2020). It is important to cite the Brazilian Health Ministry published a technical note on COVID-19 and pregnancy on March 25 2020.

Based on available evidences until this moment reporting no difference of clinical course, as well as rates of complications and evolution to severe diseases of pregnant compared to young adults; it was recommended that the COVID-19 diagnostic in pregnant women follow the protocol for the general adult population, as the prenatal care for all asymptomatic pregnant women.

However, it is highlighted the importance the prevention of agglomerations, best hygiene practices and home screening and isolation of suspected cases of flu syndrome. Also, despite the literature shows the unlikely vertical transmission of SARS-CoV-2, they suggests it is prudent to perform morphological ultrasonography in the second trimester in mothers with SARS-CoV-2 infection, when available, since the data in infected women in the first trimester of pregnancy are not available (BRASIL - Ministério da Saúde, 2020).

Taken together, we currently face a pandemic with a novel virus, and considerable uncertainty remains regarding SAR-CoV-2 infections and consequences of infection during pregnancy. Hence, most of Human Reproduction Societies are restrictive suggesting to postpone embryo transfer independently of confirmation or suspicion of COVID-19 and suspend all cycle's initiations, with rare exceptions. However, whilst every effort must be made to reduce services over coming weeks or maybe months, it is necessary to think forwards towards a resumption of services and a number of questions need to be answered around the management of ART: Should we cancel all ART cycles at this moment? Should we keep the treatments and postpone all embryo transfers? Should we keep only embryo transfers for couple whose success of treatment can be impaired or those who desire transfer the embryos?

Concluding Remarks

Based on most recent epidemiologic data on COVID-19 and pregnancy, there is no evidence to suggest increased risk for mothers or foetuses. It appears that the course of disease after infection with SARS-CoV-2 in pregnant women does not differ from that in other young adults. Moreover, recent evidence suggests no association of vertical transmission and malformations, and the management of pregnant patients should be individualized based on obstetrical indications and maternal/foetal health status. It is important to consider that the current COVID-19 pandemic causes psychological stress and anxiety in pregnant women, which may exert adverse effects. Furthermore, it is important to emphasize the recommendations regarding social isolation and quarantine as issued by health authorities in order to avoid further spreading of SARS-CoV-2. Therefore, deciding between initiating/resuming or postponing assisted reproductive treatments depends more strongly on social isolation than on COVID-19 and its potential effects during pregnancy, bearing in mind potential emotional effects on patients. However, considering the lack of knowledge regarding SARS-CoV-2 pathogenesis during pregnancy, the current pandemic requires caution and human reproduction societies generally recommended postponing embryo transfers of current cycles and do not initiate any new cycles, with rare exceptions. Nevertheless, we must be alert to new evidence, which can change these recommendations at any time, in order to adjust the management of assisted reproductive treatments.

Acknowledgments

The authors gratefully acknowledge the contributions of the team of Monteleone Centro de Reprodução Humana, São Paulo, Brazil, for technical and emotional support with patients and procedures during the COVID-19 pandemic.

REFERENCES

1. ASRM - American Society for Reproductive Medicine COVID-19: Suggestions On Managing Patients Who Are Undergoing Infertility Therapy Or Desiring Pregnancy. 2020a. [Acessed 21.03.2020]. Available at: https://www.asrm.org/news-and-publications/news-and-research/press-releases-and-bulletins/COVID-19-suggestions-on-managing-patients-who-are-undergoing-infertility-therapy-or-desiring-pregnancy/

2. ASRM - American Society for Reproductive Medicine Patient Management and Clinical Recommendations During the Coronavirus (COVID-19) Pandemic. 2020b. https://www.asrm.org/news-and-publications/COVID-19/statements/patient-management-and-clinical-recommendations-during-the-coronavirus-COVID-19-pandemic

3. BRASIL - Ministério da Saúde. Secretaria de Atenção Primária à Saúde. Departamento de Ações Programáticas Estratégicas. Coordenação-Geral de Ciclos da Vida. Coordenação de Saúde das Mulheres SEI/MS - 0014128689. Nota Técnica nº 6/2020-COSMU/CGCIVI/DAPES/SAPS/MS: ATENÇÃO ÀS GESTANTES NO CONTEXTO DA INFECÇÃO SARS-COV-2. 2020

4. Chan, J.F, Yuan, S., Kok, K,H,, To KK, Chu, H., Yang, J., Xing F, Liu J, Yip, C.C., Poon, R.W., Tsoi, H.W., Lo SK, Chan, K.H., Poon VK, Chan WM, Ip JD, Cai JP, Cheng VC, Chen, H., Hui CK, et al.(2020).A familial cluster of pneumonia associated with the 2019 novel coronavirus indicating person-to-person transmission: a study of a family cluster. Lancet. 2020;395:514–523. doi: 10.1016/S0140-6736(20)30154-9. [PMC free article] [PubMed] [CrossRef] [Google Scholar]

5. Chen, W., Wang, Q,, Li YQ, Yu, HL, Xia, YY, Zhang M.L, Qin Y, Zhang, T. Peng, Z.B., Zhang, R.C., Yang, X.K., Yin, W.W., An, Z.J., Wu, D., Yin, Z.D., Li, S., Chen, Q.L., Feng, L.Z., Li ZJ, Feng, Z.J. (2020). Early containment strategies and core measures for prevention and control of novel coronavirus pneumonia in China. 395:809–815. doi: 10.1016/S0140-6736(20)30360-3. [PubMed] [CrossRef] [Google Scholar]

6. Chen, S., Huang, B., Luo, D.J., Li, X., Yang, F., Zhao, Y., Nie, X., Huang, B.X. (2020).Pregnant women with new coronavirus infection: a clinical characteristics and placental pathological analysis of three cases. Zhonghua Bing Li Xue Za Zhi. 2020c;49(E005) doi: 10.3760/cma.j.cn112151-20200225-00138. [PubMed] [CrossRef] [Google Scholar]

7. Chen, D., Yang, H., Cao, Y., Cheng, W., Duan, T., Fan, C., Fan, S., Feng, L, Gao, Y,, He F, He J, Hu Y, Jiang Y, Li Y, Li J, Li X, Li X, Lin K, Liu C, Liu J, et al. (2020).Expert consensus for managing pregnant women and neonates born to mothers with suspected or confirmed novel coronavirus (COVID-19) infection. Int J Gynaecol Obstet. 2020d doi: 10.1002/ijgo.13146. [Epub ahead of print] [PubMed] [CrossRef] [Google Scholar]

8. Drosten, C., Gunther, S., Preiser, W., van der Werf S., Brodt, H.R., Becker, S., Rabenau, H., Panning, M., Kolesnikova, L., Fouchier, R.A., Berger, A., Burguiere, A.M., Cinatl, J., Eickmann, M., Escriou, N., Grywna, K., Kramme S, Manuguerra JC, Muller S, Rickerts V, et al.(1976). Identification of a novel coronavirus in patients with severe acute respiratory syndrome. N Engl J Med. 2003;348:1967–1976. doi: 10.1056/NEJMoa030747. [PubMed] [CrossRef] [Google Scholar]

9. European Centre for Disease Prevention and Control Coronavirus disease. 2020. https://www.ecdc.europa.eu/en

10. ESHRE - European Society of Human Reproduction and Embryology Coronavirus COVID-19: ESHRE statement on pregnancy and conception. 2020. [21.03.2020]. Available at: https://www.eshre.eu/Press-Room/ESHRE-News#CoronaStatement27feb.

11. Fan, C, Lei, D., Fang, C., Li, C., Wang, M., Liu, Y., Bao, Y., Sun, Y., Huang, J., Guo. Y., Yu, Y., Wang, S. Perinatal Transmission of COVID-19 Associated SARS-CoV-2: Should We Worry? Clin Infect Dis. 2020:ciaa226–ciaa226. doi: 10.1093/cid/ciaa226. [Epub ahead of print] [PMC free article] [PubMed] [CrossRef] [Google Scholar]

12. Goodnight, W.H., Soper, D.E.(2005). Pneumonia in pregnancy. Crit Care Med. 2005;33:S390–S397. doi: 10.1097/01.ccm.0000182483.24836.66. [PubMed] [CrossRef] [Google Scholar]

13. Guo, Y.R., Cao, Q.D., Hong, Z.S., Tan, Y.Y., Chen, S.D., Jin HJ, Tan, K.S., Wang, D.Y., Yan, Y., (2020).The origin, transmission and clinical therapies on coronavirus disease 2019 (COVID-19) outbreak - an update on the status. Mil Med Res. 2020;7:11–11. doi: 10.1186/s40779-020-00240-0. [PMC free article] [PubMed] [CrossRef] [Google Scholar]

14. Hellewell, J., Abbott, S., Gimma, A., Bosse, N.I., Jarvis, C.I., Russell, T.W., Munday, J.D., Kucharski, A.J, Edmunds, W.J. (2020) Centre for the Mathematical Modelling of Infectious Diseases C-WG, Funk S, Eggo RM. Feasibility of controlling COVID-19 outbreaks by isolation of cases and contacts. Lancet Glob Health. 2020;8:e488–e496. doi: 10.1016/S2214-109X(20)30074-7. [PMC free article] [PubMed] [CrossRef] [Google Scholar]

15. Hui, D,S., E IA,, Madani, T.A., Ntoumi, F., Kock, R., Dar, O., Ippolito, G., McHugh, T.D., Memish, Z.A., Drosten, C., Zumla, A., Petersen, E.. (2020).The continuing 2019-nCoV epidemic threat of novel coronaviruses to global health - The latest 2019 novel coronavirus outbreak in Wuhan, China. Int J Infect Dis. 2020;91:264–266. doi: 10.1016/j.ijid.2020.01.009. [PMC free article] [PubMed] [CrossRef] [Google Scholar]

16. IFFS - International Federation for Fertility Societies UPDATES AND RESOURCES RELATED TO THE CORONAVIRUS PANDEMIC AND COVID-19. 2020. https://www.iffsreproduction.org/general/custom.asp?page=COVID-19

17. Jamieson, D.J., Honein, M.A., Rasmussen, S.A., Williams, J.L., Swerdlow, D.L., Biggerstaff, M.S., Lindstrom, S., Louie, J.K., Christ, C.M., Bohm, S.R., Fonseca, V.P., Ritger, K.A., Kuhles, D.J., Eggers, P., Bruce, H., Davidson, H.A., Lutterloh, E., Harris, M.L, Burke, C., Cocoros, N,, et al. (2019). Novel Influenza A (H1N1) Pregnancy Working Group. H1N1 2009 influenza virus infection during pregnancy in the USA. Lancet. 2009;374:451–458.

18. Jamieson, D.J, Theiler RN, Rasmussen, S.A. (2006).Emerging infections and pregnancy. Emerg Infect Dis. 2006;12:1638–1643. doi: 10.3201/eid1211.060152. [PMC free article] [PubMed] [CrossRef] [Google Scholar]

19. Khan, S., Siddique, R., Shereen, M.A., Ali, A., Liu, J., Bai, Q., Bashir, N., Xue, M. (2020). The emergence of a novel coronavirus (SARS-CoV-2), their biology and therapeutic options. J Clin Microbiol. 2020 doi: 10.1128/JCM.00187-20. [Epub ahead of print] [PMC free article] [PubMed] [CrossRef] [Google Scholar]

20. Ksiazek, T.G., Erdman, D., Goldsmith, C.S., Zaki, S..R., Peret, T., Emery, S., Tong, S., Urbani, C., Comer, J.A,, Lim, W., Rollin, P.E., Dowell, S.F., Ling, A.E., Humphrey, C.D., Shieh, W.J., Guarner, J., Paddock, C.D., Rota, P., Fields B, DeRisi J, et al. (2003). A novel coronavirus associated with severe acute respiratory syndrome. N Engl J Med. 2003;348:1953–1966. doi: 10.1056/NEJMoa030781. [PubMed] [CrossRef] [Google Scholar]

21. Li Q, Guan X, Wu P, Wang X, Zhou L, Tong Y, Ren R, Leung KSM, Lau EHY, Wong JY, Xing X, Xiang N, Wu Y, Li C, Chen Q, Li D, Liu T, Zhao J, Li M, Tu W, et al. (2020) Early Transmission Dynamics in Wuhan, China, of Novel Coronavirus-Infected Pneumonia. N Engl J Med. 2020;382:1199–1207. doi: 10.1056/NEJMoa2001316. [

22. Liang, H., Acharya, G. (2020). Novel corona virus disease (COVID-19) in pregnancy: What clinical recommendations to follow? Acta Obstet Gynecol Scand. 2020;99:439–442. doi: 10.1111/aogs.13836. [PubMed] [

23. Liu, J., Zheng, X., Tong, Q., Li W, Wang, B., Sutter, K., Trilling, M., Lu, M., Dittmer, U., Yang, D. (2020). Overlapping and discrete aspects of the pathology and pathogenesis of the emerging human pathogenic coronaviruses SARS-CoV, MERS-CoV, and 2019-nCoV. J Med Virol. 2020a;92:491–494. doi: 10.1002/jmv.25709. [PMC free article] [PubMed] [CrossRef] [Google Scholar]

24. Liu, D., Li L, Wu, X., Zheng, D., Wang, J., Yang, L., Zheng C. (2020).Pregnancy and Perinatal Outcomes of Women With Coronavirus Disease (COVID-19) Pneumonia: A Preliminary Analysis. AJR Am J Roentgenol. 1-6. 2020b doi: 10.2214/AJR.20.23072. [PubMed] [CrossRef] [Google Scholar]

25. Liu, Y., Chen, H., Tang, K., Guo, Y. (2020).Clinical manifestations and outcome of SARS-CoV-2 infection during pregnancy. J Infect. 2020c:S0163-4453(20)30109-2. doi: 10.1016/j.jinf.2020.02.028. [Epub ahead of print] [PMC free article] [PubMed] [CrossRef] [Google Scholar]

26. Lu R, Zhao X, Li J, Niu P, Yang, B., Wu, H., Wang, W., Song, H., Huang, B., Zhu, N., Bi, Y., Ma, X., Zhan, F., Wang L, Hu, T., Zhou, H., Hu, Z., Zhou, W., Zhao, L., Chen, J, et al. (2020).Genomic characterisation and epidemiology of 2019 novel coronavirus: implications for virus origins and receptor binding. Lancet. 395:2020–2020. 565–574. doi: 10.1016/S0140-6736(20)30251-8. [PMC free article] [PubMed] [CrossRef] [Google Scholar]

27. Niud, Y., Xu, F. (2020).Deciphering the power of isolation in controlling COVID-19 outbreaks. Lancet Glob Health. 2020;8:e452–e453. 0.1016/S2214-109X(20)30085-1. [PMC free article] [PubMed] [Google Scholar]

28. Novel Coronavirus Pneumonia Emergency Response Epidemiology Team The epidemiological characteristics of an outbreak of 2019 novel coronavirus diseases (COVID-19) in China. Zhonghua Liu Xing Bing Xue Za Zhi. 2020;41:145–151. doi: 10.3760/cma.j.issn.1001-0939.2020.03.003. [PubMed] [CrossRef] [Google Scholar]

29. Rashidi, F., Simbar, M. (2020). Coronavirus Pandemic and Worries during Pregnancy; a Letter to Editor. Arch Acad Emerg Med. 2020;8:e21. [PMC free article] [PubMed] [Google Scholar]

30. Rothe, C., Schunk, M., Sothmann, P., Bretzel, G., Froeschl, G., Wallrauch, C., Zimmer, T., Thiel, V., Janke, C., Guggemos, W., Seilmaier, M., Drosten, C., Vollmar, P., Zwirglmaier, K., Zange, S., Wolfel, R., Hoelscher, M. (2020) Transmission of 2019-nCoV Infection from an Asymptomatic Contact in Germany. N Engl J Med. 2020;382:970–971. doi: 10.1056/NEJMc2001468. [PMC free article] [PubMed] [CrossRef] [Google Scholar]

31. SBRA - Sociedade Brasileira de Reprodução Assistida. REDLARA - Red LatinoAmericana de Reproducion Assistida Reprodução Assistida e COVID-19 | nota conjunta SBRA e REDLARA2020. https://sbra.com.br/noticias/reproducao-assistida-e-COVID-19-nota-conjunta-sbra-e-redlara/

32. SBRH - Sociedade Brasileira de Reprodução Humana COVID-19: Acompanhamento de pacientes submetidas às terapias de reprodução assistida ou que desejam engravidar. 2020. https://www.sbrh.org.br/?p=5013

33. Schwartz, D.A, Graham, A.L. (2020) Potential Maternal and Infant Outcomes from (Wuhan) Coronavirus 2019-nCoV Infecting Pregnant Women: Lessons from SARS, MERS, and Other Human Coronavirus Infections. Viruses. 2020;12(2):E194. doi: 10.3390/v12020194. [PMC free article] [PubMed] [CrossRef] [Google Scholar]

34. Spiteri, G., Fielding J, Diercke, M., Campese, C., Enouf, V., Gaymard, A., Bella, A., Sognamiglio, P., Sierra Moros, M.J., Riutort, A.N., Demina, Y.V., Mahieu, R., Broas, M., Bengner, M., Buda, S., Schilling, J., Filleul, L., Lepoutre A, Saura C, et al. (2020).First cases of coronavirus disease 2019 (COVID-19) in the WHO European Region, 24 January to 21 February 2020. Euro Surveill. 2020;25:2000178–2000178. doi: 10.2807/1560-7917.ES.2020.25.9.2000178. [PMC free article] [PubMed] [CrossRef] [Google Scholar]

35. Sun, P., Lu, X., Xu, C., Sun, W., Pan, B. (2020).Understanding of COVID-19 based on current evidence. J Med Virol. 2020 doi: 10.1002/jmv.25722. [Epub ahead of print] [PMC free article] [PubMed] [CrossRef] [Google Scholar]

36. Wang, X., Zhou, Z, Zhang, J., Zhu, F., Tang, Y., Shen, X., (2020).A case of 2019 Novel Coronavirus in a pregnant woman with preterm delivery. Clin Infect Dis. 2020a:ciaa200–ciaa200. doi: 10.1093/cid/ciaa200. [Epub ahead of print] [PMC free article] [PubMed] [CrossRef] [Google Scholar]

37. Wang, S., Guo, L, Chen, L, Liu, W., Cao, Y., Zhang, J., Feng, L (2020). A case report of neonatal COVID-19 infection in China. Clin Infect Dis. 2020b:ciaa225–ciaa225. doi: 10.1093/cid/ciaa225. [Epub ahead of print] [PMC free article] [PubMed] [CrossRef] [Google Scholar]

38. Wen, R., Sun, Y., Xing, Q.S..(2020).A patient with SARS-CoV-2 infection during pregnancy in Qingdao, China. J Microbiol Immunol Infect. 2020:S1684–1182(20)30061-X. doi: 10.1016/j.jmii.2020.03.004. [Epub ahead of print] [PMC free article] [PubMed] [CrossRef] [Google Scholar]

39. WHO - World Health Organization Preterm birth. 2018. https://www.who.int/news-room/fact-sheets/detail/preterm-birth

40. WHO - World Health Organization Coronavirus disease 2019 (COVID-19) Situation Report - 41. 2020a. https://www.who.int/docs/default-source/coronaviruse/situation-reports/20200301-sitrep-41-COVID-19.pdf?sfvrsn=6768306d_2

41. WHO - World Health Organization Coronavirus disease (COVID-19) technical guidance: Surveillance and case definitions. 2020b. https://www.who.int/emergencies/diseases/novel-coronavirus-2019/technical-guidance/surveillance-and-case-definitions

42. WHO - World Health Organization Novel Coronavirus (COVID-19) Situation. 2020c. [25.03.2020]. https://experience.arcgis.com/experience/685d0ace521648f8a5beeeee1b9125cd

43. WHO - World Health Organization Report of the WHO-China Joint Mission on Coronavirus Disease 2019 (COVID-19) 2020d. https://www.who.int/docs/default-source/coronaviruse/who-china-joint-mission-on-COVID-19-final-report.pdf

44. Wong, S.F., Chow, K.M., Leung, T.N., Ng, W.F., Ng, T.K., Shek, C.C., Ng, P.C., Lam, P.W., Ho, L.C., To, W.W., Lai, S.T., Yan, W.W., Tan. (2004). P.Y. Pregnancy and perinatal outcomes of women with severe acute respiratory syndrome. Am J Obstet Gynecol. 2004;191:292–297. doi: 10.1016/j.ajog.2003.11.019. [PMC free article] [PubMed] [CrossRef] [Google Scholar]

45. Wu Z, McGoogan, J.M. (2020). Characteristics of and Important Lessons From the Coronavirus Disease 2019 (COVID-19) Outbreak in China: Summary of a Report of 72314 Cases From the Chinese Centre for Disease Control

and Prevention. JAMA. 2020 doi: 10.1001/jama.2020.2648. Epub ahead of print] [PubMed] [CrossRef] [Google Scholar]

46. Zaki, A.M, van Boheemen S, Bestebroer, T.M., Osterhaus, A.D, Fouchier, R.A. (2012). Isolation of a novel coronavirus from a man with pneumonia in Saudi Arabia. N Engl J Med. 2012;367:1814–1820. doi: 10.1056/NEJMoa1211721. [PubMed] [CrossRef] [Google Scholar]

47. Zhang, L., Jiang, Y., Wei, M., Cheng, B.H., Zhou XC, Li J, Tian, J.H, Dong, L, Hu. R.H. (2020). Analysis of the pregnancy outcomes in pregnant women with COVID-19 in Hubei Province. Zhonghua Fu Chan Ke Za Zhi. 2020;55:E009. doi: 10.3760/cma.j.cn112141-20200218-00111. [PubMed] [CrossRef] [Google Scholar]

48. Zhao S, Lin Q, Ran J, Musa SS, Yang G, Wang W, Lou Y, Gao D, Yang L, He D, Wang, M.H.(2020). Preliminary estimation of the basic reproduction number of novel coronavirus (2019-nCoV) in China, from 2019 to 2020: A data-driven analysis in the early phase of the outbreak. Int J Infect Dis. 2020;92:214–217. doi: 10.1016/j.ijid.2020.01.050. [PMC free article] [PubMed] [CrossRef] [Google Scholar]

49. Zhou P, Yang XL, Wang XG, Hu B, Zhang L, Zhang W, Si HR, Zhu Y, Li B, Huang CL, Chen HD, Chen J, Luo Y, Guo H, Jiang RD, Liu MQ, Chen Y, Shen XR, Wang X, Zheng XS, et al.(2020). A pneumonia outbreak associated with a new coronavirus of probable bat origin. Nature. 2020;579:270–273. doi: 10.1038/s41586-020-2012-7. [PMC free article] [PubMed] [CrossRef] [Google Scholar]

50. Zhu H, Wang L, Fang C, Peng S, Zhang L, Chang G, Xia S, Zhou W.(2020)Clinical analysis of 10 neonates born to mothers with 2019-nCoV pneumonia. Transl Pediatr. 2020;9:51–60. doi: 10.21037/tp.2020.02.06. [PMC free article] [PubMed] [CrossRef] [Google Scholar]

3. Psycho-Emotional Care In A Neonatal Unit During The COVID-19 Pandemic

[1]Denise Streit Morsch[a] , Zaira Aparecida de Oliveira Custódio[b] , Zeni Carvalho Lamy[c,*]

Arduous times. Although the COVID-19 pandemic caused by SARS-CoV-2 has, until now, affected relatively few newborns (NB),[1] it has induced intense and disorganizing changes for neonatal care, influencing the bonding and neurosensory protection practices so hard-won over the past years.[2] With the presence of SARS-CoV-2, the current context requires distancing and reduced movement of people. Namely, it demands the reformulation of procedures and practices, leading to the need for new strategies to ensure care. Published documents suspended the visits from grandparents, siblings, and other individuals who comprised the support network, guaranteeing the exclusive access to the asymptomatic mother and/or father, after daily and safe checks at the entry to the Neonatal Intensive Care Unit (NICU).[3,4]

The challenge for neonatal teams is ensuring the safety of the NB, the NB's parents, and their own, without, however, departing from the basic principles of humanized care, which have guided the neonatal care in Brazil.[2] It is essential to understand and fulfill the requirements imposed by this moment in the world to ensure the needed adaptations, aiming at protecting the trinomial NB, family, and health team. To this end, it is important to consider care, regarded herein as intensive, focusing on supporting the NB, the NB's parents, and the health team. The experiences of countries that first faced this disease have shown this concern. Wang et al. reported that, in neonatal units, the stress of parents and the staff is high, and that social workers and psychologists must assist both.[5]

Intervention Strategies Targeted At Newborns For Routine Care In Neonatal Units

In times of social distancing, the parents' unrestricted access to and presence in the neonatal unit are hindered. Many situations might lead to the parents' absence; for instance, mothers and/or fathers who are symptomatic, tested positive, or had contact with someone infected with SARS-CoV-2, those with other children and/or family members in the risk group, who live far or have transport difficulties, among others.[3] According to Canvasser (*apud* Furlow), the effects of separating mothers and babies have been devastating.[6] Moments of crisis require deliberated, flexible, and unique attitudes. These changes involve the work of the entire team in a process of cooperation and mutual support. Keeping the same professionals in the care of each NB, on each shift, gives the patient a reference to recognize the routine care, the voice and touch of each professional, acting as a source of safety and trust in the face of so many changes. Mathelin[7] emphasizes the importance of the way of touching the NB, responding to their gaze, and "addressing them, as a human addressing another human, filled with feelings, thoughts, and desires." Being fully with the NB in such a delicate moment

[1] Corresponding author. E-mail: zenilamy@gmail.com (Z.C. Lamy). aNational Consultant of the Kangaroo Method, Ministry of Health, Brasília DF, Brazil. bHospital Universitário, Universidade Federal de Santa Catarina, Florianópolis, SC, Brazil. cPublic Health Department, Universidade Federal do Maranhão – São Luís, MA, Brazil. Received on May 08, 2020

of their lives is a compassionate attitude, as well as a neonatal health intervention that promotes their development. The offer of holding and handling each baby is a source of not only biological but also emotional support. The inner availability of the professional emerges upon the affection, the gaze, the gestures, and all aspects involved in the care relation. Besides this bodily contact with the NB, the professional uses verbal contact by describing what is happening. The words give the NB a meaning to what they are living. Introducing ourselves, explaining the care that will be carried out, and telling the NB where they are and why their parents are not with them allow them to recognize their personal history.[8] By using the spoken word, we give the NB an understanding of what they are experiencing in a situation of sickness and separation from their mother, father, and family.[9]Maternal death is another troublesome situation for babies.Cyrulnik[10] explains that an early loss in the life of little ones leads to catastrophe when there is no emotional substitute.

When an attachment figure disappears, a huge part of their sensory world vanishes. The baby's biological surroundings permanently lose their auditory, tactile, olfactory, and visual stimuli because the other is no longer present. Words must come into action once again, bringing, along with the narrative, the presence of another family caregiver. The intent is not leaving the baby alone, without the surroundings marked by family culture. The number of professionals who provide care for the NB should be the lowest possible. Support to the family and especially the interaction between the team and the family member who will take over the NB's care should be guaranteed. Staying beside the NB, looking at them, speaking softly, and supporting their body provide the necessary integration experience in moments of extreme vulnerability, and, according to the paediatrician and psychoanalyst Winnicott,[11] ensure the NB's well-being.

Intervention Strategies Targeted At Families For Routine Care In Neonatal Units

The entire team is responsible for facilitating the presence of the mother and/or father, whenever possible, and supporting them so they can also offer this outline of senses and meanings to the baby, stimulating the NB emotionally and using words to situate what they are experiencing. In the parents' absence, the team must ensure communication. Cell phone use in the neonatal unit, which has always been restricted, can be an important tool in this moment of crisis, shortening the distance between the family and the baby. However, its entry in the neonatal unit must be done with caution, rigorously complying with the rules of each location. Wrapping the device in plastic film after cleaning it has been recommended. A routine of contact mediated by the team might be established through recorded or read messages, which can also be proposed to siblings and other family members, such as grandparents. Photos and/or video records, short descriptions about how the baby is behaving, their traits, and routine can be sent to the parents.

When present, parents may be encouraged to capture images with their cell phones to share with the family, and the team must instruct them on how to clean the device and that their records should not involve other babies, families, or the team. Special interventions should be planned in the case of death in this context, which makes the situation even harder and sadder. Everything that has been built to facilitate the connection and the mourning process will have to be adapted at this moment, when the pain of separation between the family and the baby is unimaginably high.

How to experience the separation caused by death when the closeness was limited or virtually non-existent? How to deal with this pain when it is not possible to see, touch, dress, hold a vigil for the baby? This has become the reality of parents who lost their NB children to this pandemic.

Mourning rituals are suspended, and supportive physical contact is not recommended. Wakes have fixed, minimal, and insufficient time.

The impossibility of ritualizing the child's death will leave deep scars in parents and relatives. Cyrulnik10 highlights: "When the losses are neither accepted nor signified, the mourner can only withdraw to lessen their suffering. In this case, the loss is not mourning but a hole in the soul, an emptiness without representation." This situation leads to great psychic distress and can be traumatic, resulting in depressive disorders, anxiety, post-traumatic stress, and complicated grief, as described by Muza et al.12 It will be up to the neonatal unit professionals to assist the parents and relatives who lost their babies without even knowing them.

We suggest some actions that could be performed, considering the uniqueness of each mother and father, their family values, as well as the desire to carry them out: providing photos and videos of the NB alive; reading or playing messages from the family to the NB; instructing the parents to explain the conditions of the NB to other family members; after death, asking the parents to bring clothes and/or a small toy to accompany the baby. If possible, the family members who live in the same household can gather and perform a mourning ritual for the NB. It might be important to advise them not to rush to dispose of clothes and furniture they prepared for their child, allowing themselves time to prepare for this moment. The team can also deliver identification cards that belonged to the baby and a report written by the professionals who looked after the NB during their stay in the neonatal unit, with accounts of special situations. It is also essential to give family members the opportunity of returning to talk with the team, if they so wish, a few days after death, offering information and support

Care Strategies For The Caregivers

The neonatal unit staff is facing a huge emotional challenge. The strategies discussed in this editorial increase this challenge. However, empathizing with other humans, enabling them to experience an expression of love in such a painful moment of their lives, can generate a feeling of fulfilment and peace with what could be provided, given the real restrictions imposed. It is crucial to give voice to the health team and their requests. Used to well-defined protocols, the professionals face something still unknown. Comings and goings between different hospitals and the risk of infection or of transmitting the disease to family members lead to gruelling routines of care, hygiene, and equipment donning and doffing, often exceeding their shifts and the time for them to go back home. Team discussion and the support of the psychology and social service departments are important for the staff to be confident in their decisions regarding recent rules. Dialogues with other professionals who understand and validate their intentions are essential.

All these issues are present in the expressions and the frequent pleadings of health professionals in social networks: "We stay here for you, please stay at home for us." We share these concerns, fears, and fatigue. We believe that the support between professionals makes a difference. We can feel it when a hand reaches out to help handle a tube, place catheters, in the head that rests on another's shoulder to have a better view of the baby. Also, pay attention to the NB's body responding to your handling. Look out for expressions of comfort when you treat them. Neither you nor these babies will ever forget these experiences; they will be fleeting but intense memories, offering a shared holding. Moreover, take care of your own body. Accept suggestions about exercises that can be performed in the neonatal unit environment.

Minutes of silent or guided meditation that trigger breathing awareness and mindfulness, as well as the repetition of mantras or prayers connected to your beliefs, are practices that have proven to be beneficial in promoting relaxation, concentration, and anxiety relief.

When returning home, repeat this routine of exercises, meditation, and breathing. In your home environment, allow yourself to do what you want to do, eat or cook your favourite food, put on comfortable clothes, dance, sing, acknowledge that you are the comfort and peace these human beings need. You can speak with the NB, who still has no words. You understand their messages, conveyed by the body under your care. You welcome the parents at this delicate moment. You will also discover ways to take better care of yourselves in these demanding days because you are free to seek the best paths in life dynamics. We are thankful for the work you do. Thankful for your resilience and the teachings you share with our NB and their families.

REFERENCES

1. World Health Organization [homepage on the Internet]. Clinical management of severe acute respiratory infection (SARI) when COVID-19 disease is suspected [cited 2020 Apr 27]. Available from: https://www.who.int/publications-detail/ clinical-management-of-severe-acute-respiratory-infectionwhen-novel-coronavirus-(ncov)-infection-is-suspected

2. Brazil - Ministério da Saúde. Secretaria de Atenção à Saúde de Ações Programáticas e Estratégicas. Atenção humanizada ao recém-nascido: Método Canguru: manual técnico / Ministério da Saúde. 3ª ed. Brasília: Ministério da Saúde; 2017.

3. Brazil - Ministério da Saúde. Secretaria de Atenção Primária à Saúde. Nota Técnica nº 10/2020-CO-CAM/CGCIVI/DAPES/ SAPS/MS. Atenção à saúde do recém-nascido no contexto da infecção pelo novo Coronavírus (SARS-CoV-2). Brasília: Ministério da Saúde; 2020.

4. Sociedade Brasileira de Pediatria - Departamento Científico de Neonatologia. Prevenção e abordagem da infecção por COVID-19 em mães e recém-nascidos, em HospitaisMaternidades. Rio de Janeiro: SBP; 2020.

5. Wang. J, Qi H, Bao L, Li F, Shi Y, (2020).National Clinical Research Centre for Child Health and Disorders and Pediatric Committee of Medical Association of Chinese People's Liberation Army. A contingency plan for the management of the 2019 novel coronavirus outbreak in Neonatal Intensive Care Units. Lancet Child Adolesc Health. 2020;4:258-9. https://doi.org/10.1016/S2352-4642(20)30040-7 Psycho-emotional care and COVID-19 4 Rev Paul Pediatr. 2020;38:e2020119

6. Furlow, B.(2020). US NICUs and donor milk banks brace for COVID19. Lancet Child Adolesc Health. Epub 2020 Apr 1. https:// doi.org/10.1016/S2352-4642(20)30103-6

7. Mathelin, C. O Sorriso da Gioconda: (1999). clínica psicanalítica com os bebês prematuros. Rio de Janeiro: Companhia de Freud.

8. Szejer, M. A(1999). escuta psicanalítica de bebês em maternidade. São Paulo: Casa do Psicólogo.

9. Dolto, F.(2007). As etapas decisivas da infância. São Paulo: Martins Fontes.

10. Cyrulnik, B. (2009). De corpo e alma a conquista do bem-estar. São Paulo: Martins Fontes.

11. Winnicott, D.W. (2000). Observação de bebês em uma situação estabelecida. In: Winnicott DW. Da pediatria à psicanálise: textos selecionados. Rio de Janeiro: Francisco Alves; 2000. p. 149-64.

12. Muza, J.C., Sousa, E.M., Arrais, A.R., Iaconelli, V. (2013). Quando a morte visita a maternidade: atenção psicológica durante a perda perinatal. Psicol Teor Prat. 2013;15:34-48

CHAPTER 14

ORAL HEALTH IN THE AGE OF COVID-19

1. Access To Oral Health In Primary Care Before And After The Beginning Of The COVID-19 Pandemic In Brazil

[1]Edson Hilan Gomes de Lucena[1] Aldelany Ramalho Freire[1]

Deborah Ellen Wanderley Gomes Freire[1]Elza Cristina Farias de Araújo[1]

Gabriela Nazaré Wanderley Lira[1]Arella Cristina Muniz Brito[1]

Wilton Wilney Nascimento Padilha[1]Yuri Wanderley Cavalcanti[1]

[1] Department of Clinical and Social Dentistry.
Federal University of Paraíba. João Pessoa-PB, Brazil.

ABSTRACT

This study compared the access to oral health in primary care, before and after the beginning of the COVID-19 pandemic in Brazil. An observational study with a cross-sectional ecological design was carried out, using data from the Health Information System for Primary Care (SISAB). Data regarding the number of Oral Health Teams (OHT), Oral Health Coverage in Primary Care (OHC), number of First Programmatic Dental Consultations (FPDC), and number of visits due to dental abscess and toothache were collected. Data were collected by state as consolidated of the first quarter (January to April) of 2019 and of 2020. The median of the difference (MD) and the percentage of variation (%V) were obtained for each variable. Data were compared by Wilcoxon test ($\alpha<0,05$). An increase in the number of OHT was observed in 25 states (MD=45, %V=6.13%, p<0.001), whilst the OHC increased in 17 states (MD=1.01, %V=1.62%, p=0.035) between the 2019 and 2020. We also verified a significant reduction in the number of FPDC (MD=- 42,806, %V=-38.70%, p<0.001), as well as in the number of visits due to dental abscess (MD=-1,032, % V=-29.04%, p=0.002) and due to toothache (MD=-14,445, %V=-32.68%, p<0.001). Although an expansion of OHT and OHC between 2019 and 2020 was verified, access to oral health in primary care has decreased due to the COVID-19 pandemic.

INTRODUCTION

The first cases of COVID-19, a respiratory infection caused by the new coronavirus (SARS-CoV-2), were reported on December 29, 2019 in the Wuhan province, China. The rapid and exponential increase in the number of cases of the disease indicates that COVID-19 is more contagious than

[1] Correspondence to:
Edson Hilan Gomes de Lucena, DDS, MSc, PhD.
Departamento de Clínica e Odontologia Social. Universidade Federal da Paraíba.
DCOS/CCS/UFPB. Cidade Universitária, Campus I. João Pessoa-PB, Brasil.
58051-900 edson.lucena@academico.ufpb.br

previous epidemics such as Severe Acute Respiratory Syndrome (SARS-CoV) and Middle East Respiratory Syndrome (MERS-CoV), which makes it more lethal in absolute numbers. After its discovery, the virus spread rapidly throughout the world and on March 11th, 2020, the World Health Organization (WHO) declared the COVID-19 pandemic (1-3).In Brazil, the first case was confirmed on February 25th, being the first country to report a COVID-19 case in Latin America. On March 20th, the country acknowledged the occurrence of community transmission of the disease, and from then on, the Ministry of Health recommended measures of social isolation for the entire population (4-7). Social isolation measures are indicated in cases where it is no longer possible to identify all of those who were infected or their contacts in time to delay the spread of the disease (8). This type of intervention involves measures from social distancing, such as closing schools and cancelling public events, to completely blocking activities in a city (7,9). However, Brazil is currently considered the centre of the epidemic, which can be attributed to the fact that official government communication has not fully adhered to a series of isolation measures recommended by WHO (10).

The government chose to invest mainly in the hospital network, neglecting the strengthening of the primary health care, which may favour the collapse of the health system before the increasing trend of COVID-19 cases (11).The changes in the country's epidemiological scenario during the COVID-19 pandemic affected not only professionals who provide direct health assistance related to this disease, but other health professionals and the population that uses this service. For dental care, according to the Technical Note No. 9/2020, the main orientation of the Ministry of Health is to suspend elective care, maintaining emergency cases that must be performed individually in order to prevent the spread of the virus (12). Such measures taken to protect professionals and users of health services will also have an impact on the indicators of these services, such as access and resolution indicators, in addition to contributing to an increase in the restrained demand.

The frequency of dental care records within on the e-SUSAB individual dental care form can identify the impact that the COVID-19 pandemic can have on the offer of oral health services and indicators in Brazil (13). The e-SUSAB individual dental care form includes the registration of the First Programmatic Dental Consultation (PCOP) and Emergency Care. These parameters can then be used as indicators of the population's access to oral healthcare services. Given the above, this study aimed to compare the access to oral health in primary care of the Unified Health System (SUS), before and after the beginning of the COVID-19 pandemic in Brazil.

MATERIAL AND METHODS

This is an observational, descriptive, and analytical study, with a cross-sectional ecological design, which used data from public reports of the Health Information System for Primary Care (SISAB)of the Ministry of Health of Brazil. Data regarding the number of Oral Health Teams (OHT), Oral Health Coverage in Primary Care (OHC), number of First Programmatic Dental Consultations (FPDC), and number of visits due to dental abscess and toothache were collected by state. Data were collected and analysed as consolidated of the first four months (January to April) of 2019 and 2020, the period considered before and after, respectively, the beginning of the COVID-19 pandemic in Brazil. Data were collected on 15th of June 2020.Initially, for each study variable, the median difference (MD) and the percentage of variation (%V) were calculated. Data were then compared using the Wilcoxon non-parametric test, considering the 95% confidence interval and the 5% statistical significance. The data were tabulated and analysed using the Statistical Package for Social Sciences software (IBMSPSS, v.24, IBM, Chicago, IL).

This is an observational, descriptive, and analytical study, with a cross-sectional ecological design, which used data from public reports of the Health Information System for Primary Care (SISAB)[1] of the Ministry of Health of Brazil. Data regarding the number of Oral Health Teams (OHT), Oral Health Coverage in Primary Care (OHC), number of First Programmatic Dental Consultations (FPDC), and number of visits due to dental abscess and toothache were collected by state. Data were collected and analysed as consolidated of the first four months (January to April) of 2019 and 2020, the period considered before and after, respectively, the beginning of the COVID-19 pandemic in Brazil. Data were collected on 15th of June 2020.Initially, for each study variable, the median difference (MD) and the percentage of variation (%V) were calculated. Data were then compared using the Wilcoxon non-parametric test, considering the 95% confidence interval and the 5% statistical significance. The data were tabulated and analysed using the Statistical Package for Social Sciences software (IBMSPSS, v.24, IBM, Chicago, IL).

RESULTS

The comparative data between the January-April of 2019 and January-April of 2020 are shown in Table 1. An increase in the number of OHT was observed in 25 states ($p<0.001$), whilst the OHC increased in 17 states ($p=0.035$) between 2019 and 2020 (Table 1). We also verified a reduction in the number of FPDC ($p<0.001$), as well as in the number of visits due to dental abscess ($p=0.002$) and toothache ($p<0.001$) (Table 1).

DISCUSSION

Considering the high risk of contagion of COVID-19 in dental offices, there was a recommendation throughout the country for the elective care to be suspended, giving priority only to those considered urgency and emergency (14,15).

However, the present study showed a reduction in the number visits due to dental abscesses and toothache, considered of urgency and emergency. In addition, there was a reduction in the number of first programmatic dental consultations. Although the number of oral health teams and oral health coverage in Primary Care has increased during the same period, the findings of this study show the first negative impacts of the pandemic on access to public oral healthcare services in Brazil.

It is necessary to consider that the COVID-19 pandemic has a direct impact on the behaviour of patients in the search for dental care. In view of the recommendations for social isolation, some individuals are concerned about leaving home to seek the service, resulting in a reduction in the number of visits and seeking only in cases of extreme necessity. In addition, the population lacks clarity about what would be a dental urgency and emergency, with pain being a frequently referred symptom (16). A study conducted in China showed a 38% drop in the number of patients seen at a dental emergency service, with a significant reduction in demand of non-urgent cases in the pandemic period (17).In a recent pre-pandemic scenario, Brazil showed an increase in the number of OHT, although accompanied by a drop in the quantity of FPDC, between 2015 and 2017 (18). A reduction in the OHC in Primary Care was also observed as of 2016 (19). Factors such as political instability and freezing of investments in health provided by the advance of austerity policies have

---

[1] (https://egestorab.saude.gov.br/paginas/acessoPublico/relatorios/relatoriosPublicos.xhtml).

had a negative impact on access to oral health care in recent years (19,20). These effects, when added to the impacts of the pandemic, result in a worrying panorama. The frequency of FPDC four months of COVID-19 pandemic was similar to that observed during one-month 2003, when the number of OHT was seven times lower.

The need to adapt to new dental care routines, as well as the high costs of personal protective equipment, can impact the reduction in the number of dental care procedures (21,22). Thus, even in the face of a still rising contamination curve in Brazil, it is possible to suggest that oral health care will face thoughtful challenges during and after the COVID-19 pandemic. Although the main focus is given to the hospital environment during this period, the strengthening of primary care as a whole is essential to face these implications (11). The results of this investigation indicate that the expansion of the assistance network has not yet been affected by the pandemic. Although oral health coverage is still far from reaching the entire Brazilian population, it is known that the public health system serves the majority of the most vulnerable population (10,23). Therefore, setbacks in the expansion of the Unified Health System dental care could contribute to an increase in oral health inequities (11,19). The reduction in the number of first programmatic dental consultations would be expected, once health services were advised to only assist to urgent and emergency demands (14). However, the data in this study point out the assistance to dental abscess and toothache cases reduced significantly during the first four months of the COVID-19 pandemic in Brazil.

These indicators do not mean that the dental urgency and emergency cases did not exist, but it is suggested that such cases were not assisted by the public health sector. It is necessary for health services to prepare themselves adequately for returning elective care and effective resolution of dental urgency/emergency cases.

The increase in restrained demand in oral health can represent a serious setback for the country's oral health epidemiological scenario. Tools such as telemedicine could be used by professionals in the healthcare network with the objective of providing access to information and guidance by a health professional, without disrespecting social isolation (24). In addition to the purchase materials and equipment, it is also necessary to adapt the infrastructure of some health centres. In this sense, greater government investments in the health area are needed to enable the continuity of dental care within the Unified Health System. This study has limitations regarding the use of secondary data, obtained from a health information system. Although these data may be influenced by the quality of registration, it must be recognized that they are official information from the Ministry of Health of Brazil. Future investigations should consider a longer period of analysis, which makes it possible to verify the fluctuation of the indicators in the periods before, during and after the pandemic. The results of this study should be used by health managers and professionals to adapt the dental care provision routines, as well as by the population in general, which must demand the continued expansion of dental care within the Unified Health System.

CONCLUSION

Although there was an expansion of OHT and OHC between 2019 and 2020, access to oral health in primary care was reduced due to the COVID-19 pandemic in Brazil. This phenomenon is likely to impact negatively the epidemiological data of oral health in Brazil.

REFERENCES

1. Al-Jabir, A., Kerwan, A., Nicola, M., Alsafi, Z., Khan, M., Sohrabi, C., et al. (2020)Impact of the Coronavirus (COVID-19) pandemic on surgical practice - Part. Int J Surg. 2020; 79:168-179. doi:10.1016/j.ijsu.2020.05.022

2. Chinese Centre for Disease Control and Prevention. The Epidemiological Characteristics of an Outbreak of 2019 Novel Coronavirus Diseases (COVID-19) — China, 2020. China CDC Weekly, 2020, 2(8): 113-122. doi: 10.46234/ccdcw2020.032.

3. Rothan, H.A., Byrareddy, S.N. (2020). The epidemiology and pathogenesis of coronavirus disease (COVID-19) outbreak. J Autoimmun. 2020; 109:102433. doi:10.1016/j.jaut.2020.102433

4. BRASIL, MINISTÉRIO DA SAÚDE. Ministério da Saúde declara transmissão comunitária nacional. 2020a. Available at: https://www.saude.gov.br/noticias/agencia saude/46568ministerio-da-saude-declara-transmissao-comunitaria-nacional Accessed on: May 16[h] 2020.

5. Croda Rosa, Posenato, G.L.(2020) Resposta imediata da Vigilância em Saúde à epidemia da COVID-19. Epidemiol. Serv. Saúde. 2020; 29(1): e2020002. https://doi.org/10.5123/s167949742020000100021.

6. Rodriguez-Morales A.J., Gallego, V., Escalera-Antezana, J.P., Méndez, C.A., Zambrano, L.I., Paredes CF, et al. COVID-19 in Latin America: The implications of the first confirmed case in Brazil. Travel Med Infect Dis. 2020;101613. doi:10.1016/j.tmaid.2020.101613.

7. Schuchmann, A.Z., Schnorrenberger, B.L., Chiquetti, M.E., Gaiki, R.S., Raimann, B.W., Maeyama, M.A. (2020). Isolamento social vertical X Isolamento social horizontal: os dilemas sanitários e sociais no enfrentamento da pandemia de COVID-19. Braz. J. Hea Rev.2020; 3(2):3556-3576. https://doi.org/10.34119/bjhrv3n2-185.

8. Wilder-Smith A, Freedman, D.O. (2020). Isolation, quarantine, social distancing and community containment: pivotal role for old-style public health measures in the novel coronavirus (2019nCoV) outbreak. J Travel Med. 2020;27(2):taaa020. doi:10.1093/jtm/taaa020

9. Wilder-Smith A, Chiew, C.J., Lee, V.J. (2020). Can we contain the COVID-19 outbreak with the same measures as for SARS? Lancet Infect Dis. 2020;20(5):e102-e107. doi:10.1016/S14733099(20)30129-8.

10. Ribeiro, F., Leist, A., (2020). Who is going to pay the price of COVID-19? Reflections about an unequal Brazil. Int J Equity Health. 2020;19(1):91. doi:10.1186/s12939-020-01207-2

11. Souza, C.D.F., Gois-Santos, V.T., Correia, D.S., Martins-Filho, P.R., Santos, V.S., (2020). The need to strengthen Primary Health Care in Brazil in the context of the COVID-19 pandemic. Braz Oral Res. 2020;34:e047. doi:10.1590/1807-3107bor-2020.vol34.0047

12. BRASIL. Nota Técnica Nº 9/2020 de março de 2020. COVID-19 e o atendimento odontológico no SUS. Brasília, DF, 2020b. Available at: http://www.crosp.org.br/uploads/arquivo/ab69d79b87d04780af08a70d8cee9d70.pdf Accessed on: June 16[h] 2020.

13. BRASIL, MINISTÉRIO DA SAÚDE. e-SUS Atenção Básica: Manual Sistema com Coleta de Dados Simplificada: CDS. Brasília, DF, 2013. Available at: http://189.28.128.100/dab/docs/portaldab/documentos/manual_CDS_ESUS_1_3_0.pdf Accessed on: June 17[h], 2020.

14. BRASIL, AGÊNCIA NACIONAL DE VIGILÂNCIA SANITÁRIA. Nota Técnica GVIMS/GGTES/ANVISA Nº 04/2020, de 08 de maio de 2020. Brasília, DF, 2020 Available at: http://portal.anvisa.gov.br/documents/33852/271858/Nota+T%C3%A9cnica+n+04- 2020+GVIMS-GGTES-ANVISA/ab598660-3de4-4f14-8e6f-b9341c196b28   Accessed on:June 16[h] 2020.

15. Conselho Federal de Odontologia. Recomendações AMIB/CFO para enfrentamento da COVID-19 na Odontologia. Brasília, DF, 2020. Available at: http://website.cfo.org.br/wpcontent/uploads/2020/03/AMIB_CFO-Recomendac%CC%A7o%CC%83es.pdf Accessed on: June 17[h], 2020.

16. Macek, M.D., Cohen, L.A., Reid, B.C., Manski, R.J. (2004). Dental visits among older U.S. adults, 1999: the roles of dentition status and cost. J Am Dent Assoc. 2004;135(8):1154-1165. doi:10.14219/jada.archive.2004.0375

17. Guo, H., Zhou, Y., Liu, X., Tan, J., (2020) The impact of the COVID-19 epidemic on the utilization of emergency dental services. J Dent Sci. 2020;10.1016/j.jds.2020.02.002. doi:10.1016/j.jds.2020.02.002

18. Chaves, S.C., Almeida, A.M., Reis, C.S., Rossi, T.R., Barros, S.G. (2018). Política de Saúde Bucal no Brasil: as transformações no período 2015-2017. Saúde em Debate. 2018;42:76-91. doi: 10.1590/0103-11042018S206.

19. Rossi, T.R., Sobrinho, L., Chaves, S.C., Martelli, P.J. (2019).Crise econômica, austeridade e seus efeitos sobre o financiamento e acesso a serviços públicos e privados de saúde bucal. Ciência & Saúde Coletiva. 2019 Nov 25;24:4427-36. doi:10.1590/1413-812320182412.25582019.
20. Melo, E.A., Mendonça, M.H., Oliveira, J.R., Andrade, G.C. (2018) Mudanças na Política Nacional de Atenção Básica: entre retrocessos e desafios. Saúde em Debate. 2018;42:38-51. doi: 10.1590/0103-11042018s103.
21. Meng. L, Hua F, Bian Z. (2020). Coronavirus Disease 2019 (COVID-19): Emerging and Future Challenges for Dental and Oral Medicine. J Dent Res. 2020; 99(5):481-487.
22. Ge Z, Yang L, Xia J, Fu, X., Zhang, Y., (2020). Possible aerosol transmission of COVID-19 and special precautions in dentistry. Zhejiang Univ-Sci B (Biomed & Biotechnol). 2020; 21(5):361-368
23. Bastos, L.F., Hugo, F.N., Hilgert, J.B., Cardozo, D.D., Bulgarelli, A,F., Santos, C.M. (2019) Access to dental services and oral health-related quality of life in the context of primary health care. http://dx.doi.org/10.1590/1807-3107bor-2019.vol33.0018.
24. Caetano. R, Silva, A.B., Guedes, A.C.C.M, Paiva, C.C.N., Ribeiro, G.R., Santos, D,L., et al . (2020) Challenges and opportunities for telehealth during the COVID-19 pandemic: ideas on spaces and initiatives in the Brazilian context. Cad Saúde Pública. 2020;36(5): e00088920. https://doi.org/10.1590/0102-311x00088920.
    a.

Table 1 – Data regarding the number of Oral Health Teams (OHT), Oral Health Coverage in Primary Care (OHC), number of First Programmatic Dental Consultations (FPDC), and number of visits due to dental abscess and toothache in Brazil, from January to April 2019 and 2020. Differences were detected by the average percentage of variation, median of difference and statistical comparison (Wilcoxon test).

Variables	January to April 2019	January to April 2020	Average percentage of variation between 2020-2019	Median of the difference between 2020-2019	p-value
Number of OHT	28,018	29,662	6.13%	45	<0.001
OHC	52.59%	53.40%	1.62%	1.01	0.035
FPDC	4,081,355	2,437,646	-38.70%	-42.806	<0.001
Dental abscess	138,549	92,197	-29.04%	-1.032	0.002
Toothache	1,846,995	1,177,208	-32.68%	-14.445	<0.001

OHT: Oral Health Team; OHC: Oral Health Coverage in Primary Care; FPDC: First Programmatic Dental Consultations.

2. Rational Perspectives on Risk and Certainty for Dentistry During the COVID-19 Pandemic

Eugenio Beltrán-Aguilar, DMD, MPH, MS, DrPH, DABDPH
Habib Benzian, DDS, PhD, MScDPH *
Richard Niederman, DMD

ABSTRACT

Clinical dental practice exposes the dental team and patients to infectious airborne disease agents, due to the close contact during clinical care, and the infectious aerosols from most dental procedures. The U.S. Centres for Disease Control and Prevention (CDC), the American Dental Association (ADA) and other organizations developed recommendations to address the specific risk profile of SARS-CoV-2 transmission, adding additional protective measures to established standard precautions. When deciding on re-opening of dental services it is important to remember that so far, no reliable data on work-related infection risk for dental personnel are available. Combined with other uncertainties it seems prudent to follow four key principles: 1) All patients should be considered as potentially infectious; 2) procedures generating aerosols should be avoided, limited or closely managed; 3) infection control should be increased according to recommendations; 4) PPE measures should be maximized. Dental teams must follow ethical principles in providing the best possible and safe dental care. Yet, as business owners, they are facing existential impacts from reduced patient visits and loss of income resulting from service limitations. Reconciling the conflict of risking their life or their livelihood under the COVID-19 pandemic is not a welcome or easy choice. Decisions must be based on best possible evidence, and need to be revisited as the pandemic, and economic conditions change. COVID-19 also unmasked the challenges of access and financial coverage for dental care in the U.S. Sustainable preparation for future pandemics should consider reforms towards a more equitable system with better coverage.

Rational Perspectives on Risk and Certainty for Dentistry During the COVID-19 Pandemic

The Risk of Infection in Dentistry

The practice of dentistry exposes dental health professionals and patients to infectious disease agents.[1] The risk is considered to be higher in dental practices than in other health care settings, mainly because there is close and prolonged contact between provider and patient. In addition, most dental procedures generate aerosols that are contaminated with a patient's saliva, blood, other secreta, or tissue particles.[2] To control this risk, the U.S. Centres for Disease Control and Prevention (CDC) and other organizations developed recommendations and protocols based on the principle of standard precautions.[3, 4] The fundamental elements in these recommendations are the use of physical barriers between patient and provider, instrument sterilization, and environmental reprocessing.SARS-CoV-2, the virus causing COVID-19, is transmitted primarily through respiratory droplets and aerosols when an infected person coughs, sneezes, or talks.[5, 6] In addition, there is evidence that pre-symptomatic or asymptomatic persons can transmit the virus. COVID-19 is of particular concern for dental settings because of aerosol-creating dental procedures.[5, 6] To address this, the CDC developed "Interim infection prevention and control guidance for dental settings during COVID-19".[7] The CDC document states that the unique characteristics of the dental setting warrant special infection control considerations.

In line with this, the Occupational Safety and Health Administration (OSHA) developed a COVID-19 workplace guidance document[8] and an additional update entitled "Dentistry Workers and Employers"[1]OSHA places dental health care providers in the "very high exposure risk" category in their recommendations for preparing workplaces for COVID-19, along with doctors, nurses, paramedics, and emergency medical technicians who perform aerosol-generating procedures on known or suspected COVID-19 patients. The CDC and OSHA, therefore, both stipulate that dental practices require enhanced precautions to protect the clinical team and patients from aerosols generated during clinical care. In addition, the CDC confirmed that care for dental emergencies should be provided at all times during a pandemic, but take into account the specific local risk scenarios.[9]

The Current Status of COVID-19 Among Dental Health Care Providers

The CDC summarizes data from state health departments on SARS-CoV-2 infection among health care workers using a standardized case form. The CDC form does not differentiate between types of health care workers; specific information on COVID-19 among dental health care personnel is therefore not available. The CDC published a summary report on the characteristics of U.S. health care personnel diagnosed with COVID-19 in the United States through April 9, 2020.[10] While only 16 percent of all reported total infections contained data on whether the reported individual was a health care professional (HCP), 19 percent of HCP were reported as positive. From this group, 55 percent mentioned contact with a COVID-19 patient only in the health care setting, and the remainder in other settings. Among those infected, 2%-5% were admitted to ICU, and 0.3%-0.8% died. The CDC report warns that these numbers underestimate both, the infection and mortality rates, due to missing data and lack of information on the nature of interaction with suspected and/or confirmed COVID-19 patients. These data do support the CDC's and OSHA's guidance that health care workers face an enhanced infection risk during care provision. It is essential to understand that the lack of reported COVID-19 infections among dental health care personnel should not be taken as evidence for low or negligible risk for those working in dental settings. Rather, the CDC report supports the guidance documents that dental personnel are at high infection risk in a droplet or aerosol-generating environment.

---

[1] https://www.osha.gov/SLTC/COVID-19/dentistry.html).

Dental Services During The U.S Response To COVID-19

To reduce infection spread during the COVID-19 pandemic, the CDC recommended that dental care providers delay elective ambulatory care visits, aligned with the recommendations for medical services.[7] The American Dental Association (ADA), similar to other professional national and global organizations, developed a set of guidance and advice documents aligned with the CDC and OSHA recommendations.[11] In addition, the ADA also published clear definitions of dental emergencies to guide dentists in their decisions.[12] The majority of U.S. dental practices complied with the CDC, OSHA, and ADA advice by offering only emergency services or closing completely.[13] Currently, and in contrast to CDC, OSHA, and ADA guidance, states are beginning to lift restrictions on small businesses and dental practices, leaving the decision to re-open to the individual practice owners. While dental professional organizations are developing pre-opening recommendations, the question for dental professionals remains whether it is safe to provide care in dental practices, and what changes will be required to balance the need for care and the risks of doing so.[11, 14]

What We Know About COVID-19 Infection Risk in Dental Settings

Central to ongoing discussions around the re-opening of dental services is the evaluation of infection risk. In the absence of more detailed information, assessments of COVID-19 infection risk are done by extrapolation. Extrapolation is common in clinical and public health practice when knowledge and emergency context are rapidly evolving.[15] Such rapid recommendations or guidelines are often labelled as "interim." That said, there are a number of facts that can provide a sound basis from which principles for clinical care during the COVID-19 pandemic can be derived:

1) All patients should be considered potentially infectious

Transmission of SARS-Cov-2 can occur in pre-symptomatic or asymptomatic patients. In these encounters, medical history or body temperature offer no assurance of identifying infected individuals. Reliable and valid testing prior to dental care is currently not an option at this point in time because false-negative results cannot be ruled out. Also, vaccinations are not available, and the status of immunity after an infection is unclear. The only realistic and safe approach is to apply the principle of standard precautions. This means that, for now, all patients must be considered potentially infectious for airborne disease transmission and should be treated with equal and uniform precaution measures.

2) Droplets And Aerosols Are The Primary Sources Of Infection

COVID-19 is, therefore, an airborne infection because the primary sources of infection for SARSCoV-2 are droplets and aerosols containing the virus. The practice of dentistry produces aerosols and droplets, involves direct contact with potentially infected mucosa, and comprises procedures that may induce gagging or coughing of patients, all carried out in close proximity to the patient's mouth and nose.[16]Dental practice exposes dental health personnel to these infectious droplets and aerosols. Eliminating aerosol-generating procedures is the best protection. However, if care is acutely required and droplets are unavoidable, donning a comprehensive set of personal protective equipment (PPE) will reduce the risk of transmission. Such PPE is also used by respiratory therapists to intubate COVID-19 patients in health care settings. Other unique procedures for dentistry such as rubber dam, high-power suction, and physical barriers between patients and providers, may further reduce, but not eliminate the risk.

Airborne Infections May Require Higher Infection Control Measures Than Standard Precautions

The 2003 CDC recommendations for infection control focused on bloodborne pathogens, including hepatitis and HIV, and were later updated to address risk reduction of airborne pathogens like tuberculosis.[3, 17] The latter guideline requires airborne infection isolation rooms (AIIR) using negative pressure ventilation to reduce airborne transmission risk. However, dental operatories are generally not designed as AIIR. Current clinical evidence indicates that for aerosol generating procedures, enhanced PPE alone (handwashing, gloves, goggles, face shields, N95 face masks, and protective gowns), without AIIR, may reduce risk of transmission by approximately 90%.[18] Thus, a high-risk of transmission persists without AIIR, and infection with airborne pathogens cannot be ruled out.

Personal Protective Equipment (PPE) Required For Dental Care Should Be As Safe As Possible

The CDC interim guidance for aerosol-generating dental procedures during dental emergencies recommends the use of the highest level of PPE when treating COVID-19 patients (CDC, 2020). These recommendations are the same for health care providers in intensive care units looking after infected patients. With the remaining uncertainties about transmission risk beyond the evidence above, it is an ethical imperative to assume that all dental patients should be considered as potentially infectious. In acting with the principle of not doing any harm, maximum protective measures should be taken. Combined with the design limitations of dental operatories to appropriately and safely handle the risk of SARS-Cov-2 transmission, any consideration about providing dental care other than interventions that do not generate aerosols must be made with utmost caution.

Reconciling Risks And Uncertainties With Safety And Increasing Service Challenges

Based on our current knowledge, the COVID-19 pandemic will change the way dental services are provided. Aerosols need to be controlled, while PPE measures and patient triage procedures need to be enhanced. The possible availability of a vaccine in the mid-term provides only limited assurance because it will take time to reach effective vaccination rates and resurgence of COVID-19 or other viral outbreaks are expected.[19] Every practicing clinician, patients, staff, families, communities, and professional dental associations are at a crucial point of the pandemic. Dental health personnel are obliged to follow the ethical principle of providing the best possible dental care, including the elimination of potential risks and harms. At the same time, as owners of private practices or as health care companies providing dental services, they are facing existential impacts from reduced patient visits and loss of income resulting from service limitations or practice closures. Reconciling the conflict of risking their life or their livelihood in the context of the COVID-19 pandemic is not a welcome or easy choice. Decisions in this context must be based on scientific evidence or sound guidance when the evidence is still evolving. Solutions and compromises need to be revisited as the pandemic, and economic conditions change.[15] A pandemic is a highly dynamic process with differing scenarios within a country or state. Containment measures may entail that strict service limitations are required in one location or circumstance, but not in another, or that conditions for re-opening of services vary depending on the pandemic evolution over time. For some settings, just the availability of PPE may be a major constraining factor. Whatever the scenario, it will have domino effects with serious impacts on all oral health stakeholders. These changes will include dental supplies and manufacturers, the insurance industry, dental education, and research. Thus, there is an immediate and existential need for dentistry to develop rapid response protocols that limit the impact of this pandemic through the continued provision of safe dental care that minimizes risk and avoids procedures with aerosols.

The concept of SAFE Dentistry (Safe Aerosol-free Emergent Dentistry) may be a step in this direction.[20] The pandemic has also unmasked inequities that characterize access to dental care and financial coverage in the U.S. From this perspective, a better, more equitable system that ensures everyone's health and safety is needed. The profession needs to strive towards a future of oral health care that addresses population oral health needs, includes reliable surveillance to assess risk and outcomes, as well as improves preparedness and risk protection, while defining the best policy options for the current and future pandemics.

Author Affiliation

Eugenio Beltrán-Aguilar, DMD, MPH, MS, DrPH, DABDPH
Adjunct Professor, Department Epidemiology & Health Promotion, Associate Director Epidemiology & Surveillance, WHO Collaborating Centre Quality Improvement & Evidence-based Dentistry, College of Dentistry, New York University, 433 First Avenue, New York 10010 NY, United States.

Habib Benzian, DDS, PhD, MScDPH *
Research Professor, Department Epidemiology & Health Promotion, Associate Director Global Health & Policy, WHO Collaborating Centre Quality Improvement & Evidence-based Dentistry, College of Dentistry, New York University, 433 First Avenue, New York 10010 NY, United States, Senior Research Fellow, Global Health Centre, Geneva Graduate Institute for Policy Studies. Chemin Eugène-Rigot
2A, 1211 Geneva, Switzerland, habib.benzian@graduateinstitute.ch ORCID: 0000-0003-3692-4849

Richard Niederman, DMD
Professor & Chair, Department Epidemiology & Health Promotion, Director, WHO Collaborating Centre Quality Improvement & Evidence-based Dentistry, College of Dentistry, New York University, 433 First Avenue, New York 10010 NY, United States.

REFERENCES

1. Cully, C, Samaranayake, L.P. (2016).Emerging and changing viral diseases in the new millennium. Oral Dis. 2016;22(3):171-179.
2. Harrel, S.K., Molinari, J., (2004) Aerosols and splatter in dentistry: a brief review of the literature and infection control implications. J Am Dent Assoc. 2004;135(4):429-437.
3. Kohn, W.G., Collins, A.S., Cleveland, J.L, Harte, J.A, Eklund, K.J, Malvitz, D.M. (2003) Guidelines for infection control in dental health-care settings--2003. MMWR Recomm Rep. 2003;52(RR-17):1-61.
4. Centres for Disease Control and Prevention (CDC). Summary of infection prevention practices in dental settings: Basic expectations for safe care. Atlanta: CDC, US Dept of Health and Human Services; 2016
5. Peng, X., Xu X, Li Y, Cheng L, Zhou X, Ren B.(2020).Transmission routes of 2019-nCoV and controls in dental practice. Int J Oral Sci. 2020;12(1):9.
6. Meng, L, Hua., F., Bian. (2020). Coronavirus Disease 2019 (COVID-19): Emerging and Future Challenges for Dental and Oral Medicine. J Dent Res. 202022034520914246.
7. Centres for Disease Control and Prevention (CDC). Dentistry: Interim infection prevention and control guidance for dental settings during the COVID-19 response (27 April 2020).
8. Occupational Safety and Health Administration (OSHA), Department of Labor. Guidance on preparing workplaces for COVID-19 (OSHA 3990-02 2020). Available at: www.osha.gov/Publications/OSHA3990.pdf.
9. Centres for Disease Control and Prevention (CDC). Framework for healthcare systems providing non-COVI-19 clinical care during the COVID-19 pandemic (12 March 2020).
10. Centres for Disease Control and Prevention (CDC), COVID-19 Response Team. Characteristics of health care personnel with COVID-19 - United States, February 12-April 9, 2020. MMWR Morb Mortal Wkly Rep. 2020;69(15):477-481.
11. American Dental Association (ADA). Return to work interim guidance toolkit (29 April 2020).
12. American Dental Association (ADA). What constitutes a dental emergency? (27 March 2020
13. American Dental Association (ADA). COVID-19: Economic impact on dental practices (Summary results, accessed 30 April 2020). Available at: https://bit.ly/2K8hU16.
14. Casamassimo. P, Castellano. J., Conte. C., Czerepak, C., Jacobson, B., Lee, J., Miller, J.,(2020) Younger L. Re-emergence Pediatric Dentistry Practice Checklist: A guide for re-entry into practice for pediatric dentists during the COVID-19 pandemic (28 April 2020). Available from: https://www.aapd.org/Forbidden?ReturnUrl=%2fabout%2fabout-aapd%2fnewsroom%2fchecklist%2f.
15. Kowalski, S.C., Morgan, R.L., Falavigna, M., Florez, I.D., (2018) Etxeandia-Ikobaltzeta I, Wiercioch W, Zhang Y, Sakhia F, Ivanova L, Santesso N, Schünemann HJ. Development of rapid guidelines: Systematic survey of current practices and methods. Health Res Policy Syst. 2018;16(1):61.
16. Gamio L. The workers who face the highest coronavirus risk. New York Times. 15 March 2020
17. Cleveland, J.L., Robison, V.A., Panlilio, A.L. (2009).Tuberculosis epidemiology, diagnosis and infection control recommendations for dental settings: an update on the Centres for Disease Control and Prevention guidelines. J Am Dent Assoc. 2009;140(9):1092-1099.
18. Verbeek, J.H., Rajamaki, B., Ijaz, S., Sauni, R., Toomey, E., Blackwood, B., Tikka, C,, Ruotsalainen, J.H., Kilinc Balci, F.S. (2020) Personal protective equipment for preventing highly infectious diseases due to exposure to contaminated body fluids in healthcare staff. Cochrane Database Syst Rev. 2020;4:CD011621.
19. Moore, K.A, Lipstich, M., Barry, H., Osterholm, M. (2020) COVID-19: The CIRDAP Viewpoint. Part 1:
20. The future of the COVID19 pandemic - lessons learned from pandemic influenza. Minneapolis: Centre for Infectious Diseases Reserach and Policy (CIDRAP), University of Minnestota; 2020
21. Benzian, H, Niederman, R. (2020). A dental response to the COVID-19 pandemic - Safe Aerosol-Free Emergency (SAFE) Dentistry (DOI: 10.20944/preprints202005.0104.v1). Preprints. 20202020050104.

3. Dental Care And The COVID-19 Pandemic: The Precautionary Principle And The Best Available Evidence

Cassiano Kuchenbecker Rösing[1]
Juliano Cavagni[2]
Gerson Pedro José Langa[3]
Thais Mazzetti[4]
Francisco Wilker Mustafa Gomes Muniz[5]

ABSTRACT

The precautionary principle is part of evidence-based healthcare. However, since it is not always based in the most qualified evidence, it is frequently questioned. The emergence of a highly contagious disease, with increased levels of morbimortality, an acute respiratory syndrome, the so-called Coronavirus Disease 2019 (COVID-19), led health professionals to look for the best alternatives to save lives. In this sense, the precautionary principle was evocated.

The precautionary principle is used both preventively and therapeutically when knowledge about how to manage problems/diseases/conditions that are especially life-threatening. The aim of this short communication is to make a reflection about the precautionary principle, the dental profession and COVID-19. It is important to have in mind that in such a disease, guidelines, protocols and approaches can change very fast, since a continuous evaluation of all policies is mandatory.

INTRODUCTION

Evidence-based healthcare has been considered the current paradigm for all health professions [1]. This movement started with evidence-based medicine and spread for all health approaches. In such paradigm, the best available evidence should be used to treat individuals. This means that the so-called authority-based healthcare is increasingly questioned.

Dentistry has a considerable difference from Medicine, since the majority of the situations faced by the profession does not have death as an outcome. Death is undoubtedly a true outcome. In Dentistry, with some exceptions, the loss of a tooth is one of the most typical true outcomes [2]. Of course, patient-related outcome measures are also true outcomes (e.g, masticatory function, aesthetics, oral health-related quality of life, among others) and have to be always considered. The paradigm of evidence-based dentistry combines three fundamental aspects: the best available evidence, the expertise of the professional and patient values and preferences. All of these aspects should be taken into consideration in the decision-making processes.

However, there are some situations in which the best available evidence is of low quality or, even, inexistent. In 2020, a pandemic emerged: The Coronavirus Disease 2019 (COVID-19). It has been responsible for a very high number of deaths worldwide. The contamination with the SARS-CoV-2 (coronavirus) generates a strong respiratory syndrome, which, especially for the older adults and for those with chronic diseases has high mortality rate [3]. Therefore, different preventive and therapeutic measures have been advocated. Some of the measures are not based on high quality evidence and others might even not have any support. Their indication is frequently based in the so-called precautionary principle [4]. The present article aims at making a deep thought about the precautionary principle in dental care, especially taking into consideration the COVID19 pandemic.

The Precautionary Principle – Definition and Reflections

The precautionary principle is a preventive concept.

Traditionally, it comes from epidemiological studies that identify potential risk factors and, even without the complete proof, start to be part of the preventive policies [4]. It is used when the evidence neither clearly supports nor refutes the hypothesis. Of course, the inclusion of an action on the preventive policy needs to be under continuous and close surveillance, up to the moment in which the evidence supports or discards the measure. Figure 1 summarizes the precautionary principle in the context of evidence-based healthcare. One very important situation in the use of the precautionary principle is that the adverse events are also taken into consideration [5]. Moreover, the nature and morbimortality of the situation under consideration is of utmost importance. The precautionary principle is much more useful in situations in which morbimortality is high, which is specifically the case with COVID-19 [4].

In addition to preventive measurements, the precautionary principle is useful in therapeutic approaches. For example, in some types of cancer, a therapy starts to be used even before statistically significant differences are observed in comparison to a control group [6]. However, in such situations, in the same manner that in preventive approaches, a close surveillance of the positive and negative effects is mandatory. It is very important that the ones understanding, advocating or even analysing the precautionary principle are aware of the fact that uncertainty is present in these situations in various levels [4]. Evidence-based healthcare tries to rule out uncertainty with the best possible means, however when life is threatened, higher levels of uncertainty need to be tolerated. In this respect, one situation that needs to be strengthened is that the "absence of evidence is not evidence of absence". This means that when you do not have evidence in a specific situation, it does not support that this situation is useless or does not work. This is a very popular epidemiological sentence that needs to be always taken into consideration both in the decision-making process as well as in the planning and censuring of research projects. Sometimes it is not ethical not to perform a study, if there is no evidence to it, just because of an individual's belief. So, the precautionary principle is also used with proposals that, if continued under adequate surveillance, will be accepted or refuted. On the other hand, one very important situation comes with the precautionary principle.

This is: which is the outcome of the problem/disease/condition? If the outcome is death, high levels of handicap, or similar situations, evidence of less quality might support the approaches until a definitive answer is achieved. However, this is not adequate if the problem/disease/condition does not have a very harmful outcome. In Dentistry, the precautionary principle is, therefore, very limited [5].

One argument frequently comes into the picture: "if it does not harm, why not to use it?". This is completely inadequate in evidence-based healthcare, unless specific reasons are raised to use the precautionary principle. Several points of view are extremely critical to the precautionary principle, especially due to the misuse of it. Some reports even put it in a perspective of a scientific fallacy or incoherence. Clearly, this is not a situation that has only one side.

A more comprehensive understanding of the principle is mandatory, with a critical analysis of every situation involving the precautionary principle.

An Analysis Of COVID-19

The pandemic of COVID-19 probably started in China and has spread worldwide [7]. This is a highly contagious disease that inputs high levels of uncertainty for healthcare professionals. This is mainly related to the fact that it is a new disease and lack of knowledge exacerbates the situation. The present study was written between May 20th and June 5th, 2020. This is of high importance to be highlighted, since even during this 2-week interval, several situations changed and the information is being updated sometimes more than once a day. It is known that the pandemic has reached all continents of the world and that in absolute numbers of death, the United States of America and Brazil are the countries with high figures [8, 9]. It is estimated that more than 370 thousand people died worldwide up to the end of May 2020 and that the number of infected people is of more than 6.2 million [10]. Research is emerging from different countries and it seems that keeping social distance is one of the measurements that decreases infectivity [11, 12].

This is also of importance, since a flattening of the curve may be possible, allowing the health systems to get prepared to it. Together with the uncertainty of any kind of approach comes the need for governmental investment worldwide, which elicits high levels of polemics. The World Health Organization is trying to lead the understanding process of the pandemic and has already declared that we are facing a public health emergency, with the need of conjunct efforts from every citizen of every country [10]. Based on the precautionary principle (since no evidence was available for this specific disease), different protective measures utilized collateral evidence trying to protect the populations and the continuous evaluation of such measurements constitutes the current best available evidence. As in any situation in evidence-based healthcare, the methods used to evaluate anything are essential. In this respect, data on prevalence is not available.

This is due to the fact that different countries have different protocols for testing individuals, different ways of counting for death causes, etc. It is probable that a significant number of deaths by COVID-19 were not reported as such, especially due to under notification or even due to lack of testing of the dead individuals. Some countries with more established healthcare systems have better forms of notifications. For example, in the United States of America, a public-private partnership for community-based testing is happening. In Germany, there is a private partnership for testing. Additionally, patients can go to a hospital to test, and in case of a high demand of testing, medical students in universities are also able to perform these tests.

One point that needs to be analysed is that associations between some measures and elevation or flattening of the disease curve are available. Social isolation has been demonstrated to be effective [11]. The use of masks has been proposed [13], but the World Health Organization does not recommend the use of mask for healthy individuals, except for health workers or for individuals with direct contact with a sick person [14]. CDC recommends the use of cloth face coverings associated with hand washing, or hand sanitizer with at least 60% alcohol, social distancing (at least 1.8m), clean and disinfection of surfaces [15]. Another interesting situation that cannot be forgotten is that a hypothesis of a possible positive effect of chloroquine and hydroxychloroquine in patients with COVID19 was raised. This was a first hypothesis that led to a wrong understanding by parts of the healthcare systems. If in one hand a possible interesting effect was demonstrated, on the other the evidence was very weak and mainly observational.

After some weeks of usage by those that understood the potential benefits would be worth, studies are not confirming such benefit. On the contrary, it seems that the posed risks are very high [16]. Therefore, in a very short period of time, higher quality evidence transformed a possibility of treatment in an inadequate approach. The reality is that we are facing an unknown disease, with high level of mortality and that direct qualified evidence is not available neither for prevention nor for treatment. In this respect, taking into consideration the idea of the precautionary principle, measures based on collateral evidence might be taken and need continuous evaluation in order to, if proven consistently beneficial, become part of established protocols and, in case of not a proven benefit or a demonstration of important adverse effects, to be banned from the strategies.

The Precautionary Principle, COVID-19 And Oral Care

In the context of COVID-19, Dentistry is facing a new challenge. Similar to professionals that work in intubation of infected patients, dental professionals deal with an important situation regarding aerosol. Saliva is contaminated and a source of infection both for health professionals as well as for other patients that are in the same environment. The literature also suggests that salivary glands could be a potential reservoir for the virus [17]. Also, it should be highlighted that elective procedures should be limited at this time point of the pandemic. This means that maintenance visits, for example are probably postponed. Despite that, Centre of Diseases Control and Prevention (CDC) (USA) removed the recommendation to postpone elective procedures in May 18th [18]. In Brazil, there are different recommendations, varying for each state. Clinicians must be updated about the local current policies. They all depend on the numbers of infected people and the capacity of the health system.

One important information that has to be given for the population is that oral hygiene methods should be even emphasized, in order to avoid, to the best possible means, the necessity of urgent dental care or, even, deterioration of oral health [19].On the other hand, there are cases in which in-office dental care is unavoidable, such as individuals with pain, spontaneous bleeding, dental trauma, etc [19]. In these situations, biosafety is fundamental. In this respect, Dentistry has a lot to teach other professions. However, traditional biosafety measurements are probably not enough. Hence, evidence-based approaches should be preferred. Moreover, part of the decisions will not be evidence-based or, at least, not based on the best quality evidence. But one has to decide and, taking into consideration the best available direct or collateral evidence, guidelines should be constructed. Different organizations have worked on this topic and, up to the moment of the present article, some recommendations were made by them. CDC and ADA recommendations include previous contact with the patients for COVID-19 screening, avoid non-emergent dental care when the patient has COVID-19 symptoms, limit the number of companions whenever possible, minimize the number of patients in the waiting room and check the patient's temperature before dental care [18, 20]. One example of the included suggested procedures is rinsing with H_2O_2. For this suggestion, direct evidence is not available. The potential of H_2O_2 in reducing viral load is an example of the use of the precautionary principle. However, this needs continuous evaluation. Since evidence-based Dentistry also relies on patient participation, it is very important to clearly inform the individuals seeking dental care about the whole situation and have it in a signed written informed consent.

Final Remarks

In the moment of the writing of the present article, very little high-quality evidence was available for prevention and treatment of COVID-19. The precautionary principle should be, therefore, used. However, caution needs to be taken and continuous surveillance necessary. Science has to be mature to take steps further and steps back, with the main aim of healthcare, which is the well-being of humanity.

Affiliations

1) Department of Periodontology, Federal University of Rio Grande do Sul, Porto Alegre, Rio Grande do Sul, Brazil. E-mail: ckrosing@hotmail.com; telephone: +5551995119123. ORCID: 0000-0002-8499-5759.
2) Department of Periodontology, Federal University of Rio Grande do Sul, Porto Alegre, Rio Grande do Sul, Brazil. E-mail: jcavagni@hotmail.com; telephone: +55519995911703. ORCID: 0000-0003-0062-6604.
3) Department of Periodontology, Federal University of Rio Grande do Sul, Porto Alegre, Rio Grande do Sul, Brazil. E-mail: gerson_pedro002@hotmail.com; telephone: +55519982391908. ORCID:
4) Post-graduation program in Dentistry, Federal University of Pelotas, Pelotas, Rio Grande do Sul, Brazil. E-mail: thmazzetti@gmail.com; telephone: +55539984552970. ORCID: 0000-0001-6877-2099.
5) Department of Periodontology, Federal University of Pelotas, Pelotas, Rio Grande do Sul, Brazil. E-mail: wilkermustafa@gmail.com; telephone: +5553991253611.
    ORCID: 0000-0002-3945-1752.

Acknowledgments

This study was financed in part by the Coordenação de Aperfeiçoamento de Pessoal de Nível Superior - Brasil (CAPES) - Finance Code 001. All other funding was self-supported by the authors. The authors report no conflict of interest.

Figure legend

Figure 1. Summary of the evidence-based healthcare and precautionary principle.

REFERENCES

1. Dodson, T.B. (1997). Evidence-based medicine: its role in the modern practice and teaching of dentistry. Oral Surg Oral Med Oral Pathol Oral Radiol Endod 1997; 83(2):192-197.
2. Hujoel, P.P., DeRouen, T.A. (1995). A survey of endpoint characteristics in periodontal clinical trials published 1988-1992, and implications for future studies. J Clin Periodontol 1995; 22(5):397-407.
3. Wang, X., Fang, X., Cai, Z., Wu, X., Gao, X,, Min J, et al. (2020). Comorbid Chronic Diseases and Acute Organ Injuries Are Strongly Correlated with Disease Severity and Mortality among COVID-19 Patients: A Systemic Review and Meta-Analysis. Research (Wash D C) 2020; 2020:2402961.
4. Resnik, D.B. (2004). The precautionary principle and medical decision making. J Med Philos 2004; 29(3):281-299.
5. Tickner, J., Coffin, M., (2006). What does the precautionary principle mean for evidence-based dentistry? J Evid Based Dent Pract 2006; 6(1):6-15.
6. Weiss, N.S. (2006). When can the result of epidemiologic research not eliminate the need to invoke the precautionary principle? J Evid Based Dent Pract 2006; 6(1):16-18.

7. Zhu, N., Zhang, D., Wang, W., Li, X., Yang, B., Song, J., et al. (2020). A Novel Coronavirus from Patients with Pneumonia in China, 2019. N Engl J Med 2020; 382(8):727-733.

8. de Souza Ferreira, L.P., Valente, T.M., Tiraboschi, F.A., da Silva, G.P.F. (2020). Description of COVID-19 Cases in Brazil and Italy. S.N. Compr Clin Med 2020; 2020:1-4.

9. Team, C.C.-R. Characteristics of Health Care Personnel with COVID-19 - United States, February 12-April 9, 2020. MMWR Morb Mortal Wkly Rep 2020; 69(15):477481.

10. World Health Organization (WHO). Coronavirus disease (COVID-2019) situation reports 2020 [Available from: https://www.who.int/emergencies/diseases/novel-coronavirus-2019/situation-reports]. [Accessed on May 31, 2020].

11. Nussbaumer-Streit, B, Mayr. V., Dobrescu, A.I., Chapman, A., Persad, E., Klerings, I., et al. (2020). Quarantine alone or in combination with other public health measures to control COVID-19: a rapid review. Cochrane Database Syst Rev 2020; 4:CD013574.

12. Duczmal, L.H., Almeida, A.C.L, Duczmal, D.B., Alves, C.R.L, Magalhães, F.C.O, Lima, M.S., et al (2020).. Vertical social distancing policy is ineffective to contain the COVID-19 pandemic. Cad Saude Publica 2020; 36(5):e00084420.

13. Prather, K.A., Wang, C.C., Schooley, R.T. (2020).Reducing transmission of SARS-CoV-2. Science 2020; eabc6197. doi: 10.1126/science.abc6197.

14. World Health Organization (WHO). When and how to use masks. 2020 [Available from: https://www.who.int/emergencies/diseases/novel-coronavirus-2019/advice-forpublic/when-and-how-to-use-masks]. [Accessed on May 31, 2020].

15. Centres for Disease Control and Prevention (CDC). How to Protect Yourself & Others 2020 [Available from: https://www.cdc.gov/coronavirus/2019-ncov/preventgetting-sick/prevention.html]. [Accessed on May 31, 2020].

16. Mehra, M.R., Desai, S.S., Ruschitzka, F., Patel, A.N. Hydroxychloroquine or chloroquine with or without a macrolide for treatment of COVID-19: a multinational registry analysis. Lancet 2020; S0140-6736(20): 31180-31186.

17. Xu, J., Li, Y., Gan, F., Du, Y., Yao, Y. (2020). Salivary Glands: Potential Reservoirs for COVID-19 Asymptomatic Infection. J Dent Res 2020: 22034520918518.

18. Centres for Disease Control and Prevention (CDC). Guidance for Dental Settings[Available from: https://www.cdc.gov/coronavirus/2019-ncov/hcp/dentalsettings.html#Management].[Accessed on May 31, 2020].

19. Pereira, L.J., Pereira, C.V., Murata, R.M., Pardi, V., Pereira-Dourado, S.M. Biological and social aspects of Coronavirus Disease 2019 (COVID-19) related to oral health. Braz Oral Res 2020; 34:e041.

20. American Dental Association (ADA). Return to Work Interim Guidance Toolkit (Updated 5/7/2020)

21. [Available from: https://success.ada.org/en/practicemanagement/patients/infectious-diseases-2019-novel-coronavirus?utm_source=adaorg&utm_medium=globalheader&utm_content=coronavir us&utm_campaign=COVID-19]. [Accessed on June 1st, 2020].

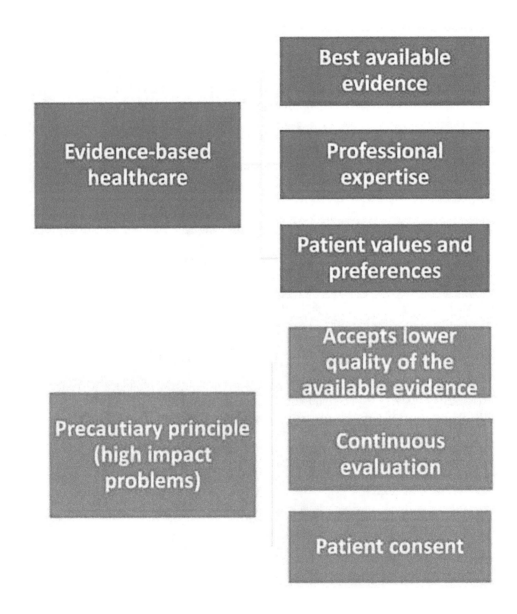

Figure 1. Summary of the evidence-based healthcare and precautionary principle.

4.Salivary Glands, Saliva And Oral Presentations In COVID-19 Infection

Marlus da Silva Pedrosa
[1]Departament of Biomaterials and Oral Biology, School of Dentistry,
University of São Paulo, SP, Brasil.

Carla Renata Sipert
[2]Departament of Restorative Dentistry (Endodontics), School of Dentistry,
University of São Paulo, SP, Brasil.

Fernando Neves Nogueira[1]
[1]Departament of Biomaterials and Oral Biology, School of Dentistry,
University of São Paulo, SP, Brasil.

ABSTRACT

Since the outbreak of the novel coronavirus disease 2019 (COVID-19) caused by SARSCoV-2, several published reports in the scientific literature called attention to the oral cavity as the potential route of infection, the implications for dental practice and the use of saliva in the diagnose of the COVID-19. Here, we would like to review the available literature on the salivary glands and saliva in the context of SARS-CoV-2 infection. A brief discussion of the oral manifestations is also presented.

INTRODUCTION

The first description of human coronavirus was published in 1965 [1]. It has generally been thought that coronaviruses could cause a future disease outbreak [2]. Since 2002, beta coronaviruses (CoV) have caused SARS-CoV in 2002-2003, MERS-CoV in 2012, and the newly emerged SARS-CoV-2 in December 2019 [3]. The first case of a novel coronavirus disease 2019 (COVID-19), caused by SARS-CoV-2, was reported in Wuhan city, China [4].Even though has been considerable debate on the origin of the COVID-19 causative virus, reports show that it is not a purposefully manipulated virus [4,5].The SARS-CoV-2 is highly transmitted from man to man through close contact with infected patients, leading to rapid global spread by infected travellers from China [6,7]. Also, substantial undocumented infections were found to facilitate the rapid dissemination ofCOVID-19 [6].

---

[1] Corresponding Author: Fernando Neves Nogueira
Department of Biomaterials and Oral Biology - School of Dentistry - University of São Paulo (USP)
Av. Prof. Lineu Prestes, 2227 – Cidade Universitária São Paulo – SP – Brazil – 05508-900
Phone/Fax: 55-11-30917849 E-mail: fnn@usp.br

On January 30, 2020, the World Health Organization (WHO) declared that COVID-19 is a public health emergency of international concern [6,7] as it is killing thousands of people worldwide. According to the most recent data from the Johns Hopkins Coronavirus Resource Centre (coronavirus.jhu.edu/), the global number of confirmed cases of COVID-19 was 5.432.512 with 345.375 deaths on May 25.Several published reports had drawn attention to the oral cavity as the main route of infection [8], the implications for dental practice [9] and the potential use of saliva in the diagnose of the COVID-19 [10,11]. A recent communication suggested the hyposalivation as responsible for exposing patients to a higher risk of getting coronavirus disease [12]. Besides, taste loss was reported in COVID-19-positive patients [13]. Here, we would like to critical review the available literature on the salivary glands and saliva in the context of SARS-CoV-2 infection. A brief discussion of oral manifestations is also presented.

SARS-CoV-2 infection

The SARS-CoV-2 uses angiotensin-converting enzyme-2 (ACE2) as an important receptor for entry into target cells and replication. SARS-CoV-2 employs the cellular transmembrane serine protease 2 (TMPRSS2) for spike protein priming and that inhibition of TMPRSS2 could at least partially protect against SARS-CoV-2 infection [14]. In addition, the viral spike protein of SARS-CoV-2 appears to be dependent of sialic acid-rich proteins and gangliosides GM1 [15]. Gangliosides are glycosphingolipids containing sialic acid found in mammalian tissues but are most abundant in the brain [16]. The gangliosides GM1 are primarily recognized as an essential component of membrane rafts, which play an important role in many cellular processes, including pathogen entry [17].

Salivary Glands and Saliva

The three pairs of major (submandibular, parotid and sublingual) and minor salivary glands secrete saliva in the mouth. Saliva presents diverse functions, including lubrication, initiation of digestion, and immunity [18]. It is a biofluid rich in water, ions, and several protein groups, including mucins, which are proteins glycosylated, and most have high sialic acid content [19]. Also, a range of disease biomarkers are recognized in saliva [20].The expression of SARS-CoV-2 has been detected in the oral epithelium [8] and in cough out [10,21] and swabs of human saliva [22]. These studies point to the importance of saliva for diagnostic strategies. It is worth to note, however, that the source of the virus in some studies were not investigated [10,21]. In one study, the tongue of each patient was lifted, and saliva was collected directly from the submandibular duct, which drains saliva from each bilateral submandibular and sublingual gland [23]. Interestingly, the expression of SARS-CoV-2 was found in four out of 31 (12.90%) COVID-19 patients [23]. Another important finding of the study of Chen and Colleagues [23] was that expression of SARS-CoV-2 was higher in critically-ill patients (3/4), which suggested the virus invasion due to high viral loads or destroyed salivary glands at the late stage of the disease. Additionally, analysis of ACE2 in human organs showed a high expression of ACE2 in minor salivary glands [24]. Besides the high content of sialic acids in salivary mucin, the salivary glands were shown to present gangliosides GM1 [25] and TMPRSS2 [26]. Overall, the literature suggests that SARS-CoV-2 could infect salivary glands [23]. Given the actual body of evidence, it is not possible, however, to make speculations regarding them as reservoirs for SARS-CoV-2.

Hyposalivation

The salivary gland secretion is dependent on several factors, including temperature, circadian rhythm and intensity, and type of taste and on chemosensory, masticatory, or tactile stimulation [20]. Hyposalivation, the reduction of unstimulated salivary flow rate, is a common finding in patients mainly reported as a consequence of the use of medication and psychological processes [27].Dry mouth was shown to be manifested in a relatively high proportion of COVID19 patients [23]. A recent communication has drawn attention to hyposalivation as responsible for exposing patients to a higher risk of getting coronavirus disease (COVID19) once the presence of many proteins with antiviral properties in saliva could be reduced [12]. Interestingly, the SARS-CoV-2 infection is more severe in individuals over 50 years of age and with the presence of associated comorbidities such as diabetes, cardiovascular problems and diseases involving the nervous system [28-30]. It is known that salivary flow reduces with age and is not explained based on medications used by older adults [31]. Besides, diabetes and medications for systemic disorders have also been associated with hyposalivation [32,33]. It is known that infectious and inflammatory processes might also lead to hyposalivation and, thus, the possibility of qualitative and quantitative disturbances in saliva secretion by SARS-CoV-2 infection in the salivary gland should not be discarded.

Taste Disorders

Taste disorders have been reported in a variety of clinical problems [34]. Amblygeustia, a diminished sensitivity of taste, was shown to be manifested by a relatively high proportion of COVID-19 [23]. In a study in which patients with influenza like symptoms underwent Covid-19 testing, smell and taste loss were reported in 68% (40/59) and 71% (42/59), respectively, of COVID-19-positive patients suggesting that chemosensory dysfunction should be considered when screening symptoms [13].Low salivary rate and disturbances in salivary biomarkers were suggested to cause xerostomia [35,36], which has been associated with taste sensorial complaints. Moreover, oral neuropathy or neurological transduction interruption induced by salivary compositional alterations is responsible for oral sensory complaints and loss of taste function [37,38]. Possible taste alterations as result of the direct effect of SARS-CoV-2 infection in sensory neurons or other components of the peripheral gustatory system should also be considered.

Oral Findings

It is known that the oral cavity may exhibit manifestations of underlying diseases such as oral ulcerations, gingival bleeding, glossitis, oral pain, or halitosis [39]. Viral infections usually manifest as either ulceration or blistering presentation of oral tissues [40,41]. A case report suggested that recurrent oral ulcers could be an inaugural symptom of COVID-19 [42]. Also, a report of three cases showed that pain and intraoral manifestations such as oral ulcers or blisters before seeking medical advice was a common finding in COVID-19 [43]. Thus, it was encouraged to perform intraoral examinations in patients suspected of SARS-CoV-2 [43]. As these oral findings are still new in the literature, their occurrence may vary significantly among COVID-19 patients and, thus, the associated systemic diseases and/or poor oral health may be a contributory factor to the oral presentations. Given the possibility of immunocompromised statuses of the patients, it is also possible that the oral manifestations may be related to other viruses or bacteria.

CONCLUSION

The Sars-CoV-2 infection is responsible for several events in the mouth. Studies, however, are necessary to understand the real role of salivary glands and saliva in COVID-19 patients.

Financial Support
This study was supported by the São Paulo Research Foundation (No. 2019/14556-7) and scholarship from the Coordenação de Aperfeiçoamento de Pessoal de Nível Superior - Capes.

Author's Contributions
MSP contributed to the conception and design, performed the analysis and interpretation, wrote the manuscript and final approval of the version to be submitted.
CRS contributed to analysis and interpretation, critically revised the manuscript and final approval of the version to be submitted.
FNN contributed to conception and design, performed the analysis and interpretation, critically revised the manuscript, and final approval of the version to be submitted.

Conflict of Interest:

The authors declare no potential conflicts of interest concerning the authorship and/or publication of this article.

REFERENCES

1. Tyrrell, D. Bynoe, M. (1965). Cultivation of a novel type of common-cold virus in organ cultures. British medical journal. 1965;1(5448):1467.
2. Cui, J. Li, F,, Shi Z-L. (2019). Origin and evolution of pathogenic coronaviruses. Nature reviews Microbiology. 2019;17(3):181-92.
3. Ou X, Liu Y, Lei X, Li P, Mi D, Ren L, et al. (2020). Characterization of spike glycoprotein of SARS-CoV-2 on virus entry and its immune cross-reactivity with SARS-CoV. 2020;11(1):1620. doi: 10.1038/s41467-020-15562-9.
4. Zhang Y-Z, Holmes, E.C. (2020). A Genomic Perspective on the Origin and Emergence of SARS-CoV-2. Cell. 2020;181(2):223-7. doi: https://doi.org/10.1016/j.cell.2020.03.035.
5. Andersen, K.G., Rambaut, A., Lipkin, W.I, Holmes, E.C, Garry, R.F. (2020). The proximal origin of SARS-CoV-2. Nature medicine. 2020;26(4):450-2.
6. Li R, Pei, S. (2020). Substantial undocumented infection facilitates the rapid dissemination of novel coronavirus (SARS-CoV-2). 2020;368(6490):489-93. doi: .1126/science.abb3221.
7. Zheng, J. (2020).SARS-CoV-2: an Emerging Coronavirus that Causes a Global Threat. International journal of biological sciences. 2020;16(10):1678-85. Epub 2020/04/01. doi: 10.7150/ijbs.45053.
8. Xu H, Zhong L, Deng J, Peng J, Dan H, Zeng X, et al.(2020). High expression of ACE2 receptor of 2019-nCoV on the epithelial cells of oral mucosa. International Journal of Oral Science. 2020;12(1):1-5.
9. Meng, L., Hua, F., Bian, Z. (2020). Coronavirus disease 2019 (COVID-19): emerging and future challenges for dental and oral medicine. Journal of Dental Research. 2020;99(5):481-7.
10. To KK-W, Tsang OT-Y, Yip CC-Y, Chan K-H, Wu T-C, Chan JM-C, et al.(2020). Consistent detection of 2019 novel coronavirus in saliva. Clinical Infectious Diseases. 2020.

11. Sabino-Silva, R., Jardim, A.C.G., Siqueira, W.L.(2020). Coronavirus COVID-19 impacts to dentistry and potential salivary diagnosis. Clinical Oral Investigations. 2020:1-3.

12. Farshidfar, N, Hamedani, S. (2020).Hyposalivation as a potential risk for SARS-CoV-2 infection: Inhibitory role of saliva. Oral Diseases. 2020.

13. Yan, C.H., Faraji, F., Prajapati, D.P., Boone, C.E, DeConde, A.S., editors. (2020). Association of chemosensory dysfunction and Covid-19 in patients presenting with influenza-like symptoms. International Forum of Allergy & Rhinology; 2020: Wiley Online Library.

14. Hoffmann, M., Kleine-Weber, H., Schroeder, S., Krüger, N., Herrler, T., Erichsen, S., et al. (2020). SARS-CoV-2 cell entry depends on ACE2 and TMPRSS2 and is blocked by a clinically proven protease inhibitor. Cell. 2020.

15. Fantini. J., Di Scala, C., Chahinian H, Yahi, N. (2020). Structural and molecular modeling studies reveal a new mechanism of action of chloroquine and hydroxychloroquine against SARS-CoV-2 infection. International journal of antimicrobial agents. 2020:105960.

16. Schnaar, R (2020). Chapter Three - The Biology of Gangliosides. In: Baker DC, editor. Advances in Carbohydrate Chemistry and Biochemistry. 76: Academic Press; 2019. p. 113-48.

17. Schnaar, R.L., Gerardy-Schahn, R., Hildebrandt, H. (2014). Sialic acids in the brain: gangliosides and polysialic acid in nervous system development, stability, disease, and regeneration. Physiological reviews. 2014;94(2):461-518. Epub 2014/04/03. doi: 10.1152/physrev.00033.2013.

18. Suzuki, A., Iwata, J. (2018). Molecular Regulatory Mechanism of Exocytosis in the Salivary Glands. International journal of molecular sciences. 2018;19(10):3208.

19. Shogren, R., Gerken, T.A., Jentoft, N. (1989).Role of glycosylation on the conformation and chain dimensions of O-linked glycoproteins: light-scattering studies of ovine submaxillary mucin. Biochemistry. 1989;28(13):5525-36.

20. Proctor, G.B. (2000).The physiology of salivary secretion. Periodontology 2000. 2016;70(1):11-25. Epub 2015/12/15. doi: 10.1111/prd.12116.

21. To KK-W, Tsang OT-Y, Leung W-S, Tam AR, Wu T-C, Lung DC, et al. (2020). Temporal profiles of viral load in posterior oropharyngeal saliva samples and serum antibody responses during infection by SARS-CoV-2: an observational cohort study. The Lancet Infectious Diseases. 2020.

22. Zhang, W., Du R-H, Li B, Zheng, X-S., Yang, X-L., Hu, B. (2020). et al. Molecular and serological investigation of 2019-nCoV infected patients: implication of multiple shedding routes. Emerging microbes & infections. 2020;9(1):386-9.

23. Chen L, Zhao J, Peng J, Li X, Deng X, Geng Z, et al. Detection of 2019-nCoV in Saliva and Characterization of Oral Symptoms in COVID-19 Patients. Available at SSRN 3556665. 2020.

24. Xu J, Li Y, Gan F, Du Y, Yao Y. (2020). Salivary Glands: Potential Reservoirs for COVID19 Asymptomatic Infection. Journal of Dental Research. 2020:0022034520918518.

25. Nowroozi, N., Kawata, T., Liu, P. Rice, D., Zernik, J.H. (2001) High β-galactosidase and ganglioside GM1 levels in the human parotid gland. Archives of Otolaryngology–Head & Neck Surgery. 2001;127(11):1381-4.

26. Vaarala, M.H., Porvari, K.S, Kellokumpu, S., Kyllönen, A.P, Vihko, P.T. (2001). Expression of transmembrane serine protease TMPRSS2 in mouse and human tissues. The Journal of pathology. 2001;193(1):134-40.

27. Bergdahl, M. Bergdahl, J.(2007).Low unstimulated salivary flow and subjective oral dryness: association with medication, anxiety, depression, and stress. Journal of dental research. 2000;79(9):1652-8.

28. Fu L, Wang B, Yuan T, Chen X, Ao Y, Fitzpatrick, T. et al.(2020). Clinical characteristics of coronavirus disease 2019 (COVID-19) in China: a systematic review and metaanalysis. Journal of Infection. 2020.

29. Cascella, M., Rajnik, M., Cuomo, A., Dulebohn, S.C., Di Napoli, R. (2020) Features, evaluation and treatment coronavirus (COVID-19).Statpearls [internet]: StatPearls Publishing; 2020.

30. Zhou, F., Yu, T., Du, R., Fan, G., Liu, Y., Liu, Z., et al. (2020). Clinical course and risk factors for mortality of adult inpatients with COVID-19 in Wuhan, China: a retrospective cohort study. The lancet. 2020.

31. Affoo, R.H, Foley, N, Garrick, R, Siqueira, W.L, Martin, R.E.(2015). Meta-Analysis of Salivary Flow Rates in Young and Older Adults. Journal of the American Geriatrics Society. 15;63(10):2142-51. Epub 2015/10/13. doi: 10.1111/jgs.13652.

32. Lopez-Pintor, R.M, (2016). Casanas E, Gonzalez-Serrano J. Xerostomia, Hyposalivation, and Salivary Flow in Diabetes Patients. 2016;2016:4372852. doi: 10.1155/2016/4372852.

33. Navazesh, M., Brightman, V.J., Pogoda, J.M.(1996). Relationship of medical status, medications, and salivary flow rates in adults of different ages. Oral surgery, oral medicine, oral pathology, oral radiology, and endodontics. 1996;81(2):172-6. Epub 1996/02/01. doi: 10.1016/s1079-2104(96)80410-0.

34. Doty, R.L.(2019). Systemic diseases and disorders. Handbook of clinical neurology. 2019;164:361-87. Epub 2019/10/13. doi: 10.1016/b978-0-444-63855-7.00021-6.

35. Romero, A.C., Ibuki, F.K., Nogueira, F.N.(2012). Sialic acid reduction in the saliva of streptozotocin induced diabetic rats. Archives of Oral Biology. 2012;57(9):1189-93.

36. Farsi, N.M.(2007). Signs of oral dryness in relation to salivary flow rate, pH, buffering capacity and dry mouth complaints. BMC oral health. 2007;7(1):15.

37. Hershkovich, O., Nagler, R.M. (2004). Biochemical analysis of saliva and taste acuity evaluation in patients with burning mouth syndrome, xerostomia and/or gustatory disturbances. Archives of oral biology. 2004;49(7):515-22.

38. Henkin, R.I. (1999).Decreased parotid saliva gustin/carbonic anhydrase VI secretion: an enzyme disorder manifested by gustatory and olfactory dysfunction. The American journal of the medical sciences. 1999;318(6):380-91.

39. Gaddey, H.L.(2017). Oral manifestations of systemic disease. Gen Dent. 2017;65(6):23-9. Epub 2017/11/04.

40. Santosh, A.B.R, Muddana, K. (2020). Viral infections of oral cavity. Journal of Family Medicine and Primary Care. 2020;9(1):36.

41. Pedrosa, M., de Paiva, M., Oliveira, L., Pereira, S., da Silva C, Pompeu, J. (2017). Oral manifestations related to dengue fever: a systematic review of the literature. Australian dental journal. 2017;62(4):404-11.

42. Chaux-Bodard, A-G., Deneuve, S., Desoutter, A.(2020) Oral manifestation of COVID-19 as an inaugural symptom? Journal of Oral Medicine and Oral Surgery. 2020;26(2):18.

43. Martín Carreras-Presas C, Amaro Sánchez, J., López-Sánchez A.F., Jané-Salas, E,, Somacarrera Pérez, M.L. (2020). Oral vesiculobullous lesions associated with SARS-CoV-2 infection. Oral Diseases. 2020. doi: https://doi.org/10.1111/odi.13382.

5. Coronavirus Disease (COVID-19): Characteristics In Children And Considerations For Dentists Providing Their Care

Sreekanth Kumar Mallineni, Nicola P. Innes, Daniela Procida
Raggio Mariana Pinheiro Araujo, Mark D. Robertson,
Jayakumar Jayaraman

ABSTRACT

The emergence of the novel virus severe acute respiratory syndrome coronavirus 2 (SARS-CoV-2) causing coronavirus disease (COVID-19) has led to a global pandemic and one of the most significant challenges to the healthcare profession. Dental practices are focal points for cross-infection, and care must be taken to minimise the risk of infection to, from, or between dental care professionals and patients. The COVID-19 epidemiological and clinical characteristics are still being collated but children's symptoms seem to be milder than those that adults experience. It is unknown whether certain groups, for example children with comorbidities, might be at a higher risk of more severe illness. Emerging data on disease spread in children, affected by COVID-19, have not been presented in detail. The purpose of this article was to report current data on the paediatric population affected with COVID-19 and highlight considerations for dentists providing care for children during this pandemic. All members of the dental team have a professional responsibility to keep themselves informed of current guidance and be vigilant in updating themselves as recommendations are changing so quickly.

1. INTRODUCTION

At the beginning of 2020, the novel virus severe acute respiratory syndrome coronavirus 2 (SARS-CoV-2) appeared, causing the coronavirus disease (COVID-19). The emerging virus has resulted in a global pandemic declared a Public Health Emergency of International Concern (PHEIC) by the World Health Organization (WHO) Director-General on the recommendation of the International Health Regulations (2005) Emergency Committee.[1] The case detection rate is changing daily and can be tracked in almost real time.[2] As of 31 March 2020, 19:50 hours (Central Standard Time), the number of confirmed cases was 857 487 and reported deaths were 42 106 with 169 418 recovered patients.[2]

The first case of a dentist being tested positive for COVID-19 was reported on 23 January 2020 at the Department of Preventive Dentistry in the Wuhan University Dental Hospital. Eventually, the transmission of disease to eight other oral healthcare professionals was identified.[3] The characteristics of epidemiological spread and clinical manifestations of COVID-19 in children have not yet been thoroughly elucidated. This article reports current data on the paediatric population affected with COVID-19 and emphasises the importance of following locally, regionally, and nationally relevant safety measures to protect dental care professionals as well as the child patient, whilst providing clinical care for the obviously affected children and those potential carriers of the infection. We emphasise that, in a rapidly changing pandemic landscape, practitioners must actively, regularly seek and use reputable and reliable sources of information on managing child patients that are appropriate for their own region and circumstances.

2 COVID-19

2.1. Clinical Characteristics Of COVID-19 In Children

The clinical symptoms of COVID-19 are still being documented and collated, although the majority of affected patients exhibit symptoms including a dry cough which is usually accompanied by fever.[4] Difficulty in breathing, fatigue, and other less typical symptoms can also occur.[5, 6] Signs and symptoms include different stages as asymptomatic, mild, moderate, severe, and critical.[7] Children tend to present with similar but milder symptoms to adults. To date, 3092 paediatric cases have been reported to have tested positive, and 1412 children were suspected of having been infected with COVID-19. A survey of 1391 children in China found 171 (12.3%) cases tested positive for SARS-CoV-2.[8] An analysis of more than 2000 child patients with suspected or confirmed COVID-19 in Hubei, China, found that over 90% presented as asymptomatic or with mild to moderate symptoms.[9] A summary of paediatric cases reported with COVID-19 is presented in Table 1.[7, 9-45] These numbers are likely to be under-representative, as there is not universal testing of the whole population for the presence of COVID-19. An overall fatality rate of 1.36%-15% has been reported across all patients with COVID-19.[46] As of 31 March 2020, seven fatalities have been reported in paediatric population due to COVID-19. These are an infant in Chicago,[47] a minor child in New York,[48] a 12-year-old boy in Belgium,[49] a 13-year-old boy in England,[50] a 14-year-old boy in China,[7] a 16-year-old girl in France,[51] and a 17-year-old boy in Los Angeles.[52]

Table 1. Summary of reported paediatric cases on COVID-19 (as of 31 March 2020)

Authors	Country	No. of cases reported	Age range
Bi et al9	China	20	-
Cai et al10	China	10	3 m to 11 y
CDC11	USA	123	<19 y
Chan et al 12	China	1	<1 y
Chang et al13	China	1	10 y

Authors	Country	No. of cases reported	Age range
Chen et al14	China	9	<1 y
Chen et al15	China	4	<1 y
Choe et al16	South Korea	480	0-19 y
Cui et al17	China	1	<1 y
D'Antiga18	Italy	3	-
Dong et al7	China	731	7 y (median)
Dong et al19	China	1	<1 y
Fan et al20	China	2	<1 y
Henry et al21	International	82	10 y
Ji et al22	China	2	>15 y
Kam et al23	Singapore	1	<1 y
Li et al24	China	5	10 m to 6 y
Liu et al25	China	6	1-7 y
Liu et al26	China	4	-
Livingston and Bucher27	Italy	270	<18 y
Lou et al28	China	3	6 m to 8 y
Lu et al29	China	171	-
Mizumoto et al30	Japan	10	0-19 y
Pan et al31	China	1	3 y
Qiu et al32	China	36	0-16 y

Authors	Country	No. of cases reported	Age range
Tang et al33	China	26	1-13 y
Wang et al34	China	1	<1 y
Wang et al35	China	1	<1 y
Wang et al36	China	34	7 y (median)
Wei et al37	China	9	<1 y
Wu et al38	China	965	<19 y
Xia et al39	China	20	-
Xing et al40	China	3	5 and 6 y
Xu et al41	China	2	10 to 11 y
Yu et al42	China	7	<1 y
Zeng et al43	China	3	<1 y
Zhang et al44	China	34	1 m to 12 y
Zhu et al45	China	10	s<1 y

- Abbreviations: CDC, Centre for Disease Control and Prevention; m, months; USA, United States of America; y, years.

2.2 The Child Patient In The Dental Setting

Because of the long incubation period (2-14 days)[6] for everyone, and because children can be asymptomatic or present with mild, nonspecific symptoms, all child patients and parents should be considered as potential carriers of SARS-CoV-2 unless proved otherwise. COVID-19 can be transmitted through direct and indirect contact, mainly via respiratory droplets and splatter from saliva and blood through contact with mucous membranes and contaminated fomites. [53,54]

This leaves dental professionals in potentially high-risk situations. Many dental treatments are aerosol generating procedures (AGPs), which have been associated with the transmission of acute respiratory infections.[55] In addition, dental settings are more likely to have a high number of potentially contaminated surfaces such as dental chairs, their handles, the spittoon, and dental instruments after carrying out a treatment which are possible routes of transmission. [3]

SARS-CoV-2 virus can persist on surfaces for up to 72 hours, [56] and all clinic surfaces should be disinfected using chemicals recommended for eliminating SARS-CoV-2. Universal precautions should be routinely followed in dental clinics.

They are critical for avoiding the transmission of SARS-CoV-2 virus to children as well as transmission from infected children to healthcare professionals. An infection prevention checklist should be used, including administrative measures, infection prevention education and training, dental healthcare personnel safety, programme evaluation, hand hygiene, personal protective equipment (PPE), respiratory hygiene/cough etiquette, sharps safety, safe injection practices, sterilisation and disinfection of patient-care items and devices, environmental infection prevention and control, and dental unit water quality.[57,58]

2.3 Country-Specific Approaches And Recommendations

The WHO has described a pandemic as having six different phases. [59]

Countries will be in different phases at different times; therefore, it is not possible to give universal guidelines, so following local updated guidelines are essential. All the above applies to child patients during the acute phase of COVID-19 pandemic, and the treatment choices and planning may vary during the next phases. Countries have put different measures in place for the overall delivery of dental care even during the 'Widespread Human Infection' phases of the pandemic leading up to the peaks of infection. These vary from those where dental practices remain open but there are screening activities and additional cross-infection measures.

These measures generally seem to fit for countries who managed to contain the disease spread quite quickly as seen in Singapore, for example where isolation and testing were put in place within a very short space of the infection being suspected as being present in the country. [60] At the other end of the spectrum, some countries have closed all dental practices. Some, such as the UK, have all cases triaged by telephone and attending only for very basic treatment in designated centres. In Brazil, The National Health Surveillance Agency (ANVISA) has recommended that only emergency and urgent dental care should be performed (from 20 March 2020), and all private offices have to stop elective treatments. Dental professionals (primary and secondary care) that work for the National Health Service (SUS) have been allocated to help other health professionals in the fast-track for COVID-19.[61] Between these two examples, there are a myriad of service delivery models. There are a number of country-specific measures currently in place. For example, in the United States (US), Telephone Health (Telehealth) systems have been introduced, and United States Department of Health and Human Services has relaxed the Health Insurance Portability and

Accountability Act (HIPAA) regulations in order to enable free and transparent Telehealth services to patients during the COVID-19 public health emergency. **62** In Brazil, the Ministry of Health has also implemented regulations for Telehealth services to reduce disease transmission. 63 Even though countries may be limiting dental care to only emergency provision, the recommendations between countries may differ.

There are some differences between recently published documents on urgent non-emergency, and emergency dental procedures by the American Dental Association, 64 and the UK Scottish Dental Clinical Effectiveness Practice guidelines.65 The American Academy of Paediatric Dentistry has also produced an algorithm specific to managing children with emergency dental conditions .**66, 67** As yet, it is difficult to give standard recommendations regarding personal protective equipment (PPE). The use of N-95 respirator masks in the United States and use of filtering facepiece respirator (often known as FFP) masks in Europe are strongly indicated in managing children but this is not a universal recommendation across all countries.**68** The evidence is lacking for mask use in some areas.**69** The recommendations provided by the Centre for Disease Control and Prevention (CDC) or other local guidelines that may supersede these should be strictly followed when placing on and removing personal protective equipment used for treating children infected by COVID-19.**58**

2.4 The Role of Guidelines And Professional Judgement

Guidance cannot ever cover all possible circumstances, and professional judgement must be exercised to make decisions around whether or not to provide treatment. Treatment should only be provided adhering to local, regional, and national guidelines as far as possible and, in the opinion of the dental professional, when it is safe for child patients, their accompanying carer, and for the dental team. During this COVID-19 pandemic, universal infection control procedures are of utmost importance with extreme vigilance and championing required by all. Globally, many primary and secondary dental services have been suspended, with many countries providing telephone-based triage systems to identify those patients requiring urgent or emergency intervention. **59, 63** Where dental professionals must offer assessment and/or treatment on a face-to-face basis, they should record all precautions that have been put in place to reduce the risk of cross-infection during treatment and evidence comprehensive risk assessment completion. This includes managing the risk from the treatment itself by carrying out the least invasive treatment possible, and avoiding AGPs.57, 68

Healthcare guidance is being updated with alarming frequency, and confusion as to how best to proceed in a care setting is both evident and widespread. It is of the highest importance that all members of the dental team acknowledge and act upon their professional responsibility to ensure they are absolutely contemporary in their understanding of current guidance. Additionally, dental teams should be familiar with treatment options that minimise or eliminate AGPs—many of which are founded on contemporary cariology, well documented in the scientific literature, and minimally invasive by their nature. It must also be appreciated that pandemic experience and staging will differ geographically. Once practice restrictions begin to be eased, continued management of dental disease with contemporary dentistry through minimally interventive concepts and other non-AGPs, whilst viral transmission risk remains high, will be pertinent.

These include atraumatic restorative treatment (ART),**70** sealing in carious lesions using fissure sealants,**71** silver diamine fluoride,**72** selective caries removal,**73** and the Hall Technique.**74** The importance of toothbrushing with fluoridated toothpaste to prevent tooth decay developing should continue to be emphasised during contact with patients, and there are opportunities being taken for dentists to carry out telephone and video consultations with parents to promote positive oral health behaviours.

3. CONCLUSIONS

Although reported clinical manifestations of COVID-19 in children are generally less severe than those of adult patients, young children, and particularly infants, remain vulnerable to infection and pose a significant transmission risk. Dental teams must ensure they remain current in their understanding of local, regional, and national guidance in a climate of uncertainty and frequent change to optimise safety for dental care providers and patients. Dentists who treat children during this pandemic should enact universal infection control procedures to the highest standard and champion this behaviour through their teams. Opportunities to promote preventive dental behaviours should be taken. Contemporary, minimally invasive procedures that minimise or eliminate aerosol generation should be employed where intervention is indicated throughout the pandemic, and in future as and when practice restrictions ease.

REFERENCES

1. World Health Organization. https://www.who.int/news-room/detai l/30-01-2020-state ment-on-the-secon d-meeti ng-of-the-inter natio nalhealt h-regul ation s-(2005)-emerg ency-commi ttee-regar ding-the-outbr eak-of-novel -coron aviru s-(2019-ncov). Accessed March 30, 2020.
2. Coronavirus Resources Centre, Johns Hopkins University of Medicine.
3. Meng L, Hua F, Bian Z. Coronavirus disease 2019 (COVID-19): emerging and future challenges for dental and oral medicine. *J Dent Res*;2020. https://doi.org/10.1177/00220 34520 914246
4. Peng X, Xu X, Li Y, Cheng L, Zhou X, Ren B. Transmission routes of 2019-nCoV and controls in dental practice. *Int J Oral Sci*. 2020;12:9.
5. Lauer SA, Grantz KH, Bi Q, et al. The incubation period of coronavirus disease 2019 (COVID-19) from publicly reported confirmed cases: estimation and application. *Annals Int Med*. 2020. https:// doi.org/10.7326/M20-0504
6. Huang C, Wang Y, Li X, et al. Clinical features of patients in-fected with 2019 novel coronavirus in Wuhan. *China. Lancet*. 2020;395(10223):497-506.
7. Dong Y, Mo X, Hu Y, et al. Epidemiological characteristics of 2143 pediatric patients with 2019 coronavirus disease in China. *Pediatrics*. 2020. https://doi.org/10.1542/peds.2020-0702
8. Lu X, Zhang L, Du H, et al. SARS-CoV-2 Infection in Children. *N Engl J Med*. 2020. https://doi.org/10.1056/NEJMc2 005073
9. Bi Q, Wu Y, Mei S, et al. Epidemiology and Transmission of COVID-19 in Shenzhen China: analysis of 391 cases and 1,286 of their close contacts. *medRxiv*. 2020. https://doi. org/10.1101/2020.03.03.20028423
10. Cai J, Xu J, Lin D, et al. A Case Series of children with 2019 novel coronavirus infection: clinical and epidemiological features. *Clin Infect Dis*. 2020. https://doi.org/10.1093/cid/ciaa198
11. Bialek S, Boundy E, Bowen V, et al. Severe outcomes among patients with coronavirus disease 2019 (COVID-19) — United States, February 12–March 16, 2020. *MMWR Morb Mortal Wkly Rep*. 2020;69(12):343-346.
12. Chan JF, Yuan S, Kok KH, et al. A familial cluster of pneumonia associated with the 2019 novel coronavirus indicating person-to-person transmission: a study of a family cluster. *Lancet*. 2020;395(10223):514-523.
13. Chang D, Lin M, Wei L, et al. Epidemiologic and clinical characteristics of novel coronavirus infections involving 13 patients outside Wuhan, China. *JAMA*. 2020;323(11):1092.
14. Chen H, Guo J, Wang C, et al. Clinical characteristics and intrauterine vertical transmission potential of COVID-19 infection in nine pregnant women: a retrospective review of medical records. *Lancet*. 2020;395(10226):809-815.
15. Chen C, Cao M, Peng L, et al. Coronavirus disease-19 among children outside Wuhan, China. *Lancet Child Adolesc Health*. 2020. http://dx.doi.org/10.2139/ssrn.3546071
16. Choe YJ. Coronavirus disease-19: The First 7,755 Cases in the Republic of Korea. *medRxiv*. 2020.
17. Cui Y, Tian M, Huang D, et al. A 55-day-old female infant infected with COVID 19: presenting with pneumonia, liver injury, and heart damage. *J Infect Dis*. 2020. https://doi.org/10.1093/infdi s/jiaa113
18. D'Antiga L. Coronaviruses and immunosuppressed patients. The facts during the third epidemic. *Liver Transpl*. 2020. https://doi. org/10.1002/lt.25756

19. Dong L, Tian J, He S, et al. Possible vertical transmission of SARS-CoV-2 from an infected mother to her newborn. *JAMA*. 2020. https://doi.org/10.1001/jama.2020.4621

20. Fan C, Lei D, Fang C, et al. Perinatal transmission of COVID-19 associated SARS-CoV- 2: Should we worry? *Clin Infect Dis*. 2020. https://doi.org/10.1093/cid/ciaa226

21. Henry BM, Oliveira MHS. Preliminary epidemiological anal-ysis on children and adolescents with novel coronavirus disease 2019 outside Hubei Province, China: an observational study utilizing crowdsourced data.

22. Ji LN, Chao S, Wang YJ, et al. Clinical features of pediatric patients with COVID-19: a report of two family cluster cases. *World J Pediatr*. 2020. https://doi.org/10.1007/s12519 -020-00356 -2. [Epub ahead of print].

23. Kam KQ, Yung CF, Cui L, et al. A well infant with coronavirus disease 2019 (COVID-19) with high viral load. *Clin Infect Dis*. 2020. https://doi.org/10.1093/cid/ciaa201

24. Li W, Cui H, Li K, Fang Y, Li S. Chest computed tomography in children with COVID-19 respiratory infection. *Pediatr Radiol*. 2020. https://doi.org/10.1007/s0024 7-020-04656 -7

25. Liu H, Liu F, Li J, Zhang T, Wang D, Lan W. Clinical and CT imaging features of the COVID-19 pneumonia: focus on pregnant women and children. *J Infect*. 2020. https://doi.org/10.1016/j. jinf.2020.03.007

26. Liu W, Zhang Q, Chen J, et al. Detection of COVID-19 in children in early January 2020 in Wuhan, China. *N Engl J Med*. 2020. https:// doi.org/10.1056/NEJMc 2003717

27. Livingston E, Bucher K. Coronavirus Disease 2019 (COVID-19) in Italy. *JAMA*. 2020.

28. Lou XX, Shi CX, Zhou CC, Tian YS. Three children who recovered from novel coronavirus 2019 pneumonia. *J Paediatr Child Health*. 2020. https://doi.org/10.1111/jpc.14871

29. Lu X, Zhang L, Du H, et al. SARS-CoV-2 Infection in Children. *N Engl J Med*. 2020. https://doi.org/10.1056/NEJMc 2005073

30. Mizumoto K, Omori R, Nishiura H. Age specificity of cases and attack rate of novel 2 coronavirus disease (COVID-19). *medRxiv*. 2020. https://doi.org/10.1101/2020.03.09.20033142

31. Pan X, Chen D, Xia Y, et al. Asymptomatic cases in a family cluster with SARS-CoV-2 infection. *Lancet Infect Dis*. 2020. https:// doi.org/10.1016/S1473 -3099(20)30114 -6

32. Qiu H, Wu J, Hong L, Luo Y, Song Q, Chen D. Clinical and epidemiological features of 36 children with coronavirus disease 2019 (COVID-19) in Zhejiang, China: an observational cohort study. *Lancet Infect Dis*. 2020.

33. Tang A, Xu W, Shen M, et al. A retrospective study of the clinical characteristics of COVID-19 infection in 26 children. *medRxiv*. 2020. https://doi.org/10.1101/2020.03.08.20029710

34. Wang S, Guo L, Chen L, et al. A case report of neonatal COVID-19 infection in China. *Clin Infect Dis*. 2020.

35. Wang X, Zhou Z, Zhang J, Zhu F, Tang Y. Shen X. A case of 2019 Novel Coronavirus in a pregnant woman with preterm delivery. *Clin Infect Dis*. 2020. https://doi.org/10.1093/cid/ciaa200

36. Wang XF, Yuan J, Zheng YJ, et al. Clinical and epidemiological characteristics of 34 children with 2019 novel coronavirus infec-tion in Shenzhen. *Zhonghua Er Ke Za Zhi*. 2020;58:E008.

37. Wei M, Yuan J, Liu Y, Fu T, Yu X, Zhang ZJ. Novel coronavirus infection in hospitalized infants under 1 year of age in China. *JAMA*. 2020. https://doi.org/10.1001/jama.2020.2131

38. Wu Z, McGoogan JM. Characteristics of and important lessons from the coronavirus disease 2019 (COVID-19) outbreak in China. *JAMA*. 2020. https://doi.org/10.1001/jama.2020.2648

39. Xia W, Shao J, Guo Y, Peng X, Li Z, Hu D. Clinical and CT features in paediatric patients with COVID-19 infection: different points from adults. *Pediatr Pulmonol*. 2020. https://doi.org/10.1002/ ppul.24718

40. Xing Y, Ni W, Wu Q, et al. Prolonged presence of SARS-CoV-2 in feces of paediatric patients during the convalescent phase.

41. Xu XW, Wu XX, Jiang XG, Xu KJ, Ying LJ, Ma CL. Clinical findings in a group of patients infected with the 2019 novel coronavirus (SARS-Cov-2) outside of Wuhan, China: retrospective case series. *BMJ*. 2020.

42. Yu N, Li W, Kang Q, et al. Clinical features and obstetric and neonatal outcomes of pregnant patients with COVID-19 in Wuhan, China: a retrospective, single-centre, descriptive study. *Lancet Infect Dis*. 2020.

43. Zeng L, Xia S, Yuan W, et al. Neonatal Early-Onset Infection With SARS-CoV-2 in 33 Neonates Born to Mothers With COVID-19 in Wuhan, China. *JAMA Pediatr*. 2020. https://doi.org/10.1001/jamap ediat rics.2020.0878

44. Zhang SC, Gu J, Chen Q, Deng N. Clinical characteristics of 34 children with coronavirus disease-2019 in the West of China: a multiple-centre case. *medRxiv*. 2020. https://doi. org/10.1101/2020.03.12.20034686

45. Zhu H, Wang L, Fang C, et al. Clinical analysis of 10 neonates born to mothers with 2019-nCoV pneumonia. *Transl Pediatr*. 2020;9(1):51-60.

46. Sun P, Lu X, Xu C, Sun W, Pan B. Understanding of COVID 19 based on current evidence. *J Med Virol*. 2020.

47. Illinois Department of Public Health. http://dph.illino is.gov/news/ publi c-healt h-offic ials-annou nce-first -death -infan t-coron aviru s-disease. Accessed March 29, 2020.

48. National Broadcasting Corporation, New York. https://www.nbcne wyork.com/news/local /nyc-virus -death s-leap-from-0-to-776in-15-days-emerg ency-hospi tal-help-arriv es-monda y/23503 57/. Accessed March 30, 2020.

49. The Daily Mail. https://www.daily mail.co.uk/news/artic le-81713 01/12-year-old-infec ted-coron aviru s-dies-Belgi um.html. Accessed March 31, 2020.

50. The Daily Mail. https://www.daily mail.co.uk/news/artic le-81732 53/Boy-13-dies-testi ng-posit ive-coron aviru s-Londo n-hospi talfundr aiser -says.html. Accessed March 31, 2020.

51. The Sun. https://www.thesun.co.uk/news/11268 073/frenc h-girlyoung est-coron aviru s-victi m-cough /.

52. Teenager's Death in California is linked to Coronavirus. The New York Times. https://www.nytim es.com/2020/03/24/us/ca-lif ornia -coron aviru s-death -child.html. Accessed March 30, 2020.

53. To KK, Tsang OT, Yip CC, et al. Consistent detection of 2019 novel coronavirus in saliva. *Clin Infect Dis.* 2020.

54. Fan C, Lei D, Fang C, et al. Perinatal transmission of COVID-19 associated SARS-CoV- 2: Should we worry? *Clin Infect Dis.* 2020. https://doi.org/10.1093/cid/ciaa226

55. Tran K, Cimon K, Severn M, Pessoa-Silva CL, Conly J. Aerosol generating procedures and risk of transmission of acute respiratory infections to healthcare workers: a systematic review. *PLoS ONE.* 2012;7:e35797.

56. van Doremalen N, Bushmaker T, Morris DH, et al. Aerosol and surface stability of SARS-CoV-2 as compared with SARSCoV-1. *New Eng J Med.* 2020. https://doi.org/10.1056/NEJMc 2004973

57. Smales FC, Samaranyake LP. Maintaining dental education and specialist dental care during an outbreak of a new coronavirus infection. Part 2: Control of the disease, then elimination. *Br Dent J.* 2003;195:679-681.

58. Personal Protective Equipment. Centre for Disease Control and Prevention.

59. World Health Organization Pandemic Phase Descriptions.

60. Dental Council of Singapore. https://www.healt hprof essio nals.gov. sg/sdc. Accessed March 30, 2020.

61. Brazil National Health System (Sistema Unico de Saude). Fast-track for primary care in places with community transmission.. http://maism edicos.gov.br/image s/fluxo_bolso_17mar 20_3.pdf. Accessed March 31, 2020.

62. Notification of Enforcement Discretion for Telehealth Remote Communications During the COVID-19 Nationwide Public Health Emergency. https://www.hhs.gov/hipaa /for-profe ssion als/speci al-topic s/emerg ency-prepa redne ss/notif icati on-enfor cemen t-discr etion -teleh ealth /index.html. Accessed March 31, 2020.

63. Brazil National Health System (Sistema Unico de Saude). Dental care during COVID-19. http://websit e.cfo.org.br/wp-con-tent/uploa ds/2020/03/COVID -19_ATEND IMENT O-ODONT OLOGI CONO-SUS.pdf.

64. American Dental Association. What constitutes a medical emergency? https://succe ss.ada.org/~/media /CPS/Files /Open%20Fil es/ADA_COVID 19_Dental_Emerg ency_DDS.pdf?_ga=2.23641 9265.19784 197.15848 91239 -19709 75310.15848 91239. Accessed March 30, 2020.

65. Scottish Dental Clinical Effectiveness Program. http://www.sdcep. org.uk/wp-conte nt/uploa ds/2020/03/SDCEP -MADP-COVID -19guide -300320.pdf. Accessed March 31, 2020.

66. American Academy of Pediatric Dentistry. https://www.aapd. org/about /about -aapd/news-room/covid -19/. Accessed March 30, 2020.

67. Meyer BD, Casamassimo P, Vann WF Jr. An algorithm for managing emergent dental conditions for children. *J Clin Pediatr Dent.* 2019;43:201-206.

68. Smales FC, Samaranyake LP. Maintaining dental education and specialist dental care during an outbreak of a new coronavirus infection. Part 1: a deadly viral epidemic begins. *Br Dent J.* 2003;195:557-561.

69. Centre for Evidence Based Medicine, University of Oxford. https:// www.cebm.net/covid -19/what-is-the-effic acy-of-stand ard-facemasks -compa red-to-respi rator -masks -in-preve nting -covid -type-respi rator y-illne sses-in-prima ry-care-staff /. Accessed March 30, 2020.

70. De Amorim RG, Frencken JE, Raggio DP, Chen X, Hu X, Leal SC. Survival percentages of atraumatic restorative treatment (ART) restorations and sealants in posterior teeth: an updated systematic review and meta-analysis. *Clinical Oral Invest.* 2018;22:2703-2725.

71. Schwendicke F, Jäger AM, Paris S, Hsu LY, Tu YK. Treating pitand-fissure caries: a systematic review and network meta-analysis. *J Dent Res.* 2015;94:522-533.

72. Seifo N, Cassie H, Radford JR, Innes NP. Silver diamine fluo-ride for managing carious lesions: an umbrella review. *BMC Oral Health.* 2019;19:145.

73. Li T, Zhai X, Song F, Zhu H. Selective versus non-selective removal for dental caries: a systematic review and meta-analysis. *Acta Odontol Scand.* 2018;76:135-140.

74. Innes NP, Evans DJ, Stirrups DR. Sealing caries in primary molars: randomized control trial, 5-year results. *J Dent Res.* 2011;90:1405-1410.

CHAPTER 15

EVALUATING COVID-19 INDUCED MENTAL HEALTH CONCERNS

1. The Impact Of COVID-19 On Brazilian Mental Health Through Vicarious Traumatization[1]

Antonio de P. Serafim, 0 Priscila D. Gonç‚alves,
Cristiana C. Rocca, Francisco Lotufo Neto
Departamento e Instituto de Psiquiatria, Hospital das Clı́nicas,

Pandemics and epidemics affect physical health and compromise psychosocial integrity, generally resulting in a high level of psychological suffering and psychosocial maladjustment. People facing the novel coronavirus (COVID-19) outbreak tend to be more susceptible to alterations in physical (not necessarily related to clinical symptoms), cognitive, behavioural and emotional aspects.[1] Worldwide actions against COVID-19 have focused primarily on efforts to contain the acceleration of peak contamination, involving social isolation and the dissemination of prevention guidelines. Although the need to include mental health care in these emergency policies has been highlighted by China,[2] few countries have formally integrated it into their emergency plan. In addition, the operationalization of policies to address this unprecedented mental health crisis must be established globally.Social isolation tends to provoke psychological reactions, as evident in increased anxiety, stress and irritability levels, the appearance of fears (based on real or subjective information) and confused thinking; such emotional conditions negatively impact an individual's ability to make coherent decisions.[1,2] In this context, pandemics require emergency actions that consider a wide range of possible psychological outcomes. In the current global situation, the specific stressors of the COVID-19 outbreak have affected both the general population and professionals who are working in direct patient care, as well as those who are not on the front lines, who can suffer from what is called indirect traumatization.[3,4]

Attention must be paid to mental health aspects of the frontline health team. However, the concept of "indirect traumatization" requires that attention should also be paid to the general public, due to the growing volume of information, both official and that of low scientific value. The fear of becoming infected, dying, or contaminating family members has already been reported in the COVID-19 literature[1] and can result in accentuated demand for mental health services. Some dysfunctional reactions and behaviours (i.e., self-medicating, abusing alcohol or other substances, compulsions, impulsivity, and depressive and anxious symptoms) are also observed after catastrophic situations. Furthermore, the symptoms of individuals diagnosed with a mental disorder may become exacerbated due to the stressful environment, changes in personal and family life, as well as in treatment routine. n this current pandemic, there is a general scenario of concern for everyone's safety, including people infected with COVID-19. These concerns must be considered as a premise for assistance programs (including online programs), which can provide a space for the population to speak openly about their concerns and/or fears (real, subjective and imaginary).

[1] Braz J Psychiatry. 2020 xxx-xxx;00(00):000-000 doi:10.1590/1516-4446-2020-0999

Thus, mental health care and psychosocial well-being programs that consider possible indirect traumatization are needed to mitigate its impact on mental health, as well as to respond to the increased demand for care during this outbreak.[5] Mental health policies are as needed as much as physical health care policies and can provide a valuable service, as has been stated in recent literature[1] which shows that the existence of support programs makes coping more appropriate and safer. This will certainly help reduce acute mental health problems.

How to cite this article: Serafim AP, Gonc͵alves PD, Rocca CC, Lotufo Neto F. The impact of COVID-19 on Brazilian mental health through vicarious traumatization. Braz J Psychiatry. 2020;00:000-000. http://dx.doi.org/10.1590/1516-4446-2020-0999

REFERENCES

1. Zhang, J., Wu W, Zhao, X., Zhang ,W. (2020).Recommended psychological crisis intervention response to the 2019 novel coronavirus pneumonia outbreak in China: a model of West China Hospital. Precis Clin Med. 2020;3:3-8.
2. Bao Y, Sun Y, Meng S, Shi J, Lu L. (2020).2019-nCoV epidemic: address mental health care to empower society. Lancet. 2020;395:e37-8.
3. Li., Ge J, Yang M, Feng J, Qiao M, Jiang R, et al. (2020).Vicarious traumatization in the general public, members, and non-members of medical teams aiding in COVID-19 control. Brain Behav Immun. 2020 Mar 10. pii: S0889-1591(20)30309-3. doi: 10.1016/j.bbi.2020.03.007. [Epub ahead of print]
4. Lai, J. Ma, S., Wang Y, Cai Z, Hu J, Wei N, et al. (2020).Factors associated with mental health outcomes among health care workers exposed to coronavirus disease 2019. JAMA Netw Open. 2020;3:e203976. 5 Duan L, Zhu G. Psychological interventions for people affected by the COVID-19 epidemic. Lancet Psychiatry. 2020;77:300-2.

2. First Study On Mental Distress In Brazil During The COVID-19 Crisis

Stephen X. Zhang
Associate Professor, University of Adelaide

Yifei Wang[1]
Doctoral Researcher, Tongji University

Asghar Afshar Jahanshahi
Associate Professor, Pontificia Universidad Católica del Perú (PUCP)

Jianfeng Jia
Professor, Northeastern University

Valentina Gomes Haensel Schmitt
Associate Professor, University of Lima

ABSTRACT

Objective: We aim to provide the first evidence of mental distress and its associated predictors among adults in the ongoing COVID-19 crisis in Brazil. **Methods:** We conducted a primary survey of 638 adults in Brazil on March 25–28, 2020, about one month (32 days) after the first COVID-19 case in South America was confirmed in São Paulo. **Results:** In Brazil, 52% (332) of the sampled adults experienced mild or moderate distress, and 18.8% (120) suffered severe distress. Adults who were female, younger, more educated, and exercised less reported higher levels of distress. Everyone's distance from the Brazilian epicentre of São Paulo interacted with age and workplace attendance to predict the level of distress. The "typhoon eye effect" was stronger for people who were older or attended their workplace less. The most vulnerable adults were those who were far from the epicentre and did not go to their workplace in the week before the survey. **Conclusion:** Identifying the predictors of distress enables mental health services to better target finding and helping the more mentally vulnerable adults during the ongoing COVID-19 crisis.

---

[1] Corresponding author: Stephen X. Zhang: stephen.x.zhang@gmail.com; Phone: +61 8 8313 9310; Fax: +61 8 8223 4782; Address: Nexus10 Tower, 10 Pulteney St, Adelaide SA 5000, Australia

INTRODUCTION

The first case of COVID-19 in South America appeared in São Paulo in Brazil on February 26, 2020. While the initial cases were imported from Italy to São Paulo – the economic engine of Brazil with a metropolitan population of 22 million, COVID-19 quickly spread across Brazil, reaching 2,433 cases in a month. As cases spread, so did the distress associated with the virus.[1,2] Research is starting to identify the potential breakout of large-scale mental health issues.[3-6] Early evidence from China revealed the prevalence of mental health issues among adults during the COVID-19 out-break.[7-9] Despite the early evidence from China, countries vary in their medical systems and resources, cultures, the COVID-19 situation, and their restrictive measures,[10] and hence research can identify the predictors of mental health in individual countries to enable effective identification of mentally vulnerable groups during the COVID-19 crisis.[11] This paper aims to provide the first evidence of mental distress and its predictors among adults in Brazil during the COVID-19 crisis. Building from early research evidence on mental health in China and Iran, where the COVID-19 outbreak occurred earlier,[7,8,11] we explore several predictors of distress during the COVID-19 crisis in Brazil. We examine individuals' distance from São Paulo – the city most affected by COVID-19 in Brazil. As the COVID-19 crisis continues to impact Brazil, we hope this research identifies useful predictors to help mental health professionals to be more targeted in locating the more mentally vulnerable individuals in the COVID-19 outbreak to provide timely assistance online or via telephone.

METHODS

Contexts

The first confirmed case of COVID-19 in South America was a Brazilian who returned from Italy to São Paulo on February 21, 2020.[12] São Paulo is the biggest city and the economic centre of Brazil. Due to its centrality in the Brazilian transportation network, São Paulo also became a centre for the spread of COVID-19 in Brazil.[13] São Paulo had the highest number of confirmed cases in Brazil and was the first city in Brazil to implement a lockdown in an attempt to slow down the spread of the virus on March 22.

Study Design and Participants

About one month after the first COVID-19 case in Brazil, we conducted an online cross-sectional survey on March 25–28, 2020. During the survey dates, the total confirmed cases in Brazil increased from 2,433 to 3,904, and deaths increased from 57 to 114. On March 25, São Paulo accounted for more than a quarter of the total confirmed cases in Brazil, and this proportion increased to one third on March 28. The survey was approved by Tongji University, and we pretested the survey with five adults from Brazil (not included in the main sample). The survey was voluntary, and we promised the participants confidentiality and anonymity of their responses. A total of 638 adults from various parts of Brazil completed our survey.

Measures

We assessed the participants' socio-demographic characteristics, including gender, age, educational level, the number of children under 18 years old, geographic location, whether they were COVID-19 positive, their exercise hours per day during the past week, and their workplace attendance.

Using the participants' location, we calculated their individual distance from São Paulo, the epicentre of COVID-19 in Brazil, and their distance from the epicentre ranged from 0 to 3,318 km. We assessed distress using the COVID-19 Peritraumatic Distress Index (CPDI)[14], which was specifically designed to capture distress during the COVID-19 outbreak. CPDI consists of 24 questions, with the possible score ranging from 4 to 100 (normal: 4–27, mild or moderate: 28–51, severe: 52–100). We had the survey back translated from English to Portuguese. The Portuguese version of the survey can be found in the online appendix. The CPDI had a Cronbach's alpha of 0.87 in the Brazil sample.

RESULTS

Descriptive Findings

Table 1 presents the descriptive findings of the sampled adults. Of the sample, 57.7% (368) were female, 78.7% (502) reported negative for COVID-19, 0.9% (6) reported positive, and 20.4% (130) were unsure whether they had COVID-19. In terms of exercise during the past week, 57.7% of the participants had not exercised; 21.9%, 6.9% and 5.2% of the participants reported exercising 1, 2 and 3 hours per day during the past week respectively; and 4.1% reported exercising more than 5 hours per day. The participants reported their workplace attendance by answering the question "how many days did you actually go to work in your office in the past week?". Of the sample, 60.0% (383) of participants were not in the office at all in the past week, while 28.8% (184) were in the office for fewer than five days last week, 7.9% (50) went to the office for five days, and the remaining 3.3% (21) went for six or seven days. The mean (SD) score of CPDI in the sample was 37.64 (15.22), higher than the CPDI of 23.65 (15.45) reported in China from January 31 to February 10, 2020.[14] The difference in the mean values between the samples in Brazil and China is 14.33 (t=23.07; p<0.0001; 95% CI: 12.80 to 15.18). The mean CPDI of sampled adults in Brazil is also significantly higher than the mean CPDI of 34.54 (14.92) of adults in Iran on February 28–30, 2020 (t=4.09; p<0.0001; 95% CI: 1.61 to 4.59).[11] Based on the cut-off values of distress in CPDI, 52.0% of sampled adults in Brazil experienced mild or moderate distress, and 18.8% experienced severe distress, compared to 47.0% and 14.1% in Iran and 29.3% and 5.1% in China respectively.

Predictors of individuals' COVID-19 Peritraumatic Distress Index (CPDI)

Females experienced more distress than males (β=-8.43, p=0.000, 95% CI: -10.73 to -6.13). Even though COVID-19 has a higher fatality rate in the elderly, younger people reported a higher level of distress (β=-2.79, p=0.000, 95% CI: -4.03 to -1.53). Adults who were more educated (β=1.93, p=0.000, 95% CI: 1.01 to 2.86) and exercised less (β=-1.47, p=0.000, 95% CI: -2.19 to -0.75) reported a higher level of distress. Family size (p=0.164) and workplace attendance (p=0.634) failed to predict CPDI directly.We analysed the relationship between individuals' distance from the epicentre and CPDI, as well as how this relationship was contingent on their age and the number of days in their workplace during the past week. The relationship between individuals' distance from the epicentre and their distress depended on individuals' age (Model 1 of Table 1). First, in Brazil we do observe a "typhoon eye effect" – mental health issues increase with distance from the epicentre, akin to a typhoon, where the effect is stronger in the periphery than in the centre. This typhoon eye effect was stronger for older adults (β=1.16, p=0.049, 95% CI: 0.00 to 2.31). We further broke down the typhoon eye effect by adults' age brackets. The relationship between the distance from the epicentre and distress was significantly positive among older adults (e.g. 46–55 years old: β=2.33, p=0.033, 95% CI: 0.19 to 4.46; 56–65 years old: β=3.49, p=0.025, 95% CI: 0.43 to 6.54; above 65 years old: β=4.65, p=0.026, 95% CI: 0.55 to 8.75).The relationship between the distance from the epicentre and distress was also contingent on the number of days that the adults went to their workplace during the past week. The number of days in the workplace attenuated the typhoon eye effect in terms of distress (β=-0.99, p=0.016, 95% CI: -1.79 to -0.19), as shown in Model 2 of Table 1. This relationship was significantly positive for adults who did not go to their workplace at all (β=2.09, p=0.025, 95% CI: 0.26 to 3.93), showing the typhoon eye effect. However, this relationship was not significant for adults who went to their workplace for one to five days last week. In particular, the typhoon eye effect (distress increases over distance) turned into the ripple effect (distress decreases over distance) for those who went to their workplace every single day in the last week (β=-4.83, p=0.050, 95% CI: -9.65 to -0.01).

Predicted scores of individuals' COVID-19 Peritraumatic Distress Index (CPDI)

Figure 1(a) shows the predicted scores of CPDI by gender, age, education, family size, workplace attendance, and distance from the epicentre. The 95% confidence intervals of CPDI in many groups based on these predictors were higher than the cut-off value of moderate distress at 28. For instance, adults who were female (mean=41.16, 95% CI: 39.70 to 42.61), aged 18–25 (mean=40.94, 95% CI: 39.14 to 42.74), highly educated (individuals with a doctorate degree, mean=42.12, 95%CI: 39.78 to 44.45), and exercised little (for those who did not exercise: mean=39.05, 95% CI:37.77 to 40.33) all had moderate distress. Since individuals' distance from the epicentre interacted with their age to predict CPDI level, we plotted the CPDI level based on the interaction of these two factors in Figure 1(b). Individuals aged 18–25 years and who were in the epicentre reported the highest level of distress (mean=41.40, 95% CI: 38.72 to 44.08), and those who were above 65 years old and were 3,300 km from the epicentre in Brazil reported the second highest level of distress (mean=40.94, 95% CI: 30.01 to 51.86). The least distressed group were people older than 65 in the epicentre (mean=28.35, 95% CI: 23.93 to 32.77). Similarly, Figure 1(c) shows the CPDI level based on the interaction between individuals' distance from the epicentre and their workplace attendance. The most vulnerable groups during the COVID-19 outbreak were those who were far from the epicentre and did not go to their workplace during the past week (e.g. at 3,300 km from the epicentre: mean=43.06, 95% CI: 38.16 to 47.95; at 2,200 km from the epicentre: mean=40.96, 95% CI: 37.98 to 43.95). The distress level was the lowest among people who lived 3,300 km from the epicentre and attended their workplace every day during the past week (mean=24.68, 95% CI: 11.55 to 37.81).

DISCUSSION

Our findings reveal a high prevalence of distress among adults during the early stage of the COVID-19 crisis in Brazil. Over half (52.0%) of the adults experienced moderate psychological distress and 18% experienced severe distress. The mean of CPDI of adults in Brazil was also worse than the means in China and Iran. Individuals who were female, younger, more educated, or exercised less had more distress. It is worth noting that two predictors of distress in Brazil, age and education, did not predict distress in the samples in Iran. The distance from the epicentre is emerging as an interesting predictor of mental health in the crisis literature, and this study found the distance effect depended on individuals' age and workplace attendance.

The positive association between the distance from the epicentre and distress, i.e. the "typhoon eye effect", was significant only in age groups of 46 years and above.

This result might be because the mortality of COVID-19 varies by age group. The typhoon eye effect was significant only among participants who did not attend their workplace. Surprisingly, the effect reversed to become a ripple effect for those who attended their workplace every single day in the last week. There are possible explanations from many perspectives, including the meaning and fulfilment associated with work, more potential social interactions from going out to work, and less time and dependence on information from online and social media.

The key contributions of this research are to help identify the predictors of those who are more vulnerable mentally during the COVID-19 crisis to enable more targeted mental health services.

We found gender, age, education, exercise, and distance from the epicentre all predicted distress in adults in Brazil during the COVID-19 crisis. In particular, this study shows the predictive effect of the distance from the epicentre varied depending on the age and workplace attendance of each individual. The findings that age and workplace attendance attenuated, and even reversed, the typhoon eye effect is particularly noteworthy to the literature and mental health service providers. There are several limitations of this study. First, our sampling is not nationally representative, because our aim was to provide rapid evidence on mental health and its predictors to enable rapid screening of the mentally vulnerable in the ongoing COVID-19 outbreak in Brazil. It is worth investigating if the level and the predictors of mental health change as the outbreak continues. Second, Brazil is a large country, and we sampled individuals from 0 to over 3,000 km from São Paulo to cover various regions in Brazil. It remains to be seen to what extent distance from the epicentre is a factor in other countries, most of which are smaller and have their own distinct geographical features.[8]In conclusion, this study provides the first empirical evidence of mental distress and its predictors in adults in Brazil during the COVID-19 crisis. We hope this research not only helps mental health professionals but also encourages more research on mental health conditions and predictors during the COVID-19 crisis in Brazil, Latin America, and beyond.[15]

REFERENCES

1. Duan, L., & Zhu, G. (2020). Psychological interventions for people affected by the COVID-19 epidemic. The Lancet Psychiatry, 7(4), 300-302.
2. Fisher, D, Wilder-Smith, A. (2020). The global community needs to swiftly ramp up the response to contain COVID-19. The Lancet, v. 395, p. 1109.
3. Santos, C.F. Reflections about the impact of the SARS-COV-2/COVID-19 pandemic on mental health. Braz J Psychiatry. 2020;00:000-000. http:// dx.doi.org/10.1590/1516-4446-2020-0981

4. Silva, A.G, Miranda, D.M., Diaz, A.P, Telles, A.L.S, Malloy-Diniz, L.F., Palha, A.P. (2020).Mental health: why it still matters in the midst of a pandemic. Braz J Psychiatry. 2020;00:000-000. http:// dx.doi.org/10.1590/1516-4446-2020-0009

5. Ornell, F., Schuch, J.B., Sordi, A.O., Kessler, F.H.P. (2020)."Pandemic fear" and COVID-19: mental health burden and strategies. Braz J Psychiatry. 2020;00:000-000. http://dx.doi.org/10.1590/15164446-2020-0008

6. Correa, H. Malloy-Diniz LF, Silva, A.G. (2020). Why psychiatric treatment must not be neglected during the COVID-19 pandemic. Braz J Psychiatry. 2020;00:000-000.

7. Zhang SX, Wang Y, Rauch A, Wei F. (2020).Unprecedented disruption of lives and work: Health, distress and life satisfaction of working adults in China one month into the COVID-19 outbreak. Psychiatry Res 2020; 288: 112958. https://doi.org/10.1016/j.psychres.2020.112958

8. Zhang, S.X., Huang, H, Wei F. (2020). Geographical Distance to the Epicentre of COVID-19 Predicts the Burnout of the Working Population: Ripple Effect or Typhoon Eye Effect? Psychiatry Res 2020: 112998. https://doi.org/10.1016/j.psychres.2020.112998

9. Wang, C., Pan, R., Wan, X., Tan, Y., Xu, L., Ho, C. S., & Ho, R. C. (2020). Immediate psychological responses and associated factors during the initial stage of the 2019 coronavirus disease (COVID-19) epidemic among the general population in china. International Journal of Environmental Research and Public Health, 17(5), 1729.

10. Fisher. D, Wilder-Smith, A. (2020). The global community needs to swiftly ramp up the response to contain COVID-19. Lancet (London, England) 2020; 395: 1109–10.

11. Jahanshahi, A.A., Dinani, M.M., Madavani, A.N., Li, J., Zhang, S.X. (2020). The distress of Iranian adults during the COVID-19 pandemic - More distressed than the Chinese and with different predictors. medRxiv 2020; : 2020.04.03.20052571.

12. Ester, C.S, Nuno, R,F. (2020).First cases of coronavirus disease (COVID-19) in Brazil, South America (2 genomes, 3 March 2020).

13. Rodriguez-Morales, A.J., Gallego, V., Escalera-Antezana, J.P., et al. (2020).COVID-19 in Latin America: The implications of the first confirmed case in Brazil. Travel Med Infect Dis 2020; : 101613.

14. Qiu J, Shen, B., Zhao, M., Wang, Z., Xie, B., Yifeng, Xu. (2020).A nationwide survey of psychological distress among Chinese people in the COVID-19 epidemic: implications and policy recommendations. Gen Psychiatry 2020; 33: 1–6.

15. Cohen, J., & Kupferschmidt, K. (2020). Strategies shift as coronavirus pandemic looms. Science, 367(6481): 962–963.

Table 1. Descriptive findings and predictors of COVID-19 Peritraumatic Distress Index (CPDI)

Variables	Description	Parameter estimates (95% CI)	
		Model 1	Model 2
CPDI (COVID-19 Peritraumatic Distress Index)		42.04*** (35.94 to 48.13)	38.21*** (32.72 to 43.70)
Normal range (4–27)	186 (29.2%)		
Mild or moderate distress (28–51)	332 (52.0%)		
Severe distress (52–100)	120 (18.8%)		
Gender			
Female	368 (57.7%)	Reference group	Reference group
Male	269 (42.2%)	-8.43*** (-10.73 to -6.13)	-8.36*** (-10.65 to -6.06)
Other	1 (0.1%)	18.95 (-8.69 to 46.59)	19.87 (-7.75 to 47.48)
Age			
18–25	118 (18.5%)		
26–35	206 (32.3%)		
36–45	156 (24.4%)	-2.79*** (-4.03 to -1.53)	-1.92*** (-2.76 to -1.07)
46–55	86 (13.5%)		
56–65	56 (8.8%)		
> 65	16 (2.5%)		
Educational level			
Elementary school	13 (2.0%)		
Middle school	1 (0.1%)		
High school	109 (17.1%)		
Vocational/technical school	47 (7.4%)	1.93*** (1.01 to 2.86)	2.06*** (1.14 to 2.99)
Bachelor	342 (53.6%)		
Master	78 (12.3%)		
Doctorate	48 (7.5%)		
Number of children under 18 years old			
0	423 (66.3%)		
1	131 (20.5%)		
2	67 (10.5%)	0.35 (-0.96 to 1.67)	0.32 (-0.99 to 1.62)
3	12 (1.9%)		
4	1 (0.1%)		
5 and above	4 (0.7%)		
Exercise hours per day in the past week			
0 hours	368 (57.7%)		
1 hour	140 (21.9%)		
2 hours	44 (6.9%)		
3 hours	33 (5.2%)	-1.47*** (-2.19 to -0.75)	-1.50*** (-2.22 to -0.78)
4 hours	15 (2.3%)		
5 hours	12 (1.9%)		
More than 5 hours	26 (4.1%)		
Number of days attending the workplace in the past week			
0 days	383 (60.0%)		
1 day	64 (10.0%)	-0.45 (-1.05 to 0.16)	0.26 (-0.59 to 1.11)
2 days	68 (10.7%)		

3 days	34 (5.3%)		
4 days	18 (2.8%)		
5 days	50 (7.9%)		
6 days	15 (2.4%)		
7 days	6 (0.9%)		
Distance from the epicentre	638 (100%)	-2.31 (-5.79 to 1.16)	2.09* (0.26 to 3.93)
Interaction			
*Distance from the epicentre *Age*	638 (100%)	1.16* (0.00 to 2.31)	
*Distance from the epicentre * Number of days working in the workplace*	638 (100%)		-0.99* (-1.79 to -0.19)

Figure 1(a). Predicted value of CPDI (COVID-19 Peritraumatic Distress Index)

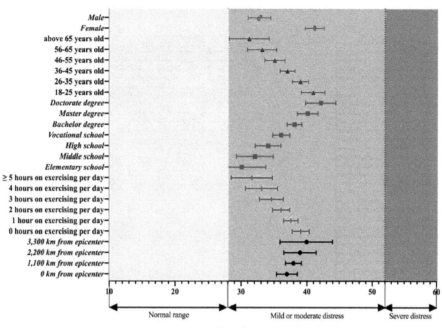

COVID-19 Peritraumatic Distress Index

Figure 1(b). Predicted value of CPDI (COVID-19 Peritraumatic Distress Index) by individuals' distance from the epicenter and age bracket

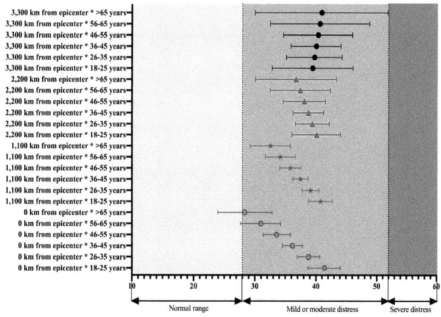

COVID-19 Peritraumatic Distress Index

Figure 1(c). Predicted value of CPDI (COVID-19 Peritraumatic Distress Index) by individuals' distance from the epicenter and workplace attendance

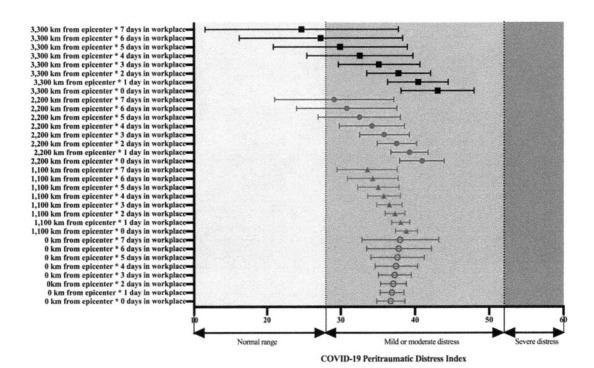

COVID-19 Peritraumatic Distress Index

3. Mental Health And Online Information During The COVID-19 Pandemic

Marileila Marques Toledo[1*] and Edson da Silva[2]

As the number of confirmed cases of deaths from COVID-19 grows fast, the health team and the general public are facing psychological suffering, including anxiety, depression, stress, anguish [1-3], boredom, loneliness, anger [4] and suicide [5-6]. These problems worsen when added to the consequences of the misinformation overload, which has spread uncertainty, fear, anxiety and racism on the internet on a scale never seen in previous epidemics, such as severe acute respiratory syndrome (SARS), Middle East respiratory syndrome (MERS) and Zika [7]. In each new epidemic, not only a new virus circulates, but also a huge flow of fear, anxiety and uncertainty. The COVID-19 epidemic highlights and expresses forms of contemporary fear.

A person's imagination makes him recognize a concrete threat posed by the virus that is capable of infecting him, and also an abstract threat, which he cannot see but which has the potential to cause harm [8]. Many people are exposed to the current pandemic against their will and are obliged to continue their daily lives, even though they know that the other people they encounter on transportation, at work, in public or collective spaces and in their own families may spread a disease that has no specific treatments yet. This type of fear is worse because the person is faced with a threat that he believes he cannot control. In the COVID-19 scenario, fear seems to circulate and spread easier and faster than the new coronavirus, and there may be a greater number of frightened people than physically ill people [8]. In the absence of specific medical treatment and vaccination for COVID-19, coronavirus transmission can be controlled through behavioural changes.

To do this, it is necessary to systematically monitor and understand how different individuals perceive risk and what leads them to act according to that risk [9]. With high levels of fear driven by information about the disease and its consequences, individuals may not think clearly and rationally when reacting to COVID-19 [10], therefore becoming more vulnerable.

In general, in this pandemic moment, the emotional reactions associated with stress are manifested in multiple ways, among which there may be an increase in fear, stress and anxiety when dealing with the disease; concern for one's own health and the health of people in one's family or social environment; changes in eating and physical activity patterns that often lead to reduced sleep or insomnia; changes in the cognitive aspect with attention and memory deficit, for example; worsening of chronic health problems and their comorbidities; and adoption of health risk behaviours, with greater use of alcohol, cigarettes and other drugs [11]. Fear, demotivation and often panic reactions affect the mental health of health professionals who are at the forefront of the fight against COVID-19, making them more vulnerable to physical illness, indisposition and decreased immunity. Facing behavioural changes that affect mental health worldwide, researchers are looking for strategies to understand and deal with new challenges.

An example was the development and validation of a research instrument called the Fear of COVID-19 Scale (FCV-19S), which will complement the clinical performance in preventing the spread of the virus and treating COVID-19 cases. This scale was validated in Iran, has robust psychometric properties and was suggested by the authors as a reliable and valid research tool for assessing fear of COVID-19, both in the general population and among individuals [10]. Another strategy focusing on mental health care in the face of the pandemic was the creation of the "Conexão Fiocruz Brasília" project by the Oswaldo Cruz Foundation (Fiocruz) in March 2020. This involves producing videos about the new coronavirus, with free transmission on the institution's various networks. The digital material is free to reproduce, download and share, thereby spreading correct information with high-quality content in Brazil [12].

Misinformation and fear of being hit by the new coronavirus have also affected emergency situations that require immediate intervention from the audience, for example, a cardiac arrest that takes place in a public place. A 60-year-old Chinese man suffered cardiac arrest outside a hospital next to a restaurant in Sydney. People did not help him for fear that the man was infected with the new coronavirus. Cardiopulmonary resuscitation manoeuvres were only initiated in the hospital environment, and the man did not survive [13]. Gao and Zheng [14] showed a high prevalence of mental health problems positively associated with frequent exposure to social media during the pandemic. The Chinese government provided mental health services through a variety of channels, including a hotline, online consultation, an online course and outpatient consultation.

In view of this, the authors suggest that governments, health systems and the media combat mental health problems related to COVID-19, using social media platforms to monitor and filter false information, in addition to promoting accurate information and reliable sources, such as the WHO and the Centres for Disease Control and Prevention (CDC, United States), among other organizations [14]. Another important aspect to highlight in this theme is understanding how the social dynamics related to COVID-19 shared on social media have played a fundamental role in the spread of information and misinformation.

This form of communication has the potential to influence people's behaviour and change the effectiveness of measures implemented by governments in situations like the current one. In this sense, the understanding of the social dynamics behind the consumption of informative content and social media is a relevant issue, since it can help to design more efficient epidemic models, responsible for social behaviour and put into practice more efficient communication strategies in this moment of health crisis [15]. There is an urgent need to combat the fear, rumours and panic that affect the mental health of the general population and of health professionals in the times of COVID-19. To avoid fear among the population, it is important that governments and health organizations like the WHO develop strategies to teach people to check the quality of what they read, especially in the case of health information. In addition, the health team must take an active role in combating disinformation. In view of this scenario, several sources of information have been established at the international [16-21] and national [22-27] levels. Brazil offers a series of digital informational content over the internet, including websites, social networks, applications, telehealth and WhatsApp, and other sources and information services prepared to clarify various aspects related to COVID-19. Provision of mental health support is likely to help people maintain their psychological wellbeing and deal with acute and post-acute events more favourably. Some examples of mental health services available online include texting, chatting, telephone, video conferencing, self-help platforms, forums and psychoeducation [28]. Such strategies can mitigate misinformation, which has led to mental health impairment, in addition to expanding the field of research in the area of health communication in facing the pandemic. In summary, the COVID-19 has and is likely to affect people worldwide. Feeling under pressure with anxiety, depression, stress, anguish, boredom, loneliness and anger is a likely experience for many people in this situation.

In addition, the excess of online information about COVID-19 on the internet can be a threat to mental health. Thus, ensure that good quality communication and accurate information updates, because, managing our mental health and psychosocial well-being during this time is very important. Therefore, all of us around the world, need working together as one community can help to create solidarity in addressing COVID-19 together.

Conflicts of interest

None declared; the authors have no conflicts of interest.

REFERÊNCIAS

1. Xiang Y T, Yang Y, Li W, Zhang L, Zhang Q, Cheung T, Ng CH. (2020).Timely mental health care for the 2019 novel coronavirus outbreak is urgently needed. Lancet Psychiatry 2020) 7(3): 228-229.
2. Kang L, Li Y, Hu S, Chen M, Yang C, Yang BX, Chen J. (2020). The mental health of medical workers in Wuhan, China dealing with the 2019 novel coronavirus. Lancet Psychiatry 2020; 7(3):e14.
3. Lai, J., Ma S, Wang, Y., Cai Z, Hu J, Wei, N., Tan, H. (2020). Factors associated with mental health outcomes among health care workers exposed to Coronavirus disease 2019. JAMA open 2020; 3(3): e203976-e203976.
4. Ornell, F., Schuch, J.B., Sordi, A.O., Kessler, F.H.P. (2020)."Pandemic fear" and COVID-19: mental health burden and strategies. Braz J Psychiatry 2020; (AHEAD).
5. Goyal, K., Chauh, P., Chhikar, K., Gupta, P., Singh, M.P. (2020). Fear of COVID 2019: First suicidal case in India! Asian Psychiatr 2020; 49:101989. .
   Montemurro, N. (2020).The emotional impact of COVID-19: from medical staff to common people. Brain, Behav immune 2020; doi:10.1016/j.bbi.2020.03.032.
6. Pulidom, C.M., Ruiz-Eugenio, L., Redondo-Sama G, Villarejo-Carballido, B. (2020).A New Application of Social Impact in Social Media for Overcoming Fake News in Health. Int J Environ Res Public Health 2020; 17(7):2430.
7. Colectiva, S. (2020).Miradas sobre el COVID-19 desde la salud colectiva. Virus 2020; 8:03.
8. Betsch, C., Wieler, L.H., Habersaat, K.. (2020). Monitoring behavioural insights related to COVID-19.
   Lancet 2020.
9. Ahorsu DK, Lin CY, Imani V, Saffari M, Griffiths MD, Pakpour AH. The Fear of COVID-
   19 Scale: Development and Initial Validation. Int J Ment Health Addict 2020;
10. Sociedade Brasileira de Diabetes. Estresse e enfrentamento. Diabetes na era COVID-19: https://www.diabetes.org.br/covid19/estresse-e-enfrentamento/. (acessado em 15/Abr/2020).
11. da Fiocruz Brasília, A. D. C. (2020). Conexão Fiocruz Brasília: o novo Coronavírus e nossa saúde mental.
12. Scquizzato, T., Olasveengen, T.M., Ristagno, G., Semeraro, F. (2020). The other side of novel coronavirus outbreak: fear of performing cardiopulmonary resuscitation. Resuscitation 2020.
13. Gao J, Zheng P, Jia Y, Chen H, Mao Y, Chen S, Dai J. Mental Health Problems and Social Media Exposure During COVID-19 Outbreak. Available at SSRN 3541120.
14. Cinelli, M., Quattrociocchi, W., Galeazzi, A., Valensise, C.M., Brugnoli, E., Schmidt, A.L., Scala, A. (2020).
    The COVID-19 social media infodemic. 2020; arXiv preprint arXiv:2003.05004.
15. Johns Hopkins University. Coronavirus Resource Centre. https://coronavirus.jhu.edu/(acessado em 15/Abr/2020).
16. Centres or Disease Control and Prevenction. Coronavirus (COVID-2019).
    https://www.cdc.gov/coronavirus/2019-ncov/index.html. (acessado em 15/Abr/2020).

17. European Centre for Disease Prevention and Control. COVID-19. https://www.ecdc.europa.eu/en/COVID-19-pandemic. (acessado em 15/Abr/2020).
18. World Health Organization. Coronavirus disease (COVID-2019) situation reports.

   https://www.who.int/emergencies/diseases/novel-coronavirus-2019/situation-reports.

   (acessado em 15/Abr/2020).
19. World Health Organization. Coronavirus disease (COVID-19) Pandemic. https://www.who.int/emergencies/diseases/novel-coronavirus-2019 (acessado em 15/Abr/2020).
20. Pan American Health Organization. Coronavirus Disease (COVID-19). https://www.paho.org/en/tag/coronavirus-disease-COVID-19 (acessado em 15/Abr/2020).
21. Fundação Oswaldo Cruz. COVID-19. Informações para pesquisadores. https://portal.fiocruz.br/coronavirus-2019-ncov-informacoes-para-pesquisadores. (acessado em 15/Abr/2020).
22. Plataforma Integrada de Vigilância em Saúde, Ministério da Saúde. Notificação de casos pelo novo coronavírus (COVID-2019). http://plataforma.saude.gov.br/novocoronavirus/ (acessado em 15/Abr/2020).
23. Ministério da Saúde. Coronavírus e novo coronavírus: o que é, causas, sintomas, tratamento e prevenção. https://www.saude.gov.br/saude-de-a-z/coronavirus (acessado em 13/Abr/2020).
24. Ministério da Saúde. Saúde sem Fake News. https://www.saude.gov.br/fakenews. (acessado em 15/Abr/2020).
25. O NOVO CORONAVÍRUS e a nossa saúde mental. Diretor: Assessoria de Comunicação da Fiocruz Brasília, Produção: Fiocruz Brasília. Brasília: Fiocruz, 2020. 1 arquivo MP4 (2mim 08s), son., colour.
26. CONEXÃO FIOCRUZ BRASÍLIA: O novo coronavírus nas redes. Diretor: Assessoria de Comunicação da Fiocruz Brasília, Produção: Fiocruz Brasília. Brasília: Fiocruz, 2020. 1 arquivo MP4 (126 min.), son., colour. Disponível em: https://www.arca.fiocruz.br/handle/icict/40499.
27. Zhou, X., Snoswell, C. L., Harding, L. E., Bambling, M., Edirippulige, S., Bai, X., & Smith, A. C. (2020). The role of telehealth in reducing the mental health burden from COVID-19. Telemedicine and e-Health.

4. Evaluation of Fear and Peritraumatic Distress During COVID-19 Pandemic in Brazil

Alberto Abad[1]*, Juliana Almeida da Silva[2,9], Lucas Emmanuel Pedro de Paiva Teixeira[3], Mayra Antonelli-Ponti[4], Sandra Bastos[5], Cláudia Helena Cerqueira Mármora[6], Luis Antonio Monteiro Campos[7], Scheila Paiva[8], Renato Leonardo de Freitas[9,10,11]**, José Aparecido Da Silva[12]

ABSTRACT

COVID-19 pandemic continues to spread exponentially worldwide, especially in America. By mid-June, 2020, Brazil is one of the most affected countries with more than one million cases and up to 50,000 deaths. This study aims to assess the fear and peri-traumatic stress during the COVID-19 pandemics in Brazil, to enhance infection control methods, appropriate interventions, and public health policies. A cross-sectional survey has been conducted from April 12th to 18th using the Peri-Traumatic Distress Scale (CPDI) and the Fear Scale (FCV-19S) aiming to measure the peri-traumatic stress and fear as psychological reactions during the COVID-19 pandemic. For that purpose, an online spreadsheet was used to send the questionnaire and scales to a sample of 1844 participants as a collecting information tool. Both scales showed a correlation factor of (r=0,660). Results highlight significant gender differences as in both scales women's mean scores are higher showing that it is paramount that women's voices were represented in policy spaces as socially constructed gender roles place them in a strategic position to enhance multi-level interventions (primary and secondary effects of COVID-19), equitable policies, and new approaches to control the pandemic.

INTRODUCTION

The coronavirus disease pandemic (COVID-19) emerged in Wuhan, China, in late 2019; by the start of 2020, it had spread to a dozen countries. Since then, the number of cases has continued to escalate exponentially worldwide. Nowadays, Brazil is one of the most affected countries, as the disease has spread to all five regions of the country – at the start of the present study (19 June 2020), there were 1,038,568 confirmed COVID-19 cases, including 49,090 deaths and 520,360 recoveries. From a bioecological approach, previous research on pandemics has revealed a profound and wide range of psychosocial impacts on people during outbreaks of the infection. On a micro level, people are likely to experience fear of falling sick or dying themselves, feelings of helplessness, and stigma (Wang et al. 2020), health threats to oneself and loved ones, and higher chances of being afflicted by mood swings, depression, irritability, anxiety, fear, anger, insomnia, changes in appetite or subjective well-being (Abad, Da Silva, das Neves Braga, Medeiros, De Freitas, Coimbra & Da Silva, 2020). On a meso level, pandemics are further associated with severe disruptions of routines, separation from family and friends, school closure, shortages of food and medicine, wage loss, and social isolation (due to quarantine or other social distancing programs). Additionally, with fear of infection as the health care system could not cope with the COVID-19 pandemic (Choi et al, 2020; Taylor, 2019). Also, on a macro level, the impact on cultural, political, and socioeconomic factors should be considered, as COVID-19 pandemics has influenced education, unemployment, and quality of work. No one can predict how things will evolve in the coming months, nor when a return to some semblance of 'normal' activity might resume (Danese et al. 2020). People from different countries experience various levels of stress, fear, or anguish. As an example, fear in China during the pandemic differs from that in Iran, Italy, and Spain, indicating the need to study mental health predictors in specific countries during the COVID-19 to effectively identify, track, and assist those people most susceptible to mental health problems (Jahanshahi et al, 2020; Maza et al, 2020; Qiu et al, 2020; Wang et al, 2020).

Consequently, and as a result of a collaboration involving a group of Brazilian and foreign researchers interested in the effects of the impact and the varied psychological states caused by the rapid spread of COVID-19 around the world, was created the research project "Physical, Psychological, and Cognitive reactions to Covid19", approved by the Research Ethics Committee (CEP) of Federal University of Alfenas (UNIFAL-MG) (process number: 4.128.627). The project is divided into six modules, each one aiming to assess, or measure, some particular dimension of a psychological state derived from the COVID-19 pandemics: psychological reactions to pandemics; psychological vulnerability factors; social isolation, the role of the media and the dissemination of coronavirus-19; effective ways to deal with psychological problems; and, the implications for public health policies, including appropriate interventions for risk communication. Besides contributing to Brazilian literature about COVID-19 pandemics, this study aims to assess the fear and peri-traumatic stress during the COVID-19 contagion in Brazil, to enhance infection control methods, appropriate interventions, and public health policies.

METHODS

As the first module of the research project entitled Physical, Psychological, and Cognitive reactions to COVID-19, a cross-sectional survey was conducted from April 12th to 18th aiming to measure the peri-traumatic stress and fear as psychological reactions during the COVID-19 pandemics. For that purpose, an online spreadsheet (Google Forms) was used to send the questionnaire and scales to the participants as a collecting information tool. Before answering the questionnaire, candidates read and accepted the Participant Consent Form that explained the objective and nature of the study and showed they could refuse to answer any question and withdraw at any time from the research. Originally, 1875 participants were reached, but researchers had to exclude 31 incomplete questionnaires possibly because of internet slow-down access during the questionnaire fill-out making the final sample of 1844 people. Participants first answered a socio-demographic survey that included specific questions about chronic disease prevalence and social isolation levels during the Covid19 pandemic. Then, we assessed distress by the Peri-Traumatic Distress Index (CPDI), designed as a self-report questionnaire that measures depression, anxiety, avoidance, compulsive behaviour, specific phobias, cognitive change, physical symptoms, and loss of social functioning (Qiu, Shen, Zhao, Wang, Xie & Xu, 2020).

The twenty-four questions were presented in a Likert format in five categories of responses (never, occasionally, sometimes, often, most of the time). According to the authors, scores range from 0 to 100 indicating mild to moderate distress (between 28 and 51) and severe distress (≥52). CPDI content has been validated by Psychiatrists from the Shanghai Mental Health Centre considering its Cronbach's alpha 0.95 (p<0.001) (Qiu, Shen, Zhao, Wang, Xie & Xu, 2020).

We measured fear with the COVID-19 Fear scale (FCV-19S) presented in a Likert format in five categories of responses (strongly disagree, disagree, neither agree nor disagree, agree, strongly agree). It consists of a seven-item unidimensional scale with robust psychometric properties (Cronbach's alpha internal consistency 0.82) reliable and valid in assessing and relieving fears of COVID-19 among individuals (Ahorsu, Lin, Imani, Saffari, Griffiths & Pakpour, 2020). Scores range from 7 to 35 indicating levels of fear: normal (7 – 16); mild to moderate (17 – 26); and severe (27 – 35). The authors authorized us to use the FCV-19S and CPDI scales in the research.

We translated and adapted them to the Brazilian Portuguese language. We used descriptive statistics as data analysis method: CPDI and FCV-19S average scores, male and female frequency ranges, and the coefficient correlation of the scales (Pearson's r).

RESULTS AND DISCUSSION

We first assessed the characteristics of the participants (gender, age, marital status, number of children, education level, job status, and social isolation levels during COVID-19 pandemic) Out of the sample, 643 participants (34.9%) declared chronic disease prevalence, standing out suffering, or psychological disorder indicators (16.1%). This is relevant because the COVID-19 pandemic outbreak not only hurts physically but also psychologically as it disrupts lives, causes public panic, mental health distress (Bao, Sun, Meng, Shi & Lu, 2020), pathological anxiety, post-traumatic stress, and depression (Veer, Riepenhausen, Zerban, Wackerhagen, Engen, Puhlmann, ... & Mor, 2020). From a COVID-19 control strategy perspective, it is also highlighted the hypertension levels (10.4%) since non-communicable diseases (hypertension, diabetes, cardiovascular and chronic obstructive pulmonary illnesses) are correlated with the need for intensive care units (Fernandes, 2020) in a delicate political, economic, and social context that reflects the importance of flattening the curve of infections due to the fragility of the health systems and high contagion rates (Abad, Da Silva, das Neves Braga, Medeiros, De Freitas, Coimbra & Da Silva, 2020).it is possible to build a rough profile of the participants: single (48.7%) woman (79.8%), with an average of 36.2 years of age, with up to one child (75.7%), with a college degree (complete or incomplete 89.7%), working (69.5%) with health insurance (69.4%) and in social isolation during the pandemic (87.0%). The profile is psychologically significant because, although men and women are similar in many ways, it matches the biological, behavioural, and cognitive differences between genders that influence the health care approach in terms of manifestation, epidemiology, and pathophysiology widespread diseases (Regitz-Zagrosek, 2012).

As gender dimensions of the pandemic are both physical and socially constructed, affecting the sexes differently (Smith, 2019), women are perceived as being more aware of their need for healthcare, more adherent to counselling and treatment, and likely, seeking healthcare more often than men (Rugema et al., 2019) that explains the higher number of female answers of this and other surveys (Lauri Korajlija & Jokic- Begic, 2020). Furthermore, since health services availability, governance structures, and emergency responders interactions, all have gender dimensions (Smith, 2019) and considering that gender roles and stigma affect adherence to counselling and treatment (Rugema et al, 2019) it is possible to infer that women could be of utmost importance to control the spread of the coronavirus infection, and consequently, improving global health security (Wenham, Smith & Morgan, 2020).

In that sense, it is of utmost importance to include women's voices and knowledge in decision making, preparedness, and response to the pandemic, as there is an insufficient women's representation in global COVID-19 policy spaces (Wenham, 2020). The findings show the gender frequency scores of the Peritraumatic Distress Scale (CPDI) and the Fear In both scales, women's mean scores are higher; women's CPDI frequency scores are predominantly on the mild and severe distress frequency levels (47.3% and 27.2%) while men rely on normal and mild levels (41.6% and 48.4%). Similarly, most women's FCV-19S frequency scores are at a mild level (44.5%), while men's scores are at a normal level (68.8%). Still, women's scores are higher (15.4%) than men (4.8%) at a severe level. Results indicated that female gender was associated with increased anxiety, depression, and stress.

This finding is in line with the results of previous studies that have consistently found an association between female gender and increased psychological distress (Olagoke, Olagoke & Hughes, 2020; Maza et al, 2020; Wang et al, 2020; Qio et al, 2020). In this regard, the "Mental Health in the UK and COVID-19" report indicated that increased depression, anxiety, and stress were associated with being younger and female during the pandemic (Jia, Ayling, Chalder, Massey, Broadbent, Coupland & Vedhara, 2020). The scores are in harmony with results of a nationwide survey of psychological distress among Chinese people in the COVID-19 where female respondents showed significantly higher psychological distress and more likely to develop post-traumatic stress disorder than their male counterparts (Ahorsu, Lin, Imani, Saffari, Griffiths & Pakpour, 2020; Jia, Ayling, Chalder, Massey, Broadbent, Coupland & Vedhara, 2020). Besides, Brazilian CPDI gender mean scores (41.1 and 33.2) in our research are higher than Chinese ones (24.87 and 21.41) (Ahorsu, Lin, Imani, Saffari, Griffiths & Pakpour, 2020).

Gender differences (higher levels of fear and distress among female respondents) could be interpreted as a social construction. It is possible that men, because not openly expressing their fears of the COVID-19, would not follow the preventive sanitary recommendations that the World Health Organization (WHO) uses to manage the spread of the coronavirus infection (WHO, 2008): minimizing the risk communication efforts of the authorities and media, not following hygiene practices, and social distancing – risk factors of the pandemic control.

CPDI scale shows that anxiety, exhaustion, and attention deficit were the factors with higher scores with important gender differences. Women showed higher levels of anxiety as they answered about feeling anxious during the pandemic as often (30.5%) and most of the time (23.7%). Men, on the contrary, showed lower levels of anxiety as they felt it often (21.2%) and most of the time (13.6%). A study with 2766 volunteers, Maza et al., (2020) assessed anxiety during the pandemic.

Results showed high levels as ranges varied from medium (81.3%), high (7.2%) and extremely high(11.5%) associated with young age, female gender, family members infected with COVID-19, and a history of stressful situations and medical problems (Maza et al., 2020).Considering that women frequently take on most of the burden and risk of Health care providers' roles at home, often with little external support (Smith, 2019), the fourteenth question of the scale that measures the exhaustion factor (I feel tired or even exhausted) showed big differences between genders: men had lower scores as they never (20.7%) or occasionally (26.4%) felt tired or even exhausted during the pandemic, while women felt that way often (22.5%) and most of the time (27.9%). Moreover, schools' closure has a differential effect on women, who provide most of the informal care within families (Smith, 2019). The question of the scale, measuring the attention Deficit factor, showed significant differences between genders: men's scores were lower as they never (20.9%) or occasionally (29.8%) found it hard to concentrate during the social isolation, whereas women's answers were often (19.9%) and most of the time (24.8%). These results could be associated with the higher levels of exhaustion showed by women during the pandemic and the cognitive differences between genders (Regitz-Zagrosek, 2012). From the FCV-19S we could highlight two questions with significant gender differences on their answers: the first (I am most afraid of coronavirus-19), 74.1% of women agreed to be most afraid of coronavirus-19, while 34.8% of men selected those answers. The second question (It makes me uncomfortable to think about coronavirus19), 66.2% of women agreed to felt uncomfortable thinking about the coronavirus-19, while 26.1% of men opted for those answers. Finally, CPDI and FCV-19S scales showed a correlation factor of (r= 0,660)Also, correlations between the FCV-19S scale and CPDI's question S3 (I feel terrified from imagining myself or my family being infected) showed an even higher relationship (r= 0,728). It is relevant to mention that this study has some limitations. First, although the participants were people for any region of Brazil, this survey should not be taken as a national sample; secondly, as most of the respondents had an incomplete or complete college degree, it does not reflect most of the Brazilian population.

CONCLUSION

CPDI and FCV-19S results show gender difference scores as a response to the pandemic. It is paramount that women's voices were represented in policy spaces as socially constructed gender roles place them in a strategic position to enhance multilevel interventions (primary and secondary effects of COVID-19), equitable policies, and new approaches to control the pandemic.

Authors' contribution: A. Abad, L.E.P.P. Teixeira, Juliana A. da Silva and R.L. de Freitas elaborated, analysed, and wrote the manuscript; José A. da Silva participated in the created, elaborated the project and revised the manuscript; S. Paiva, S. Bastos, C.H.C. Mármora, L.A.M. Campos and M. Antonelli-Ponti, revised the manuscript.

[1] Psychology Graduate Program, Federal University of Juiz de Fora (UFJF), Juiz de Fora, MG, Brazil.

[2] Laboratory of Neuroanatomy and Neuropsychobiology, Department of Pharmacology, Ribeirão Preto Medical School of the University of São Paulo (FMRP-USP), Ribeirão Preto, 14049-900, São Paulo, Brazil.

[3] Institute of Motricity Sciences, Federal University of Alfenas (UNIFAL-MG), Alfenas, Minas Gerais, Brazil.

[4] Laboratory of Studies and Research in Social Economy, University of São Paulo at Ribeirão Preto, SP, Brazil.

[5] Otorhinolaryngology Institute (ISBO), São Paulo, SP. Brazil

[6] Department of the Old, Adult and Maternal-infant, School of Physical Therapy, Graduate Program in Psychology, Federal University of Juiz de Fora (UFJF), Juiz de Fora, Minas Gerais, Brazil.

[7] Master's Program in Psychology, Catholic University of Petrópolis, Petrópolis, Brazil. Department of Psychology, Pontifical Catholic University of Rio de Janeiro, Rio de Janeiro, Brazil

[8] Psychology Graduate Program, Federal University of Juiz de Fora (UFJF), Juiz de Fora, MG, Brazil. Department Speech Therapy of Federal University of Sergipe (UFS), Lagarto, SE, Brazil.

[9] Behavioural Neurosciences Institute (INeC), Av. do Café, 2450, Monte Alegre, Ribeirão Preto, 14050220, São Paulo, Brazil.

10. Laboratory of Neurosciences of Pain & Emotions and Multi-User Centre of Neuroelectrophysiology, Department of Surgery and Anatomy, Ribeirão Preto Medical School of the University of São Paulo, Av. Bandeirantes, 3900, Ribeirão Preto, São Paulo, Brazil.

11. Biomedical Sciences Institute, Federal University of Alfenas (UNIFAL), Minas Gerais, Brazil.

[12] Laboratory of Psychophysics, Perception, Psychometrics, and Pain University of São Paulo

REFERENCES

Abad, A., da Silva, J., das Neves Braga, J., Medeiros, P., de Freitas, R., Coimbra, N. and da Silva, J. (2020) Preparing for the COVID-19 Mental Health Crisis in Latin America—Using Early Evidence from Countries that Experienced COVID-19 First. Advances in Infectious Diseases, 10,40-44.

Ahorsu, D. K., Lin, C. Y., Imani, V., Saffari, M., Griffiths, M. D., & Pakpour, A. H. (2020). The Fear of COVID-19 Scale: Development and Initial Validation. International Journal of Mental Health and Addiction, 1-9.

Olagoke, A. A., Olagoke, O. O. & Hughes, A. M. (2020). Exposure to coronavirus news on mainstream media: The role of risk perceptions and depression.

British Journal of Health Psychology, e12427. https://doi.org/10.1111/bjhp.12427

Bao, Y., Sun, Y., Meng, S., Shi, J., & Lu, L. (2020). COVID-19 epidemic: address mental health care to empower society. The Lancet, 395(10224), e37-e38. https://doi.org/10.1016/S0140-6736(20)30309-3

Choi, E. P. H., Hui, B. P. H., & Wan, E. Y. F. (2020). Depression and anxiety in Hong Kong during COVID-19. International journal of environmental research and public health, 17(10), 3740. https://doi.org/10.3390/ijerph17103740

Danese, S., Cecconi, M., & Spinelli, A. (2020). Management of IBD during the COVID-19 outbreak: resetting clinical priorities. Nature Reviews Gastroenterology & Hepatology, 17(5), 253-255. https://doi.org/10.1038/s41575-020-0322-8

Fernandes, H. The Main Risk Factors for the Number of Serious or Critical Cases of COVID-19: How is the Health of Brazilians? Preprints 2020, 2020050143. https://doi.org/10.20944/preprints202005.0143.v1

International Labour Organization. (2020). COVID-19 and the world of work: Impact and policy responses.

Jahanshahi, A. A., Dinani, M. M., Madavani, A. N., Li, J., & Zhang, S. X. (2020). The distress of Iranian adults during the COVID-19 pandemic-More distressed than the Chinese and with different   predictors. medRxiv.

Jia, R., Ayling, K., Chalder, T., Massey, A., Broadbent, E., Coupland, C., & Vedhara, K. (2020). Mental health in the UK during the COVID-19 pandemic: early observations. medRxiv. https://doi.org/10.1101/2020.05.14.20102012

Lauri Korajlija, A., & Jokic-Begic, N. (2020). COVID-19: Concerns and behaviours in Croatia.   British Journal of Health Psychology.https://doi.org/10.1111/bjhp.12425

Li, S., Wang, Y., Xue, J., Zhao, N., & Zhu, T. (2020). The impact of COVID-19 epidemic declaration on psychological consequences: a study on active weibo users. International Journal of Environmental Research and Public Health, 17(6), 2032. https://doi.org/10.3390/ijerph17062032

Mazza, C., Ricci, E., Biondi, S., Colasanti, M., Ferracuti, S., Napoli, C., & Roma, P. (2020). A nationwide survey of psychological distress among italian people during the COVID-19 pandemic: Immediate psychological responses and associated factors. International Journal of Environmental Research and Public Health, 17(9), 3165.

National Academies of Sciences, Engineering, and Medicine. (2020). Rapid Expert Consultations for the COVID-19 Pandemic: March 14, 2020–April 8, 2020. Washington, DC: The National Academies Press.

Qiu, J., Shen, B., Zhao, M., Wang, Z., Xie, B., & Xu, Y. (2020). A nationwide survey of psychological distress among Chinese people in the COVID-19 epidemic: implications and policy recommendations. General psychiatry, 33(2).

Regitz-Zagrosek, V. (2012). Sex and gender differences in health. EMBO reports, 13(7), 596-603.

Rugema, L., Persson, M., Mogren, I., Ntaganira, J., & Krantz, G. (2019). A qualitative study of healthcare professionals' perceptions of men and women's mental healthcare seeking in Rwanda. Journal of Community Psychology.

Smith J. (2019). Overcoming the "tyranny of the urgent": integrating gender into disease outbreak preparedness and response. Gender Develop 2019; 27: 355–69. https://doi.org/10.1080/13552074.2019.1615288

Taylor, S. (2019). The Psychology of Pandemics: Preparing for the Next Global Outbreak of Infectious Disease. Cambridge Scholars Publishing.

Veer, I. M., Riepenhausen, A., Zerban, M., Wackerhagen, C., Engen, H., Puhlmann, L., ... & Mor, N. (2020). Mental resilience in the Corona lockdown: First empirical insights from Europe. https://doi.org/10.31234/osf.io/4z62t

Wang, D., Hu, B., Hu, C., Zhu, F., Liu, X., Zhang, J., ... & Zhao, Y. (2020).

Clinical characteristics of 138 hospitalized patients with 2019 novel coronavirus– infected   pneumonia in Wuhan, China. Jama, 323(11), 1061-1069. https://doi.org/10.1001/jama.2020.1585

Wenham, C., Smith, J., & Morgan, R. (2020). COVID-19: the gendered impacts of the outbreak. The Lancet, 395(10227), 846-848. https://doi.org/10.1016/S0140-6736(20)30526-2

World Health Organization. (2008). WHO outbreak communication planning guide. Geneva.

Zhang, S. X., Wang, Y., Rauch, A., & Wei, F. (2020). Unprecedented disruption of lives and work: Health, distress and life satisfaction of working adults in China one month into the COVID-19 outbreak.   Psychiatry research, 112958.

5. COVID-19 Pandemics And Mental Health: In Times Like These, We Learn to Live Again

Mariana Piers, Luz William Berger

The scenario of pandemics is one of the most dreaded and alarming by mankind. Unfortunately, this is the scenario we are facing now. During a period of pandemics, many situations can be overwhelming, not only related directly to the primary disease, but also related to the measures needed to be taken to combat it, and also its aftermath. Pandemic-related stressors may come in many ways. Uncertainty and anticipated fear, excessive (and possibly fake or misguided) information, psychological and social distress, fear of death or serious illness, loss of close ones, economical societal burden and personal financial difficulties are only a few examples of stressful situations that come along with the pandemics[1,2]. Considering the prolonged and sustained nature of a pandemic, encompassing exposure to multiple potentially traumatic events during a significant period, it could be considered a type of complex trauma[3-5].

History has already shown that psychiatric morbidity is another dreadful outcome from an epidemic. The SARS (severe acute respiratory syndrome) epidemic in 2003 victimized more than 700 individuals, mostly in Asian countries. Up to 45% of SARS survivors that needed hospitalization had at least one psychiatric diagnosis in the immediate discharge from the hospital, including depression, anxiety disorders, and posttraumatic stress disorder (PTSD) symptoms. Even long-term post-discharge evaluations (e.g. 30 months after discharge) showed persistent psychiatric morbidity among SARS patients, mainly PTSD, depressive disorders and anxiety-spectrum disorders[6,7].

After the 2014/2015 Ebola virus outbreak in Africa, many psychiatric and Psychosocial problems arose, such as stigma and isolation, and also psychiatric disorders in the general population and among health care workers, including PTSD, depression and anxiety disorders[8,9].

The Middle East Respiratory Syndrome (MERS) in 2015, which had a high mortality rate (about 20%) caused hundreds of people – and entire villages and cities – to be intensively isolated. During the period of isolation due to the MERS epidemic, more than 40% of the general population reported emotional distress.

Among patients, almost 50% reported significant symptoms of anxiety[10]. It is to be expected that the COVID-19 pandemics will have several psychiatric short- and long-term consequences as well. COVID-19 pandemics is triggering psychological distress and psychiatric problems. Individual characteristics such as culture, economic status, coping mechanisms, previous psychiatric or psychological issues, personal degree of exposure to the risk of contamination, actual development of the disease and/or loss of close persons are some of the factors that influence psychological response to such unusual and uncertain times.

In a societal level, access to accurate and legitimate information, availability of medical services, governmental and medical measures to contain the spread of infection (e.g. quarantine and social isolation) and general psychosocial condition of the community may influence the collective response to the outbreak[9,11-13]. But not all is bad. Human resilience is a powerful force, and it sometimes can overcome the hardest of problems. The majority of the population will present healthy mental health responses to the traumatic events experienced during the pandemic. Peoples' ability to cope, to endure, to recover and to rebuild can even be strengthened in such difficult times. Some individuals may report increased feelings of gratitude, greater appreciation for friends and family, increased care for mental and physical health, stronger beliefs and faith, and even a sense of personal growth[1,14,15].

Recommendations for a better mental health outcome include strategies to enhance individual and collective resilience, intense psychiatric surveillance in individual and community levels, and identification and referral of individuals ate greater risk for development and intensification of psychiatric disorders. Providing accurate and reliable information to the population about the disease and the measures taken to combat it, promoting access to quality health care services, and implementing social and financial aid to the most needed are key features to prevent psychiatric morbidity.

Also, combating stigmatization and social isolation of those who had the disease or lost someone close to it, stimulation of initiating and maintaining adequate psychiatric and psychological treatments, and implementing strong psychosocial interventions are key factors for enhancing the chances of a healthy psychiatric response from the COVID-19 pandemic[1,4,16,17]. Finally, quoting Ali Ibn Abi Talib, the supposed cousin and son-in-law of Muhammad, "Do not let your difficulties fill you with anxiety, after all it is only in the darkest nights that stars shine more brightly"[18].

AFFILIATIONS

Federal University of Rio de Janeiro (UFRJ), Institute of Psychiatry (IPUB),
Rio de Janeiro, RJ, Brazil.Address for correspondence: Mariana Luz. Universidade Federal do Rio de Janeiro, Instituto de Psiquiatria. Av. Venceslau Brás, 71, Fundos – 22290-140 – Rio de Janeiro, RJ, Brasil. E-mail: marianaluzpsi@gmail.comLuz MP, Berger W

REFERENCES

1. Perrin, P.C., McCabe, O.L, Everly, G.S, Links, J.M. (2020). Preparing for an influenza pandemic: mental health considerations. Prehosp Disaster Med. 2009;24(3):223-30.
2. Taylor, S. (2020). The Psychology of Pandemics: Preparing for the Next Global Outbreak of Infectious Disease. Newcastle upon Tyn: Cambridge Scholars Publishing; 2019.J Bras Psiquiatr.
3. Maercker, A, Brewin, C.R., Bryant, R.A, Cloitre, M., van Ommeren, M., Jones, LM, et al. (2020).Diagnosis and classification of disorders specifically associated with stress: proposals for ICD-11. World Psychiatry. 2013;12(3):198-206.
4. Bao, Y., Sun, Y., Meng, S., Shi, J., Lu, L. (2020). 2019-nCoV epidemic: address mental health care to empower society. Lancet. 2020;395(10224):e37-8.
5. World Health Organization (WHO). International statistical classification of diseases and related health problems. 11th ed. Geneva: WHO; 2019.
6. Mak, I.W.C., Chu, C.M., Pan, P.C, Yiu, M.G.C, Chan, V.L. (2020). Long-term psychiatric morbidities among SARS survivors. Gen Hosp Psychiatry. 2009;31(4):318-26.
7. Tucci, V. Moukaddam, N., Meadows, J., Shah, S., Galwankar, S.C., Kapur, G.B. (2020).The forgotten plague: Psychiatric manifestations of Ebola, Zika, and emerging infectious diseases. J Glob Infect Dis. 2017;9(4):151-6.
8. Mohammed, A., Sheikh, T.L., Poggensee, G., Nguku, P., Olayinka, A., Ohuabunwo, C, et al. (2020).Mental health in emergency response: lessons from Ebola. Lancet Psychiatry. 2015;2(11):955-7.
9. Shultz, J.M., Baingana, F., Neria, Y. (2020).The 2014 Ebola outbreak and mental health: current status and recommended response. JAMA. 2015;313(6):567-8.

10. Jeong, H., Yim, H.W., Song, Y.J., Ki, M., Min, J.A., Cho, J., et al. (2020).Mental health status of people isolated due to Middle East Respiratory Syndrome. Epidemiol Health. 2016;38:e2016048.

11. Liu. D, Ren, Y., Yan, F., Li, Y., Xu, X., Yu, X, et al. (2020).Psychological Impact and Predisposing Factors of the Coronavirus Disease 2019 (COVID-19) Pandemic on General Public in China. 2020. Available at: https://ssrn.com/abstract=3551415.

12. Liu, N., Zhang, F., Wei, C., Jia, Y., Shang, Z, Sun, L, et al. (2020). Prevalence and predictors of PTSS during COVID-19 Outbreak in China Hardest-hit Areas: Gender differences matter. Psychiatry Res. 2020;287:112921.

13. Thurackal. B.J, Chith, E.N., Mascarenhas, P. (2020).The Outbreak of Novel Coronavirus in India: Psychological Impact. Available at: https://ssrn.com/abstract=3562062.

14. Greenberg, N., Docherty, M., Gnanapragasam, S., Wessely, S. (2020).Managing mental health challenges faced by healthcare workers during COVID-19 pandemic. BMJ. 2020;368:m1211.

15. Paladino, L, Sharpe, R.P., Galwankar, S.C., Sholevar, F., Marchionni, C., Papadimos, T.J, et al. (2020). Reflections on the Ebola public health emergency of international concern, part 2: the unseen epidemic of posttraumatic stress among health-care personnel and survivors of the 20142016 Ebola outbreak. J Glob Infect Dis. 2017;9(2):45-50.

16. Ho, C., Chee, C., Ho, R. (2020).Mental Health Strategies to Combat the Psychological Impact of COVID-19 Beyond Paranoia and Panic. Ann Acad Med Singapore. 2020;49(3):155-60.

17. World Health Organization (WHO). Mental health and psychosocial considerations during the COVID-19 outbreak, 18 March 2020. Geneva: WHO; 2020.

18. Poonawala, K. (2020). "ALĪ B. ABĪ ṬĀLEB I. Life," Encyclopaedia Iranica, Online Edition, 1982. Available at: http://www.iranicaonline.org/articles/ali-b-abi-taleb#

CHAPTER 16

EDUCATION DURING COVID-19

1. The Impact of Coronavirus on Learning

The closure of schools can lead to malnutrition, as children miss school-provided meals. It can also drive higher dropout rates, while the already high unemployment rates among the youth are likely to increase during the pandemic. These factors may have long-term effects on the accumulation of human capital. The rapid spread of COVID-19 in Brazil imposes pressing challenges to the country's education policy. According to the WHO, over 180 thousand schools have been closed in an attempt to contain the virus. Teachers are having to learn how to deliver their lessons online. Governments must provide tools for remote learning and internet connectivity. The situation is also unprecedented for parents, who must become learning instructors, and for 47 million students, who are having to adapt to a new routine. At the same time, they are weathering an increase on student-parent socioemotional stress, as well as an adverse income shock. By far, the biggest challenge is coordinating all these fronts and keeping students learning.

Without Coordinated Actions, Learning Gaps Tend to Rise as Students are Out of School.

Especially for the most vulnerable, school closures can mean disrupted learning processes and increased dropout rates. Even for those that are able to continue learning, parental support varies critically according to the family background (both quantitatively and qualitatively), according to the international literature.[1] Loose interactions between students and teachers during the pandemic interrupt the regular learning progress, particularly when teachers are replaced by parents with low levels of education. Besides, students from highly vulnerable households dealing with the job market dilemma can see little reason to return to school once the system reopens. According to evidence from learning poverty indicators, 42.2 percent of children in Brazil are unable to read and understand short age-appropriate texts by the age 10. Despite the relevance of all foundational skills, focusing on reading is justified because (i) it is an easily understood measure; (ii) reading is a student's gateway to learning in every other area; and (iii) it is a proxy for foundational learning in other subjects.

---

[1] Guryan, Jonathan, Erik Hurst, and Melissa Kearney. 2008. "Parental Education and Parental Time with Children." Journal of Economic Perspectives, 22 (3): 23-46.

Table 1: Simulated Impacts of School Closures on Learning Poverty (index)

Indicator	Baseline (2017)	12.5% Schoolyear equivalent	25% SYE	37.5% SYE
Learning Poverty (%)	42,2	43,5	44,8	46,1
Out-of-School	4,8	4,8	4,9	5
Below Minimum Proficiency	39,3	40,6	41,9	43,2

Source: World Bank.

Table 1 shows that school closures in Brazil may raise learning poverty levels by 2.6 percentage points to 44.8 percent. Additionally, in the short term, the proportion of children not enrolled in school may increase 0.1 percentage point and reach 4.8 percent among primary-school-aged children. If mitigation strategies are partially successful—for example, with 50 percent effectiveness—the impact will be reduced by half. Brazil has steadily decreased learning poverty in recent years by an average of 3 percentage points per year. However, with the spread of the coronavirus, the education system could backtrack the equivalent of one year on this recent progress. These results are clearly a lower-bound estimate, as they do not include the effects of income loss in both learning and school dropout rates throughout the entire educational cycle, especially in secondary and tertiary education. The first measure being implemented by governments during the pandemic was to replace face-to-face with remote learning. An effective and inclusive implementation of this strategy depends heavily on existing infrastructure.

In addition, it is important to ask whether teachers are prepared to teach remotely, and how technologies are combined. One example is the state of Amazonas, one of the most well-equipped states for remote learning. They combined Aula em Casa (a home-schooling program that broadcasts educational content on open television via satellite) with social media lives and apps. Other similarly impactful strategies come from Piauí, Paraná, Distrito Federal and Maranhão (using television), and Pernambuco and Rio de Janeiro (through online platforms).

Figure 1: Learning Poverty, SAEB
(learners under the learning poverty baseline, 2017)

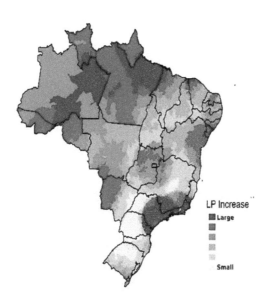

LP Increase
■ Large
■
■
▨
▨
Small

National and Subnational Governments Have Been Implementing Different Combinations of Education Policies, but Inclusiveness Remains a Challenge.

Teachers' previous experience in the use of technology for learning is another critical factor. In other words, effective remote learning and teacher training in the pedagogical use of technology are complementary policies. However, initiatives aimed at this are still to be fully explored. In Brazil, data from **SAEB 2017** (a national learning assessment) indicate that 60 percent to 70 percent of teachers consider technology training as "highly necessary". Distrito Federal has been delivering training to public school teachers on how to use online platforms. It is crucial to encourage further parental engagement while children are studying from home.

Keeping parents involved is even more important during the COVID-19 pandemic—especially if the focus is on reducing inequalities. Vulnerable families are likely to spend less time home schooling their children than non-vulnerable families.

Therefore, one awareness-raising option is to use traditional platforms, such as radio or television, to broadcast programs reinforcing the importance of parental support during the pandemic, while encouraging information sharing and creating mobile apps to motivate parents. Households must also be structurally prepared to replace regular classes with home schooling. In addition to socioeconomic gaps, several inequalities should be considered, including differences in internet connectivity among regions, and among households located in rural and urban areas. The state of São Paulo has engaged with local internet providers to substantially reduce connection costs to make it more affordable for vulnerable families. Other potential strategies to confront structural difficulties include using available devices, such as mobile phones, or computers/ tablets at school. Class suspensions also affect the social safety net generated by schools. For many children, the only regular and healthy meal of the day takes place at school. In addition, women, who tend to be the primary caregiver in many households, end up overwhelmed by accumulating remote working and childcare responsibilities during a pandemic. As mentioned earlier, Law 13,987/2020 has recently been enacted by the federal government, allowing the resources originally allocated to providing school meals in all public schools (under the National School Meals Program—PNAE) to be used to buy basic food baskets for disadvantaged families. Before this change, municipalities such as Recife were already distributing food baskets to the families of vulnerable students. One way to illustrate these aspects is by considering an index of student vulnerability to school closures.

Figure 2:Student vulnerability, per municipality(Index, 2017)

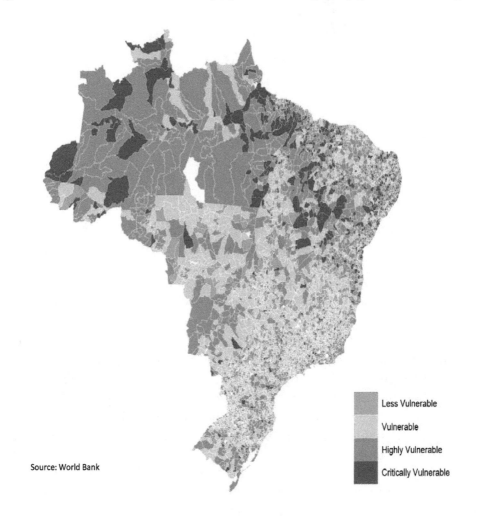

Source: World Bank

Figure3:Student vulnerability per state(Index, 2017)

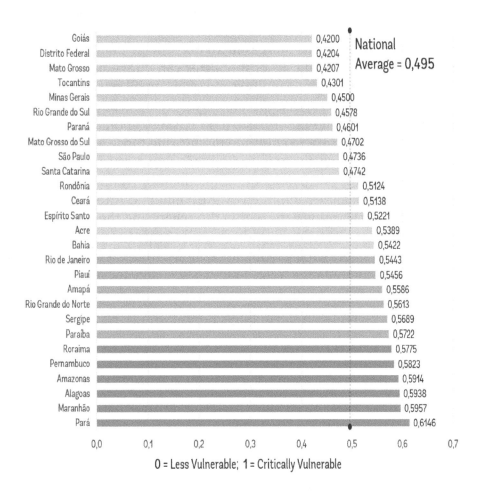

0 = Less Vulnerable; 1 = Critically Vulnerable

With this purpose, figures 2and 3 present a student vulnerability index based on (i) the availability of meals at schools; (ii) whether teachers use internet or technology in the classroom; (iii) whether the family supports their education; (iv) the incidence of students working; and (v) past dropouts. The index is ordinal and assumes that low-performing students that dropped out in the past are more vulnerable to the pandemic when school meals are cut, their teachers are less prepared for remote teaching, and their families are less engaged in home schooling (as compared with students in the opposite situation). Additional mitigating efforts should be undertaken in municipalities located in the North and Northeast. According to the student Vulnerability index, the top six states where students are most vulnerable are Pará, Maranhão, Alagoas, Amazonas, Pernambuco and Roraima, which are more than 0.1 point above the national average (weighted by the number of students). The six states where students are least vulnerable are Goiás, Mato Grosso, Distrito Federal, Tocantins, Minas Gerais and Rio Grande do Sul. However, it is important to note that the index shows data at municipal level, and vulnerabilities within a state must also be taken into account.

Another Challenge Will Start When Schools Reopen.

A safe school reopening strategy is key. The first step for a post-pandemic strategy is establishing reopening protocols that enable all students to return safely to school. In the case of the Ebola epidemic in Africa, for example, dropouts increased 18 percentage points among vulnerable girls[1]. In order to prevent that from happening, several policies can nudge families toward taking their children back to school. One option is to send text messages to all parents whose children fail to return to school.[2]Another way of attracting the most vulnerable groups is by conditioning Bolsa Família cash transfers or the distribution of basic food baskets upon children's return to school. Once they are back, it will be necessary to continue monitoring those at risk of dropping out. This can be done by setting early warning systems and introducing discussion groups to alleviate the mental health shocks caused by the pandemic. Implementing remedial learning programs is fundamental to address the inequalities amplified by the pandemic. After students return to school, the priority must be to mitigate learning gaps within the school and the network. For such, schools can apply standardized exams to all students, and introduce remedial policies based on the results. Examples of activities are small tutoring groups for lagging students; redeployment of teachers, prioritizing specific grades and students; and implementing shorter and more flexible technical programs for students.

[1] Bandiera, Oriana, Niklas Buehren, Markus Goldstein, Imran Rasul and Andrea Smurra. 2018. "The Economic Lives of Young Women in the Time of Ebola: Lessons from an Empowerment Program", mimeo UCL.

[2] Bursztyn. L, and L. Coffman. 2012. "The Schooling Decision: Family Preferences, Intergenerational Conflict, and Moral Hazard in the Brazilian Favelas," Journal of Political Economy 120: 359-97.

2.Back To School After COVID-19 Lockdown In Brazil

Alberto Abad[1]

Psychology Postgraduate Programme,
Federal University of Juiz de Fora (UFJF), Juiz de Fora, MG, Brazil.

Thaís Marques Abad[2]

Federal University of Pará (UFPA), Belém, PA, Brazil

ABSTRACT

South America has become the new epicentre of the coronavirus, especially in Brazil where the disease continues to spread exponentially across the country. This text aims to analyse the psychosocial factors of COVID-19 on back to school strategies in Brazil from a bioecological perspective. At the microsystem level, the population is experiencing different levels of stress and fear; at the mesosystem level, changes in routines, separation from family and friends, and closure of schools; and at the macrosystem level, national guidelines to control the pandemic, institutional standards on a national and international scale. Therefore, the main focus for the success of school return must be in the prevention of contagion and with physical and psychological health, and should not only consider the demands of curricula, financial or administrative management. For this reason, it is paramount that greater female representativeness is increased in decision-making levels of the meso and macrosystem, regarding the resumption of school and academic activities in the pandemic period, since the number of female leaders in decision-making, is still insufficient.

INTRODUCTION

South America has become the new epicentre of the coronavirus, especially in Brazil where the disease continues to spread exponentially across the country; on the date of writing this article Brazil sums up more than two million confirmed cases and eighty-six thousand deaths. As Brazil has not yet reached the peak of the pandemic (WHO, 2020), from a bioecological perspective (Bronfenbrenner & Morris, 2006), the psychosocial impacts of COVID-19 could be viewed at different levels of analysis: at the microsystem level, the population is experiencing different levels of stress and fear as the pandemic has disrupted lives, triggered public panic, and changed the routine (Bao et al., 2020), affecting not only physically but also psychologically (Abad et al., 2020a; Jahanshahi et al., 2020; Jia et al., 2020; Li et al., 2020; Qiu et al., 2020); at the mesosystem level, changes in routines, separation from family and friends, closure of schools, etc. (Zhang et al., 2020);

---

[1] alberto.abad@ich.ufjf.br
tmabad74@gmail.com

and at the macrosystem level, national guidelines to control the pandemic, institutional standards on a national and international scale (Smith, 2019; Taylor, 2019; Bao et al., 2020). Therefore, this text aims to analyse the psychosocial factors of COVID-19 on back to school strategies in Brazil from a bioecological perspective.

METHODS

The proposed methodology is of a descriptive type supported by bibliographic research, which included books and periodical publications that address the current studies on psychosocial factors of COVID-19 disease. To achieve the objective, the ERIC[1] and Web of Science[2] databases were chosen, as well as PsycNET (https://psycnet.apa.org). These sources of information were chosen for their relevance to the areas of Education and/or Psychology. The main original publications were read and analysed. To access these texts, electronic searches were performed in important sources of information for the areas of Education and Psychology, such as: Institutional Repository UFJF, PsycINFO, Fundación Dialnet, Educational Resources Information Centre (ERIC, Institute of Education Sciences) and Google Scholar

DISCUSSION

From a macrosystem view, Brazil faces the health crisis in a delicate social, economic and political context characterized by a lack of national leadership that offers clear guidelines to control the pandemic (the president minimizing the pandemic as a "little flu", absence for the last two months of a National Health Minister in Brazil, lack of doctors and personnel with technical knowledge of health at Brazil´s Health

Ministry, conflicting and contradictory messages from government spokespersons related to the impact and severity of the pandemic, use of medications not recommended by the World Health Organization (WHO) (Chloroquine and Hydroxychloroquine), shortages of basic inputs for the patient care, etc. – increasing the rates of contagion and weakening the Brazilian Health System. At this juncture, each State of the Federation had to face the challenges of COVID-19 pandemic with local strategies, primarily related to hospital care, social distance indexes, population lockdown, commercial restrictions, and educational institutions closures (mesosystem) mostly without support from the Federal Government (macrosystem) and out of sync with other States and regions. Lockdown and School closure have been useful measures of pandemic control at national and international levels, however, there is substantial evidence that the transmission of the infection has increased again in several countries after its reopening, which leads to the belief that there is no of a consensus between governments and technical health professionals on what would be the appropriate time for this reopening (Viner et al., 2020). Furthermore, lockdown (mesosystem) has possibly contributed to the development of psychological or cognitive disorders (microsystem) such as depression, anxiety, fear, anger, mood swings, changes in appetite, and insomnia in part of the population (Abad et al., 2020a).Consequently, planning for the reopening of schools, besides considering COVID-19's contagion prevention should also focus on the psychological health of professionals and the target audience of education. It is pivotal that

---

[1] (https://eric.ed.gov/)
[2] (www.webofknowledge.com)

reopening strategies consider the appropriate methods that the WHO uses to control the spread of infection, since there are still no specific vaccines or antiviral therapies for COVID-19 (WHO, 2008). Schools must also count on with: health professionals and a building and logistics structure that brings together with favourable hygiene conditions; not all Brazilian public schools have such adequate structures, like many, due to the lack of sanitary structure, have difficulties in controlling daily contagions such as chickenpox, flu, and even simple pediculosis control. We have identified several macro and mesosystem mental risk factors related to the return to school of education professionals.

The first, (mesosystem factor) is related to the overload of online work during the pandemic and the burn-out syndrome (Afonso & Figueira, 2020) as a significant portion of this group continued to work at home during compulsory confinement, developing their usual work activities and carrying out new activities linked to digital inclusion, causing a work overload at a time when several of these professionals were forced to link their pedagogical functions to domestic tasks carried out more frequently than usual to avoid spreading the disease in the home environment. All these tasks developed amid a health, economic, political and social crisis (macrosystem factor) that are undoubtedly inducing physical and mental exhaustion, and eventually triggering the burn-out syndrome. In a research that aimed to assess peri-traumatic stress (CPDI Scale), and fear (FCV-19S Scale) of the Brazilian population during lockdown (Abad et al., 2020b), researchers concluded that gender roles are essential to analyse psychological reactions during the pandemic, on both scales, the average scores of women were higher; this finding is psychologically significant because, although women and men are analogous in many ways, it reflects the cognitive and behavioural differences of the genders that influence how health care related to manifestation, epidemiology, and pathology is approached (Regitz-Zagrosek, 2020).

The female gender is conceived as more aware of the importance of medical assistance and more adherent to health counselling and treatment (Rugema et al., 2020). In this sense, due to social gender constructs, male gender might not openly express his fears of COVID-19 and does not follow the preventive health recommendations that WHO determines to manage the spread of coronavirus infection (WHO, 2008), that is, to minimize the risks of the pandemic and not to follow hygiene and social distancing practices.

In the study, the highest female scores in the scales were exhaustion and attention deficit, results that agree with the fact that women often assume most of the burden and risk of health care and hygiene (Smith, 2019), protection, educational and emotional assistance for children, assistance, and care for their parents, spouses, and friends usually with little intra and extra family support. Besides, the closure of schools, during mandatory confinement, has a differential effect for the female gender specifically for education professionals since they frequently carry out the monitoring and educational guidance both in their families (Smith, 2019) and of their students.

Therefore, the return to face-to-face classes for many teachers means both the fear of being infected or infecting their family and their social circle; furthermore, they are concerned with their adaptation to the new pedagogical strategies, and with fulfilling more strenuous working hours. In these conditions, how emotionally do these professionals get in the current scenario? These workers are usually more subject to progressive deterioration of their physical and mental health (Martins, 2007) both before and during the pandemic, so it is not uncommon for them to have emotional and psychosomatic illnesses arising from working conditions (stress, irritability, lack of sleep, eating disorders, among others), it is even observed that these professionals are among those with the highest incidence of cases of the burn-out syndrome (Afonso & Figueira, 2020).

The emotional health of education professionals is directly related to the good performance of their work functions in the reopening of school units, especially during the pandemic. It is worth mentioning that students also share the same effects of confinement (anxiety, fear, stress, and exhaustion), so these implications can influence, as well as their teachers, the behaviour that will act on the return to school. Fear of contagion can even determine whether they want to, or their parents allow them, to return to face-to-face classes.

Thus, for the mesosystem, the return of students represents a challenge, since they must adapt to new behavioural learning: correct use and hygiene of protective masks and the habit of social distancing, frequent care with personal hygiene, constant asepsis of materials and personal objects used in the school environment, avoid sharing personal objects and school materials.

However, another portion of students will represent an even greater challenge for returning to face-to-face classes, the students are the target audience of Special Education (disabilities, global developmental disorders, gifted and talented children) since they are people with specific behaviour patterns and routines that are likely to present many difficulties and resistance to the adaptation to new pandemic control protocols. Such students should not have their needs neglected during the reopening of face-to-face classes, so specific strategies must be devised to meet this demand since the legal provisions advocate an inclusive education to be respected even in pandemic times. These new behaviours are a challenge, since children and adolescents, from Latin- American countries and especially from the northern region of Brazil are culturally accustomed to physical contact. To avoid this work overload and possible failure of the school reopening motivated by an increase in the number of cases of COVID-19 in Brazil and Latin American countries, leading again to the closure of educational institutions,
it will be essential that each school unit has at least one professional of fixed health in each shift (psychologist, health agent, medical school or nursing student) and that the responsibility for the risks or the success of the return to face-to-face classes do not rest solely under the tutelage of education professionals, who historically have already suffered work, emotional and financial overloads worsened since the beginning of cases of contagion by the coronavirus.

CONCLUSION

A vital question of going back to school is not when to open, but how to do it and keep them safely open. The main focus for school return success must be contagion prevention and the physical and psychological health care of students and teachers. It is extremely important to make decisions related to school return, which protect students, control the infection contagion speed, and, consequently, improve the overall mental health of students (Wenham, Smith & Morgan, 2020). Therefore, going back to school should not only consider the demands of curricula, financial, or administrative management. Since the number of female leaders around the world is still insufficient, it is paramount to increase their decision-making representativeness on the mesosystem level (back to school strategies and protocols) and the macrosystem level (educational and health public policies). In short, women in general, and teachers, for their roles in society, are in a strategic position to improve interventions, equitable policies, and new approaches to control the COVID-19 pandemic.

REFERENCES

Abad, A. , da Silva, J. , das Neves Braga, J. , Medeiros, P. , de Freitas, R. , Coimbra, N. and da Silva, J. (2020a). Preparing forthe COVID-19 Mental Health Crisis in Latin America—Using Early Evidence from Countries that Experienced COVID-19 First. Advances in Infectious Diseases, 10, 40-44. https://doi.org/10.4236/aid.2020.103005

Abad, A., da Silva, J. A., de Paiva Teixeira, L. E. P., Antonelli-Ponti, M., Bastos, S., Mármora, C. H. C., ... & da Silva, J. A. (2020b). Evaluation of Fear and Peritraumatic Distress during COVID-19 pandemic in Brazil. https://doi.org/10.1590/SciELOPreprints.890

Afonso, P., & Figueira, L. (2020). Pandemia COVID-19: Quais são os Riscos para a Saúde Mental? Revista Portuguesa de Psiquiatria e Saúde Mental, 6(1), 2-3. https://www.revistapsiquiatria.pt/index.php/sppsm/article/view/131

Bao, Y., Sun, Y., Meng, S., Shi, J., & Lu, L. (2020). COVID-19 epidemic: address mental health care to empower society. The Lancet, 395(10224), e37-e38.

Bronfenbrenner, U., & Morris, P. (2006). The Bioecological Model of Human Development. Chapter 14 in Learner, R (Ed) Handbook of Child Psychology, Volume 1 Theoretical Models of Human Development. https://doi.org/10.1002/9780470147658.chpsy0114

Jahanshahi, A. A., Dinani, M. M., Madavani, A. N., Li, J., & Zhang, S. X. (2020). The distress of Iranian adults during the COVID-19 pandemic-More distressed than the Chinese and with different predictors. medRxiv.https://doi.org/10.1016/j.bbi.2020.04.081

Jia, R., Ayling, K., Chalder, T., Massey, A., Broadbent, E., Coupland, C., & Vedhara, K. (2020). Mental health in the UK during the COVID-19 pandemic: early observations. medRxiv. https://doi.org/10.1101/2020.05.14.20102012

Li, S., Wang, Y., Xue, J., Zhao, N., & Zhu, T. (2020). The impact of COVID-19 epidemic declaration on psychological consequences: a study on active weibo users. International Journal of Environmental Research and Public Health, 17(6), 2032.https://doi.org/10.3390/ijerph17062032

Martins, M. D. G. T. (2007). Sintomas de stress em professores brasileiros. Revista Lusófona de Educação, (10), 109-128. http://www.scielo.mec.pt/scielo.php?script=sci_arttext&pid=S1645-72502007000200009

Qiu, J., Shen, B., Zhao, M., Wang, Z., Xie, B., & Xu, Y. (2020). A nationwide survey of psychological distress among Chinese people in the COVID-19 epidemic: implications and policy recommendations. General psychiatry, 33(2).https://doi.org/10.1136/gpsych-2020-100213

Regitz-Zagrosek, V. (2012). Sex and gender differences in health. EMBO reports, 13(7), 596-603. https://doi.org/10.1038/embor.2012.87

Rugema, L., Persson, M., Mogren, I., Ntaganira, J., & Krantz, G. (2019). A qualitative study of healthcare professionals' perceptions of men and women's mental healthcare seeking in Rwanda. Journal of Community Psychology.https://doi.org/10.1002/jcop.22308

Smith J. (2019). Overcoming the "tyranny of the urgent": integrating gender into disease outbreak preparedness and response. Gender Develop 2019; 27: 355–69.

Taylor, S. (2019). The Psychology of Pandemics: Preparing for the Next Global Outbreak of Infectious Disease. Cambridge Scholars Publishing: UK.

Viner, R., et al. (2020). School closure and management practices during coronavirus outbreaks including COVID-19: a rapid systematic review. The Lancet Child & Adolescent Health. https://doi.org/10.1016/S2352-4642(20)30095-X

Wenham, C., Smith, J., & Morgan, R. (2020). COVID-19: the gendered impacts of the outbreak. The Lancet, 395(10227), 846-848.https://doi.org/10.1016/S0140-6736(20)30526-2

World Health Organization. (2008). WHO outbreak communication planning guide. Geneva.
World Health Organization. (2020). Coronavirus disease (COVID-19). Situation Report –   153. https://www.who.int/docs/default-source/coronaviruse/situationreports/20200621-covid-19-sitrep-153.pdf?sfvrsn=c896464d_2

Zhang, S. X., Wang, Y., Rauch, A., & Wei, F. (2020). Unprecedented disruption of lives and work: Health, distress and life satisfaction of working adults in China one month into the COVID-19 outbreak. Psychiatry research, 112958.https://doi.org/10.1016/j.psychres.2020.112958

3. Social Distancing Effects On The Teaching Systems And Teacher Education Programmes In Brazil: Reinventing Without Distorting Teaching

Martha Maria Prata- Linhares[a], Thiago da Silva Gusmão Cardoso[b,c], Derson S. Lopes-Jr[d] and Cristina Zukowsky-Tavares[b]

[a]Institute of Education, Exact and Natural Sciences, Federal University of Triangulo Mineiro, Uberaba, Brazil; [b]Graduate Programm in Health Promotion, Adventist University of São Paulo, São Paulo, Brazil; [c]Graduate Program in Childhood and Adolescence Education and Health, Federal University of São Paulo, São Paulo, Brazil; [d]LPM People and Marketing Laboratory, University of Campinas, Campinas, Brazil

ABSTRACT

Brazil has marked social asymmetries, which have an impact on the impoverishment of basic educational proficiencies. We present a snapshot in a cross-sectional documentary study that registered the risk of distorting educational processes even more intensely, due to the easing of political and pedagogical decision- making. Planning and thinking about how to keep our teachers and students learning during the isolation and the post-pandemic period, implies the redesigning of education scenarios, searching for balance in teaching and in the use of technologies and resources. Until now, we have noticed an enlarged reproduction of pre-existing educational asymmetries. People who live in a situation of social vulnerability and digital exclusion are facing many more difficulties in the isolation period, as well as in managing to keep learning, than those in better financial conditions and with broadband internet access. It is a time that requires collective reinvention, bringing together policies and practices in a resolutive and equitable way

INTRODUCTION

After the start of COVID-19 community transmission in the Brazilian territory, social isolation and distancing measures rapidly became harsher and more real in the country (Brasil 2020d). In a country, the size of a continent, with approximately 210 million inhabitants (IBGE, 2018), marked by economic and social inequalities, responses to the health crisis may lead to quite divergent educational consequences. Nearly 1.5 billion young people from 165 countries are out of school, corresponding to 87% of the world's student population. This unprecedented educational crisis calls for responses from teachers, administrators and families, supported by public policies based on citizen-centred solutions (UNESCO, 2020). Despite being on the same planet, countries have differing and unequal conditions, which makes them react differently to the pandemic. The article presents a snippet of the three months of restrictions imposed by the COVID-19 triggered social isolation in Brazil and its effects on teaching systems and teacher education programmes. Initially, a retrospective of the set of actions taken and their implications is presented to understand the current teaching scenario in the country. Then, the immediate effects of the crisis on teaching, the organisation of some higher education institutions and their respective teacher education programmes are addressed. Finally, we discuss the impacts on the practice/theory relationship in teacher education.

How The Brazilian Government Handled The Pandemic Related Challenges

On 3 February 2020, human infection by the novel coronavirus was declared a nationally important public health emergency in Brazil (Brasil 2020d). On 16 March, the Emergency Operations Committee of the Ministry of Education met for the first time to initiate actions to prevent the spread of the novel coronavirus in the school system. On 17 March 2020, the first death by COVID-19 was recorded in the country (Ministério da Saúde. Brasil 2020), and based on recommendations from the ministry, state and municipal governments decided to adopt ever more restrictive horizontal social isolation measures. This implied the suspension of classes at all education levels, from basic to higher.

From that date, the Ministry of Education decreed the replacement of classroom classes for remote classes, for as long as social isolation endured, for public higher education institutions, members of the federal education system (Brasil 2020b). On 18 March 2020, the National Education Council (CNE), a subordinate body of the Ministry of Education, saw it necessary to reorganise academic activities, as a result of actions to prevent the spread of COVID-19 in educational systems and institutions at all levels, stages and modes.

On 1 April 2020, the Ministry of Education established rules for the school year in basic education and higher education. They suspended the mandatory 200 days in school in basic education, as long as the 800 hours of classes provided for by the annual calendar were fully met (Brasil 2020d). The effects of the pandemic triggered an immediate reaction, suspending degree courses in federal higher education. In May 2020, 78.8% of students, including those doing teacher education were facing suspended activities (see http://portal.mec.gov.br/ coronavirus/).

On 1 June, the National Education Council (CNE, 2020), granted autonomy to Brazilian education systems, establishing that the reorganising of the school calendar was to be the responsibility of each education system. The Council's report establishes that in order to reschedule school days at the end of the pandemic, institutions will be able to use unanticipated time slots, like recesses and Saturdays, and when necessary, may add hours to the daily timetable. In addition, it recommended which activities and non-face- to-face media may be used (digital media, including WhatsApp, Facebook, Instagram, etc.), video classes, educational videos, virtual platforms, television or radio programmes, printed educational material given to parents or guardians, among others. However, with regard to early childhood education, no standard was provided for remote teaching, despite the emergency situation. The National Education Council also authorised internships in teacher education courses to be done in the remote format, with student teachers working with the final years of lower secondary and upper secondary education, in public and private schools.

In spite of this normative body, the effects of COVID-19 in higher education and teacher education programmes vary a lot among Brazilian educational institutions. Most recommendations were aimed at the adoption of remote classes; however, not all regions and communities in the country have equal access to the internet or have remote teaching infrastructure. Inequalities related to digital exclusion already existed, but the crisis caused by social distancing has dramatically worsened the situation, representing an important vulnerability factor in relation to the virus, with strong losses in educational performance (Beaunoyer, Dupéré, and Guitton 2020).

Transition to remote teaching and the effects on teachers

There is an enormous gap between the resources available for public and private educational institutions to implement the so-called remote education. Although 79.9% of Brazilians live in homes with an internet connection, the main form of access is by mobile phones (99.2%), and only 48.1% use computers. Average per capita income is an indicator of the type of resources available in a household. In 2018, the average per capita income for households without a computer or tablet was BRL 957; for homes in which there was at least one gadget, the average was BRL 2,404 (IBGE 2018). In addition to the difference in resources available for public and private educational institutions to implement remote education, another challenge to fully adopting non-face -to-face pedagogical and teaching activities is teacher education in this format. Before the COVID-19 crisis, Brazilian teachers already referred to the difficulties of integrating digital resources in educational practice at different levels of education (Loureiro, Cavalcanti, and Zukowsky-Tavares 2019; Prata-Linhares and Arruda 2017).

It is clear that this difficulty and lack of education in teaching totally mediated by technological resources have demanded great effort from teachers, causing insecurity, and changes in teaching habits and routine (Instituto Península 2020). A survey on the feelings and perception of 7,773 Brazilian teachers from public and private basic education institutions, during the coronavirus pandemic in Brazil, revealed that 88% of the professionals interviewed had never taught classes, using the non-face-to-face format, before social distancing. Furthermore, the vast majority of teachers, 83.4%, feel little or not prepared at all to teach remotely. Early childhood teachers are the ones who feel least prepared for virtual/online education (89%). In upper secondary education, this percentage is lower, with 77% of teachers not feeling prepared to tackle non-classroom teaching (Instituto Península 2020).

The difficulty faced by basic and higher education teachers in using digital means for teaching is pointed out in a survey entitled 'Professional challenges in times of COVID-19'. Out of the 996 Brazilian workers, who answered the survey during April, 283 (28.41%) identified themselves as education professionals, with 34 managers, 65 higher education professors and 113 basic education teachers. Education professionals had an average age of 41, 75% were women, 34.5% had master's and doctoral degrees, 24.14% of them experienced wage reduction and 5% had lost their jobs in the first months of the pandemic. Sixty-two per cent of those working as teachers, pointed out a gap in training focused on the use of different digital interface platforms, which made remote teaching extremely difficult. Despite this, 70.2% of education professionals showed enthusiasm in learning new technologies, even if 77.5% of them pointed out that their workload increased during the pandemic. Furthermore, 61.4% indicated that students seemed to be more absent in remote classes, than in face-to-face lessons, showing even more the value of teacher education in digital technologies, mitigating negative developments in the acquisition of basic educational proficiencies.

A previous survey with higher education professors, some of them in charge of basic education teacher training, revealed data that helped further clarify teacher education challenges during the social distancing period. Pimenta, Prata-Linhares, and Melo (2019) studied professors from different areas, including teacher trainers from 16 higher education institutions located in 10 cities in three Brazilian geographic regions: the Central-West, Southeast and South. The survey results reveal that less than 40% of the professors declared having some type of knowledge in media literacy. Basically, media literacy comprises of skills and capacities such as knowing how to access information, moving onto more complex processes like critically assessing the information accessed, and having knowledge on content production using different languages and platforms. Although important, knowing how to use digital technologies is not enough. The survey also revealed teachers' lack of knowledge vis-à-vis deontological ethics and copyright licences, such as Creative Commons (Pimenta, Prata-Linhares, and Melo 2019).

In addition to teachers, students and their families are affected by remote education measures. Another survey, conducted with 1,476 students, from all levels of basic education in public and private schools revealed that 45.06% of pupils in public primary and lower secondary education were not even contacted by schools during the social isolation period. This figure did not reach 1% in private schools. Another worrying datum revealed by the survey was that 41.86% of the students were found to have the unsuitable infrastructure for remote learning (internet access and housing conditions). In addition, in relation to student perception, 22.76% of them considered themselves as not having the right psycho-pedagogical conditions for remote education (they feel terrible and have no family support to do school activities) (PPGED-SO, 2020). These data have repercussions on teachers' daily routines, as they now have to deal with the demand for psychological support from students, but are often unable to reach them.

Reorganisation of higher education and initial teacher education

The effects of this crisis on education are still unpredictable. Although the inclusion process is growing in Brazil, the country is still far from any figure that could mean a reality, where all children and adolescents are in school and with access to education.

Only 60% of young Brazilians attending upper secondary education are doing so at the correct age; out of every 100 students who enrol in school, only 76 finish primary and lower secondary education, and 59 conclude upper secondary education. Approximately 20% of young people, aged 18 to 24, attend higher education. In addition, 1.7 million young people, aged 15 to 18, do not study, nor work (INEP, 2018, 2019). Teacher education curricula were already in the process of being changed in this context, before the pandemic. However, as most of these young people with difficulties in connecting to education come from low socio-economic classes, social isolation can enhance inequalities of access and permanence at all levels of education. Public and private higher education institutions, responsible for initial teacher education, respond differently to the threat of social distancing imposed by the pandemic.

This initial social distancing period in three higher education institutions has been described, as an example: Adventist University of São Paulo (UNASP), Federal University of Triângulo Mineiro (UFTM) and University of Campinas (UNICAMP). On 13 March, Adventist University of São Paulo, a community institution located in the state of São Paulo, set up a crisis management committee for actions against Covid-19 in its three campuses. The institution published a note on its website on 15 March, suspending all classroom academic activities, with only a few essential services, such as security, janitorial and academic management, remaining active. Immediately, students were informed that classes would be resumed in one week, but remotely and keeping to the same timetable for daytime and night-time courses. Teachers received a week- long intensive training course, on the use of the virtual platform Moodle, and the Zoom video-conferencing application. Afterwards, all activities started being conducted remotely, including classes, meetings, end of course dissertation supervision and master's examination boards. The workload was kept the same, and the faculty's wages were paid in full.

Important pedagogical questions arose during this period, which were the subject of specific training during the following weeks, such as what to do with students who do not have access to the internet, how to manage absences, adjust subjects to the new online teaching model, stimulate students' attention and motivation during classes, and carry out assessments, among others. Some measures have been taken for each of these issues. Regarding students' internet access, a questionnaire was built to survey the situation and synchronous classes were recorded and made available on the virtual platform, for later access by students. To encourage motivation, active methodologies discussed in the training were implemented. In relation to absences, it was decided that each case would be analysed later, with the necessary flexibility, due to the difficulties of access reported or not by the students. Finally, examinations started to be discussed with training on the virtual platform to be used in the assessment-related activities like seminars, tests, reviews, case discussions and reports, among others.

Internships, part of the undergraduate initial teacher education at Adventist University of São Paulo, were split equally between activities monitored in the online environment and face-to-face. However, the 50% mandatory face-to-face activities are waiting for the end of the pandemic to be concluded. Teaching sequences and plans were outlined for distance activities, in addition to a study of the common curricular national base and teaching resources. Federal University of Triângulo Mineiro, an institution located in the state of Minas Gerais, started its remote ventures on 15 March 2020, suspending all undergraduate academic events and activities. Soon after, the COVID-19 management committee was created to guide academic actions during the virus containment period. Hence, temporary measures were established in the institution, with a view to reducing personal exposure and interaction between people in the academic community.

Despite the Ministry of Education authorising face-to-face classes to be replaced with remote lessons, until 1 June, Federal University of Triângulo Mineiro had not started remote teaching activities in undergraduate courses. Thus, all undergraduate courses in initial teacher education have gone without classes, including internships.

In postgraduate courses, master's and doctoral degrees, face-to-face classes were replaced by the remote format and examination boards, supervision and meetings continued to take place normally, mainly via the Google Meet tool. Teachers were invited and encouraged to participate in non-classroom teaching. It was not a mandatory activity, but they are having the opportunity of learning through practice, from more experienced teachers. The institution already used the Moodle learning platform environment and its use was intensified.In the first two months of social isolation, the institution promoted internal discussions, suspending the academic calendar of undergraduate courses, thus, interrupting all classes and internships in teacher education programmes. After internal discussions and a questionnaire, forwarded to students to ascertain whether they were able to continue their academic activities, an additional period was proposed, keeping in mind the least possible loss to students and faculty. This proposal has yet to be implemented.

During this period, there has been a significant increase in lives and podcasts created by teachers for teachers and student teachers in initial and continuing education. The themes addressed are in context with social isolation and the use of technologies in education, touching on Brazilian social history, balance and mental health, gender relations, concepts in education, active methodologies and others. The videos are available on YouTube.Federal University of Triângulo Mineiro is a public, free of charge institution. In the federal university universe, until 1 June 2020, only 21.2% of them had continued their undergraduate classes which implies that initial teacher education courses are going without lessons.[1] The University of Campinas is a public state, free of charge institution, located in the state of São Paulo. On 13 March, it adopted measures to face the pandemic, suspending classroom teaching activities. With the support of the Educational Technologies Management Group (GGTE) and the Teaching and Learning Support Space, they offered activities such as the production of podcasts and video lessons, and the use of educational platforms.

They also allocated financial resources for hybrid teaching improvement projects. Undergraduate students have access to synchronous classes and solve problems related to the studied topic on the digital platform. Google Meet is the official tool used, but not the only one. In relation to postgraduate activities, faculty has been using several technologies to support remote teaching. For example, students receive lists of subjects for prior study, and later, meetings are scheduled on Skype or Google Meet. All activities have been maintained by faculty members and students. Examination boards continue to take place, usually via Google Meet. To assist in the migration process to remote education, the institution has created the Digital Teaching Support Space, where faculty members with more experience in digital tools and information technology staff help teachers still facing difficulties. Despite the institution keeping initial teacher education undergraduate courses going through the remote format, but with internships suspended, pedagogy students claim they do not have the right conditions to ensure their full access to classes and pedagogical activities (Assembléia dos estudantes de Pedagogia 2020).

The suspension of internships in teacher education courses is also due to difficulties schools and teachers have faced in implementing non-classroom learning activities. In the state of Minas Gerais, as well as São Paulo, the municipal and state education secretariats took measures in relation to basic public education. They prepared booklets with guidelines for families, availability of digital books and granted recess to students in the first years of schooling. They created virtual spaces for this period and organised educational materials in all areas of knowledge, to be worked on at home via Google Classroom, and an application designed for content monitoring. Television is also being used to show video lessons during this period.

However, teachers and family members had access related difficulties due to lack of knowledge and basic work infrastructure (computer and broadband internet), which resulted in social inequities (Zhang 2015). Therefore, the families also received printed material and food vouchers. Nonetheless, there are testimonies stating that after two months, some students have yet to receive these resources. Social asymmetries and unequal school results are understood to have been intensified during this period in São Paulo, as well as Minas Gerais, presenting several challenges to be overcome collectively in the post-pandemic phase. Despite the difficulties faced by teachers and pupils, refresher and continuous education courses for faculty members and students registered an increase in interest. In addition, the number of courses created by the Ministry of Education grew. AVAMEC, the Ministry of Education's virtual learning environment, offers free courses for student and professional teachers. The platform registered record access in recent months, with over 340 thousand in March alone. The environment has 1,244 distance learning classes and 179 thousand registered users. At the end of the course, if the person meets all the requirements, they receive a document stating they concluded the workload. This document may be used in the education

---

[1] (see <http://portal.mec.gov.br/coronavirus/>),

network for professional advancement and help the student teacher prove to the university that they have finished the course (see http://educacaoconectada.mec.gov.br/). These courses provide learning opportunities in the education of teachers and student teachers during the isolation period, and despite not being enough, they are alternatives for continuing studies for undergraduate students.

Internships And The Theory And Practice Relationship In Initial Teacher Education

As schools have had their face-to-face classes suspended, discussions related to the internship are underway in undergraduate teacher education courses, so that theoretical lessons may be held remotely. Then, after the social distancing period is over, the internship would move onto its practical component. There is a risk of aggravating the lack of contextualisation of teacher education in schools (Marcondes, Leite, and Ramos 2017) and the difficulties still faced in Brazil and other countries, in uniting practice and theory in teacher education. (Gatti et al. 2014; Fontoura 2018; Craig and Orland-Barak 2015; Flores 2017; Loureiro, Cavalcanti, and Zukowsky-Tavares 2019; Veiga 2010). Another issue is fragmenting internships in initial teacher education, which could trigger a superficial experience in the theory and practice relation (Gatti et al. 2019). Even during the social distancing period, these are challenges that still need to be overcome.

Final considerations

Before the COVID-19 pandemic, Brazilian education was already in crisis. Social distancing brought this crisis to the forefront, providing an opportunity for reflection. Trends are not destinations, and the option from now on is to continue or transform what is there. In this context of severity, which the country's education systems are going through, and taking into account the available variables, the responsibility to discuss possible scenarios, where education is not distorted by the undergoing changes, becomes essential. Knowledge building processes are defended, which without ignoring the need for appropriating technological advances of its times, focus on expanding the human potential to communicate, interact, create and problematise for full development. By distortion, we refer to the adoption of basic education teaching completely mediated by digital technologies and without discussions, planning and continuing teacher education.

Finally, the distortion in teaching work and training, without its protagonism, is a matter of concern. Experts are saying that with the school calendar resuming, this will imply an increase in working hours, a growing demand for emotional support for students and their families, further burdening the teaching profession, which in Brazil is one of the riskiest professions vis-à-vis mental illness and symbolic violence (Cortez et al. 2017).

On the other hand, the crisis may drive the reinvention of education, in a way never seen before. The most important changes are those resulting from an intellectual utopia, which makes a political utopia possible (de Santos 2014). When educational policies for this period have been criticised, as having resulted in the exclusion of poor young people from the education systems and challenged teachers to guarantee access to quality education, claims present for a long time in the Brazilian educational crisis are brought up. Claims for democratising and improving access to education, in the sense of promoting profound changes in school curricula and teacher education, public policies and roles of teachers, students and educational managers.

The community, as a joint horizontal political organisation may be part of this educational reinvention and renewal movement. Indeed, hopes are placed in academic communities, which have awakened from the lethargy of years of financial disinvestment and political and social disengagement. After all, more than ever, it is in times of crisis that choices are made about the paths to be taken, opting for the distorting teaching track or collective reinvention.

Disclosure statement

No potential conflict of interest was reported by the authors.

REFERENCES

Assembléia dos estudantes de Pedagogia. 2020. Carta à direção da Faculdade de Educação da Unicamp. 25 de maio de 2020.

Beaunoyer, E., S. Dupéré, and M. J. Guitton. 2020. "COVID – 19 and Digital Inequalities: Reciprocal Impacts and Mitigation Strategies." *Computers in Human Behavior* 111: 01–9. doi:10.1016/j. chb.2020.106424.

Brasil. 2020a. "Ministério da Saúde. Portaria MS/GM nº 188, de 3 de fevereiro de 2020. Declara Emergência em Saúde Pública de importância Nacional (ESPIN) em decorrência da Infecção Humana pelo novo Corona vírus (2019-nCoV) [Internet]." Brasília, DF: Diário Oficial da União 2020 fev. 4; Seção Extra:1. Accessed 13 May 2020. http://www.in.gov.br/web/dou/-/portaria-n- 188-de-3-de-fevereiro-de–2020–241408388

Brasil. 2020b. "Ministério da Educação. Portaria n. 343 de 17/03/2020." Accessed 13 May 2020. http:// www.planalto.gov.br/CCIVIL_03/Portaria/PRT/Portaria%20nº%20343-20-mec.htm

Brasil. 2020c. "Portaria nº 454, de 20 de março de 2020. Declara, em todo o território nacional, o estado de transmissão comunitária da corona vírus (COVID-19)." Diário Oficial da União.

Brasil. 2020d. "Ministério da Educação. Medida Provisória 934 de 1º de abril de 2020." Accessed 13 May. http://www.planalto.gov.br/ccivil_03/_ato2019-2022/2020/Mpv/mpv934.htm

Conselho Nacional de Educação (CNE). 2020. "Parecer nº 05/2020, de 28 de abril de 2020." Accessed 13 May. http://portal.mec.gov.br/index.php?option=com_docman&view=download&alias= 145011-pcp005-20&category_slug=marco-2020-pdf&Itemid=30192

Cortez, P. A., M. V. R. Souza, L. O. Amaral, and L. C. A. Silva. 2017. "A saúde docente no trabalho: apontamentos a partir da literatura recente." *Cadernos de Saúde Coletiva. Rio de Janeiro* 25 (1): 113–122. doi:10.1590/1414-462x201700010001.

Craig, C.J. and Orland-Barak, L. (2015), "International Teacher Education: Promising Pedagogies Introduction", International Teacher Education: Promising Pedagogies (Part B) (Advances in Research on Teaching, Vol. 22B), Emerald Group Publishing Limited, pp. 1–5. https://doi.org/ 10.1108/S1479–368720150000025045 de Santos, B. S. 2014. *Direitos humanos, democracia e desenvolvimento*. 1 ed. São Paulo: Cortez. Flores, M. A. 2017. "Practice, Theory and Research in Initial Teacher Education: International Perspectives." *European Journal of Teacher Education* 40 (3): 287–290. doi:10.1080/ 02619768.2017.1331518.

Fontoura, H. A. 2018. "Narratives by Initial Teachers: stories about Experiences and Challenges." *Education and Self Development* 13 (2): 10–18. doi:10.26907/esd13.2.02.

Gatti, B. A., E. S. S. de Barreto, M. E. D. André, and P. C. Almeida. 2019. *Professores do Brasil: novos cenários de formação*. Gatti, A., Barreto. Brasília: UNES.

Gatti, B. A., M. E. D. Andre, N. A. S. Gimenes, and L. Ferragut. 2014. "Um estudo avaliativo do Programa Institucional de Bolsa de Iniciação à Docência (PIBID)." *Coleção Textos FCC (Impresso)* 41: 4–117.

Instituto Brasileiro de Geografia e Estatística. (IBGE). 2018. "PNAD Contínua TIC 2018: Internet chega 79,1% dos domicílios do país." Accessed 28 May. https://agenciadenoticias.ibge.gov.br/agencia- sala-de-imprensa/2013-agencia-de-noticias/releases/27515-pnad-continua-tic-2018-internet- chega-a-79-1-dos-domicilios-do-pais

Instituto Nacional de Estudos e Pesquisas. INEP. 2018. *Censo da educação superior 2018: resumo técnico*. Brasília: Instituto Nacional de Estudos e Pesquisas Educacionais Anísio Teixeira.

Instituto Nacional de Estudos e Pesquisas. INEP. 2019. *Censo da educação básica 2019: resumo técnico*. Brasília: Instituto Nacional de Estudos e Pesquisas Educacionais Anísio Teixeira.

Instituto Península. 2020. "Sentimento e percepção dos professores brasileiros nos diferentes estágios do Corona vírus no Brasil." *Março de 2020*. Accessed June 3. https://institutopeninsula. org.br/wp-content/uploads/2020/05/Covid19_InstitutoPeninsula_Fase2_at%C3%A91405-1.pdf

la Velle, L. 2019. "The Theory–practice Nexus in Teacher Education: New Evidence for Effective Approaches." *Journal of Education for Teaching* 45 (4): 369–372. doi:10.1080/02607476.2019.1639267.

Loureiro, A. C., C. C. Cavalcanti, and C. Zukowsky-Tavares. 2019. "Concepções docentes sobre o uso das Tecnologias na Educação." *Revista Novas Tecnologias na Educação. RENOTE* 17 (3): 468–477.

Marcondes, M. I., V. A. Leite, and R. K. R. Ramos. 2017. "Theory, Practice and Research in Initial Teacher Education in Brazil: Challenges and Alternatives." *European Journal of Teacher Education* 40 (3): 326–341. doi:10.1080/02619768.2017.1320389.

Ministério da Saúde. Brasil. 2020. "Secretaria de Vigilância em Saúde." *Especial: doença pelo corona vírus 2019*. Bol. Epidemiológico [Internet]. 2020 abr. [citado 2020 abr. 7];7(spe):1–28. Accessed 13 May. https://portalarquivos.saude.gov.br/images/pdf/2020/April/06/2020-04-06-BE7-Boletim- Especial-do-COE-Atualizacao-da-Avaliacao-de-Risco.pdf

Pimenta, M. A. A., M. M. Prata-Linhares, and T. R. Melo. 2019. "Professores universitários, competência midiática e autoscopia." In *Competências Midiáticas em Cenários Brasileiros*, edited by G. Borges and M. B. da Silva, 109–136. 1 ed. Juiz de Fora: Ed. da UFJF.

Prata-Linhares, M., and R. Arruda. 2017. "Inovação e integração das tecnologias digitais na docência universitária: conceitos e relações." *Reflexão e Ação* 25 (2): 250–268. doi:10.17058/rea.v25i2.8843.

Programa de Pós-graduação em Educação - PPGED-SO. 2020. "Condições e dinâmica cotidiana e educativa na RMS (Região Metropolitana de Sorocaba/SP) durante o afastamento social provocado pelo corona vírus. Relatório técnico-científico de pesquisa. UFSCAR, Sorocaba." Accessed June 3. http://www.ppged.ufscar.br/pt-br/arquivos-1/relatorio-de-pesquisa-educacao -e-coronavirus-na-reg-de-sorocaba-ufscar-26-05-2020pdf.pdf

United Nations Educational, Scientific and Cultural Organization (UNESCO). 2020. Accessed 13 May. https://pt.unesco.org/news/no-dia-da-educacao-unesco-chama-atencao-urgencia-acoes- enfrentamento-apos-impacto-da-COVID-19

Veiga, I. P. A. 2010. *A aventura de formar professores*. 2 ed. Campinas: Papirus.

Zhang, M. 2015. "Internet Use that Reproduces Educational Inequalities: Evidence from Big Data."

4.Brazilian School Feeding During The COVID-19 Pandemic

Ana Carla Bittencourt Reis *
University of Brasilia

Mara Lúcia Castilho
Federal Institute of Brasilia

Ana Paula Melo Mariano
State University of Santa Cruz

Edilson de Souza Bias
University of Brasilia

ABSTRACT

School feeding is part of for million students' routine worldwide. Schools' closure during the COVID-19 pandemic brought to the fore the challenge of providing food for children and adolescents by alternative means, through food programs, whether governmental or otherwise. In Brazil, approximately 40.1 [1] million children and adolescents enrolled in basic public education were affected and went without their daily meal during this period. To provide them food, most local governments chose to transfer financial resources to their parents. The challenge of knowing if children are receiving these meals adequately during school closures, which can be lengthy, is the target of this study. The current situation in the 27 Brazilian federated entities regarding the transfer of funds and delivery of meals is presented herein. A monitoring model is proposed for children and adolescents to be followed during the pandemic, in order to guarantee their adequate nutrition.

INTRODUCTION

The first case of COVID-19 was recorded in December 2019, in the city of Wuhan, China [2]. In Brazil, the first recorded cases were in February 2020 [3], and, among the measures taken to contain the spread of the pandemic, social distancing has been widely adopted as a non-pharmaceutical measure. Other measures taken include the closure of educational institutions at all levels, followed by restaurants, offices, and commerce in general, in addition to others. As of April 2020, school closures during the pandemic, affected approximately 197 countries and 1.6 billion children and adolescents [4]. Of this number, there are currently about 352 million that are no longer receiving meals at school, and for many, these are the only meals of the day [4]. There are countries with a significant number of students regularly benefiting from school meals that are being affected by this pandemic, such as: India (approximately 90.4 million), Brazil (40.1 million),

United States (30 million), Egypt (11 million), Nigeria (9.8 million), South Africa (9.2 million), Turkey (6.1 million), Colombia (4 million), Peru (2.3 million), Bolivia (2.3 million), Ethiopia (2.5 million), and Argentina (1.6 million) [1].

Providing food is one of the functions performed by a school, in addition to others, such as education, socialization, and care for children and adolescents [5]. Maintaining a healthy diet is crucial for preserving the general well-being of a population. A good nutritional status is directly related to proper development and growth in childhood, better immune response, less risk of developing diseases, and is fundamental for recovery, in cases of infection [6,7]. School feeding programs work under the auspices of promoting Food and Nutritional Security (SAN) and it is in this context that the school environment is the fundamental and strategic space for promoting SAN, since it provides meals and also helps in the formation of healthy eating habits. The benefit of school meals is incalculable, because healthy eating is a way of providing child development through adequate nutrition, improving cognitive ability, as well as contributing to reducing school dropout rates. Therefore, in countries with great social difficulties, such as Brazil, Mexico, Ecuador and Ghana, for example, many children rely on schools as their main source of food [8]; and, during this pandemic, the lack of food can impair the development of these children and adolescents and contribute to increased school dropout rates [9].It is worth mentioning that the more precarious a child's food situation is, that is, the more vulnerable the family structure is to supplying basic needs, the greater the importance of school [5] for filling this deficiency.

In addition, in situations of social vulnerability, school meals constitute an indirect income for families, and this can contribute to overall family income. [10]. In the article, "Mitigating the effects of the COVID-19 pandemic on food and nutrition of schoolchildren," UNESCO mentions the transfer of money to families affected by the closure of educational institutions, via the card normally used to acquire school supplies. According to this article, the amount of the transfer varies according to the daily number of meals that children usually receive in schools [11]. The Brazilian government passed Law 13,987/20 in order to guarantee the distribution of food to the families of students in public schools (from zero to 17 years old), whose classes were suspended during the new coronavirus pandemic [12] through the National School Feeding Program - PNAE. However, little is known about the effectiveness of the adopted measures. When seeking to know more about this process on the websites of Brazilian state education departments, little information was found on this topic, or on the number of children and adolescents benefiting from this measure, which among other reasons, influenced the motivation of this research. In light of the above, and in addition to promoting a discussion about this important and urgent problem, this work aims to: present the types of transfer (food and/or cash rations) carried out by Brazilian state authorities to children and adolescents who are away from school; and propose strategies for monitoring and controlling the use of these transfers by families, in order to mitigate the risks arising from the lack of food for these students during the COVID-19 pandemic.

THE ROLE OF SCHOOL FEEDING PROGRAMS

As illustrated in Figure 1, schools play at least four roles that reflect their importance in the lives of children, adolescents, family members, and to society as a whole. At the heart of this context, especially when considering cognitive development, education is driven by: socialization, through which children and adolescents can develop their socio-emotional skills; care, that is being a safe place where parents can leave their children to be able to work; and, finally, through food, because in many cases this is the only food meeting the nutritional standards necessary for development and health that children and adolescents manage to obtain. There is a complexity in fulfilling the objectives of each of these school roles during this pandemic, which has further challenged educators, governments, schools, and families. In Brazil, public schools are specifically represented by the model in Figure 1, as they play a fundamental role in the development, training and care of children and adolescents, especially in view of their vulnerability within their social environments, and who in most cases, come from low-income families and difficult social conditions

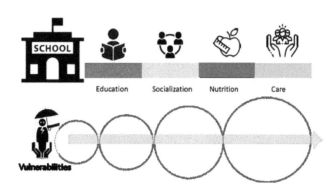

Figure 1. Role of the school in the student's life. Adapted from [5]

During the pandemic, alternatives to classroom education such as distance teaching and remote monitoring have been implemented to reduce the impacts upon cognitive development as a consequence of material expected to be otherwise taught throughout the school year. The care and socialization offered by the school are factors to be discussed, and the impact of the closure of schools upon these factors is very large. However, social distancing makes it difficult to make decisions about measures that address their mitigation. The subject of this study, school food, has been addressed as a relevant issue and it is necessary to assess whether the measures taken for this purpose reflect the urgency to solve this problem.Even before the pandemic, much research was carried out to assess the benefits of school meals upon the lives of students. Previous studies have already shown the positive effects of school feeding programs on the development of verbal fluency in malnourished children [13].

Additionally, Jomaa, McDonnell, and Probart [14] presented a bibliographic survey of articles published over the span of 20 years evaluating school feeding programs and, based on these articles, analysed the impact of school feeding programs on the lives of children and adolescents. This research revealed a relative positive effect of school meals on student enrolment and dropout rates, when compared to students not covered by these programs. In Latin America, the Food and Agriculture Organization of the United Nations (FAO) encourages countries to develop their school feeding programs. In the United States, there are at least two care programs aimed at vulnerable children, such as the School Nutrition Program, a school nutrition program aimed at offering free meals to children from needy families, and the Farmers Market Nutrition Program (FMNP), a special supplementary nutrition program for women, babies, and children. Another program of great relevance is the World Food Program (WFP), a worldwide initiative that serves about 17.3 million school children with meals and snacks [WFP].Brazil counts on the PNAE (National School Feeding Program), a social program linked to the Education Ministry (implemented in 1955) that seeks to guarantee students enrolled in public schools and philanthropic entities an adequate and healthy meal. Other alternatives to promote nutrition for children and adolescents have been developed as well, such as micronutrient fortified co okies produced in Vietnam that, according to research, have reduced the prevalence of anaemia and improved the status of iron intake [15].

SCHOOL FEEDING PROGRAMS DURING COVID-19

Without school feeding programs during the COVID-19 pandemic, thousands of children are subject to starvation. As of April, regarding strategies for the provision of school meals during this pandemic, of the approximately 197 countries with schools closed during this period, 10 of them have implemented programs for the transfer of cash rations to families, 47 are providing take-home food rations, 9 have placed programs on hold, and 16 are adopting mixed strategies [1]. However, the provision of food or other assistance to supply school meals does not guarantee that children are, in fact, being fed. [4].In addition to Brazil, other countries that have also provided financial assistance to families include: The United States, through the Supplemental Nutritional Assistance Program (SNAP); Peru, with the transfer of cash rations through the Qali Warma National School Food Program; and many others. According to the WFP, at least 10 countries have adopted a strategy of transferring cash rations to family members in order to mitigate this problem. This is a measure that can be effective; however, other difficulties can be faced by families, such as bearing the costs of preparing food, which can be a difficult task under a scenario of high unemployment.

- Maintain flexibility and responsiveness to changes in the food supply and in the distribution and provision of nutrition services, while ensuring compliance with COVID-19 protocols.
- Use available resources to protect food and nutritional security for school children.

- Build upon existing welfare structures to cover vulnerable school children.
- Ensure that food and nutritional needs of vulnerable children are taken into account when designing any large-scale national response to COVID-19.
- Plan for the future reopening of schools, if possible, with specific benchmarks.

The expected duration of the pandemic is strongly related to the development of new drugs and a possible vaccine [16]. It is not yet clear how long schools will be closed as a measure to reduce or contain the contamination resulting from COVID-19, or if there will be episodes of intermittent opening and closing. This leads to a discussion of the sustainability and effectiveness of initiatives carried out. With regard to school feeding programs, the measures adopted need to be adapted to these scenarios. For example, school closures in situations similar to the current pandemic were used during the H1N1 outbreak as a non-pharmaceutical containment measure [17], which, according to these authors, contributed to a decrease in the spread of the disease. However, in Brazil in 2009, only a few states postponed returning to classes by 15 days in the second semester of the academic year [18], with no extended school closures as in 2020.Short-term harm to students' health as a result of missed meals during the pandemic may include fatigue and a reduced immune response, which makes children and adolescents more vulnerable to contracting infectious agents such as viruses, bacteria, etc., and consequently to developing diseases, which can worsen their condition because of a deficient immune response. In the long term, this harm can affect psychological, physical, and emotional development [19].

As mentioned, Federal Law 13,987/20 has the clear objective of guaranteeing the distribution of food to the families of students whose schools are closed. When the Law was enacted, the government of the Federal District opted for the distribution of food allowances to the parents of students from public schools14. However, little has been disclosed about the monitoring of this mitigation measure. Information regarding this initiative in the Federal District of Brazil can be found on the website of the State Bureau for Education of the Federal District (SEEDF) [20] and, as disclosed by this site, during the three phases of funds released, only 69,848 families are benefiting, or 106,435 students. No information was found regarding criteria for the distribution of food allowances or the percentage of families receiving benefits, in relation to the total number of students enrolled in the public-school system of the Federal District. Still, even for those who receive government assistance, it is necessary to analyse its effectiveness in relation to the needs of children, in view of the nutritional requirements presented by schools, as these requirements cannot be guaranteed at home.

Chart 1 (Appendix 1) presents data on the benefits related to school meals provided by each of the Brazilian states and the Federal District to the families of students during the cessation of classes due to the pandemic, and available on the websites of the 27 State Departments of Education of each federated entity (retrieved between June 6 and June 8, 2020). We sought to identify the number of families and students receiving some type of benefit, the value and type of the benefit transferred, the form of transfer or delivery, and the eligibility criteria for such procedure. It should be noted that most of the information presented in Chart 1 was found in press releases from the State Education Bureaus. Despite the assistance provided to students, whether in the form of prepared meals, meal kits, or financial aid, some issues still need to be addressed, such as: the actual destination of the aid (whether the students will personally benefit from this assistance), the nutritional content and amount of food in the meal kits, and the difficulties that the family can face in receiving the benefit and preparing food.

PROPOSED MODEL FOR MONITORING, FOLLOW-UP, AND CONTROL

This work presents a proposed model for monitoring, accompanying, and controlling the financial aid benefits received by children and adolescents during the COVID-19 pandemic. The model was outlined for the situation in Brazil, referencing the public policies adopted by that country and its social conditions. However, it is understood that it can also be used as a basis for other places to intervene in this process, in order to ensure that students receive adequate food during the pandemic. In Brazil, the family health community agent (currently more than 200,000) is very common, whose role is to assist the poorest communities with the objective of promoting health surveillance, primary care and community health [21]. During this pandemic, these agents could monitor families and, regarding children and adolescents, contribute to the monitoring, not only of their health, but also of food intake. This monitoring could employ the use of telemedicine, and involve the following actors: families, schools, government, and health agents (Figure 2). The latter can be replaced by another actor, to be defined by the government, to fulfill this role.

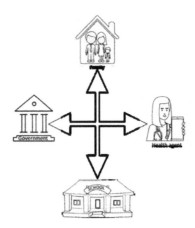

Figure 2. School feeding model during the COVID-19 pandemic.

The proposed monitoring needs to follow a checklist with issues to be observed within the family, in order to provide an understanding of the nutritional status of the child or adolescent. At the same time, it's important to invest in geographic intelligence, aiming to map and monitor the areas of greatest vulnerability; locate all families that are linked to the receipt of benefits from this food program, and perform, through random selection, the verification of the effectiveness of this process, including the use of web applications to monitor and receive information from all those involved who are not receiving the aid. Registrations must follow the active surveillance model. The implementation of this model should provide data, to support the government in understanding the effectiveness of the school feeding program during the pandemic, so that adjustments and adaptations can be made in favour of the students' nutritional requirements

CONCLUSIONS

In times of pandemic, children's nutrition is a crucial aspect to be discussed by society, given that, for many, school is the central point of daily support. Ensuring that food reaches children and is consumed by them is difficult for governments to monitor, since food or the financial aid to purchase it is delivered to families, and the lack of control over the correct distribution and use of this food makes it difficult to know its effectiveness in mitigating this problem. Monitoring strategies need to be effective and family health agents could assist the government, using means similar to telemedicine, based on information provided by competent departments.

Therefore, to contribute to the transparency of the use of public resources, it is necessary to develop research on the conditions throughout the Brazilian regions, and also to use of geographic intelligence tools that allow spatial monitoring, linked to active surveillance mechanisms, within the concept of participatory control of public funds, using information collection platforms to: know if the distribution of this benefits to families is effective and if children are receiving the food referred to in the Law and the PNAE; know what food is consumed by children and young people during this period and the number of meals eaten daily by them, with the help of family health agents; subsidize the government with information necessary to outline strategies for monitoring and following the diet of these children and adolescents during the pandemic.

In this way, it would be possible to contribute not only to the debates regarding the fulfilment of this role by the school, and aggravated by the pandemic, but also to know the effectiveness of public policies adopted during this period of emergency declared by the federal and state governments.

* ***Correspondence:*** Dra. Ana Carla Bittencourt Reis, anacarlabr@unb.br

REFERENCES

1. Global Monitoring of School Meals During COVID-19 School Closures. World Food Programme (WFP). (2020). https://cdn.wfp.org/2020/school-feeding-map/index.html [Accessed June 7,2020]
2. Imai N, Cori A, Dorigatti I, Baguelin M, Donnelly C. A., Riley S, Ferguson N. M. Report 3: Transmissibility of 2019-nCoV. *Imperial College London* (2020). Available at: https://fpmag.net/wp-content/uploads/2020/01/Imperial-2019-nCoV-transmissibility.pdf
3. BRASIL. Ministério da Saúde. (2020). https://www.saude.gov.br/noticias/agenciasaude/46435-brasil-confirma-primeiro-caso-de-novo-coronavirus [Accessed Mai 14, 2020]
4. Mert Er. World Food Programme Insight. School feeding at home. (2020). https://insight.wfp.org/school-feeding-at-home-95ff24a2c78 [Accessed June 03, 2020].
5. Pesquisadores associados. Observatório PrEpidemia. Relatório Técnico 01. Volta às aulas no Distrito Federal durante a pandemia de COVID-19. (2020) https://www.prepidemia.org/notaserelatorios-tecnicos [Accessed June 10, 2020].
6. Minussi, Bianca Baptisti, et al. "Grupos de risco do COVID-19: a possível relação entre o acometimento de adultos jovens "saudáveis" e a imunidade / COVID-19 risk groups: the possible relationship between the impairment of healthy young adults and immunity". *Brazilian Journal of Health Review* (2020) 3.2: 3739-3762. https://doi.org/10.34119/bjhrv3n2-200
7. World Health Organization (WHO). Technical Report Series, 394, Healthy Diet. (2015). https://www.who.int/nutrition/publications/nutrientrequirements/healthydiet_factsheet394.pdf[Accessed June 09, 2020].
8. Lesley, D., Alice, W., Carmen, B., & Donald, B. (2016). *Global school feeding sourcebook: lessons from 14 countries.* Imperial College Press. Available at: http://www.worldscientific.com/worldscibooks/10.1142/P1070
9. United Nations World Food Programme (WFP). (2020). https://www.wfp.org/ [Accessed May 10, 2020].
10. School feeding in times of COVID-19. What can governments do? (2020). https://centrodeexcelencia.org.br/wp-content/uploads/2020/04/SchoolFeedingCOVID_EN.pdf[Accessed May 10, 2020].
11. Mitigating the effects of the COVID-19 pandemic on food and nutrition of schoolchildren. (2020). https://www.unicef.org/media/68291/file/Mitigating-the-Effects-of-the-COVID-19Pandemic-on-Food-and-Nutrition-of-school-children.pdf [Accessed May 10, 2020].
12. BRASIL, Law n° 13.987 de 7 de abril de 2020.http://www.planalto.gov.br/ccivil_03/_ato2019-2022/2020/lei/l13987.htm [Accessed June 05, 2020]
13. Ann-Marie K. Chandler, Susan P. Walker, Kevin Connolly, Sally M. Grantham-McGregor,
14. School Breakfast Improves Verbal Fluency in Undernourished Jamaican Children, *The Journal of Nutrition* (1995)125:4, 894–900, https://doi.org/10.1093/jn/125.4.894
15. Lamis H Jomaa, Elaine McDonnell, Claudia Probart, School feeding programs in developing countries: impacts on children's health and educational outcomes, *Nutrition Reviews* (2011) 69:2, 83–98, https://doi.org/10.1111/j.1753-4887.2010.00369.x
16. Hieu, N., Sandalinas, F., De Sesmaisons, A., Laillou, A., Tam, N., Khan, N., . . . Berger, J. Multi-micronutrient-fortified biscuits decreased the prevalence of anaemia and improved iron status, whereas weekly iron supplementation only improved iron status in Vietnamese school children. *British Journal of Nutrition* (2012) 108:8, 1419-1427. https://doi.org/10.1017/S0007114511006945
17. Food in a time of COVID-19. *Nature plants,* (2020) 6:5, 429.https://doi.org/10.1038/s41477020-0682-7
18. Wu, Joseph T et al. "School closure and mitigation of pandemic (H1N1) 2009, Hong Kong."*Emerging infectious diseases.* (2010) 16:3, 538-41. https://doi.org/10.3201/eid1603.091216
19. Niconielo, B. Gripe suína na escola (2019)https://sites.google.com/site/agestaoeducacional/artigo/h1n1 [Accessed April 30, 2020]. [19] Dunn CG, Kenney E, Fleischhacker SE, Bleich SN. Feeding Low-Income Children during the COVID-19 Pandemic. *N Engl J Med.* (2020) 382:18, e40. https://www.nejm.org/doi/full/10.1056/NEJMp2005638
20. Secretaria de Estado de Educação (2020) http://www.se.df.gov.br/bolsa-alimentacao-2/[Accessed June5, 2020].
21. Ministério da Saúde. O trabalho do agente comunitário de saúde. (2009). Available at: http: // 189.28.128.100/dab/docs/publicacoes/geral/manual_acs.pdf.

5. Concerns of Health-Related Higher Education Students in Brazil Pertaining to Distance Learning During the Coronavirus Pandemic

Renan Morais Peloso[1], Fernanda Ferruzzi[2],
Aline Akemi Mori[2], Daiane Pereira Camacho[3],
Lucimara Cheles da Silva Franzin[4],
Ana Paula Margioto Teston[5],
Karina Maria Salvatore Freitas[11]

ABSTRACT

This survey aimed to assess the concerns of students of health-related higher education in Brazil regarding distance learning during the coronavirus pandemic. A Google Forms anonymous questionnaire was sent by WhatsApp Messenger to students at a private university. Seven hundred and four students answered the questionnaire (566 female, 138 males, mean age = 23.09 years), reflecting approximately a third of the students in health-related disciplines. Students reported feeling anxious due to the pandemic. Most of the students agreed with having the ability to continue education through distance learning, but relatively few of them enjoyed it. Also, students were concerned that learning of clinical material and professional training would be impaired, and they were afraid of failing the year of education. Health-related higher education private institutions in Brazil should focus on reassessing and prioritizing their policies and protocols and include a detailed plan for the future.

INTRODUCTION

The spread of the novel coronavirus (SARS-CoV-2), which causes the disease known as COVID-19, emerged in Wuhan, China, in late December 2019, and is a pandemic according to the World Health Organization (WHO). To date (June 12, 2020), the coronavirus pandemic accounts for more than 7,400,000 people infected worldwide, and these numbers are increasing each day, including more than 418,000 deaths (World Health Organization, 2020). Brazil is currently in a critical situation, with the second highest number of officially reported coronavirus cases in the world

[11]Department of Orthodontics, Ingá University Center UNINGÁ, Maringá, Brazil
[2]Department of Prosthetic Dentistry, Ingá University Center UNINGÁ, Maringá, Brazil
[3]Department of Biomedicine, Ingá University Center UNINGÁ, Maringá, Brazil
[4]Department of Pediatric Dentistry, Ingá University Center UNINGÁ, Maringá, Brazil
[5]Department of Pharmacy, Ingá University Center UNINGÁ, Maringá, Brazil
Karina M. S. Freitas, Department of Orthodontics, Ingá University Center UNINGÁ, Rod PR 317, 6114, Maringá, PR 87035-510, Brazil.
Email: kmsf@uol.com.br

(more than 770,0000) and with the third highest number of deaths (40,919; John Hopkins University, 2020). In addition, Brazil is likely to have many more cases of COVID-19 than is officially reported by the government due to a paucity of testing and long waits to confirm the results. Further, Brazil demonstrates a continuing steep incline of cases.

Most governments around the world have temporarily closed educational institutions to in-person instruction in an attempt to contain the spread of COVID-19. Education has changed dramatically, with the distinctive rise of e-learning, whereby teaching is undertaken remotely and on digital platforms. In Brazil, all private institutions adopted the distance learning protocol to avoid a halt in educational activities. Distance learning is not commonly used in the health-related higher education courses and programs in Brazil, as the curricula require clinical training and professional socialization. It is challenging for faculty and students to introduce distance learning strategies in an educational program suddenly, without prior preparation and training.

In Brazil, while the substitution of face-to-face with digital media classes was authorized during the pandemic, the substitution of professional clinical practices for internships and laboratories has been prohibited. There was no educational or administrative contingency plan for moving to distance learning for such clinical practices. Further, many of the Brazilian educational institutions were not technologically prepared. Little is known about student concerns regarding emergency remote learning and its impact on their higher education. A survey was administered to assess the concerns of students of health-related higher education courses in Brazil regarding distance learning during the coronavirus pandemic.

METHODS

Survey items assessed personal information, feelings regarding the coronavirus pandemic, distance learning, and the impact of distance learning on their higher education course performance The level of anxiety/stress due to the pandemic was evaluated by a numerical rating scale (Johnson, 2005)[1]. The survey was anonymous and created using Google Forms. The link was sent to students by WhatsApp Messenger, from May 2 to May 7, 2020, at a relatively early stage of the pandemic in Brazil. An attempt was made to reach 1000 (one half) of the students who attended the participating private university from among the health-related disciplines: Dentistry, Medicine, Biomedicine, Physical Therapy, Physical Education, Pharmacy, Psychology, Nutrition, Nursing and Veterinary Medicine. The answers obtained were tabulated in Excel, for statistical analysis. Descriptive statistics was calculated. This study was approved by the Ethics Research Committee of the Ingá University Center UNINGÁ (protocol n. 4.017.346).

RESULTS

The response rate was 70.4% (n = 704). The mean age of the participants was 23.09 years (s.d. = 6.28). Most of the students were females (80.4%); 19.6% were males. These gender differences are representative of the student composition in the health-related disciplines at the university. Only 2% reported symptoms of COVID-19. A total of 48.2% of the students were anxious, and 19.5% were afraid of suffering from the disease. The mean level of self-reported anxiety was 6.18 (s.d. = 2.58; out of 10), indicating moderate but not severe anxiety. With respect to the quarantine, 81.8% were going out just when necessary, 9.7% were not respecting the quarantine and 8.5% were not leaving

---

[1] (Appendix 1). (0=no anxiety/stress/concern to 10 = extremely anxious/stressed/concerned)

home. Most of the students (51.4%) agreed with the substitutability of education through distance learning, 37.6% partially agreed and only 10.9% disagreed. However, only 24.1% enjoyed distance learning; 42% partially enjoyed it.

A minority of the students (31.8%) were following classes and did not have trouble understanding content, while 40.1% had some difficulty and 24.6% had great difficulty and reported that their learning was impaired. Only 3.5% were not following the distance learning activities. When asked about how the quarantine might affect their higher education courses, more than 70% of the students were concerned that their learning of clinical and professional training would be impaired. More than 50% were concerned about evaluation of their learning and were afraid they would fail the year, and 45% were concerned that their learning of conceptual material would be worse than in-person learning. Still, most of the students believed the distance activities were consistent with the content taught, helped to consolidate and improve learning, and that the frequency of instruction was adequate. The greatest difficulties involved establishing a study routine (33.4%), learning without the presence of the faculty (26.0%), consolidating the learning (24.4%) and finding time to access the material (16.2%). Only 21% percent of the students wanted distance online activities to continue after quarantine.

DISCUSSION

Although our sample was small considering the number of students in health-related higher education in Brazil, it is representative, since most institutions in the country are private, and most graduate courses in the health field were included in the sample. The gender and age breakdown were similar to other institutions. Further, all private institutions were suddenly facing the same challenge of distance learning, without prior training. It is not possible to suddenly replace traditional teaching strategies with internet classes and hope that everything will remain the same. While online learning has increased a great deal, there were few Brazilian institutions and faculty well-prepared to use technologies for e-learning in health-related courses. In Brazil, as in other countries, an economic recession is expected. At the present time, to avoid further damage to the country's economy, some business activities are gradually returning, which could be a mistake at this stage of the pandemic in Brazil. Optimists believe that in-person instruction at universities will be able to resume in the next semester, but others believe there may be a delay of a year or more. It is possible that many potential students will postpone attending university (waiting for the return of in-person instruction), or those that do attend online may find prospects for employment after graduation more limited.

Distance learning requires a high level of self-discipline from students to achieve good standards and to prevent dropout (Gorbunovs et al., 2016). Our study showed that the most common difficulty mentioned was establishing a study routine. Distractions and the absence of a specific place to study can make home study difficult. The universities in Brazil have to train their faculty, so that they are competent and comfortable in using e-learning as a central teaching strategy (Turkyilmaz et al., 2019). Technological innovation has not only impacted social change in recent years but has been the prime driver of educational transformation (Sinclair et al., 2015). Health-related higher education in Brazil should focus on reassessing and prioritizing their policies and protocols and the future plan should include distance learning.

Limitations of the study includes the recruitment of participants from a single private university in Brazil and the cross-sectional design. In addition, the survey was carried out at a relatively early stage of the pandemic in Brazil (at the beginning of May 2020), and this may not reflect student perceptions later on as the pandemic causes more problems for patients, health care professionals and institutions. Still, this study is important as it contributes to a pool of such higher education system student concern evaluations around the world. Institutions of higher education may be able to learn from each other's experience during COVID-19 pandemic and transform learning activities for the future in times of emergency.

REFERENCES

Gorbunovs, A., Kapenieks, A., Cakula, S. (2016). Self-discipline as a key indicator to improve learning outcomes in elearning environment. Procedia Social and Behavioral Sciences, 231, 256–262.

John Hopkins University . (2020). COVID-19 dashboard by the center for systems science and engineering (CSSE) at johns Hopkins university. Retrieved June 12, 2020, from https://coronavirus.jhu.edu/map.html

Johnson, C. (2005). Measuring pain. Visual analog scale versus numeric pain scale: What is the difference? Journal of Chiropractic Medicine, 4(1), 43–44. https://doi.org/10.1016/S0899-3467(07)60112-8

Sinclair, P., Kable, A., Levett-Jones, T. (2015). The effectiveness of internet-based e-learning on clinician behavior and patient outcomes: A systematic review protocol. JBI Database of Systematic Reviews and Implementation Reports, 13(1), 52–64. https://doi.org/10.11124/jbisrir-2015-1919

Turkyilmaz, I., Hariri, N. H., Jahangiri, L. (2019). Student's perception of the impact of e-learning on dental education. Journal of Contemporary Dental Practice, 20(5), 616–621.

World Health Organization . (2020). Coronavirus disease 2019 (COVID-19) situation report – 144. https://www.who.int/docs/default-source/coronaviruse/situation-reports/20200612-COVID-19-sitrep-144.pdf?sfvrsn=66ff9f4f_4

6. Distress Among Brazilian University Students Due To The COVID-19 Pandemic: Survey Results And Reflections

Carlos Von Krakauer Hübner PhD. Marcella de Lima Bruscatto,,
Rafaella Dourado Lima

ABSTRACT

The first case of infection with the new coronavirus was identified in December 2019 in Wuhan, China. In March, the World Health Organization (WHO) defined the disease epidemic as a pandemic. Thus, a quarantine was imposed by many governments. As a consequence, and given that epidemiological outbreaks of infectious diseases, such as COVID-19, are associated with psychological disorders and symptoms of mental illness, researchers at the Shanghai Mental Health Centre have created the COVID-19 Peritraumatic Distress Index (CPDI), in which the results are obtained: normal, mild/moderate distress and severe distress. The main objective of the study was based on the application of CPDI, in order to identify the health and well-being of Brazilian students from different undergraduate courses at the Pontifical Catholic University of São Paulo (PUC/SP) during the COVID-19 pandemic and to test the hypothesis that medical students suffer more than students from other courses. The research is based on a cross-sectional observational study, in which we applied, using Google Forms[R], the questions contained in CPDI, along with demographic data: age, sex, educational institution, undergraduate course and school year. The Index was applied online for seven days in which a total of 654 valid responses were obtained: 501 (76.6%) female and 149 (22.8%) male. Regarding age, 333 students (50.91%) were 17-20 years old, 279 (42.66%) between 21-25, 30 (4.59%) between 26-30 and 12 (1.84%) between 31-50. The results indicate that the participants reported significant psychological distress, according to the CPDI score. Practically 90% (87.92%) of the students experienced suffering, while only 12.08% did not suffer. The study provides the first empirical evidence on the level of psychological distress in Brazilian university students during the COVID-19 pandemic. Also, it suggests support and monitoring of university students during and after the pandemic, with effective and efficient intervention in their mental health.

SPREAD OF COVID-19 WORLDWIDE

Experiences of affected countries, as well as evolution of the disease and the number of deaths in the world show an association between measures that were implemented by the State and Government through health preventive authorities and rigor with which they were incorporated by the population, as well as their impact on coping and progressing cases of the disease (Figure 2).

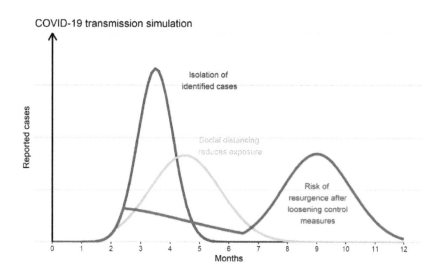

Figure 2 – Illustration of the COVID-19 transmission curve and its relationship with the population's adoption of hygiene, social restriction and non-agglomeration measures.[25] **Belo Horizonte, Minas Gerais, Brazil, 2020.**

What we have observed, however, is that even though the Ministry of Health reinforces the relevance of adopting such measures on a daily basis, its compliance at first showed a new learning for the population, above all, regarding the restriction or social distancing, threatened in part by the risk of increased unemployment, drop in income and/or often by minimizing the potential risk of the pandemic. These behaviours could decrease effectiveness of measures and increase the risk of resurgence of cases,[25] as shown in Figure 2. Efforts by health and political authorities in the states to encourage the population to stay at home to achieve a flattening of the curve and less circulation of the virus have been verified, as well as review of some recommendations.

In this setting of daily learning and monitoring of each case in the states and in the country, until April 18, 2020, by following the growth curve of cases in Brazil compared to other countries, it is possible to verify that the growth line shows itself differently from the devastating situation recorded in Italy, Spain, and the United States (Figure 3, left panel).[11-12] However, in the initial phase, a similar evolution can be seen in such countries, but which over time has distanced, possibly due to the impact of greater population compliance and strengthening of state policies for social restriction. The evolution of COVID-19 cases in Brazil in relation to some countries in Latin America (Figure 3, right panel) shows a prominent progression curve, followed by Peru, Chile and Ecuador. This figure shows the daily evolution of the infection, after each country has notified at least ten cases.[26]From the rapid evolution, world statistics consolidated by John Hopkins University, in the United States, until April 18, 2020, point out that after 39 days of recognition by WHO of the outbreak as a pandemic. The world registered 2,317,758 cases and 159,509 deaths, affecting 185 countries and regions worldwide.[26]

The total number of confirmed cases increased from 100 thousand to 200 thousand, with an interval of twelve days. Six days later, it exceeded 400 thousand cases, reaching more than 800 thousand seven days later; and, went from 500 thousand to 1 million in seven days, and passed the 2 million infected people 13 days later, showing a high speed in the doubling of the number of cases worldwide.[26]

On the other hand, it is necessary to consider a certain difference in spread of infections in each country in a particular way, worldwide. The evolution of the doubling time of cases of the new coronavirus is shown in Figure 4, prepared considering information dated April 18, 2020.[27]

Therefore, it appears that, for instance, the estimated speed of duplication of cases, until March 24, for Canada and the United States (US), should occur every two and a half days. However, on April 7, this time increased to around seven days, showing a reduction in the speed of the spread, although it keeps these countries on alert for the total number of cases.[27] Colombia and Brazil, in the same interval, behaved differently, increasing the doubling time, that is, decreasing the speed of spread of the infection, until March 29 and 30, respectively. However, until April 3, this speed was higher for Brazil, reaching a doubling interval slightly higher than four days, showing the need to reinforce measures to contain the epidemic, seeking effective arrest of its advance. Until the end of the interval, on April 18, in general the times for doubling cases increased, showing a reduction in the speed of infections dissemination; in Mexico, Bolivia, Peru and Brazil the cases would be duplicated in up to 8 days, and the other countries in figure 4 showed duplication intervals of more than eleven days, up to eighteen days in the case of Colombia.

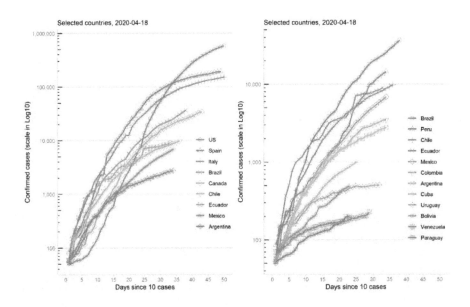

Figure 3 – Daily evolution curve for notified COVID-19 cases in Brazil, compared to other countries, from ten confirmed cases.[26] Belo Horizonte, Minas Gerais, Brazil, 2020.

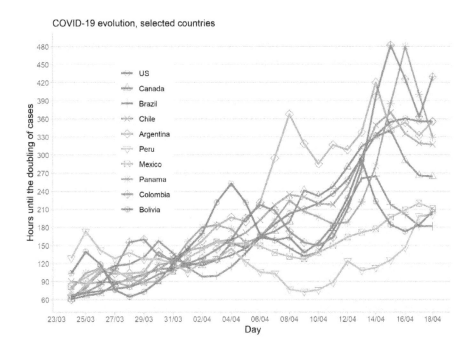

Figure 4 – Time distribution of doubling the number of COVID-19 cases in Brazil, compared to other countries.[27] Belo Horizonte, Minas Gerais, Brazil, 2020.

EPIDEMIC CONTROL

The COVID-19 outbreak is still new and its duration uncertain. Thus, reducing exposure to the virus is necessary to control/delay spread of the disease and negative impacts, such as increased mortality and degradation of the economic and social situation. Experiences from countries that adopted measures such as social distancing and early suspension of classes, Singapore, South Korea and Japan, point out that immediate implementation of these measures as well as rigorous management of cases and mass diagnoses influenced the course of transmissibility, resulting in a lower number of deaths. Singapore, for instance, on February 17, 2020, recorded the largest number of confirmed cases outside mainland China. However, it immediately implemented control measures such as isolating all suspected or confirmed cases in rooms with negative pressure; training and re-education of health professionals to use personal protective equipment; use of respirators and air purifiers; monitoring of isolation teams for COVID-19 symptoms with thermal scanners to track fever; and investment in single-use equipment such as disposable bronchoscopes for bronchoscopy and percutaneous tracheostomy.[28]

And even though there was an increase in cases in the last week, until April 18, Singapore recorded eleven deaths and 5,992 confirmed infections.[26] South Korea, which had its first case registered on January 20, 2020, adopted contact management between suspects and infected people for epidemiological investigation. It also implemented a system for assessing the risk of exposure among people in all places where there were confirmed cases (after the onset of symptoms) and classified the contact persons based on that risk. In addition, to eliminate the possibility of exposure to infection in the places visited by the confirmed patient, it performed appropriate disinfection of areas that could harbour environmental contamination.[29] Thus, systematic investigations were successful due to a rigorous control process based on scientific principles and continuous feedback assessment cycles to contain the outbreak. Although there were more than 10,600 patients as of April 18, new infections have been abruptly reduced in recent weeks.[26] Japan carried out a rigorous surveillance between the time from the onset of the disease in a primary (suspected) case to its manifestation in a secondary (infected) case to understand the transmissibility of the disease.[30-31] With the mapping of suspect/infected data, it was initially possible to control spread and transmissibility from substantial pre-symptomatic transmissions and early isolation of people with COVID-19 in a population of 120 million. As a result, as of April 18, 2020, cases reached 10,300, with a total of 222 deaths.[26] The Chinese special administrative region of Hong Kong, where 7.5 million people live, which shares a land border with the rest of China, recorded 1,024 cases and four deaths on April 18, 2020.[26] In this setting, WHO and experts agree that early detection of cases is a fundamental factor to contain the spread of a virus.

CONCLUSION

The involvement of the whole society in the conscious adoption of preventive measures against COVID-19 requires a change in individual and collective behaviour at that moment, immediately and rigorously. In this pandemic setting, it is possible to learn that its course and impacts in Brazil depend on the collaborative effort of all, government, families, and citizens. The world reality still points to a situation of great attention and can support choices of the path to be followed to face this critical moment, in order to allow interference in the rapid evolution of COVID-19.

REFERENCES

1. Word Health Organization. Considerations for quarantine of individuals in the context of containment for coronavirus disease (COVID-19): Interim guidance [Internet]. Geneva (CH); 2020 [cited 2020 Mar 24]. Available from: https://apps.who.int/iris/handle/10665/331299

2. Chang Le, Yan Y, Wang L. (2020).Coronavirus disease 2019: Coronaviruses and blood safety. Transfus Med Rev [Internet]. 2020 Feb 21 [cited 2020 Mar 23]. Available from: https://dx.doi.org/10.1016/j. tmrv.2020.02.003

3. Shang, J., Wan, Y., Liu, C., Yount, B., Gully, K., Yang. Y., et al(2020). Structure of mouse coronavirus spike protein complexed with receptor reveals mechanism for viral entry. PLoS Pathog [Internet]. 2020 [cited 2020 Mar 23];16(3):e1008392. Available from: https://dx.doi.org/10.1371/journal.ppat.1008392

4. Li R, Pei S, Chen, B., Song, Y., Zhang, T., Yang W, et al. (2020). Substantial undocumented infection facilitates the rapid dissemination of novel coronavirus (SARS-CoV2). Science [Internet]. 2020 Mar 16 [cited 2020 Mar 21]. Available from: https://www.ncbi.nlm.nih.gov/pubmed/32179701

5. Kampf G, Todt T, Pfaender S, Steinmann E. (2020).Persistence of coronaviruses on inanimate surfaces and their inactivation with biocidal agents. J Hosp Infect [Internet]. 2020 [cited 2020 Mar 22];104(3):246-51. Available from: https://dx.doi.org/10.1016/j.jhin.2020.01.022

6. Tian, H., Liu, Y., Li, Y., Wu, C.H, Chen, B., Kraemer, M.U.G, et al. (2020).The impact of transmission control measures during the first 50 days of the COVID-19 2 epidemic in China. MedRxiv [Internet]. 2020 Mar 10 [cited 2020 Mar 23]. Available from: https://dx.doi.org/10.1101/2020.01.30.20019844

7. Kim, J.Y., Choe PG, Oh Y, Oh KJ, Kim J, Park SJ, et al. (2020).The first case of 2019 novel coronavirus pneumonia imported into Korea from Wuhan, China: implication for infection prevention and control measures. J Korean Med Sci [Internet]. 2020 [cited 2020 Mar 21];10;35(5):e61. Available from: https://dx.doi.org/10.3346/jkms.2020.35.e61

8. World Health Organization. Rational use of personal protective equipment (PPE) for coronavirus disease (COVID-19): interim guidance [Internet]. Geneva (CH); 2020 [cited 2020 Mar 23]. Available from: https://apps.who.int/iris/handle/10665/331498

9. Ministério da Saúde (BR). Portaria nº 454, de 20 de março de 2020: declara, em todo o território nacional, o estado de transmissão comunitária do coronavírus (COVID-19). Diário Oficial da União [Internet]. 2020 Mar 20 [cited 2020 Mar 26]; 1:1. Available from: http://www.in.gov.br/en/web/ dou/-/portaria-n-454-de-20-de-marco-de-2020-249091587

10. Valente, J. (2020).COVID-19: governo declara transmissão comunitária em todo o país. Agência Brasil [Internet]. 2020 Mar 20 [cited 2020 Mar 21]. Available from: https://agenciabrasil.ebc.com.br/ saude/noticia/2020-03/COVID-19-governo-declara-transmissao-comunitaria-em-todo-o-pais

11. Vetter, P., Guitart C, Lotfinejad N, Pittet D(2020).. Understanding the emerging coronavirus: what it means for health security and infection prevention. J Hosp Infect [Internet]. 2020 Mar 4 [cited 2020 Mar 17];104(4):440-8. Available from: https://dx.doi.org/10.1016/j.jhin.2020.02.023

12. Remuzzi A; Remuzzi, G. (2020). COVID-19 and Italy: what next? Lancet [Internet]. 2020 Mar 13 [cited 2020 Mar 24];395:1225-8 Available from: https://doi.org/10.1016/S0140-6736(20)30627-9

13. European Centre for Disease Prevention and Control. Considerations relating to social distancing measures in response to the COVID-19 epidemic [Internet]. Stockholm (SW); 2020 Mar 23 [cited 2020 Mar 23]. Available from: https://www.ecdc.europa.eu/en/publications-data/considerationsrelating-social-distancing-measures-response-COVID-19-second

14. World Health Organization. Critical preparedness, readiness and response actions for COVID-19 [Internet]. Geneva (CH); 2020 [cited 2020 Mar 18]. Available from: https://www.who.int/emergencies/ diseases/novel-coronavirus-2019/technical-guidance/critical-preparedness-readiness-andresponse-actions-for-COVID-19

15. World Health Organization. 2019 Novel coronavirus (2019-nCoV): strategic preparedness and response plan [Internet]. Geneva (CH); 2020 [cited 2020 Mar 17]. Available from: https://reliefweb. int/report/world/2019-novel-coronavirus-2019-ncov-strategic-preparedness-and-response-plandraft-3

16. European Centre for Disease Prevention and Control Rapid risk assessment: Novel coronavirus disease 2019 (COVID-19) pandemic: increased transmission in the EU/EEA and the UK: sixth update [Internet]. Stockholm (SW); 2020 Mar 12 [cited 2020 Mar 17]. Available from: https:// www.ecdc.europa.eu/en/publications-data/rapid-risk-assessment-novel-coronavirus-disease2019-COVID-19-pandemic-increased

17. Oliveira, A., De Paula, A., Souza, M., Silva, A. (2020).. Adesão à higiene de mãos entre profissionais de um serviço de pronto atendimento. Rev Med [Internet]. 2016 [cited 2020 Mar 20];95(4):162-7. Available from: https://dx.doi.org/10.11606/issn.1679-9836.v95i4p162-167

18. Amorim, C..S..V, Pinheiro, I.F., Vieira, V.G., Guimarães, R.A., Nunes, O.S., Marinho, T.A. (2020). Hand hygiene and influenza prevention: knowledge of health students. Texto Contexto Enferm [Internet]. 2018 [cited 2020 Apr 3];27(4):e4570017. Available from: https://dx.doi.org/10.1590/0104-070720180004570017

19. European Centre for Disease Prevention and Control. Interim guidance for environmental cleaning in non-healthcare facilities exposed to SARS-CoV-2 [Internet]. Stockholm (SW); 2020 Feb 18 [cited 2020 Apr 2]. Available from: https://www.ecdc.europa.eu/en/publications-data/interimguidance-environmental-cleaning-non-healthcare-facilities-exposed-2019

20. Van Doremalen, N, Bushmaker, T., Morris, D.H., Holbrook, M.G., Gamble, A., Williamson, B.N. Aerosol and surface stability of SARS-CoV-2 as compared with SARS-CoV-1. N Engl J Med [Internet]. 2020 Mar 17 [cited 2020 Mar 23];382:1564-7. Available from: https://dx.doi.org/10.1056/NEJMc2004973

21. Gostic, K., Gomez, A.C, Mummah, R.O., Kuchars. (2020). ki AJ, Lloyd-Smith JO. Estimated effectiveness of symptom and risk screening to prevent the spread of COVID-19. Elife [Internet]. 2020 Feb 24 [cited 2020 Mar 18];2020;9:e55570 Available from: https://dx.doi.org/10.7554/eLife.55570

22. Hellewell, J., Abbott, Gimma, A., Bosse, N.I., Jarvis ,C.I, Russel, T.W., et al. Feasibility of controlling COVID-19 outbreaks by isolation of cases and contacts. Lancet Glob Health [Internet]. 2020 [cited 2020 Mar 15];8(4):e486. Available from: https://www.thelancet.com/journals/langlo/article/ piis2214-109x(20)30074-7/fulltext

23. Agência Nacional de V.(2020). igilância Sanitária (BR). Nota técnica GVIMS/GGTES/ANVISA nº 04/2020: orientações para serviços de saúde: medidas de prevenção e controle que devem ser adotadas durante a assistência aos casos suspeitos ou confirmados de infecção pelo novo coronavírus (SARS-CoV-2) [Internet]. Brasília, DF(BR); 2020 [cited 2020 Mar 23]. Available from: http://portal. anvisa.gov.br/documents/33852/271858/nota+t%c3%a9cnica+n+04-2020+gvims-ggtes-anvisa/ ab598660-3de4-4f14-8e6f-b9341c196b28

24. Ministério da Saúde (BR). Máscaras caseiras podem ajudar na prevenção contra o Coronavírus [Internet]. Brasília, DF(BR);2020 [cited 2020 Apr 3]. Available from: https://www.saude.gov. br/noticias/agencia-saude/46645-mascaras-caseiras-podem-ajudar-na-prevencao-contra-ocoronavirus

25. Anderson, R.M., Heesterbeek, H., Klinkenberg, D., Hollingsworth, T.D. (2020).How will country-based mitigation measures influence the course of the COVID-19 epidemic? Lancet [Internet]. 2020 [cited 2020 Apr 4];395(10228):931-34. Available from: https://www.thelancet.com/journals/lancet/article/ piis0140-6736(20)30567-5/fulltext

26. Dong, E, Du, H, Gardner, L. An interactive web-based dashboard to track COVID-19 in real time. Lancet Infect Dis [Internet]. 2020 Feb 27 [cited 2020 Apr 3]. Available from: https://dx.doi. org/10.1016/S1473-3099(20)30120-1

27. Abbott, S., Hellewell, J., Munday, J.D., Chun, J.Y., Thompson, R.N. Bosse., NI, et al. (2020).Temporal variation in transmission during the COVID-19 outbreak. CMMID Repository [Internet]. 2020 Mar 2 [cited 2020 Apr 2]. Available from: https://cmmid.github.io/topics/covid19/current-patterns-transmission/ global-time-varying-transmission.html

28. Liew, M.F, Siow, W.T., MacLaren, G,, See KC. Preparing for COVID 19: early experience from an intensive care unit in Singapore. Crit Care [Internet]. 2020 [cited 2020 Mar 26];24(1):83. Available from: https://dx.doi.org/10.1186/s13054-020-2814-x

29. COVID-19 National Emergency Response Centre, Epidemiology & Case Management Team, Korea Centres for Disease Control & Prevention. Contact Transmission of COVID-19 in South Korea: novel investigation techniques for tracing contacts. Osong Public Health Res Perspect [Internet]. 2020 [cited 2020 Mar 25];11(1):60-3. Available from: https://dx.doi.org/10.24171/j. phrp.2020.11.1.09

30. Kakimoto, K, Kamiya, H., Yamagishi, T., Matsui, T., Suzuki, M., Wakita, T (2020).. Initial investigation of transmission of COVID-19 among crew members during quarantine of a cruise ship: Yokohama, Japan, February 2020. MMWR Surveill Summ. [Internet]. 2020 [cited 2020 Mar 18];69(11):312-3. Available from: https://dx.doi.org/10.15585/mmwr.mm6911e2

31. Nakazawa, E., Ino H, Akabayashi, A. (2020). Chronology of COVID-19 cases on the Diamond Princess cruise ship and ethical considerations: a report from Japan. Disaster Med Public Health Prep [Internet]. 2020 Mar 24 [cited 2020 Mar 20]. Available from: https://dx.doi.org/10.1017/dmp.2020.50

7. Science-Based Education And Mental Health After COVID-19 Pandemic.

Mônica Naves Barcelos[1,2], Priscila Medeiros[3,4],
Carla Benedita da Silva Tostes[5],
Juliana Almeida da Silva[3], Josie Resende Torres da Silva[2],
Jorge Gelvane Tostes[5],Norberto Cysne Coimbra[3,], José Aparecido da Silva[6,7], Marcelo Lourenço da Silva[2],Renato Leonardo de Freitas[1,4*1]

ABSTRACT

In response to the outbreak of the novel Severe Acute Respiratory Syndrome Coronavirus-2 (SARS-CoV-2), pathogen of the new coronavirus disease (COVID-19), several sectors and social activities have been affected, including education. At first, it is explained that educators and students can feel fragile during and after the SARSCoV-2 outbreak. Subsequently, it is discussed that their relationship ought to be carefully established given the triggering of psychological and neuropsychiatric effects arising from neural coding and plasticity processes, which result in the formation of positive and negative memories in the short to long term. Finally, it is pointed out that the SARS-CoV-2 pandemic generates a need for adequacy and adaptation for the significant attention to students during the re-starting of studies, given that possible disorders of sensory modulation and involvement of limbic brain areas triggered in situations of risk of death, potential or real threat, can happen. It is assumed that at times of the SARS-CoV-2 pandemic, in addition to preserving life, one of the challenges is the behavioural (re)organisation, which includes habits from the educational context that need to contemplate a scientific perspective, seeking to transform the consequences of the pandemic fear on opportunities to reinforcement of familiar links. In the context of modern rationality, the SARS-CoV-2 pandemic is also a period to think about the relationship between scientific knowledge and common sense. With this logic, neurosciences can develop a new format for the teaching-learning process, so that educators and students experiencing the pandemic threatening do not manifest psychological distress and secondary consequences. Therefore, education can be considered a central space in decision-making in the face of SARS-CoV-2 pandemic. In this sense, the urgency of a multidisciplinary strategies development is highlighted, connecting the synergy between neurosciences and education after the COVID-19 pandemic.

---

[1] *Corresponding author: Prof. Dr. Renato Leonardo de Freitas: Biomedical Sciences Institute, Federal University of Alfenas (UNIFAL), Alfenas, MG, Brazil and Laboratory of Neurosciences of Pain & Emotions and Multi-User Centre of Neuroelectrophysiology, Department of Surgery and Anatomy, Ribeirão Preto Medical School of the University of São Paulo, Av. Bandeirantes, 3900, Ribeirão Preto, São Paulo, Brazil. E-mail: defreitas.rl@gmail.com

1. INTRODUCTION

At the end of 2019, precisely in mid-December in Wuhan, China, cases of pneumonia with unknown cause began to appear. After performing evaluations of patients with the disease, a new type 2 of Coronavirus (SARS-CoV-2), RNA enveloped virus, was discovered that cause respiratory, hepatic, enteric and neurological new coronavirus disease (COVID-19) (1).

After contamination in China, the virus has spread rapidly around the world to the point of being considered a pandemic by the World Health Organisation (WHO) (2). The SARS-CoV-2 has a viral evolution with high pathogenicity and high transmissibility (1). Outbreaks like this promote possibilities of transformations within several places and social activities (3).

The pandemic and its consequences on education

The unusual situation caused by the SARS-CoV-2 pandemic affects and exposes educators and learners to weaknesses and potentialities to raise the need for criteria that provides support to face up the new conditions. The cognitive development criterion is the result of different stimuli and synaptic activation into the hippocampus and cerebral cortex, crucial aspects for teaching-learning. However, research indicates that several types of coronavirus can invade the central nervous system (CNS) (4).In other terms, we might consider the possible occurrence of viral transmission in the encephalon, reached after intranasally viral infection, through synaptic contacts in the sensorial system and neurotropism (5). As taken along this way, coronavirus can attack the teaching-learning process by weakening educators and learners who can experience a range of negative emotions, affecting mood and behavioural skills when dealing with the information about the COVID-19.

Fear And Anxiety As Risk Factors For Triggering Psychiatric Disorders During The COVID 19 Pandemic

The need for social isolation caused by the COVID-19 pandemic, combined with global uncertainty related to SARS-CoV-2, has generated a lot of tension and suffering. Although the world has already experienced other similar events, nothing was reported until now in proportions and speed of spread like the current pandemic (6). In the face of so many changes and uncertainties, natural reactions arise, such as unconditioned and conditioned fear and chronic anxiety itself, which, to a certain extent, provide care and prevention, but which can reach unbearable or even dysfunctional or pathological levels. In this scenario, prophylactic social isolation causes several risks to mental health (7). Isolation has been a strategy adopted aiming to mitigate the spread of the virus and was adopted at other critical times. However, it is also known that the longer we are isolated, the greater the risks of suffering from psychiatric illnesses (8). It is still necessary to consider the fact that during pandemics, attention is focused on the pathogen and its inherent biological risk, measures to be taken for prevention, containment action and medical protocols for the treatment of the disease.

As a result, psychological and psychiatric implications secondary to the pandemic phenomenon, at the individual and collective levels, tend to be underestimated and neglected (9, 10).Reynolds et al.

(11) reported that during social isolation a constellation of psychopathological symptoms may appear, such as depressed mood, irritability, anxiety, fear, anger, insomnia, among others, remaining long-term consequences for mental health. Hawryluck et al. (12) reported that even three years after a period of isolation, there was still a greater risk for alcohol abuse, symptoms of post-traumatic stress disorder and depression.

The most significant areas of activation during social anxiety disorder are the following: bilateral amygdaloid complex, the left medial temporal lobe encompassing the entorhinal cortex, the left medial aspect of the inferior temporal lobe encompassing perirhinal cortex and the Para hippocampal gyrus, the right anterior cingulate cortex in human beings, according to Hattingh et al. (13). The amygdala complex, the entorhinal cortex, the cingulum gyrus and the hippocampus and Para hippocampal gyrus are connected to the limbic system the main encephalic system related to the organisation of emotions in human beings and in other mammals. Additionally, the right brain hemisphere specific thinning was found in the frontal, temporal, parietal and insular cortices of individuals with social anxiety disorder (14). Shigemura et al. (15) reported that patients infected with COVID-19 (or suspected of being infected) may experience intense emotional and behavioural reactions, such as fear, boredom, loneliness, anxiety, insomnia or anger, symptoms already reported in conditions of epidemics occurring in the past (BROOKS et al.,2020).

In a pandemic, fear increases the levels of anxiety and stress in healthy individuals and intensifies the symptoms of those with pre-existing psychiatric disorders (15). However, little is known about individuals affected by their reactions based on fear of infectious disease. In China, the initial focus of the current pandemic, high levels of depression, post-traumatic stress, anxiety and insomnia have occurred among health professionals (16, 17) and their patients infected by COVID-19 (18), but the extent to which these psychological conditions are attributable to coronavirus anxiety has not been determined. Corroborating these concerns, in a recent study using 775 adults citizens living in the United States of America, individuals functionally impaired by the fear and anxiety of the coronavirus exhibited greater hopelessness, suicidal ideation, spiritual crisis and problems with alcohol/drug abuse than those who were anxious, but they did not have dysfunctional anxiety because of COVID-19 (19).

In previous research on the hurricane and flood, as well as other infectious disease epidemics, adverse psychological reactions covering anxiety, acute stress, addictive behaviours and symptoms of post-traumatic stress disorder, along with increased suicide and depression stood out in the population during and after these threatening events (20). Thus, it is believed that they will certainly occur in the current COVID-19 pandemic. Another important point, based on the observation of previous events, is that during pandemics, the number of people whose mental health is affected tends to be greater than the number of people affected by the infection itself. Previous tragedies have shown that the implications for mental health can last longer and have a higher prevalence than the epidemic or pandemic itself and that the psychosocial and economic impacts (15).

It is believed that fear can be the centre of many of these conditions because it is one of the most basic and primordial human emotions. Fear is a primitive emotion that is considered conservative in the animal kingdom (21). In the pandemic, there are still feelings of helplessness and loss of a fundamental sense of security, financial stability and the ability to predict a better future. The fear of infection, of being contaminated in the environment or contact with people evokes more and more distrust, avoidance and withdrawal, thus reducing our social interactions and restricting opportunities for contact and social support, which are very important for adaptive behaviour (22). Fear is composed of several variables and determinants and the study of neurobiological structures involved in its genesis is complex. One of the particularities associated with stress, fear and anxiety is the generalisation phenomenon that can have an adaptive value. However, overgeneralisation is inadequate and is one of the main characteristics of mental disease such as post-traumatic stress disorder (23). In this understanding, the maladaptive generalisation of fear occurs when an abnormal stimulus-response gradient emerges to produce defensive behaviours in environments or clues that are not explicitly associated with threat or danger (24). Concerning the possibility of exposure to triggering stimuli, it is estimated that up to 50 to 60% of the North American population may be exposed to at least one traumatic event in life (25) and although most individuals recover from the traumatic experience, about 10 to 30% develop post-traumatic stress disorder and, although pharmacological and psychotherapeutic treatment is often effective, 20 to 30% of patients with this condition do not respond to conventional therapies (26).

 So, at the current juncture, if a large number of people tend to experience clinically significant fear and anxiety during an outbreak of infectious disease (27) (TAYLOR, 2019) and if there is a massive exposure of the whole society to potentially traumatic events, as in the case of COVID-19 pandemic, there is a risk that many people will develop anxiety disorders such as post-traumatic stress disorder. Thus, it is crucial that health professionals understand the psychological risks of those with this specific condition (28). But if, on the one hand, as described by Dong and Bouey (29), fear and anxiety are common psychological responses during disasters and other similar situations, the entire population is more vulnerable to the development of mental disease in these critical events, especially the anxiety disorders.

These mental disorders are classified, according to the 5th edition of the Diagnostic and Statistical Manual of mental disorders (DSM-5), into a generalised anxiety disorder, panic disorder, agoraphobia, separation anxiety disorder, social anxiety disorder, specific phobias and selective mutism (30). Corroborating concerns about the onset of these mental disorders, Batelaan et al. (31) noted that there is evidence that anxiety disorders increase the incidence of cardiovascular diseases by 52% and that the severity of anxiety symptoms would be directly associated with functional impairment (32). Supporting these findings, it is understood that, in an attempt to preserve its homeostasis, the body reacts with adaptive responses, mediated by neuroendocrine and neuronal defensive activity, involving the autonomic nervous system and activation of the Hypothalamus-Pituitary-Adrenal axis (HHA) and the release of cortisol. The functional abnormalities of this axis alter the response to stressful events, contributing to the development of anxiety disorders (33).

In acute anxiety, the activation of the HHA axis is adaptive. On the contrary, in chronic anxiety, this mechanism fails, the HHA axis remains activated and impairs coping mechanisms, in addition to inducing low tolerance to chronic stress (34). Chronic stress, on the other hand, has consequences for cognitive and emotional processing and is associated with changes in brain plasticity, can affect the immune system, increase the risk for developmental diseases, impairment of negative feedback from the HHA axis, decrease in neurotrophic factors, among others (34). Thus, the literature already has robust evidence of a role played by stress in the development of psychiatric disorders in both laboratory animal (35) and in human experimental models (36), in addition to contributing to the appearance or worsening of clinical conditions.

In extreme cases, these mental health problems can lead to suicidal behaviour. It is well established that about 90% of global suicides are due to mental disorders such as depression (37). Based on these findings and experience in previous pandemics, such as Severe Acute Respiratory Syndrome Coronavirus-1 (SARS-CoV-1) in 2003 when the suicide rate among the elderly increased in Hong Kong during and after the pandemic (38, 39), the present issue is relevant and must be considered with due seriousness.

Although until now the effects of COVID-19 on mental health have not been studied systematically, it is expected to produce significant effects due to public reactions already observed (40). Observing this reaction and in previous experiences, the National Health Commission of China has taken important steps and issued a notification stipulating guidelines for emergency interventions in cases of psychosocial disasters, in order to reduce the psychosocial impacts of the COVID-19 outbreak, with teams composed of psychiatrists, mental health professionals and psychological support hotlines (41).

According to these concerns, the Department of Mental Health and Psychoactive Substances of the World Health Organisation (2) has published a document with recommendations aimed at mental health and psychosocial well-being by placing psychiatrists and psychologists to assist other health professionals, patients and the general public to understand the possible effect of COVID-19 and help their patients, families and the general public. Supporting the same line of reasoning of the need to implement efforts to care for the mental health of the population in the pandemic, Gao et al., (2020) presented the result of a survey conducted in China, where they concluded that there is a high prevalence of health problems mental disorders, such as depression and anxiety, which were associated with massive exposure to social media during the COVID-19 outbreak. They highlighted the need to combat the spread of false news and the importance of circulating reliable information. Besides, they demonstrated that the implementation of measures such as mental health services through different channels is extremely important. In conclusion,

it is important to highlight the panorama of uncertainty, insecurity and isolation experienced by humanity as a catalyst for emotions and different feelings such as fear, anxiety and sadness. This whole scenario is favourable to the emergence of mental disorders, especially those with a spectrum of anxiety and mood, or even exacerbation of the condition in people who already have it. Against this background, there is a need for a more careful examination of authorities and health professionals in addition to the symptoms caused by COVID-19, especially concerning the mental health of the population

Psychological Effects Caused By The Pandemic On Educators And Learners

In developing autonomy to conduct studies in times of COVID-19, one should consider that, in the encephalon, there are three levels of attention behaviour formation: the alert state; focus and concentration. The alert state is the initial condition for concentration in the teaching-learning process, as well as the adequacy and adaptation of educators and learners to the new physical and social context. Furthermore, the teaching-learning process must be permeated by motivation. Motivation is reflected in attention and memory. With the maintenance of the alert state, one reaches the focus and consequently, the concentration (42, 43).During and after the COVID-19 pandemic, the relationship between educators and learners must be carefully established before neural processes of coding and plasticity, which result in the formation of positive and negative memories, from short to long term (44).The multidisciplinary study of cognitive and socio-affective processes in teaching-learning can benefit from the concept of function modularity, i.e. the notion that motivation, attention and memory comprise a set of skills and abilities mediated by different modules of the nervous system, which function independently, but cooperatively, for the development of autonomy and conduction of studies during and after the COVID-19 pandemic threat. In this follow-up, attention should also be paid to somatisation regarding the manifestation of physical symptoms resulted from

psychological effects.

. Pharmacological Management On The Attention Deficit Hyperactivity Disorder (ADHD): Relation In COVID-19 Pandemic

Attention Deficit Hyperactivity Disorder (ADHD) is a neurobiological condition of genetic and environmental influences, which can set in early development (period inside the womb). It is characterised by a behaviour that goes to the extreme of inattention, restlessness and impulsiveness in a level that would not be expected for more advanced stages of the child development. That disorder can affect the person during adulthood (45). ADHD affects 5.3% of children and adolescents and 2.5% of adults, worldwide (46). The occurrence of that disorder increases the death rate, school difficulties and drug abuse, in addition to worsening job placement (45).

In the case of the COVID-19 outbreak, schools in China are closed and students are restricted to staying at home. Primary and secondary schools in China open official online educational sites to allocate students to continue education (47). Most parents of these children are required to have educational responsibility, in addition to dealing with all of children's emotional and behavioural problems 24 hours a day, 7 days a week.

The most effective current treatment for adults and children with ADHD is stimulating medications. Inattention and hyperactivity symptoms respond more to medications, but a person with the disorder often has several other associated problems that require interventions, such as psychoeducation, psychotherapy (48).Zhang and colleagues (49) investigated conditions related to the mental health of children with ADHD during the COVID-19 outbreak. During the outbreak of COVID19, ADHD symptoms in children were significantly worse compared to normal. These findings alerted the importance of focusing on special vulnerable groups during the outbreak. Attention is needed to identify an appropriate approach for children with ADHD in terms of disaster risk reduction activities.

5.School Environment Interventions Based On Complementary And Integrative Practices

The resumption of activities must be not only based on the fulfilment of the school curriculum but also support for psychological and social care. Psychological problems, when left untreated, can affect family Relationships, academic performance, and social functioning (50).

Furthermore, childhood mental health problems often continue into adulthood and lead to decreased productivity, increased substance abuse, and substantial economic burden to the individual and society (51, 52). Conventional medical treatments are based on pharmaceutical drugs and psychological therapy (53). However, the use of alternative and complementary therapies (manipulative/body techniques and practices based on attention, music therapy, etc.), can be an important adjunct treatment and or minimise the adverse effects themselves caused by pharmaceutical drugs (54, 55). There is evidence that therapies can help children reduce ADHD/ ADD symptoms, autism, anxiety, depression, and stress (56, 57).

Many studies have suggested mindfulness-based practices (e.g., yoga, tai chi, qigong, and meditation) may be a beneficial adjunct to the treatment of mental health problems, particularly mood and anxiety disorders improving quality of life (58). Mindfulness, the "intentional, accepting, and non-judgmental focus of one's attention on the emotions, thoughts, and sensations occurring in the present moment" (59). Practices like yoga and mindfulness-based procedures can positively impact the body in many ways, to increase alertness and positive feelings, and decrease negative feelings of aggressiveness, depression and anxiety (60, 61).

A study showed the effect of mindfulness and yoga on quality of life for elementary school students and teachers indicate that both benefit on intervention. The students who received the intervention demonstrated significantly greater improvement in the psychosocial and emotional quality of life compared with their peers who received standard care (62).There is evidence that one of the mechanisms through which yoga improves mood in major depressive disorder is by increasing the activity of the GABA system (63). Yoga practitioners have increased functions on Superior Parietal Lobule and Supramarginal Gyrus of the cerebral cortex (64). Long-term Ashtanga Yoga practice decreased regional glucose metabolism in the medial temporal cortex, striatum, and brainstem (65). In brainstem is situated the main output of the encephalic aversion system, the periaqueductal grey matter (PAG), whose activation elicits unconditioned fear and panic attack-like behaviour (66). Meditation and Yoga also was associated with a significantly lower right amygdala volume (67). Both PAG and amygdaloid complex neurons are also spontaneously activated in a threatening situation (68). Another non-pharmacological intervention is the music therapy has always played crucial roles in the regulation of emotions and facilitating human well-being, resulting in elevated stress threshold and enhanced immunity, for improving quality of life and reducing anxiety (56, 69, 70). There is evidence that music produces analgesia and depresses abnormal brain neural activity (71).Thus, considering the real benefits of integrative and complementary therapies, the absence of side effects and the possibility of being applied in the school environment, it is interesting to show that its use can be an additional tool in improving post-pandemic education.

7. DISCUSSION

7.1Neurosciences And Education In Times Of Pandemic

The neurosciences applied to education aims to justify that the criterion of affective development influences the criterion of cognitive development, such as attention and memory. Therefore, there has been an important process of evidence on the importance of skill and capacity building mainly in the last decades, as well as the formulation and implementation of scientific actions to educational activity (72). This perspective faced to the COVID-19 pandemic and after its passage supports educators and learners in issues regarding mental health.

In brief logical reasoning, the engagement of brain areas involved with emotions, such as the limbic system, associated with the possibility of viral transmission between neurons, damages the release process of important neurotransmitters such as glutamate and acetylcholine (excitatory), GABA and dopamine (inhibitors), in addition to serotonin (excitatory and inhibitory) and glial cells (which respond to environmental stimuli). Thus, it is assumed that SARS-CoV-2 may affect brain networks (or circuits) making them less effective, reflecting in afferent and efferent projections fundamental to the learning path (73). In this sense, pedagogical practices can be conducted and supported by the application of scientific knowledge, as to be a source of further progress. In this regard, the opening of discussion spaces beyond content and discipline sets the triad between information support on COVID-19, socio-affective and cognitive processing. For the prescription of the integral development of educators and learners, the equilateral conservation of this triangle during and after the COVID-19 pandemic, goes against the multidisciplinary perspective, based on the fact that positive or negative stimuli weaken or enhance the associative neuroplasticity, which involves connectivity, regulation and neural modulation (74).

7.2. Role of Neuroeducation during the pandemic

The triad of informational, cognitive and socio-affective support during the COVID-19 pandemic awakens to the importance of scientific education (75). Information about the outbreak can generate problems, difficulties, disorders, and disruptions in the teaching-learning process that can gradually produce persistent changes in the behaviour of educators and learners. Thus, to be meaningful, the relationship between educators and learners must mutually produce appropriate responses adapted to sensory and emotional stimuli to maintain the appropriate alert state for the content transmitted during the pandemic (76).

7.3. Role of post-pandemic neuroeducation

Faced with a complex reality where confinement is the main prophylactic means to prevent the virus spreading (2, 77), educators and learners develop new behaviours of adaptation and appropriateness, where physiological transformations are produced in response to the outbreak. From fear to courage (and vice-versa), the process of resistance or "struggle" to confront the COVID-19, demands cognitive-affective attention to contain the exponential increase of fears and insecurities that generate psychic suffering.

In times of COVID-19, besides the preservation of life, one of the challenges is, therefore, the behavioural reorganisation, that is, habits that, in the educational context, must contemplate a scientific perspective, seeking to transform the consequences of the pandemic into opportunities.

In this sense, neurosciences present neuroplasticity as the maximum law (43), a property that can prepare educators and students for confrontations and conflicts triggered during and after the COVID-19 pandemic. Moreover, through the adverse conditions that are being exposed, the development and prevalence of abilities and skills demand the need to build autonomy for the conduct of studies, based on the fact that teaching-learning is a dialectical process in which, for example, memory losses can be confused with attention losses, and vice-versa (78). In the context of modern rationality, the COVID-19 pandemic is also a time to think about the relationship between scientific knowledge and common sense. Thus, neurosciences can develop a new path along the teaching-learning process, so that educators and learners who go through the pandemic do not manifest psychic suffering and secondary consequences, such as anxiety and depression (79).

A virus like SARS-CoV-2 cannot benefit from weaknesses, but be seen by potentialities, as a gateway to a new world, whose human evolution overcomes the resilient way of feeling, remembering and making decisions. In other words, it is necessary to carry out an education that enables educators and learners to understand reality through science.

8. CONCLUSION

Because SARS-CoV-2 is not yet fully known, emotions such as fear and anxiety are usually conceived. Therefore, during this critical scenario within society, the validation of knowledge is fundamental for the creation of better methodologies, strategies and tactics for teaching-learning. In other words, the relationship between educators and learners, with ethical and humanitarian commitment, must permeate values of scientific thought. Education is, therefore, a central space in decision making while facing COVID-19. In this regard, we emphasise the need for a multidisciplinary development, involving the synergy between neurosciences and education.

AFFILIATION

[1]Biomedical Sciences Institute, Federal University of Alfenas (UNIFAL), Alfenas, MG, Brazil.
[2]Institute of Motricity Sciences, Federal University of Alfenas, Alfenas, MG, Brazil
[3]Laboratory of Neuroanatomy and Neuropsychobiology, Department of Pharmacology, Ribeirão Preto Medical School of the University of São Paulo (FMRP-USP), Ribeirão Preto, São Paulo, Brazil.
[4]Laboratory of Neurosciences of Pain & Emotions and Multi-User Centre of Neuroelectrophysiology, Department of Surgery and Anatomy, Ribeirão Preto Medical School of the University of São Paulo, Ribeirão Preto, São Paulo, Brazil.
[5]Itajubá Medicine School, Itajubá, MG, Brazil.
[6]Laboratory of Psychophysics, Perception, Psychometrics, and Pain, Department of Psychology, Ribeirão Preto School of Philosophy, Sciences and Literature of the University of São Paulo, Ribeirão Preto, SP, Brazil. [7]Department of Psychology, Federal University of Juiz de Fora (UFJF), MG, Brazil.

REFERENCES

1   Zhu N, Zhang D, Wang W, Li X, Yang B, Song J, et al. A Novel Coronavirus from Patients with Pneumonia in China, 2019. N Engl J Med. 2020;382(8):727-33.

2   Eurosurveillance Editorial T. Note from the editors: World Health Organization declares novel coronavirus (2019-nCoV) sixth public health emergency of international concern. Euro Surveill. 2020;25(5):200131e.

3   Hirschfeld K. Microbial insurgency: Theorizing global health in the Anthropocene. The Anthropocene Review. 2019;7(1):3-18.

4   De Felice FG, Tovar-Moll F, Moll J, Munoz DP, Ferreira ST. Severe Acute Respiratory Syndrome Coronavirus 2 (SARS-CoV-2) and the Central Nervous System. Trends in neurosciences. 2020;43(6):355-7.

5   5. Li Y-C, Bai W-Z, Hashikawa T. The neuroinvasive potential of SARS-CoV2 may play a role in the respiratory failure of COVID-19 patients. Journal of Medical Virology. 2020;92(6):552-5. 6. Chiyomaru K, Takemoto K. Global COVID-19 transmission rate is influenced by precipitation seasonality and the speed of climate temperature warming. medRxiv. 2020:2020.04.10.20060459.

6   Afonso P. The Impact of the COVID-19 Pandemic on Mental Health. 2020. 2020;33(5):2.

7   Wu D, Yang T, Rockett IR, Yu L, Peng S, Jiang S. Uncertainty stress, social capital, and suicidal ideation among Chinese medical students: Findings from a 22-university survey. Journal of health psychology. 2018:1359105318805820.

8   Tucci V, Moukaddam N, Meadows J, Shah S, Galwankar SC, Kapur GB. The Forgotten Plague: Psychiatric Manifestations of Ebola, Zika, and Emerging Infectious Diseases. Journal of global infectious diseases. 2017;9(4):151-6.

9   Morens DM, Fauci AS. Emerging Infectious Diseases: Threats to Human Health and Global Stability. PLOS Pathogens. 2013;9(7):e1003467.

10   Reynolds DL, Garay JR, Deamond SL, Moran MK, Gold W, Styra R. Understanding, compliance and psychological impact of the SARS quarantine experience. Epidemiol Infect. 2008;136(7):997-1007.

11   Hawryluck L, Gold WL, Robinson S, Pogorski S, Galea S, Styra R. SARS control and psychological effects of quarantine, Toronto, Canada. Emerg Infect Dis. 2004;10(7):1206-12.

12   Hattingh CJ, Ipser J, Tromp SA, Syal S, Lochner C, Brooks SJ, et al. Functional magnetic resonance imaging during emotion recognition in social anxiety disorder: an activation likelihood meta-analysis. Frontiers in human neuroscience. 2012;6:347.

13   Syal S, Hattingh CJ, Fouché JP, Spottiswoode B, Carey PD, Lochner C, et al. Grey matter abnormalities in social anxiety disorder: a pilot study. Metabolic brain disease. 2012;27(3):299309.

14   Shigemura J, Ursano RJ, Morganstein JC, Kurosawa M, Benedek DM. Public responses to the novel 2019 coronavirus (2019-nCoV) in Japan: Mental health consequences and target populations. Psychiatry and Clinical Neurosciences. 2020;74(4):281-2.

15   Lai J, Ma S, Wang Y, Cai Z, Hu J, Wei N, et al. Factors Associated With Mental Health Outcomes Among Health Care Workers Exposed to Coronavirus Disease 2019. JAMA Network Open. 2020;3(3):e203976-e.

16   Xiang Y-T, Yang Y, Li W, Zhang L, Qinge Z, Cheung T, et al. Timely mental health care for the 2019 novel coronavirus outbreak is urgently needed. The Lancet Psychiatry. 2020;7.

17   Li B, Yang J, Zhao F, Zhi L, Wang X, Liu L, et al. Prevalence and impact of cardiovascular metabolic diseases on COVID-19 in China. Clin Res Cardiol. 2020;109(5):531-8.

18   Lee S. Coronavirus Anxiety Scale: A brief mental health screener for COVID-19 related anxiety. Death Studies. 2020;44:1-9.

19   Norris F. Psychosocial Consequences of Natural Disasters in Developing Countries:

20   What Does Past Research Tell Us About the Potential Effects of the 2004 Tsunami? 2006.

21   Adolphs R. The biology of fear. Current biology : CB. 2013;23(2):R79-R93.

22   Bonanno GA. Meaning making, adversity, and regulatory flexibility. Memory. 2013;21(1):150-6.

23   Dunsmoor JE, Paz R. Fear Generalization and Anxiety: Behavioural and Neural Mechanisms. Biological psychiatry. 2015;78(5):336-43.

24   Asok A, Kandel ER, Rayman JB. The Neurobiology of Fear Generalization. Frontiers in Behavioural Neuroscience. 2019;12(329).

25   Merikangas KR, He JP, Burstein M, Swanson SA, Avenevoli S, Cui L, et al. Lifetime prevalence of mental disorders in U.S. adolescents: results from the National Comorbidity Survey Replication--Adolescent Supplement (NCS-A). Journal of the American Academy of Child and Adolescent Psychiatry. 2010;49(10):980-9.

26   Reznikov R, Bambico FR, Diwan M, Raymond RJ, Nashed MG, Nobrega JN, et al. Prefrontal Cortex Deep Brain Stimulation Improves Fear and Anxiety-Like Behaviour and Reduces Basolateral Amygdala Activity in a Preclinical Model of Posttraumatic Stress Disorder. Neuropsychopharmacology. 2018;43(5):1099-106.

27   Taylor S. The Psychology of Pandemics: Preparing for the Next Global Outbreak of Infectious Disease: Cambridge Scholars Publishing; Edição: Unabridged edition; 2019. 178 p.

28   Asmundson G, Taylor S. How health anxiety influences responses to viral outbreaks like COVID-19: What all decision-makers, health authorities, and health care professionals need to know. Journal of Anxiety Disorders. 2020;71:102211.

29   Dong L, Bouey J. Public Mental Health Crisis during COVID-19 Pandemic, China. Emerg Infect Dis. 2020;26(7).

30   Association AP. Highlights of Changes From DSM-IV to DSM-5.Diagnostic and Statistical Manual of Mental Disorders. DSM Library: American Psychiatric Association; 2013.

31   Batelaan NM, Seldenrijk A, Bot M, van Balkom AJ, Penninx BW. Anxiety and new onset of cardiovascular disease: critical review and meta-analysis. The British journal of psychiatry : the journal of mental science. 2016;208(3):223-31.

32   McKnight PE, Monfort SS, Kashdan TB, Blalock DV, Calton JM. Anxiety symptoms and functional impairment: A systematic review of the correlation between the two measures. Clinical psychology review. 2016;45:115-30.

33   Faravelli C, Lo Sauro C, Godini L, Lelli L, Benni L, Pietrini F, et al. Childhood stressful events, HPA axis and anxiety disorders. World journal of psychiatry. 2012;2(1):13-25.

34   Prenderville J, Kennedy P, Dinan T, Cryan J. Adding fuel to the fire: The impact of stress on the ageing brain. Trends in neurosciences. 2015;38:13-25.

35 Brydges NM, Whalley HC, Jansen MA, Merrifield GD, Wood ER, Lawrie SM, et al. Imaging conditioned fear circuitry using awake rodent fMRI. PloS one. 2013;8(1):e54197-e.

36 Nolte T, Guiney J, Fonagy P, Mayes LC, Luyten P. Interpersonal stress regulation and the development of anxiety disorders: an attachment-based developmental framework. Frontiers in behavioural neuroscience. 2011;5:55-.

37 Mamun MA, Griffiths MD. A rare case of Bangladeshi student suicide by gunshot due to unusual multiple causalities. Asian journal of psychiatry. 2020;49:101951.

38 Cheung YTD, Chau P, Yip P. A revisit on older adult suicides and Severe Acute Respiratory Syndrome (SARS) epidemic in Hong Kong. International journal of geriatric psychiatry. 2008;23:1231-8.

39 Chan S, Chiu F, Lam C, Leung P, Conwell Y. Elderly suicide and the 2003 SARS epidemic in Hong Kong. International journal of geriatric psychiatry. 2006;21:113-8.

40 Li W, Yang Y, Liu ZH, Zhao YJ, Zhang Q, Zhang L, et al. Progression of Mental Health Services during the COVID-19 Outbreak in China. International journal of biological sciences.2020;16(10):1732-8.

41 Lu D, Jennifer B. Public Mental Health Crisis during COVID-19 Pandemic, China. Emerging Infectious Disease journal. 2020;26(7).

42 Geng F, Redcay E, Riggins T. The influence of age and performance on hippocampal function and the encoding of contextual information in early childhood. NeuroImage. 2019;195.

43 James L. McGaugh FB-R, Roberto A. Prado-Alcalá. Plasticity in the Central Nervous System: Learning and Memory. 1 ed: Routledge; 2019. 216 p.

44 Cross ZR, Santamaria A, Kohler MJ. Attention and Emotion-Enhanced Memory: A Systematic Review and Meta-Analysis of Behavioural and Neuroimaging Evidence. bioRxiv. 2018:273920.

45 Pediatrics AAo. Clinical practice guideline: diagnosis and evaluation of the child with attention-deficit/hyperactivity disorder. American Academy of Pediatrics. Pediatrics. 2000;105(5):1158-70.

46 Wang LJ, Lee SY, Yuan SS, Yang CJ, Yang KC, Huang TS, et al. Prevalence rates of youths diagnosed with and medicated for ADHD in a nationwide survey in Taiwan from 2000 to 2011. Epidemiology and psychiatric sciences. 2017;26(6):624-34.

47 Chen P, Mao L, Nassis GP, Harmer P, Ainsworth BE, Li F. Returning Chinese school-aged children and adolescents to physical activity in the wake of COVID-19: Actions and precautions. J Sport Health Sci. 2020:S2095-546(20)30049-1.

48 Kolar D, Keller A, Golfinopoulos M, Cumyn L, Syer C, Hechtman L. Treatment of adults with attention-deficit/hyperactivity disorder. Neuropsychiatric disease and treatment. 2008;4(2):389-403.

49 Zhang J, Shuai L, Yu H, Wang Z, Qiu M, Lu L, et al. Acute stress, behavioural symptoms and mood states among school-age children with attention-deficit/hyperactive disorder during the COVID-19 outbreak. Asian journal of psychiatry. 2020;51:102077.

50 Kessler RC, Foster CL, Saunders WB, Stang PE. Social consequences of psychiatric disorders, I: Educational attainment. The American journal of psychiatry. 1995;152(7):1026-32.

51 Reeves WC, Strine TW, Pratt LA, Thompson W, Ahluwalia I, Dhingra SS, et al. Mental illness surveillance among adults in the United States. MMWR supplements. 2011;60(3):1-29.

52 Smit F, Cuijpers P, Oostenbrink J, Batelaan N, de Graaf R, Beekman A. Costs of nine common mental disorders: implications for curative and preventive psychiatry. The journal of mental health policy and economics. 2006;9(4):193-200.

53 Bennett S, Shafran R, Coughtrey A, Walker S, Heyman I. Psychological interventions for mental health disorders in children with chronic physical illness: a systematic review. Archives of disease in childhood. 2015;100(4):308-16.

54 Edwards E, Mischoulon D, Rapaport M, Stussman B, Weber W. Building an evidence base in complementary and integrative healthcare for child and adolescent psychiatry. Child and adolescent psychiatric clinics of North America. 2013;22(3):509-29, vii.

55 Park C. Mind-body CAM interventions: current status and considerations for integration into clinical health psychology. Journal of clinical psychology. 2013;69(1):45-63.

56 Chang C, Tsai G, Hsieh CJ. Psychological, immunological and physiological effects of a Laughing Qigong Program (LQP) on adolescents. Complementary therapies in medicine. 2013;21(6):660-8.

57 Uebel-von Sandersleben H, Albrecht B, Rothenberger A, Fillmer-Heise A, Roessner V, Sergeant J, et al. Revisiting the co-existence of Attention-Deficit/Hyperactivity Disorder and Chronic Tic Disorder in childhood—The case of colour discrimination, sustained attention and interference control. PloS one. 2017;12(6):e0178866.

58 Hagen I, Nayar US. Yoga for Children and Young People's Mental Health and WellBeing: Research Review and Reflections on the Mental Health Potentials of Yoga. Frontiers in psychiatry. 2014;5:35.

59 Zgierska A, Rabago D, Chawla N, Kushner K, Koehler R, Marlatt A. Mindfulness meditation for substance use disorders: a systematic review. Substance abuse. 2009;30(4):266-94.

60 Miller JJ, Fletcher K, Kabat-Zinn J. Three-year follow-up and clinical implications of a mindfulness meditation-based stress reduction intervention in the treatment of anxiety disorders. General hospital psychiatry. 1995;17(3):192-200.

61 de Bruin EI, Formsma AR, Frijstein G, Bögels SM. Mindful2Work: Effects of Combined Physical Exercise, Yoga, and Mindfulness Meditations for Stress Relieve in Employees. A Proof of Concept Study. Mindfulness. 2017;8(1):204-17.

62 Bazzano AN, Anderson CE, Hylton C, Gustat J. Effect of mindfulness and yoga on quality of life for elementary school students and teachers: results of a randomized controlled schoolbased study. Psychology research and behaviour management. 2018;11:81-9.

63 Streeter CC, Gerbarg PL, Brown RP, Scott TM, Nielsen GH, Owen L, et al. Thalamic Gamma Aminobutyric Acid Level Changes in Major Depressive Disorder After a 12-Week Iyengar Yoga and Coherent Breathing Intervention. Journal of alternative and complementary medicine (New York, NY). 2020;26(3):190-7.

64 Wadden KP, Snow NJ, Sande P, Slawson S, Waller T, Boyd LA. Yoga Practitioners Uniquely Activate the Superior Parietal Lobule and Supramarginal Gyrus During Emotion Regulation. Frontiers in integrative neuroscience. 2018;12:60.

65 van Aalst J, Ceccarini J, Schramm G, Van Weehaeghe D, Rezaei A, Demyttenaere K, et al. Long-term Ashtanga yoga practice decreases medial temporal and brainstem glucose metabolism in relation to years of experience. EJNMMI Research. 2020;10.

66 Coimbra NC, De Oliveira R, Freitas RL, Ribeiro SJ, Borelli KG, Pacagnella RC, et al. Neuroanatomical approaches of the tectum-reticular pathways and immunohistochemical evidence for serotonin-positive perikarya on neuronal substrates of the superior colliculus and periaqueductal gray matter involved in the elaboration of the defensive behaviour and fearinduced analgesia. Experimental neurology. 2006;197(1):93-112.

67 Gotink RA, Vernooij MW, Ikram MA, Niessen WJ, Krestin GP, Hofman A, et al. Meditation and yoga practice are associated with smaller right amygdala volume: the Rotterdam study. Brain Imaging Behav. 2018;12(6):1631-9.

68 Paschoalin-Maurin T, dos Anjos-Garcia T, Falconi-Sobrinho LL, de Freitas RL, Coimbra JPC, Laure CJ, et al. The Rodent-versus-wild Snake Paradigm as a Model for Studying Anxiety- and Panic-like Behaviours: Face, Construct and Predictive Validities. Neuroscience. 2018;369:336-49.

69 Abrams A. Music, cancer, and immunity. Clinical journal of oncology nursing. 2001;5(5):222-4.

70 Hatem T, Lira P, Mattos S. The therapeutic effects of music in children following cardiac surgery. Jornal de pediatria. 2006;82:186-92.

71 Metcalf CS, Huntsman M, Garcia G, Kochanski AK, Chikinda M, Watanabe E, et al. Music-Enhanced Analgesia and Antiseizure Activities in Animal Models of Pain and Epilepsy: Toward Preclinical Studies Supporting Development of Digital Therapeutics and Their Combinations With Pharmaceutical Drugs. Frontiers in neurology. 2019;10:277.

72 Thomas MSC, Ansari D, Knowland VCP. Annual Research Review: Educational neuroscience: progress and prospects. Journal of child psychology and psychiatry, and allied disciplines. 2019;60(4):477-92.

73 Purves D. Brains: how they seem to work: Ft Press; 2010.

74 de Sousa LB, de Oliveira Sá IS, de Oliveira ARSM, de Carvalho MdG, de Souza Teixeira MM. Neuroeducation: An Approach to Brain Plasticity in Learning. Amadeus International Multidisciplinary Journal. 2019;4(7):86-104.

75 Carey S. Cognitive science and science education. American psychologist. 1986;41(10):1123.

76 de Tienda Palop L. The Role of the Emotions in Moral Neuroeducation.Moral Neuroeducation for a Democratic and Pluralistic Society: Springer; 2019. p. 61-75.

77 Belasco AGS, Fonseca CDd. Coronavirus 2020. Revista Brasileira de Enfermagem.2020;73(2).

78 Davis JL. Brain Structure, Learning, and Memory: Routledge; 2019.

79 DE FREITAS RLN-B, Mônica; MEDEIROS, Priscila de. Neurociência das emoções, da aprendizagem e do comportamento autolesivo.: FMIT; 2019.

CHAPTER 17

THE EFFICACY OF LOCKDOWNS

1. Determinants of Physical Distancing During The COVID-19 Epidemic In Brazil: Effects From Mandatory Rules, Numbers Of Cases And Duration Of Rules

Rodrigo Fracalossi de Moraes[1]

Institute for Applied Economic Research (IPEA)

ABSTRACT

During the COVID-19 pandemic, physical distancing is being promoted to reduce the disease transmission and pressure on health systems. Yet, what determines physical distancing? Through a panel data analysis, this article identifies some of its determinants. Using a specifically built index that measures the strictness of physical distancing rules in the 27 Brazilian states, this paper isolates the effect of mandatory physical distancing rules from other potential determinants of physical distancing. The article concludes that physical distancing is influenced by at least three variables: the strictness of mandatory physical distancing rules, the number of confirmed cases of COVID-19, and the duration of rules. Evidence also indicates that the effect of physical distancing measures is relatively stronger than that of the number of cases – physical distancing is determined proportionally more by mandatory policies than people's awareness about the severity of the epidemic. These results have at least two policy implications. First, governments should adopt mandatory measures in order to increase physical distancing – rather than expect people to adopt them on their own. Second, the timing of adopting them is important, since people are unlikely to comply with them for long periods of time.

1. INTRODUCTION

What determines physical distancing? In the context of an epidemic in which there are no better alternatives to reduce the transmission of a disease and no effective treatment, the answer to this question might determine government policies to contain an epidemic.

If people practice physical distancing voluntarily, based on the severity of the epidemic or out of a sense of social responsibility, strict physical distancing measures would be largely unnecessary.

However, if people respond to mandatory restrictions (closing nonessential shops, suspending classes, suspending mass gatherings, etc), governments should adopt these non-pharmaceutical interventions (NPIs) in order to contain an epidemic. Maloney & Taskin (2020) [1] argued that the COVID-19 pandemic *per se* led to voluntary demobilization and that this effect is stronger than that of NPIs, what was observed in all but the poorest countries. This finding was reinforced by case

---

[1] rodrigo.moraes@ipea.gov.br   ORCID: 0000-0001-5751-3593

studies on the US and Sweden, where evidence indicates that physical distancing increased *before* mandatory measures were adopted. The causal mechanism could be not only the fear of getting infected but also empathy for those most vulnerable to the virus (2) or people's belief in science (3). If this is true, lifting restrictive measures during the epidemic would not have a great impact, as people would practice physical distancing anyway. From a different angle, Engle, Stromme, and Zhou (2020) [2], Brzezinski et al. (2020) [3], Painter and Qiu(2020) [4] and Anderson et al (2020). [5] demonstrated that mandatory physical distancing measures in the United States significantly increased the probability of someone staying at home. In addition, physical distancing levels may depend on the length of restrictions on people's mobility: the longer they last the higher the costs for people to stay at home, reducing their probability of complying with physical distancing rules. Frequent extensions may also create confusion and frustration, leading people to reduce levels of compliance, something that was observed in Italy (8).

Through a panel data analysis, this paper seeks to answer the question of what influences physical distancing during the COVID-19 pandemic. It looks at the effects of mandatory physical distancing rules, numbers of COVID-19 cases, and the duration of mandatory rules on the levels of physical distancing in Brazil. As physical distancing policies in Brazil were implemented mainly by states (27 in total, including the Federal District), comparing their policies and respective outcomes might indicate the extent to what mandatory policies are necessary to increase physical distancing in the context of an epidemic. Evidence presented in this article suggests that levels of physical distancing are positively correlated with the strictness of mandatory restrictions and the severity of the epidemic, as well as negatively correlated with the number of days since the first mandatory measures were adopted.

2. METHOD AND DATA

In order to identify some of the potential determinants of physical distancing levels during the COVID-19 pandemic in Brazil I conducted a panel data analysis (using a balanced panel) covering the period 22 Mar – 24 May 2020. I created a daily series for all variables starting from 22 Mar, when all Brazilian states had reported at least one case of COVID-19. The model has the following variables and uses the following data sources.

Dependent Variable: Physical Distancing

The Brazilian geolocation company In Loco generates data on daily levels of physical distancing discriminated by state, using data collected through apps in over 60 million smartphones in Brazil. The company monitors movement trends, producing data similar to those of Google Mobility Reports. In Loco uses various apps, including those of the main telecommunication companies, retailer stores, banks, etc. in Brazil (9). Data is aggregated into the 'social distancing index', which is used here as a proxy for physical distancing, a method used in previous research (10,11). The index has values expressed in percentages (in a scale of 0% to 100%), in which 100% is a hypothetical situation in which the whole population stays at home for a whole day. In the model, I use rolling averages (7 days) to minimize the effect of short-term variations.

Independent Variables: Strictness of Mandatory Physical Distancing Rules

I created an index that measures the strictness of physical distancing rules, which I have called the *physical distancing rules index* (PDI). This index is composed of six variables, measuring: whether mass gatherings, as well as cultural, sport or religious activities are suspended; whether bars, pubs, restaurants and similar places are closed; whether non-essential shops are closed; whether non-essential industries are closed; whether classes are suspended; and whether there are restrictions on passenger transportation. Each of these variables represents a type of agglomeration of people that may be restricted by NPIs: if these activities were all suspended, the aggregate effect should be a broad reduction in the number of agglomerations. For each of these variables, values of 2, 1 or 0 were assigned depending on whether suspension or restriction was full, partial or non-existent. As the sum of the values would vary between 0 and 12 (there are six variables), the index's values were adjusted to be between 0 and 10 (a more intuitive scale), in which 10 is the greatest level of restriction.

Table 1:Variables of the index

# of the variable	Description of the variable	Values
1	Mass gatherings and cultural, sport or religious activities	2 = Full suspension
2	Bars, pubs, restaurants and similar places	1 = Partial
3	Non-essential shops	suspensionor
4	Non-essential industries	restriction
5	Classes	0 = No suspensionor
6	Public transportation	restriction

- Information used to code the values of these variables come from open sources, especially legal documents from state governments, complemented by news from local media. Details are in the appendix and in Moraes (12,13). The original dataset is in Moraes (14).

This index has at least one caveat: its values are a non-weighted sum of the variables, regardless of how much the activities they measure produce in terms of agglomerations. This could be corrected by an index with weighted variables, but this would require data about how much different activities produce agglomerations of people (Not available) or arbitrary assumptions.

2. Number of Cases of COVID-19

A high number of cases should make people more aware of the epidemic or more afraid of getting infected, which is likely to influence their behaviour. In the model, I use rolling averages (7 days) to compensate for random factors affecting the number of reported cases in a given day. For example, cases during weekends and bank holidays take longer to be reported to the Ministry of Health (which consolidates data from all Brazilian states). Underreporting is of course a problem, but the high correlation between the number of cases and the number of deaths (0.80) indicates that underreporting rates did not vary substantially over time. Number of deaths were not used in the model due to a high number of observations with a value of zero: in a log scale these observations would either be discarded or have arbitrary values, which is likely to bias results. Data for this variable come from Brazil's Ministry of Health.

3. Duration of Physical Distancing Rules

Levels of physical distancing should be negatively correlated with the number of days since mandatory physical distancing rules were introduced. The longer the rules last the less likely people are to comply with them (holding everything else constant), which should occur for a few reasons: their savings (in case they have them) were all spent; people are looking for jobs or need to increase their income; social isolation produces stress; or people may seek to escape from domestic abuse. In the model, this variable is measured by the number of days since the first mandatory physical distancing rule was introduced in a given state.

4. Levels of Development

In poorer places people should be less likely to practice physical distancing as they are less likely to have savings and more likely to have informal jobs, reducing incentives for them to stay at home. This variable is measured through GDP per capita, which has a substantial variation in Brazil: between R$ 12,800 a year in the poorest state (Maranhão) and R$ 80,500 in the richest one (Distrito Federal). The interpretation of results for this variable should be cautious though as it is likely to capture the effect of others: lower levels of GDP per capita are associated with a lower number of ICU beds, a lower percentage of people living in urban areas, a lower population density, less access to reliable information and a lower educational level, which might all influence levels of physical distancing. Data for this variable come from the Brazilian Institute of Geography and Statistics (IBGE).

5. Health Infrastructure

In places with limited health infrastructure, people should have more incentives to practice physical distancing as they would be less likely to have healthcare available. In the model, this is measured by the number of ICU beds per 100,000 people. Data for this variable come from Brazil's Ministry of Health (DATASUS).

6. Political Party or Coalition In Power

The ideology of a government in power might indicate people's willingness to practice physical distancing. A stronger sense of social responsibility might be more common among left-wing people, so that voters who elected left-wing candidates would be more likely to practice physical distancing. In contrast, people who elected right-wing candidates might put more emphasis on their freedom of going and coming, making them less likely to practice physical distancing. In the model there are three values for this variable: 0 for a left-wing party or coalition; 1 for a centrist party or coalition; or 2 for a right-wing party or coalition.

7. Population Density

People living in places with a high population density have a greater risk of getting infected and infecting others, creating more incentives for people to stay at home. In the model, this is measured by the log of the population density. Data for this variable come from the Brazilian Institute of Geography and Statistics (IBGE).

RESULTS AND DISCUSSION

As observed in Figure 1, values of the PDI are highly and positively correlated with values of the social distancing index, suggesting that these two phenomena are associated.

Figure 1
Physical distancing rules index (PDI) and social distancing index, 11 Mar-21-May (only business days)

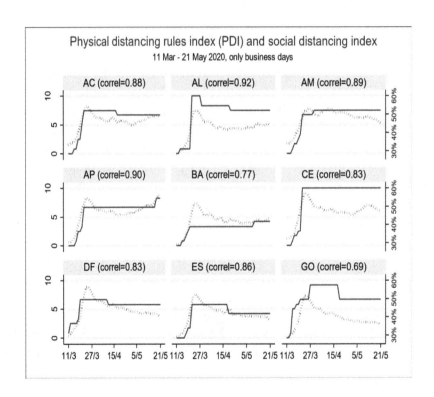

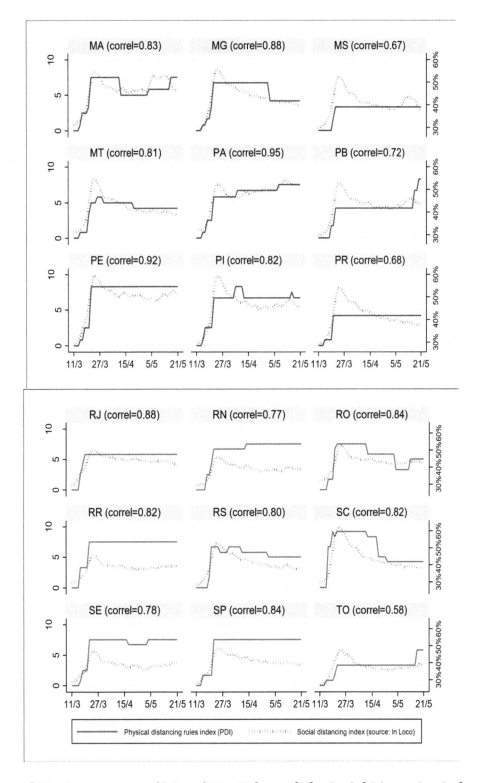

Centred-Moving Averages (3 Days) For Values of The Social Distancing Index.

AC: Acre, AL: Alagoas, AM: Amazonas, AP: Amapá, BA: Bahia, CE: Ceará, DF: Distrito Federal, ES: Espírito Santo, GO: Goiás, MA: Maranhão, MG: Minas Gerais, MS: Mato Grosso do Sul, MT: Mato Grosso, PA: Pará, PB: Paraíba, PE: Pernambuco, PI: Piauí, PR: Paraná, RJ: Rio de Janeiro, RN: Rio Grande do Norte, RO: Rondônia, RR: Roraima, RS: Rio Grande do Sul, SC: Santa Catarina, SE: Sergipe, SP: São Paulo, TO: Tocantins.

Yet, there is substantial variation across states, suggesting that other variables also determine levels of physical distancing. Moreover, physical distancing's decrease over time was on average higher than the decrease in the strictness of mandatory physical distancing rules. This is puzzling because it coincided with rising numbers of cases and deaths due to COVID-19, which should make people comply more – rather than less – with physical distancing rules. This indicates that the length of legal rules of physical distancing may be negatively correlated with levels of physical distancing.

Results from a panel data analysis indicate that levels of physical distancing depend on the strictness of mandatory physical distancing rules, on the number of confirmed cases of covid19 and on the number of days since the first mandatory measures were introduced. As observed in table 2, the coefficients of these three variables were similar across different models.

An increase of one additional unit in the PDI (which has a scale of 0 to 10) is expected to increase physical distancing by about 0.8 percentage point. The effect of an increase in the number of cases is also significant: one additional unit increases physical distancing by about 0.9 percentage point. Yet, it is important to consider that one unit in the log scale represents an increase of about 3 times in the number of cases per 100,000 people. Consequently, an increase of 3 times in the number of cases have an effect only slightly stronger than the effect of increasing one additional unit in the strictness of mandatory physical distancing rules.

The duration of mandatory physical distancing measures is also statistically significant: holding everything else constant, an additional day of physical distancing mandatory rules decreases physical distancing by about 0.2 percentage point. This implies that keeping physical distancing levels constant over time requires an increase in the strictness of physical distancing rules or other measures that increase physical distancing.

Table 2 :Determinants of physical distancing in Brazil (22 March – 24 May 2020)

Social distancing index (0-100%)	(1)	(2)	(3)	(4)	(5)	(6)
Physical distancing rules index (PDI)	0.799*** (0.055)	0.788*** (0.054)	0.799*** (0.055)	0.799*** (0.055)	0.799*** (0.055)	0.799*** (0.055)
Number of days	-0.194*** (0.007)	-0.195*** (0.006)	-0.194*** (0.007)	-0.194*** (0.007)	-0.194*** (0.007)	-0.194*** (0.007)
Log cases	0.926*** (0.075)	0.945*** (0.074)	0.926*** (0.075)	0.926*** (0.075)	0.926*** (0.075)	0.926*** (0.075)
Log GDP per capita			1.008** (0.298)			
ICU beds				0.048** (0.014)		
Ideology					0.048 (0.445)	
Log population density						0.287** (0.085)
Constant	49.287*** (0.533)	49.166*** (0.600)	39.118*** (3.239)	48.362*** (0.682)	49.287*** (0.533)	49.370*** (0.524)
State dummies	Yes	No	Yes	Yes	Yes	Yes
# of observations	1.725	1.725	1.725	1.725	1.725	1.725
R^2	0.772	0.544	0.772	0.772	0.772	0.772

The numbers of the models are indicated at the top row. Physical distancing rules index (PDI): strictness of mandatory physical distancing rules; number of days: days since the first mandatory physical distancing rules was adopted; log cases: log of the number of new confirmed cases; Log GDP per capita: log of the GDP per capita; ICU beds: number of ICU beds per 100,000 people; ideology: ideology of the political party or coalition in power (left-wing, centre or right-wing); log population density: log of the population density.

Data indicates that GDP per capita might have an influence but it does not add predictive power to the model. Due to a high or medium correlation of GDP per capita with the number of ICUs per 100,000 people (correl=0.82), the ideology of the political party/coalition in power (correl=-0.50), and population density (correl=0.34), separate models with each of these variables were built. The number of ICU beds and population density were significant but did not increase the predictive power of the models, and the political party (or coalition) in power was not statistically significant. The R^2 values for models with state dummies should be interpreted with caution as they are inflated by the use of these dummies. The R^2 of 0.54 in model 2 indicates a good predictive power of the model, suggesting that more than 50% of the variation in physical distancing levels is caused by the strictness of physical distancing rules, the number of confirmed COVID-19 cases, and the length of mandatory physical distancing measures.

There are at least three limitations in these models. First, the physical distancing rules index captures only the suspension or restriction of activities, not including measures that are also essential to contain an epidemic, such as awareness campaigns, mandatory use of EPI, cash transfers (which encourages people to stay at home), or the enforcement of legal rules.

Second, the models do not capture overall social norms, which may lead people to stay at home more in certain states than in others. Third, there is variation over time for the independent variables of interest (strictness of physical distancing rules, number of COVID-19 cases, and number of days since mandatory measures were introduced), but not for the other covariates, either because there was no daily data available or because they only change substantially over larger periods of time. Therefore, the results for population density, GDP per capita, ideology and ICU beds should be interpreted with caution. These findings do not imply that similar results should be found in other countries, as there might be specific determinants in Brazil not captured in this model. Among others, the federal government encouraged people not to respect physical distancing and sought to undermine states' policies of physical distancing, which is likely to have influenced people's behaviour (15).

CONCLUSIONS

This paper was an attempt to estimate the determinants of physical distancing levels. Results show that mandatory physical distancing rules and the number of confirmed COVID-19 cases are positively correlated with physical distancing levels, while the duration of rules are negatively correlated with them. It also shows that the effect of physical distancing mandatory rules is relatively stronger than the effect of the number of cases, suggesting that people respond more to mandatory rules of physical distancing than to the severity of the epidemic.

These findings have at least two policy implications. First, increasing physical distancing to high levels requires governments to adopt mandatory measures, especially when numbers of cases and deaths are not high. For a variety of reasons, a substantial part of the population seems to have a risk-taking behaviour, which might result from economic needs, cultural or psychological traits, or influence from pandemic-negationists. Second, evidence indicates that mandatory physical distancing rules have an 'expiry date': for a variety of reasons people's compliance with mandatory rules decrease over time, even if the number of cases and deaths from COVID-19 increases. This implies that the 'timing' for adopting mandatory measures is important, as compliance with rules might decrease when it is most needed. This also implies that keeping levels of physical distancing constant over time are likely to require additional mandatory restrictions, a greater enforcement or nonmandatory measures (awareness campaigns or cash transfers to people, for example).

This problem might be minimized by an on-off lockdown policy, as suggested by Scherbina,[7] which may not be the best solution from an epidemiological point of view, but necessary in some cases for practical reasons.

Acknowledgements

I would like to thank Acir dos Santos Almeida, Amanda Reis Montenegro, Flávia de Holanda Schmidt, Paulo de Tarso Linhares and an anonymous reviewer for comments and suggestions on drafts of this paper or the research project as a whole.

REFERENCES

1. Maloney WF, Taskin T. (2020). Determinants of social distancing and economic activity during COVID-19: A global view. *World Bank Policy Res Work Pap.* 2020. Available from: http://documents.worldbank.org/curated/en/325021589288466494/Determinants-ofSocial-Distancing-and-Economic-Activity-during-COVID-19-A-Global-View.

2. Pfattheicher S, Nockur L, Böhm R, Sassenrath C, Petersen MB. The emotional path to action: Empathy promotes physical distancing during the COVID-19 pandemic. [Preprint] 2020. Available from: https://psyarxiv.com/y2cg5.

3. Brzezinski A, Kecht V, Van Dijcke D, Wright AL. Belief in science influences physical distancing in response to COVID-19 lockdown policies. *Univ Chic Becker Friedman Inst Econ Work Pap.* 2020. Available from: https://bfi.uchicago.edu/working-paper/belief-inscience-influences-physical-distancing-in-response-to-COVID-19-lockdown-policies.

4. Engle S, Stromme J, Zhou A. Staying at home: mobility effects of COVID-19. *Covid Economics.* 2020; 4:86-102. Available from https://cepr.org/sites/default/files/news/CovidEconomics4.pdf.

5. Brzezinski A, Deiana G, Kecht V, Van Dijcke D. The COVID-19 pandemic: government vs. community action across the United States. *INET Oxford Work Pap.* 2020; 06. Available from: https://www.inet.ox.ac.uk/publications/no-2020-06-the-COVID-19-pandemicgovernment-vs-community-action-across-the-united-states.

6. Painter M, Qiu T.(2020). Political beliefs affect compliance with COVID-19 social distancing orders. [Preprint] 2020. Available from: SSRN 3569098.

7. Anderson RM, Heesterbeek H, Klinkenberg D, Hollingsworth TD. How will country-based mitigation measures influence the course of the COVID-19 epidemic? *The Lancet.* 2020; 395(10228):931–4.

8. Briscese G, Lacetera N, Macis M, Tonin M. Compliance with COVID-19 social-distancing measures in Italy: the role of expectations and duration. *IZA - Institute of Labor Economics Discussion Paper Series.* 2020. Available from: http://ftp.iza.org/dp13092.pdf.

9. In Loco. Mapa brasileiro da COVID-19 [Internet]. In Loco; 2020. Available from: https://mapabrasileirodacovid.inloco.com.br/pt.

10. Ajzenman N, Cavalcanti T, Da Mata D. More than words: Leaders' speech and risky behaviour during a pandemic. [Preprint] 2020. Available from: SSRN 3582908.

11. Peixoto PS, Marcondes DR, Peixoto CM, Queiroz L, Gouveia R, Delgado A, et al. Potential dissemination of epidemics based on Brazilian mobile geolocation data. Part I: Population dynamics and future spreading of infection in the states of São Paulo and Rio de Janeiro during the pandemic of COVID-19. [Preprint] 2020. Available from: https://www.medrxiv.org/content/10.1101/2020.04.07.20056739v1.

12. Moraes RF de. Medidas legais de incentivo ao distanciamento social: comparação das políticas de governos estaduais e prefeituras das capitais no Brasil. *Nota Téc - Ipea.* 2020; 16. Available from:https://www.ipea.gov.br/portal/images/stories/PDFs/nota_tecnica/200415_dinte_n_16.pdf

13. Moraes RF de. COVID-19 e medidas legais de distanciamento social: tipologia de políticas estaduais e análise do período de 13 a 26 de abril de 2020. *Nota Téc - Ipea.* 2020; 18. Available from: http://www.ipea.gov.br/portal/images/stories/PDFs/nota_tecnica/200429_nt18_covid19.pdf.

14. Moraes RF de. Índice de medidas legais de distanciamento social. Ipea; 2020. Available from: http://tinyurl.com/ipeacoronavirus.

15. Ajzenman N, Cavalcanti T, Da Mata D. More than words: Leaders' speech and risky behaviour during a pandemic. [Preprint] 2020. Available from: SSRN 3582908.

16. Scherbina A. Determining the optimal duration of the COVID-19 suppression policy: A cost-benefit analysis. [Preprint] 2020. Available from: SSRN 3562053.

2. Lockdown or Participatory Health Surveillance? Lessons From The COVID-19

Heleno Rodrigues Corrêa Filho[12 1]
Ana Maria Segall-Corrêa[3]

This issue of the journal 'Saúde em Debate' brings contributions to understand the world of collective health at the critical moment of the 2020 Coronavirus pandemic (Severe Acute Respiratory Syndrome Coronavirus 2 – Sars-Cov-2), in which the disease caused by this virus was named COVID-19. In a previous editorial, 'Saúde em Debate' expressed the prediction that the success of the Chinese model would bring inevitable criticism to the Western model of mitigation and vertical state action without direct popular participation[1].

In the second half of March 2020, the indiscriminate closure of cities (Lockdown) was discussed in Brazil, as opposed to the Chinese and Korean experience of epidemiological surveillance by popular mobilization with organization and information by the base, selective closure, and maintenance of essential services such as health, food, and survival. China was victorious. On March 3rd, 2020, the Chinese government released the first bulletin with no new cases of Coronavirus contagion. On the same day, Italy announced the death of more than 600 people, heading for the peak of the epidemic spread across the country after it started in the region of Lombardy, around the city of Milan.

Several films made in China during the surveillance and control actions revealed that entering and leaving condominiums, subways, buses, shopping venues in Wuhan were monitored by members of the Chinese Communist Party and members of Local People's Committees. These committees acted as local authorities under a central command, defining authorizations to go out for purchase of supplies and contacts of absolute necessity. One must keep in mind that essential need or service is a class concept according to which what is little for a minority is too much for many.

The control of departure, route, and arrival was done in China using social networking applications such as 'WeChat', reading of standard identification 'QR' codes by cell phones, centralizing information and analysis. The Chinese state service provided big data and computing infrastructure for collecting, storing, processing, and analysing information to control the epidemic.

If a person in Wuhan demonstrated to be infected with symptoms or signs after riding in a specific subway car or shopping in a supermarket, they would be identified as to the time, route, contacts, and close people to be called in for examinations and surveillance.

Not even George Orwell could have imagined a big brother so present with a capillary structure to control people and those carrying a lethal virus. In the same period, mortality in Korea was 7.9 per thousand (0.79%) and affected mainly the elderly and conglomerate groups in homes for the elderly. In Italy, mortality reached over 9% and went on to killing babies. The upward graphs of

[1]

1Centro Brasileiro de Estudos de Saúde (Cebes) – Rio de Janeiro (RJ), Brasil. lenocorrea@uol.com.br
2Universidade de Brasília (UnB) – Brasília (DF), Brasil.
3Fundação Oswaldo Cruz (Fiocruz) - Brasília (DF), Brasil.

cases and mortality in European countries and in Brazil made it possible to predict that, here, there would be a greater chance of reproducing the Italian model of dissemination of the COVID-19[2].

The similarity between Brazil and Italy comes from the implantation of the neoliberal model destroying public devices of health services and surveillance in Italy after 2010. What is the origin of the Italian tragedy of the Coronavirus[3,4]? In 2020, Italy completed ten years of budget cuts. It is estimated that the country had a deficit of 56,000 doctors and 50,000 nurses. In addition, between 2015 and 2020, 758 Italian health establishments were closed, including clinics, polyclinics, health centres, and hospitals.

This demolition of the public apparatus of health care and surveillance in Italy resulted from the practices called fiscal and budgetary 'austerity' of the states, required by the ECB-EEC-IMF 'Troika' (European Central Bank, European Economic Commission and the International Monetary Fund), which required governments to set aside most of the public budget to finance bank interest and public debt and limited investments, public services, and social security rights. The 'austerity' that closed the Italian public health apparatus was similar to that which came to be applied in Brazil after the failure of the coalition government (2010-2015), the legal and parliamentary *coup d'état* (2016), and the fraudulent election of the ultra-right wing in 2018.

Similar ultraliberal programs took place at the same time in Chile, Peru, Argentina, Paraguay, Ecuador, Colombia, and Bolivia, forced by the pressure of international financial and diplomatic sanctions, by media propaganda campaigns during the elections, by parliamentary coups, or by the so-called 'hybrid war', overthrowing elected governments. The Sars-Cov-2 pandemic or simply the 'new' Coronavirus of Severe Respiratory Distress Syndrome in 2019 flattened the drastic aggression of the ultraliberal model and exacerbated the capital accumulation crisis in order to force a real setback in the implementation of the 'austere States' of countries like The United Kingdom, Germany, and France.

The COVID-19 accelerated European measures to save the poor, to transfer income to informal workers and individual entrepreneurs, the sick, the elderly, and the children. Ultraliberal governments that argued that each person should save themselves began to distribute income to prevent death by starvation and acute illnesses and a wave pillaging and plundering. The US government pressured Brazil to maintain ultraliberal policies while drastically modifying its domestic Minimum Citizen Income policy, promising to distribute a minimum monthly income to all poor Americans during the pandemic. This paradoxical political movement came to Brazil in convulsion at the rising peak of the pandemic, with 400,000 cases worldwide, and 2,200 in Brazil (3/25/2020)[2].There were and still are people on the Internet defending the closing of borders with the deportation of travellers arriving from an epidemic area. It is inhumane, cruel. and epidemiologically ineffective. Closing borders is ineffective and authoritarian. It serves political and economic interests. We know that fascism does not prevent the migration of bacteria, viruses, toxic agents, smuggling, and authoritarianism. Quite the opposite. What must be done is to hire trained personnel for health surveillance and to increase the 'direct' popular participation in the right to notify, monitor the investigation, and learn about the outcome of the cases. To take in, treat if necessary, notify, investigate, and never close borders.

Travel restriction is a policy that requires departure and arrival control. It must be done with planned monitoring of necessities. People with a strict need to travel on state missions, cases of death, and logistical needs for trade in activities considered essential would travel knowing that, when leaving and arriving, they should undergo signs and symptoms control. In case of contact with the public, they would accept screening tests, if necessary, be in quarantine for the maximum incubation period – 14 days. In controlled circumstances, only people in search of repatriation would travel, those returning to their country of origin, people in search of international cooperation actions, study, migration, and work in activities also considered essential.

Italy, at the beginning of the pandemic, took a swing in the policy of social distancing[4]. Initially, it preferred to close its citizens within their old burghs, small towns in the North. Then, it decided to isolate the elderly and the poor to only later understand that the country should be stopped, allowing solely that people could leave the houses due to the need for food and medicine. Subsequently, they released departures and arrivals without the previous selective restrictions, and then returned again to the recommendations of social distancing. It is one thing to tell citizens not to leave their homes for 15 or 20 days and ask that only food and health materials circulate.

It is another thing and ineffective – to close cities, arrest migrants, and vote on laws in secret. The social control model worked by statisticians and computer science scholars has as its starting point the current situation grading different levels of effectiveness of the 'social distancing' or the 'stay home if you don't want to kill others or get sick'. Brazil sought to convince the population not to leave home. We may be successful in changing the model and reducing the speed of the epidemic with protection and 'flattening the curve'. The people will be able to understand if we can achieve a result that brings us closer to China and South Korea and distances us from what happened in Italy. We hope that the working and poor population do not have to pay for the risk in crowded buses and subways in order to serve the class that can romanticize the quarantine.

Social distancing and universal testing of asymptomatic contacts are the explanations of South Korea's success in blocking the emergence of new cases and reducing mortality to almost 100 times less than Italy. There is no point in testing IGM levels five days after suspicious contacts, signs or symptoms. Rapid testing is required for carriers of viral particles. Brazil has scientific and technological capacity to manufacture diagnostic kits. The Federal University of Bahia and the Oswaldo Cruz Foundation have developed kits on laboratory bench that did not find financing for production in industrial plants. Public funding was lacking because of the 'austere' Constitutional Amendment 95[5].

The success of universal testing has already mobilized even North American health workers. The internet list dedicated to public health called 'spiritof1848' has advocated universal testing in the USA since the end of February 2020, and the use of facial masks by people with the virus or sick people, preventing the spread to the 86% that will be asymptomatic (95% CI: [82% -90%]. Universal testing has allowed Korea to search for and isolate positive asymptomatic patients who are responsible for 55% of the transmission to new cases (95% CI: [46% -62%])[6-8].P What made a difference was to isolate positive asymptomatic patients. That in addition to the action of the gods of hygiene – water and soap. South Korea demonstrated creativity with improvised masks to avoid human contact with aerosols of saliva and human secretions in public transport, even those with reduced capacity.

In the absence of sufficient industrial production, they used everything from tights, pieces of cloth; scraps of paper towels, even cups of bras tied to the face. It became an international joke, but it worked. In March 2020, Brazil still does not have a mobilization and contingency plan for social distancing and collective and individual protection measures.

Only with the Minimum Citizen Income could it prevent the economic death of the popular economy, starvation, and violence. If nothing is done, those who do not catch the Coronavirus will catch the *'Guedesvirus'* of bankruptcy, poverty, and a lack of money for rent, food, electricity, water, and everything that ultraliberals have privatized or want to privatize. Although Brazil does not have an epidemiological health control model, whether vertical or participatory, the country has a set of authoritarian epidemiological laws, which allow the federal government to apply draconian measures without consulting and without allowing actions to defend regional or local interests[9].

The best lists of essential needs and rights of the working population under quarantine and social distancing appeared in the manifesto of the ten Brazilian Union centrals and in the '16 questions from the slums' published by the urban periphery movement[10,11]. The Brazilian Centre for Health Studies (Cebes) has guided its action of studies and translational scientific exchange between the sectors of health, economy, law, popular education, and others, with the interface formalized in the forums of institutions such as the National Health Council and the National Fronts, created to fight for health and for life[12,13].

The discussions in the various instances of the Cebes and the content of its journal 'Saúde em Debate' aim to denounce that the strategy of mitigating to await the immunization of the 'herd' (group immunity) has proved ineffective in Iran and in Italy. The cost of human lives was due to the very high rate of reproduction (Rzero or Ro) that led to serious cases of babies, children and young people, besides elderly adults, with concomitant diseases. This experience did not exist in January because of the low severity rate and proportion of asymptomatic patients, which was unknown in January 2020. Personal protective equipment has proven to be useless or to require several layers of protection, which make them unfeasible for use in the primary care network, due to the high costs of disposal and cleaning, and unavailability due to the volume of demand with the very high number of cases. The extent of this demand was also not yet known in January 2020, and became a concrete reality after the Coronavirus arrived in the Middle East and Europe, in March of the same year.

The impact of it was the extremely high mortality of nurses, assistants, and doctors in Italy, even harming the attendance of hospitals that were dismantled and without staff, with the sickening and death of a high number of health professionals. After understanding the speed of reproduction (Ro = 2.5), the high rate of asymptomatic transmitters (86%), the persistence of the virus for up to several days on furniture, hospital waste, and objects for individual and community use ('fomites' in the health dialect), the inability to reverse the acute inflammatory condition in critically ill patients who are admitted to the Intensive Care Unit (ICU), even with mechanical ventilation for up to 20 consecutive days, have changed the scenario in Europe.

They have also made Trump and Bolsonaro's strategy of letting many people die so as not to paralyze the economy equally unsustainable. We also denounce the strategy of liberating non-essential trade and activities as criminal, putting the working population at risk, in the expectation that the epidemic will be extinguished and admitting the increase in mortality of many poor people from the peripheries, who will not have access to the means that can save their lives, such as access to the ICU of the few hospitals that will be equipped. The strategy of planned suppression was imposed after the dissemination of scientific knowledge on the experience of China, South Korea, Iran, Italy, Germany, and The United Kingdom. The model adopted in the US, which suffers much resistance even there, is a murderous model of colonialist imperialism that imposes mitigation measures with commercial and banking liberation. The Brazilian government has sought to imitate such strategies since the beginning of the year 2020. If the 'liberate all' strategy wins here, we will know that the implication will be to send the people to die so that the economy, the investors, and financiers may profit, as it always happens.

REFERÊNCIAS

1 Corrêa Filho HR. A utopia do debate democrático na vigilância em saúde. Saúde debate [internet]. 2020 [acesso em 2020 fev 19]; 43(123)979-81. Disponível em: https://doi.org/10.1590/0103-1104201912300. [Links]

2 The Centre for Systems Science and Engineering (CSSE) at JHU. 2019-NCov Global Cases By Johns Hopkins CSSE - Online Accrual [Electronic Digital Media]. Baltimore - MD - USA: Johns Hopkins Whiting School of Engineering at JHU; 2020. [acesso em 2020 fev 4]. Disponível em: https://gisanddata.maps.arcgis.com/apps/opsdashboard/index.html#/bda7594740fd40299423467b48e9ecf6. [Links]

3 Nogueira K, Ruivo E, Nogueira P, et al. Em fevereiro, quando contava 17 mortos, a Itália "protegeu a economia" e cancelou isolamento. Hoje são 6 820. Diário do Centro do Mundo [internet]. 2020. [acesso em 2020 mar 26]. Disponível em: https://www.diariodocentrodomundo.com.br/em-fevereiro-quando-contava-17-mortos-a-italia-protegeu-a-economia-e-cancelou-isolamento-hoje-sao-6-820/. [Links]

4 Cimini F. Coronavírus: os 15 dias de brigas políticas que selaram o desfecho trágico da Itália. The Intercept Brasil [internet]. 2020. [acesso em 2020 mar 26]. Disponível em: https://theintercept.com/2020/03/24/coronavirus-poltica-italia/. [Links]

5 Brasil. Casa Civil. Emenda Constitucional nº 95, de 15 de dezembro de 2016 - Altera o Ato das Disposições Constitucionais Transitórias, para instituir o Novo Regime Fiscal, e dá outras providências, CLIV. Diário Oficial da União. 16 Dez 2016. [acesso em 2020 mar 26]. Disponível em: http://pesquisa.in.gov.br/imprensa/jsp/visualiza/index.jsp?data=16/12/2016&jornal=1&pagina=2&totalArquivos=368. [Links]

6 Li R, Pei S, Chen B, et al. Substantial undocumented infection facilitates the rapid dissemination of novel coronavirus (SARS-CoV2). Science. 2020. [acesso em 2020 mar 26]. Disponível em: https://static.poder360.com.br/2020/03/science-estudo-coronavirus-contagio-documentacao-16-mar-2020.pdf. [Links]

7 Silva AAM. Sobre a possibilidade de interrupção da epidemia pelo coronavírus (COVID-19) com base nas melhores evidências científicas disponíveis. Rev. bras. epidemiol. [internet]. 2020 [acesso em 2020 mar 26]; 23. Disponível em: http://www.scielo.br/scielo.php?script=sci_arttext&pid=S1415-790X2020000100100. [Links]

8 Silva AAM. Sobre a importância da ampliação da capacidade de testagem dos sintomáticos para a contenção da epidemia pela COVID-19 no Brasil. Agência Bori [internet]. [acesso em 2020 mar 26]. Disponível em: https://abori.com.br/artigos/sobre-a-importancia-da-ampliacao-da-capacidade-de-testagem-dos-sintomaticos-para-a-contencao-da-epidemia-pela-COVID-19-no-brasil/. [Links]

9 Corrêa Filho HR. Comentário à Lei do Coronavirus 2019: Uma lei autoritária sem garantias de cidadania. CEBES Portal Eletronico [internet]. [acesso em 2020 mar 26]. Disponível em: http://cebes.org.br/2020/02/comentario-a-lei-do-coronavirus-2019-uma-lei-autoritaria-sem-garantias-de-cidadania/. [Links]

10 Borges T. Coronavírus e as quebradas: 16 perguntas ainda sem resposta sobre impacto da pandemia nas periferias. Periferia em Movimento - Informação dos extremos ao centro [internet]. [acesso em 2020 mar 26]. Disponível em: https://periferiaemmovimento.com.br/coronavirus-e-as-quebradas-16-perguntas-ainda-sem-resposta-sobre-impacto-da-pandemia-nas-periferias/. [Links]

11 Central Única dos Trabalhadores. Medidas de proteção à vida, à saúde, ao emprego e à renda dos trabalhadores e trabalhadoras. [internet]. [acesso em 2020 mar 26]. Disponível em: https://www.cut.org.br/noticias/coronavirus-cut-e-centrais-vao-exigir-medidas-de-protecao-ao-emprego-e-a-renda-0d5d. [Links]

12 Centro Brasileiro de Estudos de Saúde. Cebes e a Frente Ampla em Defesa da Saúde dos Trabalhadores apoia, endossa e recomenda o posicionamento do MPT sobre a pandemia do COVID-19. [internet]. [acesso em 2020 mar 26]. Disponível em: http://cebes.org.br/2020/03/cebes-e-a-frente-ampla-em-defesa-da-saude-dos-trabalhadores-apoia-endossa-e-recomenda-o-posicionamento-do-mpt-sobre-a-pandemia-do-COVID-19/. [Links]

13 Athaide C. Propostas de medidas para reduzir os impactos da pandemia de Covid19 nos territórios das favelas brasileiras - #Afavelacontraovirus. CUFA - Central Única de Favelas [internet]. [acesso em 2020 mar 26]. Disponível em: https://www.cufa.org.br/noticia.php?n=MjYx. [Links]

Collaborators

Corrêa Filho HR (0000-0001-8056-8824)* is responsible for elaborating the manuscript. Segall-Corrêa AM (0000-0003-0140-064X)* contributed to the revision of the manuscript.

3. Would The Lockdown Really Be Necessary For The Control Of COVID-19 In Brazil?

Haniel Soares Fernandes[11]

ABSTRACT

The lockdown quarantine applied in Brazil to contain the advances of the new coronavirus pandemic equivalent to European countries without first observing their demographic, socioeconomic and cultural differences, seems to involve political issues, in addition to controlling problems public health. Therefore, it is necessary to explain a critical idea about the type of prior conduct taken by Brazil to control this pandemic through a descriptive approach that links published policies adopted with the structure of the local health system and the country's socio-economic and demographic characteristics, in addition to response to contagion. Thus, examining some facts intrinsic to the pandemic process that is installed in the world today.

INTRODUCTION

Among the various strategies advocated by the world health organization (WHO) to respond to the advancement of the corona virus in the world, are the reduction of secondary infections between close contacts, identification, isolation and care of patients early after symptoms or possible diagnosis, in addition to communicating information criticisms of risks and events to all communities combating misinformation[1]. Several countries have taken this recommendation as a basis for tackling the pandemic without even looking at how their population might react to the climate, demographic density, the economy and the number of people belonging to the risk group, as well as the age group. population age. A study concluded that to avoid further contagion with the corona virus, it would be interesting to avoid close individual contact and social gatherings in each country[2].

Coronavirus Contagion and A Possible Union Among Other Viruses

One work evaluated patients allegedly asymptomatic to COVID-19, observing them on trajectories recently reported since the beginning of 2020 and concluded that there are people who do not have symptoms who appear to have previously developed antibodies to the corona virus[3]. Therefore, at the hospital level, it is important that people who are not suspected of having COVID-19 or who have a mild respiratory disease, are evaluated if they are currently infected sub clinically (viral test)

[1] 1Estácio de Sá University, Nutrition department, Fortaleza, Ceará, Brazil
1São Gabriel da Palha College, Nutrition, mebolism and physiology in sport, Minas Gerais, Brazil
1Faculty of Economics, Administration, Actuaries and Accounting, Federal University of Ceará, Fortaleza, Ceará, Brazil

or if they have been previously infected (serological test) or both [4]. Besides that, the vulnerability to the virus includes differences between women and men with regard to primary care within families and their level of contact with risk groups [5]. Factors that must be taken into account so that the numbers cannot be overestimated with clinical errors in the diagnosis of possible contaminants. Once infected with the new coronavirus, the patient needs prompt attention and efficient treatment to control viral load. Worldwide, the combined treatment of hydroxychloroquine with azithromycin was released by the FDA (food and drug administration) in mid-February from *in vitro* tests. [6,7] and randomized controlled trials demonstrated success in use in patients with COVID-19 in the same month [8-10]. However, the Agência Nacional de Vigilância Sanitária (ANVISA) officially regulated for use in patients with COVID-19 in late March. [11].

This indicates a possible delay in control decisions with the spreading pandemic and may, perhaps, suggest a political bias for the current control of serious cases. Because, of the countries that are above Brazil in number of COVID-19 cases to date, all have a greater number of cured patients, such as Canada, Switzerland and Belgium with 4,474, 9,800 and 4,681, respectively, and greater testing rate per million inhabitants [12]. What makes it possible to create possible questions about the accuracy of the figures released, the effectiveness of the treatments performed and the quality of diagnosis made to patients with this clinical condition in Brazil, in which they need a better screening for optimal detection of the contaminated reals [13] in the midst of a possible union, as the Pan American Health Organization warns of the current epidemiological scenario, of measles, dengue and COVID-19, among others, where attention would be intensified in cases of health surveillance so that there are no misinterpretations of them [14]. Therefore, global cooperation in the sphere of public health and economic development is essential. Since, some costs can be avoided through the global cooperative investment in public health in all countries, including in Brazil, of course, in improving the quality of life and as an engine of economic growth [15].

Some Government Decisions During the New Coronavirus Pandemic

During this urgent phase of the COVID-19 pandemic, decisions must be made using the scarce data available, as scientific evidence will be gradually established as research continues. [16]. So, social distance is still important to minimize the transmission of COVID-19. Besides that, they also include high temperature and relative humidity as factors that slow down viral spread, even without knowing for sure if this pandemic decreases in summer [17]. Since, countries inserted in colder climates should be more concerned with the increase of contagion [18]. As not all countries are adept at horizontal quarantine or "lockdown" [19], perhaps Brazil could have a more holistic and coherent vision for its more than 40 million informal workers [20], who may not have economic stability to remain without moving revenue over an extended period.

The Brazilian Institute of Economics of the Getúlio Vargas Foundation (FGV Ibre) estimates that, due to the crisis of the new coronavirus, 5 million Brazilians may be laid off this quarter [21], This number was intensified due to the closing of trade as a result of the applied "lockdown", intensifying the level of unemployment in the country and joining a mass of informal and unemployed workers without the capacity to exercise labour. In parallel, to help low-income families, the state of São Paulo, with the highest number of cases of corona virus in the country, created a social program to distribute one million basic food baskets to families [22]. What seems to be inconsistent with the assumptions of social distance and with the problems that extend to education, which, with the unexpected closure of schools, can influence the increase in child poverty of low-income families [23]. Thus, a recent study proposes a cyclical strategy in which to be adjusted according to the trends in the number of cases over the weeks, making it possible to regulate the lockdown cycles when the control meets a desired demand, making the contagion number plummets even without a total and continuous blockade of the country's economy [24].

When compared to Italy, the country where the first Brazilian Coronavirus registry came from, at the Albert Einstein hospital in São Paulo on February 26 of this same year [25], and with one of the biggest outbreaks of the new coronavirus pandemic, in which it assumed a rigid process in its quarantine, Brazil has an average income per capita three times lower and substantially fewer jobs [26]. In addition to a lower population density than Europeans, 24.96 against 200.64 people per square kilometre [27]. The high-risk group, individuals over 80, with a mortality rate greater than 14% [12] preenche um parcela de 0,4% da população masculina brasileira contra 1,6% da italiana, além de 0,7% da população feminina brasileira contra 2,2% [27]. Therefore, at the level of Brazil, the action of government public policies, both in health and in the economy, could escape the bias of different countries in combating the advance of the current pandemic and have a holistic and particular view. Where, government, states and municipalities, act unilaterally in controlling the progress of COVID-19 aiming at the best way out for the country and its population.

CONCLUSION

Apparently, public policies applied in Brazil to control the new coronavirus pandemic, may contain biases from other nations. The idea of social detachment plus the application of the "lockdown" that can bring the elderly to asymptomatic people, increasing unemployment in parallel with the promotion of public policies for food distribution, ignoring factors such as tropical climate and demographic density that can reduce contagion along the poor screening of patients and the low number of tests, do not seem to provide a better accuracy in the diagnosis of those infected in the midst of a possible union with other viruses, and they can overestimate the number of people infected and killed by COVID-19.

Strengths and Limitations of This Study

Apparently, public policies applied in Brazil to control the new coronavirus pandemic may contain biases from other nations or ideological politicians. The idea of social detachment coupled with the application of the "lockdown" is in contradiction by bringing together the elderly with asymptomatic individuals, and by increasing unemployment in parallel with the promotion of public food distribution policies. Climatic and sociodemographic factors seem to have been ignored, which are factors directly linked to less contagion in the Brazilian population. The low quality screening of patients and the low number of tests, do not seem to provide a better accuracy in the diagnosis of those infected in the midst of a possible union with other viruses, which may, perhaps, lead to overestimated numbers of those contaminated and / or killed by COVID- 19. The study carried out presents limitations regarding the public policies emphasized, since they converge only in the case of Brazil, in addition to the premises that may be unknown in its performance due to selection and evaluation biases of the data collected until the creation of the work, as they may be intimately outdated during the possible reading of this paper.

REFERENCES

1. Livingston, E., Bucher, K., Rekito, A.,(2020). Coronavirus Disease 2019 and Influenza 2019-2020. *Jama.* 2020;323(12):1122. doi:10.1001/jama.2020.2633

2. Remuzzi, A., Remuzzi, G., (2020). COVID-19 and Italy: what next? *Lancet.* 2020;2:10-13. doi:10.1016/S0140-6736(20)30627-9

3. Li, Q., Guan, X., Wu, P, et al. (2020). Presumed Asymptomatic Carrier Transmission of COVID-19. *N Engl J Med.* 2020;382(13):1199-1207. doi:10.1056/NEJMoa2001316

4. Lipsitch M, Swerdlow D.L., Finelli, L. (2020). Defining the Epidemiology of COVID-19 - Studies Needed. *N Engl J Med.* 2020;382(13):1194-1196. doi:10.1056/NEJMp2002125

5. Wenham, C., Smith, J., Morgan, R., (2020). COVID-19: the gendered impacts of the outbreak. *Lancet.* 2020;395(10227):846-848. doi:10.1016/S0140-6736(20)305262

6. Mahase, E. (2020).COVID-19: six million doses of hydroxychloroquine donated to US despite lack of evidence. *BMJ.* 2020;368(March):m1166. doi:10.1136/bmj.m1166

7. Lenzer, J. (2020). COVID-19: US gives emergency approval to hydroxychloroquine despite lack of evidence. *Bmj.* 2020;369(PG-m1335-m1335):m1335-m1335. doi:10.1136/bmj.m1335

8. Chen, Z., Hu, J., Zhang, Z., et al. (2020). Efficacy of hydroxychloroquine in patients with COVID-19: results of a randomized clinical trial. *medRxiv.* 2020;7:2020.03.22.20040758. doi:10.1101/2020.03.22.20040758

9. Gautret, P., Lagier J-C, Parola, P., et al. (2020). Hydroxychloroquine and azithromycin as a treatment of COVID-19: results of an open-label non-randomized clinical trial. *Int J Antimicrob Agents.* 2020:105949. doi:10.1016/j.ijantimicag.2020.105949

10. Colson, P., Rolain, J., Lagier, J., et al.(2020).Chloroquine and hydroxychloroquine as available weapons to fight COVID-19. *Int J Antimicrob Agents.* 2020;S0924-8579. doi:https://doi.org/10.1016/j.ijantimicag.2020.105949

11. Brasil M da saude. NOTA INFORMATIVA Nº 5 / 2020-DAF / SCTIE / MS. In: *Ministério Da Saúde Secretaria de Ciência, Tecnologia, Inovação e Insumos Estratégicos Em Saúde Departamento de Assistência Farmacêu!Ca e Insumos Estratégicos.* ; 2020:9-12. https://www.saude.gov.br/images/pdf/2020/marco/30/MS---0014167392---NotaInformativa.pdf.

12. WorldoMeter. COVID-19 CORONAVIRUS PANDEMIC. https://www.worldometers.info/coronavirus/#countries. Published 2020. Accessed April 8, 2020.

13. Catherine, A., Hogan., M.D. Ms, Malaya, K., Sahoo, P., Benjamin, A., Pinsky., M.D. P. (2020). Sample Pooling as a Strategy to Detect Community Transmission of SARS-CoV-2. *JAMA Netw Open.* 2020:1-2. doi:10.1056/NEJMp2002125

14. Rodriguez-Morales, A.J., Gallego, V., Escalera-Antezana, J.P., et al.(2020).COVID-19 in Latin America: The implications of the first confirmed case in Brazil. *Travel Med Infect Dis.* 2020;(February):101613. doi:10.1016/j.tmaid.2020.101613

15. McKibbin, W.J., Fernando, R.(2020). The Global Macroeconomic Impacts of COVID-19: Seven Scenarios. *SSRN Electron J.* 2020. doi:10.2139/ssrn.3547729

16. Zhang, W., Qian, B., (2020). Correspondence Making decisions to mitigate COVID-19 with. *Lancet Infect Dis.* 2020;3099(20):30280. doi:10.1016/S14733099(20)30280-2

17. Wang, J. Tang, K., Feng, K., Lv W.(2020). High Temperature and High Humidity Reduce the Transmission of COVID-19. *SSRN Electron J.* 2020. doi:10.2139/ssrn.3551767

18. Notari, A. (2020). Temperature dependence of COVID-19 transmission. *medRxiv.* 2020:1-6. doi:https://doi.org/10.1101/2020.03.26.20044529.

19. Juliana Kaplan LF e MM-J. A third of the global population is on coronavirus lockdown — here's our constantly updated list of countries and restrictions. Business insider. https://www.businessinsider.com/countries-on-lockdowncoronavirus-italy-2020-3. Published 2020. Accessed April 8, 2020.

20. Amorim, D. Brasil tem recorde com 41,4% dos trabalhadores na informalidade. O Estado de S.Paulo. https://economia.estadao.com.br/noticias/geral,brasil-temrecorde-com-41-4-dos-trabalhadores-na-informalidade,70003071073. Published 2020. Accessed April 8, 2020.

21. Barbosa, M. 5 milhões podem entrar na fila do desemprego em apenas três meses.Correio Braziliense. https://www.correiobraziliense.com.br/app/noticia/economia/2020/04/05/internas _economia,842458/5-milhoes-podem-entrar-na-fila-do-desemprego-em-apenastres-meses.shtml. Published 2020. Accessed April 8, 2020.

22.   Pereira, F. SP vai distribuir um milhão de cestas básicas a população de baixa renda. UOL. https://noticias.uol.com.br/saude/ultimasnoticias/redacao/2020/04/07/sp-vai-distribuir-um-milhao-de-cestas-basicas-apopulacao-de-baixa-renda.htm. Published 2020. Accessed April 8, 2020.

23.   Lancker, W. Van, Parolin, Z. (2020). Comment COVID-19 , school closures , and child poverty : a social crisis in the making. *Lancet Public Heal*. 2020;2019(20):2019-2020. doi:10.1016/S2468-2667(20)30084-0

24.   Karin, O., Bar-On, Y.M., Milo T, et al. (2020).Adaptive cyclic exit strategies from lockdown to suppress COVID-19 and allow economic activity. *medRxiv*. 2020:2020.04.04.20053579. doi:10.1101/2020.04.04.20053579

25.   Arrais TA. PANDEMIA COVID-19: O CARÁTER EMERGENCIAL DAS TRANSFERÊNCIAS DE RENDA DIRETA E INDIRETA PARA A POPULAÇÃO VULNERÁVEL DO ESTADO DE GOIÁS. 2020.
      https://repositorio.bc.ufg.br/bitstream/ri/18959/5/Relatório de pesquisa - Tadeu Alencar Arrais - 2020.pdf.

26.   OECD. Brasil - OECD Better Life Index. http://www.oecdbetterlifeindex.org/pt/paises/brazil-pt/. Published 2020. Accessed April 8, 2020.

27.   Density P. Population density. Population density. https://www.populationpyramid.net/pt/densidades-populacionais/brasil/2019/.

4. 'Stay Home Without a Home'

Guya Accornero

Centre for Research and Studies in Sociology,Lisbon University Institute

Mona Harb

Department of Architecture and Design and Beirut Urban Lab, American University of Beirut

Alex F. Magalhães

Institute of Urban and Regional Planning and Research, Federal University of Rio de Janeiro

Felipe G. Santos

Department of Politics, University of Manchester

Giovanni Semi

Department of Cultures, Politics and Society, University of Turin

Samuel Stein

Graduate Centre, City University of New York

Simone Tulumello

Instituto de Ciências Sociais da Universidade de Lisboa

ABSTRACT

This updated report is from a webinar on the impact of lockdown measures put in place globally amid the COVID-19 pandemic on the right to housing and linked political struggles. Three main threads emerged from the conversation: the impacts of the pandemic are deepening pre-existing housing inequalities, while government' responses are largely insufficient; activists and contentious actors worldwide are changing their framings and repertoires to adapt to lockdown measures and attempt to radicalize their action; possibilities, albeit limited, are opening for the construction of global networks of struggle.

INTRODUCTION

This update reports from a webinar on the right to housing vis-à-vis COVID-19 lockdown measures. It took place on April 16, 2020, organized by Guya Accornero and Simone Tulumello in collaboration with the Research Committee 47, 'Social Classes and Social Movements', of the International Sociological Association.[1] Short interventions by Guya Accornero, Mona Harb, Alex Magalhães, Felipe G. Santos, Giovanni Semi and Samuel Stein kicked off the webinar, followed by two rounds of responses to questions posed by the audience via the chat of the streaming service.

The goal of the webinar was to share local and national experiences (from Portugal, Lebanon, Brazil, Spain, Italy and the USA) on how lockdown measures and particularly 'shelter in place' and 'social distancing' orders imposed by governments to slow down the spread of Coronavirus are affecting housing rights and struggles.

During the discussion, which lasted slightly more than a hour and a half, three main threads emerged: the way the COVID-19 pandemic is deepening pre-existing housing inequalities and the insufficiency of governments' responses; the reframing of local and national forms of political and activist organization; and openings for the construction of global networks of struggle. In what follows, we will summarize the discussion following these threads.

Deepening Housing Inequalities and Insufficient Government Responses

The first thread that emerged from the conversation was the perception that the impacts of the COVID-19 pandemic in the housing sector should be overtly understood as the simultaneous addition of further layers to, and the deepening of, pre-existing injustices and inequalities. In Portuguese cities, impacts may be particularly strong due to the dependency of recent economic growth to tourism and real estate, resulting in processes of displacement that have socially weakened many urban fabrics.

In Lebanon, the pandemic is piling up on a national system already affected by a long oligarchic rule, a rentier economy and a financial breakdown. In Brazil, 'staying at home' is almost impossible for the millions living in informal settlements, and an incomplete welfare system is hardly providing all the answers needed. In Italy, where 30 per cent of households already live in overcrowded conditions (compared to the European average of 15 per cent), the impacts are particularly strong for populations already made vulnerable by ten years of homelessness crises, and growing housing problems for minorities, refugees and asylum seekers.

In Spain, new problems are building on top of the long wave of evictions that started during the 2008 economic crisis continued during the following rebound USA, the COVID-19 pandemic is making more evident the explosion of homelessness in many cities, the increasing number of working poor who struggle to pay for housing, and the deadly expressions of racial capitalism. Granted, governments local or national, depending on multilevel governance arrangements in the

---

[1] The recording of the webinar is available at RC47 Youtube page: https://youtu.be/TlAWnZwqDdk.

various countries have been enacting some measures, particularly where the potential for social conflict is more acute. Evictions have been frozen and moratoria on mortgage instalments have been allowed in Portugal, Spain, Italy and several US states.[1] Portugal and Spain have allowed those tenants who have lost part of their income to suspend or postpone rent payments. Italian funds for rent/instalment subsidies have been increased.

Bailout funds for real estate investors and recipients of federal housing subsidies have been offered in the US. Select measures have been adopted virtually everywhere in support of homeless persons and households living in precarious settlements. However, we all agree that these interventions are largely insufficient to cope with the scale of the impacts of the pandemic for a number of reasons. They are not generalized, geographically and socially (for instance, protections have been particularly weak for tenants), and they have often arrived late (with many cases of evictions just before the approval of moratoria). Maybe most importantly, measures have been designed to postpone, rather than solve, growing housing problems. This is the case for temporary moratoria of evictions, but also for suspensions of rent payments when not accompanied by measures to automatically allow the renegotiation of instalments in line with income losses or the cancellation of the debts that will pile up during the emergency.

Shifting Contentious Framings and Repertoires

How did activists and other contentious actors react in the face of the impossibility of using a crucial instrument of their repertoires—that is, public space? 'Staying at home' has become both a necessity and a political argument, even as the slogan 'how to stay at home without a home?' has spread worldwide. But, once again, it has spread with significant geographical differences as pre-existing experiences and resources seem to be playing a crucial role in new struggles. Among the experiences shared, Spain seems to be the country where organization is the fiercest. Rent strikes have been called globally, but only in this country have they reached a national scale, with some 15 thousand households refusing to pay April's rent in an organized way. This is linked to the long and steady growth of housing movements, from the emergence of the Plataforma de Afectados por la Hipoteca (PAH; Platform for those Affected by the Mortgage) during the economic crisis of 2008 to the growth of tenants' unions afterwards, the strength of left-libertarian housing organizations across the country, as well as the wide coalitions built up during these years.

While Spanish movements had discussed the possibility of widespread rent strikes for many years, the outbreak of the pandemic has readied people more to take such action. In Lisbon, struggles have reorganized among two main axes. While activist groups have shifted online to keep supporting households with the greatest housing distress, activist scholars have produced reports to push governmental action. In the USA, while rent strikes are in preparation and workers fight to halt construction on luxury real estate projects for the duration of the public health crisis, mutual aid networks have re-emerged to cover gaps in institutional action through provision of relief to populations most in need. In Italy, social movements have suffered several decades of state repression. Organization has been stronger in fields other than housing, particularly logistics and delivery, that have already been at the forefront of struggles in previous years.

---

[1] In Brazil, federal laws on the matter are being discussed as we complete this report (late April 2020). In the meanwhile, the suspension of payments and evictions, the free provision of utilities to poor households, depends on the action of local authorities or judicial decisions.

In Brazil, social movements have seemed quite weak and forms of 'weak resistance', like unorganized rent strikes, have emerged even as local authorities have been stepping in. In Lebanon, with its fierce street politics against the government between 2015 and 2018, protests calling for rent strikes took place before the lockdown, but housing movements have been pretty fragmented. A crucial dimension of future struggles will be changing patterns of criminalization. On the one hand, lockdown measures criminalize any type of street politics and new forms of digital policing may be on the horizon. On the other, the moratorium on evictions and the expected delay in civil court cases after they reopen will delay, if not ultimately write off, the repressive consequences of actions like rent strikes. Extraordinary periods and social fear often encourage states to be more heavy-handed with groups challenging the status quo but these organizations have more time to strategize and prepare for this in turn.

Toward Global (Housing) Politics?

The third thread emerging from the conversation pushed by the audience in the form of questions and comments, we should admit has been an attempt at reflecting on existing openings for the construction of global activisms and networks of struggle.

Different opinions emerged about the possibility of scaling up housing struggles *per se*, as some of us see other fields of struggle like the environment and wider urban rights to be more useful in developing transnational cooperation. Others, however, pinpointed areas of potential cooperation that are emerging from the proximity of social movements with international housing studies networks, and above all from the transnational nature of housing economics. Real possibility exists, for instance, to create international networks of tenants of global institutional investors and funds as the exploitation of the very ambiguities of the socio-spatial organization of capital has long been a strategy of radical politics.

We all agreed, however, that, to fully exploit such openings, it is crucial that we build relations with other fields of struggle. Some are directly connected with housing—above all, urban planning and mobility and others connected more loosely. One such indirect connection lies in the unexpected ecological impacts of the pandemic, as people in some of the most industrialized areas of the planet experience, even through the hardships of lockdowns, fresh air and bits of nature offered by wild animals wandering in the streets. This may create a space for a wider awareness of the intersection of social and ecological inequalities. We are doing anything but romanticizing the present conjuncture here. Indeed, housing, with all of its many inequalities, is a perfect space from which to understand that 'we are NOT all in this together'. Yet this seems to be a particularly fruitful moment, if anything, to visualize, and possibly make common sense of, the very contradictions of capitalism that radical movements and scholars have denounced for so long. The challenge ahead is triggering those contradictions before they or, possibly better while they are exploited to justify doubling down on long-term trajectories of increasing authoritarianism, policing and repression.

ACKNOWLEDGEMENTS

The webinar is an activity of the project 'HOPES: Housing Perspectives and Struggles (FCT, PTDC/GES-URB/28826/2017; PI: Guya Accornero), and the CIES-ISCTE-IUL Monthly Seminar on Social Movements and Political Action.

5. People Experiencing Homelessness: Their Potential Exposure To COVID-19[1]

[2]Nádia Nara Rolim Lima[a], Ricardo Inácio de Souza[b], Pedro Walisson Gomes Feitosa[c], Jorge Lucas de Sousa Moreira[c],Claudio Gleidiston Lima da Silva[c], Modesto Leite Rolim Neto[a,b,c]

[a]The Suicidology Research Group from Universidade Federal do Ceará (UFC),Fortaleza, Ceará, Brazil.
[b]School of Medicine of Juazeiro do Norte – FMJ/Estácio, Juazeiro do Norte, Ceará, Brazil.
[c]School of Medicine, Federal University of Cariri – UFCA, Barbalha, Ceará, Brazil.

ABSTRACT

Background: Insufficient housing quality is associated with stress and mental health impacts. Crowding, pollution, noise, inadequate lighting, lack of access to green spaces, and other environmental factors associated with slums can exacerbate mental health disorders, including depression, anxiety, violence, and other forms of social dysfunction. **Method**: The studies were identified using large-sized newspapers with international circulation. **Results**: Experts say that people who sleep in shelters or on the streets already have lower life expectancy, suffer from addiction, and have underlying health conditions that put them at greater risk should they develop the virus. There are just so many competing and unmet needs, which makes it much harder for homeless to contend with all of this. If exposed, people experiencing homelessness might be more susceptible to illness or death due to the prevalence of underlying physical and mental medical conditions and a lack of reliable and affordable health care. Nevertheless, without an urgent solution, people experiencing homelessness will remain in limbo. **Conclusions**: Many people living on the streets already have a diminished health condition, higher rates of chronic illnesses or compromised immune systems, all of which are risk factors for developing a more serious manifestation of the coronavirus infection. Those suffering from mental illness may have difficulty in recognizing and responding to the threat of infection. Homeless people have less access to health care providers who could otherwise order diagnostic testing and, if confirmed, isolate them from others in coordination with local health departments.

People Experiencing Homelessness: Their Potential Exposure To COVID -19

About one billion people live in slum-like conditions, making up 30% of the world's urban population. These housing facilities tend to have very little ventilation, drainage and sewage facilities; therefore, diseases spread easily (BBC, 2020). These individuals are much more susceptible to contracting COVID-19 because of cramped quarters, utensil sharing, and lack of

[1] Braz. J. Psychiatry vol.42 no.3 São Paulo May/June 2020 Epub Apr 03, 2020
[2] Correspondence author:Modesto Leite Rolim NetoSchool of Medicine,Federal University of Cariri, UFCA, Barbalha, Ceará, Brazil.Email: modesto.neto@ufca.edu.br

proper sanitation facilities (The Daily Star, 2020). It is known that depression and stress weaken our immune systems. Individuals of low incomes are disproportionately likely to suffer from poor mental health. As the coronavirus continues to unleash mayhem, we could be on an economic precipice (The Guardian, 2020a). Mental-health issues are exacerbated by the uncertainty that has been happening across the world (The Philadelphia Inquirer, 2020). Insufficient housing quality is associated with stress and mental health impacts. Crowding, pollution, noise, poor lighting, poor access to green spaces, and other environmental factors associated with slums can exacerbate mental health disorders, including depression, anxiety, violence, and other forms of social dysfunction (WHO, 2020).

Experts say that keeping hands clean is one of the easiest and best ways to prevent transmission of the new coronavirus, in addition to social distancing. However, homeless and urban poor populations that live in thousands of slums across major cities and towns, maintaining good hygiene, are nearly impossible to notice (International News, 2020). In addition to the public health implications there are deep concerns about violations of human rights (Health Affairs, 2020).

Homeless organizations have been sounding the alarm for weeks. They have been warning that the coronavirus could cause catastrophic harm to unhoused communities amid the absence of a coordinated strategy to aid people already struggling to survive in tents and overcrowded shelters (The Guardian, 2020b). Experts say that people who sleep in shelters or on the streets already have lower life expectancy, suffer from addiction, and have underlying health conditions that put them at greater risk should they develop the virus (CTV News, 2020). There are just so many competing and unmet needs, which makes it much harder for homeless to contend with all of this (Aljazeera, 2020). While some people experiencing homelessness have found refuge in local shelters, more are spread across the state, sleeping on sidewalks and under tunnels.

Many have also erected makeshift homes. Experts say the chronically ill homeless have a unique vulnerability to the new coronavirus. A number that is expected to exponentially rise in the coming days. If exposed, people experiencing homelessness might be more susceptible to illness or death due to the prevalence of underlying physical and mental medical conditions and a lack of reliable and affordable health care. Nevertheless, without an urgent solution, people experiencing homelessness will remain in limbo (The Texas Tribune, 2020).

In the midst of all the conversations about social distancing and sense of entitlement, the mental health and well-being aspect has been relatively less discussed, though it remains one of the foremost challenges for public health in these times of a new 'normal life'. It is very important for people to maintain a 'healthy' mind at this point of time and help those who are particularly vulnerable to mental health challenges. Individual with mental health disorders are by and large vulnerable to day-to-day stressful events; their ability to cope with such stressors is generally not always adequate.

This may result in them having a difficult time to cope with such situations (Citizen Matters, 2020) One of the causes here is everyday life stress. Humility, not certainty less accusation and panic — should be the order of the day (City Journal, 2020). Over half a million people are homeless in the US. Their living conditions and poor health may place them at higher risk for contracting the disease. Many homeless people who do not stay in shelters may sleep in train or bus stations, ride subways or buses or go to the waiting room of a hospital emergency department in the evening. These are places where an exposed person could contaminate doors and bathroom fixtures, chairs or other objects, providing opportunities for spreading the infection to others. Once exposed, homeless people may have a mortality risk due to other health conditions they may already have, such as diabetes, hypertension, cardiovascular disease, and increased age. Many people living on the streets already have a diminished health condition, higher rates of chronic illnesses or compromised immune systems, all of which are risk factors for developing a more serious manifestation of the coronavirus infection. Those suffering from mental illness may have difficulty in recognizing and responding to the threat of infection. Homeless people have less access to health care providers who could otherwise order diagnostic testing and, if confirmed, isolate them from others in coordination with local health departments (Next City, 2020). People experiencing homelessness are increasingly older and sicker. Many have underlying health conditions but lack access to primary-care physicians or preventive health screenings. They struggle to find public bathrooms to maintain their basic hygiene. Those who live in tent encampments or crowded shelters might be unable to keep their distance from others or self-isolate if they show symptoms (The Washington Post, 2020). They have only been invalidated by bad luck and social injustice. COVID-19 is likely to serve up even more injustice for them. Finally, it is noteworthy that this needs proper attention from a high level [in social psychiatry] (Ham & High, 2020).

CONCLUSION

Insufficient housing quality is associated with stress and mental health impacts. Homeless organizations have been sounding the alarm for weeks. They've been warning that the coronavirus could cause catastrophic harm to unhoused communities amid the absence of a coordinated strategy to aid people already struggling to survive in tents and overcrowded shelters. Depression and stress weaken our immune systems. Individuals with low incomes are disproportionately likely to suffer from poor mental health. As the coronavirus continues to unleash mayhem, we could be on an economic precipice.

REFERENCES

BBC, 2020. Coronavirus: Why washing hands is difficult in some countries. https://www.bbc.com/news/world-51929598
The Daily Star, 2020. Tough times ahead in the wake of coronavirus. https://www.thedailystar.net/opinion/open-dialogue/news/tough-times-ahead-the-wake-coronavirus-1882108

The Guardian, 2020a. We're about to learn a terrible lesson from coronavirus: inequality kills. https://www.theguardian.com/commentisfree/2020/mar/14/coronavirus-outbreak-inequality-austerity-pandemic
The Philadelphia Inquirer, 2020. Dealing with mental health and the coronavirus: 'It's triggering.' https://www.inquirer.com/health/coronavirus/coronavirus-COVID-19-philadelphia-pennsylvania-mental-health-ocd-depression-anxiety-20200320.html
WHO, 2020. Housing and health equity. https://www.who.int/sustainable-development/housing/health-equity/en/
International News, 2020. Lack of clean water for India's poor spawns virus concerns. https://www.wsav.com/news/international-news/lack-of-clean-water-for-indias-poor-spawns-virus-concerns/
Health Affairs, 2020. What Questions Should Global Health Policy Makers Be Asking About The Novel Coronavirus? https://www.healthaffairs.org/do/10.1377/hblog20200203.393483/full/
The Guardian, 2020b. 'If I get it, I die': homeless residents say inhumane shelter conditions will spread coronavirus. https://www.theguardian.com/world/2020/mar/19/if-i-get-it-i-die-homeless-residents-say-inhumane-shelter-conditions-will-spread-coronavirus
CTV News, 2020. Coronavirus outbreak among homeless would be 'devastating,' experts warn. https://www.ctvnews.ca/health/coronavirus/coronavirus-outbreak-among-homeless-would-be-devastating-experts-warn-1.4859225

Aljazeera, 2020. Homeless amid the coronavirus outbreak. https://www.aljazeera.com/news/2020/03/homeless-coronavirus-outbreak-200311121536154.html

The Texas Tribune, 2020. Staying home slows the coronavirus, but what if you're homeless? https://www.texastribune.org/2020/03/18/coronavirus-homeless-texas/

Citizen Matters, 2020. COVID-19: "Community spread could lead to proportional rise in mental illness cases". https://citizenmatters.in/community-spread-of-coronavirus-and-mental-illness-16535

City Journal, 2020. Some Coronavirus Humility. https://www.city-journal.org/coronavirus-pandemic-humility

Next City, 2020. The Coronavirus Could Hit People Experiencing Homelessness Hard. https://nextcity.org/daily/entry/the-coronavirus-could-hit-people-experiencing-homelessness-hard

The Washington Post, 2020. Follow the outbreak with Coronavirus Updates. https://www.washingtonpost.com/local/cities-struggle-to-protect-vulnerable-homeless-populations-as-coronavirus-spreads/2020/03/20/1144249c-67be-11ea-b5f1-a5a804158597_story.html

Ham & High, 2020. Coronavirus: Act now to protect homeless people warns north London doctor. https://www.hamhigh.co.uk/news/health/coronavirus-act-now-to-protect-homeless-people-warns-north-london-doctor-1-6566354

6. Intraregional Propagation of COVID-19 Cases In Pará, Brazil. Assessment of Isolation Regime To Lockdown.

Félix Lélis da Silva [a], Javier Dias Pita [b], Maryjane Diniz A. Gomes [c], Andréa P. Lélis da Silva [d], Gabriel Lélis P. da Silva [e]

[a, b, c] Federal Institute of Science and Technology of Pará – IFPA Campus Castanhal

[a, b, b] Research Group for Biosystems Management, Modeling and Experimentation GEMAbio

[d] Metropolitan Regional Hospital, Specialist in Intensive Care Unit

[e] Estácio de Sá College of Castanhal, Law undergraduate student.

ABSTRACT[1]

Due to the high incidence of COVID-19 case numbers internationally, the World Health Organization (WHO) declared a Public Health Emergency of global relevance, advising countries to follow protocols to combat pandemic advance through actions that can reduce spread and consequently avoid a collapse in the local health system. On March 18, 2020, Pará notified the first case of COVID-19. After seven weeks, the number of confirmed cases reached 4,756 with 375 deaths. Knowing that infected people may be asymptomatic, the disease symptomatology absence and the population's neglect of isolation influence the spread, and factors such as chronic pneumonia, high age, obesity, chronic kidney diseases and other comorbidities favour the mortality rate. On the other hand, social isolation, quarantine and lockdown seek to contain the intraregional contagion advance. This study analyses the dynamics of COVID-19 new cases advance among municipalities in the state of Pará, Brazil. The results show it took 49 days for 81% of the state's municipalities to register COVID-19 cases. The association between social isolation, quarantine and lockdown as an action to contain the infection was effective in reducing the region's new cases registration of COVID-19 in the short-term.

---

[1] corresponding author (s): Félix Lélis da Silva (felix.lelis@ifpa.edu.br), Javier Dias Pita (javier.pita@ifpa.edu.br), Maryjane Dias A. Gomes (maryjane.gomes@ifpa.edu.br), Andréa P. Lélis da Silva (andlelis@yahoo.com.br), Gabriel Lélis P. da Silva (biellellis@yahoo.com.br).

1. NTRODUCTION

The COVID-19 pandemic stands out as the main global health crisis (Wu et al., 2020). It started in Wuhan, China in December 2019 (Şahin, 2020; Ahmadi et al., 2020; See et al., 2020). It is a respiratory infection caused by the coronaviruses family (2019nCoV) (Prata et al., 2020). Its etiological agent is Sars-CoV-2 (Saez et al., 2020; Yang et al., 2020), which causes severe acute respiratory syndrome (SARS) (Solé at al., 2020). The viral infection presents severe clinical symptoms such as fever, dry cough, dyspnoea, and pneumonia (Coccia, 2020; Wu et al., 2020) and can cause the death of the infected (Waldecy; David; Wainesten; 2020). Flu is one of the main causes of illnesses and death in the world (Mertz et al., 2013). Epidemiological data associated with COVID-19 infection has shown different dynamics in several countries (Marson; Ortega, 2020). Several studies have shown the reverse effect of rising temperatures and the confirmed number of new cases (Zhu and Xie, 2020; Wu et al. 2020). Brazil, a country with a tropical climate, with an average annual temperature ranging from 16 to 27.4 ºC, modelled results show a negative effect on the linear relationship of temperature with the new confirmed cases number (Prata et al., 2020). Several factors have contributed to pandemic advance in Brazil, as the country, in addition to having a deficiency in the number of doctors per inhabitant, the number of ICU beds and ventilators available for urgent and emergency cases, presents several risk groups, such as: elderly over 60 years old, people with prognostic comorbidity, indigenous people and population's great genetic variation (Marson; Ortega, 2020). Government actions to mitigate the COVID-19 epidemic curve have been adopted in several countries. In Spain, according to Saez (2020), measures of social distancing led to a cases curve flattening, after the first few days the cumulative change rate in new cases decreased by an average of 3.059 percentage points daily. In Pará state, high mortality and lethality rates were reported even with social isolation, which raised the curve of new cases and directly affected hospital care due to overcrowding by infected people. On May 6, 2020, a more extreme control policy was decreed by the State of Pará government aimed at containing the pandemic advance, setting the lockdown model in the metropolitan region and neighbouring municipalities. People's traffic control measures are fundamental in controlling the pandemic progress. According to Kucharski et al. (2020), the cases' reduction of COVID-19 in Wuhan observed in February 2020, coincided with traveling control measures adopted in the region.

Therefore, it has been suggested that environmental factors and social control through social distancing tend to control the new cases and deaths numbers due to COVID-19. As well, the deficiency in the health system associated with the reduced number of intensive-care physicians, low numbers of mechanical ventilators, the minimum number of available beds, and the specific medication absence tend to compromise the diagnosed population care. It is questioned: What are the dynamics of new community cases and mortality records evolution due to COVID-19 in subtropical regions with temperatures between 20 and 35 ºC, with social distancing by quarantine and lockdown adoption?

2. MATERIALS AND METHODS

2.1 Study area

The study was carried out in 114 affected municipalities among the 144 existing in the state of Pará, North region, Brazil (Fig.1). The state has a territorial extension of 247,689,515 km² and an estimated population of 8,602,285 people, with 8,191,559 residents in urban areas and 2,389,492 in rural areas, with a population density of 6.07 inhabitants/km² and an average Human Development Index of (HDI = 0.698) (BIGS, 2020).

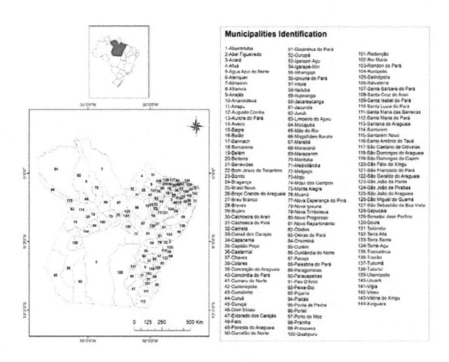

Fig. 1. State of Pará, Northern Brazil and its 144 municipalities.

2.2. Data collection

The cumulative daily number of deaths by age group and sex of COVID-19 cases in 114 municipalities in the state of Pará, with a record of infection, were obtained through the daily monitoring of technical bulletins provided by the State of Pará Public Health Secretary (SHSP, 2020). General data for Brazil and its northern region were obtained from the Secretary of Health Surveillance of the Ministry of Health (BRAZIL, 2020).

2.3. Statistical analysis

Since understanding the dynamics of infection spread can favour more effective public control policies and allow control of transmission in new regions, an exploratory data analysis (EDA) was carried out, with numerical variables described using means, standard deviations, coefficient of variation, distributions and Pareto. Weekly maps were built for the new accumulated cases, in the period of 49 days, to assess the spread of the COVID-19 pandemic in the municipalities of the state of Pará. It was used a classification method using the Jenks algorithm based on the Absolute Deviations over the Median of the Classes.

3. RESULTS AND DISCUSSION

3.1 Descriptive analysis

In Brazil, on May 5, 2020, 114,715 cases of COVID-19 were registered and 7,921 deaths, with a lethality rate of 6.8%, the Southeast and Northeast regions are the most affected counting around 75% of the registered cases (Fig 2B). The most affected regions in the country are the Southeast (64,756; 44.6%), followed by the Northeast (45,724; 31.5%) and North (23,207; 16.0%) (BRASIL, 2020). In the North, the state of Amazonas had the largest number of confirmed infected, 10,727 cases and disease lethality around 874 registered deaths. The country on May 6, 2020, registered 114,715 cases and 7,921 deaths.

In Northern Brazil, the federative units most affected on May 5, 2020, in terms of the spatial distribution of registered cases of COVID-19 with an incidence and mortality rate per 1,000,000 inhabitants, were Amazonas (2327.5 and 251.7) and Pará (627.4 and 49.5).

The capital of Pará has the highest incidence (1,816.4/1,000,000 inhabitants)and mortality (240/1,000,000 inhabitants) with a mortality rate of 9.9% (Fig. 3B).Predictive studies in Brazil report smaller records of new cases of COVID-19 at temperatures around 25.8ºC, reducing the behaviour of curve growth (Prata et al., 2020).Since SARS-CoV-2 may be vulnerable to fluctuations in environmental conditions similar to other coronaviruses (Le et al., 2020). It is important to note that climatological factors variability can interfere with the curve behaviour even at higher temperatures. The northern region of Brazil has an equatorial climate ranging from humid to semi-arid, with temperatures ranging from 20 to 35 ºC. In the state of Pará, the temperature presents spatial and seasonal homogeneity, with an average variation of 25 ºC to 35 ºC. In the region, there are two distinct periods of temperature ranges, classified as rainier between December to May and less rainy between June to November, according to rainfall variation that occurs in the Amazon. The metropolitan region of Belém city in the period between January 1, 2020, to May 5, 2020, presented temperature variation between 24 ºC to 31 ºC and relative humidity between 70 to 80%. In this period, the number of new cases and mortality due to COVID-19 has risen since the first case notification on March 18, 2020, with the first death recorded on April 1, (Fig.2).

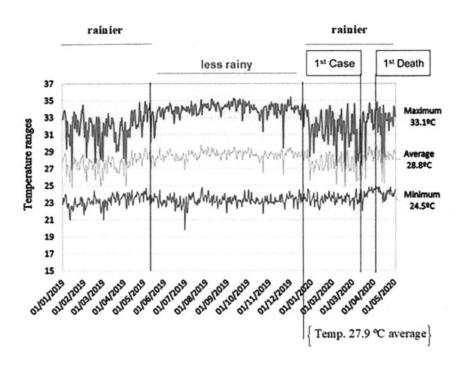

Fig. 2. Temperature behaviour (ºC), rainfall behaviour, 1st confirmed case and 1st death registration by COVID-19 in the state of Pará.

The North region was in 3rd place in cases number with approximately 16% of the confirmed cases on May 5, 2020. In the state of Pará, the outbreak of COVID-19 registered a record of 4,756 cases with an incidence rate of 788 cases in 49 days after the first infection confirmation. The first confirmed case of the disease was notified on March 18, 2020, in Belém city, capital of the state. These records occurred when the average temperature of the region, for the period considered to be the rainiest in the region, was 27.9 ºC and the air relative humidity ranging from 70 to 80%.

The first notification of death occurred on April 1, 2020, and since then the curve of new cases and deaths incidence have been frequent and registered with high rates in the region. *A priori* it is suggested that there is no inverse relationship between ambient temperature and new cases of COVID-19 in Pará in the period considered as the rainiest in the Amazon region. Therefore, there is no evidence to suppose that in regions with warm climates, low relative humidity and high rainfall variation, the cases number is lower compared to regions with moderate and/or cold climates.

Similar results were obtained by Jahangiri, Jarangiri, Njafgholipour (2020) in the transmission rate evaluation of the new coronavirus in different provinces of Iran.

The overall cases number compared to diagnosed population sex, the cumulative daily descriptive statistics of newly notified cases of COVID-19, and the age group distribution behaviour of diagnosed population with the infection since the first disease case notified in the State of Pará. The analysis was carried out after seven weeks of the first COVID-19 case recorded in Pará, being 4,756 cases reported between March 18 to May 5, 2020. Of the total, 2,420 (50.9%) diagnosed cases were men and had an average age of 45.6 years.

The women were 2,320 (48.8%) infected cases with an average age of 47.4 years. It is reported that 15 registered cases did not present notification regarding gender and were considered as unidentified. Similar results of higher COVID-19 cases prevalence in men were obtained by Chen et al. (2020) and Nikpouraghdam et al., (2020).In Pará, 75% were under 58 years old. Only 25% of infected cases were elderly and 1.6% of those diagnosed infected were children from 0 to 10 years old. Only 26 (0.5%) registered cases had no age identified and were considered in terms of registration as "unidentified". In terms of the sample of the infected population age range, negative asymmetric behaviour was identified for distribution, with ages concentration around the median of 34 years old, with 80% of cases diagnosed aged between 20 and 60 years old

In Iran, the cases concentration was between 30 and 70 years old for 79.1% of COVID19 records and approximately 39% for the elderly (Nikpouraghdam et al., 2020). Concerned with the new cases and mortality rates, the government of Pará established a decree for lockdown in the capital and additional nine municipalities to increase the social isolation index, reducing the disease spread and reducing the new cases registration number of COVID-19.The restrictive measure was initially focused on forcing social isolation in the municipalities of Belém, Ananindeua, Marituba, Benevides, Santa Bárbara do Pará, Santa Izabel do Pará, Castanhal, which form the Belém Metropolitan Region (BMR) and inland towns, such as Santo Antonio do Tauá, Vigia de Nazaré and Breves. The lockdown arises when the state of Pará registered a COVID-19 rate in the order of 51/100,000 inhabitants, higher than the national rate.

The municipalities affected by the restriction presented rates of 75/100,000 inhabitants, higher than that registered by the state. Despite the restrictions having focused on only 10 municipal regions, it is worth mentioning that when the lockdown was set, more than 70% of the municipalities forming the state of Pará already had notifications of COVID-19 cases.

The regional disease expansion and the high registration rates in the BMR have compromised the structure of the state's public and private healthcare systems due to the high demand for basic care services and the high need for more complex services involving hospitalizations and intubation of patients with aggravated cases.

In Pará state, severe cases of COVID-19 and mortality records are related to several comorbidities, the most commons are associated with heart disease, diabetes, kidney disease, pneumonia, immunodeficiency, asthma, obesity, neurological disease, haematological disease and illness hepatic; the most frequent ones being associated with heart disease and diabetes (Fig. 3). According to Chen et al. (2020), patients infected with COVID-19 tend to have associated comorbidities with one or more chronic diseases. In Iran, patients diagnosed with COVID-19 had a strong association with chronic diseases such as diabetes, chronic respiratory diseases, hypertension, cardiovascular diseases, kidney diseases and cancer, these comorbidities were also observed in cases of deaths (Nikpouraghdam et al. 2020). Similar results were verified in infected people in Wuhan, China (Wu et al., 2020), corroborating with the results occurred in this study region.

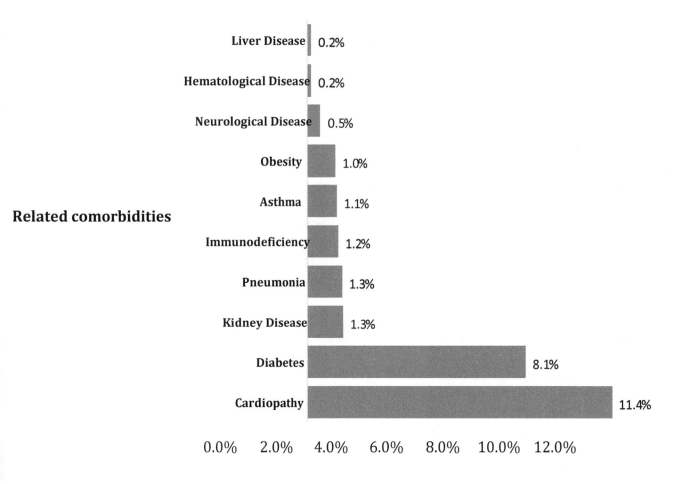

Related comorbidities

Liver Disease	0.2%
Hematological Disease	0.2%
Neurological Disease	0.5%
Obesity	1.0%
Asthma	1.1%
Immunodeficiency	1.2%
Pneumonia	1.3%
Kidney Disease	1.3%
Diabetes	8.1%
Cardiopathy	11.4%

0.0% 2.0% 4.0% 6.0% 8.0% 10.0% 12.0%

ecords

Fig. 3. Common comorbidities in diagnosed cases of COVID-19 in the state of Pará, from March 18 to May 5, 2020.

These factors associated with the precarious service capacity of hospitals and emergency care units (ECU), the insufficient health professional staff, lack of rapid tests to identify infected patients, contributed to COVID-19 advance in the region. Associated with these problems, there is still an insufficient hospital beds number available according to the State Department of Public Health of Pará. There are only 249 ICU beds available for adults care in the pandemic for a population of 7,581,051 inhabitants, which represents a ratio of 1/30,445.98 bed/inhabitants, such fact leads the system to collapse in a short period during a pandemic, contributing to the disease and the number of deaths progress. Collapsing is already experienced in paediatric clinic beds (Table 1).

Due to the risk of COVID-19 infected people promoting the disease advance through community transmission to more remote regions of the state, it is essential to understand the dynamics of disease new cases to enable decision-making regarding control, prevention, treatment of infected, identify groups of risks and enable decision making on resources allocation and allow better planning on the health system in difficult times.

Table 1: Availability and occupation of exclusive hospital beds for COVID-19 in the public healthcare system in the state of Pará.

Hospital bed type	Total	Available	% Occupation
Paediatric	1109	497	55.2
Paediatric clinical	8	8	0.0
adult ICU	249	37	85.2
Paediatric ICU	7	4	42.9
Intermediate unit	26	25	3.9
Neonatal ICU	4	1	75.0

Source: Secretary of Public Health of Pará.
https://portalarquivos.saude.gov.br/images/pdf/2020/May/09/2020-05-06-BEE15Boletim-do-COE.pdf

Results show that a week after the first notified case, only 0.82% of the municipalities had infected people, in the second week of contagion they already had 5.56%, in the third 15.3%, in the fourth 24.3%, in the fifth 46.5%, in the sixth 69.4% and the seventh week after the first notified case, there were already 81.8% of the municipalities in the state of Pará with notified COVID-19 cases (Fig.5). The highest concentration of registered cases was in the Metropolitan Region of Belém, constituted by the capital Belém, Ananindeua, Marituba, Benevides, Santa Bárbara do Pará, Santa Izabel do Pará, Castanhal. The measure of containment by social isolation in the region did not have an expected effect on the curve of new cases for the period under study, mainly due to the low rate of population adherence. However, the lockdown instituted on May 5, 2020, gave positive percentage results in the short-term on new cases registration in the following week of decreed intervention, with a 10.07% reduction compared to the accumulated record in the week previous epidemiologic.In the long-term, the reduction of the cases may be more significant, given the greater respect and adherence of the population to isolation policies.

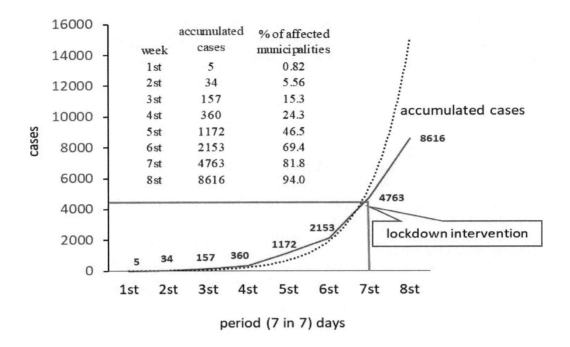

week	accumulated cases	% of affected municipalities
1st	5	0.82
2st	34	5.56
3st	157	15.3
4st	360	24.3
5st	1172	46.5
6st	2153	69.4
7st	4763	81.8
8st	8616	94.0

Fig. 4. Propagation of notified COVID-19 cases in the municipalities of the state of Pará, from March 18 to May 5, 2020, and the 1st post-lockdown period.

Efforts to prevent infected people from reaching more remote regions are important to stop disease transmission and prevent new cases (Coccia, 2020). To understand the dynamics of COVID-19 cases advance to remote regions from the capital, 7 maps were adjusted and show the weekly evolution of the accumulated cases registered in the municipalities of the state (Figures 5 to 11).

The municipalities that registered cases of infection in the first week were Belém (code 19) with 2 cases and Marabá (code 67) with 1 notified case (Fig. 5). The municipalities that did not present COVID-19 case records in the seven weeks after the first case were: Abel Figueiredo (code 2), Aveiro (code 14), Belterra (code 20), Brasil Novo (code 25), Brejo Grande do Araguaia (code 26), Cachoeira do Arari (code 30), Cumaru do Norte (code 41), Curionópolis (code 42), Eldourado dos Carajas (code 47), Faro (code 48), Araguaia Forest (code 49), Gurupá (code 52), Jacareacanga (code 60), Mojuí dos Campos (code 74), Piçarra (code 93), Plates (code 94), Rio Maria (code 102), Rurópolis (code 104), Santa Luzia do Pará (code 112), Santa Maria das Barreiras (code 111), Santana do Araguaia (code 113) Francisco do Pará (code 121), Sapucaia (code 128), Soure (code 130), Trairão (code 136) and Vitória do Xingu (code 120) (Fig.12).

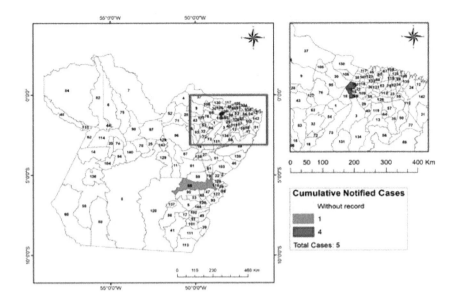

Fig. 5. Propagation of new cases of COVID-19 accumulated in the municipalities of the 288 state of Pará in the 1st week after registration of the first case in the region.

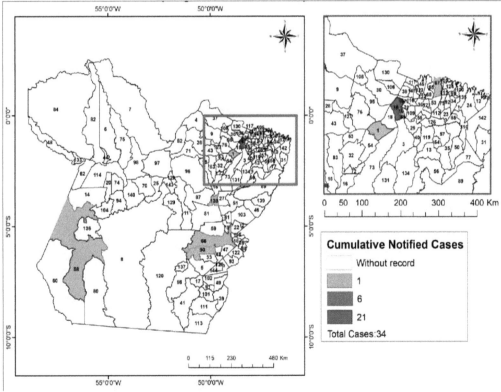

Fig. 6. Propagation of new cases of COVID-19 accumulated in the municipalities of the state of Pará in the 2nd week after registration of the first case in the region.

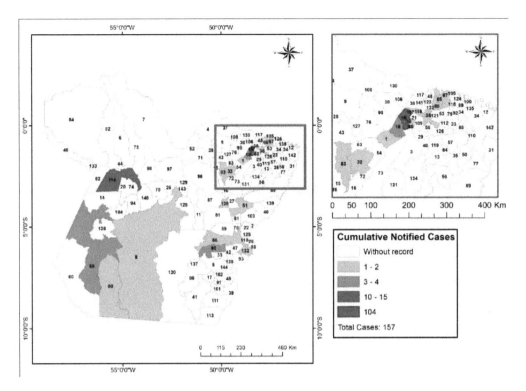

Fig. 7. Propagation of new cases of COVID-19 accumulated in the municipalities of the state of Pará in the 3rd week after registration of the first case in the region.

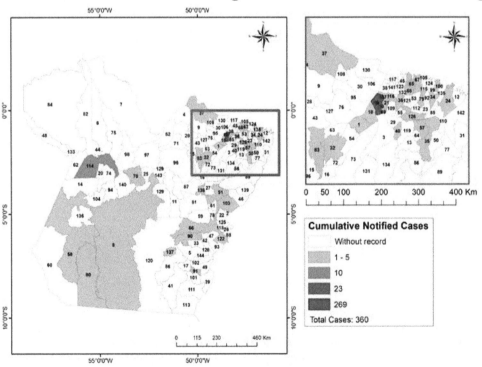

Fig. 8. Propagation of new cases of COVID-19 accumulated in the municipalities of the state of Pará in the 4th week after registration of the first case in the region.

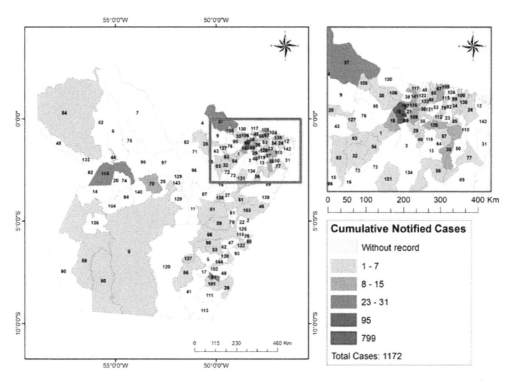

Fig. 9. Propagation of new cases of COVID-19 accumulated in the municipalities of the state of Pará in the **5th week** after registration of the first case in the region.

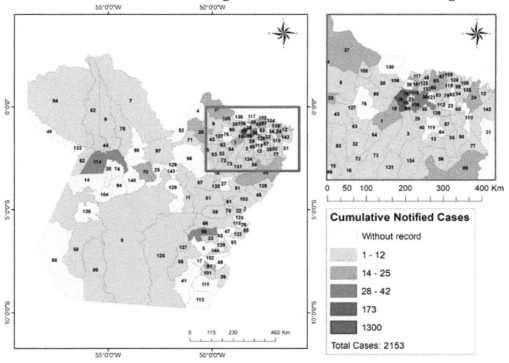

Fig. 10. Propagation of new cases of COVID-19 accumulated in the municipalities of the state of Pará in the 6th week after registration of the first case in the region.

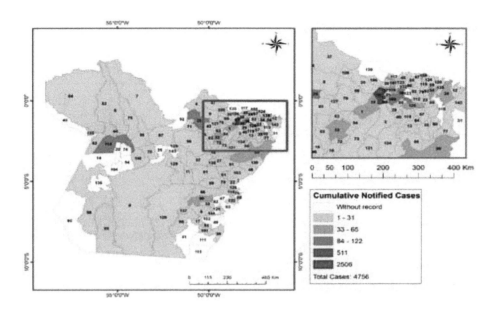

Fig. 11. Propagation of new cases of COVID-19 accumulated in the municipalities of the state of Pará in the 7ᵗʰ week after registration of the first case in the region.

4. CONCLUSIONS

Several factors can influence the spread of the virus and consequently influence the rate of incidence and mortality. In this research, the incidence rate and mortalities in Brazil and the North region were analysed, as well as the monitoring of dynamics of the COVID-19 progress for the municipalities of the state of Pará. The results indicated that 49 days were necessary to 81% out of 144 municipalities over an area of approximately 1,248,000 km² were affected by COVID-19 cases. Social isolation was not efficient to contain new cases advance, due to low population adherence. The social isolation and quarantine associated with the adoption of a strict measure of population circulation, the "Lockdown", and the mandatory use of masks in public environments were effective in reducing new cases of COVID-19 registration in the short-term.

Acknowledgments

This study was prepared with support from the Research Group for Biosystems Management, Modelling and Experimentation - GEMAbio.

REFERENCES

Ahmadi, M., Sharifi, A., Dorosti. S., Ghoushchi. S. J., Ghanbari, N. Investigation of effective climatology parameters on COVID-19 outbreak in Iran. Science of The Total Environment. 2020. v.729. DOI. https://doi.org/10.1016/j.scitotenv.2020.138705.

Brazil. Ministry of Health. Accumulated COVID-19 cases and deaths by confirmation date. Available at: https://covid.saude.gov.br/. Access date: May 9 2020.

Coccia, M. Factors determining the diffusion of COVID-19 and suggested strategy to prevent future accelerated viral infectivity similar to COVID, **Science of the Total Environment**. 2020. https://doi.org/10.1016/j.scitotenv.2020.138474.

Mertz D., Kim T. H., Johnstone J., Lam P. P., Kuster S. P., Fadel S. A. et al., Populations at risk for severe or complicated influenza illness: systematic review and meta-analysis, BMJ. 2013. DOI. https://doi.org/10.1136/bmj.f5061.

BIGS. Brazilian Institute of Geography and Statistics. Populations. Available at:

Jahangiri, M., Jahangiri, Milad., Najafgholipour, M. The sensitivity and specificity analyses of ambient temperature and population size on the transmission rate of the novel coronavirus (COVID-19) in different provinces of Iran. 2020. Science of The Total. Environment. v.728, DOI. https://doi.org/10.1016/j.scitotenv.2020.138872.

Kucharski. A. J., Russell. T. W., Diamond. C., Liu. Y., Edmunds. J., Funk. S., et al. Early dynamics of transmission and control of COVID-19: a mathematical modelling study. Lancet Infect Dis. 2020. DOI.

Le.N. K., Parikh. A. V., Brooks. J., Gardellini. J. P., Izurieta. T. R., 2020. Ecological and health infrastructure factors affecting the transmission and mortality of COVID-19

BMC Infect. Dis. https://doi.org/10.21203/rs.3.rs-19504/v1.

Marson, F. A. L., Ortega. M. M.COVID-19 in. Brazil. Pneumology. 2020. DOI. https://doi.org/10.1016/j.pulmoe.2020.04.008.

Nikpouraghdam et al. Epidemiological characteristics of coronavirus disease (COVID19) patients in IRAN: A single centre study. 2020. Journal of Clinical Virology. 2019.

SHSP. Secretary of Health of the State of Pará (SHSP). Coronavirus in Pará. Available at: https://portalarquivos.saude.gov.br/images/pdf/2020/May/09/2020-05-06-BEE15Boletim-do-COE.pdf. Date accessed: 10 May. 2020.

Prata, D. N., Rodrigues W., Bermejo, P. H. Temperature significantly changes COVID19 transmission in (sub) tropical cities of Brazil. 2020. Science of the Total Environment. v.729. 138862.DOI. https://doi.org/10.1016/j.scitotenv.2020.138862.

Saez, M., Tobias, A., Varga, D., Barceló, M. A. Effectiveness of the measures to flatten the epidemic curve of COVID-19. The case of Spain. Science of the Total Environment. 2020. v. 727. 138761. DOI. https://doi.org/10.1016/j.scitotenv.2020.138761.

Şahin, M. Impact of weather on COVID-19 pandemic in Turkey. Science of the Total Environment. 2020. v.720. DOI. https://doi.org/10.1016/j.scitotenv.2020.138810.

See. K. C., Liew, S.M., David C. E. N., et. al., COVID-19: Four Paediatric Cases in Malaysia. 2020. International Journal of Infectious Diseases. v. 94, p. 125–127. DOI. https://doi.org/10.1016/j.ijid.2020.03.049

olé et al. Guidance for the care of neuromuscular patients during the COVID-19 pandemic outbreak from the French Rare Health Care for Neuromuscular Diseases Network, Revue Neurologique. 2020.DOI.https://doi.org/10.1016/j.neurol.2020.04.004.

Waldecy. R., David. N. P., Wainesten. C. Regional determinants of the expansion of COVID-19 in Brazil. 2020, MedRxiv. doi: https://doi.org/10.1101/2020.04.13.20063925

Yang, Y., Peng, F., Wang, R., Guan, K., Jiang, T., Xu, G., Sun, J., Chang, C. The deadly coronaviruses: The 2003 SARS pandemic and the 2020 novel coronavirus epidemic in China. 2020. J. Autoimmun. 102434. Https://doi.org/10.1016/j.jaut.2020.102434

Wu Y., Jing W., Liu J., Ma Q., Yuan J., Wang Y., Du M., Liu M. Effects of temperature and humidity on the daily new cases and new deaths of COVID-19 in 166 countries. 2020. Science of the Total Environment.v.729.139051. DOI: https://doi.org/10.1016/j.scitotenv.2020.139051.

Zhu Y., Xie J., 2020. Association between ambient temperature and COVID-19 infection in 122 cities from China. 2020. Sci. Total Environ. 138201. DOI. https://doi.org/10.1016/j.scitotenv.2020.138201.

CHAPTER 18

THE IMPACT OF SOCIAL DISTANCING

1. The Impact of Early Social Distancing At COVID-19 Outbreak In The Largest Metropolitan Area Of Brazil.

Fabiana Ganem[1], Fabio Macedo Mendes[2],
Silvano Barbosa de Oliveira[1], Victor Bertollo Gomes Porto[1],
Wildo Navegantes de Araújo[2], Helder I. Nakaya[3,4],
Fredi A. Diaz-Quijano[5], Julio Croda[1,6,7,8].

ABSTRACT

We calculated the impact of early social distancing on the COVID-19 transmission in the São Paulo metropolitan area and forecasted the ICU beds needed to cope the epidemic demand by using an age-stratified SEIR model. Within 60 days, these measures would avoid 89,133 deaths.

INTRODUCTION

The COVID-19 pandemic has led to the collapse of healthcare systems in several countries (1). The virus has a higher basic reproduction number ($R0$) (i.e., the average number of secondary cases generated by a primary case when introduced in a fully susceptible population) and case fatality rate (CFR) when compared with Influenza ($R0$:2,5-3,2 and CFR:0,4-2,9% versus $R0$:1,2-2,3 and CFR:0,15%-0,25%, respectively) (2–5). Among the confirmed cases in China, 18.5% were considered severe and 25.3% of those required intensive care (2).

To tackle the spread of disease, a range of interventions have been implemented in China, including increasing test capacity, rapid isolation of suspected and confirmed cases and their contacts, social distancing measures, as well as restricting mobility (6).In Brazil, the first confirmed COVID-19 case was reported on February 26th in the São Paulo city and, since March 16th, the state of São Paulo has recommended several social distancing measures. These include recommending that older adults and individuals with underlying chronic medical conditions stay at home as much as possible; cancelling mass events; reducing public transportation; closing schools, universities and workplaces; and maintaining only essential services.

The São Paulo Metropolitan Area (SPMA), one of the most populous urban area in the world, has 7,300 ICU beds registered in the National Council of Health Establishments (Cadastro Nacional de Estabelecimentos de Saúde, CNES: http://cnes.datasus.gov.br), 2,880 of which belong to the Public Healthcare system.

As the collapse of health care systems is the major concern for most countries hit by the pandemic, non-pharmacological interventions has been recommended to flatten the epidemic curve and gain time to prepare the health system to avoid shortage of ICU beds and healthcare workers needed to treat critically ill patients (4).

THE STUDY

We evaluated the impact of early social distancing measures in the transmission of COVID-19 in the SPMA, and forecast the number of ICU beds necessary for COVID19 patients in Brazil. In 2009, the MoH established a mandatory notification for hospitalized cases of severe acute respiratory illness (SARI) through the National Disease Notification System (SIVEP-GRIPE). We retrieved all SARI cases reported on the SIVEP-GRIPE system between 26th February and 30th March. Those cases were included regardless of COVID19 confirmation as a proxy of COVID19 case. This proxy was used to calculate the time dependent reproductive number R(t) of confirmed COVID19 cases and was chosen in order to minimize the impact of shortage of RT-PCR tests. In addition, we also calculated R(t) using the daily number of COVID19 confirmed cases from the São Paulo state epidemiological records. We calculated the R(t) during one-month period in the SPMA, both, for COVID19 confirmed cases, as well as for SARI cases, and estimated the expected number of SARI cases requiring an ICU bed.

The reproductive number at the beginning of the epidemic (R0) and during the epidemic (Rt) were calculated using the package R0 R Studio (3). The expected ICU demand was calculated using an age stratified SEIR model (7), which includes compartments for individuals requiring hospitalization and intensive care. The model parameters are described in Table 1.

Considering only the confirmed cases reported by São Paulo state, the R(t) was close to 2 throughout the assessed period with a large confidence interval. (Figure 1a). Underreporting and lack of confirmatory tests for COVID19 could directly affect these

R(t) estimations. (Figure 1a). By analysing the number of SARI available in the Epidemiological Surveillance of Influenza System (SIVEP-GRIPE), we found that the social distancing measures reduced the R(t) below to 1 with a more accurate confidence interval (Figure 1b). The R0 was used in the SEIR model to forecast the ICU beds needed and the number of deaths in a scenario without social distancing measures. The R(t) of SARI cases was used to forecast the scenario with social distancing measures. We defined the ICU bed capacity for COVID-19 as 20% of the total number of ICU beds in the SPMA. In the absence of social distancing measures, the model predicts that after 30 days, COVID19 patients would demand 5,384 ICU beds, which surpasses the current ICU capacity in 130%; furthermore, in the second month the ICU bed demand would be 14 times the ICU capacity. Overall, this would result in 1,783 deaths in the first month and 89,349 in the second month. While social distancing measures are maintained, the model predicts 317 deaths in the first month and a total of 1682 in the second. This scenario does not overburden the healthcare system which represents a maximum of 76% ICU beds capacity. Using the severe cases notification systems, we identified that the social distancing measures implemented in the SPMA reduced the COVID19 R(t) to less than 1.

If a similar level of social distance is maintained in April and May, during influenza seasonality, no additional ICU beds for COVID-19 patients will be needed in the SPMA. We observed that the downward trend in hospitalized cases started on 9th March, before the intervention. This could be explained by a decrease in mobility documented since the first days of March in places like national parks, dog parks, plazas, and public gardens. According to a COVID-19 Community Mobility Report informed by Google this reduction was intensified and spread to other settings since the local government declared a state of emergency (8).

This report suggested that intervention was effectively applied, and it is consistent with the transmissibility reduction observed. Furthermore, this study indicated that social distancing measures impact should be monitored on daily based using hospitalized SARI cases, especially during the shortage of the COVID-19 confirmatory tests. The baseline scenario shows that completely relaxing social distancing results in thousands of additional deaths. Figure 2 shows that the rate of fatalities per day increases dramatically when ICU capacity is overloaded. The simulation shows a swift change in the number of deaths per day in this scenario quickly spikes from 100, a week prior the system is overloaded, to a peak of 4,160 deaths per day in less than a month. A potential limitation is that many COVID-19 patients from nearby cities usually sought for medical care in the SPMA area, which is a reference for the state of São Paulo, leading to overburden of the healthcare system even if the epidemic is controlled in the SPMA. The last week of data has not been included to minimize the impact of delay in reporting.

CONCLUSIONS

Despite the limitations, by using SARI electronic notification systems as a proxy for severe cases of COVID19 we reported a substantial decrease on the R(t) after two week of the implemented of social distance measures in the SPMA. These measures are expected to avoid 89,133 deaths within 60 days even without expanding the ICU bed capacity. Fabiana S.G. dos Santos is a biologist and PhD candidate. Her main research interest is epidemiology of infectious diseases and mathematical modelling

Author Affiliation

1 Secretariat of Health Surveillance, Department of Immunization and Communicable Diseases, Ministry of Health, Brasília, Brazil.
2 University of Brasilia, Brasília, Brazil
3 Department of Clinical and Toxicological Analyses, School of Pharmaceutical Sciences, University of São Paulo, São Paulo, Brazil
4 Scientific Platform Pasteur USP, São Paulo, Brazil
5 University of São Paulo, School of Public Health, Department of Epidemiology, Laboratório de Inferência Causal em Epidemiologia, São Paulo, SP, Brazil.
6School of Medicine, Federal University of Mato Grosso do Sul, Campo Grande, MS, Brazil.
7. Department of Epidemiology of Microbial Diseases, Yale University School of Public Health, New Haven, United States of America.
8.Oswaldo Cruz Foundation, Mato Grosso do Sul, Campo Grande, MS, Brazil.

Acknowledgments:

FADQ and JC were granted a fellowship for research productivity from the Brazilian National Council for Scientific and Technological Development – CNPq,
process/contract identification: 312656/2019-0 and 310551/2018-8, respectively. Dra. Maria Almiron, PAHO - Pan American Health Organiz

ation, Brazil Country Office for review the manuscript

REFERENCES

1. Li, Q., Guan, X., Wu, P., Wang, X., Zhou, L., Tong, Y., et al. (2020). Early Transmission Dynamics in Wuhan, China, of Novel Coronavirus-Infected Pneumonia. N Engl J Med. 2020 Jan 29;

2. Novel Coronavirus Pneumonia Emergency Response Epidemiology Team. [The epidemiological characteristics of an outbreak of 2019 novel coronavirus diseases (COVID19) in China]. Zhonghua Liu Xing Bing Xue Za Zhi Zhonghua Liuxingbingxue Zazhi. 2020 Feb 17;41(2):145–51.

3. Boëlle, P, Ansart, S, Cori, A, Valleron, A.(2011). Transmission parameters of the A/H1N1 (2009) influenza virus pandemic: a review. Influenza Other Respir Viruses. 2011 Sep;5(5):306–16.

4. Girard MP, Tam JS, Assossou OM, Kieny MP. The 2009 A (H1N1) influenza virus pandemic: A review. Vaccine. 2010 Jul;28(31):4895–902.

5. Liu, Y., Gayle, A.A., Wilder-Smith, A., Rocklöv, J. (2020). The reproductive number of COVID-19 is higher compared to SARS coronavirus. J Travel Med. 2020 Mar 13;27(2):taaa021.

6. Roosa, K., Lee, Y., Luo, R., Kirpich, A., Rothenberg, R., Hyman, J.M., et al. (2020). Real-time forecasts of the COVID-19 epidemic in China from February 5th to February 24th, 2020. Infect Dis Model. 2020;5:256–63.

7. Ferguson, N., Laydon, D., Nedjat, Gilani G., Imai, N., Ainslie, K., Baguelin, M., et al. (2020).Report 9: Impact of non-pharmaceutical interventions (NPIs) to reduce COVID19 mortality and healthcare demand [Internet]. 2020 Mar [cited 2020 Apr 5]. Available from:
   http://spiral.imperial.ac.uk/handle/10044/1/77482

8. COVID-19 Community Mobility Report [Internet]. COVID-19 Community Mobility Report.
   [cited 2020 Apr 5]. Available from: https://www.google.com/covid19/mobility

9. Park, M., Cook, A.R., Lim, J.T., Sun, Y., Dickens, B.L. (2020). A Systematic Review of COVID-19 Epidemiology Based on Current Evidence. J Clin Med. 2020 Apr;9(4):967.

TABLES

Table 1.
Parameters used in the age stratified SEIR model to forecast the ICU beds

Parameters	Values	Source
Incubation period	5.1 days	Rocha-Filho et al (8)
infectious period	1.61 day	Rocha-Filho et al (8)
Symptomatic	50%	Ferguson et al (7)
Serial interval (mean±standard deviation)	4,18±3,20	Park et al (9)
Infection Fatality Rate	0.8%	
Case Fatality Rate	1.6%	
Reproduction number	2.27	
Imported cases rate	24 cases/day	
Serial interval (mean±standard deviation)	4,18±3,20	

Fig 1 a

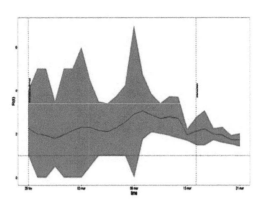

Fig 1b

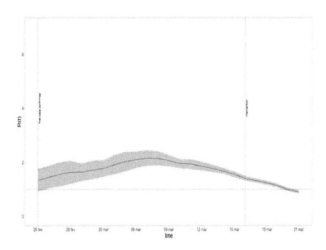

Figure 1. Time-dependent reproductive number R(t) estimated for the confirmed COVID19 cases (a), and for the SARI cases (b). Solid line corresponds to R(t), the red area of the confidence interval; the vertical dotted line represents, respectively, the date of the onset of symptoms of the first confirmed case in Brazil and date of the first social distancing measure implemented by the São Paulo state.

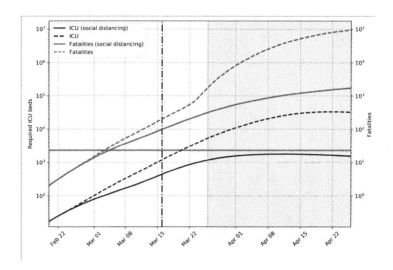

Figure 2. Estimation of the number of ICU patients (Black line) and fatalities (Red line). The solid line uses the time dependent reproductive number R(t) measured for SPMA and the dashed line represents the scenario in which no social distancing takes place. The vertical dashed line represents the date in which the local government declared a state of emergency and the horizontal grey line represents the number of available ICU beds.

2. Social Distancing Measures To Control The COVID-19 Pandemic: Potential Impacts And Challenges In Brazil

Estela M. L. Aquino[...]Raíza Tourinho dos Reis Silva Lima

ABSTRACT

The COVID-19 pandemic has challenged researchers and policy makers to identify public safety measures for preventing the collapse of healthcare systems and reducing deaths. This narrative review summarizes the available evidence on the impact of social distancing measures on the epidemic and discusses the implementation of these measures in Brazil. Articles on the effect of social distancing on COVID-19 were selected from the PubMed, medRXiv and bioRvix databases. Federal and state legislation was analyzed to summarize the strategies implemented in Brazil. Social distancing measures adopted by the population appear effective, particularly when implemented in conjunction with the isolation of cases and quarantining of contacts. Therefore, social distancing measures, and social protection policies to guarantee the sustainability of these measures, should be implemented. To control COVID-19 in Brazil, it is also crucial that epidemiological monitoring is strengthened at all three levels of the Brazilian National Health System (SUS). This includes evaluating and using supplementary indicators to monitor the progression of the pandemic and the effect of the control measures, increasing testing capacity, and making disaggregated notifications and testing results transparent and broadly available.

INTRODUCTION

Ever since the emergence in China in December 2019 of the new coronavirus, SARS-CoV-2, the virus responsible for the COVID-19 pandemic, humanity has been facing a severe global health crisis. Numerous new cases quickly appeared in Asian countries such as Thailand, Japan, South Korea and Singapore, followed by nations in Europe and in the other continents, leading the World Health Organization (WHO) to declare a public health emergency of international concern on January 30, 2020[1] and a pandemic on March 11, 2020[2]. By April 16 of this same year, 210 countries and territories worldwide had reported a total of 2.1 million confirmed cases of COVID-19,with a death toll exceeding 144,000[3]. Although the lethality of the disease caused by SARS-CoV-2 is lower than that found with other coronaviruses, its high transmissibility has led to more deaths in terms of absolute numbers than the combination of the SARS-CoV and MERS-CoV epidemics[4]. SARS-CoV-2 transmission occurs predominantly through the spread of contaminated droplets of oropharyngeal secretions from an infected individual to a disease-free person. However, the role of airborne transmission and transmission via contact with contaminated surfaces and objects, where the virus could remain active for up to 72 hours, is still unknown[5], and the role of faecal-oral transmission remains under debate[6,7]. SARS-CoV-2transmission is aggravated by its protracted mean incubation period of approximately 5-6 days (min-max: 0-24 days)[8-10], and by the fact that individuals who are asymptomatic, pre-symptomatic or with only mild symptoms are able to transmit the disease[11-13]. Although 80% of cases present as milder respiratory infections and pneumonias, the severe forms of the disease tend to affect the elderly and those with underlying chronic diseases[14], requiring hospitalization, intensive care and mechanical ventilation.

The still sparse information on the modes of transmission and the role of asymptomatic carriers in spreading SARS-CoV-2, together with the inexistence of vaccines and specific treatment options, represents a challenge to researchers, healthcare managers and governments. Non-pharmaceutical public health interventions aimed at reducing the spread of the virus and avoiding the collapse of healthcare systems, have been used to allow timely treatment of severe complications and avoid deaths. Several countries have implemented a series of interventions to reduce transmission of the virus and decelerate progression of the pandemic[15].

These include isolation of cases, encouraging hand hygiene, respiratory etiquette and the use of homemade facemasks, and implementing social distancing measures such as closing schools and universities, banning large events and mass gatherings, restricting travel and public transportation, making the public aware of the need to stay at home, and even implementing total lockdown in which individuals are only allowed out to buy food or medicines or to seek healthcare. These measures have been introduced gradually and in differing ways, to a greater or lesser extent, in the different countries, and their results probably depend on socioeconomic and cultural aspects, on the characteristics of their political and healthcare systems, and on the operational procedures used in their implementation.

The sustainability and effectiveness of these measures depend on establishing social protection and support policies for vulnerable populations, guaranteeing the survival of individuals and their families while restrictions to economic activities remain in effect. In Brazil, there are vast social and regional inequalities, with 66 million individuals living in poverty or extreme poverty and only 40% of the population in formal employment[16]. Such conditions require urgent economic measures to be implemented to guarantee a minimum income for the most vulnerable segment of the population and employment protection for salaried workers so as to ensure that a relevant proportion of the population will comply with social distancing measures. The present study aimed to analyse the impact of social distancing policies on the COVID-19 pandemic and the challenges to implementing these policies in Brazil with a view to increasing understanding in the population and to provide a basis capable of supporting managers in their decision-making.

METHODS

A total of 2,771 articles on COVID-19, published up to April 6, 2020 and listed in the PubMed databases, were screened for inclusion in this narrative review. In addition, manuscripts in the prepublication phase and available in the medRXiv and bioRvix databases or in the grey literature were also reviewed. Due to the speed of publication at the present time, articles published after the cut-off date but of the utmost relevance for Brazil were included in this review *a posteriori*. Twenty-one original or review articles focusing on control strategies and measures, particularly those on social distancing measures in different countries, were selected for inclusion. In addition to the scientific papers, federal and state legislation implemented throughout the country, specifically decrees and judicial decisions regarding social distancing, were analysed up to the cut-off date of

April 16, 2020 to summarize social distancing strategies in Brazil. Since a great number of new papers are being produced every day, the recommendations presented here are subject to change as new evidence emerges.

What are social distancing measures and what is known regarding their effect on the progression of the epidemic?

The recent discovery of SARS-CoV-2 has resulted in a colossal effort by doctors, epidemiologists and other healthcare professionals to classify individuals with symptoms such as fever, cough, breathing difficulties and loss of smell and taste as being suspected of having the disease or not. Defining a case is relevant in monitoring the progression of an epidemic and studying the effect of disease control strategies in the population. In view of the high transmissibility of individuals infected by SARS-CoV-2 (symptomatic, pre-symptomatic and asymptomatic individuals), ideally, health surveillance authorities should adopt the definition most capable of detecting the universe of cases within a population. Since this is a new disease, the definitions need to be reviewed as more detailed information on the cases investigated comes to light[17]. In Brazil, a large proportion of symptomatic SARS-CoV-2 infections fail to be diagnosed in a timely fashion; therefore, to monitor the progression of the epidemic it has been suggested that broader definitions of cases should be included in the figures, also taking into consideration additional admissions to hospital and excess deaths due to acute respiratory diseases.

Some terms have been used to refer to the control actions used in the COVID-19 epidemic. These terms are not new and refer to the non-pharmaceutical public health interventions historically adopted for the control of epidemics, particularly in the absence of vaccines and antivirals. These include, principally, isolation, quarantining, social distancing and community containment strategies[18]. *Isolation* consists of separating people who are ill from uninfected individuals to reduce the risk of transmission of the disease. To be effective, the isolation of sick individuals requires cases to be detected at an early stage and viral transmissibility of asymptomatic carriers to be very low. In the case of COVID-19, in which the incubation period is longer than that of other viruses, the high transmissibility of the disease by asymptomatic carriers limits effectiveness whenever case isolation constitutes the single or main measure[18]. In fact, there is evidence that in asymptomatic SARS-CoV-2 carriers the viral load is similar to that of symptomatic patients[19], a finding that is corroborated by reports of disease transmission involving both asymptomatic carriers and individuals with only mild symptoms[20]. Therefore, the mass use of diagnostic tests, allowing infected individuals to be identified, as adopted in Germany and South Korea, is essential for isolation to be effective.

Quarantining consists of restricting the movement of individuals who are presumed to have been exposed to a contagious disease but who are not ill, either because they were not infected or because they are still in the incubation period of the disease or even because in the case of COVID-19 they will remain asymptomatic and will fail to be identified. This can be applied at individual or group level, ensuring that exposed individuals remain in their own homes, in institutions or in other specifically designated places. Quarantine can be voluntary or obligatory. During quarantine, all individuals must be monitored for the occurrence of symptoms. If symptoms develop, the individuals must be immediately isolated and treated. Quarantining is more successful in situations in which cases are detected rapidly and their contacts can be identified and screened within a short space of time[18].

Social distancing refers to measures aimed at reducing interactions within a community, which can include infected individuals as yet unidentified, hence not in isolation. Since diseases transmitted through respiratory droplets require a certain physical proximity for contagion to occur, social distancing allows transmission to be reduced. Examples of social distancing measures that have been adopted include: the closure of schools and workplaces, closure of certain businesses, and cancellation of events to avoid mass gatherings. Social distancing is particularly useful in settings where there is community transmission of the virus, where the restriction measures imposed exclusively on known cases or on the most vulnerable segments of the population are considered insufficient to prevent new transmissions. The most extreme case of social distancing is total lockdown in which a rigorous intervention is applied to an entire community, city or region by forbidding people to leave their homes except to purchase basic supplies or to access emergency services. Lockdown enables social contact to be drastically reduced[18].

hat measures have been adopted in different countries and under what circumstances?

The first cases of this new disease began to appear in December 2019 in the Chinese city of Wuhan. There was one common source of exposure, a seafood market that also sold live animals[21]. The health surveillance authorities were alerted, and several measures began to be taken to identify the causative agent of the disease. On December 31 of that same year, China notified the WHO of the outbreak and on the following day the market where the cases had originated was closed[22]. From then onwards, an exponential increase occurred in the number of cases and community transmission was confirmed. Within a short period of time, measures were implemented to restrict travel and the circulation of people, including screening travellers for symptoms, until on January 23, 2020 total lockdown was declared in Wuhan, with no one being allowed to enter or leave the region[23]. These localized measures were followed by the implementation of similar actions in other Chinese provinces affected by the virus, in several other Asian countries, and in other countries around the world. The initial measures focused to a major extent on controlling travel at a time when the majority of cases were imported; however, the measures were progressively ramped up as community transmission was confirmed.

The first three cases of COVID-19 in Europe were recorded in France on January 24, 2020 and the first death in that continent was reported in that same country on February 15[24]. A week later, cases were registered in another eight countries. The epidemic expanded dramatically in Italy, Spain and France, where it rapidly developed into a severe health crisis with many critical cases and deaths, consequently overwhelming healthcare system resources. This accelerated the adoption of control measures, which did not occur simultaneously and varied greatly between countries and between different regions of the same country. However, over time these measures had to be ramped up and strengthened in all countries as the health crisis deteriorated. Chart 1 summarizes the main interventions adopted by selected European countries based on a study by Imperial College London. Despite some similarities, implementation of the different measures varied, even in relation to the time period between the first initiative and the announcement of total lockdown.

Chart 1. Measures to contain COVID-19 implemented in a selection of European countries affected by the disease.

Country	Date of the 1st and the 50th confirmed cases	Isolation of suspected/ confirmed cases	type of Measurement (date of the start of implementation)					time between the 50th case and the start of social distancing
			Social Distancing					
			Closure of schools and universities	Social distancing encouraged	Mass gatherings banned	total lockdown decreed		
Germany	1st:One case (local transmission) 27/01/2020 50th: 29/02/2020	Individuals with symptoms should undergo testing and then selfisolate (06/03/2020)	Nationwide (14/03/2020)	The Prime Minister recommended avoiding social interaction whenever possible (12/03/2020)	No gatherings of >1,000 people. Otherwise, regional restrictions (only until lockdown) (08/03/2020)	Meeting of more than 2 people forbidden; 1.5 meters of distance between individuals (22/03/2020)		8 days
Spain	1st:One case (imported) 31/01/2020 50th:01/03/2020	Self-isolation for 7 days if symptoms of cough or fever are present (17/03/2020)	Nationwide (13/03/2020)	Social distancing and working from home recommended (09/03/2020)	All public events banned (14/03/2020)	Nationwide lockdown (14/03/2020)		8 days
France	1st: Three cases (imported) 24/01/2020 50th: 29/02/2020	Recommended from lockdown (16/03/2020)	Nationwide (14/03/2020)	Recommended from lockdown (16/03/2020)	Events involving more than 100 people banned (13/03/2020)	The population must stay at home. Allowed out for maximum of 1 hour with a selfdeclaration form (17/03/2020)		13 days
Italy	1st: Two cases (imported) 31/01/2020 50th: 22/02/2020	Recommendation to self-isolate if symptoms are present and to quarantine if test is positive (09/03/2020)	Nationwide (05/03/2020)	People must keep at least one meter from each other and all gatherings are banned (09/03/2020)	Government bans all public events (09/03/2020)	The government closed all public venues. People should stay at home except for essential travel (11/03/2020)		12 days

United Kingdom	1st: Two cases (imported) 31/01/2020 50th: 04/03/2020	Self-isolation for 7 days if symptoms of cough and fever are present (12/03/2020)	Nationwide. Kindergartens and nurseries instructed to follow guidance to close (21/03/2020)	Warnings to avoid pubs, clubs, theaters and other public institutions (16/03/2020)	Implemented with lockdown (24/03/2020)	Meetings of more than 2 people not from the same household banned and police authorized to break them up. (24/03/2020)	12 days

Measures to contain COVID-19 implemented in a selection of European countries affected by the disease. In some countries, the first initiative was to ban mass gatherings of more than 1,000 people; however, this number was subsequently reduced to 500 and then to 50. In other countries, cinemas, restaurants, gyms and places of worship were closed. Germany determined the closure of most non-essential shops and extended the opening times of supermarkets to reduce the number of customers in the stores at the same time. In some countries, stores reserved the first hours of trading for elderly clients at a high risk of severe disease[25].

The closure of schools, a measure adopted in all countries, has been the subject of much debate. Children are rarely affected by COVID-19 and the extent to which they develop asymptomatic infections and transmit the virus is unclear. Although closing schools may have the added benefit of contributing towards ensuring that parents remain at home, this measure may affect the ability of parents, who are health professionals and whose services are of the utmost importance at this time, to work. Furthermore, other negative effects include an increase in the number of children cared for by elderly grandparents, interruption to the supply of free school meals to vulnerable children and, obviously, the fact that children would be denied their right to formal education for months at a time[25].

For these reasons, although schools in Austria, the Netherlands and the United Kingdom were closed, an exception was made for the children of key workers such as health professionals[25,26]. In the United Kingdom, vulnerable children (recipients of social care) were also allowed to attend school. In addition, the government decided that schools could provide meals to children who usually received them free of charge and announced in the media the creation of a national program of food vouchers[26].

In Singapore, although schools remained open, measures were adopted to reduce the size of classes and the number of interclass and interschool activities, while rigorous hygiene measures were implemented and recess and lunch breaks were staggered[25,27]. Countries such as the United Kingdom, the Netherlands, Sweden and the United States were initially reluctant to adopt social distancing measures[28,29], advocating the isolation of confirmed cases and of groups at greater risk. Nevertheless, as the epidemic progressed and epidemiological indicators worsened, these countries were obliged to review their policies and adopt restrictive measures already implemented in other countries. Within a context of rapid spread of the pandemic, with the number of cases and the number of deaths continuing to increase in many countries, the need for social distancing measures and measures to restrict the circulation of people became obvious, with total lockdown sometimes being necessary[30].

Measures of this nature allow time to be gained in which to organize the healthcare and epidemiological surveillance resources required to control COVID-19. In countries of continental dimensions and very large populations such as India and Brazil, social inequalities are immense and healthcare resources are chronically deficient and unequally distributed. In such countries, the adoption of more rigorous social distancing measures will be a determining factor in minimizing the imminent collapse of healthcare services and avoiding thousands of deaths as a result of lack of care for severe cases of the disease.

What scientific evidence is there on the impact of control measures on the epidemic?

Due to the speed at which the COVID-19 epidemic emerged, many of the epidemic control interventions were introduced simultaneously, and compliance differed from country to country. Therefore, it is difficult to evaluate the effectiveness of each single intervention alone. In general, the studies available involve mathematical models of disease transmission based on observed data and on the simulation of hypothetical scenarios according to which the interventions adopted would be able to reduce transmission of the virus. Simulation studies evaluate responses associated with different contexts and are useful for directing the allocation of resources and taking decisions to maximize the intervention strategies. Few studies have managed to evaluate the actual effectiveness of some of these measures in the dynamics of SARS-CoV-2 transmission.

In mid-March, investigators from Imperial College London used a mathematical model to simulate the effect of a series of epidemic control measures, implemented individually or together, in the United Kingdom (specifically Great Britain) and in the United States. The effectiveness of any single intervention seemed limited, indicating that multiple interventions must be used in conjunction to make a substantial impact in reducing transmission of the virus[31]. Combining less restrictive control measures (isolation of suspected cases, quarantining of contacts and social distancing for the elderly and those at greater risk of the disease) could reduce the peak of demand on healthcare services by two-thirds, also halving the number of deaths. Nevertheless, with this type of strategy, the COVID-19 epidemic would result in hundreds of thousands of deaths and would overwhelm healthcare services, particularly intensive care units (ICUs). For this reason, drastic measures of social distancing applied to the entire population should be the policy of choice, despite the fact that this option will depend on the feasibility of its implementation and on the social contexts[31].

China initiated a form of isolation in which all cases were hospitalized, not only those requiring hospital care, while simultaneously implementing social distancing for the entire population, resulting in a reduction in transmission. Several studies have estimated that these interventions reduced the mean rate of transmission of COVID-19,as measured by a decrease in the basic reproduction number (R0)[32] to less than 1, i.e. showing that an infected individual can infect on average less than one other person, a situation that is essential if a decrease in the incidence of cases is to be achieved[31]. A study conducted in Wuhan using COVID-19 data associated with smartphone records concluded that people's mobility was the principal factor in the spread of SARS-CoV-2, both in that city and in other provinces, before implementation of the sanitary cordon[10]. In this respect, restricting the mobility of the population can contribute to delaying the peak of the epidemic, to reducing the number of cases within a city and to avoiding transmission to other locations[10,23,33,34]. Measures involving travel restrictions from Wuhan, the quarantining of household contacts and social distancing were responsible for increasing the doubling time in the number of cases of the disease and for slowing disease spread, as measured by the R0, which decreased from 0.98 to 0.91[34]. Another study that evaluated travel restrictions in Wuhan, using COVID-19 data from within and outside this urban centre for the period from December 2019 to February 2020, found a reduction in transmission at the end of January, coinciding with the introduction of travel restrictions[35].

In addition, the closure of the airports in China, which occurred around two months after the beginning of the epidemic, led to a delay in the occurrence of new cases outside of Wuhan, both in the rest of China and internationally[23]. Nevertheless, it is estimated that reducing the number of flights by up to 90% would only result in a decrease in the number of cases in other countries if early detection, isolation and behavioural changes in the population such as hand hygiene, avoiding mass gatherings, etc., were implemented and encouraged in conjunction[23].

The reduction in the epidemic in China partially attributed to social distancing triggered the implementation of similar measures in other places. An early study using smartphone tracking data to evaluate the impact of social distancing in Italy reported a reduction of around 40% in travel between regions and a 17% reduction in the rates of social mixing (the number of devices within 50 meters of each other over a 1-hour period) following total lockdown in the country[36]. In the northern provinces, in the regions more affected by the disease, the measures implemented to control spread of the virus achieved a reduction of up to 30% in the rate of social contact[36].In an attempt to perform a broader modelling of the course of the epidemic in various countries around the world, data from China and from other high-income countries were used to model the effect of three interventions on COVID-19-related mortality[37]. A comparison was made with data from a setting in which social distancing measures were not implemented but where mass testing for COVID-19 is performed, including the isolation of cases and quarantining of contacts (measures already widely reported to be essential).

By protecting the elderly, reducing their social contacts by 60%, and reducing social contacts in the general population by 40%, there would be a huge decrease in the number of infections, admissions to hospital and deaths. A drop of up to 67% was estimated in COVID-19-related deaths (median 49%; range 23-67%), representing 20 million lives saved. Nevertheless, the effect of these strategies on reducing the number of infections in low- and medium-income countries could be less, since the elderly in those countries tend to have greater contact with the younger generations. In general, the authors of that study exert caution when discussing the actual impact of these interventions on the reduction in the number of cases of COVID-19 in these countries.

If, on the one hand, the demographic structure is characterized by a greater percentage of younger people, on the other hand, a large proportion of the population lives in conditions of social vulnerability, in overcrowded environments and homes, and consists of individuals with chronic morbidities. In settings in which the organization and capacity of the healthcare system are precarious, these factors can contribute to increasing mortality.

A study conducted in Brazil using a mathematical model to estimate the effect of social distancing measures in the greater metropolitan region of São Paulo showed that, without the adoption of social distancing measures, the capacity of the ICUs for COVID-19 would be overwhelmed by 130% in the first month and 14-fold in the second month. The model also suggested that the set of social distancing measures implemented (and their continuation up to the present time) could avoid overwhelming the healthcare system, maintaining capacity at a maximum of 76% and avoiding the death of around 90,000 individuals over the course of the epidemic[38].

Furthermore, the study recommended the use of data on admissions to hospital for severe acute respiratory syndromes (SARS) to monitor the effect of social distancing measures[38]. Another study conducted in Brazil also showed that, at the present moment, maintaining and strengthening current social distancing measures, quarantining and isolating cases, is absolutely vital to avoid the collapse of the healthcare systems in the country[39]. Other studies, still at the prepublication stage, describe similar findings, arguing that the more restrictive the measures, the more effective they are in reducing the number of affected individuals and the faster the end of the epidemic will be reached[40,41].

Finally, a rapid Cochrane review performed to evaluate the effectiveness of quarantine measures in avoiding deaths due to COVID-19 included 22 papers on epidemics such as SARS, MERS and COVID-19 published up to March 12, 2020, ten of which deal with the current epidemic[42]. The synthesis of the studies included, most of which used a mathematical model, indicated that quarantining is an effective measure to reduce the number of cases of COVID-19; however, to achieve effective control of the disease, quarantine must be implemented together with other control measures[42].Therefore, there are strong indications that the strategies used to control the spread of the epidemic are effective when the isolation of cases and quarantining of contacts are combined with a set of social distancing measures that encompass the entire population[42]. In general, data on the effectiveness of single measures are sparse[31]; however, it is extremely unlikely that they would be effective, since asymptomatic individuals, including children and adults, contribute to the chain of transmission of the disease. Furthermore, it is of the utmost importance that screening and the isolation of cases and contacts are enhanced in combination with social distancing measures[34]. Chart 2 summarizes the principal measures, and their respective impacts, as evaluated in the studies included in this narrative review.

Chart 2. Principal effects of non-pharmaceutical interventions in the COVID-19 epidemic as analyzed in the scientific literature..

Intervention Analyzed	Resulting Impact	Referência
Reducing mobility	The peak of the epidemic was delayed; there was a reduction in the number of cases within cities, and in transmission to other locations	10,23,33,34
Travel restrictions, quarantining and distancing	A reduction in R0 and an increase in doubling time	34
Travel restrictions	A reduction in transmission and in the number of cases in the country and abroad	23,35
Social distancing	A reduction in social interaction A reduction in the demand for hospital care and in the number of deaths	36 37 38,39*

What is the current epidemiological situation in Brazil and what constitutes adequate measures to control the epidemic?

Principal effects of non-pharmaceutical interventions in the COVID-19 epidemic as analysed in the scientific literature. The first case of COVID-19 in Latin America was registered in Brazil on February 25, 2020 and consisted of a 61-year old male from São Paulo who had recently returned from a trip to Lombardy in Italy. Following laboratory confirmation of COVID-19, the patient, who had mild symptoms of the disease, was given the standardized care recommended by the epidemiological surveillance authorities and told to self-isolate at home while contacts were investigated among family members, at the hospital where he received care and on the flight back from Italy. Since then, the epidemic has spread in the country and, on April 16, 2020, there were already 30,718 confirmed cases and 1,926 deaths throughout Brazil, with an incidence of 14.51/100,000 inhabitants[43]. The entire academic community was mobilized nationwide, with the creation of several national networks formed to combat COVID-19[44].

The large number of samples for laboratory testing that remained untested due to the impossibility of increasing testing capacity points to major underreporting. Although legislation regarding measures with which to tackle COVID-19 has been in place in the country since February 7, 2020, i.e. before the epidemic was officially recognized in the country, President Jair Bolsonaro has given little importance to it. In fact, he is one of the few world leaders who refuse to recognize the threat constituted by the virus. There are numerous articles in the media repeating his public statements against the measures implemented in the states and municipalities and encouraging his followers on social media sites to disobey the social distancing recommendations. An open political conflict began between the president and the then Minister of Health, Luiz Henrique Mandetta, who defended the measures recommended by the WHO and until recently supported the more rigorous measures implemented locally and regionally to control COVID-19.

At the beginning of April, following rumours regarding his imminent removal from office, which indeed occurred on April 16, Mandetta began to recommend "relaxation" of the social distancing measures implemented in the states and municipalities from April 13 onwards. In this political setting in which a serious political crisis is compounding the health crisis, control measures, including social distancing, have been implemented by the state governors and municipal mayors (and sometimes by the Judiciary), particularly in the states most affected by the epidemic.

The administrative autonomy of the states and municipalities in areas such as health, education and business, guaranteed in the federal constitution, limits the possibility of direct interference by the federal government in decisions made by local governments. This has been a subject of debate in the Supreme Court and up to the present time recognition of the autonomy of the states and municipalities with respect to the adoption of emergency measures regarding public health has been upheld.

Chart 3 describes the measures adopted in Brazil in some of the states in which the epidemic has been more severe and in Bahia, one of the first states to adopt social distancing measures. The complete Chart is presented as supplementary material (Chart S1). In general, practical measures to restrict circulation and prevent mass gatherings have already been put into practice, to greater and lesser degrees. Nevertheless, the federal government, by minimizing the importance of social distancing and publicly opposing the measures adopted in the states and municipalities, may well undermine the population's willingness to comply with them.

Chart 3. COVID-19 control measures implemented at state and federal level in Brazil, presented for a selection of Brazilian states, together with the number of notified cases per 100,000 inhabitants, updated on April 16,

Location (Notified cases/100,000 inhabitants)	Category of social distancing	Measure (government act)	effective date
Brazil (14.51)	Social distancing	Remote working for vulnerable civil servants in at-risk groups (Administrative Act19 - Ministryof Economy)	17/03
		Remote working, anticipation of individual and collective statutory leave, compensation of time and anticipation of public holidays (Provisional Act927)	22/03
Amapá (39.69)	Events	Mass gatherings banned (Judicialdecision)	29/03
	Education	Closure of all teaching establishments(Decree 1377)	17/03
	Circulation of people	Remote working for vulnerable civil servants in at-risk groups(Decree 1377)	17/03
		Mass gatherings banned (Decree 1414)	20/03
		Non-essential businesses and services closed except for deliveries (Decree 1414)	20/03
		All river transport stopped (Decree 1415)	23/03
Amazonas (36.93)	Events	Public gatherings and gatherings in public facilitiesbanned (Decree 42,061)	16/03
		Events involving more than 100 people banned (Decree 42,063)	17/03
	Education	Partial closure of state schools (Decree 42,061)	16/03
	Circulation of people	Remote working for vulnerable civil servants in at-risk groups and those with mild symptoms (Decree 42,061)	16/03
		All river transport stopped (Decree 42,087)	19/03
		Gyms and similar establishments closed (Decree 42,087)	19/03
		Circulation of all intercity bus services and tourist coaches stopped (Decree 42,098)	20/03
		All establishments involved in serving food directly to customers, as well as the leisure events industry, closed (Decree 42,099)	21/03
		Remote working for all civil servants (Decree 42,101)	23/03
		All non-essential businesses and services closed (Decree 42,101)	23/03
		Circulation of interstate bus services stopped (Decree 42,158)	04/04

COVID-19 control measures implemented at state and federal level in Brazil, presented for a selection of Brazilian states, together with the number of notified cases per 100,000 inhabitants, updated on April 16, 2020. Although no studies have yet been published on the degree to which the Brazilian population is complying with these measures, in a survey conducted by Datafolha 1,511 individuals were interviewed between April 1 and 3, with results showing that 76% were in agreement with maintaining social distancing to control the epidemic despite the economic damage resulting from these measures. Support was highest in the northeast of the country (81%) and lowest in the south (70%) (Figure 1). Nevertheless, a quarter of those interviewed reported that they had to leave their homes to go to work or to perform other activities.

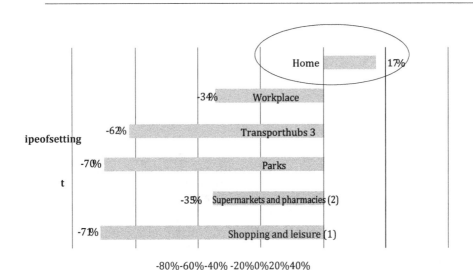

Changes in mobility compared to baseline (Sunday, February 16, 2020)

1 Restaurants, cafés, shopping malls, museums, libraries, cinemas;
2 supermarkets, grocery stores, farmers markets, specialist food shops, drug stores and pharmacies; 3 subway, bus and train stations.

Figure 1. Performance of activities of daily living during social distancing in Brazil, April 1-3, 2020 (Source: Datafolha).Source: COVID-19 Community Mobility Report (google.com/covid19/mobility)

Some indicators supplied by Google, obtained from smartphone records, suggest that there was a reduction of 70% of peoples movements in parks, of 71% in people engaging in commercial and leisure activities and of 64% in people circulating in transport hubs (Figure 2). However, as shown in the Datafolha survey, a significant proportion of the population is unable to stop working or cannot work from home and, in this respect, the reduction in mobility was of 34%.

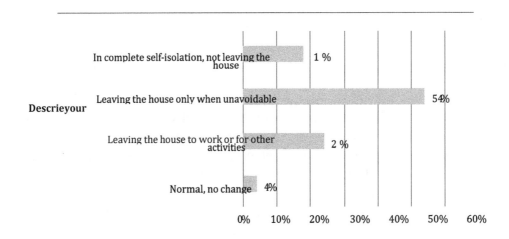

Figure 2. Changes in social mobility according to the type of setting in Brazil on March 29, 2020 in relation to February 16, 2020 (Source: COVID-19 Community Mobility Report: google.com/covid19/mobility).

Changes in social mobility according to the type of setting in Brazil on March 29, 2020 in relation to February 16, 2020[1] Despite support by the population for social distancing measures, however insufficient these may be, the Ministry of Health, on April 6 (hence still under the jurisdiction of Mandetta) expressed intention to relax these measures[45], at a time when the epidemic was still on the increase, not yet having reached its peak, even in São Paulo where the first cases in Brazil were registered. The states were recommended to transition to selective distancing if the number of confirmed cases did not exceed 50% of the capacity of the healthcare facilities already in existence prior to the pandemic. In places where the incidence rate was 50% higher than the national rate, social distancing measures should be maintained until supplies and equipment (hospital beds, personal protective equipment, mechanical ventilators and laboratory testing) and healthcare teams were sufficient available.

The decision to relax social distancing measures and the criteria adopted by the Ministry of Health should be discussed in the light of the information available in the international scientific literature, which, contrary to those proposed for Brazil, has based its decisions on monitoring the speed of transmission of the epidemic and, consequently, as a function of the increase in the number of infected individuals, the number of cases of the disease and the number of deaths. Relaxing or ending social distancing measures is a delicate issue, since maintaining control of the pandemic until a vaccine is available could require the population's routine activities of daily living to be curtailed for many months, with economic implications and consequent high costs for the lives of the population. On the other hand, the possibility has been suggested of ending the more rigorous social distancing measures, allowing some infections to occur, preferably in low-risk groups such as children or young adults so that a large part of the population gains immunity (the so-called "herd immunity").

The principal limitation in the Ministry of Health's proposed criteria for relaxing the social distancing measures is that these are based solely on the capacity of the healthcare services, as measured by indicators of the offer and structure of the services. Hence, they fail to take into consideration the surveillance and monitoring indicators of the pandemic in each one of the Brazilian municipalities such as, for example, the number of suspected and confirmed cases, the number of admissions to hospital for acute respiratory syndromes, mortality, R0 and doubling time. Furthermore, the epidemic is at different stages in the different parts of the country. As suggested by the European commission[46], the criteria for relaxing social distancing measures must include: 1) a significant decrease and stabilization for a sustained period of the number of cases and the number of admissions to hospital due to the disease; 2) sufficient health system capacity, including the occupation rate for ICUs, the availability of health care workers and medical material; 3) appropriate monitoring capacity, including large-scale testing capacity to quickly detect and isolate infected individuals and quarantine contacts, and, if possible, the application of rapid testing to monitor herd immunity.

In addition, up to the present moment, the Ministry of Health has failed to make clear what has to be taken into consideration when measuring the capacity of healthcare services, although the number of hospital beds, personal protective equipment (PPE), mechanical ventilators and laboratory testing are already covered, apparently indicating that priority is being given to the more specialized services. Given that in Brazil there are marked social and regional inequalities in the distribution of healthcare services and in access to those services, particularly those of greater

---

[1] (Source: COVID-19 Community Mobility Report: google.com/covid19/mobility).

complexity, we are aware that not everyone who needs care will receive it. Therefore, the collapse not only of hospital services but indeed of the entire healthcare network is predictable.COVID-19 control measures implemented at state and federal level in Brazil and the number of notified cases per 100,000 inhabitants, updated on April 16, 2020.Social distancing measures cannot be implemented without analysing the progression of the disease, as monitored by health surveillance measures. This is the only possible way of defining the moment at which the interventions can be temporarily relaxed for relatively short windows of time in case it becomes necessary to reintroduce measures if or when the number of cases starts to rise again[31]. The criteria adopted in various countries for relaxing social distancing measures have prioritized monitoring the speed of transmission of the virus and, as a consequence, the number of infected individuals and of existing cases.

Imperial College London proposed the systematic inclusion of data on hospital admissions in surveillance systems on which decisions to activate and deactivate social distancing are based, rather than opting for interventions of fixed duration. Measures can then be adapted for use at regional and state level. Since the pandemic does not occur in a synchronized fashion, local policies can be more effective, reaching levels of suppression comparable with those at national level, even if in effect for a shorter period. Estimates for Great Britain indicate that nationwide social distancing strategies would need to be kept in force for at least two-thirds of the time until a vaccine becomes available[31].

The experiences in China and South Korea have shown that suppression of the epidemic is possible over the short term; however, it is not known whether this is maintained over the long term and if the social and economic costs of the interventions adopted up to now could be reduced.

China, which managed to stop progression of the epidemic with social distancing measures implemented in conjunction with the isolation of cases, started to relax these measures after they had been in force for three months. This relaxing of the measures is accompanied by rigorous monitoring of the epidemiological situation so as to permit rapid reversal should the number of cases start to increase again. This will, without doubt, help direct strategies in other countries[31] Major uncertainties still remain regarding the effectiveness of the measures and to what extent the population will spontaneously adopt risk-reduction behaviour. Therefore, it is impossible to establish the precise duration of the measures, except that it will probably be several months. Nevertheless, the only certainty at the moment is that future decisions regarding the moment at which measures can be safely relaxed and for how long will have to be based on continuous and rigorous epidemiological surveillance[31].

Final Considerations and Recommendations

The COVID-19 epidemic is still on the increase in all the Brazilian states and Federal District. The political crisis, aggravated by the change in command at the Ministry of Health, introduces further uncertainties regarding the policies to be adopted by the federal government. The scientific findings presented in this review strongly suggest that, taken in conjunction, isolating cases, quarantining contacts and implementing large-scale social distancing measures, particularly those aimed at reducing social contact by at least 60%, can potentially reduce transmission of the disease. Although there is little in the literature on the subject in the particular setting of Brazil, the prior experience of countries in Asia and Europe suggests that social distancing strategies should be strengthened, should be intersectoral and must be coordinated between different government and regional agencies with the aim of reaching the end of the epidemic as quickly as possible and avoiding second and subsequent waves of the virus.

Implementation in Brazil is undoubtedly an enormous challenge. The marked social inequalities in the country, with a large percentage of the population living in a state of poverty and an increasing number of homeless people, in addition to the large prison population, may facilitate transmission and hamper the adoption of social distancing. In addition, the large proportion of informal workers means that policies of social protection and support for vulnerable segments of the population will have to be instituted to guarantee the sustainability and effectiveness of COVID-19 containment measures. Minimum income guarantees for the entire population, as well as policies that guarantee the jobs of those in the formal job market, are crucial in ensuring the survival of individuals, particularly, but not exclusively, while measures are in place that restrict economic activities. Finally, it is vital to strengthen the surveillance system at all three levels of the National Health Service. This includes: developing indicators with which to evaluate the progression of the epidemic; systematically disclosing notification data, separated by municipality and sanitary district; increasing testing capacity to identify asymptomatic, pre-symptomatic and symptomatic infected individuals, hospitalized cases and deaths resulting from COVID-19; precisely defining suspected and confirmed cases based on clinical and laboratory criteria; and continuously evaluating the implementation, effectiveness and the impact of control strategies. Only then will it be possible to provide data on which to base decision-making regarding the continuation of social distancing measures and the right moment at which to relax them.

ACKNOWLEDGMENTS

JMP is funded by the NIHR Global Health Research Program. EMLA has a CNPq Research Productivity Scholarship.

REFERENCES

1. World Health Organization (WHO). *WHO Director-General's statement on IHR Emergency Committee on Novel Coronavirus (2019-nCoV)* Geneva: WHO; 2020. [cited 2020 Apr 16]. Available from: https://www.who.int/news-room/detail/23-01-2020-statement-on-the-meeting-of-the-international-health-regulations-(2005)-emergency-committee-regarding-the-outbreak-of-novel-coronavirus-(2019-ncov)
»https://www.who.int/news-room/detail/23-01-2020-statement-on-the-meeting-of-the-international-health-regulations-(2005)-emergency-committee-regarding-the-outbreak-of-novel-coronavirus-(2019-ncov)
2. World Health Organization (WHO). *WHO Director-General's opening remarks at the media briefing on COVID-19-11 March 2020* Geneva: WHO; 2020 [cited 2020 Apr 16]. Available from:
https://www.who.int/dg/speeches/detail/who-director-general-s-opening-remarks-at-the-media-briefing-on-COVID-19---11-march-2020
» https://www.who.int/dg/speeches/detail/who-director-general-s-opening-remarks-at-the-media-briefing-on-COVID-19---11-march-2020
3. Worldometer. *Countries where COVID-19 has spread* 2020 [cited 2020 Apr 16]. Available from: https://www.worldometers.info/coronavirus/countries-where-coronavirus-has-spread/
» https://www.worldometers.info/coronavirus/countries-where-coronavirus-has-spread/
4. Mahase E. Coronavirus COVID-19 has killed more people than SARS and MERS combined, despite lower case fatality rate. *BMJ* 2020; 368:m641.
5. van Doremalen N, Bushmaker T, Morris DH, Holbrook MG, Gamble A, Williamson BN, Tamin A, Harcourt JL, Thornburg NJ, Gerber SI, Lloyd-Smith JO. Aerosol and Surface Stability of SARS-CoV-2 as Compared with SARS-CoV-1. *N Engl J Med* 2020; 382(16):1564-1567.

6. Ong SW, Tan YK, Chia PY, Lee TH, Ng OT, Wong MS, Marimuthu K. Air, Surface Environmental, and Personal Protective Equipment Contamination by Severe Acute Respiratory Syndrome Coronavirus 2 (SARS-CoV-2) From a Symptomatic Patient. *JAMA* Netw Open 2020. [Epub ahead of print]

7. Wang W, Xu Y, Gao R, Lu R, Han K, Wu G, Tan W. Detection of SARS-CoV-2 in Different Types of Clinical Specimens. *JAMA* Netw Open 2020. [Epub ahead of print]

8. Wang Y, Wang Y, Chen Y, Qin Q. Unique epidemiological and clinical features of the emerging 2019 novel coronavirus pneumonia (COVID-19) implicate special control measures. *J Med Virol* 2020. [Epub ahead of print]

9. Huang R, Xia J, Chen Y, Shan C, Wu C. A family cluster of SARS-CoV-2 infection involving 11 patients in Nanjing, China. *Lancet Infect Dis* 2020.

10. Kraemer MU, Yang CH, Gutierrez B, Wu CH, Klein B, Pigott DM, du Plessis L, Faria NR, Li R, Hanage WP, Brownstein JS. The effect of human mobility and control measures on the COVID-19 epidemic in China. *Science* 2020; pii:eabb4218.

11. Bai Y, Yao L, Wei T, Tian F, Jin DY, Chen L, Wang M. Presumed Asymptomatic Carrier Transmission of COVID-19. *JAMA Netw Open* 2020. [Epub ahead of print].

12. Tong ZD, Tang A, Li KF, Li P, Wang HL, Yi JP, Zhang YL, Yan JB. Potential Presymptomatic Transmission of SARS-CoV-2, Zhejiang Province, China, 2020. *Emerg Infect Dis* 2020; 26:5.

13. Kimball A, Hatfield KM, Arons M. Asymptomatic and Presymptomatic SARS-CoV-2 Infections in Residents of a Long-Term Care Skilled Nursing Facility - King County, Washington, March 2020. *MMWR Morb Mortal Wkly Rep* 2020; 69(13):377-381.

14. Eurosurveillance Editorial Team. Updated rapid risk assessment from ECDC on coronavirus disease 2019 (COVID-19) pandemic: increased transmission in the EU/EEA and the UK. *Euro Surveill* 2020; 25:12.

15. Kupferschmidt K, Cohen J. Can China's COVID-19 strategy work elsewhere? *Science* 2020; 367(6482): 1061-1062.

16. Instituto Brasileiro de Geografia, Estatística (IBGE). *Síntese de indicadores sociais: uma análise das condições de vida da população brasileira* Rio de Janeiro: IBGE; 2018.

17. Brasil. Ministério da Saúde (MS). [informar o título da publicação]. Brasilia: MS; 2018.

18. Wilder-Smith A, Freedman DO. Isolation, quarantine, social distancing and community containment: pivotal role for old-style public health measures in the novel coronavirus (2019-nCoV) outbreak. *J Travel Med* 2020; 27:2.

19. Zou L, Ruan F, Huang M, Liang L, Huang H, Hong Z, Yu J, Kang M, Song Y, Xia J, Guo Q. SARS-CoV-2 Viral Load in Upper Respiratory Specimens of Infected Patients. *N Engl J Med* 2020; 382(12):1177-1179.

20. Ling Z, Xu X, Gan Q, Zhang L, Luo L, Tang X, Liu J. Asymptomatic SARS-CoV-2 infected patients with persistent negative CT findings. *Eur J Radiol* 2020; 126:108956.

21. Singhal T. A Review of Coronavirus Disease-2019 (COVID-19). *Indian J Pediatr* 2020; 87(4):281-286.

22. World Health Organization (WHO). *Novel Coronavirus (2019-nCoV) Situation report-5, 25 January 2020* Geneva: WHO; 2020.

23. Chinazzi M, Davis JT, Ajelli M, Gioannini C, Litvinova M, Merler S, Piontti AP, Mu K, Rossi L, Sun K, Viboud C. The effect of travel restrictions on the spread of the 2019 novel coronavirus (COVID-19) outbreak. *Science* 2020; pii:eaba9757.

24. Spiteri G, Fielding J, Diercke M, Campese C, Enouf V, Gaymard A, Bella A, Sognamiglio P, Moros MJ, Riutort AN, Demina YV. First cases of coronavirus disease 2019 (COVID-19) in the WHO European Region, 24 January to 21 February 2020. *Euro Surveill* 2020; 25:9.

25. Cohen J, Kupferschmidt K. Countries test tactics in 'war' against COVID-19. *Science* 2020; 367(6484):1287-1288.

26. Mahase E. COVID-19: schools set to close across UK except for children of health and social care workers. *BMJ* 2020; 368:m1140.

27. Lee VJ, Chiew CJ, Khong WX. Interrupting transmission of COVID-19: lessons from containment efforts in Singapore. *J Travel Med* 2020; pii:taaa039.

28. The Lancet Respiratory Medicine. COVID-19: delay, mitigate, and communicate. *Lancet Respir Med* 2020; 8(4):321.

29. Eurosurveillance Editorial Team. Updated rapid risk assessment from ECDC on the novel coronavirus disease 2019 (COVID-19) pandemic: increased transmission in the EU/EEA and the UK. *Euro Surveill* 2020; 25:10.

30. Deshwal VK. COVID 19: A Comparative Study of Asian, European, American continent. *IJSRED* 2020; 3:2.

31. Ferguson N, Laydon D, Nedjati Gilani G, Imai N, Ainslie K, Baguelin M, Bhatia S, Boonyasiri A, Cucunuba Perez ZU, Cuomo-Dannenburg G, Dighe A. *Impact of non-pharmaceutical interventions (NPIs) to reduce COVID-19 mortality and healthcare demand. Imperial College COVID-19 Response Team* United Kingdom: Imperial College COVID-19 Response Team, 2020.

32. Barreto ML, Teixeira MG, Carmo EH. Infectious diseases epidemiology. *J Epidemiol Community Health* 2006; 60(3):192.

33. Boldog P, Tekeli T, Vizi Z, Denes A, Bartha FA, Rost G. Risk Assessment of Novel Coronavirus COVID-19 Outbreaks Outside China. *J Clin Med* 2020; 9:2.

34. Lau H, Khosrawipour V, Kocbach P, Mikolajczyk A, Schubert J, Bania J, Khosrawipour T. The positive impact of lockdown in Wuhan on containing the COVID-19 outbreak in China. *J Travel Med* 2020; pii:taaa037.

35. Kucharski AJ, Russell TW, Diamond C, Liu Y, Edmunds J, Funk S, Eggo RM, Sun F, Jit M, Munday JD, Davies N. Early dynamics of transmission and control of COVID-19: a mathematical modelling study. *Lancet Infect Dis* 2020; S1473-3099(20)30144-4.

36. Pepe E, Bajardi P, Gauvin L, Privitera F, Lake B, Cattuto C, Tizzoni M. COVID-19 outbreak response: a first assessment of mobility changes in Italy following national lockdown. *medRxiv* 2020; 2020.03.22.20039933.

37. Flaxman S, Mishra S, Gandy A. *Estimating the number of infections and the impact of non-pharmaceutical interventions on COVID-19 in 11 European countries* United Kingdom: Imperial College COVID-19 Response Team; 2020.

38. Ganem F, Mendes FM, Oliveira SB, Porto VB, Araujo W, Nakaya H, Diaz-Quijano FA, Croda J. The impact of early social distancing at COVID-19 Outbreak in the largest Metropolitan Area of Brazil. *medRxiv* 2020; 2020.04.06.20055103.

39. Canabarro A, Tenorio E, Martins R, Martins L, Brito S, Chaves R. Data-Driven Study of the COVID-19 Pandemic via Age-Structured Modelling and Prediction of the Health System Failure in Brazil amid Diverse Intervention Strategies. *medRxiv* 2020; 2020.04.03.20052498.

40. Hou J, Hong J, Ji B, Dong B, Chen Y, Ward MP, Tu W, Jin Z, Hu J, Su Q, Wang W. Changing transmission dynamics of COVID-19 in China: a nationwide population-based piecewise mathematical modelling study. *medRxiv* 2020; 2020.03.27.20045757.

41. Yang Q, Yi C, Vajdi A, Cohnstaedt LW, Wu H, Guo X, Scoglio CM. Short-term forecasts and long-term mitigation evaluations for the COVID-19 epidemic in Hubei Province, China. *medRxiv* 2020; 2020.03.27.20045625.

42. Nussbaumer-Streit B, Mayr V, Dobrescu AI, Chapman A, Persad E, Klerings I, Wagner G, Siebert U, Christof C, Zachariah C, Gartlehner G. Quarantine alone or in combination with other public health measures to control COVID-19: a rapid review. *Cochrane Database Syst Rev* 2020; 4:CD013574.

43. Rede CoVida [Internet]. *Painel Coronavírus Brasil* Salvador: Rede CoVida; 2020. [cited 2020 Apr 16]. Available from: http://www.covid19br.org » http://www.covid19br.org

44. Silva AAM. Sobre a possibilidade de interrupção da epidemia pelo coronavírus (COVID-19) com base nas melhores evidências científicas disponíveis. *Rev Bras Epidemiol* 2020; 23:e200021.

45. Brasil. Ministério da Saúde (MS). *Boletim Epidemiológico Especial 7: doença pelo coronavírus 2019* Brasília: MS; 2020.

46. European Comission. *A European roadmap to lifting coronavirus containment measures* 2020 [cited 2020 Apr 16]. Available from: https://ec.europa.eu/info/live-work-travel-eu/health/coronavirus-response/european-roadmap-lifting-coronavirus-containment-measures_en
» https://ec.europa.eu/info/live-work-travel-eu/health/coronavirus-response/european-roadmap-lifting-coronavirus-containment-measures_en

47. World Health Organization (WHO). *Coronavirus disease (COVID-2019) situation reports* Geneva: WHO; 2020.

hart 1. Measures to contain COVID-19 implemented in a selection of European countries affected by the disease.

Country	Date of the 1st and the 50th confirmed cases	Isolation of suspected/ confirmed cases	type of Measurement (date of the start of implementation)				time between the 50th case and the start of social distancing
			Social Distancing				
			Closure of schools and universities	Social distancing encouraged	Mass gatherings banned	total lockdown decreed	
Germany	1st:One case (local transmission) 27/01/2020 50th: 29/02/2020	Individuals with symptoms should undergo testing and then self isolate (06/03/2020)	Nationwide (14/03/2020)	The Prime Minister recommended avoiding social interaction whenever possible (12/03/2020)	No gatherings of >1,000 people. Otherwise, regional restrictions (only until lockdown) (08/03/2020)	Meeting of more than 2 people forbidden; 1.5 meters of distance between individuals (22/03/2020)	8 days
Spain	1st:One case (imported) 31/01/2020 50th:01/03/2020	Self-isolation for 7 days if symptoms of cough or fever are present (17/03/2020)	Nationwide (13/03/2020)	Social distancing and working from home recommended (09/03/2020)	All public events banned (14/03/2020)	Nationwide lockdown (14/03/2020)	8 days
France	1st: Three cases (imported) 24/01/2020 50th: 29/02/2020	Recommended from lockdown (16/03/2020)	Nationwide (14/03/2020)	Recommended from lockdown (16/03/2020)	Events involving more than 100 people banned (13/03/2020)	The population must stay at home. Allowed out for maximum of 1 hour with a self declaration form (17/03/2020)	13 days
Italy	1st: Two cases (imported) 31/01/2020 50th: 22/02/2020	Recommendation to self-isolate if symptoms are present and to quarantine if test is positive (09/03/2020)	Nationwide (05/03/2020)	People must keep at least one meter from each other and all gatherings are banned (09/03/2020)	Government bans all public events (09/03/2020)	The government closed all public venues. People should stay at home except for essential travel (11/03/2020)	12 days

United Kingdom	1st: Two cases (imported) 31/01/2020 50th: 04/03/2020	Self-isolation for 7 days if symptoms of cough and fever are present (12/03/2020)	Nationwide. Kindergartens and nurseries instructed to follow guidance to close (21/03/2020)	Warnings to avoid pubs, clubs, theaters and other public institutions (16/03/2020)	Implemented with lockdown (24/03/2020)	Meetings of more than 2 people not from the same household banned and police authorized to break them up. (24/03/2020)	12 days

Source: Adapted from Flaxman et al.[37] and WHO Situation Reports[47].
[28,29]

COVID-19 control measures implemented at state and federal level in Brazil, presented for a selection of Brazilian states, together with the number of notified cases per 100,000 inhabitants, updated on April 16, 2020.

Location (Notified cases/100,000 inhabitants)	Category of social distancing	Measure (government act)	effective date
Brazil (14.51)	Social distancing	Remote working for vulnerable civil servants in at-risk groups (Administrative Act19 – Ministry ofEconomy)	17/03
		Remote working, anticipation of individual and collective statutory leave, compensation of time and anticipation of public holidays (Provisional Act927)	22/03
Amapá (39.69)	Events	Mass gatherings banned (Judicial decision)	29/03
	Education	Closure of all teaching establishments(Decree 1377)	17/03
	Circulation of people	Remote working for vulnerable civil servants in at-risk groups(Decree 1377)	17/03
		Mass gatherings banned (Decree 1414)	20/03
		Non-essential businesses and services closed except for deliveries (Decree 1414)	20/03
		All river transport stopped (Decree 1415)	23/03
Amazonas (36.93)	Events	Public gatherings and gatherings in public facilities banned (Decree 42,061)	16/03
		Events involving more than 100 people banned (Decree 42,063)	17/03
	Education	Partial closure of state schools (Decree 42,061)	16/03
	Circulation of people	Remote working for vulnerable civil servants in at-risk groups and those with mild symptoms (Decree 42,061)	16/03
		All river transport stopped (Decree 42,087)	19/03
		Gyms and similar establishments closed (Decree 42,087)	19/03
		Circulation of all intercity bus services and tourist coaches stopped (Decree 42,098)	20/03
		All establishments involved in serving food directly to customers, as well as the leisure events industry, closed (Decree 42,099)	21/03
		Remote working for all civil servants (Decree 42,101)	23/03
		All non-essential businesses and services closed (Decree 42,101)	23/03
		Circulation of interstate bus services stopped (Decree 42,158)	04/04

Chart 3. COVID-19 control measures implemented at state and federal level in Brazil, presented for a selection of Brazilian states, together with the number of notified cases per 100,000 inhabitants, updated on April 16, 2020.

location (Notified cases/100,000 inhabitants)	Category of social distancing	Measure (government act)	effective date
Bahia (5.92)	Events	Events involving more than 50 people banned in cities in which there is community transmission (Decree 19,529)	17/03
		Events involving more than 50 people banned in the entire state (Decree 19,586)	28/03
	Education	Partial closure of teaching establishments (Decree 19,529)	17/03
		Complete closure of teaching establishments (Decree 19,586)	28/03
	Circulation of people	Obligatory self-isolation at home for people with symptoms of the disease (Decree 19,529)	17/03
		Docking of large vessels banned (Decree 19,529)	17/03
		Remote working for vulnerable civil servants in at-risk groups (Decree 19,528)	17/03
		Circulation of interstate buses stopped (Decree 19,528)	19/03
		Circulation of intercity transport stopped in locations in which there is community transmission - except for professional activity (Decree 19,549)	19/03
Ceará (24.95)	Events	No licenses granted for events involving more than 100 people (Decree 33,510)	16/03
		Collective activities using public facilities banned (Decree 33,510)	16/03
	Education	Total closure of all teaching establishments (Decree 33,510)	19/03
	Circulation of people	Remote working for vulnerable civil servants in at-risk groups (Decree 33,510)	16/03
		Discretionary leave for civil servants (Decree 33,519)	19/03
		Non-essential industrial activities and non-essential onsite activities in the commercial and service sectors closed(Decree 33,519)	19/03
		All beaches, rivers, lakes and swimming pools closed for visitation (Decree 33,519)	19/03
		Circulation of intercity and municipal public road transport, and subways stopped (Decree 33,519)	19/03
		Obligatory self-isolation at home for people with symptoms of the disease (Decree 33,519)	19/03
		Circulation of interstate buses stopped (Decree 33,519)	19/03
		Remote working for all civil servants able to work from home (Decree 33,536)	05/04
Federal District (22.80)	Events	No licenses granted for events involving more than 100 people (Decree 40,509)	11/03
		No licenses issued for any events (Decree 40,538)	19/03

	Education	Complete closure of all teaching establishments (Decree 40,509)	11/03
	Circulation of people	Quarantining of suspected cases and obligatory self-isolation at home for individuals with symptoms of the disease (Decree 40,475)	28/02
		Remote working for civil servants with mild symptoms (Decree 40,526)	17/03
		Non-essential on-site activities in the commercial and services sectors closed(Decree 40,538)	19/03
		Remote working for all civil servants (Decree 40.546)	23/03

it continues

Chart 3. COVID-19 control measures implemented at state and federal level in Brazil, presented for a selection of Brazilian states, together with the number of notified cases per 100,000 inhabitants, updated on April 16, 2020.

location (Notified cases/100,000 inhabitants)	Category of social distancing	Measure (government act)	effective date
Espírito Santo (18.55)	Events	All events banned except for places of worship (Decree 4599-R)	18/03
	Education	All teaching establishments closed (Decree 4597-R)	23/03
	Circulation of people	Remote working for vulnerable civil servants in at-risk groups (Decree 4599-R)	18/03
		Self-isolation for civil servants with mild flu-like symptoms (Decree 4599-R)	18/03
		All gyms and shopping malls with on-site activities closed (Decree 4600-R)	19/03
		On-site activities at bank branches stopped (Decree 4604-R)	20/03
		All commercial establishments and restaurants with on-site activities closed (Decree 4605-R)	20/03
Rio de Janeiro (21.55)	Events	Mass gatherings banned (Decree 46,970)	13/03
	Education	All teaching establishments closed (Decree 46,970)	13/03
	Circulation of people	Remote working for vulnerable civil servants in at-risk groups (Decree 46,970)	13/03
		Circulation of interstate buses with journeys originating in a state with community transmission banned (Decree 46,973)	17/03
		Free student travel pass cancelled (Decree 46,973)	17/03
		Intercity public road transport between the state capital and other cities banned (Decree 46,980)	19/03
		Air transport and docking of cruise ships coming from areas in which there is community transmission stopped (Decree 46,980)	19/03
		All beaches, rivers, lakes and pools closed for visitation (Decree 46,980)	19/03
Roraima (22.50)	Events	All events banned (Decree 28,587-E)	16/03
	Education	Partial closure of teaching establishments (Decree 28,587-E)	16/03
	Circulation of people	Circulation of intercity transport stopped (Decree 28,635-E)	23/03
		All non-essential business and service activities stopped except for deliveries (Decree 28,635-E)	23/03
		Remote working for all civil servants (Decree 28,635-E)	23/03
São Paulo (23.86)	Events	Events involving more than 500 people banned (Decree 64,862)	14/03
		Mass gatherings banned (Decree 64,864)	17/03
	Education	Partial closure of teaching establishments (Decree 64,862)	14/03
	Circulação de pessoas	Remote working for vulnerable civil servants in at-risk groups (Decree 64,864)	17/03
		Parks closed for visitation (Decree 64,879)	21/03
		All non-essential business and service activities closed except for deliveries (Decree 64,881)	24/03

Source: Datafolha (April 1-3, 2020)
Chart 4. COVID-19 control measures implemented at state and federal level in Brazil and the number of notified cases per 100,000 inhabitants, updated on April 16, 2020.

Area (Notified cases/100,000 inhabitants)	Social distancing category	Measure (Government Act)	effective date
Brazil (14.51)	Social distancing	Remote working for vulnerable civil servants in at-risk groups (Administrative Act19 - Ministry of Economy)	17/03
		Remote working, anticipation of individual and collective statutory leave, compensation of time and anticipation of public holidays (Provisional Act927)	22/03
Acre (11.29)	Events	Events involving more than 100 people banned (Decree 5,465)	17/03
	Education	Partial closure of teaching establishments (OrdinanceSEE 764)	20/03
	Circulation of people	Non-essential businesses and services closed except for deliveries (Decree 5,496)	20/03
		International and interstate transport stopped (Decree 5,496)	20/03
Alagoas (2.48)	Events	Open-air events involving more than 500 people and indoor events involving more that 100 people banned (Decree 69,501)	16/03
		Activities using public cultural facilities banned (Decree 69,501)	16/03
		Total ban on any events (Decree 69,541)	20/03
	Education	Complete closure of all teaching establishments (Decree 69,501)	23/03
	Circulation of people	Remote working for vulnerable civil servants in at-risk groups (Decree 69,502)	16/03
		Non-essential businesses, industries and services closed except for deliveries (Decree 69,502)	20/03
		Intercity road transport and subways stopped (Decree 69,502)	20/03
		All beaches and parks closed for visitation (Decree 69,502)	20/03
		Self-isolation obligatory for individuals with any flu-like symptoms(Decree 69,502)	20/03
		Discretionary leave for civil servants (Decree 69,502)	23/03
		Remote working for all civil servants able to work from home (Decree 69,577)	30/03
Amapá (39.69)	Events	Mass gatherings banned (Judicial decision)	29/03
	Education	Total closure of all teaching establishments(Decree 1,377)	17/03
	Circulation of people	Remote working for vulnerable civil servants in at-risk groups (Decree 1,377)	17/03
		Gatherings in public places banned (Decree 1,414)	20/03
		All non-essential businesses and services closed except for deliveries (Decree 1,414)	20/03
		River transport stopped (Decree 1,415)	23/03
Amazonas	Events	Public events and those using public facilities banned (Decree 42,061)	16/03

(36.93)		Events involving more than 100 people banned (Decree 42,063)	17/03
	Education	Partial closure of state teaching establishments (Decree 42,061)	16/03
	Circulation of people	Remote working for vulnerable civil servants in at-risk groups and for those with mild symptoms (Decree 42,061)	16/03
		River transport stopped (Decree 42,087)	19/03
		Gyms and similar establishments closed (Decree 42,087)	19/03
		Circulation of intercity buses and tourist coaches stopped (Decree 42,098)	20/03
		On-site food sector closed and leisure events banned (Decree 42,099)	21/03
		Remote working for all civil servants (Decree 42,101)	23/03
		All non-essential businesses and services closed (Decree 42,101)	23/03
		Circulation of interstate public road transport stopped (Decree 42,158)	04/04

it continues

Chart 4. COVID-19 control measures implemented at state and federal level in Brazil and the number of notified cases per 100,000 inhabitants, updated on April 16, 2020.

Area (Notified cases/100,000 inhabitants)	Social distancing category	Measure (Government Act)	effective date
Bahia (5.92)	Events	Events involving more than 50 people banned in municipalities in which there is community transmission (Decree 19,529)	17/03
		Events involving more than 50 people banned throughout the entire state (Decree 19,586)	28/03
	Education	Partial closure of teaching establishments (Decree 19,529)	17/03
		Total closure of teaching establishments (Decree 19,586)	28/03
	Circulation of people	Obligatory self-isolation at home for people with symptoms of the disease (Decree 19,529)	17/03
		Docking of large vessels banned (Decree 19,529)	17/03
		Remote working for vulnerable civil servants in at-risk groups (Decree 19,528)	17/03
		Circulation of interstate buses stopped (Decree 19,528)	19/03
		Intercity bus transport from cities in which there is community transmission stopped except for professional activity (Decree 19,549)	19/03
Ceará (24.95)	Events	No licenses granted for events involving more than 100 people (Decree 33,510)	16/03
		Gatherings in public spaces banned (Decree 33,510)	16/03
	Education	Complete closure of teaching establishments (Decree 33,510)	19/03
	Circulation of people	Remote working for vulnerable civil servants in at-risk groups (Decree 33,510)	16/03
		Discretionary leave for civil servants (Decree 33,519)	19/03
		All non-essential industries and non-essential on-site commercial establishments and services closed (Decree 33,519)	19/03
		All beaches, rivers, lakes and swimming pools closed for visitation (Decree 33,519)	19/03
		Intercity and metropolitan road transport and subways stopped (Decree 33,519)	19/03
		Self-isolation at home obligatory for anyone with symptoms of the disease (Decree 33,519)	19/03
		Circulation of interstate buses stopped (Decree 33,519)	19/03
		Remote working for all civil servants able to work from home (Decree 33,536)	05/04
Federal District (22.80)	Events	No licenses granted for events involving more than 100 people (Decree 40,509)	11/03
		No licenses for events granted (Decree 40,538)	19/03
	Education	Complete closure of all teaching establishments (Decree 40,509)	11/03
	Circulation of people	Quarantining of suspected cases and obligatory self-isolation at home for individuals with symptoms of the disease (Decree 40,475)	28/02

		Remote working for civil servants with mild symptoms (Decree 40,526)	17/03
		All on-site non-essential businesses and services banned (Decree 40,538)	19/03
		Remote working for all civil servants (Decree 40,546)	23/03
Espírito Santo (18.55)	Events	All events banned except for places of worship (Decree 4,599-R)	18/03
	Education	Complete closure of all teaching establishments (Decree 4,597-R)	23/03
	Circulation of people	Remote working for all vulnerable civil servants in at-risk groups (Decree 4,599R)	18/03
		Self-isolation at home for civil servants with flu-like symptoms (Decree 4,599-R)	18/03
		Gyms and shopping malls with on-site service closed (Decree 4,600-R)	19/03
		On-site service at banks stopped (Decree 4,604-R)	20/03
		Retail businesses and restaurants with on-site service closed (Decree 4,605-R)	20/03

it continues

Chart 4. COVID-19 control measures implemented at state and federal level in Brazil and the number of notified cases per 100,000 inhabitants, updated on April 16, 2020.

Area (Notified cases/100,000 inhabitants)	Social distancing category	Measure (Government Act)	effective date
Goiás (4.27)	Events	All events banned (Decree 9,633)	13/03
	Education	Complete closure of all teaching establishments (Technical note 1/2020 - SES/ GO)	18/03
	Circulation of people	Remote working for vulnerable civil servants in at-risk groups and alternating schedules for the remainder (Decree 9,634)	17/03
		Non-essential commercial establishments and services closed except for deliveries (Decree 9,637)	19/03
		Road and air transport from regions where the virus is in circulation stopped (Decree 9,638)	24/03
		Non-essential businesses closed (Decree 9,644)	25/03
Maranhão (9.77)	Events	No licenses granted for events (Decree 35,660)	16/03
		Activities involving mass gatherings banned (Decree 35,677)	21/03
	Education	Partial closure of teaching establishments (Decree 35,662)	17/03
	Circulation of people	Self-isolation at home for civil servants with mild symptoms (Decree 35,660)	16/03
		Interstate transport stopped (Decree 35,672)	21/03
		Non-essential commercial establishments and services closed except for deliveries (Decree 35,677)	21/03
		Docking of large vessels from countries in which the disease is in circulation banned (Decree 35,677)	21/03
Mato Grosso (4.28)	Events	All events banned except for those guaranteeing at least 1.5 meters between each individual present (Decree 419)	20/03

		All events banned (Decree 425)	26/03
	Education	Complete closure of all teaching establishments (Decree 425)	26/03
	Circulation of people	Remote working and alternating schedules authorized for civil servants (Decree 407)	16/03
		Bars, convenience stores, bakeries and restaurants closed except for deliveries (Decree 421)	23/03
		Intercity road transport stopped (Decree 421)	23/03
		Leisure spaces, places of worship, sports and cultural venues closed for visitation (Decree 425)	26/03
		"Vertical" isolation of infected individuals in cities with community transmission (Decree 432)	02/04
		Restrictions imposed on non-essential activities in cities with community transmission (Decree 432)	02/04
Mato Grosso do Sul (4.31)	Events	No licenses for events granted (Decree 15,396)	20/03
	Education	Partial closure of teaching establishments (Decree 15,393)	23/03
	Circulation of people	Remote working for vulnerable civil servants in at-risk groups and who have any symptom (Decree 15,391)	16/03
		Remote working for all civil servants able to work from home, with alternating schedules being an option (Decree 15,393)	20/03
		All state-run parks and sports facilities closed (Decree 15,393)	20/03
		Discretionary leave for civil servants (Decree E 29)	03/04

it continues

Chart 4. COVID-19 control measures implemented at state and federal level in Brazil and the number of notified cases per 100,000 inhabitants, updated on April 16, 2020.

Area (Notified cases/100,000 inhabitants)	Social distancing category	Measure (Government Act)	effective date
Minas Gerais (4.24)	Events	Events involving more than 30 people banned (Decision 17 of the Extraordinary COVID-19 Committee)	22/03
	Education	Partial closure of all teaching establishments (Decision 01)	18/03
		Complete closure of all teaching establishments (Decision 15)	21/03
	Circulation of people	Priority given to remote working for all civil servants and/or measures to reduce the number of employees present (Decision 02)	17/03
		Remote working for all vulnerable civil servants in at-risk groups (Decision 04)	18/03
		All interstate road, river and rail transport stopped(Decision 11)	21/03
		Remote working for all civil servants (Decision 12)	21/03
		All municipalities ordered to close businesses and services (Decision 17)	22/03
Pará (5.60)	Events	No licenses issued for events involving more than 500 people (Decree 607)	16/03
		Events involving more than 10 people banned (Decree 609)	07/04
	Education	Total closure of all state teaching establishments (Decree 607)	16/03
	Circulation of people	Possibility of remote working, particularly for vulnerable civil servants in at-risk groups (Decree 607)	16/03
		All beaches, riversides, bathing resorts, clubs, etc. closed for visitation (Decree 607)	16/03
		Gyms, bars, restaurants, nightclubs and similar types of establishment closed except for deliveries (Decree 607)	16/03
		On-site religious gatherings banned (Decree 607)	16/03
		Interstate road, sea and river transport stopped (Decree 607)	23/03
		Intercity road and sea/river transport stopped during April extended public holidays (Decree 607)	08/04
Paraíba (4.08)	Events	State-run events cancelled (Decree 40,128)	19/03
		Events in cities in which there are cases of the disease banned (Decree 40,173)	04/04
	Education	Partial closure of teaching establishments (Decree 40,128)	19/03
	Circulation of people	Alternating schedules for all civil servants and remote working for all those in at-risk groups (Decree 40,128)	19/03
		All crews from cargo ships banned from disembarking (Decree 40,135)	21/03
		All non-essential businesses and services closed except for deliveries (Decree 40,135)	21/03
		Intercity transport from major cities stopped (Decree 40,135)	21/03
		Remote working for all civil servants able to work from home (Decree 40,136)	21/03

		Reduction in service of the main ferry routes (Decree 40,135)	22/03
Paraná (7.09)	Events	Events involving more than 50 people banned (Decree 4,230)	16/03
	Education	Complete closure of all teaching establishments (Decree 4,230)	20/03
	Circulation of people	Remote working for vulnerable civil servants in at-risk groups and a reduction in working hours, alternating schedules and remote working for the remainder (Decree 4,230)	16/03
		All state road transport stopped (Decree 4,263)	20/03
		Access of non-residents to an isolated community (Ilha do Mel) banned (Decree 4,230)	21/03

it continues

Chart 4. COVID-19 control measures implemented at state and federal level in Brazil and the number of notified cases per 100,000 inhabitants, updated on April 16, 2020.

Area (Notified cases/100,000 inhabitants)	Social distancing category	Measure (Government Act)	effective date
Pernambuco (15.43)	Events	Events involving more than 500 people banned (Decree 48,809)	14/03
		Events involving more than 50 people banned (Decree 48,822)	18/03
		Activities in cultural facilities and gyms banned (Decree 48,822)	18/03
		All events banned (Decree 48,837)	24/03
	Education	Complete closure of all teaching establishments (Decree 48,810)	18/03
	Circulation of people	Docking of large vessels banned (Decree 48,809)	14/03
		Remote working for all vulnerable civil servants in at-risk groups (Decree 48,810)	17/03
		Obligatory self-isolation at home for individuals arriving from countries in which there are cases of the disease (Decree 48,822)	18/03
		All travel to an isolated community (Fernando de Noronha) and tourism there stopped (Decree 48,822)	18/03
		All crews of cargo ships banned from disembarking (Decree 48,830)	19/03
		All non-essential businesses and services closed except for deliveries (Decree 48,833)	21/03
		All access to an isolated community (Fernando de Noronha) stopped except for essential activities (Decree 48,878)	03/04
		All beaches and parks closed for visitation (Decree 48,881)	04/04
Piauí (2.77)	Events	Open-air events involving more than 100 people and indoor events for more than 50 people banned (Decree 18,884)	16/03
	Education	Partial closure of teaching establishments (Decree 18,884)	16/03
		Complete closure of all teaching establishments (Decree 18,913)	30/03
	Circulation of people	All non-essential businesses and services closed except for deliveries (Decree 18,901)	21/03
		Reduction of 50% in the flow of personnel involved in essential activities (Decree 18,902)	23/03
		Reduction in working hours for the industrial sector (Decree 18,902)	23/03
		All intercity road transport stopped (Decree 18,924)	03/04
Rio de Janeiro (21.55)	Events	Mass gatherings banned (Decree 46,970)	13/03
	Education	Complete closure of all teaching establishments (Decree 46,970)	13/03
	Circulation of people	Remote working for vulnerable civil servants in at-risk groups (Decree 46,970)	13/03
		The circulation of all interstate buses coming from states in which there is community transmission of the disease banned (Decree 46,973)	17/03
		Free student travel pass cancelled (Decree 46,973)	17/03
		All intercity road transport between the state capital and other cities cancelled (Decree 46,980)	19/03
		Air transport and docking of cruise ships from areas with community transmission of the virus stopped (Decree 46,980)	19/03
		Beaches, rivers, lakes and swimming pools closed for visitation (Decree 46,980)	19/03

it continues

Chart 4. COVID-19 control measures implemented at state and federal level in Brazil and the number of notified cases per 100,000 inhabitants, updated on April 16, 2020.

Area (Notified cases/100,000 inhabitants)	Social distancing category	Measure (Government Act)	effective date
Rio Grande do Norte (11.29)	Events	Events involving more than 100 people banned (Decree 29,524)	18/03
		Events involving more than 50 people banned (Decree 29,541)	21/03
		Events involving more than 20 people banned (Decree 29,583)	02/04
	Education	Complete closure of all teaching establishments (Decree 29,524)	18/03
	Circulation of people	Remote working for vulnerable civil servants in at-risk groups (Decree 29,512)	14/03
		All non-essential businesses and services closed except for deliveries and for open air shopping malls(Decree 29,541)	21/03
		Any establishment with artificial air circulation system closed (Decree 29,583)	02/04
Rio Grande do Sul (6.67)	Events	All events banned (Decree 55,128)	19/03
	Education	Partial closure of all teaching establishments (Decree 55,118)	17/03
		Complete closure of all teaching establishments (Decree 55,154)	01/04
	Circulation of people	Remote working for all civil servants able to work from home and alternating schedules for the remainder (Decree 55,118)	17/03
		Remote working for all vulnerable civil servants in at-risk groups (Decree 55,118)	17/03
		Interstate transport banned (Decree 55,128)	19/03
		Alternating schedules and remote working for all civil servants (Decree 55,128)	19/03
		All interstate and international road transport stopped (Decree 55,130)	21/03
		Beaches closed for visitation (Decree 55,130)	21/03
		All non-essential businesses and services stopped except for deliveries (Decree 55,128)	01/04
Rondônia (4.06)	Events	All events involving more than 5 people banned (Decree 24,887)	25/03
	Education	Complete closure of all teaching establishments (Decree 24,871)	17/03
	Circulation of people	Remote working for all civil servants able to work from home (Decree 24,871)	17/03
		Circulation of all motorcycle taxis banned (Decree 24,887)	25/03
		All flights from out of state banned (Decree 24,887)	25/03
		All non-essential businesses and services closed except for deliveries (Decree 24,887)	25/03
		The entry of all vehicles from other countries banned (Decree 24,887)	25/03
		The circulation of personnel for essential activities to be obligatorily reduced (Decree 24,887)	25/03
Roraima (22.50)	Events	All events banned (Decree 28,587-E)	16/03
	Education	Partial closure of all teaching establishments (Decree 28,587-E)	16/03
	Circulation of people	All intercity transport stopped (Decree 28,635-E)	23/03
		All non-essential businesses and services closed except for deliveries (Decree 28,635E)	23/03
		Remote working for all civil servants (Decree 28,635-E)	23/03

it continues

Chart 4. COVID-19 control measures implemented at state and federal level in Brazil and the number of notified cases per 100,000 inhabitants, updated on April 16, 2020.

Area (Notified cases/100,000 inhabitants)	Social distancing category	Measure (Government Act)	effective date
Santa Catarina (12.29)	Events	All events banned (Decree 515)	17/03
	Education	Complete closure of all teaching establishments (Decree 509)	17/03
	Circulation of people	Remote working for all vulnerable civil servants in at-risk groups (Decree 507)	16/03
		Public spaces closed for gatherings and visitation (Decree 521)	19/03
		Municipal, intercity and interstate public road transport stopped (Decree 521)	19/03
		River and sea transport for pedestrians and cyclists stopped (Decree 525)	23/03
		All non-essential businesses and services closed except for deliveries (Decree 525)	23/03
		Reduction of 50% in number of customers for essential activities (Decree 525)	23/03
		Reduction of 50% in the size of the workforce in the industrial sector - prioritizing remote working for personnel in at-risk groups and administrative staff, without affecting salaries. Charter transportation service to run at no more than 50% of capacity (Decree 525)	23/03
São Paulo (23.86)	Events	Events involving more than 500 people banned (Decree 64,862)	14/03
		Mass gatherings banned (Decree 64,864)	17/03
	Education	Partial closure of teaching establishments (Decree 64,862)	14/03
	Circulation of people	Remote working for vulnerable civil servants in at-risk groups (Decree 64,864)	17/03
		Parks closed for visitation (Decree 64,879)	21/03
		All non-essential businesses and services closed except for deliveries (Decree 64,881)	24/03
Sergipe (2.07)	Events	Open-air events involving more than 100 people and indoor events involving more than 50 people banned (Decree 40,560)	17/03
		All events banned (Decree 40,563)	20/03
	Education	Complete closure of all teaching establishments (Decree 40,560)	17/03
	Circulation of people	Cinemas, theaters and similar establishments closed (Decree 40,560)	17/03
		Remote working for all vulnerable civil servants in at-risk groups (Decree 40,560)	17/03
		All non-essential businesses and services closed except for deliveries (Decree 40,563)	20/03
		Docking of ships coming from regions where the virus is in circulation banned (Decree 40,563)	23/03
		Interstate buses from states in which the virus is in circulation stopped (Decree 40,563)	23/03

		Alternating schedules for the workforce in the commercial and industrial sectors (Decree 40,563)	20/03
		Alternating schedules and remote working for all civil servants, as well as a reduction in working hours (Decree 40,563)	20/03
		Remote working for all civil servants able to work from home (Decree 40,567)	25/03
Tocantins (1.82)	Events	All events banned (Decree 6,072)	21/03
	Education	Partial closure of all teaching establishments (Decree 6,065)	18/03
		Total closure of all teaching establishments (Decree 6,071)	19/03
	Circulation of people	Reduction in working hours and alternating schedules for civil servants (Decree 6,066)	16/03
		Nature parks closed for visitation (Decree 6,067)	17/03
		The practice of sports in state-owned venues banned (Decree 6,071)	19/03
		Remote working for vulnerable civil servants in at-risk groups (Decree 6,072)	21/03

REFERENCES

1. the EU/EEA and the UK. *Euro Surveill* 2020; 25:10.

2. Deshwal VK. COVID 19: A Comparative Study of Asian, European, American continent. *IJSRED* 2020; 3:2.

3. Ferguson N, Laydon D, Nedjati Gilani G, Imai N, Ainslie K, Baguelin M, Bhatia S, Boonyasiri A, Cucunuba Perez ZU, Cuomo-Dannenburg G, Dighe A. *Impact of non-pharmaceutical interventions (NPIs) to reduce COVID-19 mortality and healthcare demand. Imperial College COVID-19 Response Team*. United Kingdom: Imperial College COVID-19 Response Team, 2020.

4. Barreto ML, Teixeira MG, Carmo EH. Infectious diseases epidemiology. *J Epidemiol Community Health* 2006; 60(3):192.

5. Boldog P, Tekeli T, Vizi Z, Denes A, Bartha FA, Rost G. Risk Assessment of Novel Coronavirus COVID-19 Outbreaks Outside China. *J Clin Med* 2020; 9:2.

6. Lau H, Khosrawipour V, Kocbach P, Mikolajczyk A, Schubert J, Bania J, Khosrawipour T. The positive impact of lockdown in Wuhan on containing the COVID-19 outbreak in China. *J Travel Med* 2020; pii:taaa037.

7. Kucharski AJ, Russell TW, Diamond C, Liu Y, Edmunds J, Funk S, Eggo RM, Sun F, Jit M, Munday JD, Davies N. Early dynamics of transmission and control of COVID-19: a mathematical modelling study. *Lancet Infect Dis* 2020; S1473-3099(20)30144-4.

8. Pepe E, Bajardi P, Gauvin L, Privitera F, Lake B, Cattuto C, Tizzoni M. COVID-19 outbreak response: a first assessment of mobility changes in Italy following national lockdown. *medRxiv* 2020; 2020.03.22.20039933.

9. Flaxman S, Mishra S, Gandy A. *Estimating the number of infections and the impact of non-pharmaceutical interventions on COVID-19 in 11 European countries*. United Kingdom: Imperial College COVID-19 Response Team; 2020.

10. Ganem F, Mendes FM, Oliveira SB, Porto VB, Araujo W, Nakaya H, Diaz-Quijano FA, Croda J. The impact of early social distancing at COVID-19 Outbreak in the largest Metropolitan Area of Brazil. *medRxiv* 2020; 2020.04.06.20055103.

11. Canabarro A, Tenorio E, Martins R, Martins L, Brito S, Chaves R. Data-Driven Study of the COVID-19 Pandemic via Age-Structured Modelling and Prediction of the Health System Failure in Brazil amid Diverse Intervention Strategies. *medRxiv* 2020; 2020.04.03.20052498.

12. Hou J, Hong J, Ji B, Dong B, Chen Y, Ward MP, Tu W, Jin Z, Hu J, Su Q, Wang W. Changing transmission dynamics of COVID-19 in China: a nationwide population-based piecewise mathematical modelling study. *medRxiv* 2020; 2020.03.27.20045757.

13. Yang Q, Yi C, Vajdi A, Cohnstaedt LW, Wu H, Guo X, Scoglio CM. Short-term forecasts and longterm mitigation evaluations for the COVID-19 epidemic in Hubei Province, China. *medRxiv* 2020; 2020.03.27.20045625.

14. Nussbaumer-Streit B, Mayr V, Dobrescu AI, Chapman A, Persad E, Klerings I, Wagner G, Siebert U, Christof C, Zachariah C, Gartlehner G. Quarantine alone or in combination with other public health measures to control COVID-19: a rapid review. *Cochrane Database Syst Rev* 2020; 4:CD013574.

15. Rede CoVida [Internet]. *Painel Coronavírus Brasil*. Salvador: Rede CoVida; 2020. [cited 2020 Apr 16]. Available from: http://www.covid19br.org.

16. Silva AAM. Sobre a possibilidade de interrupção da epidemia pelo coronavírus (COVID-19) com base nas melhores evidências científicas disponíveis. *Rev Bras Epidemiol* 2020; 23:e200021.

17. Brasil. Ministério da Saúde (MS). *Boletim Epidemiológico Especial 7: doença pelo coronavírus 2019*. Brasília: MS; 2020.

18. European Comission. *A European roadmap to lifting coronavirus containment measures*. 2020 [cited 2020 Apr 16]. Available from: https://ec.europa.eu/info/ live-work-travel-eu/health/coronavirus-response/ european-roadmap-lifting-coronavirus-containment-measures_en

19. World Health Organization (WHO). *Coronavirus disease (COVID-2019) situation reports*. Geneva: WHO; 2020.

3. Implications of Social Distancing In Brazil In The COVID-19 Pandemic

Raquel Cristina Cavalcanti Dantas PhD[1],
Paola Amaral de Campos PhD[2], Iara Rossi MSc[2] and
Rosineide Marques Ribas PhD[2]

[1]Institute of Biotechnology, Federal University of Uberlandia, Brazil and [2]Laboratory of Molecular Microbiology, Federal University of Uberlandia, Brazil

The pandemic caused by a novel coronavirus disease, known as COVID-19, carried millions of people around the world to a state of unprecedented panic.

The World Health Organization (WHO) stated that more than one-third of the world is currently under some social distancing pattern, which is the oldest and probably one of the most effective methods for controlling infectious disease outbreaks. However, governments of many countries have difficulty implementing social distancing, particularly in developing countries such as Brazil, where income inequality is high and the national economy is fragile. Several studies in the literature, both in developed and developing countries, have demonstrated the effectiveness of social distancing in slowing the spread of COVID-19.[1,2] In a recent study, Taghrir et al[1] investigated the efficacy of mass quarantine during the pandemic and found good-quality evidence for the social distancing strategies to have been highly effective in controlling the spread of the disease. Complementing this analysis, other researchers analysed data of 8 countries extremely affected by COVID-19: China, Italy, Iran, Germany, France, Spain, South Korea, and Japan. They concluded that the rapidly increasing COVID-19 case numbers in European countries occurs due to late contention measures[2]. Therefore, social distancing is currently the most effective way to slow the spread of COVID-19.

In Brazil, the Ministry of Health recommended measures of social distancing, respiratory etiquette, and hand hygiene.[3] Social distancing measures included the closing of schools, universities, and almost all shops, except food stores and pharmacies. In addition, cafes, restaurants, clubs, gyms, museums, and other institutions across the country have closed. Public gatherings, religious services, and social and sporting events have been cancelled. Nonetheless, the number of cases for COVID-19 has continued to grow exponentially due to difficulties in establishing true and effective social distancing. In the real Brazilian context, a large number of informal workers are still working normally and there is a lack of access to information for a large part of the population regarding minimum infection prevention and control measures, including hand washing and respiratory etiquette. Although handwashing and social distancing are still the best measures to protect against the virus, the flattening the COVID-19 curve will require additional measures in developing countries, where the spreading factor of the virus are different and more complex.

In Brazil, it is essential to better understand the true prevalence of COVID-19, but the lack of mass testing is one of the main problems that make it difficult to implement measures to ensure that infected individuals are in an appropriate quarantine. Here, the physical distancing between infected and people is crucial in the high-risk group, such as the elderly and those with respiratory or chronic illnesses, to reduce the lethal effect of the pandemic. According to the WHO, wearing a surgical mask, in combination with hand hygiene and other preventative measures, is one of the prevention measures to limit the spread of SARS-CoV-2 in affected areas.[4] Cowling et al[5] demonstrated that the implementation of social distancing measures and changes in population behaviours, including use of facial masks, were associated with reduced transmission of SARS-CoV-2 in Hong Kong. In Brazil, the adoption of this equipment can be difficult due to the low adhesion or the lack of access to facial masks by the Brazilian population. Thus, the correct use of facial masks is fundamental to the effectiveness of the measure and can be encouraged and improved through education campaigns.

In Brazil, coronavirus is advancing exponentially. Although the disease has spread rapidly in large capitals, where the incidence of cases is high, COVID-19 cases are increasing in smaller cities and poorer communities as well. More than three-quarters of the confirmed cases are in southern and south-eastern regions of Brazil, which are more densely populated, including many elderly, and with tropical and subtropical climates. In addition, the economic burden that sustained distancing can impose is potentially catastrophic in Brazil and other developing countries. Furthermore, if social distancing is not effective and/or is not sustained for long enough, the healthcare system may collapse, contributing to a greater tragedy.

Acknowledgments. The authors would like to thank the Brazilian research and development agencies for supporting this article.

Financial support. This work was supported by Coordenação de Aperfeiçoamento de Pessoal de Nível Superior (CAPES), by Brazilian

Author for correspondence: Rosineide Marques Ribas, E-mail: rosi_ribas@yahoo. com.br

10.1017/ice.2020.210
National Council for Scientific and Technological Development (CNPq), and by Fundação de Amparo à Pesquisa do Estado de Minas Gerais (FAPEMIG). This letter was based on observations and reflections about the COVID-19 pandemic during studies supported by the funding agencies.

REFERENCES

1.Taghrir, M.H., Akbarialiabad, H., Ahmadi Marzaleh, M. (2020) Efficacy of mass quarantine as leverage of health system governance during COVID-19 outbreak: a mini policy review. *Arch Iran Med* 2020;23:265–267.
2.Parmet, W.E., Sinha, M.S. (2020). The law and limits of quarantine. *N Engl J Med* 2020;382(15):e28.CrossRef
3.Medidas Não Farmacológicas [in Italian]. Ministério da Saúde website. https://coronavirus.saude.gov.br/. Published 2020. Accessed April 27, 2020.Google Scholar
4.Advice on the use of masks the community, during homecare and in healthcare settings in the context of the novel coronavirus (2019-nCoV). Outbreak Interim Guidance. World Health Organization
website. https://www.who.int/publications-detail/ Published 2020. Accessed April 27, 2020.Google Scholar
5.Cowling, B.J., Ali, S.T., Ng, T.W.Y, et al. (2020).Impact assessment of non-pharmaceutical interventions against coronavirus disease 2019 and influenza in Hong Kong: an observational study. *Lancet Public Health* 2020; pii: S2468-2667(20)30090-6.CrossRef | Google Scholar

4. Vertical Social Distancing Policy Is Ineffective To Contain The COVID-19 Pandemic [1]

Luiz Henrique[2] Duczmal [3]

Alexandre Celestino Leite Almeida [4]

Denise Bulgarelli Duczmal [5]

Claudia Regina Lindgren Alves [6]Flávia Costa Oliveira Magalhães [7]

Max Sousa de Lima [6]Ivair Ramos Silva [8]

Ricardo Hiroshi Caldeira Takahashi [3]

ABSTRACT

Considering numerical simulations, this study shows that the so-called vertical social distancing health policy is ineffective to contain the COVID-19 pandemic. We present the SEIR-Net model, for a network of social group interactions, as a development of the classic mathematical model of SEIR epidemics (Susceptible-Exposed-Infected (symptomatic and asymptomatic) Removed). In the SEIR-Net model, we can simulate social contacts between groups divided by age groups and analyse different strategies of social distancing. In the vertical distancing policy, only older people are distanced, whereas in the horizontal distancing policy all age groups adhere to social distancing. These two scenarios are compared to a control scenario in which no intervention is made to distance people. The vertical distancing scenario is almost as bad as the control, both in terms of people infected and in the acceleration of cases. On the other hand, horizontal distancing, if applied with the same intensity in all age groups, significantly reduces the total infected people "flattening the disease growth curve". Our analysis considers the city of Belo Horizonte, Minas Gerais State, Brazil, but similar conclusions apply to other cities as well. Code implementation of the model in R-language is provided in the supplementary material.

INTRODUCTION

[1] Cad. Saúde Pública 2020; 36(5):e00084420

[2] CorrespondenceC. R. L. Alves Rua Tavares Bastos 287, Belo Horizonte, MG 30380-040, Brasil. lindgrenalves@gmail.com

[3] Departamento de Estatística, Universidade Federal de Minas Gerais, Belo Horizonte, Brasil.

[4] Departamento de Estatística, Física e Matemática, Universidade Federal de São João del-Rei, Ouro Branco, Minas Gerais.

[5] Departamento de Matemática, Universidade Federal de Minas Gerais, Belo Horizonte, Brasil.

[6] Departamento de Pediatria, Universidade Federal de Minas Gerais, Belo Horizonte, Brasil.

[7] Polícia Civil de Minas Gerais, Belo Horizonte, Brasil. 6 Departamento de Estatística, Universidade Federal do Amazonas, Manaus, Brasil.

[8] Departamento de Estatística, Universidade Federal de Ouro Preto, Ouro Preto, Brasil.

In Brazil, there is a widespread belief that the so-called vertical social distancing health policy, just restricting social contact with older people – and higher risk individuals –, would be enough to contain the propagation of the SARS-CoV-2 coronavirus disease (COVID-19). This idea assumes that people under the age of 60 would suffer only mild symptoms and could leave their houses to work and study during the epidemic.

However, we have observed a high number of hospitalizations, with severe cases and deaths also affecting people under 60 years old and without underlying diseases. Besides, social distancing is not a strict rule, and older people tend to make social contacts during the period, increasing the possibility of infection. Through this study, we shall use the terms "social distance" and "social isolation" interchangeably to indicate a reduction in the intensity of social contact. Social distance measures in the COVID-19 pandemic are already proving its effectiveness, reducing the number of infected people 1,2,3,4,5,6,7. Why is it important? Mainly because we want the peak of the epidemic to be minimized, to avoid overloading the health system with many people requiring intensive care simultaneously because of COVID-19 and its symptoms.

This goal of the public health services is popularly known as "flattening the curve" of cases and hospitalizations. If there are not enough hospital beds to serve everyone, many people may die from lack of care. Postponing the peak of cases would be potentially beneficial so health managers are better prepared, and so researchers can find more effective treatments. Therefore, if social distancing can reduce the peak of infected people, at the same time postponing its occurrence, many lives can be saved.

We will analyse these problems with a mathematical technique for simulating the evolution of epidemics, the SEIR-Net model, obtained from a modification of the traditional SEIR model (Susceptible-Exposed-Infected-Removed). In the SEIR model, people susceptible to infection randomly come into contact with the SARS-CoV-2 virus becoming exposed. After the incubation period, they are infected and can pass this virus at random to other susceptible people. Infected people can be asymptomatic (have few or no symptoms) or symptomatic (develop typical symptoms of COVID-19 infection). Infected people become, over time, removed (a technical term to say that they cannot infect other people and may survive or die). In this model, we use an estimate of unreported cases, based on the reported (confirmed) cases.

This extrapolation/estimation happens because it is not possible to test the entire population.

In Brazil, the estimates show at least 20 times more unreported than reported cases, and it was based on model fitting using a mathematical SEIR model for the disease spread in Minas Gerais State 8. Still, this number now is probably much higher, mainly due to the scarcity of available test kits. Our model assumes that the contact among persons follow a uniformly random pattern of interaction, and apart from the age groups, there is no spatial (geographic) restriction to social contact – which is embedded into the B transmission parameter determined empirically from the observed data at the beginning of the epidemic.

Some parameters are important in this simulation, such as the average incubation time (Z), the average infectious period (D) (for how many days the infected individual can infect others), and the fraction of asymptomatic infected individuals still capable of infecting others (although with less intensity).

An important parameter, which does not depend only on the virus, is the transmission rate (B); it depends on the country's health system and the population's living conditions. If B is high, it means that the virus tends to spread more quickly. All COVID-19 parameters used in this study were obtained from the article 9 and adapted to the observed case data from Belo Horizonte, Minas Gerais State 8. In the next section, we will build our new model SEIR-Net with social distancing and network interaction. In the following section, we will present several scenarios simulating different conditions of vertical and horizontal social distancing in Belo Horizonte and study their impact on reducing simultaneously infected people. Code implementation of the model in R-language is provided in the Supplementary Material[1]

The SEIR-Net model

The model proposed in this study is a development of the model used in Takahashi 8, and generalizes the SEIR is model proposed in Duczmal et al. 10. The recent model by Prem et al. 3 also uses the SEIR model with a partitioning of the population into groups and considers their interaction. The SEIR-Net model divides the population between n social distancing groups and uses the *F Contact Fraction Matrix*, given by:

$$F \quad \begin{pmatrix} F_{11} & \cdots & F_{1n} \\ \vdots & \ddots & \vdots \\ F_{n1} & \cdots & F_{nn} \end{pmatrix}$$

Where the entry F_{ij} indicates the contact intensity of virus transmission from an individual in the group i to an individual in the group j, where $0 \le F_{ij} \le 1$. If $F_{ij} = 1$, then the contact is not restricted, and if $F_{ij} = 0$ no individual in the group *i* can transmit the virus to any individual in the group *j*. This system connects the n groups. In our study, we will use groups formed by age groups in the city of Belo Horizonte. In future work, we will extend this idea to groups divided by income level, place of residence or work, occupation, etc. How will the COVID-19 epidemic evolve in this case? In the next section we will analyse scenarios with different structures for the F matrix.

Case Studies

In the SEIR-Net model, we can simulate social contact between groups divided by age and analyse different strategies of social distancing. The population of Belo Horizonte, with approximately 2.5 million inhabitants, has the following age distribution interpolated for 2015 0-9 years old: 11.7%; 10-24 years old: 21.8%; 25-59 years old: 52.3%; 60+ years old: 14.2%. Initially, we present a control scenario without distancing intervention. In this case, all elements Fij of the F matrix are equal to 1. In vertical distancing, only people aged 60+ years old are socially distanced. The F matrix is given by:

$$F \begin{bmatrix} 1 & 1 & 1 & c \\ 1 & 1 & 1 & c \\ 1 & 1 & 1 & c \\ c & c & c & c \end{bmatrix}$$

Where $c = 1/k$ means that contact between individuals aged 60+ years old have a *k*-fold reduced social contact with individuals of all age groups and *vice versa*. Finally, in horizontal distancing, individuals of all age groups adhere to distancing. The F matrix becomes:

[1] (http://cadernos.ensp.fiocruz.br/site/public_site/arquivo/ suppl-e00084420_6775.pdf).

$$F \begin{bmatrix} c & c & c & c \\ c & c & c & c \\ c & c & c & c \\ c & c & c & c \end{bmatrix}$$

Where the value of c depends on the social contact reduction factor. A value of $c = 1/15$ corresponds to the estimated social contact reduction factor for New York city, USA, during the end of March, with a 15-fold social contact reduction, meaning that social contact was reduced by $1 - 1/15 = 93\%$ [2]. When $c = 1$, we go back to the control scenario, with 0% of social contact reduction. As we will see, a value of $c = 0.55$ (1.8 fold, i.e., 45% reduction of social contact) for the above matrix is consistent with the observed data in Belo Horizonte.

The results of the simulations using the SEIR-Net model are presented below. The four dashed curves measure the cumulative number of individuals infected over time for each age group, according to the legend. The solid curve indicates the number of individuals from all age groups currently infected. The thin dotted horizontal lines indicate the persons for each age group, thus showing the ceiling for the accumulated possible infected persons in each group.

The numbers in parentheses indicate the approximate percentage of each age group within the population. In the control scenario (without distancing) of Figure 1, about 500,000 simultaneously infected people is the maximum reached approximately 55 days after the beginning of the epidemic. The number of infected people is extremely high for all age groups. Within the age group of 60+ years old, we would have more than 350,000 infected people accumulated over the period. In the scenario of vertical distancing, with a 4-fold (75%) reduction of social contact exclusively for the 60+ years old age group (Figure 2), about 400,000 simultaneously infected people is the maximum reached approximately 65 days after the beginning of the epidemic. The number of infected people is extremely high for all age groups. In the 60+ years old group, we would have more than 200,000 infected people accumulated.

In other age groups, virtually everyone would be infected. Horizontal distancing with the same 4-fold (75%) reduction of social contact, for all age groups, is shown in Figure 3. The epidemic does not reach significant dimensions in the first 180 days of simulation. As can be seen in Figure 4, the number of simultaneously infected people only becomes significant about 18 months later, with a relatively small number of simultaneously infected people (less than 10,000). By the end of March, the estimate was that social contact would decrease between 30% and 50% (corresponding to contact intensity between 0.50 and 0.70) in Belo Horizonte [11]. The intensity of $c = 0.55$, corresponding to $(1/0.55) = 1.8$-fold (i.e. 45%) reduction in social contact, results in the graph of Findings also indicate that the 1.8-fold reduction is not sufficient to deter the epidemic outbreak, as could be observed by the accumulated case's curves reaching more than 85% of the ceiling limit of infected persons for all groups. The peak of simultaneous infections (more than 200,000) is reached after about 105 days.

Figure 1: Control scenario without any social distancing, presented for comparison purposes.

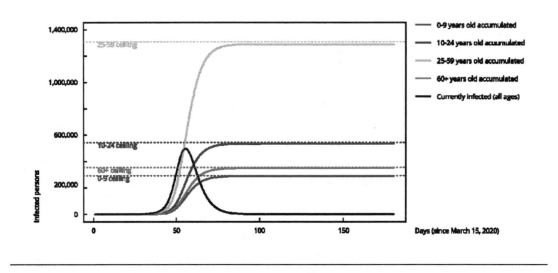

Note: age groups: 0-9 years old (12%), 10-24 years old (22%); 25-59 years old (52%); 60+ years old (14%) with no interventions.

Figure 2: Vertical distancing, only with the 60+ years old age group socially distanced (4-fold, i.e. 75% reduction).

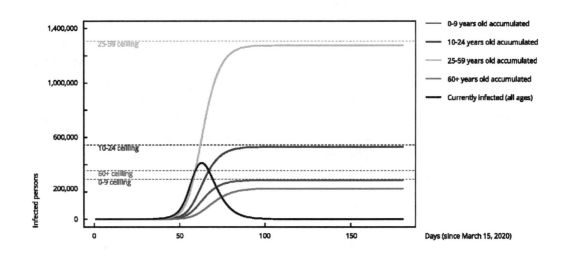

Notes: age groups: 0-9 years old (12%), 10-24 years old (22%); 25-59 years old (52%); 60+ years old (14%) with vertical isolation (4-fold (75%) reduction only for 60+ years old age group). This scenario is almost as unfavourable as the scenario in which there is no distancing at all.

Figure 3: Horizontal distancing, with a 4-fold social contact intensity factor (75% reduction) for all age groups.

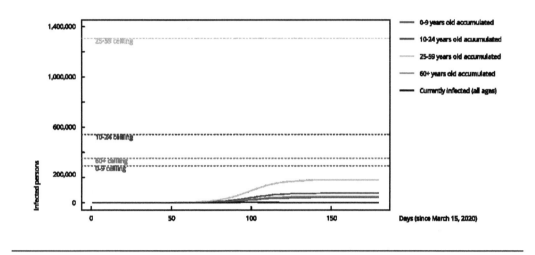

Note: age groups: 0-9 years old (12%), 10-24 years old (22%); 25-59 years old (52%); 60+ years old (14%) with horizontal isolation (4-fold (75%) reduction for all age groups). The epidemic does not reach significant levels in the first 180 days of simulation.

Figure 4

Same as the previous scenario, here displayed for five years, for the horizontal distancing, with a 4-fold social contact intensity factor (75% reduction) for all age groups.

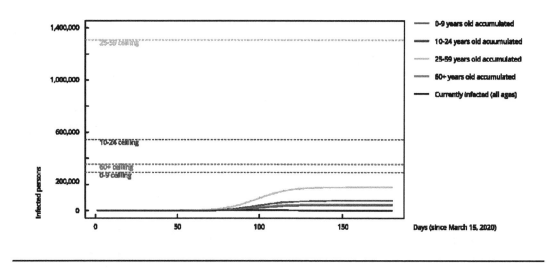

Note: age groups: 0-9 years old (12%), 10-24 years old (22%); 25-59 years old (52%); 60+ years old (14%) with horizontal isolation (4-fold (75%) reduction for all age groups). The epidemic only manifests itself in a reduced way, about 18 months later.

CONCLUSIONS

Vertical distancing is only marginally better than no social distancing at all and much worse than the horizontal distancing scenario – with an equivalent level of reduction in social contact. Vertical distancing with a 4-fold (75%) reduction in social contact only for the 60+ years old age group could not prevent a large number of older people infected (more than 200,000), with 350,000 individuals simultaneously infected. This scenario would also overload the healthcare system in Belo Horizonte. Horizontal distancing, with a similar 4-fold (75%) reduction for all age groups, should slow the surge of cases, postponing the peak for about two years. That should relieve the hospital network, reducing the number of fatal victims, allowing future interventions (vaccination, new treatments, etc.). However, this 4-fold reduction is far from being adopted by the general population. Mobility data for Belo Horizonte shows only a 1.8-fold (45%) reduction in social contact during the last two weeks, which is clearly not sufficient to deter the epidemic outbreak. An urgent effort is recommended to improve reduction of social contact through a strong horizontal distancing health policy for several months.

NOTES

Publicly available population data was used (Departamento de Informática do SUS. População residente – estudo de estimativas populacionais por município, idade e sexo 2000-2015 – Brasil. http://tabnet.datasus.gov.br/cgi/tabcgi.exe?novapop/cnv/popbr.def, accessed on 03/Apr/2020).

L. H. Duczmal and C. R. L. Alves participated in the conception and design, acquisition, analysis and interpretation of data, draft and review of the article and approval of the final version. A. C. L. Almeida, D. B. Duczmal, F. C. O. Magalhães, M. S. Lima, I. R. Silva and R. H. C. Takahashi contributed in the conception and design, acquisition, analysis and interpretation of data and approval the final version.

ADDITIONAL INFORMATION

ORCID: Luiz Henrique Duczmal (0000-0002-05774107); Alexandre Celestino Leite Almeida (00000003-3475-3863); Denise Bulgarelli Duczmal (0000-0003-2295-5820); Claudia Regina Lindgren Alves (0000-0002-0885-1729); Flávia Costa Oliveira Magalhães (0000-0002-6467-1917); Max Sousa de Lima (0000-0002-8556-7318); Ivair Ramos Silva (0000-0003-2701-8924); Ricardo Hiroshi Caldeira Takahashi (0000-0003-0814-6314).

Acknowledgments

We thank the contribution of the researchers of the UFMG-COVID19-Task Force.

REFERENCES

1. Jefferson, T., Del Mar C., Dooley, L., Ferroni, E., Al-Ansary, L.A., Bawazeer, G.A., et al. (2020). Physical interventions to interrupt or reduce the spread of respiratory viruses: systematic review. BMJ 2009; 339:b3675.
2. Bakker, M., Berke, A., Groh, M., Pentland, A.S. Moro, E. (2020). Effect of social distancing measures in the New York City metropolitan area. Boston: Massachusetts Institute of Technology; 2020.
3. Prem, K, Liu, Y., Russell, T.W., Kucharski, A.J, Eggo, R.M., Davies, N., et al.(2020).The effect of control strategies to reduce social mixing on outcomes of the COVID-19 epidemic in Wuhan, China: a modelling study. Lancet Public Health 2020; 5:E261-70.
4. Ganem, F., Mendes, F.M., Oliveira, S.B., Porto, V.N.G, Araujo, W.N., Nakaya, H.I, et al. (2020).The impact of early social distancing at COVID-19 outbreak in the largest Metropolitan area of Brazil. medRxiv 2020; 6 apr. https://www.me drxiv.org/content/10.1101/2020.04.06.20055 103v1.
5. Sanche, S., Lin, Y.T., Xu, C., Romero-Severson, E., Hengartner, N., Ke, R.,High contagiousness and rapid spread of severe acute respiratory syndrome coronavirus 2. Emerg Infect Dis 2020; [Epub ahead of print].
6. Adam D. Modeling the pandemic: the simulations driving the world's response to COVID-19. Nature 2020; 580 (Special Report). https://media.nature.com/original/magazineassets/d41586-020-01003-6/d41586-02001003-6.pdf.
7. Gallotti. R, Valle, F., Castaldo, N., Sacco, P., Domenico, M.(2004). Assessing the risks of "infodemics" in response to COVID-19 epidemics. arXiv 2020; 8 apr. https://arxiv.org/abs/2004.03997.
8. Força-Tarefa de Modelagem da COVID-19. Análise do efeito das medidas de contenção na propagação da COVID-19 em Belo Horizonte (23/03 a 29/03/2020). https://drive.google. com/file/d/1dkOfGHZBwuxiAhScRVvC2saQ w4CbjhQa/view (accessed on 03/Apr/2020).
9. Li, R., Pei, S., Chen, B., Song, Y., Zhang, T., Yang, W., et al. (2020). Substantial undocumented infection facilitates the rapid dissemination of novel coronavirus (SARS-CoV2). Science 2020; 368:489-93.
10. Duczmal, L.H., Almeida, A.C.L., Duczmal, D.B., (2020) Avaliação de cenários de isolamento social para a pandemia COVID-19 no Município de Belo Horizonte. https://drive.google.com/open?i d=1E-u3LS_Ve00k3mijpIJ6EP_z5p2WRQBt (accessed on 03/Apr/2020).
11. Mobility changes. COVID-19 Community Mobility Report 2020; https://www.gstatic. com/covid19/mobility/2020-03-29_BR_ Mobility_Report_en.pdf (accessed on 03/ Apr/2020).

5. Political Orientation And Support For Social Distancing During The COVID-19 Pandemic: Evidence From Brazil

Guilherme Ramos 1 * Yan Vieites 1 * Jorge Jacob 2 3
Eduardo B. Andrade 1

1 Fundação Getulio Vargas / Brazilian School of Public and Business Administration, Rio de Janeiro / RJ – Brazil 2 Columbia University, New York / NY – United States of America [3] University of Virginia, Charlottesville / VA – United States of America

ABSTRACT

Social distancing practices have been widely recommended to curb the COVID-19 pandemic. However, despite the medical consensus, many citizens have resisted adhering to and/or supporting its implementation. While this resistance may stem from the non-negligible personal economic costs of implementing social distancing, we argue that it may also reside in more fundamental differences in normative principles and belief systems, as reflected by political orientation. In a study conducted in Brazil, we test the relative importance of these explanations by examining whether and how support for social distancing varies according to self-identified political orientation and personal economic vulnerability.

Results show that while economic vulnerability does not influence support for social distancing, conservatives are systematically less supportive of these practices than liberals. Discrepancies in sensitivity to threats to the economic system help explain the phenomenon.

1. INTRODUCTION

As of June 10th, there were more than 7 million confirmed cases and 400 thousand fatalities due to the Coronavirus disease 2019 (COVID-19) worldwide. In response to the pandemic, international and local health agencies converged in recommending the early implementation of strict social distancing policies to curb the spread of the virus (Tabari et al., 2020; World Health Organization, 2020). However, despite the medical consensus, many citizens have been reluctant to adopt these control measures (Tanne, 2020). This research investigates the role played by political orientation in shaping attitudes and behaviors concerning social distancing policies. Political polarization is alive and well in Brazil (Samuels & Zucco, 2014). In fact, it has been on the rise over the last decades across the globe (Carothers & O'Donohue, 2019), and this trend shows no sign of stopping (Abramowitz & Saunders, 2008; Mansbridge, 2016). In the US, for instance, the share of people self-identified as liberal (i.e., left-wing) or conservative (i.e., right-wing) increased from 57% in 1992 to 65% in 2010 (Saad, 2012).

As political orientation increases in importance, preferences become more clearly divided along ideological lines. Liberals and conservatives have been shown to display different opinions on a wide variety of issues, from gun control to climate change (Gramlich & Schaeffer, 2019; VanBoven et al., 2018). Given that political orientation largely shapes opinions on public policy (Bail et al., 2018; Dimock & Carroll, 2014), people's views on social distancing may also hold a strong relationship with their position in the political spectrum.

At the heart of the discussions about the adoption of social distancing measures is the apparent trade-off between public health and economic well-being. In many regions of the world, people have ascribed to the view that due to a brutal and lasting economic impact, stringent and earlier social distancing measures could be as or even more harmful to society than softer isolation policies or no policy at all (Snooks, 2020). Although many have eventually changed their minds, a few still resist (The Lancet, 2020). While this resistance may be rooted in non-negligible personal costs of implementing social distancing, it may also reside in more fundamental differences in normative principles and belief systems. To test the relative importance of these explanations, we examine the association between support for social distancing and two measures: (a) economic vulnerability (i.e., social class and anticipated impact on one's personal finances), and (b) political orientation, which is at the core of the presumed trade-off between public health and economic well-being.

Although the health and economic consequences of social distancing may impact both liberals and conservatives alike, the latter may be much more sensitive to the possible economic effects of adopting strict social distancing measures. Unlike liberals, conservatives consider institutions such as businesses and industries as key aspects of society (Choma et al., 2014; Kerlinger, 1984).

They also tend to endorse protestant work values, which emphasize the importance of continuous hard work (Atieh et al., 1987), and oppose increased public spending (Jacoby, 2000; Rudolph & Evans, 2005), a traditional measure used to alleviate the economic losses inflicted by social distancing.

Therefore, we hypothesize that conservatives will be systematically less supportive of social distancing practices and policies than liberals. Further, this association should be, at least in part, explained by their differences in sensitivity to threats to the economic system. This research offers a number of contributions to the literature. First, while previous research has called the influence of political orientation and party identification into question (Converse, 1964; Fiorina, 2006), recent work shows that the predictive power of political orientation on policy preferences is particularly pronounced (Dimock & Carroll, 2014; Bail et al., 2018). In light of the gravity of the problem at stake and the relative consensus about its solution, the COVID-19 pandemic offers a critical test for the importance of political orientation in shaping policy support.

Second, thus far, research has emphasized the role of perceived health risks to the self to explain the relationship between political orientation and support for social distancing measures (Alcott et al., 2020; Barrios & Hochberg, 2020; Conway III et al., 2020; Painter & Qiu, 2020; Rosenfeld et al., 2020). We advance these findings by introducing a new mechanism into the discussion: sensitivity to threats to the economic system.

Finally, while evidence for the effect of political orientation on adherence to social distancing measures already exists, it is overwhelmingly based on US data. However, whether a given issue becomes politically polarized or not depends on idiosyncratic regional characteristics (McCright, Dunlap, & Marquart-Pyatt, 2016). We therefore further contribute to the literature by examining the robustness of the phenomenon in Brazil.

2. STUDY

2.1 Methods

Following a recent trend in the behavioural sciences (Nosek et al., 2018), we conducted a preregistered experimental study. Prior to analyzing the data, we submitted our hypotheses and the analytical plan to an independent registry [1]Overall, albeit not a panacea (Yamada, 2018), pre-registration is an important practice in academia insofar as it lends credibility to research by reducing questionable practices such as hypothesizing after the results are known and p-hacking (Miguel et al., 2014; Munafò et al., 2017; Nosek et al., 2018; Yamada, 2018).

As outlined in the pre-registration report, we tested the relative importance of political orientation vis-à-vis economic vulnerability (e.g., social class, anticipated impact on personal earnings) in predicting support for social distancing.

Although not anticipated in the preregistration, we conducted exploratory mediation analyses to assess whether this effect could be explained by sensitivity to threats to the economic system. The pre-registration protocol also included hypotheses about three different interventions designed to bolster support for social distancing. However, given that none of these interventions systematically swayed attitudes and behaviour, we followed the suggestions of the review team to put less emphasis on it in the paper. We detail them in the appendix.

Participants. Participants were recruited in Brazil through the authors' networks and social media between March 24th and March 27th, 2020. In exchange for their participation, they were told that we would donate R\$1 per participant to a social cause related to mitigating the impacts of COVID-19. Although 1,053 people took part in this study, only 768 of them met all the inclusion criteria established in the pre-registration. Specifically, participants were excluded from the sample if they failed to complete the study or chose the "I don't know" option in any of the dependent variables.

Procedure. Upon providing their consent, participants were randomly assigned to one of four experimental conditions, which were part of the hypothesis we elaborate in the appendix. Next, all participants proceeded to the dependent variables. First, we asked how much they supported the adoption of social distancing practices for about one month (1=strongly against, 4=strongly in favour). Second, we asked how strict the governmental social distancing policies should be (1=no policy, 4=strong and immediate policy). Third, they completed a consequential measure of the type of cause they were willing to donate the compensation for their participation (1=a cause aimed at mitigating impacts of the pandemic on health, 0=on the economy). While the first two dependent measures were attitudinal, the third one captured a consequential behaviour that reflected more explicitly the trade-off between economy and public health. Next, participants filled a socio-demographic questionnaire.

Embedded in this questionnaire was a 4-point scale of political orientation. Even though we use the labels "liberals" and "conservatives" throughout the article for the sake of consistency with the international literature, our questionnaire actually employed the meaningful terms for political orientation in Brazil "left-wing" and "rightwing," respectively (Hasson et al., 2018; Jost, Federico, & Napier, 2009).

---

[1] (https://aspredicted.org/blind.php?x=4er5ui).

This measure read "in terms of political orientation, how do you classify yourself?" (1=clearly left-wing; 4=clearly right-wing; also including an "I do not know what it means to be left- or right-wing" option). Additionally, this sociodemographic questionnaire also included: (a) a measure of anticipated impact on personal earnings in case the participant had to comply with social distancing (1=at least partially affected, 0=not affected; also including a "cannot predict" option), (b) a 5-point measure of subjective social class (1=my income is much below the average of the Brazilian population; 5=much above the average), and (c) questions about education and income, which following prior literature (Adler et al., 2000; Korndörfer, Egloff, & Schmukle, 2015), were standardized and collapsed into a single composite measure of objective social class.

While political orientation captures people's belief systems and normative principles, anticipated impact on personal earnings and social class both served as measures of economic vulnerability. Finally, we asked participants about the dimension of their personal lives that would likely be the most affected by the pandemic (1=finances, 0=health or security). We asked the same about the lives of close others (e.g., family, neighbours, community) and of people in society in general (e.g., fellow Brazilians). These variables sought to capture, respectively, relative sensitivity to threats to personal finances, to close others' finances, and to the economic system as a whole. Further, we collected measures of exposure to the Coronavirus, as well as other usual demographic questions (e.g., age, gender, ethnicity, marital status, geographic region) for descriptive purposes only. Participants were then thanked and dismissed.

Analytical Plan. We tested the effects of political orientation, social class, and anticipated impact on personal earnings on our three dependent measures: decision to donate to the health- (vs. economy-) related cause and support for social distancing practices and policies. We used logistic regressions for the donation decision variable and linear regression models for the two social distancing measures. To investigate the mediating role of relative sensitivity to threats to the economic system and compare it with the effect of threats to the self and to one's community, we conducted seemingly unrelated regressions, which allow for a simultaneous estimation of equations.

3. RESULTS AND DISCUSSION

Data description. **Table 1** displays the summary statistics. Our sample is composed by a majority of female, white and upper-class people, living in the south and southeast regions of Brazil. By the time the study was conducted, only a small percentage of the participants had been tested for COVID-19, but 16% of them knew someone who had tested positive. Further, participants seemed to be well distributed along the political spectrum. A Shapiro-Wilk test on our measure of political orientation suggests that participants followed a normal distribution (W=1.00, z=-1.49, p=.93). 4

TABLE 1 SUMMARY STATISTICS

Variables	Mean	SD	Min	Max	N
Controls					
Men	0.39	0.49	0	1	768
Age	37.81	12.46	18	72	768
White	0.79	0.41	0	1	768
Religiosity	2.86	1.48	1	5	768
Married	0.48	0.50	0	1	768
Southeast Region	0.67	0.47	0	1	768
South Region	0.20	0.40	0	1	768
Northeast Region	0.07	0.26	0	1	768
Health Sector	0.21	0.41	0	1	768
Tested for Coronavirus	0.03	0.18	0	1	768
Positive Result	0.00	0.04	0	1	768
Acquaintance Positive	0.16	0.37	0	1	768
Independent Variables					
Conservative (Scale)	2.46	0.95	1	4	747
Anticipated Impact on Earnings	0.39	0.49	0	1	543
Subjective SES	4.13	1.04	1	5	774
Objective SES	0.00	0.80	-3.70	3.84	730
Years of Education	16.66	1.82	5	18	774
Household income	14789	11322	500	40000	730
Dependent Variables					
Support Social Distancing Practices	3.49	0.74	1	4	768
Support Social Distancing Policies	3.58	0.64	1	4	768
Donation to Health (vs. economy)	0.70	0.46	0	1	768

Source: Elaborated by the authors.

Data Analyses. As mentioned before, we performed the analyses for the donation decision variable using logistic regressions, and for the two social distancing measures using linear regression models. Thus, we regressed each of these outcomes on political orientation, objective and subjective social class, and anticipated impact on personal earnings. To avoid omitted variable biases and help provide more accurate estimations, we controlled for the participants' age, gender, race, religiosity, marital status, geographic region of residence, whether s/he worked in the health sector, whether friends or family members had tested positive for COVID-19, and day of participation in the study. We present different specifications to attest to the robustness of the results. Surprisingly, neither social class nor anticipated impact on personal earnings consistently shaped support for social distancing and/or donation decisions **(see table 2)**. In sharp contrast, and consistent with our expectations, political orientation systematically predicted support for social distancing and donation decisions.

As shown in Figure 1, the more the participants self-identified as conservatives (vs. liberals), the less supportive of both social distancing practices (β=-.30, $t(498)$=-8.91, p<.001) and policies (β=-.23, $t(498)$=-7.43, p<.001) they were. They were also less likely to donate to the health-related cause (β=-.21, z=-1.85, p=.06). Importantly, among the predictors, political orientation had the strongest effect on social distancing practices and policies[1]. Overall, these findings highlight the substantial importance of political orientation in predicting support for social distancing. Interestingly, these effects outweighed the importance of economic vulnerability.

---

[1] We reran models 6 and 9 using standardized coefficients to analyze the relative importance of each variable in explaining support for social distancing. Political orientation was by far the strongest predictor ($\beta_{practices}$ = -.37; $\beta_{policies}$ = -.34). The second-strongest predictor had about half of this effect.

TABLE 2 EFFECTS OF POLITICAL ORIENTATION ON SUPPORT FOR SOCIAL DISTANCING AND DONATIONS TO THE HEALTH CAUSE

DEPENDENT VARIABLES

	Donation to Health (vs. Economy)			Support Social Distancing Practices			Support Social Distancing Policies		
	Logistic			OLS			OLS		
	(1)	(2)	(3)	(4)	(5)	(6)	(7)	(8)	(9)
Conservative	-0.34***	-0.26**	-0.21*	-0.35***	-0.38***	-0.30***	-0.23***	-0.26***	-0.23***
	(0.09)	(0.10)	(0.12)	(0.03)	(0.03)	(0.03)	(0.02)	(0.03)	(0.03)
Subjective SES		-0.14	-0.08		0.01	0.00		0.06*	0.05
		(0.13)	(0.14)		(0.04)	(0.04)		(0.03)	(0.04)
Objective SES		-0.01	0.00		-0.05	-0.03		0.00	0.00
		(0.14)	(0.15)		(0.04)	(0.04)		(0.04)	(0.04)
Anticipated Impact		-0.17	-0.17		-0.13**	-0.10		0.02	0.00
		(0.20)	(0.21)		(0.06)	(0.06)		(0.06)	(0.06)
Age			0.01			-0.00			-0.00
			(0.01)			(0.00)			(0.00)
Men			-0.06			-0.29***			-0.16***
			(0.21)			(0.06)			(0.06)
White			-0.26			0.01			0.18**
			(0.27)			(0.08)			(0.07)
Religiosity			0.03			-0.01			0.02
			(0.07)			(0.02)			(0.02)
Married			-0.54**			-0.05			-0.10
			(0.22)			(0.06)			(0.06)
Health Worker			0.24			-0.07			0.04
			(0.25)			(0.07)			(0.07)
Acquaintance Positive			0.11			-0.03			-0.05
			(0.27)			(0.08)			(0.07)
Region Effects	Yes	Yes	Yes	Yes	Yes	Yes	Yes	Yes	Yes
Time Effects	Yes	Yes	Yes	Yes	Yes	Yes	Yes	Yes	Yes
Observations	747	514	514	747	514	514	747	514	514
R-squared				0.20	0.25	0.32	0.12	0.15	0.20
Log-Likelihood	-452.32	-313.77	-308.29						
Akaike Inf. Crit.	908.64	637.53	648.57						

Note: Standard errors in parentheses. *** $p<0.01$, ** $p<0.05$, * $p<0.10$ Source: Elaborated by the authors.

FIGURE 1 (PANELS A-C) - EFFECTS OF POLITICAL ORIENTATION ON SUPPORT FOR SOCIAL DISTANCING AND DONATIONS TO THE HEALTH CAUSE

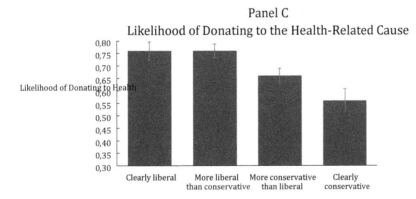

Panel A:
Support for the Practice of Social Distancing

Panel B
Support for Social Distancing Policies

Panel C
Likelihood of Donating to the Health-Related Cause

Source: Elaborated by the authors.

Economy vs. Health. As highlighted in the introduction of the paper, conservatives and liberals display fundamental differences in values and belief systems. Conservatives are likely to give more weight to the detrimental economic effects of social distancing than liberals when facing the apparent trade-off between the health-related consequences of the disease and the expected economic side effects of social distancing. The significant differences in donation preferences shown above (Figure 1 – Panel C) converge with this assumption.

Along these lines, we also examined whether the lower support for social distancing practices and policies and the lower donation rates for the health-related cause among conservatives (vs. liberals) could be explained by a greater relative sensitivity to the possible threats to the economic system. Although it is important to acknowledge that we had not anticipated this possibility in the pre-registration, our data allow us to test it empirically.

As outlined in the procedure, we collected measures assessing the participants' relative sensitivity to economic threats (finances = 1, health or security = 0) at the levels of the self, close community, and society. To analyse the relative importance of sensitivity to threats to the economic system, we conducted a series of seemingly unrelated regressions with 5,000 replications to test parallel mediation models for each of the dependent variables. The finding are and consistent with our rationale, conservatives' (vs. liberals') higher likelihood of donating to the economic-related cause was significantly mediated by relative sensitivity to economic threats to society ($\beta_{society}$=-.03, z=-3.94, bootstrap 95% CI=[-.043, -.014]), but not by economic threats to oneself or to one's community (β_{self}=-.01, z=-1.48, bootstrap 95% CI=[-.016, .002]; $\beta_{close community}$=-.01, z=-1.91, bootstrap 95% CI=[-.016, .000]). In addition, while participants' relative sensitivity to economic threats to society significantly mediated the relationship between political orientation and social distancing practices ($\beta_{society}$ =-.02, z=-3.04, bootstrap 95% CI=[-.041, -.009]), evidence for the effects in more personal levels was mixed (β_{self} =-0.02, z=-2.18, bootstrap 95% CI=[-.031, -.002]; $\beta_{close community}$=-.01, z=-1.68, bootstrap 95% CI=[-.019, .001]). Finally, the effect of political orientation on support for social distancing policies was mediated by participants' relative sensitivity to economic threats to society ($\beta_{society}$=-.02, z=-2.77, bootstrap 95% CI=[-.035, -.006]), but evidence for the effects in more personal levels failed to reach significance (β_{self}=-.01, z=-1.43, bootstrap 95% CI=[-.020, .003]; $\beta_{close community}$=-.005, z=-1.07, bootstrap 95% CI=[-.013, .004]). Taken together, these findings converge with the idea that political orientation shapes support for social distancing through more general values and belief systems rather than sheer selfish motives (i.e., a concern about the economic consequences of social distancing or the close community).

4. GENERAL DISCUSSION

The COVID-19 outbreak has engendered a staggering number of deaths worldwide. Yet, based on the argument that stringent and earlier social distancing measures could be as or even more harmful to society than softer distancing policies or no policy at all (Snooks, 2020), many citizens have shown reluctance to adhere to and/or to support social distancing, despite the medical consensus. While this resistance might be rooted in significant personal economic costs of implementing social distancing, it is also possible that the lack of support for such measures might reflect more abstract normative principles and belief systems, the core of which is political orientation (Jost et al., 2009). The current research investigated the relative importance of political orientation vis-à-vis economic vulnerability in predicting support for social distancing and consequential donation decisions. Consistent with our predictions, political orientation shaped support for social distancing above and beyond personal economic vulnerability, which, somewhat surprisingly, did not consistently influence support for social distancing. More specifically, conservatives were systematically less supportive of social distancing practices and policies when compared to their liberal counterparts. Further, in a more explicit test of the trade-off between public health and economic well-being, political orientation also predicted consequential donation decisions to a cause aimed at mitigating the health (vs. economic) impacts of the COVID-19 pandemic. Mediation analyses lent additional support for the idea that the phenomenon is rooted in abstract belief systems rather than on personal economic vulnerability.

Admittedly, we are not the first to investigate the link between political orientation and support for social distancing. Emerging research in the context of the COVID-19 pandemic has provided consistent support for the claim that political orientation predicts support for social distancing (Alcott et al., 2020; Barrios & Hochberg, 2020; Conway III et al., 2020; Painter & Qiu, 2020; Rosenfeld et al., 2020). More broadly, research on political orientation and policy support has documented that people tend to value policies favored by their own political group and to devalue policies advocated by the opposing political group (Gadarian, Goodman, & Pepinsky, 2020; Van Boven, Ehret, & Sherman, 2018). In contrast to these line of research, we focus on the role of abstract normative principles and belief systems. Further, past research has shown that whether a given issue becomes politically polarized or not depends on idiosyncratic regional characteristics (McCright, Dunlap, & Marquart Pyatt, 2016).

While the extant evidence for the effect of political orientation on adherence to social distancing measures is overwhelmingly based on US data, we move the debate away from the US by examining the robustness of the phenomenon in Brazil. Our study also has important practical implications for public communication. Conservatives tend to be less favourable toward social distancing because they are more sensitive to the economic threats to society this measure apparently imposes. While this pandemic seems to have inevitable negative consequences for the economy, previous research has shown that early and strict adoption of preventive measures (e.g., social distancing) actually have positive effects on economic growth after the pandemic, and therefore contributes to faster economic recovery (Correia, Luck, & Verner, 2020).

Thus, rather than enhancing economic depression, the adoption of social distancing measures seems to mitigate it, thereby breaking down the trade-off. Policy-makers can therefore highlight this feature in public communications in order to enhance compliance with, and support for, social distancing among conservatives.

This study does not come without limitations, however. First, our sample is not representative of the Brazilian population. Given the pressingness of the issue and the data collection restrictions imposed by the virus, the overwhelming majority of studies on the COVID-19 pandemic share this limitation (Di Lorenzo et al., 2020; Marta et al., 2020; Padala, Jendro, & Padala, 2020).

Nation-wide data collections with representative samples are therefore needed to attest to the external validity of the phenomenon. Second, our sample's strong support for social distancing suggests the existence of ceiling effects. Future research could employ alternative measures of support for social distancing to mitigate this concern.

Third, we are mindful that our data have been collected at a single time period within an unprecedented moment. Therefore, not only the results of this investigation warrant replication but also future investigations should account for potential variation in public policy guidance or social perception on the COVID-19 pandemic. Nonetheless, our findings show clearly the power of political orientation, over and above personal economic considerations, on shaping health protection attitudes and behaviour during the COVID-19 pandemic in Brazil.

REFERENCES

Abramowitz, A. I., & Saunders, K. L. (2008). Is polarization a myth?. *The Journal of Politics*, *70*(2), 542-555.

Adler, N. E., Epel, E. S., Castellazzo, G., & Ickovics, J. R. (2000). Relationship of subjective and objective social status with psychological and physiological functioning: Preliminary data in healthy, White women. *Health psychology*, *19*(6), 586.

Allcott, H., Boxell, L., Conway, J., Gentzkow, M., Thaler, M., & Yang, D. Y. (2020). *Polarization and public health: Partisan differences in social distancing during the Coronavirus pandemic* (NBER Working Paper). Cambridge, MA: The National Bureau of Economic Research.

Atieh, J. M., Brief, A. P., & Vollrath, D. A. (1987). The Protestant work ethic-conservatism paradox: Beliefs and values in work and life. *Personality and Individual Differences*, *8*(4), 577-580.

Bail, C. A., Argyle, L. P., Brown, T. W., Bumpus, J. P., Chen, H., Hunzaker, M. F., ... & Volfovsky, A. (2018). Exposure to opposing views on social media can increase political polarization. *Proceedings of the National Academy of Sciences*, *115*(37), 9216-9221.

Barrios, J. M., & Hochberg, Y. (2020). *Risk perception through the lens of politics in the time of the COVID-19 pandemic* (NBER Working Paper). Cambridge, MA: The National Bureau of Economic Research.

Carothers, T., & O'Donohue, A. (Eds.).
(2019). *Democracies divided: The global challenge of political polarization*. Washington, DC: Brookings Institution Press.

Choma, B. L., Hanoch, Y., Hodson, G., & Gummerum, M. (2014). Risk propensity among liberals and conservatives: The effect of risk perception, expected benefits, and risk domain. *Social Psychological and Personality Science*, *5*(6), 713-721.

Converse, P. E. (1964). "The Nature of Belief Systems in Mass Publics." In D. E. Apter (Ed.), *Ideology and Its Discontents* (pp. 206-261). New York, NY: The Free Press of Glencoe.

Conway III, L. G., Woodard, S. R., Zubrod, A., & Chan, L. (2020, April 13). Why are conservatives less concerned about the coronavirus (COVID-19) than liberals? Testing experiential versus political explanations. *PsyArXiv*.

Correia, S., Luck, S., & Verner, E. (2020, June 05). Public Health Interventions Do Not: Evidence from the 1918 Flu (Working Paper). *SSRN*.

Di Lorenzo, G., Toniolo, P., Lurani, C., Foresti, L., & Carrisi, C. (2020). Evaluating the adequacy of Prima COVID-19 IgG/IgM Rapid Test for the assessment of exposure to SARS-CoV-2 virus. *medRxiv*.

Dimock M, Carroll D. (2014). *"Political polarization in the American public: How increasing ideological uniformity and partisan antipathy affect politics, compromise, and everyday life"*. Washington, DC: Pew Research Center.

Fiorina, M. F. P., Abrams, S. J. & Pope, J. C. (2006). *Culture War? The Myth of a Polarized America* (2nd ed.). New York, NY: Pearson Longman.

Gadarian, S. K., Goodman, S. W., & Pepinsky, T. B. (2020, March 27). Partisanship, health behavior, and policy attitudes in the early stages of the COVID-19 pandemic (Working Paper). *SSRN*.

Gramlich, J. & Schaeffer, K. (2019). *"7 facts about guns in the U.S."*. Washington, DC: Pew Research Center.

Hasson, Y., Tamir, M., Brahms, K. S., Cohrs, J. C., & Halperin, E. (2018). Are liberals and conservatives equally motivated to feel empathy toward others?. *Personality and Social Psychology Bulletin*, *44*(10), 1449-1459.

Jacoby, W. G. (2000). Issue framing and public opinion on government spending. *American Journal of Political Science*, 750-767.

Jost, J. T., Federico, C. M., & Napier, J. L. (2009). Political ideology: Its structure, functions, and elective affinities. *Annual review of psychology*, *60*, 307-337.

Kerlinger, F. (1984). *Liberalism and conservatism: The nature and structure of social attitudes*. Hillsdale, NJ: Lawrence Erlbaum.

Korndörfer, M., Egloff, B., & Schmukle, S. C. (2015). A large scale test of the effect of social class on prosocial behavior. *PloS one*, *10*(7), e0133193.

Lancet, T. (2020). COVID-19: learning from experience. *Lancet (London, England)*, *395*(10229), 1011.

Loewenstein, G., Read, D., & Baumeister, R. F. (Eds.). (2003). *Time and decision: Economic and psychological perspectives of intertemporal choice*. New York, NY: Russell Sage Foundation.

Mansbridge. (2016, March 11). *Three reasons political polarization is here to stay. The Washington Post*. Retrieved from https://www.washingtonpost.com/ news/in-theory/wp/2016/03/11/three-reasonspolitical-polarization-is-here-to-stay/ Marta, I., Mirjana, Đ., Aleksandar, K., Filip, M., Kristina, N., Tamara, P., ... Irena, T. (2020). Serbian Citizens' Opinion on the COVID-19 Epidemic. *South Eastern European Journal of Public Health (SEEJPH)*.
Retrieved from https://doi.org/10.4119/seejph-3459 McCright, A. M., Dunlap, R. E., & Marquart-Pyatt, S. T. (2016). Political ideology and views about climate change in the European Union. *Environmental Politics*, *25*(2), 338-358.

Miguel, E., Camerer, C., Casey, K., Cohen, J., Esterling, K. M., Gerber, A., ... Van der Laan, M. (2014). Promoting transparency in social science research. *Science*, *343*, 30-31.

Munafò, M. R., Nosek, B. A., Bishop, D. V. M., Button, K. S., Chambers, C. D., du Sert, N. P., ... Ioannidis, J. P. A. (2017). A manifesto for reproducible science. *Nature Human Behavior* 1, 1-9.

Nosek, B. A., Ebersole, C. R., DeHaven, A. C., and Mellor, D. T. (2018). The preregistration revolution. *Proceedings of the National Academy of Sciences*, *18*, 201708274.

O'Donoghue, T., & Rabin, M. (2015). Present bias: Lessons learned and to be learned. *American Economic Review*, *105*(5), 273-79. Padala, P. R., Jendro, A. M., & Padala, K. P. (2020). Conducting clinical research during the COVID-19 Pandemic: Investigator and participant perspectives. *JMIR Public Health and Surveillance*, *6*(2), e18887.

Painter, M., & Qiu, T. (2020, April). Political beliefs affect compliance with COVID-19 social distancing orders (Working Paper) *SSRN*.

Rosenfeld, D. L., Rothgerber, H., & Wilson, T. (2020). Politicizing the COVID-19 pandemic: Ideological differences in adherence to social distancing. *PsyArXiv*.

Rudolph, T. J., & Evans, J. (2005). Political trust, ideology, and public support for government spending. *American Journal of Political Science*, *49*(3), 660-671.

Saad, L. (2012). "Conservatives Remain the Largest Ideological Group in U.S.". Retrieved from http://www.gallup.com/poll/152021/conservativesremain-largest-ideological-group.aspx

Samuels, D., & Zucco, C., Jr. (2014). The power of partisanship in Brazil: Evidence from survey experiments. *American Journal of Political Science, 58*(1), 212-225.

Snooks, G. D. (2020). *Fight the Virus (COVID-19), Not the Economy!. Institute of Global Dynamic Systems* (Working Paper, 20). Canberra, Australia: Institute of Global Dynamic Systems.

Tabari, P., Amini, M., Moghadami, M., Moosavi, M. (2020). International Public Health Responses to COVID-19 Outbreak: A Rapid Review. *Iranian Journal of Medical Sciences*, 45(3), 157-169.

Tanne, Janice Hopkins (2020), "COVID-19: cases grow in US as Trump pushes promise of a malaria drug." *BMJ (Clinical research ed.), 368*, m1155.

Van Boven, L., Ehret, P. J., & Sherman, D. K. (2018). Psychological barriers to bipartisan public support for climate policy. *Perspectives on Psychological Science, 13*(4), 492-507.

World Health Organization (2020, January), "Household transmission investigation protocol for 2019-novel coronavirus (2019-nCoV) infection," *EarlyInvestigations-2019*, 1-31.

Yamada, Y. (2018). How to crack pre-registration: Toward transparent and open science. *Frontiers in psychology, 9*, 1831.pandemic," Technical Report, National Bureau of Economic Research 2020.

6.Figures and Tables

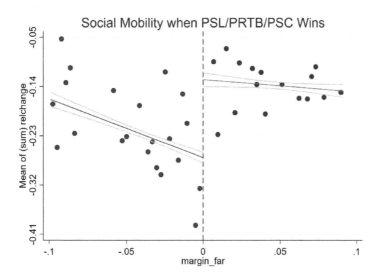

Figure 1: Change in Relative Social Mobility

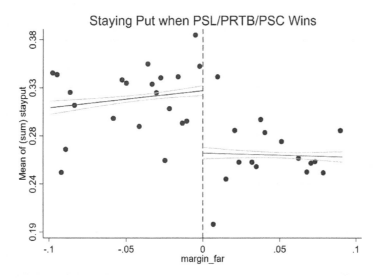

Figure 2: Proportion Staying Within Regional Boundaries

Notes: These figures plot social mobility measures against the forcing variable, which is the margin of victory of three Bolsonaro-affiliated parties (PSC, PRTB, and PSL) in the 2016 mayoral elections. Each point represents the average value of the outcome in a bin containing 20 municipalities. The solid line plots predicted values on the unbinned raw data, with separate linear trends estimated on either side of the 0% threshold. The dashed lines show 95% confidence intervals.

Table 1: Effect of Close Victories on Social Mobility

	RelativeSocialMobility	StayingPut
	(1)	**(2)**
Sharp RD Estimate	0.108***	-0.041***
	(0.03)	(0.011)
State Fixed Effects	Yes	Yes
Date Fixed Effects	Yes	Yes
Mean of Dependent Variable	-0.182	0.293
Observations	26431	26431
Estimation Bandwidth	± 0.208	± 0.258

*Each regression discontinuity estimate is from a separate local linear regression on either side of the threshold with the specified bandwidth. Robust standard errors clustered at the municipality level in parentheses. All columns include state and date fixed effects. * 10%, ** 5%, *** 1% significance levels.*

Table 2: Effect of Close Victories on Social Mobility: By Party

	RelativeSocialMobility	StayingPut
	(1)	(2)
Panel A: PSC Victory		
Sharp RD Estimate	0.076**	-0.039***
	(0.033)	(0.134)
State Fixed Effects	Yes	Yes
Date Fixed Effects	Yes	Yes
Mean of Dependent Variable	-0.164	0.288
Observations	16575	16575
Estimation Bandwidth		
Panel B: PRTB Victory		
Sharp RD Estimate	0.223***	-0.113***
	(0.012)	(0.008)
State Fixed Effects	Yes	Yes
Date Fixed Effects	Yes	Yes
Mean of Dependent Variable	-0.271	0.328
Observations	4392	4392
Estimation Bandwidth		
Panel C: PSL Victory		
Sharp RD Estimate	0.088***	-0.037***
	(0.014)	(0.008)
State Fixed Effects	Yes	Yes
Date Fixed Effects	Yes	Yes
Mean of Dependent Variable	-0.196	0.303
Observations	5464	5464

*Each regression discontinuity estimate is from a separate local linear regression on either side of the threshold with the specified bandwidth. Robust standard errors clustered at the municipality level in parentheses. All columns include state and date fixed effects. * 10%, ** 5%, *** 1% significance levels.*

CHAPTER 19

INCARCERATED AND ISOLATED BY COVID-19

1. COVID-19 Spells Disaster For Brazil's Overcrowded Prisons As First Inmate Death Recorded

Fernanda Canofre[1]

Brazil registered its first COVID-19-related death in a jail on April 17, stoking fears that the disease could devastate the country's overcrowded,[2] unsanitary, and large – the third-largest[3] in the world, in fact — prison system. According to Brazil's National Prison Department, by April there were currently 125 suspect cases of COVID-19 in Brazil's prisons. On March 31, the number of suspect cases was 74[4]. The first three confirmed cases[5] of the disease in the prison system were recorded on April 9. By April 20, Brazil had registered 2,575 deaths and over 40,000 confirmed cases of COVID-19, according to[6] the country's Ministry of Health. Numbers could be a lot higher as testing capacity has been limited.[7] A study by Imperial College London[8] released in late March estimates that between 44,000 (if social isolation is enforced) and 1.1 million (with no restrictions) people could die from the disease in Brazil, a country of 210 million. Brazil's prison system has long faced criticism for its severe overcrowding and unhealthy conditions. Bug infestations are common, as well as chronic shortages of hygiene products and healthcare – 31 percent[9] of the country's prison units don't have in-house doctors, according to data by the Prosecutor's Office, obtained by newspaper Folha de S. Paulo. Experts estimate that there is a 300,000 vacancy shortage[10] in the prison system overall.

The Prison Pastoral (Pastoral Carcerária), a branch of the Catholic Church that provides social, legal, and health assistance Brazil's jails, did a survey with its employees, inmates' family, prison workers, lawyers, judges, public defendants, and members of social organizations about the new coronavirus. Their conclusions[11] were published on April 9: 377 people (31,35 percent) said that yes, there are suspected cases of coronavirus in prisons, while 207 (17,2 percent) claim there aren't. 621 people (51,5 percent) didn't know how to answer whether such cases exist or not. Regarding confirmed cases, 245 people (20,4 percent) claimed to have knowledge about people inside the prison system infected with the new coronavirus, while 222 (18,5 percent) said they didn't know concrete cases. Once again, a significant number of people replied they didn't know how to answer the question: 736, or 61,2 percent. Justice and Public Security Minister Sergio Moro, the former federal judge who became famous for heading Operation Car Wash[12], said on April 13 that "everything is under control"[13]

---

[1] Journalist, with a master's degree in History, was born in a crossing land in the southern part of Brazil..

[2] https://globalvoices.org/2017/07/06/whats-it-like-to-live-in-a-brazilian-prison-cell-cramped-dirty-and-dangerous-to-your-health/

[3] http://agenciabrasil.ebc.com.br/geral/noticia/2020-02/brasil-tem-mais-de-773-mil-encarcerados-maioria-no-regime-fechado

[4] https://noticias.uol.com.br/cotidiano/ultimas-noticias/2020/03/31/coronavirus-casos-suspeitos-em-presidios-do-brasil.htm

[5] https://globalvoices.org/2017/07/06/whats-it-like-to-live-in-a-brazilian-prison-cell-cramped-dirty-and-dangerous-to-your-health/

[6] https://covid.saude.gov.br/

[7] https://covid.saude.gov.br/

[8] https://noticias.uol.com.br/ultimas-noticias/agencia-estado/2020/03/28/brasil-pode-ter-ao-menos-44-mil-mortes-isolar-so-idosos-eleva-n-para-529-mil.htm

[9] https://www1.folha.uol.com.br/equilibrioesaude/2020/03/31-das-unidades-prisionais-do-pais-nao-oferecem-assistencia-medica.shtml

[10] https://agenciabrasil.ebc.com.br/geral/noticia/2020-02/brasil-tem-mais-de-773-mil-encarcerados-maioria-no-regime-fechado

[11] https://carceraria.org.br/combate-e-prevencao-a-tortura/pastoral-carceraria-divulga-dados-de-questionario-sobre-coronavirus-nas-prisoes

[12] https://en.wikipedia.org/wiki/Operation_Car_Wash

[13] https://noticias.uol.com.br/politica/ultimas-noticias/2020/04/13/moro-apesar-de-casos-de-covid-19-em-prisoes-situacao-esta-sob-controle.htm

inside Brazil's prisons. In March, he had assured the population[1] that there was "no reason for unfounded fears [when it comes to] prisons", and added:

"There is an environment of relative safety in the prison system regarding the coronavirus, because of the prisoners' very condition of being isolated."

Brazilian prisons have long been prone to epidemics. According to an exclusive report by Agência Pública[2], a non-profit media outlet from Brazil, there were more than 10,000 confirmed cases of tuberculosis in the country's prisons in 2018. That means there were over 1,400 cases of the disease per 100,000 people inside prisons – while outside, there were only 40 per 100,000 at the time of the research. Professor Carla Machado, from the Federal University of Minas Gerais, who was interviewed in the article, says that it is only a matter of time until the new coronavirus starts spreading uncontrollably in the prison system. Her colleague, professor and physician Dirceu Greco, added:

"Overcrowding makes for the ideal conditions for any biological agent transmissible by air. The lack of supplies is another factor: people don't have water and soap. And, of course, the lack of healthcare, medical care, nurses and social assistance"

To avoid such a deadly scenario, governors of almost all 26 Brazilian states and the Federal District have granted home arrest to prisoners who are under "semi-open regime" (a type of arrest regime in which the inmate goes out to work but sleeps in the prison), and to those who belong to at-risk groups. They have also suspended all visitation and delivery of food and hygiene kits by families. Initially, that measure triggered revolt among inmates – hundreds fled[3] a São Paulo prison on March 16 – as many Brazilian prisons rely on supplies provided by the inmates' relatives. On a statement,[4] Prison Pastoral denounced that prisons in the northern state of Amazonas had provided rotten food to its inmates, and added:

"We ask: how do you prevent diseases from entering a prison, such as coronavirus, or how do you reduce symptoms – or allow the cure – without healthy food, hygiene and cleaning products?"

OVER-INCARCERATION

Brazil has long struggled with coming up with alternative criminal punishment to stop prison overcrowding. With the pandemic, measures such as revaluation of preventive arrests — 253,963 people currently in jail in the country still haven't had a trial — are among the recommendations by the National Justice Council (CNJ) in order to avoid a disaster. A note by the Criminal Justice Network (Rede Justiça Criminal),[5] a group of several organizations, emphasizes the importance of adopting precautionary measures:

"The alarming growth of new cases of coronavirus, in a global level, expose the intensity of social, racial and economic vulnerabilities in Brazil. In prison, the situation aggravates itself exponentially"

---

[1] https://istoe.com.br/para-moro-sistema-prisional-e-relativamente-seguro-apesar-do-coronavirus/
[2] https://apublica.org/2020/03/em-alerta-por-coronavirus-prisoes-ja-enfrentam-epidemia-de-tuberculose/
[3] https://ponte.org/prisoes-de-sp-promovem-maior-onda-de-rebelioes-desde-2006/
[4] https://carceraria.org.br/combate-e-prevencao-a-tortura/pandemia-do-coronavirus-expoe-brutalidade-do-carcere
[5] https://redejusticacriminal.org/wp-content/uploads/2020/03/2020_03_17-Nota-sobre-Coronavi%CC%81rus-RJC_versa%CC%83o-final-1.pdf

2. COVID-19 In Prisons:
An Impossible Challenge for Public Health?

Alexandra Sánchez[1] [2]Luciana Simas
Vilma Diuana, Bernard Larouze

Brazil has 748,000 prison inmates [1], 50,000 of whom in the state of Rio de Janeiro alone, who are practically absent from the public debate on COVID-19. But is it possible to imagine more favourable conditions for the spread of SARS-CoV-2, a virus with airborne and person-to-person transmission, in a population confined to overcrowded cells with poor ventilation and limited access to running water? According to estimates in the general population, one infected individual transmits the virus to two to three others. Given the conditions in Brazilian prisons, based on estimates, one case can infect 10 other inmates. Thus, in a cell holding 150 prisoners, 67% will be infected within 14 days, and 100% will be infected in 21 days. The majority of the infected individuals (80%) will either remain asymptomatic or develop mild forms of the disease, 20% will evolve to more serious forms requiring hospitalization, whose 6% will require intensive care [2]. In this context, measures to confront COVID-19 should be anticipated in order not to lose control of the situation. To predict the pandemic's evolution in Brazilian prisons, the reference should not be European prisons, where the virus' spread has been limited, since European prison cells normally hold no more than four inmates each, and in better conditions of health and hygiene. The pandemic hit Brazil when the country's prison health system was already weakened and overcrowded, with high mortality from potentially curable infectious diseases like tuberculosis.

Furthermore, the prison population includes elderly inmates and/or those with diseases associated with evolution to the severe and fatal forms of COVID-19, such as diabetes, cardiopathies, hypertension, renal failure, asthma, HIV/AIDS, and tuberculosis. Pregnant women and mothers with children are also part of this group because of their increased vulnerability. In this scenario, legal decarceration measures are urgent and necessary to reduce the system's overcrowding, which reaches the absurd rate of 300% in some Brazilian prisons. The pandemic requires rapid responses, especially in low-income countries with inhumane conditions and high incarceration rates. Decarceration is a key measure in the response to COVID-19 [3,4,5]. However, there is intense debate on a false dichotomy: on the one hand, a view of public security that sees a major risk of releasing inmates, and on the other, the perceived and real risk of infection and death from COVID-19 in incarcerated persons. Some have opposed the decarceration *measures* in Recommendation n. 62/2020 of the Brazilian National Council of Justice [6], which provides for the possibility of house detention and case reviews as a protective measure during this pandemic, for individuals accused of non-violent or non-threatening crimes. As the Brazilian Supreme Court has stated repeatedly, health in the country's prisons is the State's responsibility [7,8], and inmates have the right, under the

---

[1] All contributors are affiliated to the:
Escola Nacional de Saúde
Pública Sergio Arouca,
Fundação Oswaldo Cruz, Rio de Janeiro, Brasil.
[2] Correspondence A. Sánchez. alexandrarsanchez@gmail.com

Brazilian Unified National Health System (SUS), to the same conditions for prevention and care as the rest of the population, as provided by the Federal Constitution, the Criminal Execution Act, the National Policy for Comprehensive Healthcare for the Prison Population, and various international legal provisions such as the United Nations Minimum Rules for the Treatment of Prisoners [2]. However, most of the official documents dealing with the COVID-19 pandemic in Brazil fail to mention the prison population or only mention it generically.

Meanwhile, the main recommendations for prevention in the general population, such as social distancing and hand hygiene, have proven extremely difficult to enforce in the country's prisons.

The strategies for COVID-19 prevention cannot be limited, as in many states, to a ban on visits, suspension of transfers between prison facilities, and interruption of group activities like sports, work, classes, and religious meetings. A contingency plan is essential for prisons to adjust and implement the measures recommended for the general population. However, the prison population is not mentioned in either the state [9] or municipal contingency plans in Rio de Janeiro [10,11], as in other states, which provide details on the procedures and roles of various levels and agencies for the prevention, detection, and confirmation of suspected cases of COVID-19, clinical care, and epidemiological surveillance. This omission reveals the de facto exclusion of the prison population from public policies established for the general population, thus violating the principles of the universal health system, with negative effects on healthcare and access to the necessary inputs for confronting the pandemic in the prisons, such as diagnostic tests and personal protective equipment (PPE), but also on epidemiological surveillance strategies. All of these factors favour the invisibility of COVID-19 inside the prison walls.

It is thus urgent and necessary for Rio de Janeiro to effectively include the 46 intramural primary healthcare units, the Penal Sanatorium, and the Prison Emergency Care Department in the state epidemiological surveillance system as reporting units in order for health professionals in the primary health services to promptly and electronically report cases of flu syndrome as suspected cases of COVID-19, according to the criteria established for the general population [9,10,11] and the Joint Resolution by the Rio de Janeiro State Health Department and Department of Correctional Facilities [12].

In addition, due to the prison system's characteristics and the high potential for the spread of COVID-19, the system should be included as a sentinel unit alongside the other 10 existing units, distributed across the five health program areas in the city of Rio de Janeiro, in order to monitor the evolution and dynamics of the pandemic's spread in the various prison units.

In the context of overcrowded prisons, rigorous surveillance to promptly identify COVID-19's introduction in the prison units and rapid blockade of transmission are essential to avoid mass spread of the infection.

Thus, the 14-day quarantine implemented in Rio de Janeiro for all new prisoners before being assigned to the various prison units is important for controlling transmission, so long as asymptomatic incoming prisoners are maintained separately from symptomatic ones.

Since Brazil's prisons lack the infrastructure to allow isolation in individual cells, in order to isolate suspected cases in the prison population, cohort isolation is recommended [13]; that is, prisoners with the same characteristics (suspected/confirmed cases) should be isolated by groups in different areas. Whether incoming or veteran inmates,

it is extremely important for all prisoners with even mild symptoms consistent with COVID-19 to be tested as quickly as possible with RT-PCR, and to be isolated if they test positive. Influenza vaccination is a key priority, reducing the incidence of influenza and thus decreasing the number of symptomatic persons to be tested for COVID-19.

Thus, testing of prison inmates, prison guards, and health staff with flu symptoms should be a priority for dealing with the pandemic in the prisons. However, thus far, prison inmates are not considered a priority for testing suspected cases, and even those who have died with suspicion of COVID-19 have not been tested post-mortem. Therefore, the purported absence of suspected or confirmed cases and deaths from COVID-19 in prisons in the state of Rio de Janeiro, as announced on April 14 by the prison system's administration, should be questioned due to the systematic failure to perform diagnostic testing [14]. The lack of clarity on the clinical management of suspected cases is another delicate issue. For the general population, every patient with symptoms of a common cold or flu syndrome should be managed as a possible case of SARS-CoV-2, according to the Brazilian Ministry of Health guidelines.

Cases classified as mild should remain in isolation for 14 days starting at the onset of symptoms, and serious cases should be referred to the urgency regulation system (*"Vaga Zero"*) [9,11]. For the prison population, the procedures are currently limited to isolation, with no operational definition of patient flows [14]. In case prisoners are not released, those belonging to the risk group should be assigned to an independent prison wing, with cells holding only a small number of inmates, reinforcing measures to prevent transmission and with regular medical care to reduce the likelihood of SARS-CoV-2 infection and to ensure treatment of the individual's underlying illness. This would guarantee adequate care, given the overload on the health system resulting from COVID-19 and the preventive work leave of healthcare staff included in this same risk group. In prison, the perceived risk to health and life from COVID-19, the restrictions on circulation inside the prison walls, and the interruption of work, educational, and religious activities tend to aggravate tensions, with strong emotional implications [15]. The suspension of family visits exacerbates the inmates' feeling of isolation and insecurity, generating concern over the health and lives of family members (How are they? What might be happening to the them?) and their own welfare (Will I get sick? Will we receive medical care, or are we simply going to die in here?).

To mitigate the feeling of loss of control and anxiety resulting from this situation, prisoners need to be informed on the strategies adopted by the prison administration for protection, prevention, and healthcare, and especially for them to maintain communication with their families, through letters, telephone calls, and other means provided by the institution for this purpose.

It is also important to avoid stigmatization and violence against individuals identified as possible coronavirus carriers. In this scenario, information for health personnel and security staff, the availability of PPE, diagnostic testing, influenza vaccination, and adjustment of COVID-19 risk prevention practices are indispensable, besides preventive work leave for those belonging to the risk group. Various countries have experienced constant difficulty in access to information on the COVID-19 situation inside prisons.

There are cases of prison guards and inmates who test positive or have symptoms, which are only revealed extra-officially by the media, third sector organizations, families, or prison staff [4]. Key roles have been played by the justice system's oversight agencies (especially the Offices of the Public Prosecutor and Public Defender) and civil society (such as the Mechanism to Prevent and Combat Torture) to determine the real epidemiological situation and ensure that the recommended measures are actually enforced. Further according to the World Health Organization (WHO), clinical decisions must be made by health professionals and should not be ignored or overridden by prison staff. The COVID-19 pandemic cannot justify restrictions that constitute torture or cruel, inhumane, or degrading treatment, nor should the pandemic be used to impede independent inspections by international or national agencies [2]. It is a mistake to believe that the total blockade of prisons, with prisoners' collective isolation and limitation of information on the situation inside prison walls, will avoid the spread of COVID-19 in the prison system. It is ethically imperative to implement totally transparent strategies to deal with the pandemic, including evidence-based care and surveillance, with measures similar to those recommended for the general population in order to avoid the risk of a humanitarian tragedy, more than ever placing prisons at the epicentre of necropolitics.

REFERENCES

1. Departamento Penitenciário Nacional, Ministério da Justiça. Levantamento nacional de informações penitenciárias. Atualizado em 09/04/2020. https://app.powerbi.com/vie w?r=eyJrIjoiZ-TlkZGJjODQtNmJlMi00OTJhL WFlMDktNzRlNmFkNTM0MWI3Iiwid CI6ImViMDkwNDIwLTQ0NGMtNDNm Ny05MWYyLTRiOGRhNmJmZThlM (accessed on 14/Apr/2020).
2. WHO Regional Office for Europe. Preparedness, prevention and control of COVID-19 in prisons and other places of detention. Interim guidance; 15 March 2020. http://www.euro. who.int/__data/assets/pdf_file/0019/434026/ Preparedness-prevention-and-control-of- COVID-19-in-prisons.pdf?ua=1 (accessed on 14/Apr/2020).
3. Amon, J.J.(2020). COVID-19 and detention: respecting human rights. Health and Human Rights Journal 2020; 23 mar. https://www.hhrjournal. org/2020/03/COVID-19-and-detention-respect ing-human-rights/ (accessed on 12/Apr/2020).
4. European Prison Observatory. COVID-19: what is happening in european prisons? http://www.prisonobservatory.org/upload/ 25032020European_prisons_during_covid19. pdf (accessed on 14/Apr/2020).
5. Assembleia da República. Lei nº 9 de 10 de abril de 2020. Regime excecional de flexibilização da execução das penas e das medidas de graça, no âmbito da pandemia da doença COVID-19. Diário da República Eletrónico 2020. https:// dre.pt/home/-/dre/131338919/details/maxi mized.
6. Conselho Nacional de Justiça. Recomendação no 62, de 17 de março de 2020. Recomenda aos Tribunais e magistrados a adoção de medidas preventivas à propagação da infecção pelo novo coronavírus – COVID-19 no âmbito dos sistemas de justiça penal e socioeducativo. https:// www.cnj.jus.br/wp-content/uploads/2020/03/ 62-Recomendação.pdf (accessed on 14/Apr/ 2020).
7. Supremo Tribunal Federal. Tema 365: responsabilidade do Estado por danos morais decorrentes de superlotação carcerária. RE 580252. http://portal.stf.jus.br/processos/detalhe.as p?incidente=2600961.
8. Supremo Tribunal Federal. Tema 592: em caso de inobservância do seu dever específico de proteção previsto no art. 5o, inciso XLIX, da Constituição Federal, o Estado é responsável pela morte de detento. RE 841526.
9. Secretaria de Estado de Saúde do Rio de Janeiro. Plano de contingência da atenção primária à saúde para o coronavírus no Estado do Rio de Janeiro. https://www.saude.rj.gov.br/aten cao-primaria-a-saude/noticias-saps/2020/03/ atualizacao-plano-de-contingencia-da-aps-pa ra-o-coronavirus-no-estado-do-rio-de-janeiro
10. Secretaria Municipal de Saúde do Rio de Janeiro. Resolução SMS no 4.330, de 16 de março de 2020. Diário Oficial do Município do Rio de Janeiro 2020; 18 mar.
11. Secretaria Municipal de Saúde do Rio de Janeiro. Resolução SMS no 4.330, de 16 de março de 2020. Anexo I à Resolução SMS no 4.330, de 16 de março de 2020. Nota técnica da Assessoria Especial – Atenção Primária à Saúde. Orientações sobre a prevenção e manejo da transmissão e infecção pelo novo coronavírus (SARS-CoV-2) e organização dos serviços de atenção primária à saúde do Município do Rio de Janeiro (atualizada em 26/03/2020). Diário Oficial do Município do Rio de Janeiro 2020; 27 mar.
12. Secretaria de Estado de Saúde do Rio de Janeiro; Secretaria de Estado de Administração Penitenciária do Rio de Janeiro. Resolução Conjunta SES/SEAP no 736 de 16 de março 2020. Promove recomendações para prevenção e controle de infecções pelo novo coronavírus (COVID-19) a serem adotadas nas unidades prisionais do Estado do Rio de Janeiro. Diário Oficial do Estado do Rio de Janeiro 2020; 17 mar.
13. Ministério da Justiça e Segurança Pública; Ministério da Saúde. Portaria Interministerial no 7, de 18 de março de 2020. Dispõe sobre as medidas de enfrentamento da emergência de saúde pública previstas na Lei no 13.979, de 6 de fevereiro de 2020, no âmbito do Sistema Prisional. Diário Oficial da União 2020; 18 mar.
16. Mecanismo Estadual de Prevenção e Combate à Tortura do Rio de Janeiro. Relatório parcial sobre impactos do COVID-19 no Sistema Prisional do Rio de Janeiro. Informações adicionais até o dia 10 de abril de 2020. Fundação Oswaldo Cruz. Saúde mental e atenção psicossocial na pandemia COVID-19. Recomendações gerais. ttps://www.fiocruzbrasilia.fiocruz.br/wp-.

3. COVID-19 Is Increasing The Power Of Brazil's Criminal Groups

Ryan Berg

American Enterprise Institute

Andrea Varsori

Urban Violence Research Network.

BACKGROUND

Data from various states suggest that COVID-19 lockdowns have done little to reduce the use of violence by criminal groups in Brazil. What has changed is governance, with criminal actors adapting to coronavirus by imposing curfews, restricting movement, promoting public-health messages, and discouraging price gouging – alongside their usual practices of extortion and drug trafficking. Such changes in violence and governance indicate that Brazil's non-state armed groups continue to augment their power, and these gains may well persist once the pandemic has receded.

INTRODUCTION

The COVID-19 pandemic has shaken the world and paralysed most national economies. And this is true even of illicit economies, with many criminal organisations seeing their freedom of action and profits squeezed[1] as borders close worldwide. Yet the pandemic has also provided some non-state actors with opportunities to augment their power[2], as the case of Brazil reveals.

Violence And Governance As Proxies Of Power

The growing power of Brazil's criminal groups during the pandemic can best be viewed through two lenses: violence and governance. Both serve as excellent proxies for the power of criminal groups and, fortunately, both are measurable despite the current lockdown. Levels of violence serve as a good proxy of criminal groups' power because violence is an essential ingredient of their claims to legitimacy. Some of Brazil's criminal groups, such as the Primeiro Comando da Capital (PCC, First Capital Command) have the capacity to influence[3] the country's homicide rates due to their control over sanctioning of murders and over residents views on what constitutes "legitimate" use of force. While the control exercised by Brazil's criminal groups is periodically enforced by violence that produces fear and intimidation, violence is also useful for spreading informal governance in the marginalised areas where they operate. By maintaining a monopoly on the "legitimate" use of violence, Brazil's criminal groups shape behavioural norms and expectations. Governance serves as

---

[1] https://www.occrp.org/en/blog/11905-cocaine-corona-how-the-pandemic-is-squeezing-italian-crime-groups
[2] https://www.foreignaffairs.com/articles/americas/2020-04-21/pandemic-could-bring-power-latin-americas-criminal-gangs
[3] https://pesquisa-eaesp.fgv.br/sites/gvpesquisa.fgv.br/files/arquivos/pax.pdf

a useful proxy because Brazil's criminal groups often dominate neighbourhoods in the urban periphery and provide governance functions[1] in communities that are poorly served – if served at all – by state institutions. In normal times, they might mimic states and provide key public goods, such as trash collection and basic infrastructure, cable TV and electricity provision, and even justice and policing services. In an example suggestive of the mutually reinforcing nature of violence and governance, the holding of criminal tribunals[2] shows how armed groups can ruthlessly apply disciplinary power through a literal monopoly on violence.

Criminal Violence Under Lockdown In Brazil

With respect to violence, the data indicates a likely increase in its use by Brazil's criminal groups during state-level lockdowns, as seen in both homicides and lethal crimes (a broader indicator that subsumes homicides). While both are rough indicators of criminal violence, a rise in these two rates makes a decrease in gang-related murders unlikely.

In most Brazilian states, the COVID-19 lockdown started around mid-March. Examining homicide and lethal crime rates for the month of April is therefore the best option when analysing trends in violence under anti-pandemic measures. While several important states have yet to disclose data for April, figures are already available for Ceará, Rio Grande do Norte[3], and Pernambuco[4]. The governors of these states ordered the closure of all non-essential businesses in quick succession between 18 and 24 March.

In Ceará[5] and Rio Grande do Norte, a decrease in the number of lethal crimes in March (respectively -21.8% and -12.5%)[6] was followed by an increase in April (+22% and +12.7%)[7]. In Pernambuco, the trend has been the opposite[8]: an increase in March (+22.4%) followed by a decrease in April (-11.4%). Nevertheless, even with the lockdown, April saw more lethal crimes than February (+8.5%), as well as slightly more than April 2019[9]. Data from these states makes a decrease in gang-related violence unlikely. Notably, in the aforementioned states, rival criminal groups are battling for control of criminal markets and territory. This is especially the case in Ceará, where drug trafficking routes to Europe have been disputed by four criminal factions[10] since the mid-2010s. Although homicide rates fell considerably in 2019[11], a police strike in February led to a spike in homicides.

A new spike was registered in April 2020, during the lockdown. More specifically, murders have been clustered in the poorer peripheries of the capital Fortaleza, where inter-gang violence is very common. Rio de Janeiro state, historically beset by rivalries amongst criminal factions and friction

[1] https://www.cambridge.org/core/journals/journal-of-latin-american-studies/article/dynamics-of-criminal-governance-networks-and-social-order-in-rio-de-janeiro/C69DCE555949A535D2ECE7399C49B4C6

[2] https://www.cambridge.org/core/journals/latin-american-politics-and-society/article/myth-of-personal-security-criminal-gangs-dispute-resolution-and-identity-in-rio-de-janeiros-favelas/30F5284538717D1365EE2558C75A6BEC

[3] https://agorarn.com.br/cidades/governo-do-rn-ja-publicou-20-decretos-de-combate-a-covid-19-confira-o-que-eles-dizem/

[4] https://g1.globo.com/pe/pernambuco/noticia/2020/03/20/coronavirus-governo-de-pernambuco-determina-fechamento-de-comercio-servicos-e-obras-de-construcao-civil.ghtml

[5] https://www.sspds.ce.gov.br/wp-content/uploads/sites/24/2020/05/01-CVLI-Estat%C3%ADsticas-Mensais.pdf

[6] http://www.tribunadonorte.com.br/noticia/crimes-no-rn-reduzem-em-mara-o/476667

[7] http://www.tribunadonorte.com.br/noticia/homica-dios-aumentam-28-durante-o-ma-s-de-abril-no-rn/478751

[8] http://www.sds.pe.gov.br/images/indicadores/CVLI/CVLI_MENSAL_POR_REGI%C3%83O_COM_ENFRENTAMENTO.pdf

[9] http://www.sds.pe.gov.br/images/media/1559159212_04 - Informe Mensal da Conjuntura Criminal - Abril de 2019.pdf

[10] https://noticias.uol.com.br/cotidiano/ultimas-noticias/2018/02/25/estrategico-para-o-trafico-ceara-vira-centro-de-distribuicao-de-drogas-e-esconde-guerra-de-faccoes.htm

[11] https://g1.globo.com/ce/ceara/noticia/2019/11/13/ceara-registra-queda-de-522percent-no-numero-de-homicidios-em-2019-diz-secretaria-da-seguranca.ghtml

with police paramilitary groups, also saw a rise in recorded homicides in March[1], and this has increase has been linked to several intense turf wars[2]. Between March 13 and April 9 alone, turf wars have been reported in nine different areas[3], eight of which are within Rio's metropolitan region. Thus, the lockdown does not seem to deter the use of violence by criminal groups where longstanding rivalries exist.

Criminal Governance Under Lockdown In Brazil

With respect to governance, Brazil's criminal groups have also proven to be nimble and adaptive during the pandemic. So far, they have imposed curfews[4], utilised mobile loudspeakers to broadcast public-hygiene announcements, and gone door-to-door to ensure compliance with quarantine measures. Criminal factions have postponed large social gatherings, such as the frequent dance parties staged for local entertainment.

Limited state presence in the favelas meant that the then Health Minister Luiz Henrique Mandetta was left with no other option but to dialogue[5] with criminal groups to promote public health and negotiate safe passage for public health personnel. In a sign of their growing power, criminal groups have distributed personal protective equipment[6] and repurposed precursor chemicals used in the production of drugs to manufacture "hand sanitiser[7]". Criminal factions also managed to steal[8] a shipment of 15,000 coronavirus tests and 2,000 units of personal protective equipment from an airport in São Paulo; these would have been sold and distributed had they not been recovered by Brazilian authorities.

Criminal factions in Rio favelas such as Rocinha and Vidigal are effectively prohibiting entry to outsiders,[9] which serves both to slow transmission of the virus and also to maintain the gangs' socioeconomic role as providers. In the face of scarcity, Brazilian criminal groups have sought to control [10]the price of goods on the open market by threatening violence against vendors to prevent price gouging. That said, the factions' daily bread of extortion[11] continues in all of its usual forms, as does the trafficking of drugs.

Despite coronavirus-induced trade disruptions, Brazil's criminal groups continue to export illicit narcotics to their top destination, Europe, and seizures[12] are up 20 per cent this year when compared to the same period of last year. The isolation and anxiety associated with social distancing measures have also led to increased international demand for illicit narcotics, with widespread

[1] http://www.ispvisualizacao.rj.gov.br/

[2] https://oglobo.globo.com/rio/isolamento-social-nao-altera-numeros-de-homicidios-registrados-em-marco-no-estado-do-rio-segundo-isp-24369592

[3] https://extra.globo.com/casos-de-policia/trafico-milicia-disputam-favelas-no-rio-em-meio-pandemia-de-coronavirus-24350795.html

[4] https://g1.globo.com/rj/rio-de-janeiro/noticia/2020/03/23/coronavirus-traficantes-e-milicianos-impoem-toque-de-recolher-em-comunidades-do-rio.ghtml?fbclid=IwAR0dUuMXvlDiSAIFEs9XkmEG4FCkuT_b5upQp3zfBPZ6uvsjUasCOido23s

[5] https://www.terra.com.br/vida-e-estilo/saude/ministerio-dialoga-com-o-trafico-e-a-milicia-diz-mandetta,90e4627d550049272f8242e7b94c75e9qwxjeix4.html

[6] https://www.theguardian.com/world/video/2020/apr/21/bolsonaro-wont-help-with-coronavirus-so-brazils-favelas-helping-themselves-video

[7] https://amp.theguardian.com/world/2020/mar/25/brazil-rio-gangs-coronavirus

[8] https://veja.abril.com.br/brasil/policia-prende-suspeitos-de-furtar-15-mil-testes-de-coronavirus-em-sp/

[9] https://www.terra.com.br/noticias/coronavirus/coronavirus-trafico-proibe-turistas-em-favelas-do-rio,fe51c0a4cb56352a96bda95e0acd642amrqlvjve.html?fbclid=IwAR0UbpiAL5BwXJC3w-mgn0-Hk2NBSu5Mkimln3huOHei2zr1w2dzJqzkRtI

[10] https://g1.globo.com/rj/rio-de-janeiro/noticia/2020/03/26/traficantes-ameacam-comercio-em-favelas-do-rio-contra-o-aumento-de-preco-do-alcool-gel.ghtml

[11] https://g1.globo.com/rj/rio-de-janeiro/noticia/2020/04/17/milicia-obriga-reabertura-do-comercio-para-recolher-taxa-em-comunidades-do-rj.ghtml

[12] https://www.reuters.com/article/us-health-coronavirus-eu-drugs/europe-flooded-with-cocaine-despite-coronavirus-trade-disruptions-idUSKBN22C1TY

panic buying despite rising prices[1]. Finally, the pandemic has augmented the governance power of criminal groups in another critical domain: prisons. Many of Brazil's top criminal groups[2] are based in prisons, with top leaders incarcerated and the prison experience remaining central to group identity. Even in normal times, criminal groups fill the gaps in the state's paltry delivery of essential goods and services throughout the country's decrepit prison facilities, and they have leveraged their power[3] even further during the pandemic. With the virus spreading rapidly through overcrowded jails and normal rights (like visiting hours) often being curtailed, criminal groups have gone so far as to take prison guards hostage[4] in order to demand better conditions, sometimes even leading massive prison escapes[5]. Overall, COVID-19 has given Brazil's criminal groups a new swagger. Trends in violence and criminal governance indicate that Brazil's non-state armed groups continue to augment their power, and these gains may well endure once the pandemic recedes. When the country reopens completely, state and federal authorities are likely to encounter a highly altered landscape in which they have lost considerable ground in their fight against criminal factions.

Andrea Varsori is a co-coordinator of the Urban Violence Research Network (UVRN).
Posted In: COVID19 | Society

Ryan Berg is a Research Fellow in Latin America Studies at the American Enterprise Institute (AEI).

---

[1] https://theconversation.com/how-coronavirus-is-changing-the-market-for-illegal-drugs-134753

[3] https://www.foreignaffairs.com/articles/americas/2020-05-05/latin-americas-prison-gangs-draw-strength-pandemic
[4] https://www.reuters.com/article/us-brazil-prison-rebellion/prisoners-take-guards-hostage-in-brazils-coronavirus-hit-manaus-idUSKBN22E0KB
[5] https://agenciabrasil.ebc.com.br/geral/noticia/2020-03/sao-paulo-tem-rebeliao-em-quatro-presidios-e-fuga-de-presos-no-litoral

4.The Pandemic in Prison:
Interventions and *Overisolation*

Sérgio Garófalo de Carvalho
Universidade Federal da Bahia

Andreia Beatriz Silva dos Santos
Universidade Estadual de Feira de Santana Médica do Sistema Penitenciário

Ivete Maria Santos
Universidade Federal da Bahia Médica do Sistema Penitenciário da Bahia

ABSTRACT

Prison health is, in its essence, public health. The COVID-19 pandemic poses a great threat to the world and has shown that preventing the disease escalation in prisons integrates the novel corona virus clash in society in general. Up to this moment, the most effective known measure to curb the disease spread is social isolation. Nevertheless, in penal institutions, often overcrowded, social isolation becomes difficult to carry out and, when it happens, it takes the enclosed population to *overisolation*, with consequences to their mental health. Besides, prisoners suffer with clogged up environment, lack of materials for personal hygiene, poor basic sanitary conditions and difficulties in accessing health services. In order to reduce the disease spread, several countries are taking measures such as definite or temporary release of prisoners and visiting restrictions. This paper deals with a narrative review on the pandemic effects in prisons and how government and civil society have organized themselves in order to reduce the disease consequences at those places. The text has been divided into three sections: the first with literature review on the current health theme; the second discusses how different countries have been dealing with the prison situation in the pandemic context, and, the last part focuses on how the Brazilian Penal System has reacted to the new disease.

INTRODUCTION

The outbreak of the disease (COVID-19) caused by the novel coronavirus (SARS-CoV-2) in China gained global prominence and was declared a pandemic by the World Health Organization (WHO) on March 11, 2020. As there are no specific treatments and vaccines available to control the disease, the COVID-19 pandemic represents a major threat to public health worldwide, requiring prevention actions, such as social isolation and strengthening hygiene measures[1].

The potential for transmission of the virus is already known when indoors and with agglomerations. Mizumoto and Chowell[2] described the epidemiological evolution within an Asian cruise, in which the average number of reproductions in the confined environment reached values close to 11, which is higher than the estimates reported in the dynamics of community transmission in China and

Singapore, ranging from 1.1 to 7. On this ship, cases went from 1 to 454 in just 16 days. The Spanish flu affected about a quarter of all prisoners; a much higher prevalence compared to data from the general population[3]Criminal institutions confer a confinement imposed by a judicial authority and are surrounded by stigma and vulnerability[4]. Confinement within a prison unit is distinct from other types, such as cruises, schools, quarantine, which are voluntary isolations, while in prison freedom is unwittingly curtailed. In this sense, when applied to the prison context, the isolation measure results in a superposition of confinements, which we call *overisolation.*

Many prisons in Brazil and in the world are overcrowded, offering little space in relation to what is recommended for adequate distancing. Of the countries, 59% have prison occupancy rates that exceed the reported capacity[5]. With this, the possibility is high that the corona virus is rapidly transmitted within the criminal institutions. In a single day in February, China recorded 200 contaminated in one of its prisons, when the curve of infections was already falling in the country[6]. In addition to being a risk for people deprived of liberty, a high prevalence of viral respiratory infections in prison populations can serve as a potential source of infection for the general population. This is because prisons are porous institutions, such as the borders of countries in the globalized world[7]. Through prison officers, workers, visitors, prisoners released and transferred, corona virus can pass through the bars of the prison system and be transmitted to local communities[8]. By definition, prison health is public health and should be treated as such by governments and the scientific community. Thus, this article is a narrative review on the SARS-CoV-2 and the prison population, in order to gather what has been published on the subject in health journals and elucidate the theme, with the aim of reinforcing the need to guarantee fundamental human rights to people deprived of liberty and safeguarding the health of the population in general. For better reading and understanding of the subject, this publication is divided into the following topics: the state of the art on COVID-19 and the prison population; COVID-19 prevention measures in prisons worldwide; coping with the novel coronavirus in the Brazilian prison system and final considerations.

THE STATE OF ART ABOUT COVID-19 AND PRISON POPULATION

To carry out this narrative review, articles published until April 25, 2020 in health journals were researched. Texts in English, Spanish and Portuguese and in any formats, such as editorials, comments, correspondence, opinions, empirical studies and others were included. The search took place in two databases, PubMed and Google Scholar, the search strategy is in Table 1. A total of 605 results were found and, after reading the title and/or abstract, 13 articles remained for complete reading. No formal quality assessment was performed, but the important methodological characteristics were considered when interpreting the results presented here narratively.

In PubMed, 3,710 articles were found in the search for the descriptor "COVID-19", but only six publications (0.16%) addressing the pandemic in the prison context. Of the 13 articles included in this review, only one is an original study. In Table 2, you can see the description of these works. Social distancing is practically impossible in correctional facilities, where individuals live in confinement in overcrowded and poorly ventilated environments, share bathrooms and showers, as well as common areas such as cafeterias, patios and classrooms[10]. Hand hygiene is hampered by policies that limit access to soap, and many prisons restrict alcohol intake, fearing that people have ingested it[14].

Populations deprived of liberty have an increased prevalence of infectious diseases, such as HIV infections and hepatitis C virus (HCV)[7]. Inequities in social determinants of health that affect groups that are disproportionately liable to incarceration - racial and sexual minorities, people with mental disorders or psychoactive substance use, individuals without access to the health system or education lead to higher concentrations of some diseases in incarcerated populations[7]. The risk for a person deprived of liberty to develop tuberculosis in Brazil is 30 times higher than the general Brazilian population[21]. Infectious diseases account for about 17.5% of deaths in prisons[11].

In addition to the difficulties related to the physical and social structures mentioned above, there are administrative challenges, largely caused by the lack of mismanagement of financial resources[14], which may hinder the access of possible prisoners with COVID-19 to adequate health care in case of need for advanced support. The rights of all affected persons must be respected, and all public health measures should be implemented without discrimination of any kind[18]. All the revised publications highlight the urgent need to take measures to prevent SARS-CoV2 in prison environments, it is necessary to consider chains as reservoirs that can lead to the resurgence of the epidemic, if it is not adequately treated in these facilities[7]. Therefore, three premises must be fulfilled: the entry of the virus into penitentiaries should be postponed as much as possible; if it is already in circulation, it must be checked and, finally, prisons must prepare to deal with those who develop COVID-19[7]. Given the epidemiological dynamics of COVID-19, in the absence of any intervention, among inmates, the outbreak is considerably more severe than in the general population, requiring more hospitalization and leading to more deaths.

The peak of the epidemic within a penal institution, according to mathematical modeling[20], is considerably earlier, occurring 63 days earlier than the peak of infections in the community. The same study[20] showed that postponing the arrest of 90% of individuals from groups at risk to COVID-19 would reduce the mortality of the disease in prisons by 56.1%. Although only 1.5% of the prison population is elderly in Brazil[22], incarceration itself degrades people's health, leaving them more vulnerable to infection and severe infection results. There is consensus that an effective action to mitigate the evolution of the pandemic in correctional environments is the release, temporary or definitive, of prisoners. For example, Iran has released 70,000 individuals so far incarcerated[7]. Two articles[10,13] that discuss the current situation of immigrants imprisoned in the United States advocate releasing all individuals who do not pose a threat to local security, and to momentarily cease the policy of incarceration against illegal immigration adopted in recent years. Yang and Thompson[11] suggest that sentences for people tried with misdemeanours are alternatives to deprivation of liberty.

The WHO[18] recommends that individuals who make up the risk group for COVID-19 leave prisons if they do not pose a danger to society. An important argument for this measure is raised by the assumption[20] that the interruption of the arrest of individuals for minor crimes, with the overall reduction of arrests by approximately 83%, would result in 71.8% fewer infections in the incarcerated population. This strategy[20] would also lead to 2.4% fewer infections among employees and 12.1% in the community in general. Public policies to mitigate inequality must follow the judicial decisions of release of these people, since many graduates of the prison system do not have family and social support. This can lead to the desired opposite effect with the release of these individuals and they become carriers and transmitters of SARS-CoV-2 while searching for income, housing, or even, to compose the population in street situation[16].

Stephenson[15] recalls that in California and New York, the government is renting hotel rooms to some of those prisoners released.

Thus, freeing imprisoned individuals should be an intersectoral action, involving public power, social assistance, NGOs, health services and the judiciary. If, however, the only measure is to reduce the size of the prison population, there will be a neglect of countless other things that must be done[17]. Mitigation strategies in detention centres should be complemented by routine screening and containment procedures. This involves screening all people entering the facility, including new inmates, employees, visitors and suppliers, quarantined those who are positive for exposure to the novel coronavirus[10].Other measures are suggested in the revised bibliography.

Yang and Thompson[11] suggest intensifying health education for inmates and prison workers. Everyone should receive training on how to identify signs of COVID-19 and ways to prevent the disease. Suspension of visits from family and lawyers and reduction of transfers are proposed by Akiyama, Spaulding and Rich[7], also suggesting that teleconference be applied in these cases in order to reduce emotional isolation. Cleaning and disinfection of the environments, as well as purchase of toiletries and masks must be carried out by the government[12,14]. In the revised publications, it was also said that the measures should take and account that the psychological reactions of people deprived of liberty may differ from those observed in people who observe social distancing in the community, since, in prison, there will be a *overisolation*. The unintended consequences of these mitigation policies should be considered. The recent rebellions in Italian prisons have revealed the potential for negative psychological impact of emergency policies aimed at reducing the spread of SARS-CoV-2 in criminal institutions[14]. Therefore, the growing need for emotional and psychological support, transparent awareness and sharing of information about the disease and the guarantee that continuous contact with family will be maintained[18], so that people deprived of liberty can collaborate in pandemic mitigation strategies.

COVID-19 IN PRISONS IN THE WORLD

This review aims to show that, despite what has been done by people deprived of liberty in the current pandemic, it is still insufficient and marginalizing. In 2018, there were more than 10 million people deprived of liberty worldwide[23], largely in poor sanitary conditions, with little access to health services and in overcrowded institutions. The prison population of several countries, as well as graduates of the penal system, suffers from stigma[4], abandonment of public power and what the philosopher Mbembe calls necropolitics[24], based on a State of Exception, in which it has the power to dictate who should live and who should die, desizing from the subject his political status and, if not actively taking his life, exposing him to death.

For information on how different countries are dealing with the pandemic in the prison context, information contained in the Prison Insider initiative[25], created by the founder of the International Observatory of Prisons, has been reviewed and summarized. The site gathers up to-date information on various aspects of prisons in the world and currently has an area focused on the novel coronavirus. It should be noted, however, that there is a limitation of this information, since not all countries or organizations make the data available and, when they do, it is not in real time.

As of May 5, 2020, there were 145 countries with data presented and a total of 23,019 records of SARS-CoV-2 infections, with the United States being the first, with more than 17,000 people deprived of their freedom infected[25]. On the other hand, there are complaints in several countries of lack of transparency in data[26,27].

The supervision by activists, international organizations and parliamentarians have been compromised[27-28] under the pretext of reducing access to prisons due to COVID-19. Concern stemmed from concern that in Syria the regime may be using the pandemic to get rid of prisoners, hardening repression against them[29], and similarly, Palestinian prisoners have been more exposed to the new virus in Israeli prisons[30].

Figure 1 shows the measures practiced by several countries, summarized through our review of the Prison Insider initiative[24]. Something that could be effective was reported only 5 of the 145 countries reviewed[25]: mass testing of trapped individuals.

The two most practiced measures are the suspension or reduction of visits and the release of prisoners. It should be noted, however, that even though there are large numbers of prisoners being released, the institutions still fall short of holding so many people. There are reports that the excess of prisoners, coupled with the fear of falling ill and the suspension of visits in various locations has caused rebellions in various penal institutions around the world. To exemplify: in Luxembourg, there were reports of a hunger strike[31]. In Italy, rebellions have been reported in several areas of the country[32]. In Argentina, there have been at least one death and several injured as a result of riots[33].The effervescence that occurred in prisons may be associated with the little health quality information passed on to inmates. Few countries reported having invested

in health education, given the context of the pandemic. WHO[18] stresses the importance of providing adequate information and legal guarantees to people deprived of liberty in order to reassure them and their families. If, on the one hand, prisoners must be protected by efficient public health policies, on the other, they actively participate in the fight against SARS-CoV-2. Several countries have reported that the prison population is voluntarily working on the making of masks to be distributed in health services and in the community. In Guatemala, a young prisoner reported to the report while wearing masks: "If I was able to harm Guatemala in the past, today I want to make up for my mistakes."[34].

COPING WITH CORONAVIRUS IN THE BRAZILIAN PRISON SYSTEM

In Brazil, the health needs of people deprived of liberty are under the responsibility of the State, as provided for by the Criminal Execution Law – LEP[35], but policies have also been implemented for the inclusion of the prison population within the SUS. In 2014, the National Policy for Integral Health Care of the Private Person of Liberty [36] (PNAISP) was instituted, whose objective is focused on ensuring the care of people deprived of liberty at all levels of complexity, expanding and organizing from the forms of financing of prison health teams to the main health actions for people arrested.

A challenge for prison systems around the world, COVID-19, whose most effective treatment is in the prevention of their transmission, individual hygiene and collective spaces, ventilated environments and social isolation[1], exposes the precariousness of prisons in Brazil. This challenges managers to ensure the effectiveness of the actions foreseen in the PNAISP, as well as for health professionals who are on the front line in prisons to organize themselves in the face of the risks of an explosion of cases and deaths. In 2019, there were 1,422 prisons in Brazil, of which 49% are destined for the detention of provisional prisoners and 79% are overcrowded[22]. Half of the prison institutions do not have a doctor's office. According to the National Penitentiary Department[22], in the same year, there were 755,274 people deprived of liberty in the country, of which 31% are provisional prisoners.

Brazil complied with the measures proposed by WHO[18] in relation to the population deprived of liberty through Recommendation 62/2020 of the National Council of Justice (CNJ)[37]. This involves incarceration and non-imprisonment measures, in addition to other sanitary actions, detailed in Table 3. Recommendation 62/2020[37] considers as belonging to the risk group: elderly; pregnant women; people with chronic, respiratory or immunosuppressive conditions. In addition to the above recommendations, the Brazilian Society of Family and Community Medicine issued a document stressing the need for other measures: educational actions, combating fake news, individual and collective hygiene, hygiene of environments, providing information to family members and hygiene of hygiene material of safety professionals, involving actions for prisoners and various prison professionals[38].As of May 11, 2020, there were 603 cases of COVID-19 confirmed in Brazilian prisons, resulting in 23 deaths[22]. With only 20 days, the numbers jumped from 1 to more than 100 in Brazil[39]. Despite the recommendations and efforts of civil society, much remains to be done. A religious entity working in prisons disclosed the data that 65.9% of food and hygiene materials sent by family members were not entering prisons[40]. The same religious organization cites the lack of transparency and PPE, in addition to poor hygiene conditions, such as the report that 35 prisoners would be using the same toothbrush[41]. It is noteworthy that of the 603 cases of COVID-19 in Brazilian prisons, 444 (74%) are in the Penitentiary Complex of Papuda[42], in the Federal District, an institution that houses many imprisoned politicians and criminals with greater purchasing power. The data may evidence an inequality in the Penitentiary System that reproduces that of society in general, in which there is more access to tests for the novel coronavirus when it occupies a position of social or financial privilege.

FINAL CONSIDERATIONS

The PNAISP and the recommendations of the CNJ, adapted to the reality of each place are significant initiatives in the health care of people deprived of liberty and give visibility to this problem sensitive and relevant to public health, considering that, because they are porous institutions, the injuries that affect prisons are not restricted to it. Coping with COVID-19 in Brazilian prison institutions, as in much of the world, is a challenge, in view of the precariousness that characterizes them, the result of chronic disregard of public authorities and civil society, which give prisoners an illegitimate worsening of the formal sentence, such as the denial of basic sanitary conditions, such as access to drinking water. In this sense, in times of pandemic, the prison scenario is aggravated by the overlapping of problems, pre-existing and new, that require more aggressive sanitary measures, such as the suspension of visits and others, which result in *overisolation*, which, in addition, can affect the mental health of people deprived of liberty. Pandemic containment measures taken around the world reveal that there is a consensus on releasing prisoners and suspending visits, but other actions are put aside, such as health education and mass testing in the prison population, which could help in epidemiological projections, given that they are closed and controlled groups. Another consensus is that the lack of health data available on this population prevents the adoption of more effective measures. Scientific publications related to COVID-19, as well as other infectious diseases, in the prison population are scarce, pointing to a possible lack of interest in this theme by the scientific community, which may result from the stigma and difficulty of access to this group. Given the above, the pandemic for the novel corona virus has been playing a revealing role in the unhealthy and inhuman conditions aimed at the recovery of human beings.

May the public authorities, civil society and the scientific community take something positive from the current public health crisis in order to change the fate of vulnerable populations!

Acknowledgment

Thanks to Professor Hélio Marques da Silva, for translating the article, and to Richard Luiz Eduardo and Antônio Teixeira, for their contributions.

REFERENCES

1. Jin, Y., Yang., H, Ji., W, Wu, W., Chen, S., Zhang, W., Duan, G. (2020). Virology, Epidemiology, Pathogenesis, and Control of COVID-19. Viruses. 2020 Mar 27;12(4):E372.
2. Mizumoto, K., Chowell, G. (2020). Transmission potential of the novel coronavirus (COVID19) onboard the diamond Princess Cruises Ship, 2020. Infect Dis Model. 2020 Feb 29;5:264-270.
3. Finnie, T.J., Copley, V.R., Hall, I.M., (2014).Leach S. An analysis of influenza outbreaks in institutions and enclosed societies. Epidemiol Infect. 2014 Jan;142(1):107-13.
4. Goffman, E.(1982). Estigma: notas sobre a manipulação da identidade deteriorada. Rio de Janeiro: Zahar; 1982.
5. World prison brief online database [Internet]. 2020. Occupancy level (based on official capacity); [cited 2020 Apr 30]; Available from: https://www.prisonstudies.org/highest-to-lowest/occupancylevel?field_region_taxonomy_tid=All
6. NPR [Internet]. 2020 Feb 21. Coronavirus Found In China Prisons, As Cases Spike In South Korea; [cited 2020 Apr 30]; Available from: https://www.npr.org/2020/02/21/808002924/coronavirus-found-in-china-prisons-ascases-spike-in-south-korea
7. Akiyama, M.J., Spaulding, A.C., Rich, J.D. (2020). Flattening the Curve for Incarcerated Populations - COVID-19 in Jails and Prisons. N Engl J Med. 2020 Apr 2.
8. Sylverken, A., El-Duah, P., Owusu, M., Yeboah, R., Kwarteng, A., Ofori, L., Gorman, R., Obiri-Danso, K., Owusu-Dabo, E. (n..d. Burden of respiratory viral infections among inmates of a Ghanaian prison.
9. Simpson, P.L., Butler, T.G. (2020) COVID-19, prison crowding, and release policies. BMJ. 2020 Apr 20;369:m1551.
10. 10-Meyer JP, Franco-Paredes C, Parmar P, Yasin F, Gartland M. COVID-19 and the coming epidemic in US immigration detention centres. Lancet Infect Dis. 2020 Apr 15:S1473-3099(20)30295-4.
11. Yang H, Thompson JR. Fighting COVID-19 outbreaks in prisons. BMJ. 2020 Apr 2;369:m1362.
12. Kinner SA, Young JT, Snow K, Southalan L, Lopez-Acuña D, Ferreira-Borges C, O'Moore É. Prisons and custodial settings are part of a comprehensive response to COVID-19. Lancet Public Health. 2020 Apr;5(4):e188-e189.
13. Keller A.S, Wagner B.D. (2020). COVID-19 and immigration detention in the USA: time to act. Lancet Public Health. 2020 May;5(5):e245-e246.
14. Wurcel, A.G., Dauria, E., Zaller, N, Nijhawan. A., Beckwith, C., Nowotny, K., BrinkleyRubinstein, L. (2020). Spotlight on Jails: COVID-19 Mitigation Policies Needed Now. Clin Infect Dis. 2020 Mar 28:ciaa346.
15. Stephenson, J. (2020).COVID-19 Pandemic Poses Challenge for Jails and Prisons. InJAMA Health Forum 2020 Apr 1 (Vol. 1, No. 4, pp. e200422-e200422). American MedicalAssociation.
16. Gorman, G., Ramaswamy, M. (2020). Detained during a pandemic: A postcard from the Midwest. Public Health Nurs. 2020 May;37(3):325-326.
17. 17-Rubin, R. (2020) The challenge of preventing COVID-19 spread in correctional facilities. JAMA. 2020 Apr 7.
18. World Health Organization. Preparedness, prevention and control of COVID-19 in prisons and other places of detention (2020), Interim guidance 15 March 2020.
19. Liebrenz, M., Bhugra, D., Buadze, A., Schleifer, R., (2020).Caring for persons in detention suffering with mental illness during the COVID-19 outbreak. Forensic science international. Mind and law. 2020;1.

20. Lofgren, E., Lum, K., Horowitz, A., Madubuowu, B., Fefferman, N.. The Epidemiological Implications of Incarceration Dynamics in Jails for Community, Corrections Officer, and Incarcerated Population Risks from COVID-19. medRxiv. 2020 Jan 1.

21. Mabud, T.S., Alves, M.D., Ko, AI, Basu, S., Walter, K.S., Cohen, T., Mathema, B., Colijn, C., Lemos, E., Croda, J., Andrews. J.R.,(2019) Evaluating strategies for control of tuberculosis in prisons and prevention of spillover into communities: An observational and modeling study from Brazil. PLoS medicine. 2019 Jan;16(1).

22. DEPEN [Internet]. 2017 Jun 30. INFOPEN; [cited 2020 May 11]; Available from: http://depen.gov.br/DEPEN/depen/sisdepen/infopen

23. Walmsley, R. (2018). International World Prison Population List. Institute for Criminal Policy Research (ICPR)..

24. 24-Mbembe A. (2019) Necropolitics. Duke University Press; Oct 25.

25. Prison Insider [Internet]. [place unknown]; 2020 May 05. Coronavirus : la fièvre des prisons; [cited 2020 May 5]; Available from: https://www.prisoninsider.com/articles/coronavirus-la-fievre-des-prisons

26. The Marshall Project [Internet]. [place unknown]; 2020 Mar 17. As COVID-19 Measures Grow, Prison Oversight Falls; [cited 2020 May 1]; Available from: https://www.themarshallproject.org/2020/03/17/as-COVID-19-measures-grow-prisonoversight-falls.

27. Sobesednik [Internet]. [place unknown]; 2020 Mar 31. Vladimir Osechkin: I'm afraid that prison statistics on COVID-19 are falsified; [cited 2020 May 1]; Available from: https://sobesednik.ru/obshchestvo/20200331-vladimir-osechkin-boyus-chtot?fbclid=IwAR3Bi0kBBpFujMihl1XnyFFXqsuD9rXBg5iH_1ppwE3Ry8bjmLBZUL CENYwvid-19-measures-grow-prison-oversight-falls.

28. France 3 [Internet]. [place unknown]; 2020 Apr 16. Coronavirus : le député LFI Ugo Bernalicis conteste son interdiction de visiter la prison de Sequedin; [cited 2020 May 1]; Available from: https://france3-regions.francetvinfo.fr/hauts-defrance/coronavirus-depute-lfi-ugo-bernalicis-conteste-son-interdiction-visiter-prisonsequedin-1817236.html.

29. Syria Direct [Internet]. [place unknown]; 2020 Apr 14. Coronavirus: The Syrian regime's novel weapon against detainees; [cited 2020 May 4]; Available from: https://syriadirect.org/news/coronavirus-the-syrian-regime%E2%80%99s-novelweapon-against-detainees/.

30. Middle East Monitor [Internet]. [place unknown]; 2020 Apr 14. Israel's jail conditions will kill Palestinian prisoners before coronavirus does; [cited 2020 May 4]; Available from: https://www.middleeastmonitor.com/20200414-israels-jail-conditions-will-killpalestinian-prisoners-before-coronavirus-does/#comment-4876974513.

31. RTL [Internet]. [place unknown]; 2020 Mar 31. 30 inmates embark on hunger strike following protests; [cited 2020 May 2]; Available from: https://today.rtl.lu/news/luxembourg/a/1493481.html.

32. Prison Insider [Internet]. [place unknown]; 2020 Mar 12. Italie : révoltes dues au coronavirus, douze prisonniers décédés; [cited 2020 May 2]; Available from: https://www.prison-insider.com/articles/italie-revoltes-dues-au-coronavirus-douzeprisonniers-decedes?referrer=%2Fpreview.php%2Farticles%2Fcoronavirus-la-fievredes-prisons.

33. Clarín [Internet]. [place unknown]; 2020 Mar 23. Un muerto en un motín en dos cárceles de Santa Fe: reclaman medidas de seguridad por el coronavirus; [cited 2020 May 7]; Available from: https://www.clarin.com/policiales/graves-disturbios-carcelessanta-fe-reclaman-medidas-seguridad-coronavirus_0_z6ZWKbGfp.html.

34. CNN [Internet]. [place unknown]; 2020 Mar 27. Coronavirus en Guatemala: Jóvenes fabrican al menos 5.000 mascarillas desde la prisión; [cited 2020 May 6]; Available from: https://cnnespanol.cnn.com/video/coronavirus-mascarillas-jovenes-prisionciudad-guatemala-pandemia-pkg-digital-orig-michelle-mendoza/.

35. BRASIL. LEI Nº 7.210, de 11 de julho de 1984. Institui a Lei de Execução penal. 2010.

36. BRASIL. Portaria Interministerial n. 1, de 02 de janeiro de 2014. Institui a Política Nacional de Atenção Integral à Saúde das Pessoas Privadas de Liberdade no Sistema Prisional (PNAISP) no âmbito do Sistema Único de Saúde (SUS). Diário Oficial da União. 2014.

37. Conselho Nacional de Justiça. Recomendação nº 62, de 17 de março de 2020. Recomenda aos Tribunais e magistrados a adoção de medidas preventivas à propagação da infecção pelo novo coronavírus - COVID-19 no âmbito dos sistemas de justiça penal e socioeducativo. https://www.cnj.jus.br/wp-content/uploads/2020/03/62-Recomendação.pdf (acessado em 14/Abr/2020).

38. SBMFC [Internet]. 2020 Mar 25. Medidas e orientações para o enfrentamento da COVID-19 nas prisões; [cited 2020 Apr 29]; Available from: https://www.sbmfc.org.br/wp-content/uploads/2020/03/Medidas-eorientac%CC%A7o%CC%83es-para-o-enfrentamento-a-COVID-%E2%80%93-19nas-priso%CC%83es.pdf.

39. Ponte [Internet]. 2020 Apr 28. Casos de coronavírus em prisões vão de 1 a 107 em 20 dias, com 7 mortes; [cited 2020 Apr 8]; Available from: https://ponte.org/casos-deCOVID-19-em-prisoes-vao-de-1-a-107-em-20-dias-com-7-mortes/.

40. Pastoral Carcerária [Internet]. 2020 Apr 09. Pastoral Carcerária divulga dados de questionário sobre coronavírus nas prisões; [cited 2020 May 6]; Available from: https://carceraria.org.br/combate-e-prevencao-a-tortura/pastoral-carceraria-divulgadados-de-questionario-sobre-coronavirus-nas-prisoes.

41. Pastoral Carcerária [Internet]. 2020 Apr 22. Pastoral Carcerária divulga relatos e denúncias sobre o sistema carcerário em tempos de pandemia; [cited 2020 May 6]; Available from: https://carceraria.org.br/combate-e-prevencao-a-tortura/pastoralcarceraria-divulga-relatos-e-denuncias-sobre-o-sistema-carcerario-em-tempos-depandemia.

42. Correio Braziliense [Internet]. 2020 May 11. Número de presos infectados pelo coronavírus na Papuda chega a 444; [cited 2020 May 14]; Available from: https://www.correiobraziliense.com.br/app/noticia/cidades/2020/05/11/interna_cidade sdf,853723/numero-de-presos-infectados-pelo-coronavirus-na-papuda-chega-a-444.shtml.

Database search strategy

PubMed	Google Scholar
(((((((((((((((((((((prison[Title/Abstract]) OR (prisons[Title/Abstract])) OR (jail[Title/Abstract])) OR (emprisionment[Title/Abstract])) OR (in jail[Title/Abstract])) OR (arrest[Title/Abstract])) OR (arrested[Title/Abstract])) OR (detention[Title/Abstract])) OR (custody[Title/Abstract])) OR (confinement[Title/Abstract])) OR (cage[Title/Abstract])) OR (in cage[Title/Abstract])) OR (quod[Title/Abstract])) OR (chokey[Title/Abstract])) OR (choky[Title/Abstract])) OR (gaol[Title/Abstract])) OR (entanglement[Title/Abstract])) OR (accouchement[Title/Abstract])) OR (constrain[Title/Abstract])) OR (ewer[Title/Abstract])) OR (captivity[Title/Abstract])) AND (((((coronavirus[Title/Abstract]) OR (SARS-COV-2[Title/Abstract])) OR (coronaviruses[Title/Abstract])) OR (COVID-19[Title/Abstract])) OR (pandemy[Title/Abstract]))	☐ Coronavirus AND prisons ☐ COVID-19 AND prisons

Publications included in the review

Title	Authors	Publication type	Journal
COVID-19, prison crowding, and release policies[9]	Simpson PL, Butler TG.	Editorial	BMJ
COVID-19 and the coming epidemic in US immigration detention centres[10]	Meyer JP, Franco-Paredes C, Parmar P, Yasin F, Gartland M.	Comment	Lancet Infect Dis
Fighting COVID-19 outbreaks in prisons[11]	Yang H, Thompson JR.	Letter	BMJ
Flattening the Curve for Incarcerated Populations — COVID-19 in Jails and Prisons[7]	Akiyama MJ, Spaulding AC, Rich JD.	Perspective	N Engl J Med.
Prisons and custodial settings are part of a comprehensive response to COVID-19[12]	Kinner SA, Young JT, Snow K, et al.	Comment	Lancet Public Health
COVID-19 and Immigration Detention in the USA: Time to Act[13]	Keller AS, Wagner BD.	Comment	Lancet Public Health
Spotlight on Jails: COVID-19 Mitigation Policies Needed Now[14]	Wurcel AG, Dauria E, Zaller N, et al.	Correspondence	Clin Infect Dis.
COVID-19 Pandemic Poses Challenge for Jails and Prisons[15]	Stephenson, J.	Comment	JAMA Health Forum
Detained during a pandemic: A postcard from the Midwest[16]	Gorman G, Ramaswamy M.	Editorial	Public Health Nurs.
The challenge of preventing COVID19 spread in correctional facilities[17]	Rubin, R.	Perspective	JAMA
Preparedness, prevention and control of COVID-19 in prisons and other places of detention[18]	World Health Organization.	Technical document	World Health Organization
Caring for persons in detention suffering with mental illness during the COVID-19 outbreak[19]	Liebrenz, M., Bhugra, D., Buadze, A. e Schleifer, R.	Comment	Forensic science international. Mind and law
The Epidemiological Implications of Incarceration Dynamics in Jails for Community, Corrections Officer, and Incarcerated Population Risks from COVID-19[20]	Lofgren, E., Lum, K., Horowitz, A., Madubuowu, B., & Fefferman, N.	*Preprint:*Mathematical Modelagem	medRxiv

Measures to combat the novel coronavirus in the Brazilian Penal System

Extrication
Reassessment of socio-educational measures for adolescents with: progression from hospitalization to semi-freedom; temporary suspension or remission of the measure. Preference given to: pregnant, lactating, indigenous or disabled; hospitalized in units with reduced capacity or in units without health care.
Reassessment of sentences of provisional prisons that have exceeded 90 days or that are related to crime without violence or serious threat to the person.
Reassessment of provisional arrests of people in the risk group or prisoners in units without medical assistance.
Consider regime progression for people in a at-risk group or who are in overcrowded prisons or without health care.
In the absence of space for adequate isolation, placing the person arrested with suspicion or confirmation of COVID-19 under house arrest.
No entrapment
Alternative socio-educational measures and suspension of provisional hospitalizations for adolescents whose offense did not incurred violence. Preference given to: pregnant, lactating, indigenous or disabled; hospitalized in units with reduced capacity or in units without health care.
House arrest for people arrested for child support debt.
Maximum exceptionality of new pretrial detention orders, observing the protocol of the health authorities.
Other measures
Suspension of the duty of periodic submission to the court of persons on provisional release.
Extension of the period of return or postponement of the granting of the temporary exit benefit.
Restriction or reduction of visits to prisoners.
Temporary replacement of prison officers who are part of the risk group.
Education campaigns on the novel coronavirus.
Increased frequency of cleaning of cells and common spaces.
Avoid shared transportation of people deprived of liberty.
Screening of prisoners, staff and visitors.
Supply of personal protective equipment (PPE) to employees.
Uninterrupted supply of water to persons deprived of liberty and public servants of the units.
Isolation of suspected or confirmed cases in prison.

Figure 1: Measures to combat the new coronavirus in prisons worldwide

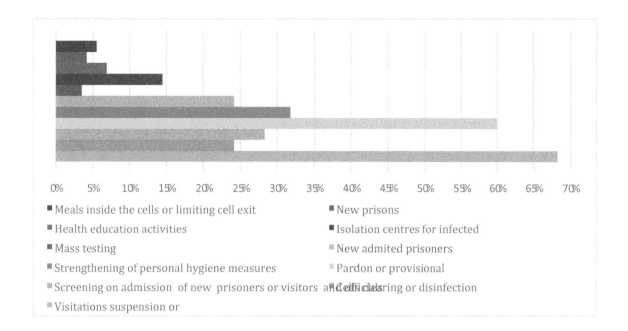

- Meals inside the cells or limiting cell exit
- Health education activities
- Mass testing
- Strengthening of personal hygiene measures
- Screening on admission of new prisoners or visitors and officials
- Visitations suspension or
- New prisons
- Isolation centres for infected
- New admited prisoners
- Pardon or provisional
- Cells clearing or disinfection

CHAPTER 20

MITIGATING COVID-19

1. Fast Deployment of COVID-19 Disinfectant From Common Ethanol of Gas Stations In Brazil

RodneyItiki1 Prithwiraj Roy Chowdhury

Department of Electrical and Computer Engineering, University of North Carolina at Charlotte, 9201 University City Blvd, Charlotte, NC28223-0001, United States

ABSTRACT

Objectives: Coronavirus COVID-19 is spreading very fast in Brazil, requiring innovative strategies for the fast deployment of disinfectants. Panic in population triggered by COVID-19 has caused a shortage of alcohol-based hand sanitizers and disinfectants in many cities of Brazil. Despite the governmental reaction against the outbreak, a risk of shortage of disinfectants still exists. The objective of this research is to investigate an alternative method for the fast deployment of alcohol-based disinfectants to protect the population against COVID-19.**Methods and Results**: This research highlights the feasibility of disinfectant production from common ethanol available in Brazilian gas stations, as a last resort. A four-by-one (4:1) ratio of common alcohol diluted in water meets the minimum requirements set by health agencies for the alcoholic concentration of disinfectants. Risks factors on alcohol dilution process are associated with corresponding measures of risk mitigation for public health and safety. Conclusions and Perspectives: This research proposes a process for the production and deployment of ethanol-based disinfectant from gas stations. However, the implementation is not timely possible for the COVID-19 pandemic due to complexities in the productive process. For the post-COVID-19 period, the authors give three perspectives: (a) future investigation of human dermal toxicity of common ethanol, (b) establishment of a program for the ethanol decontamination, and (c) countries such as the US, Sweden, Thailand, and Colombia to rethink their energy policy for the adoption of biofuel E100 (ethanol and water) instead of E85 (blend of ethanol, gasoline, and water), as part of their biodefense strategy.

INTRODUCTION

The first steps to contain the outbreak of COVID-19 in Brazil started during the first semester of 2020. Many health organizations instruct the public to wash hands with soap and water or making use of hand sanitizers with alcohol content [1], [2], [3], [4]. Alcohol-based hand sanitizers are helpful in reducing the frequency of illness [5,6]. However, a panic of the public due to the coronavirus outbreak, reported in the news, caused a shortage of alcohol-based hand sanitizers in Brazil. The COVID-19 outbreak is spreading globally, including Latin America [7], [8], [9]. The author of this paper takes an out-of-box perspective of the COVID-19 pandemic by proposing a process for the shortage of alcohol-based disinfectants in Brazil as last resort solution for the scarcity of COVID-19 disinfectants, presenting the timeline of facts of regulatory agency decisions concerning alcohol in parallel with the fast speed of COVID-19 outbreak in Brazil, and define health and safety policy for alcohol-based disinfectant deployment as a last resort.

A Brief Overview of The Infrastructure For Ethanol-Fuel Distribution In Brazil

In 1975, the Brazilian federal government introduced the National Alcohol Program (Proalcool) to increment the consumption of ethanol by mixing it with gasoline to propel common gasoline vehicles [10,11]. In the period of 1979 to 1985, during the second oil shock, the Proalcool program incentivized the construction of alcohol distilleries. The automotive sector, at the same time, focused on the manufacturing of cars powered exclusively by ethanol [12].In 2018, the total production of ethanol was 33.1 million of cubicle meters, being 23.7 million of hydrous ethanol [13]. Decades of experience in the production, storage, and distribution of ethanol for vehicles have also led to a currently vast and well-established infrastructure of gas stations throughout Brazilian territory [13]. In 2018, the total number of gas stations in Brazil was 40,021 [13]. Most of the gas stations in Brazil are currently equipped with fuel dispensers to pump ethanol fuel into vehicles [13]. Despite the vast availability of ethanol in gas stations in Brazil, only one type of ethanol-based product has a potential for the production of COVID-19 disinfectant. Table 1 summarizes ethanol-based fuels commercialized in Brazil and specifications according to material safety data sheets [14], [15], [16], [17].

Table 1. Comparison between Common Ethanol, Additive Ethanol, E85,

Usual name	Common Ethanol (E100)	Hydrous Ethanol with additive	Anhydrous alcohol with gasoline
Synonyms	Ethyl Alcohol without additive, or Reference Hydrous Ethanol	Ethyl Alcohol with additive	Ethyl Alcohol with gasoline (E85)
Chemical Composition	Ethyl Alcohol (92.6 – 93.8% min. 94.6% max) Water (remaining) Gasoline trace (30 mL/L max.)	Ethanol (92.6 – 93.8 %) Water (6.2 – 7.4 %) Additive (0.03-0.06% m)	Anhydrous alcohol (85%) Gasoline (15%)
COVID-19 disinfection application	Under consideration in this research	Not appropriate for COVID-19 disinfection due to harmful additive	Not appropriate for COVID-19 disinfection due to high content of gasoline
Carcinogenicity	Not expected in the product	Additive (category 2)	Not considered carcinogenic for humans, according to the International Agency for Research on Cancer. (IARC).
Material Safety Data Sheet	[14,15]	[16]	[17]

Common ethanol shows potential for use as COVID-19 disinfectant due to the absence of additive and gasoline. However, the concentration of ethyl alcohol is above 92.6%. This concentration is not usual in the common practice of disinfection in the technical literature [18,19]. An adjustment of concentration would turn common ethanol into a regular and effective disinfectant to COVID-19.

The infrastructure for ethanol distribution in other countries of the world

The three largest ethanol-producing countries are the US (56%), Brazil (28%), and the European Union (5%) [20]. Most of the ethanol refineries in the US are in the Mid-West region [20]. The US has around 4,500 gas stations offering E85 and other flex fuels [20]. The American flex vehicle runs with a seasonal-dependent blend of ethanol and gasoline [20]. Gas stations pump two types of mixture: E85 Summer (74% ethanol and 26% gasoline) and E85 Winter (82% of ethanol and 18% gasoline) [21]. E85, despite the existing distribution infrastructure, cannot be used as a disinfectant.

In Europe, Sweden is the leading country in the ethanol-fuel consumption with 1,695 gas stations for E85 [22]. Ethanol fuel E85 (approximately 85% ethanol and 15% gasoline) and E70 Winter (70% of ethanol and 30% gasoline) are commercially available [23].

Ethanol fuel ED95 (approximately 84.36% ethanol, 4.44% water, and 11.20% additive) are used in trucks and buses in Sweden [22,24]. An alternative ethanol fuel called 5%GE (approximately 89.3% ethanol, 4.75% water, 0.95% Lauric acid, and 5% Glycerol ethoxylate) is being investigated in the technical literature [24]. Due to the presence of gasoline or additive, despite the existing infrastructure of gas stations in Sweden, E85 and ED95 fuel cannot be used as a disinfectant.

India, Thailand, Colombia, Mexico, Australia, and Guatemala cultivates approximately 32% of the world's sugarcane crop, a raw material for ethanol and sugar production. In India, despite the great potential for ethanol production, a huge demand by its internal market make unfeasible, in the short term (2020), the blending of ethanol in the gasoline for concentration above E50 [25]. During the COVID-19 pandemic, India implemented repurposing of the existing industrial capacity of private liquor companies for the production of ethanol-based sanitizers. However, such repurposing was unlikely quick enough because the supply chains become affected in the pandemic [26,27]. Similarly, repurposing of breweries for ethanol-based sanitizers has proceeded in the US, Canada, European Union, and the United Kingdom [28].

Thailand is expanding the utilization of ethanol fuel E85 for transportation [29]. Colombia is planning to introduce E85 in its markets in 2030 [30,31]. The literature review shows that some countries, such as the US, Sweden, Thailand, and Colombia, have the infrastructure and plans for the production and distribution of ethanol fuel E85. One of the significant barriers for E100 distribution infrastructure was that a flex-vehicle required a small independent tank for the injection of gasoline into the motor engine during the start of a vehicle on E100 [32]. A new technology of injectors provides preheating of the E100 for the cold start of the vehicle, allowing start without gasoline injection system [32]. Such new technology opens new opportunities for the widespread adoption of ethanol fuel E100 in these countries.

Method For Adjustment Of Ethanol Concentration For Usage As COVID-19 Disinfectant

Health agencies around the world diverge on the minimum ethyl alcohol concentration. Brazilian Federal Ministry of Health recommends the same as the World Health Organization, i.e., 70% concentration of ethyl alcohol [4].

Table 2. Different Recommendations of Health Agencies For Alcohol Concentration

Health Agencies	Recommendations in March 2020	Recommendations after March 2020
Centresfor Disease Control and Prevention (CDC)	Minimum 60% ethanol or minimum 70% isopropanol [3]	hand sanitizers with 60% to 95% alcohol [33]
World Health Organization (WHO)	At least 60% alcohol-based hand sanitizers, or 70% for small objects [1,2]	After May 15, 2020, proceed surface cleaning followed by 70% - 90% ethanol [34]
Brazilian Federal Ministry of Health	It may (not must) be 70% alcohol concentration [4]	It may (not must) be 70% alcohol concentration [4]
Brazilian Federal Counsel of Chemistry	minimum 60% and a maximum 80% are also effective, according to some studies. [35]	minimum 60% and a maximum 80% are also effective, according to some studies. [35]
ANVISA	It is illegal commercialization of liquid ethyl alcohol one-liter bottle for the public in supermarkets and drug stores if the concentration is above 54%, except for 70%.[36]	It is illegal commercialization of liquid ethyl alcohol one-liter bottle for the public in supermarkets and drug stores if the concentration is above 54%, except for 70%.[36]. After May 26, 2020, proceed cleaning with 70% alcohol or neutral detergent cleaning, followed by 60% to 90% alcohol [37].

Assuming that the alcohol-based disinfectant must meet the requirements of the Brazilian Federal Ministry of Health, the process of disinfectant production must result in a possible 70% of alcohol concentration [4]. This percentage number suggests that the ratio of 4:1 would closely meet the recommendations of the Brazilian Federal Ministry of Health, leading to a concentration calculation of:(1)Concentration(4:1dilution)=$4 \times 0.926/5 = 74.1\%$. According to the material safety data sheet (MSDS) of the common ethanol, there is a tolerance of 92.6 % to 94.6% in the composition of ethyl alcohol in the common ethanol product [14,15].The common ethanol can reach up to 94.6% maximum concentration due to tolerance of the productive process. In this case, the dilution process would result in 75.68% maximum concentration, assuming the evaporation of ethyl alcohol negligible in the dilution process.

RESULTS AND RISKS

The resulting concentration of the 4:1 dilution process is 74.1%. For ANVISA, commercialization of 74.1% ethanol for the public is illegal because it exceeds 70% [36]. However, 74.1% ethanol concentration is within the 60% - 90% range, also recommended by ANVISA for surface cleaning [37]. The 74.1% ethanol concentration is also within the 60% to 80% effective range of the Brazilian Federal Council of Chemistry [35]. It is also close to 78.2% and 80% ethanol concentration for disinfection reported in the technical literature [18,19,5]. In June 2020, a literature review shows that SARS-CoV-2 is efficiently inactivated by ethanol concentrations ranging from 60% to 95% (v/v) or from 70% and 91.3% (v/v) [38]. SARS-CoV-2, the pathogen of COVID-19 pandemic, is not a bacteria. Concentrations not exceeding 80% for high contact time necessary to achieve an efficient bactericidal activity are disregarded by the Federal Drugs Administration [38] A perspective for health and safety policy should include the mitigation of these risks because it is part of the strategy of pandemic fatalities minimization. However, the implementation of clinical trials for dermal toxicity and a perspective formulation of a health and safety policy for alcohol-based disinfectants is under the constraint of time, since the COVID-19 pandemic continues to spread at fast speed. A timeline of facts gives the context of challenges during a pandemic.

The 4:1 Dilution of Common Ethanol In Water For COVID-19 Disinfection Brings Some Risks For The Population

The handling of common ethanol by non-qualified public brings risks to their health and safety. Table 3 indicates some of them.

Table 3. Health and safety risks of common alcohol handling to the public

Risk classification	Description	Effect	Mitigation of risk
Health	Public buying inappropriate type of ethanol, for example, ethanol with additive or with gasoline	Inhalation of additive or gasoline	Adequate training of gas station personnel to make the consumer buy the appropriate product (common ethanol).
Health	Inadequate handling of common ethanol during pumping or dilution	Inhalation of alcohol	Adequate training of gas station personnel to pump common ethanol in certified fuel canister and leaving space in it for water addition for alcohol dilution.
Health	Possibility of the presence of a maximum 0.5% of methanol in the common ethanol composition, even though officially prohibited by the Brazilian Petroleum Agency [39]	Skin irritation	Clinical trials for dermal toxicity are needed.
Safety	Blending of common ethanol in unsafe ventilation conditions	Explosion or fire during the dilution process of a flammable material	Water filling prior to the pumping of common ethanol to the certified can.
Safety	Over usage of alcohol-based disinfectant on large areas [40]	Formation of an explosive atmosphere classified area [14].	Adequate instruction to the public not to spread the disinfectant on a large scale in poorly ventilated areas.

The Timeline of Facts Concerning COVID-19 And Regulatory Agencies In Brazil

ANVISA, the Brazilian federal agency for health surveillance, is in charge of decisions concerning public health in Brazil. In March 17, 2020, ANVISA issued the Resolution 347, allowing compounding pharmacies to prepare and commercialize six types of alcohol-based products: (a) ethyl alcohol 70% in 50 ml bottles for non-institutional customer, (b) glycerinated ethyl alcohol 80% in 50 ml bottles for non-institutional customer, (c) gel alcohol, (d) glycerinated isopropyl alcohol 75% in 50 ml bottles for non-institutional customer, (e) hydrogen peroxide in 10 volume, and (f) chlorhexidine digluconate 0.5% [41].On March 17, 2020, the total number of COVID-19 cases confirmed in Brazil was 234 [42].

Despite helping to improve the supply of COVID-19 disinfectants and antiseptics, it is questionable if such measures are too late and too short against the fast COVID-19 outbreak. The compound pharmacies in Brazil, after the ANVISA resolution, still have to start up the production process to make 70% alcohol available to the customers. The progression of the COVID-19 outbreak over time is a constraint to the success of all levels of public governance to minimize the impact on the health system. Some aspects of the ANVISA resolution 347 [41], particularly to the ethyl alcohol 70% in 50 ml bottles, seem in harsh contrast to products available in online sales in the US.

Table 4 Shows The Differences In Bottle Volume.

Table 4. Alcohol sale advertised to the public in the US, in March 2020

Online sale	Product	Bottle volume
Amazon.com (USA)	Laboratory-Grade Denatured Ethyl Alcohol, 95%, 500mL - The Curated Chemical Collection - Not for Use on Body or Skin	500 ml
Amazon.com (USA)	Laboratory-Grade Denatured Ethyl Alcohol, 95%, 1L The Curated Chemical Collection	1000 ml
Amazon.com (USA)	Blending of common ethanol in unsafe ventilation cond Amazon Brand - Solimo 70% Ethyl Rubbing Alcohol First Aid Antiseptic, 16 Fluid Ounces (Pack of 12)	473 ml
Amazon.com (USA)	Denatured Alcohol 200-1 Gallon (128 oz.)	3,785 ml

ANVISA established the prohibition of liquid alcohol with more than 54% concentration for sale to non-institutional customers in 2002. The ban on liquid alcohol resulted in a sharp decrease of 60% in the occurrence of burnings caused by flammable ethanol [43].
However, the supply of alcohol for the public seems to be at the highest priority during a pandemic. On March 21, 2020, the ANVISA resolution gave 180 days of permission for commercialization of 70% liquid ethanol produced by industries in bottles of one liter [36]. Even with the recently

approved regulation, a delay is expected from the beginning of the alcohol production process to the actual availability of bottles in the supermarket shelves.

In a race against time, the number of confirmed cases of COVID-19 in Brazil on March 21 reached 904 [44]. On April 23, and May 26, 2020, ANVISA published alternatives for ethanol-based disinfectants [45,37]. Table 5 summarizes the ANVISA recommendations for disinfectants of surfaces and objects for COVID-19. ANVISA informed that the virus is inactivated by alcohol 70% and chlorine [37].

Table 5. ANVISA Recommendations For The Disinfection Of Surfaces And Objects.

April 23, 2020 [45]	May 26, 2020 [37]
Ethanol 70%	Neutral detergent cleaning followed by alcohol: 60% to 90% in water solution v/v
Sodium hypochlorite at 0.5%	Neutral detergent cleaning followed by inorganic active chlorine-releasing compounds (e.g., sodium, calcium and lithium hypochlorites): 0.02% to 1.0%;
Bleaches containing hypochlorite (sodium, calcium) at 2-3.9%	Neutral detergent cleaning followed by inorganic active chlorine-releasing compounds (e.g., sodium, calcium and lithium hypochlorites): 0.02% to 1.0%;
Iodinepovidone (1%)	-
Hydrogen peroxide 0.5%	-
Peracetic acid 0.5%	Neutral detergent cleaning followed by peracetic acid: 0.5% (note: can be used in combination with hydrogen peroxide);
Quaternary ammonium, e.g. Benzalkonium Chloride 0.05%	Neutral detergent cleaning followed by quaternary ammonium: from 1000 to 5000 ppm;
Phenolic compounds	-
Disinfectants commonly used with virucidal action.	-
-	Neutral detergent cleaning followed by organic active chlorine-releasing compounds (e.g. dichloroisocyanuric acids - DCCA and trichloroisocyanuric - TCCA: 1.9% to 6.0%;
-	Neutral detergent cleaning followed by potassium monopersulfate: 1%;
-	Glucoprotamine: 0.5 to 1%;
-	Polymeric biguanide (PHMB): as recommended by the manufacturer.

On April 23, 2020, Brazil reported 43,079 confirmed cases and 2,741 deaths by COVID-19; on May 26, 2020, 363,211 confirmed cases and 22,666 deaths [46,47]. On May 19, 2020, the Brazilian National Oil Regulatory Agency published a technical note not recommending the use of common ethanol from gas stations as COVID-19 disinfectant due to the risk of contamination by toxic products, such as methanol, gasoline, diesel during the production, transportation, and storage process.

Additionally, the common ethanol may have traces of organic salts based on sulphur, iron, sodium, and potassium, whose ingestion or contact with skin and mucous membranes is harmful to health [48].On May 19, 2020, Brazil reported 241,080 confirmed cases and 16,118 deaths by COVID-19 [49].

DISCUSSIONS

Soap and water cleaning is recommended by most health organization guidelines [1], [2], [3], [4]. However, not all people in the world has an abundant supply of clean water, paper towel, and washing stations. People living in precarious shelters (slums) may not have adequate sanitary installations. Sharing cloth towels can facilitate virus spreading. Washing stations with automatic water faucet and motorized dispensers for contactless paper towel release are not commonplace in the developing countries. Soap cleaning may require scrub sponge for rinsing and rubbing, gloves for hand protection, and more paper for drying. Water spill over during the cleaning may cause mould proliferation. On the other hand, ethanol spares water, sponge, and a large quantity of paper towel supply because it mostly self-dissipate from the surface by volatility and evaporation.

It may not be just a matter of convenience but the only practical solution for the most impoverished strata of the society. Also, ethanol from gas stations is available in an outdoor environment, as opposed to soap, sponge, gloves, and paper towels, which usually are in indoor sales point, exposing consumers to community spread of COVID-19.The COVID-19 pandemic caused an extra peak demand for all types of personal protective equipment and cleaning products [26]. Panic about the unknown life threat caused widespread hoarding disorder.

The consumer may not have a choice between soap and accessories (water, sponge, paper towel) or ethanol-based disinfectant since all types of cleaning products become scarce in the sales points during a pandemic. This research aims at an alternative method for peak extra-supply of ethanol-based disinfectant. The last resort strategy happens when it is better to choose a non-perfect but acceptable alternative than doing nothing.

An example of last resort strategy is exemplified by the CDC decision for optimization of supply of facemasks for health care professionals (HCP) under crisis management [26]. Unavailability of facemasks urges CDC to recommend HCP to use homemade masks (e.g., bandana, scarf) for the care of patients with COVID-19 as a last resort [50].The COVID-19 pandemic caused a fast shortage of personal protective equipment [26,51]. The disinfectant supply suffered the same shortcomings. However, the ethanol fuel E100 currently has risks of toxic contaminants, according to the Brazilian National Oil Regulatory Agency [48].The risk of toxic methanol in the common ethanol composition is easily eliminated by thorough quality auditing on gas stations by the Brazilian Oil Regulatory Agency, and proper punishment for violation of conformity. The Brazilian Oil Regulatory Agency prohibits the addition of methanol on fuel since 2018 [39]. The assessment of compliance of ethanol fuel in gas stations is monthly reported by the Brazilian Oil Regulatory Agency [52]. Very few cases of methanol in E100 fuel were reported in recent months.

In May 2020, for instance, just one non-conformity related to methanol content exceeding 0.5% was detected out of 1,558 samples from different gas stations in Brazil [52]. The elimination of other contaminants, described by Talita and colleagues in [21], may require major intervention on the production process, which would not be timely possible in this COVID-19 pandemic.

CONCLUSIONS AND PERSPECTIVES

The author of this paper proposes a process for the production of 74.1% alcohol-based disinfectant obtained by a 4:1 ratio dilution of common ethanol of gas stations in Brazil in water. However, the proposal is not timely possible due to the complexities of the ethanol production, transportation, and storage process. It seems unfeasible in a short period to eliminate all risks of toxicity from contaminants pointed out by the Brazilian Oil Regulatory Agency. For this reason, three relevant perspective recommendations emerge from the post-COVID-19 period.

Firstly, the scientific community is urged to investigate the human toxicity potential by dermal exposure to the ethanol fuel E100 from gas stations. The National Regulatory Oil Agency are urged to investigate the risks, challenges, and the economic feasibility of improving the quality of ethanol fuel E100 within the parameters of acceptable dermal toxicity. Secondly, the fast deployment of ethanol-based disinfectants from gas stations may be one course of action of a national biodefense strategy against pandemics and biological attacks.

A program for decontamination of ethanol E100, if proved technically and economically feasible, should involve the participation of the health regulatory agency, and the oil regulatory agency, in the context of a national biodefense strategy. Finally, the perspective of future pandemics like COVID-19 or biological war can make other governments in the world to rethink about ethanol fuel E100 as a new standard for dual-use fuel, instead of E85. Countries like the US, Sweden, Thailand, and possibly in Colombia, major ethanol consumers or producers, may improve their biodefense strategy by adopting the ethanol E100 as their biofuel standard.

REFERENCES

[1] World Health Organization, Key Messages and Actions for COVID-19 Prevention and Control in Schools. March; 2020, Geneva, Switzerland. https://www.who.int/docs/default-source/coronaviruse/key-messages-andactions-for-COVID-19-prevention-and-control-in-schools-march-2020.pdf?sfvrsn=baf81d52_4 (accessed on Mar 23, 2020).

[2] World Health Organization, Infection prevention and control during health care when novel coronavirus (nCoV) infection is suspected, Interim guidance 19 March; 2020, Geneva, Switzerland. https://www.who.int/publicationsdetail/infection-prevention-and-control-during-health-care-when-novel-coronavirus-(ncov)-infection-is-suspected20200125 (accessed on Mar 23, 2020).

[3] Centres for Disease Control and Prevention, CDC Statement for Healthcare Personnel on Hand Hygiene during the Response to the International Emergence of COVID-19; 2020, USA. https://www.cdc.gov/coronavirus/2019-ncov/infection-control/hcp-hand-sanitizer.html (accessed Mar 23, 2020).

[4] Adriana MT, Marcelo OB, Francisco AF, Protocolo de tratamento do novo coronavirus (2019-nCoV). Brazilian Ministry of Health; 2020. https://portalarquivos2.saude.gov.br/images/pdf/2020/fevereiro/05/Protocolo-de-manejoclinico-para-o-novo-coronavirus-2019-ncov.pdf (accessed on Mar 23, 2020).

[5] Nils-Olaf H, Claudia H, Michael W, Günter K, Axel K, Effectiveness of alcohol-based hand disinfectants in a public administration: Impact on health and work performance related to acute respiratory symptoms and diarrhoea.BMC Infectious Diseases, 10, 250; 2010. DOI: 10.1186/1471-2334-10-250.

[6] Chris L, Nikunj M, Beryl O, Jim G, Washing our hands of the problem. J. Hosp. Infect.; Vol. 104, Issue 4, 2020, pp. 401-403, 2020. https://www.sciencedirect.com/science/article/pii/S0195670120301092.

[7] Amy M, The race to unravel the biggest coronavirus outbreak in the United States. Nature 579; 2020, 181-182, doi: 10.1038/d41586-020-00676-3.

[8] Alfonso JRM, Jaime ACO, Estefanía GO et al., Clinical, laboratory and imaging features of COVID-19: A systematic review and meta-analysis. Travel Med. Infect. Di., 101623, 2020. https://doi.org/10.1016/j.tmaid.2020.101623.

[9] Cristian B, Patricia A, Susana L et al, The next big threat to global health? 2019 novel coronavirus (2019-nCoV): What advice can we give to travellers? Interim recommendations January 2020, from the Latin-American society for Travel Medicine (SLAMVI), Travel Med. Infect. Di., 33; 2020, 101567, https://doi.org/10.1016/j.tmaid.2020.101567.

[10] Jose APO, The policymaking process for creating competitive assets for the use of biomass energy: the Brazilian alcohol programme. Renew. Sust. Energ. Rev., 6, Issues 1–2; 2002, pp. 129-140. https://doi.org/10.1016/S1364-0321(01)00014-4.

[11] João L, Maria SMA, Christiano PC et al.; Analyses and perspectives for Brazilian low carbon technological development in the energy sector. Renew. Sust. Energ. Rev., 15, Issue 7; 2011, pp. 3432-3444, ISSN 1364-0321,https://doi.org/10.1016/j.rser.2011.04.022.

[12] Julieta APR, Sonia SPM, Ildo LS, Genesis and consolidation of the Brazilian bioethanol: A review of policies and incentive mechanisms. Renew. Sust. Energ. Rev., 14, Issue 7; 2010, pp. 1874-1887, https://doi.org/10.1016/j.rser.2010.03.041.

[13] Ministry of Mining and Energy of the Brazilian National Agency of Petroleum; Anuario Estatistico Brasileiro do Petroleo, Gas Natural e Biocombustiveis 2019. Brazil, ISSN 1983-5884; 2019. http://www.anp.gov.br/arquivos/central-conteudos/anuario-estatistico/2019/2019-anuario-versao-impressao.pdf (accessed on Mar 23, 2020).

[14] Petrobras, Ficha de Informações de Segurança de Produto Químico – FISPQ – Etanol Hidratado Combustivel EHC. 2020, Brazil. http://www.br.com.br/wcm/connect/6fad4419-69ca-47f1-aabb-b507d1980d19/fispq-combetanol-etanol-hidratado-combustivelehc.pdf?MOD=AJPERES&CVID=mKJNQFV (accessed on Mar 23, 2020).

[15] Brazilian National Agency of Petroleum, Natural Gas and Biofuel, Resolution ANP number 764. Official Diary of the Union, Dec 21; 2018, Brazil. http://legislacao.anp.gov.br/?path=legislacao-anp/resolanp/2018/dezembro&item=ranp-764-2018 (accessed on Mar 23, 2020).

[16] Petrobras, Ficha de Informações de Segurança de Produto Químico – FISPQ – Etanol Hidratado Aditivado Petrobras Grid. 2020, Brazil. http://www.br.com.br/wcm/connect/91bd4b12-3841-4845-9bcc-9f2ab21eac4d/fispqcomb-etanol-ehc-petrobrasgrid.pdf?MOD=AJPERES&CVID=mN9MYKR&CVID=mN9MYKR&CVID=mN9MYKR&CVID=mN9MYKR&CVID=mN9MYKR&CVID=mN9MYKR&CVID=mN9MYKR&CVID=mN9MYKR&CVID=mN9MYKR&CVID=mN9MYKR&CVID=mN9MYKR&CVID=mN9MYKR&CVID=mN9MYKR (accessed Mar 23, 2020).

[17] Petrobras, Ficha de Informações de Segurança de Produto Químico – FISPQ – Etanol E85. ; 2020, Brazil. http://www.br.com.br/wcm/connect/0a074cd5-abb8-4700-a6c6-dc5698b1a613/fispq-comb-etanol-etanole85.pdf?MOD=AJPERES&CVID=mKJNteK&CVID=mKJNteK&CVID=mKJNteK&CVID=mKJNteK&CVID=mKJNteK&CVID=mKJNteK&CVID=mKJNteK&CVID=mKJNteK&CVID=mKJNteK&CVID=mKJNteK&CVID=mKJNteK&CVID=mKJNteK&CVID=mKJNteK (accessed on Mar 23, 2020).

[18] Suchomel M, Gnant G,Weinlich M, Rotter M, Surgical hand disinfection using alcohol: the effects of alcohol type, mode and duration of application. J. Hosp. Infect., 71, Issue 3; 2009, pp. 228-233, https://doi.org/10.1016/j.jhin.2008.11.006.

[19] Nils-Olaf H, Günter K, Harald L, Axel K, Effect of a 1 min hand wash on the bactericidal efficacy of consecutive surgical hand disinfection with standard alcohols and on skin hydration. Int. J. Hyg. Envir. Heal.,, 209, Issue 3; 2006, Pages 285-291. https://doi.org/10.1016/j.ijheh.2006.01.002.

[20] Renewable Fuels Association, 2019 Ethanol Industry Outlook - Power with Renewable Energy, RFA, 2019, pp.1-36. https://ethanolrfa.org/wp-content/uploads/2019/02/RFA2019Outlook.pdf. (accessed on Jun 23, 2020).

[21] Talita Dias da Silva et al., Secondary particles formed from the exhaust of vehicles using ethanol-gasoline blends increase the production of pulmonary and cardiac reactive oxygen species and induce pulmonary inflammation, Environmental Research, Volume 177, 2019, 108661. https://doi.org/10.1016/j.envres.2019.108661.

[22] André Månsson, Alessandro Sanches-Pereira, Sebastian Hermann, Biofuels for road transport: Analysing evolving supply chains in Sweden from an energy security perspective, Applied Energy, Vol. 123, 2014, pp. 349-357, https://doi.org/10.1016/j.apenergy.2014.01.098.

[23] Trifa M. Ahmed, Christoffer Bergvall, Roger Westerholm, Emissions of particulate associated oxygenated and native polycyclic aromatic hydrocarbons from vehicles powered by ethanol/gasoline fuel blends, Fuel, Vol. 214,2018, pp. 381-385, https://doi.org/10.1016/j.fuel.2017.11.059.

[24] R. Munsin, Y. Laoonual, S. Jugjai, M. Matsuki, H. Kosaka, Effect of glycerol ethoxylate as an ignition improveron injection and combustion characteristics of hydrous ethanol under CI engine condition, Energy Conversion and Management, Vol. 98, 2015, pp. 282-289, https://doi.org/10.1016/j.enconman.2015.03.116.

[25] P. Sakthivel, K.A. Subramanian, Reji Mathai, Indian scenario of ethanol fuel and its utilization in automotive transportation sector, Resources, Conservation and Recycling, Vol. 132, 2018, pp. 102-120, https://doi.org/10.1016/j.resconrec.2018.01.012.

[26] Sudip Bhattacharya, Md Mahbub Hossain, Amarjeet Singh, Addressing the shortage of personal protective equipment during the COVID-19 pandemic in India-A public health perspective, AIMS Public Health, 2020, 7(2), pp. 223-227. http://dx.doi.org/10.3934/publichealth.2020019

[27] Rajvikram Madurai Elavarasan, Rishi Pugazhendhi, Restructured society and environment: A review on potential technological strategies to control the COVID-19 pandemic, Science of The Total Environment, Vol. 725, 2020, 138858, https://doi.org/10.1016/j.scitotenv.2020.138858.

[28] Euan L. Thomson, Andrew R. Bullied, Production of Ethanol- Based Hand Sanitizer in Breweries During the COVID- 19 Crisis, MBAA TQ, vol. 57, no. 1, 2020, pp. 47–52. https://www.mbaa.com/publications/tq/tqPastIssues/2020/PublishingImages/TQ%E2%80%9057%E2%80%901%E2%80%900417%E2%80%9001.pdf

[29] Juan Arturo Castañeda-Ayarza, Luis Augusto Barbosa Cortez, Final and B molasses for fuel ethanol production and some market implications, Renewable and Sustainable Energy Reviews, Vol. 70, 2017, pp. 1059-1065, https://doi.org/10.1016/j.rser.2016.12.010.

[30] Miguel Angel Gonzalez-Salazar, Mauro Venturini, Witold-Roger Poganietz, Matthias Finkenrath, Manoel Regis L.V. Leal, Combining an accelerated deployment of bioenergy and land use strategies: Review and insights for a post-conflict scenario in Colombia, Renewable and Sustainable Energy Reviews, Vol. 73, 2017, pp. 159-177,https://doi.org/10.1016/j.rser.2017.01.082.

[31] Miguel Angel Gonzalez-Salazar et al., Development of a technology roadmap for bioenergy exploitation including biofuels, waste-to-energy and power generation & CHP, Applied Energy, Vol. 180, 2016, pp. 338-352,https://doi.org/10.1016/j.apenergy.2016.07.120.

[32] R.J. Pearson, J.W.G. Turner, 3 - Using alternative and renewable liquid fuels to improve the environmental performance of internal combustion engines: key challenges and blending technologies, Editor(s): Richard Folkson, Alternative Fuels and Advanced Vehicle Technologies for Improved Environmental Performance, WoodheadPublishing, 2014, pp. 52-89, https://doi.org/10.1533/9780857097422.1.52.

[33] Centres for Disease Control and Prevention, Interim Infection Prevention and Control Recommendations for Healthcare Personnel During the Coronavirus Disease 2019 (COVID-19) Pandemic, Update June 19, 2020, USA. https://www.cdc.gov/coronavirus/2019-ncov/hcp/infection-controlrecommendations.html?CDC_AA_refVal=https%3A%2F%2Fwww.cdc.gov%2Fcoronavirus%2F2019-ncov%2Finfection-control%2Fcontrol-recommendations.html (accessed on Jun 23, 2020).

[34] World Health Organization, Cleaning and disinfection of environmental surfaces in the context of COVID-19,May 2020, pp.1 – 8, Geneva, Switzerland. https://www.who.int/publications/i/item/cleaning-and-disinfection-ofenvironmental-surfaces-inthe-context-of-COVID-19 (accessed on Jun 23, 2020)

[35] Conselho Federal de Quimica, Nota Oficial (atualizada) esclarecimentos sobre álcool gel caseiro, limpeza deeletrônicos e outros. March 18; 2020, Brazil. http://cfq.org.br/noticia/nota-oficial-esclarecimentos-sobre-alcool-gelcaseiro-higienizacao-de-eletronicos-e-outros/(accessed on Mar 23, 2020).

[36] ANVISA, Nota da Anvisa sobre álcool líquido 70%. March 21; 2020, Brazil. http://portal.anvisa.gov.br/en_US/noticias/-/asset_publisher/FXrpx9qY7FbU/content/nota-da-anvisa-sobre-alcoolliquido-70/219201?inheritRedirect=false&redirect=http%3A%2F%2Fportal.anvisa.gov.br%2Fen_US%2Fnoticias%3Fp_p_id%3D101_INSTANCE_FXrpx9qY7FbU%26p_p_lifecycle%3D0%26p_p_state%3Dnormal%26p_p_mode%3Dview%26p_p_col_id%3Dcolumn-2%26p_p_col_count%3D1 (accessed on Mar 23, 2020).

[36] ANVISA, Perguntas & Respostas, 4º ed., Brasília, May 26, 2020, http://portal.anvisa.gov.br/documents/219201/4340788/Perguntas+e+Respostas+GGTES.pdf/7fce6e91-cf99-4ec2-9d20-1fb84b5a6c38 (accessed on Jun 23, 2020)

[37] Alberto Berardi et al., Hand sanitisers amid COVID-19: A critical review of alcohol-based products on the market and formulation approaches to respond to increasing demand, International Journal of Pharmaceutics, Vol.584, 2020, 119431. https://doi.org/10.1016/j.ijpharm.2020.119431.

[38] Agencia Nacional do Petroleo, Gas Natural e Biocombustiveis, Resolution ANP number 740 of August 15,2018. Union Official Diary, 2018, Brazil. http://legislacao.anp.gov.br/?path=legislacao-anp/resolanp/2018/agosto&item=ranp-740-2018 (accessed on Mar 23, 2020).

[39] Yonghong X, Mili ET, Taking the right measures to control COVID-19. The Lancet Infectious Diseases; 2020.https://doi.org/10.1016/S1473-3099(20)30152-3.

[40] ANVISA, Resolution of the Collegiate Directory number 347 of March 17; 2020. Union Official Diary, Brazil. http://portal.anvisa.gov.br/documents/10181/5809525/%281%29RDC_347_2020_COMP.pdf/89527ffe-7cab-479a9e1a-944aaa661475 (accessed on Mar 23, 2020).

[41] World Health Organization, Coronavirus disease 2019 (COVID-19) Situation Report – 57. March 17, 2020, Geneva, Switzerland, https://www.who.int/docs/default-source/coronaviruse/situation-reports/20200317-sitrep-57-COVID-19.pdf?sfvrsn=a26922f2_4 (accessed on Mar 23, 2020).

[42] Tibola J, Barbosa E, Renck LI, Guimarães FSV, Kroeff MS, Pereima MJL, The liquid alcohol in Brazilian current context. Burns, 33, Issue 1, Supplement, pp. S19; 2007. https://doi.org/10.1016/j.burns.2006.10.048.

[44] World Health Organization, Coronavirus disease 2019 (COVID-19) Situation Report – 62 - Data as reported by national authorities by 21 March, 2020, Geneva, Switzerland; 2020. https://www.who.int/docs/defaultsource/coronaviruse/situation-reports/20200322-sitrep-62-COVID-19.pdf?sfvrsn=f7764c46_2 (accessed on Mar 23, 2020).

[45] ANVISA, Nota Técnica Nº 34/2020/SEI/COSAN/GHCOS/DIRE3/ANVISA, April 23, 2020, http://portal.anvisa.gov.br/documents/219201/4340788/SEI_ANVISA+-+0976782+-+Nota+T%C3%A9cnica.pdf/1cdd5e2f-fda1-4e55-aaa3-8de2d7bb447c

[46] World Health Organization, Coronavirus disease 2019 (COVID-19) Situation Report – 94, April 23; 2020, Geneva, Switzerland. https://www.who.int/docs/default-source/coronaviruse/situation-reports/20200423-sitrep-94-covid19.pdf?sfvrsn=b8304bf0_4 (accessed on Jun 23, 2020).

[47] World Health Organization, Coronavirus disease 2019 (COVID-19) Situation Report – 127, May 26; 2020, Geneva, Switzerland. https://www.who.int/docs/default-source/coronaviruse/situation-reports/20200526-COVID-19-sitrep-127.pdf?sfvrsn=7b6655ab_8 (accessed on Jun 23, 2020).

[48] Agencia Nacional do Petroleo, Gas Natural e Biocombustiveis, Coronavírus: riscos dos usos inadequados de etanol combustível, May 19, 2020. http://www.anp.gov.br/noticias/5768-coronavirus-riscos-dos-usos-inadequados-de-etanol-combustivel (accessed on Jun 23, 2020).

[49] World Health Organization, Coronavirus disease 2019 (COVID-19) Situation Report – 120, May 19; 2020, Geneva, Switzerland. https://www.who.int/docs/default-source/coronaviruse/situation-reports/20200519-COVID-19-sitrep-120.pdf?sfvrsn=515cabfb_4 (accessed on Jun 23, 2020).

[50] Centres for Disease Control and Prevention, Strategies for Optimizing the Supply of Facemasks. CDC; 2020, USA. https://www.cdc.gov/coronavirus/2019-ncov/hcp/ppe-strategy/face-masks.html (accessed on March 23, 2020).

[51] Donald RJ Singer, Health policy and technology challenges in responding to the COVID-19 pandemic, Health Policy and Technology, Volume 9, Issue 2, 2020, Pages 123-125, https://doi.org/10.1016/j.hlpt.2020.04.011.

[52] Agencia Nacional do Petroleo, Gas Natural e Biocombustiveis, Boletim de Monitoramento da Qualidade dos Combustíveis, May, 2020, http://www.anp.gov.br/publicacoes/boletins-anp/boletim-de-monitoramento-da-qualidadedos-combustiveis. (accessed on Jun 23, 2020).

TRANSMISSION OF COVID-19 AND MEASURES TO PREVENT ITS SPREAD

The term "virus" comes from Latin, understood as "poison" or "toxin". They are mostly 20-300 nm in diameter, have a genome consisting of one or more nucleic acid molecules (DNA or RNA), covered by a protein wrapper formed by one or more proteins, and by a complex envelope in a lipid bilayer.[2] Coronaviruses are enveloped positive-RNA viruses, and have a unique replication strategy, which makes it possible to vary their pathogenicity and ease of adaptation in different environments.[2] SARS-CoV-2 comes from a new strain identified in 2019 and, because it has not yet been isolated in humans, the measures to be implemented to face the pandemic are aimed at destroying the virus, preventing rapid transmission from person to person.[1-3]

SARS-CoV-2 transmission from person to person occurs through autoinoculation in mucous membranes (nose, eyes or mouth) and contact with contaminated inanimate surfaces, which has increasingly called attention to the need for rapid and preventive adoption of human protection measures to prevent contamination of persons.[5] For this reason, one of the most important measures for preventing transmission refers to hand hygiene, considered a low-cost and high-effectiveness measure, since hands are the main vehicle of cross-contamination.

Countless studies point to inadequate adoption of this practice among professionals during care for patients in health services.[5,11-13] Admittedly, the practice of hand hygiene by rubbing with water and soap reduces the occurrence of preventable infections, reducing morbidity and mortality in health services.[14-18] However, the complexity involved in complying with this measure is great, and can often be related to factors such as human behaviour, including false perceptions of an invisible risk, underestimation of individual responsibility and lack of knowledge, behaviours that can interfere with compliance with preventive measures.[16-18] People have emphasized compliance with this measure and its importance, but, in addition to the difficulties mentioned, some barriers that should not exist are still part of institutional realities, such as lack of sinks and supplies such as soap and water or even paper in public places that are characterized by high handling and contact of people, transit of escalators, toilets, buses, subways etc., as well as in communities without regular water and sewage supply.

Due to the potential of the virus to survive in the environment for several days, facilities and areas potentially contaminated with SARS-CoV-2 must be cleaned before being reused, with products containing antimicrobial agents known to be effective against coronaviruses.[13,17] Although there is a lack of specific evidence of its effectiveness against SARS-CoV-2, cleaning with water and household detergents and common disinfectant product use are considered sufficient for general household cleaning.[19-20] In hospital, several antimicrobial agents have been tested against different coronaviruses such as isopropanolol, povidone-iodine, ethanol, and sodium hypochlorite.[5,14]

Some of the active ingredients, for instance, sodium hypochlorite and ethanol, are widely available in non-medical and non-laboratory environments, which contributes to population access.[5,14] Evidence points out that surfaces that were cleaned with 70% alcohol had an expected disinfecting effect for two types of coronaviruses (mouse hepatitis virus and transmissible gastroenteritis virus) after one minute of contact, compared to 0.06% of sodium hypochlorite.[19] Tests carried out with SARS-CoV showed that sodium hypochlorite is effective at a concentration of 0.05% to 0.1% after five minutes when it is mixed with a solution containing SARS-CoV.[5,14] A study analysed surface stability of SARS-CoV-2, compared to SARS-CoV-1, the closest related human coronavirus.[5] The result of the experimental study is illustrated in Chart 1.

Chart 1 – Persistence of coronaviruses on inanimate surfaces.
Belo Horizonte, Minas Gerais, Brazil, 2020.

Type of surface	Persistence
Steel	48 hours
Metal	5 days
Paper	4-5 days
Glass	4 days
Plastic	< 5 days
Silicone rubber	5 days
Latex Glove	< 8 hours

Source: Adapted from Kampf et al.5

The results indicated that the virus can remain viable and infectious on surfaces from hours to days (depending on the inoculum), reinforcing the importance of hand hygiene after contact with inanimate environments and surfaces. This is most likely because the droplets of viruses that cause respiratory infections are expelled by coughing and sneezing, and a single droplet can easily contain an infectious dose. Furthermore, social distancing is also among the priorities of institutions to decrease transmission of SARS-CoV-2. Separation minimizes contact between potentially infected and healthy individuals, or between groups with high rates of transmission and or those with no or low levels, in order to delay the peak of the epidemic and lessen the magnitude of its effects, to protect assistance capacity clinic.[8] Isolation effectiveness depends on some epidemiological parameters, such as the number of secondary infections generated by each new infection and the proportion of transmissions that occur before the onset of symptoms.[14-15] These measures are justified due to the risk that asymptomatic people who remain in the community may infect others until their isolation, which makes it a challenge to control the pandemic. Based on this premise, Figure 1 shows the main public health measures to be adopted early to reduce the impact of the pandemic.

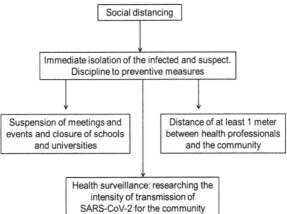

Figure 1 - Flowchart of measures to contain the circulation of the new coronavirus aiming at reducing the impact of the pandemic by COVID-19.[13] Belo Horizonte, Minas Gerais, Brazil, 2020.

A study that evaluated the case isolation effectiveness concerning COVID-19 control showed that isolation may be sufficient for its control over a period of three months, having been more effective when there was low transmission, before the onset of symptoms.[21] However, isolation, without adequate preventive measures, may be considered insufficient to control the outbreak. Thus, society/community, at this moment, is alerted to the importance of correct hand hygiene technique, mask use and surface hygiene measures that jointly prevent spread of the virus.[8,22]

Surgical mask use by patients reduces aerosol transmission, when in contact with suspected people of COVID-19 and with mild respiratory symptoms, since arrival at the health service, at the isolation site and during circulation within the service (transport from one area/sector to another), avoiding touching the mask, eyes, mouth and face as much as possible.[22-23]This measure can limit the spread of respiratory diseases, including the new coronavirus.

However, only mask use is insufficient to provide safe level of protection in isolation and should always be associated with those already referred to as hand hygiene, especially before and after using masks. It should also be remembered that wearing masks when not indicated can generate unnecessary costs and create a false sense of security, inducing negligence to other measures, such as hand hygiene and cleaning of inanimate surfaces potentially contaminated with SARS-CoV -2.[22-23]

For performing procedures in patients with suspected or confirmed infection with (SARS-CoV-2), which generates aerosols, such as procedures that induce cough, intubation or tracheal aspiration, invasive and non-invasive ventilation, cardiopulmonary resuscitation, manual ventilation before intubation, sputum induction, nasotracheal sample collections, healthcare professionals must use respiratory protection masks with minimum efficiency in the filtration of 95% of particles up to 0.3 μ (type N95, N99, N100, PFF2 or PFF3).[8,23]

Procedures that can generate aerosols should preferably be performed in a respiratory isolation unit with negative pressure and a Hepa filter (high efficiency particulate arrestance).

In the absence of this type of unit, patients should be placed in a room with closed doors (and open windows) and restrict the number of professionals during these procedures.[23]To use respirators or mask N95 or PFF2, it must be considered that the equipment must be properly adjusted to the face. How they are uses, handled and stored must follow the manufacturer's recommendations, also the accessory must never be shared among professionals.

The following checks of the components must be made before use, including strips and material of the nasal bridge, to ensure its fit and sealing: visually inspect the N95 mask to determine if its integrity has been compromised (damp, dirty, torn, dented or creased masks cannot be used). It is also important to note that the surgical mask should not be superimposed on the N95 mask or equivalent, as, in addition to not guaranteeing protection from filtration or contamination, it can also lead to the waste of another Personal Protective Equipment (PPE), which can be very damaging in this pandemic setting.[23]

Another relevant aspect is that exceptionally, in situations of lack of supplies and to meet the demand of the COVID-19 epidemic, the N95 mask or equivalent can be reused by the same professional, provided that mandatory steps are taken to remove the mask without contamination. inside. To minimize the contamination of the N95 mask or equivalent, if available, a face shield can be used. Also, if the mask is intact, clean and dry, it can be used several times during the same shift by the same professional (up to 12 hours or as defined by the Hospital Infection Control Commission - HICC - of the health service).[23] To remove the mask, the side elastics must first be removed, and the inner surface must not be touched. After removal, the mask must be packed in a paper bag or envelope with the elastics out, to facilitate the removal of the mask for new use. Plastic bag use, however, may contribute to the mask remaining moist and potentially contaminated. Another aspect to be highlighted is about its cleaning, after use, these cannot be cleaned or disinfected for later use and when wet they lose their filtration capacity.[23]

On the other hand, with the indication of mask use for health professionals, there was a rush to pharmacies to acquire these by the general population, which has generated a shortage for health services, in the care of patients with COVID-19. On April 2, 2020, the Ministry of Health of Brazil began to recommend the use of masks made of cotton, non-woven-textiles, among others, for the population in contact with suspects at home and that needs to go out to perform activities that may require contact with other people, so that masks act as a mechanical barrier.[24] However, attention must be paid to the other preventive measures already recommended, such as social distancing and keeping hands away from the eyes, nose and mouth, in addition to proper hand hygiene.

This indication is justified by the fact that the tissue mask can reduce the spread of the virus by asymptomatic or pre-symptomatic people who may be transmitting the virus without knowing it, but it does not protect the individual who is using it, as it has no filtering capacity of microorganisms. It should be noted that its use must be individual, and cannot be shared, and that, in health services, fabric masks should not be used under any circumstances, considering the provisions of Technical Note 4/2020, of the Brazilian National Surveillance Sanitary Agency (ANVISA – correspondent to US' FDA).[24] This measure favours the potential for contagion of people to happen, gradually, without the occurrence of a peak in the curve. Therefore, it contributes for the health system to be able to effectively care for those who are contaminated, with availability of equipment and personnel, without the overload found in the experience of other countries, due to the high number of infected in a short period of time.[4,11]

The other preventive and professional protection components must be aligned to the type of contact and procedure to be performed and to the vestment for assistance to the suspected patient/ carrier of COVID-19 and include the use of gloves, cloak/apron, goggles or protection facial, hat and apron.

The cloak or apron (minimum weight of 30 g/m^2) must be used to avoid contamination of the skin and clothing of professionals, who, after removal, needs to wash their hands.[23] Waterproof apron should be used to care for people suspected or infected by SARS-Cov-2.[23] Professionals should assess the need for the use of a waterproof coat or apron (minimum weight 50 g/m^2) depending on the patient's clinical condition (vomiting, diarrhoea, orotracheal hypersecretion, bleeding, etc.).

The cloak or apron must have long sleeves, a mesh or elastic cuff and a rear opening. In addition, it must be made of good quality material, non-toxic.[23] It is recommended that the impermeable cloak or apron, after use, be considered contaminated, and should be removed and discarded as an infectious residue after performing the patient's procedure with COVID-19 before leaving the isolation room.[8,23]

However, in a considerable part of places far from large centres in Brazil, the aprons available at the institutions are made of fabric, not disposable. In these cases, however, at this time of the pandemic, it is necessary that after use, it is sent immediately to the laundry, and its reuse is not recommended during new appointments. Contamination risk and spread may increase in the case of apron reuse, increasing the demand for beds destined to more serious cases and even removal of health professionals due to their contamination. As for the use of procedure gloves, they must also be discarded before professionals leave the isolation room of patients. In addition, long-barrelled rubber glove use should be implemented for support personnel, such as cleaning professionals.[23] Care and attention of all professionals is essential for the premise that glove use does not replace hand hygiene and that the areas around patients, infected or not, such as tables and bedside rails, are considered contaminated. The areas should not be touched with gloves, in order not to favour spread of the virus in the environment.

Thus, glove use inappropriately, especially in isolation sites with more than one patient with COVID-19, may cause cross-contamination among patients, favouring increased morbidity.

REFERENCES

1. World Health Organization. Statement on the second meeting of the International Health Regulations (2005) Emergency Committee regarding the outbreak of novel coronavirus (2019-nCoV) [Internet]. Geneva: World Health Organization; 2020 [cited 2020 Mar 27]. Available from: Available from: https://www.who.int/news-room/detail/30-01-2020-statement-on-the-second-meetingof-the-international-health-regulations-(2005)-emergency-committee-regarding-the-outbreak-of-novel-coronavirus-(2019-ncov)
» https://www.who.int/news-room/detail/30-01-2020-statement-on-the-second-meetingof-the-international-health-regulations-(2005)-emergency-committee-regarding-the-outbreak-of-novel-coronavirus-(2019-ncov)
2. Ministério da Saúde (BR). Portaria MS/GM n. 188, de 3 de fevereriro de 2020. Declara Emergência em Saúde Pública de importância Nacional (ESPIN) em decorrência da Infecção Humana pelo novo Coronavírus (2019-nCoV) [Internet]. Diário Oficial da União, Brasília (DF), 2020 fev 4 [citado 2020 mar 27]; Seção 1:1. Disponível em: Disponível em: http://www.in.gov.br/web/dou/-/portaria-n-188-de-3-de-fevereiro-de-2020-241408388
» http://www.in.gov.br/web/dou/-/portaria-n-188-de-3-de-fevereiro-de-2020-241408388
3. Croda JHR, Garcia LP. Resposta imediata da Vigilância em Saúde à epidemia da COVID-19. Epidemiol Serv Saúde [Internet]. 2020 [citado 2020 Mar 26];29(1):e2020002. Disponível em: Disponível em: https://doi.org/10.5123/s1679-49742020000100021
» https://doi.org/10.5123/s1679-49742020000100021
4. Anderson RM, Heesterbeek H, Hollingsworth TD. How will country-based mitigation measures influence the course of the COVID-19 epidemic? Lancet [Internet]. 2020 Mar [cited 2020 Mar 27];395(10228):931-4. Available from: Available from: https://doi.org/10.1016/S0140-6736(20)30567-5
» https://doi.org/10.1016/S0140-6736(20)30567-5
5. Qualls N, Levitt A, Kanade N, Wright-Jegede N, Dopson S, Biggerstaff M, et al. Community mitigation guidelines to prevent pandemic influenza - United States, 2017. MMWR Recomm Rep [Internet]. 2017 Apr [cited 2020 Mar 27];66(1):1-32. Available from: Available from: https://doi.org/10.15585/mmwr.rr6601a1
» https://doi.org/10.15585/mmwr.rr6601a1
6. Source: Adapted from: CDC. Interim pre-pandemic planning guidance: community strategy for pandemic influenza mitigation in the United States-early, targeted, layered use of nonpharmaceutical interventions. Atlanta, GA: US Department of Health and Human Services, CDC; 2007. https://stacks.cdc.gov/view/cdc/11425.» https://stacks.cdc.gov/view/cdc/11425
7. van Doremalen N, Bushmaker T, Morris DH, Holbrook MG, Gamble A, Williamson BN, et al. Aerosol and Surface Stability of SARS-CoV-2 as Compared with SARS-CoV-1. N Engl J Med [Internet]. 2020 Mar [cited 2020 Mar 27]. Available from: Available from: https://www.nejm.org/doi/full/10.1056/NEJMc2004973. » https://www.nejm.org/doi/full/10.1056/NEJMc2004973
8. Centre for Disease Control and Prevention (USA). Departamento f Health & Human Services. Interim pre-pandemic planning guidance: community strategy for pandemic influenza mitigation in the United States: early, targeted, layered use of nonpharmaceutical interventions [Internet]. [Washington, D.C.]: Centre for Disease Control and Prevention; 2007 [cited 2020 Mar 27]. 108 p. Available from: Available from: https://www.cdc.gov/flu/pandemic-resources/pdf/community_mitigation-sm.pdf
» https://www.cdc.gov/flu/pandemic-resources/pdf/community_mitigation-sm.pdf
9. Freitas ARR, Napimoga M, Donalisio MR. Análise da gravidade da pandemia de COVID-19. Epidmiol Serv Saúde. No prelo 2020.
10. Centre for Disease Control and Prevention (USA). Implementation of mitigation strategies for communities with local COVID-19 transmission [Internet]. [Washington, D.C.]: Centre for Disease Control and Prevention; 2019 [cited 2020 Mar 27]. 10 p. Available from: Available from: https://www.cdc.gov/coronavirus/2019-ncov/downloads/community-mitigation-strategy.pdf
» https://www.cdc.gov/coronavirus/2019-ncov/downloads/community-mitigation-strategy.pdf
11. Markel H, Stern AM, Navarro JA, Michalsen JR, Monto AS, Di Giovanni C. Nonpharmaceutical influenza mitigation strategies, US communities, 1918-1920 pandemic. Emerg Infect Dis [Internet]. 2006 Dec [cited 2020 Mar 27];12(12):1961-4. Available from: Available from: https://doi.org/10.3201/eid1212.060506. » https://doi.org/10.3201/eid1212.060506
12. Teh B, Olsen K, Black J, Cheng AC, Aboltins C, Bull K, et al. Impact of swine influenza and quarantine measures on patients and households during the H1N1/09 pandemic. Scand J Infect Dis [Internet]. 2012 Apr [cited 2020 Mar 27];44(4):289-96. Available from: Available from: https://doi.org/10.3109/00365548.2011.631572
» https://doi.org/10.3109/00365548.2011.631572
13. Kraemer MU, Yang CH, Gutierrez B, Wu CH, Klein B, Pigott DM, et al. The effect of human mobility and control measures on the COVID-19 epidemic in China. Science [Internet]. 2020 Mar [cited 2020 Mar 27]:eabb4218. Available from: Available from:

https://science.sciencemag.org/content/early/2020/03/25/science.abb4218

» https://science.sciencemag.org/content/early/2020/03/25/science.abb4218

14. Governo do Estado do Rio de Janeiro. Secretaria de Estado da Casa Civil e Governança. Decreto n. 46.970, de 13 de março de 2020. Dispõe sobre medidas temporárias de prevenção ao contágio e de enfrentamento da propagação decorrente do novo coronavírus (COVID-19), do regime de trabalho de servidor público e contratado, e dá outras providências [Internet]. Diário Oficial do Estado do Rio de Janeiro, Rio de Janeiro (RJ), 2020 mar 13 [citado 2020 mar 27]. Disponível em: Disponível em: http://www.fazenda.rj.gov.br/sefaz/content/conn/UCMServer/path/Contribution%20Folders/site_fazenda/Subportais/Portal-GestaoPessoas/Legislações%20SILEP/Legislações/2020/Decretos/DE-CRETO%20Nº%2046.970%20DE%2013%20DE%20MARÇO%20DE%202020_MEDIDAS%20TEMPORÁRIAS%20PRE-VENÇÃO%20CORONAVÍRUS.pdf?lve

» http://www.fazenda.rj.gov.br/sefaz/content/conn/UCMServer/path/Contribution%20Folders/site_fazenda/Subportais/Portal-GestaoPessoas/Legislações%20SILEP/Legislações/2020/Decretos/DE-CRETO%20Nº%2046.970%20DE%2013%20DE%20MARÇO%20DE%202020_MEDIDAS%20TEMPORÁRIAS%20PRE-VENÇÃO%20CORONAVÍRUS.pdf?lve

15. Governo do Distrito Federal (BR). Decreto n. 40.550, de 23 de março de 2020. Dispõe sobre as medidas para enfrentamento da emergência de saúde pública de importância internacional decorrente do novo coronavírus, e dá outras providências [Internet]. Diário Oficial do Distrito Federal, Brasília (DF), 2020 mar 23 [citado 2020 mar 27]; Edição Extra, Disponível em: Disponível em: http://www.sinj.df.gov.br/sinj/Norma/ed3d931f353d4503bd35b9b34fe747f2/Decreto_40520_14_03_2020.html

» http://www.sinj.df.gov.br/sinj/Norma/ed3d931f353d4503bd35b9b34fe747f2/Decreto_40520_14_03_2020.html

16. Prefeitura de São Paulo (SP). Casa Civil. Decreto n. 59.283, de 16 de março de 2020. Declara situação de emergência no Município de São Paulo e define outras medidas para o enfrentamento da pandemia decorrente do coronavírus [Internet]. São Paulo: Prefeitura; 2020 [citado 2020 mar 27]. Disponível em: Disponível em: https://leismunicipais.com.br/a/sp/s/sao-paulo/decreto/2020/5929/59283/decreto-n-59283-2020-declara-situacao-de-emergencia-no-municipio-de-sao-paulo-e-defineoutras-medidas-para-o-enfrentamento-da-pandemia-decorrente-do-coronavirus

» https://leismunicipais.com.br/a/sp/s/sao-paulo/decreto/2020/5929/59283/decreto-n-59283-2020-declara-situacao-de-emergencia-no-municipio-de-sao-paulo-e-defineoutras-medidas-para-o-enfrentamento-da-pandemia-decorrente-do-coronavirus

17. Governo do Estado de Santa Catarina. Decreto n. 515, de 17 de março de 2020. Declara situação de emergência em todo o território catarinense, nos termos do COBRADE nº 1.5.1.1.0 - doenças infecciosas virais, para fins de prevenção e enfrentamento à COVID-19, e estabelece outras providências [Internet]. Florianópolis: Governo do Estado de Santa Catarina; 2020 [citado 2020 mar 27]. Disponível em: Disponível em: https://www.sc.gov.br/images/Secom_Noticias/Documentos/VERS%C3%83O_ASSI-NADA.pdf

» https://www.sc.gov.br/images/Secom_Noticias/Documentos/VERS%C3%83O_ASSINADA.pdf

18. Governo do Estado de São Paulo. Decreto n. 64.881, de 22 de março de 2020. Decreta quarentena no Estado de São Paulo, no contexto da pandemia do COVID-19 (Novo Coronavírus), e dá providências complementares [Internet]. São Paulo: Governo do Estado de São Paulo; 2020 [citado 2020 mar 27]. Disponível em: Disponível em: https://www.saopaulo.sp.gov.br/wp-content/uploads/2020/03/decreto-quarentena.pdf

» https://www.saopaulo.sp.gov.br/wp-content/uploads/2020/03/decreto-quarentena.pdf

19. Armitage R, Nellums LB. COVID-19 and the consequences of isolating the elderly. Lancet Public Health [Internet]. 2020 Mar [cited 2020 Mar 27];pii:S2468-2667(20)30061-X. Available from: Available from: https:/doi.org/10.1016/S2468-2667(20)30061-X

» https:/doi.org/10.1016/S2468-2667(20)30061-X

2. Non-Pharmaceutical Interventions For Tackling The COVID-19 Epidemic In Brazil[1]

Leila Posenato Garcia[1] Elisete Duarte

[1]Instituto de Pesquisa Econômica Aplicada,
Diretoria de Estudos e Políticas Sociais, Brasília, DF, Brazil

[2]Secretaria de Vigilância em Saúde do Ministério da Saúde, Coordenação-Geral de Desenvolvimento da Epidemiologia em Serviço, Brasília, DF, Brazil

COVID-19 was detected in Wuhan, China, in December 2019. In view of the growing number of cases, deaths and affected countries, on January 30th 2020 the World Health Organization (WHO) declared the event to be a Public Health Emergency of International Concern.[1] In Brazil, the epidemic was declared a Public Health Emergency of National Concern on February 3rd 2020.[2,3] Following notification of over 110,000 cases and 4,000 deaths in countries on all continents, on March 11th 2020 WHO declared that COVID-19 had become pandemic.

In the absence of prior immunity in the human population and with no vaccine against SARS-CoV-2, the causative agent of COVID-19, its highly virulent nature means that case numbers grow exponentially. Nonpharmaceutical interventions (NPIs) are indicated in this context, aimed at inhibiting transmission between humans, slowing the spread of the disease and consequently reducing and delaying the peak of its occurrence on the epidemiological curve.[4] In this way, it is possible to reduce instantaneous demand for health care and mitigate the consequences of the disease for people's health, including minimizing associated morbidity and mortality (Figure 1).[57]

---

[1] Epidemiol. Serv. Saude, Brasília, 29(2):e2020222, 2020

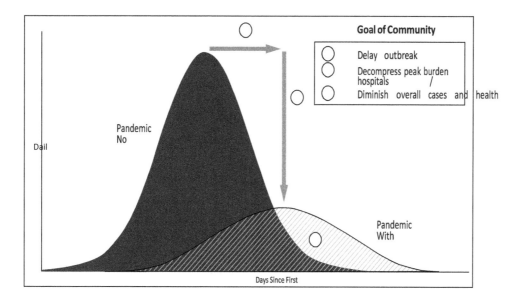

Figure 1 – Hypothetical epidemic curve showing the normal course of the epidemic and flattening of the curve expected by adopting non-pharmaceutical interventions Source: Adapted from Centres for Disease Control and Prevention (CDC), 2007.

NPIs are public health measures with personal, environmental and community scope. Individual measures include hand hygiene, respiratory etiquette and social distancing. In turn, social distancing involves case isolation, quarantine of contacts and the voluntary practice of not frequenting places where many people are gathered together.[5] Another personal measure is the use of masks, recommended for people with confirmed or suspected coronavirus and their carers. WHO recommends that asymptomatic people should not use masks, due to lack of evidence as to their effectiveness in reducing influenza transmission, apart from giving a false sense of protection. Furthermore, there are no studies on the effectiveness of mask use by asymptomatic people for preventing COVID-19 transmission.

Environmental measures refer to rooms being well ventilated and exposed to the sun, as well as routine cleaning of indoor environments and other surfaces, these being procedures that help to eliminate the virus.[5] SARS-CoV-2, like the influenza virus, can remain stable outside the human body, in aerosols and on various surfaces for up to three days, as in the case of plastic and stainless steel.[7] Special attention must be paid to cleaning elevator buttons, handrails, public transport hand straps, door handles, card terminal buttons, smartphones, workstations, among other objects and surfaces which, if contaminated, can contribute to spreading viruses.

Community measures are actions taken by managers, employers and/or community leaders to protect the population.

They include restricting access to schools, universities, community gathering places, public transport, as well as other places where large numbers of people gather, such as social and sports events, theatres, cinemas and commercial establishments, which are not characterized as providing essential services.[5] The starting time and duration of the various community NPIs will influence their impact. It is a considerable challenge to determine the best time to start such interventions, as if they are implemented too soon this can result in economic and social hardships without any benefit for public health and, over time, can result in "intervention fatigue" and the population ceasing to commit to the intervention. On the other hand, implementation once the disease has become widespread can limit the benefits for public health.

It needs to start soon enough to prevent the initial sharp rise in the number of cases, and last for long enough to cover the peak of the expected epidemic curve.[5] In view of the knowledge gaps inherent to a new disease and considering the similarity between the behaviour patterns of SARS-CoV-2 and the viruses that cause pandemic influenza, the strategies adopted in pandemic influenza contingency plans are being considered for the COVID-19 pandemic.

The guidelines of the United States Centres for Disease Control and Prevention (CDC) on pandemic influenza mitigation, indicate that the time to start interventions should be based on assessments of disease severity.[8] Assessment of COVID-19, in accordance with the CDC Pandemic Severity Assessment Framework (PSAF), has indicated that the disease has high transmissibility and clinical severity.[9] In view of the severity of the disease and the intensity of community transmission, the use of community NPIs to mitigate the COVID-19 pandemic is justified.[10] Measures such as home quarantine for infected people, social distancing and reduction in public gatherings, such as church services, as well as closing schools, were implemented during the 1918-1919 influenza pandemic in several cities in the United States.[11]

During the 2009 influenza pandemic, home quarantine was found to be feasible and achieved good uptake in Australia.[12] The experience of China suggests that NPIs, which included strict lockdown measures, such as those adopted in the city of Wuhan with effect from January 23rd 2020, contributed to suppressing the COVID-19 epidemic in that country.[4, 13]

On February 6th 2020, Brazil enacted Law No. 13979 which makes provisions for measures to address the COVID-19 epidemic and lists the community NPIs that can be adopted. The country's Federative Units began to adopt these measures with effect from the second week of March 2020. Examples include the state of Rio de Janeiro (Decree No. 46970, dated March 13th 2020),[14] the Federal District (Decree No. 40520, dated March 14th 2020),[15] the city of São Paulo (Decree No. 59.283, dated March 16th 2020)[16] and the state of Santa Catarina (Decree No. 515, dated March 17th 2020)[17] which, subsequently, approved new decrees establishing stricter measures. It is expected and desirable that actions to fight the epidemic will be reviewed and altered as it unfolds.

It's noteworthy that the state of São Paulo, the country's most populous state, adopted rigorous quarantine measures with effect from March 24th 2020.[18]

It should be highlighted that for some NPIs to be implemented, conditions of vulnerability peculiar to population subgroups need to be taken into consideration, such as street dwellers, people deprived of liberty, the institutionalized elderly,[18] people living in overcrowded households, households without adequate ventilation or without running water, migrants, people with special needs, people who live alone, among others. Moreover, adopting these measures has important impacts on everyday activities, on people's lives and on society. For example, children stop going to school, their studies are interrupted, and they lose their access to school meals. Restricting social contact can have consequences for people's mental and physical health, particularly in the case of children and the elderly.[4, 19]

Workers may be stopped from going to work, may need to alter their routines so as to work from home, or may lose their jobs or sources of income. Women and children in particular become more vulnerable to domestic and intrafamily violence. People, families, companies and countries are also expected to face economic losses. Within this context, it is fundamental for the Brazilian National Health System (SUS) and the other areas of the social protection system to work together in an articulated manner, so as to favour people's uptake of NPIs and minimize the detrimental impacts of community measures. Protecting public health must guide decisions to be taken by government managers. It is fundamental for these decisions to be based on the best available evidence and for them to be communicated in a transparent manner in order to gain the population's trust. Guidance given by authorities and people's uptake of NPIs will be determining factors for the course of the COVID-19 epidemic in Brazil.

INTRODUCTION

On the world stage, although distant from our daily lives, the beginning of 2020 was characterized by an outbreak of a mysterious pneumonia caused by a variation of coronavirus, whose first case was reported in December 2019 in the city of Wuhan, China.[1] The increase in the number of cases quickly characterized the infection as an outbreak, so that, at the end of January 2020, the World Health Organization (WHO) declared the situation as a public health emergency of international interest.[1] This is a virus isolated for the first time in 1937, and in 1965 was described as coronavirus, due to its profile under microscopy, similar to a crown.[2] Between 2002 and 2003, the WHO reported 774 deaths due to Severe Acute Respiratory Syndrome (SARS-CoV). In 2012, 858 deaths from Middle East Respiratory Syndrome (Mers-CoV) were confirmed in Saudi Arabia, both complications caused by members of the coronavirus family.[2]

Eight years later, 2019-2020, the world found the mutating RNA virus expanding, especially asymptomatically, as an emerging infection, with milder symptoms than SARS-CoV and Mers-CoV, but with greater transmissibility, thus generating considerable impacts on health systems.[1]

Most people are infected with coronavirus throughout their lives, especially children, in which case α-coronavirus 229E and NL63, β-coronavirus OC43 and HKU1 are recognized.[2] However, they can occasionally cause serious respiratory diseases in the elderly and the immunocompromised.[2-3] From virus isolation in initial cases, researchers identified genetic mutation in a spike surface protein, which the virus uses to attack the human organism and multiply.[3] Little by little, information about its incubation period, between two and ten days, and of propagation through contaminated droplets, hands and surfaces were described in the literature.[4-5] Immediately, the news reports recorded increase in infected people, deaths, and high rate of contamination in Wuhan, where the first control measures included suspension of public transport, closure of entertainment venues, prohibition of public meetings, cleaning of buildings, streets and compulsory home restrictions on all citizens.[6] Spread of cases to other geographic areas has been greatly accelerated due to globalization and lack of knowledge to adopt restrictive measures for travellers. There were many questions and few answers at first, a direct and active mobilization by WHO to monitor cases and virus spread to all continents. Then, by the results of the first researches, the picture was outlined with human-human transmission of n-COVID-19.[7]

In this setting, WHO declared COVID-19 a pandemic on March 11, 2020, and instituted essential measures for prevention and confrontation. They included hand washing with soap and water whenever possible and alcohol gel use in situations where access to water and soap is not possible. They also recommended avoiding touching the eyes, nose and mouth, and protecting people around them when sneezing or coughing, with the adoption of a cough etiquette, by using a flexed elbow or disposable handkerchief.[8] Moreover, the WHO indicated maintaining social distancing (minimum of one meter), avoiding crowding and using a mask in case of flu or infection by COVID-19, or if a health professional in caring for suspected/infected patients.[8] In Brazil, on February 3, 2020, it was declared, through Ordinance 188 from the Ministry of Health, a public health emergency of national importance, corresponding to a risk classification at level 3, due to human infection with the new coronavirus (SARS-CoV-2). This action aimed to favour that administrative measures were taken with greater agility so that the country began to prepare itself to face the pandemic, although at the time there was still no record of a confirmed case.[9] The first case of infection in Brazil was notified by the Ministry of Health on February 26, in the city of São Paulo, and the entire country from that moment on went on alert. Hand hygiene measures and cough etiquette were reinforced.[10]

However, the advance of the disease has been rapid, evolving in less than thirty days of cases imported for community or sustainable transmission. Imported cases are those in which it is possible to identify the origin of the virus, in general, when a person acquires it on trips abroad, at first, coming from countries like China and Italy.[10] In community transmission, the origin of the disease can no longer be identified, in addition to asymptomatic cases that come to represent a greater risk, considering that they spread the virus effectively.[10] In this new context of transmission at the national level, we witnessed, in parallel, estimates based on mathematical models proposed by researchers, and progression of COVID-19 cases in countries whose entry of the virus occurred in the period prior to notification in Brazil. In this perspective, this paper set out to analyse the COVID-19 pandemic, what we have (re) learned from the world experience of adopting prevention measures recommended by the WHO, as well as the epidemiological overview in the world, in Latin America and in Brazil.

3.New Development: 'Healing At A Distance' Telemedicine And COVID-19

Higor Leite, Ian R. Hodgkinson &Thorsten Gruber

ABSTRACT

In extreme circumstances such as pandemics, the presence of patients in hospital emergency departments becomes untenable. Healthcare professionals and organizations worldwide are leaning on technology as a crucial ally to deal with the COVID-19 outbreak. This article focuses on the positive impact of telemedicine for helping service provision, from enabling virtual triage to mitigating the negative psychological effects of social isolation. The authors discuss the challenges and opportunities to telemedicine practices. This article explains how telemedicine and other e-healthcare technologies can benefit people, medical staff and healthcare systems. One of the main challenges for telemedicine in many countries is the lack of regulations. The authors call on policy-makers to facilitate wider implementation of e-healthcare technologies, while considering issues of inclusiveness, privacy and data protection. The article informs managers about the use of new technologies. Examples are provided of e-healthcare technologies implemented during the COVID-19 pandemic, for example in terms of healthcare capacity and providing support to people affected by quarantine.

INTRODUCTION

Bubonic plague (1347–1351), yellow fever (1800s), the Spanish flu (1918–1919), and now COVID-19 have been collectively responsible for fatalities across the globe. Unlike historical pandemics, healthcare management of the COVID-19 pandemic can draw on new technologies for prevention, initial symptoms triage, self-isolation, quarantine and, ultimately, the return to social interaction. The article presents the challenges and opportunities of healing at a distance using telemedicine practices for e-healthcare. Pandemics provoke panic, fear, and motivate people to seek help across public healthcare systems creating service waves that can trigger further problems for the service ecosystem, such as overcrowded emergency departments in hospitals, which struggle to handle high demand and constrained capacity. This becomes a vicious cycle, as according to Gainer (2020), the excessive presence of patients in emergency departments creates even greater contamination in populations. While face-to-face interactions undoubtedly play a central role in the physician–patient relationship (Duffy & Lee, 2018), this is untenable in managing pandemics. This raises a key dilemma for healthcare professionals and organizations: how to provide healthcare without physical interactions with patients. In response, in this article we discuss how health professionals and the wider healthcare system can adopt telemedicine in the collective fight against COVID-19.

Telemedicine: Healing At A Distance

Technology can be adopted to mitigate extreme exogeneous shocks, such as natural disasters and diseases (Hollander & Carr, 2020; Lurie & Carr, 2018). Telemedicine represents the use of technology in healthcare to enable 'healing at a distance' (Strehle & Shabde, 2006). In e-healthcare, telemedicine provides a new means to support and promote long-distance clinical care, education, and healthcare, from first response to recovery with low cost and extensive coverage. Public administrations around the world, such as Australia, the USA and the UK, are investing in telemedicine to manage COVID-19, with the specific aim to reduce the volume of patients interacting with emergency departments and, in turn, halt the spread of the virus.

As an illustration, the Australian Department of Health (2020) are enabling medical staff to deliver services via telemedicine, encouraging citizens to access health services remotely to reduce the risk of exposure to COVID-19. Similarly, the NHS in the UK is providing online consultation in designated areas to avoid patient visits to general practitioners (NHS, 2020). These initiatives align with recommendations to implement triage via telemedicine before people enter healthcare facilities, to limit unnecessary healthcare visits (CDC, 2019).

These illustrations are examples of how telemedicine might engender the safety of patients and physicians, while simultaneously providing an effective frontline service to the citizenry (Gavidia, 2020).Other telemedicine approaches to identify and track infected sub-populations and areas, as well as provide self-assessment capabilities, are telemedicine apps. An illustration from the Brazilian government is the 'Coronavírus SUS' app. If the app-facilitated diagnosis indicates likely infection, patients are referred to the nearest emergency department or healthcare facility for testing, improving the efficiency and effectiveness of the traditional healthcare setting. The Brazilian app also serves to provide evidence-based insights as to the spread of a pandemic, reducing the prevalence of fake news and, consequently, helping to reduce panic (Ministry of Healthcare, 2020).

The combination of prevention, triage and information in one app has become a telemedicine tool, reducing demands on the public healthcare system in Brazil and, in turn, helping to avoid the collapse of the healthcare system; a similar initiative is being explored in the USA (Guardian, 2020a). Similarly, in the UK, King's College London, together with Guy's and St Thomas' hospitals, have developed an app (C-19 COVID Symptom Tracker, 2020) that takes citizens one minute per day to self-report their health condition. Citizens are asked to provide information such as their location, age, gender and any existing medical conditions. They then can report daily whether they feel healthy and, if not, can answer questions covering a wide range of symptoms, including the classic COVID-19 symptoms such as coughs and fever, but also non-traditional symptoms such as fatigue, diarrhoea, chest pain, lack of taste and confusion. New symptoms will be added to the list of symptoms if the app reveals that citizens report them in clusters across the country (*Guardian*, 2020 *b*). Data from the app means that it is possible to identify how fast the virus is spreading in an area; where the high-risk 'hotspot' areas are; and who is most at risk, by gaining more accurate understanding of how symptoms are linked to underlying health conditions (C-19 COVID Symptom Tracker, 2020).

The key use of telemedicine in these illustrations is to have a thorough understanding of the current healthcare situation in the country and also provide healthcare from a distance, without diminishing the quality of care, to enable more successful prevention without face-to-face interaction and the inherent dangers of traditional service provision.

Further preventative measures to protect people from contamination, and to flatten the COVID-19 'curve', include limited social interactions or minimal physical interaction during quarantine and self-isolation (CDC, 2020; Phend, 2020). However, the quarantine or self-isolation period has the potential to create loneliness and overwhelm vulnerable groups in the community. Individuals who have experienced periods of social isolation have reported problems such as anxiety, fear and depression and, in some cases, have developed symptoms of post-traumatic stress disorder (American Psychological Society, 2020; WHO, 2020). These negative psychological effects, and the further strain on healthcare systems that they may create, can be mitigated with the use of digital platforms such as video-chats to enable social interactions (Bowers, 2020). By extension, such platforms enable further telemedicine opportunities in the form of psychotherapy sessions via video, for example. The Australian government is providing mental health professional support through telemedicine during the COVID-19 pandemic, which again serves to ensure delivery of core services to those in need while significantly reducing (and in some case complete removal) of face-to-face treatment in hospitals (Australian Department of Health, 2020).

Telemedicine: Challenges and Opportunities

Telemedicine provides a new approach for wider e-healthcare to help combat the COVID-19 pandemic (Smith et al., 2020); however, there are a number of challenges to its implementation. In Brazil, for instance, the Federal Medical Council has deemed the practice of telemedicine (between patient and physician) as not legal (CFM, 2019). Similarly, in most states in the USA the use of telemedicine is severely constrained by regulatory bodies. Such barriers are in contradiction to recent actions taken by governments to halt the spread of COVID-19, which have focused on telemedicine implementation and usage. In the USA, for example, some federal rules have been waived to make it easier for physicians to provide care remotely, i.e. to adopt telemedicine (Archambault, 2020; Fung & Luhby, 2020).

Technologies for e-healthcare support require adequate bandwidth to support the transmission of data, images and sound. Consequently, access to broadband is essential for telemedicine in e-healthcare. This factor raises challenges for people living in rural areas, those without access to the internet, or vulnerable groups who cannot afford this service (Correa & Pavez, 2016; Smith et al., 2020). Moreover, engagement with telemedicine initiatives might be challenging for some citizens and they will need training in the use of new technologies and software connected to the internet (Ahlqvist, 2015). Data privacy and protection is also a critical issue to the success of telemedicine and e-healthcare. The privacy and protection of a patient's data must be paramount, and this issue has been raised as a core challenge by scholars and practitioners in the telemedicine field (Hit Consultant, 2020; Spencer & Patel, 2019). Finally, there are several telemedicine opportunities emerging for e-healthcare, including wearables, artificial intelligence, machine learning, 5G optimization, and Big Data, which have the potential to benefit patients, medical staff and healthcare organizations (*American Journal of Managed Care*, 2020; Chiaraviglio et al., 2017). Such technologies provide not just the opportunity to help ease the impact of critical events, such as pandemics or natural disasters, but provide a platform to rethink traditional healthcare practices and facilitate a transition to e-healthcare as the norm.

CONCLUDING REMARKS

This article has outlined how healthcare professionals and organizations are adopting telemedicine practices to 'flatten the infection curve' of COVID-19. We do not suggest that the technology of telemedicine itself is the panacea to improve healthcare, as the challenges in this sector are many. Nevertheless, embedding telemedicine into healthcare practices during the COVID-19 pandemic is proving beneficial to citizens, patients, medical professionals and healthcare organizations alike. We urge policy-makers worldwide to take advantage of the telemedicine experiences reported during this outbreak to allow the practices of e-healthcare under laws of privacy and data protection. Finally, we hope that this article motivates future work and prompts a significant reflection on telemedicine and healing at a distance.

REFERENCES

1. Ahlqvist, E. (2015). Digital inclusion in Sweden done in the "Digidel way". *The IFLA Library is IFLA's Institutional Repository* . [Google Scholar]
2. American Journal of Managed Care . (2020). https://www.ajmc.com/press-release/annual-ajmc-health-it-issue-covers-machine-learning-telehealth-portable-licensure.Accessed 12 February 2020. [Google Scholar]
3. American Psychological Society . (2020). https://www.apa.org/practice/programs/dmhi/research-information/social-distancing.Accessed 15 March 2020. [Google Scholar]
4. Archambault, J. (2020). *Forbes*: https://www.forbes.com/sites/theapothecary/2020/03/17/coronavirus-requires-telehealth-update-from-congress-and-states/#7146bd9da55a.Accessed 17 March 2020. [Google Scholar]
5. Australian Department of Health . (2020). https://www.health.gov.au/sites/default/files/documents/2020/03/COVID-19-national-health-plan-primary-care-bulk-billed-mbs-telehealth-services_0.pdf.Accessed 17 March 2020. [Google Scholar]
6. Bowers, L. A. (2020). *Operators using telehealth, live-streaming, video-chatting in this time of COVID-19*. https://www.mcknightsseniorliving.com/home/columns/editors-columns/operators-using-telehealth-live-streaming-video-chatting-in-this-time-of-COVID-19/.Accessed 18 March 2020. [Google Scholar]
7. C-19 COVID Symptom Tracker . (2020). https://covid.joinzoe.com/ Accessed 24 March 2020. [Google Scholar]
8. CDC . (2019). https://www.cdc.gov/coronavirus/2019-ncov/downloads/community-mitigation-strategy.pdf Accessed 10 February 2020. [Google Scholar]
9. CDC . (2020). https://www.cdc.gov/coronavirus/2019-ncov/index.html.Accessed 15 March 2020. [Google Scholar]
10. CFM . (2019). https://portal.cfm.org.br/index.php?option=com_content&view=article&id=28096:2019-02-22-15-13-20&catid=3.Accessed 9 March 2020. [Google Scholar]
11. Chiaraviglio, L. , Blefari-Melazzi, N. , Liu, W. , Gutiérrez, J. A. , Van De Beek, J. , Birke, R. , Chen, L. , Idzikowski, F. , Kilper, D. , Monti, P. , & Bagula, A. (2017). Bringing 5G into rural and low-income areas: Is it feasible? *IEEE Communications Standards Magazine* , *1* (3), 50–57. doi: 10.1109/MCOMSTD.2017.1700023[Crossref], [Google Scholar]
12. Correa, T. , & Pavez, I. (2016). Digital inclusion in rural areas: A qualitative exploration of challenges faced by people from isolated communities. *Journal of Computer-Mediated Communication* , *21* (3), 247–263. doi: 10.1111/jcc4.12154[Crossref], [Web of Science ®], [Google Scholar]
13. Duffy, S. , & Lee, T. H. (2018). In-person health care as option B. *N Engl J Med* , *378* , 104–106. doi: 10.1056/NEJMp1710735[Crossref], [PubMed], [Web of Science ®], [Google Scholar]
14. Fung, B. , & Luhby, T. (2020). *CNN*: https://edition.cnn.com/2020/03/14/politics/telehealth-us-federal-response-coronavirus/index.html.Accessed 15 March 2020. [Google Scholar]
15. Gainer, H. (2020). *How telehealth will help fight COVID-19 outbreak* https://www.uab.edu/news/health/item/11172-how-telehealth-will-help-fight-COVID-19-outbreak.accessed 13 March 2020. [Google Scholar]
16. Gavidia, M. (2020). https://www.ajmc.com/focus-of-the-week/telehealth-during-covid19-how-hospitals-healthcare-providers-are-optimizing-virtual-care Accessed 15 march 2020. [Google Scholar]

17. Guardian . (2020a). https://www.theguardian.com/us-news/2020/mar/16/coronavirus-testing-website-trump-promised-verily.Accessed 17 March 2020. [Google Scholar]
18. Guardian . (2020b). https://www.theguardian.com/australia-news/live/2020/mar/24/coronavirus-live-news-updates-us-trump-uk-lockdown-global-deaths-cases-covid19-latest-update Accessed 24 March 2020. [Google Scholar]
19. Hit Consultant . (2020). https://hitconsultant.net/2020/03/13/coronavirus-COVID-19-considerations-tele-health-providers/#.Xm9wg2Viyi4.Accessed 14 March 2020. [Google Scholar]
20. Hollander, J. E. , & Carr, B. G. (2020). Virtually perfect? Telemedicine for COVID-19. *New England Journal of Medicine* . [Crossref], [PubMed], [Web of Science ®], [Google Scholar]
21. Lurie, N. , & Carr, B. G. (2018). The role of telehealth in the medical response to disasters. *JAMA Intern Med* , *178* , 745–746. doi: 10.1001/jamainternmed.2018.1314[Crossref], [PubMed], [Web of Science ®], [Google Scholar]
22. Ministry of Healthcare . (2020). - https://www.saude.gov.br/o-ministro/928-saude-de-a-a-z/coronavirus.Accessed 15 March 2020. [Google Scholar]
23. NHS . (2020). https://www.nhs.uk/using-the-nhs/nhs-services/the-nhs-app/help/online-consultations/.Accessed 5 March 2020. [Google Scholar]
24. Phend, C. (2020). https://www.medpagetoday.com/infectiousdisease/covid19/85306.Accessed 12 March 2020. [Google Scholar]
25. Smith, A. C. , Thomas, E. , Snoswell, C. L. , Haydon, H. , Mehrotra, A. , Clemensen, J. , & Caffery, L. J. (2020). Telehealth for global emergencies: Implications for coronavirus disease 2019 (COVID-19). *Journal of Telemedicine and Telecare* . [Crossref], [PubMed], [Web of Science ®], [Google Scholar]
26. Spencer, A. , & Patel, S. (2019). Applying the data protection act 2018 and general data protection regulation principles in healthcare settings. *Nursing Management* , *26* , 1. doi: 10.7748/nm.2019.e1806[Crossref], [Google Scholar]
27. Strehle, E. M. , & Shabde, N. (2006). One hundred years of telemedicine: Does this new technology have a place in paediatrics? *Archives of disease in childhood* , *91* (12), 956–959. doi: 10.1136/adc.2006.099622[Crossref], [PubMed], [Web of Science ®], [Google Scholar]
28. WHO . (2020). https://www.who.int/docs/default-source/coronaviruse/mental-health-considerations.pdf?sfvrsn=6d3578af_.8 accessed 15 March 2020. [Google Scholar]

Public Utilization of Face Masks in Brazil During COVID-19 Pandemic Outbreak: Temporal Trend Analysis

Bernanda Maria Vieira Pereira-Ávila, Eliã Pinheiro Botelho,
Fernanda Garcia Bezerra Góes, Elucir Gir,
Laelson Rochelle Milanês Sousa,
Natália Maria Vieira Pereira Caldeira,
Ana Cristina de Oliveira e Silva, Simon Ching Lam

ABSTRACT

Background: The coronavirus disease 2019 (COVID-19) has recorded approximately 8.6 million confirmed. cases and more than 450.000 deaths worldwide. As of today, Brazil remains the second most affected country, with more than 1 million confirmed cases and more than 50,000 related deaths. This study aimed to evaluate the temporal trend of the frequency of face mask use among Brazil's general population. **Method**: A cross-sectional survey method was adopted in this study. Online survey regarding sociodemographic and protective personal measures against COVID-19 was used to collect data. Data were collected from April 17 to May 15, 2020. The frequency of face mask use was divided into five categories: "never," "rarely," "sometimes," "frequently," and "always." Joinpoint regression model was employed to analyze the daily percentage change (DPC) of each category. Ethics aspects were considered.

Results: A total of 14,756 volunteers comprised the study sample. The "frequently" and "aways" categories represented 71% of the sample, with the former being superior to the latter (39.4% vs. 31.6%, respectively). Temporal trend analysis showed two trend periods for all categories. The "never," "rarely," and "sometimes" categories decreased in the first period and stabilized in the second period. Conversely, the "frequently" and "always" categories showed an upward trend. Like other categories, the "frequently" category had stabilized in the second period. However, the "always" category still showed an increasing trend in the second period. The association analysis results showed a decrease in the use of face masks in women, postgraduate people, those aged above 35 years, and those earning more than seven times the federal monthly income minimal wage. However, the use of masks increased among young people and those with elementary to graduate degrees. The "always" use of face masks increased in the south and decreased in the southeast of Brazil.

Conclusion: The preponderance of the "frequently" category and the slow DPC in the second trend period of the "always" category suggest the necessity of further enforcement of the use of face masks in Brazil. The adaptation of this new habit among Brazilians is time demanding, and thus strategies must be implemented in a more natural way.

BACKGROUND

The novel coronavirus SARS-CoV-2 (COVID-19) has reported approximately 12 million confirmed cases and more than 550,000 deaths worldwide. As of today, Brazil's Ministry of Health has confirmed more than 1,7 million COVID-19 cases and more than 69,000 related deaths. Consequently,

Brazil has been recognized as the second most affected country by the pandemic after the United States (US) [1–2].Given the COVID-19 pandemic outbreak, the use of face masks has been proposed as an effective means of protection against the virus that is transmitted primarily through respiratory droplets. The Centers for Disease Control and Prevention (CDC) guidance includes the use of N95 mask or higher-level respirators to health professionals and surgical or cloth masks to the general population [3]. The efficacy level of
N95, medical, and homemade masks regarding human-to-human virus transmission prevention is 99.98%, 97.14%, and 95.15%, respectively [4]. Simulation models for the impact of the use of face masks in the pandemic in New York and Washington (US) have suggested that community-wide utilization of face masks could reduce the risks of COVID-19,including transmission, hospitalizations, and deaths [5]. Another study supported this claim by showing an extremely lower incidence of COVID-19 in an administrative region of Hong Kong that implemented community-wide utilization of face masks than the countries doing differently, such as Spain, France, Italy, and Germany [6]. In addition to personal protection against COVID-19, the utilization of face masks reminds the people of the severity of the disease and highlights the importance of social distancing [7].Given the internal political conflicts in Brazil and the insufficient evidence on face mask efficiency meanwhile, the public use of face masks started to implement on April 2, 2020, three weeks after the ⊠rst100 cases [8–9].
However, the number of COVID-19 cases and deaths are still increasing even with this implementation. The notification of new COVID-19 cases has increased rapidly up to 1,329.04% from April 2 to May 15(1,071 and 15,305 cases, respectively). On June 29, 2020, a total of 24,052 new confirmed cases were reported to the Ministry of Health, corresponding to an increase of 2,145.75% since April 2, 2020 [2]. This continuously increasing number suggests a low adherence of the public to the use of face masks. Therefore, this study aims to analyze the changes in the frequency of public utilization of face masks during this pandemic, within the period after federal implementation.

METHODS

Study Design and Settings

A cross-sectional survey study was conducted and participated by Brazilians adult. Brazil is known as the largest country in South America surrounded by the Atlantic Ocean on the east coast. The country's population is approximately 250million. Brazil is divided into five main political regions: north, northeast, midwest, south, and southeast. It is surrounded by ten other countries (Uruguay, Paraguay, Argentina, Peru, Bolivia, Colombia, Venezuela, Suriname, Guiana, French Guiana). It makes clearly the importance of bringing under control the COVID-19 in Brazil. The results of this study provide implications to health authorities to implement new strategies and evaluate the already implemented ones to eliminate COVID-19 in Brazil.

Study Sample and Variables

Convenience sampling was used to select the study sample, which was composed of adult people aged above 18 years. The specific adult population projection in 2019 (159,095,000) was used as the basis to calculate the sample size, considering 1.2% margin of error and 99% of confidence interval. Although the result provided a sample size of 11,556 adult people, a total of 14,756 volunteers had participated in this study. The following variables were collected from the online survey: dates of answering the survey, age, sex, province of residency, monthly income, schooling, occupations, marital status, and the frequency of facemask use. The frequency of face mask use was divided into five categories: never, rarely, sometimes, frequently, and always.

The respondents were also asked if they consider their occupation at risk for SARS-CoV-2transmission/infection, if they had close contact with someone diagnosed with COVID-19, if they consider themselves vulnerable to the virus infection, and if they developed feelings of fear toward it.

Data Collection Procedure

Data were collected online from April 17 to May 15, 2020 via social media (Facebook, Twitter, Instagram, WhatsApp, and e-mail), employing online survey through Google forms. The survey was validated by a committee of experts. Afterwards, a pilot test participated by 20 people was conducted on each region. This study was widely disseminated in all regions in Brazil. All volunteers read and accepted the free and informed consent terms included in the Google Forms. All ethics aspects were considered.

Statistical Analysis

Data were first analyzed descriptively considering absolute (n) and relative (%) frequencies. Then, the joinpoint regression model was employed to analyze changes in relative frequency of face mask use during the period of this study. The daily frequency for each category was calculated according to the total of people that responded to the survey in that day. In the temporal trend analysis, the categories of frequency were taken as dependent variables and the days as independent variable. The best fitting joinpoint regression model was accessed by Monte Carlo permutation test, which employed 4,999 permutations. The daily percentage change (DPC), 95% confidence interval (95% CI) and p-value were considered for each category. Trends were considered increasing or decreasing if the DPC is positive or negative, respectively, and $p < 0.05$. Otherwise, they were considered stationary.

We employed the chi-squared test to verify the level of association among outcome variables with the periods identified in joinpoint regression for the category of "always." We grouped the outcome variables in each one of the trend periods before applying the association test (April 17–25 and April 25 to May15). Then, we applied binary logistic regression to all association with $p < 0.20$ to estimate the probabilities associated with the frequency of face masks use in each trend period. We considered Odds Ratio (OR), 95% confidence intervals, and $p < 0.05$ as statistically significance.

RESULTS

The study sample was composed by 14,756 people. Most of them were female (75.4%), single (47.0%), postgraduate (43.5%), from the northeast region (39.2%), and had jobs out of the health field (58.0%). The sample averaged age was 35years old (SD = 13.0), with minimal and maximum ages of18 and 88 years, respectively. For the frequency of face mask use, the following values were the absolute and relative (%) frequencies for each category: never = 700 (4.7%), rarely = 902 (6.1%), sometimes = 2,674 (18.1%), frequently = 5,814 (39.4%), and always = 4,666 (31.6%). Table 2 **Figure 1** show the joinpoint analysis results. All categories had two trend periods. The "never," "rarely," and "sometimes" categories had downward trends in the first period and became stabilized in the second one. Conversely, the "frequently" and "always" categories had an upward trend in the first period. However, the "frequently" category had a stable trend in the second period, and the "always" category had a slow increasing trend.

Table 2 – Temporal trend analysis of Mask usage frequencies (n = 14.756). Brazil, 2020

Face-mask usage frequency	Periods	DPC (%)	CI 95%	p-valor
Never	17 April – 13 May	-9.93	-11.6 - -8.3	0.000
	13–15 May	82.07	-42.5–476.7	0.309
Rarely	17 April – 11 May	-6.76	-8.0 - -5.5	0.000
	11–15 May	17.73	-4.9–45.07	0.120
Sometimes	17 April – 08 May	-2.17	-3.3 - -1.1	0.000
	08–15 May	-4.42	-8.9–0.3	0.070
Frequently	17–23 April	4.45	2.2–6.7	0.000
	23 April – 15 May	0.37	0.2–1.4	0.200
Always	17–25 April	6.95	3.1–10.1	0.000
	25 April – 15 May	1.23	0.3–2.1	0.004

The initial association analysis results among the outcome variables with the two trend periods identified in the "always" category. In the second period, an increase in the frequency of face mask use was observed among males, singles, young people, and those living in the north, midwest, northeast, and south regions. The same phenomenon was observed in people with elementary to graduate degrees and those with low rental income. An increase in the frequency of face mask use was observed among people who have low-risk jobs, those did not experience close contact with a sick person, and those who did not express vulnerability to the virus or fear about acquiring the disease.

All variables were submitted to binary logistic regression to estimate the association probabilities among them with both periods in the "always" category. The variables associated to both trend periods were gender, age, region, monthly income, occupation considered at risk for virus infection, and feelings of vulnerability to virus. In the second period, an increased frequency of face mask usage was observed in ages 18–34 years (1.5x) and in the south region (2x). A decreased chance was observed to the following predictors: women (1.8x), those aged above 35 years (1.5x), those living in the southeast region (8.0x), those who had a postgraduate degree (7.0x), those who earned seven times the monthly minimal income (2.2x), those who worked in job positions considered at risk for COVID-19 (1.9x), and those expressing vulnerability and feelings of fear toward the disease (1.7x**).**

DISCUSSION

This study is the first to evaluate the use of face masks in Brazil. Our results show an increase in the frequency of face mask usage by Brazilians during the COVID-19 pandemic outbreak. This finding maybe due to the preventive mediatic campaign against COVID-19 promulgated and implemented by the health authorities. Media campaigns are efficient on promulgating information and stimulating the adherence to protective measures against COVID-19 [10]. The level of knowledge about COVID-19 is directly correlated with face mask use and other personal protective measures, which has been observed in Malaysia and China [11–12]. In our study, the "frequently" and "always" categories have represented 71% of the sample. However, the ideal "always" category is only 31.6%. The temporal trend analysis results show that women did not always wear face masks in the second trend period. This result corroborates with previous studies [12–13]. In China, a study with 10,304 volunteers showed that although women practice more protective measures against COVID-19 during the pandemic, only males have shown an upward trend [13]. This finding can be explained by the quarantine restrictions implemented by the Health Ministry in Brazil. After the school activities were interrupted, most women stopped their jobs to take care of their children, thereby decreasing their exposure to the virus. Given that women are less vulnerable to the virus, their frequency of face mask use is also lesser to that of men.

Discrepancies among regional implementations of face mask use were also observed. In the second period, an increasing trend was observed in the south region, whereas a decreasing trend was observed in the southeast region. The north region had the lowest frequency in both trend periods. Among all the regions, the south and north regions were the least and the most affected by COVID-19, respectively. The regional discrepancies in COVID-19 incidence are still evident today [2]. The following facts are also considered: 1) regional developmental differences: the south and southeast regions are the richest, whereas the north and northeast regions are the poorest; 2) provincial implementation of protective measures against COVID-19 were conducted at different times, and they started only when the Ministry of Health recommended the use of homemade masks in public places on April 2, 2020 [9]; and 3) wrong previews about the stabilization of COVID-19 curve transmission have been promulgated in the southeast region, which could have influenced the loosening of the use of face masks.

The continuous use of face masks increased among the youth in the second period and decreased in people aged above 35years. A study in Pakistan showed the same result and suggested that young people have higher knowledge regarding prevention practices than the adults [14]. However, 42% of our sample is composed of health professionals, and 55.02% of them assumed older than 35years old. Like other countries, Brazil has experienced scarcity in face masks and other personal protective equipment (PPE). Consequently, health workers are often working without proper medical gear and attire. Health professionals' long and stressful work and the scarcity of PPE in the national level have increased their feelings of vulnerability and fear of acquiring the virus [15].

Health workers could also have influenced the faster DPC observed in the first period than that of the second one (6.95% vs. 1.23%, respectively). By contrast, the slower DPC in the second period suggests a low gradual adherence of the population in general to face masks. This hypothesis corroborates with the increase of face mask use in people earning low monthly income and those with lower degrees compared with the ones in the first period.The internal political conflicts in Brazil and the spread of fake news still influence the willingness of the public to adopt the promoted protective measures against COVID-19. The general population in Brazil remains clueless about the pandemic situation they are currently experiencing, and no specific guidelines are given to them to stop further transmission of the virus [18–20]. Negative assumptions and fake news regarding the risks of wearing face masks were widely disseminated during the second period (April 25 to May 15) [21–22]. In addition, utilization of face masks is not a cultural habit in Brazil, and it is never needed that much before. Strategies must be implemented with congruences among policymakers and local authorities to incorporate this new habit in the daily routine of the general population and reinforce the importance of face masks [19–22].The study sample is limited by the convenience method used in this study and by the limitation on response rate. Finally, the participants may have also provided socially desirable responses.

Table 5
– Binary logistic regression to category mask-usage "always". Brazil. 2020
–

Variables	Mask usage	
	OR (IC95%)	p-value
Female	0.55 (0.45–0.66)	< 0.001
35 years and over	0.65 (0.49–0.86)	< 0.001
Northeast region	0.63 (0.49–0.81)	< 0.001
South region	2.28 (1.64–3.1)	< 0.001
Southeast region	0.12 (0.09-015)	< 0.001
High school	0.34 (0.13–0.89)	0.026
Graduated	0.26 (0.10–0.66)	0.005
Postgraduated	0.13 (0.05–0.33)	< 0.001
Monthly income		
1–2	0.58 (0.35–0.95)	0.029
3–4	0.48 (0.29–0.79)	0.004
5–6	0.53 (0.32–0.88)	0.014
> 7	0.45 (0.27–0.74)	0.002
Occupation at risk to COVID-19	0.52 (0.45–0.62)	< 0.001
Vulnerability feeling about getting COVID-19	0.57 (0.38–0.87)	0.008

CONCLUSION

Policymakers and local authorities need to reinforce further the frequent use of face masks to the public in addition to other protective personal measures to combat COVID-19. Although 71% of the sample fell under the "frequently" and "always" categories, the ideal "always" category was still lower than the "frequently" category. In addition, more than 29% were not using face masks at all. This finding was alarming given that SARS-CoV-2 could be easily transmitted from one person to another. Providing PPE and better work conditions to health workers were extremely important and long overdue. Brazil had the highest number of health professionals that died by COVID-19. The government should recognize the scholarly efforts and prioritize public health to eliminate COVID-19 and avoid its second and subsequent waves.

Abbreviations

DPC Daily Percentage Changes

CI confident Interval

PPE Personal Protective Equipment

US United States

Declarations

Ethical approve and consent to participate

This research project was submitted and approved by the National Research Ethic Committee under recording number CAAE: 30572120.0.0000.0008. Report: 4.094.626. Our sample was composed by Brazilian general population aged over 18 years old and all volunteers read and accepted the consent form.

Availability of data and materials

All tables and the figure were constructed by the authors. Restrictions apply to the availability of these data, which were used under license for the current study, and so are not publicly available.

Funding

This study was financial supported by the Brazilian National Research Council (CNPq; grant 401371/2020-4).

REFERENCES

1. Center for Disease Control and Prevention. Coronavirus Disease 2019 (COVID-19) – Situation Report – 151. https://covid19.who.int (2020). Acessed 09 Jul 2020.

2. BRASIL. CORONAVIRUS. https://covid.saude.gov.br (2020). Acessed 09 Jul 2020.

3. Center for Disease Control and Prevention. Coronavirus Disease 2019 (COVID-19).

https://www.cdc.gov/coronavirus/2019-ncov/hcp/using-ppe.html (2020). Acessed 07 Jul 2020.

4. Ma QX, Zhang HL, Li GM, Yang RM, Chen, JM. Potential utilities of mask-wearing and instant hand hygiene for fighting SARS-CoV-2. J Med Virol. 2020;1-5.

5. Eikenberry SE, Mancuso M, Iboi E, Phan Tin, Eikenberry K et al. To mask or not to mask: Modeling the potential for face mask use by the general public to curtail the COVID-19 pandemic. Infect Dis Model.2020;5:293-308.

6. Cheng VCC, Wong SC, Chuang VWM, So SYC, Chen JHK et al. The role of community-wide wearing of face mask for control of coranvirus disease 2019 (COVID-19) epidemic due to SARS-CoV-2. J Infec.2020. 81(1):107-114.

7. Jhon. Facial mask: a necessity to beat COVID-19. Build Environ. 2020;175:106827.

8. The Lancet. COVID-19 in Brazil: "So what?". Lancet. 2020;395:1641.

9. Brasil. Máscaras caseiras podem ajudar na prevenção contra o coronavírus. 2020.

https://www.saude.gov.br/noticias/agencia-saude/46645-mascaras-caseiras-podem-ajudar-na-prevencao-contra-o-coronavirus (2020). Acessed Jun 18 2020.

10. Jørgensen F J, Bor A, Petersen, MB. Compliance Without Fear: Predictors of Protective Behavior During the First Wave of the COVID-19 Pandemic. PsyArXiv. 2020;1-61.

11. Azlan AA, Hamzah MR, Sem TJ, Ayub SH, Mohamad E. Public knowledge, attitudes and practices toward COVID-19: A cross-sectional study in Malaysia. PLOS ONE. 2020.

12. Zhong B, Luo W, Li H, Zhang Q, Liu X, Li W et al. Knowledge, attitudes, and practices towards COVID-

19 among Chinese residents during the rapid rise period of the COVID-19 outbreak: a quick online cross-sectional survey. Int J Biol Sci. 2020;16(10):1745-1752.

13. Huang Y, Wu Q, Wang P, Xu Y, Wang L, Zhao Y et al. Measures undertaken in China to avoid COVID-19 infection: Internet-based, cross-sectional survey study.

14. Hayat K, Rosenthal M, Xu S, Arshed M, Li P, Zhai P et al. View of Pakistani residents toward Coronavirus Disease (COVID-19) during a Rapid Outbreak: A rapid online survey. Int J Environ Res Public Health. 2020;17(10):3347.

15. Miranda FMD, Santana LL, Pizzolato AC, Saquis LMM. Working conditions and the impact on the health of nursing professionals in the context of COVID-19. Cogitare enferm. 2020;23:e72702.

16. Ribeiro R, Leist A. Who is going to pay the price of COVID-19? Reflections about an unequal Brazil Int J Equity Health. 2020;19:91.

17. Mandetta LH, Baia-da-Silva DC, Brito-Sousa JD, Monteiro WM, Lacerda MVG. COVID-19 in Brazil:advantages of a socialized unified health system and preparation to contain cases. Rev Soc BrasMed Trop. 2020; 53: e20200167.

18. Croda J, Oliveira WK, Frutuoso RL, Mandetta LH, Baia-da-Silva DC, Brito-Sousa JD et al . COVID-19 in Brazil: advantages of a socialized unified health system and preparation to contain cases. Rev SocBras Med Trop. 2020; 53: e20200167.

19. Orso D, Federici N, Copetti R, Vetrugno L, Bove T. Infodemic and the spread of fake news in the COVID-19-era, Eur J Emerg Med. 2020; XXX:00–00

20. Brasil. Ministério da Saúde. https://www.saude.gov.br/component/tags/tag/novo-corona-virus-fake-news (2020). Acessed 18 Jun 2020.

21. Oliveira AC, Lucas TC, Iquiapaza RA. What has the COVID-19 pandemic taught us about adopting preventive measures? Texto Contexto Enferm. 2020;29:e20200106.

Table 1

− Sociodemographic charaterization of the study voluntaries (n = 14,756). Brazil, 2020.

Variables	n (%)
Sex	
Male	3623 (24.6)
Female	11133 (75.4)
Marital status	
Single	6929 (47.0)
Married	6658 (45.1)
Divorced	939 (6.4)
Widower	230 (1.6)
Age	
18–34	7708 (52.2)
35+	7048 (47.8)
Brazilian Region	
North	1346 (9.1)
Northeast	5784 (39.2)
Midwest	1762 (11.9)
Southeast	4475 (30.3)
South	1389 (9.4)
Schooling	
Elementary school	184 (1.3)
High school	2662 (18.0)
Graduated	5489 (37.2)
Postgraudated	6421 (43.5)

Health professional	
No	8564 (58.0)
Yes	6192 (42.0)

*Brazilian monthly income (minimum wage)
= R$1045,00 or U$199,43

Variables	n (%)
Monthly income (minimal wage)*	
< 1	548 (37)
1 a 2	3247 (22.0)
3 a 4	3756 (25.5)
5 a 6	2433 (16.5)
7+	4610 (31.2)
No income	162 (1.1)

*Brazilian monthly income (minimum wage) = R$1045,00 or U$199,43

Table 3

– Face mask usage category "always" association with sociodemographic variables in the two temporal trend periods (n = 4,666). Brazil, 2020

Variables	Temporal trend periods (n 4.666)		p-value
	April 17-April 25 n(%)	April 25 May 15 n(%)	
Sex			
Male	272 (14.3)	738 (26.7)	0.000
Female	1632 (85.7)	2024 (73.3)	
Marital status			
Single	658 (34.6)	1627 (58.9)	0.000
Married	1024 (53.8)	972 (35.2)	
Separated/Divorced	191 (10.0)	111 (4.0)	
Widower	31 (1.6)	52 (1.9)	
Age (years)			
18–34	657 (34.5)	1842 (66.7)	0.000
35+	1247 (65.5)	920 (33.3)	
Brazilian Region			
North	117 (6.1)	373 (13.5)	0.000
Northeast	617 (32.4)	1235 (44.7)	
Midwest	166 (8.7)	400 (14.5)	
Southeast	915 (48.1)	259 (9.4)	
South	89 (4.7)	495 (17.9)	
Schooling			
Elementary	6 (0.3)	52 (1.9)	0.000

	April 17-April 25	April 25 May 15	
High school	192 (10.1)	661 (23.9)	
Graduate	506 (26.6)	1213 (43.9)	
Postgraduate	1200 (63.0)	836 (30.3)	
Monthly income (minimum wage)			
< 1	24 (1.3)	156 (5.6)	0.000
Variables	**Temporal trend periods (n 4.666)**		**p-value**
	April 17-April 25 **n(%)**	**April 25 May 15** **n(%)**	
1–2	286 (15.0)	783 (28.3)	
3–4	461 (24.2)	715 (25.9)	
5–6	358 (18.8)	397 (14.4)	
> 7	763 (40.1)	670 (24.3)	
No income	12 (0.6)	41 (1.5)	

Table 2 – Temporal trend analysis of Mask usage frequencies (n = 14.756). Brazil, 2020

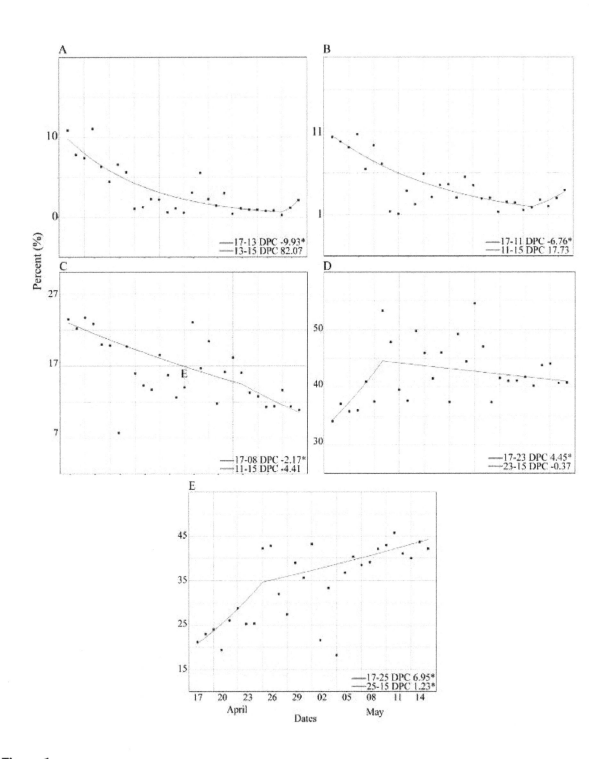

Figure 1

4. The Most Prominent Antiviral Pharmaceuticals Used Against COVID-19 And Their Perspectives

[1] Nelson Durán1,2*

[1]Laboratory of Urogenital Carcinogenesis and Immunotherapy, Department of Structural and Functional Biology, University of Campinas, Campinas, SP, Brazil

Wagner J. Fávaro[1]*

[2]Nanomedicine Research Unit (Nanomed), Federal University of ABC (UFABC), Santo André, SP, Brazil.

ABSTRACT

Many well-known commercial pharmaceuticals have been used in the therapy against SARS-CoV-2, although in a random and experimental way, since this use is only based on the knowledge about culture cells *in vitro*. But, it is widely known that it is not correlated with assays *in vivo* conducted with in animals or with clinical trials in humans. Knowledge about treatments applied to previous pandemic infections caused by viruses such as MERS and SARS may be the most interesting strategy used to screen products with potential to act against SARS-CoV-2. Mechanistic aspects of virus infections and antiviral action mechanisms were herein analysed based on the assumption that these commercial pharmaceuticals can eliminate the virus. Perspectives about these procedures, as well as about finished clinical trials and the ones yet in progress, were also addressed in the current study.

INTRODUCTION

The large number of clinical trials carried out to research likely therapies against COVID-19 emphasizes both the necessity and ability of the scientific community to generate high-quality proof, even during the COVID-19 pandemic. Unfortunately, treatments applied so far were not fully efficient (Sander et al., 2020).It is well-known that inflammatory caspases represent a key function in innate immunity, since they reproduce cytosolic signals and induce dual responses (Jorgensen and Miao, 2015). Two important targets can be used to eliminate viruses, mainly SARS-CoV-2; the first one is pyroptosis, which is an important process triggered by caspase-1 - which activates and releases pro-inflammatory cytokines such as interleukin-18 (IL-18) and IL1β. In addition, caspase-11 or caspase-1 are capable of activating some type of lytic, programmed cell death. Pyroptosis acts

[1] *Correspondence: Prof. Nelson Durán (E-mail: nelsonduran1942@gmail.com) and Prof. Wagner J. Fávaro (E-mail: favarowj@unicamp.br).

by removing the reproduction site of intracellular pathogens, like bacteria or viruses, and it makes them susceptible to phagocytosis and to be destroyed by subsidiary phagocytes. However, in several cases, abnormal systemic activation of pyroptosis *in vivo* can lead to sepsis. Emphasizing the ability of inflammasome recognition of viral infections, several pathogens have improved its abilities to prevent or disrupt pyroptosis (Durán and Fávaro, 2020a). These observations are also found in many other diseases (Ma et al., 2018; Liang et al., 2020) such as cancer (Durán and Fávaro, 2020b) and cardiovascular diseases (Zeng et al., 2019). The other target lies on RNA-dependent RNA polymerase (RdRp) because SARS-CoV-2 is a strand RNA virus, whose propagation is based on multiple subunit reproduction or/and transcription complex of viral proteins (Ziebuhr, 2005).

Although there are many other targets that can be used against SARS-CoV-2 (e.g., blocking the host target TMPRSS2 (ACE2 receptor), three of the most important ones (pyroptosis, RNA-dependent polymerase and nucleocytoplasmic trafficking of viral proteins), which are associated with pharmaceuticals used nowadays, will be addressed in the current study.

Pyroptosis

Recently, Zhao and Zhao (2020) have investigated PRRs (pattern recognition receptors) such as LRR, PYD and NACHT domains. These PRRs present protein-3 inflammasome, which is a complex consisted of the NOD-like receptor protein-3 - NLRP3 (NOD domain (nucleotide-binding oligomerization) NOD-like receptor NLRP3), which, in its turn, is the transcriber of apoptosis connected speck-like protein (ASC) and caspase-1.

This kind of complex is crucial to hosts' defence against microbes since it stimulates IL-1β and IL-18 release and triggers pyroptosis, as previously mentioned. NLRP3 is capable of recognizing a whole diversity of PAMPs (pathogen-connected molecular patterns) and DAMPs (danger-connected molecular patterns) generated through viral replication; this process activates the NLRP3 inflammasome which is really of antiviral immunological responses and makes viral eradication possible. Unfortunately, many viruses use very sophisticated strategies to prevent the immune system from attacking the NLRP3 inflammasome (Sollberger et al., 2014). Few viruses have been reported to inhibit NLRP3 inflammasome stimulation to avoid innate immunity and enhance viral replication. The virus is capable of suppressing either the adjustment or the stimulation of NLRP3 inflammasome through a direct/indirect interaction. Influenza virus NS1, paramyxovirus V and measles virus inhibit NLRP3 inflammasome induction and diminish IL-1β release.

This interaction of viral protein and NLRP3 avoid self-oligomerization and, at the same time, the enrolment of ASC, culminating in the blocks inflammasome activation (Zhao and Zhao, 2020).Yang et al. (2020) conducted a study focused on investigating the history and epidemiology of SARS and emphasized several points, such as pathogenesis, epidemiology, clinical features, diagnosis and guidance of individuals infected with SARS-CoV-2.

At the first coronavirus contamination stage, epithelial and dendritic cells are activated and present a cluster of chemokines and pro-inflammatory cytokines, such as interleukins (IL-2, IL-6, IL-8, IL-1β), tumour necrosis factor (TNF), interferons (IFN-α/β), C-C motif chemokines and IP-10, among others. All these pro-inflammatory factors are modulated by the immune system. Thereby, excessive generation of all these chemokines ad cytokines accelerates disease progress. Interleukin IL-10 is generated by T-helper-2 (Th2) and has antiviral activity; however, SARS-CoV-2 infection is capable of significantly inhibiting it (Zhang et al., 2020a).

Thus, patients contaminated with SARS-CoV-2 present raised serum IL-1β levels (Huang et al., 2020), which is a strong symptom of cell pyroptosis. This factor may indicate that cell pyroptosis induction is implicated in the pathogenesis of SARS-CoV-2infected patients. It is well-known that both non-classical and classical pyroptosis indication can trigger IL-1β release, a fact that should be further investigated in SARS-CoV-2-associated pneumonia patients. Besides, both leukopenia and lymphopenia are observed in pneumonia patients, most SARS-CoV-2-contaminated patients show lymphopenia, that likely indicates that lymphocytes may be susceptible to cell pyroptosis throughout infection processes.

Chen et al. (2020a) have found the same conduct in many patients with SARSCoV-2-associated pneumonia; nearly all patients who died presented lymphopenia (Durán and Favaro, 2020a; and references therein). Interestingly, Chang et al. (2020) reported that all assessed patients with confirmed SARS-CoV-2 diagnosis have recovered and presented scarcely elevated contents of inflammatory markers like the number of lymphocytes; all these facts were confirmed by Lipi and Plebani (2020) and Henry et al (2020). Besides, based on current data, SARS-CoV-2 presumably immunomodulatory effects leads to cell pyroptosis, mainly in lymphocytes, due to NLRP3 inflammasome induction. Steps involved in the induction of the signalling linking NLRP3, IL-18, IL-1β, and gasdermin D were suggested (Yang, 2020; Yang et al., 2020a).

A study review provided the pathophysiology of SARS-CoV-2 contamination and described the SARS-CoV-2/immune system interaction, as well as the sequential aid of dysfunctional immune responses to infection progression. Based on the current knowledge about coronavirus infections, the authors of the aforementioned study have pointed out the participation of these strategies in potential therapies focused on attacking viral infection and/or immunomodulation (Tay et al., 2020). Many immunosuppressive therapies contributed at limiting immune-mediated damage in COVID-19 patients are at different evolution stages.

Trials conducted with corticosteroids (e.g., prednisolone) to treat COVID-19 are currently in progress, although this class of therapy was not suggested during the 2003 SARS epidemic.

An assay at clinical trial level, focused on testing the effectiveness of tocilizumab, a IL-6 antagonist is also in progress; sarilumab is also under investigation. Many others clinical trials are studying the effects of targeting granulocyte–macrophage colony-stimulating factor (GM-CSF), incorporating the application of gimsilumab, lenzilumab and namilumab. Cytosorb is another complement therapy that operates by absorbing a wide spectrum of cytokines, PAMPs and DAMPs with the view to reduce their circulating levels and improve immunopathology. Thalidomide is a pharmaceutics with immunomodulatory qualities; it has also been effectively administered to patient with COVID-19.

Thus, two clinical trials have been recently implemented to test thalidomide potential to diminish lung injury. TNF (tumour necrosis factor) antagonism was indicated, although not tested, in SARS-CoV-contamination cases, but not in patients with COVID-19. An open-label, non-randomized study indicated that the combination of hydroxychloroquine (well known, antimalarial agent) and azithromycin (common antibiotic) might be useful to patients with acute COVID-19. While hydroxychloroquine's effect on direct virus suppression, as well as its anti-inflammatory and immunomodulatory activities are known, if these mechanisms play a role against COVID-19 remains unclear (Tay et al., 2020, and references therein). A scarcity of clinical information with ribavirin for SARSCoV-2 means its therapeutic function must be inferred from other nCoV information (Sander et al., 2020). Nitazoxanide was effective as antiviral activity *in vitro* against MERS and SARS-CoV-2 (Rossignol, 2016; Wang et al., 2020a).

Awaiting further evidence, immunodulatory effect and the antiviral activity and safety profile of nitazoxanide requires further investigating it as alternative treatment for SARS-CoV-2. Another pharmaceutical called ivermectin has also appeared in some studies. A phase-III clinical trial focused on investigating ivermectin effectiveness against dengue virus infection was conducted in Thailand; results have shown that this pharmaceutical was safe and reduced the serum levels of viral NS1 protein, although it did not show significant clinical benefit to the investigated patients (Yamasmith et al., 2018).

It is known that extensive cytokine release due to immune system's reaction to viral contamination can lead to cytokine explosion and sepsis, which may lead to death in approximately 30% of severe COVID-19 cases. Uncontrolled inflammation condition lead to multiple organ injuries, which, in their turn, may lead to organ failure, mainly in hepatic, renal and cardiac functions. Patients contaminated with SARS-CoV who evolved to renal failure have died. Contrary, patients whose recruited cells healed the lung contamination, showed immunological response retreat and were healed. Meanwhile, dysfunctional immune reaction was observed in some cases due to cytokine explosion aimed at regulating extensive inflammation. Critical COVID-19 patients in need of rigorous hospital care presented exacerbated parameters such as significantly high G-CSF (granulocyte colony-stimulating factor) blood plasma levels, interleukins, such as IL-2, 7 and 10, IP-10, MCP1 and MP1α (inflammatory protein 1α from macrophage) and NTF (tumour necrosis factor). The IL-6 cytokine levels in these cases were also high, which led to higher death than survival rates. Importantly, there was a wide macrophage content of inflammatory monocyte from FCN1+ in the Broncho-alveolar material extracted from individuals with serous, although not mild, COVID-19. Likewise, individuals at advanced disorder stage have shown significant incidence of inflammatory monocytes (CD14+CD16+) in their peripheral blood in comparison to patients with mild COVID19. These cellular systems release inflammatory cytokines and lead to cytokine explosion, incorporating MCP1, MIP1α, and IP-10 (Tay et al. 2020, and references therein).

Some of the main COVID-19 trials were carried out with the following compounds: Chloroquine, hydroxychloroquine, nitazoxanide, thalidomide, ivermectin, remdesivir and favipiravir (pro-drugs) and prednisolone/dexamethasone (Figure 1).

Chloroquine and Hydroxychloroquine

Chloroquine is a potent NLRP3 inflammasome-pathway inhibitor. Therefore, it can suppress mature IL-1β and IL-18 production and enhance the survival rates of patients with endotoxic shock by suppressing NLPR3 inflammasome activation, as well as IL-1β and IL-18 maturation. In addition, the inhibitory process of chloroquine on NLRP3 inflammasome activation comprises the inhibition of NLRP3, IL-1β, and IL-18 transcription by restricting in NF-κB and MAPK pathways, as well as the inhibition of NLRP3 complex assembly by restraining K+ efflux and ASC speck formation (see Figure 2).These results indicate that chloroquine might be an auspicious therapy against LPS-induced endotoxin shock and other type of disease depending of NLRP3 inflammasome-related diseases (Chen et al., 2017). Hydroxychloroquine has anti-inflammatory activity on Th17-related cytokines (IL-6, 17, and -22) in healthy subjects, as well as in rheumatoid arthritis (RA) systemic andlupus erythematosus (SLE) patients (da Silva et al., 2013).

According to Borba et al. (2020), high (600 mg x 2 day) and low (450 mg x 2 day) chloroquine doses delivered for 10 days, in association with azithromycin and oseltamivir, were not safe enough to assure the continuation of the study group. Chloroquine did not show any apparent benefit to patients' lethality rate. COVID-19 patients hospitalized in metropolitan New York, who was treated with hydroxychloroquine, azithromycin, or both, did not shown significant differences in in hospital mortality rate in comparison to patients who were not subjected to these treatments.

But, the interpretation of these observations may have been restricted by the observational design (Rosenberg et al., 2020). Based on another study conducted with hospitalized patients with COVID-19, hydroxychloroquine treatment was not related to either significantly lower or higher risk of patient intubation or death.

The main analysis did not find important association between hydroxychloroquine administration and patient intubation or death. Results in multiple sensitivity analyses were similar and it was necessary conducting randomized regulated trials with hydroxychloroquine in individuals with COVID-19 infection (Geleris etal., 2020).However, France, Belgium and Italy and recently USA have recently expressed their objection about administration of hydroxychloroquine to treat COVID-19 cases and banned its use. All of these countries were not the first to reject the use of this medicine. The World Health Organization (WHO) excluded the global trial with hydroxychloroquine a few days ago due to safety concerns. Similarly, Oxford University has paused a global trial a week after its implementation[1] Nowadays, confusing data about hospital treatment were reported including a retracted paper posteriorly by Lancet (Mehra et al., 2020) and reopened the controversy about chloroquine use. However, health professionals are aware that this pharmaceutical is not safe to be used in an indiscriminate manner.

Nitazoxanide

Since nitazoxanide uncouples mitochondrial electron transport, the current study took into consideration the chance that mitochondrial effects, apart from DNA leakage, might intervene the antiviral responses. The defeat of pan-caspase inhibitor z-VAD (Selleckchem) in blocking nitazoxanide antiviral activities debates against pyroptosis or apoptosis; both of them can be interced by mitochondrial factors and are key elements of the nitazoxanide mechanism (Hickson et al., 2018). Besides to its antiviral activity (Antony et al., 2020), nitazoxanide suppress the generation of pro-inflammatory cytokines TNF, IL-2, IL-4, I-5, IL-6, IL-8 and IL10 in peripheral blood mononuclear cells (PBMCs). Mice subjected to oral administration of nitazoxanide *in vivo* have reduced plasma IL-6 levels by 90% in comparison to vehicle treated mice. The relevancy of all of the data to humans has not yet been investigated, however, these information indicate that nitazoxanide can enhance outcomes in patients infected with MERS-CoV by inhibiting the overproduction of pro-inflammatory cytokines such as IL-6 (Rossignol et al., 2016). Clinical trials focused on investigating monotherapy with nitazoxanide are currently in progress (Clinical Trials. gov. Identifier NCT04348409-Aciduz-Brazil; NCT04343248-Romak Lab.-USA and NCT04359680-Romak Lab.-USA).

Thalidomide

Studies conducted *in vitro* or *in vivo* have shown that thalidomide damages the synthesis of TNF-α (tumour necrosis factor alpha). It raises peripheral blood CD8+ T cells, IL-12 levels, IFN-γ generation and cytotoxic activity. According to the study *in vitro* by Tabata et al. (2015), thalidomide was capable of decreasing IL-1β and IL-6 expression in human lung epithelial cells and helped

---

[1] (https://www.wionews.com/world/covid-19-france-italy-and-belgium-ban-usage-ofhydroxychloroquine-301449) (accessed on May 28th, 2020).

preventing emphysema. A study conducted with animals has shown that thalidomide notably mitigated pulmonary fibrosis, oxidative stress and inflammation in mice's lungs.

Similarly, thalidomide has decreased the production of TNF-α, IL-1β, IL-6, and modifying growth factor-β.Dogs with transplanted lung had better corticosteroids

in early postoperative immunosuppression after the transplantation due to decreased incidence of pneumonia. Besides, it was published that thalidomide had anti-fibrotic effects against bleomycin-induced pulmonary fibrosis in rats. The anti-inflammatory activity of thalidomide on lung injury induced by H1N1 influenza virus in mice have shown that thalidomide significantly improved their survival rate, reduced the infiltration of inflammatory cells, as well as cytokine (e.g., IL-6, TNF-α), and chemokine (chemokine ligand 5, C-X-C motif chemokine 10) levels, and inhibited p-NFκB p6 activation. A combination of thalidomide and low-dose glucocorticoid therapy against COVID-19 has shown beneficial results (Dastan et al., 2020; and references therein).Thalidomide has inhibited pro-inflammatory cytokine IL-1 secretion by human primary keratinocytes and monocytes in a dose-dependent manner. Besides, this pharmaceutical also diminished the liberation of pro-angiogenic growth factor FGF2 and of several other proteins.

The secretion of all these proteins demands caspase-1 activity. Proteolytic enzyme itself is activated by multimeric innate immune complexes called inflammasomes. Then, thalidomide has inhibitory effects on NLRP3 inflammasome, since it blocks caspase-1activity (Keller et al., 2009; Thi and Hong, 2017).A positive-COVID-19 patient treated with lopinavir/ritonavir and, subsequently, with thalidomide, did not show any results.

Laboratorial analyses showed a high increased C-reactive protein (CRP) level, and cytokine levels (interleukin IL-6, IL-10 and interferon (IFN)-γ),as well as significantly decreased T cell absolute value (including CD4 + T cells, CD8 + T cells,NK cells and B cells). Six days after thalidomide treatment implementation, IL-6, IL-10 and IFN-γ cytokine levels returned to the normal range. Besides its ability to inhibit cytokine release and regulate immune functions, thalidomide can be used to relax COVID-19 patients for reducing their oxygen consumption and alleviate digestive symptoms. Therefore, thalidomide may shed new light on an adjuvant treatment strategy focused on this potentially lethal viral disease. It is necessary conducting a randomized controlled trial focused on investigating the effectiveness of thalidomide use, in association with low-dose glucocorticoid therapy, to treat COVID-19 pneumonia (Chen et al., 2020). Actually, a clinical trial is lready in course.[1]

Methylprednisolone and Dexamethasone

inhaled corticosteroids diminish the number of inflammatory cells (e.g., eosinophils, T-lymphocytes, mast and dendritic cells) at cellular level in any disease affecting individuals' airways.

Corticosteroid activity relies on suppressing the recruitment of inflammatory cells in patients' airways by inhibiting the generation of chemotactic intermediates and adherence molecules and by suppressing the subsistence of inflammatory cells (e.g., T-lymphocytes, eosinophils, mast cells) in the airways. Epithelial cells are the major action site of inhaled corticosteroids (ICS), since they can inhibit several activated inflammatory genes in airway epithelial cells and the epithelial unity is recovered by normal ICS (Figure 3). Mucosal inflammation is overall rapidly inhibited due to significant reduction in the number of perceptible eosinophils within six hours; such an inhibition

---

[1] (Clinical trial.gov:NCT04273529-China).

is linked to reduced airway hyper responsiveness. The reversal of this stage may take months to reach a threshold that may indicate improved structural changes in airways (Barnes, 2010).

Overall, corticosteroids dissipate through the cell membrane and link to glucocorticoid receptors (GRα) in the cytoplasm; next they translocate to the nucleus cell and trigger molecular effects. A GR homodimer is linked to a GRE (glucocorticoid response element) located in the promotor region of genes susceptible to steroids; this association is connected, or not, to gene transcription.

Genes activated by corticosteroids comprise genes encoding anti-inflammatory proteins such as secretory leukoprotease inhibitor, β2-adrenergic receptors and the mitogen-activated protein kinase phosphatase1 (MKP-1), which suppresses MAP kinase routes.

These outcomes may enable the anti-inflammatory activity of corticosteroids. GR association with negative GREs may inhibit gene transcription; assumingly, this inhibition may play a key role in influencing many of the collateral effects caused by corticosteroids (Barnes, 2010). Systemic treatments with glucocorticoids were largely applied to patients infected with coronavirus (SARS-COV) who developed severe respiratory complications during the SARS epidemic in 2003.

The administration of pulsed high-dose methylprednisolone enabled clinical enhancement in SARS patients. A female patient subjected to bone marrow transplant due to acute myeloid leukemia was infected with SARS; she was subjected to treatment with oral prednisolone and ribavirin, which improved her lymphopenia, modified transaminases, chest X-ray and computed tomography results very fast (Lam et al., 2004). Interleukin-8, monocyte chemoattractant protein-1 and Th1 chemokine interferon-g-inducible protein-10 levels have decreased after 5-8 days of glucocorticoid therapy. Nevertheless, some data showed that pulsed doses of methylprednisolone presented high-risk factor associated with increased 30-day mortality. Besides, an observational study has shown that glucocorticoid treatment application in patients with MERS (Middle East respiratory syndrome coronavirus MERS-CoV) was associated to delay respiratory syndrome.

However, the clinical therapeutics of systemic glucocorticoid therapy in patients with COVID-19 is not actually evident; thus, the systemic use of glucocorticoids, or not, in severe COVID-19 cases demands further investigation (Qin et al., 2020, and references therein). However, a recent study has shown that glucocorticoids used in combination with antibiotics have significantly diminished the viral infection. In this case, patients with severe COVID-19 pneumonia presented significantly increased number of inflammatory markers such as C-reactive protein (CRP), IL-6 and ferro protein (FER), which corresponded to the inflammatory reaction stage.

Wang et al. (2020b) suggested that once the secondary infection happens in patients with severe COVID-19 pneumonia, besides methylprednisolone doses, full-dose antibacterial drugs (e.g. cephalosporin) should be immediately added to the treatment. Data have shown that this treatment was related to faster decrease in CRP and IL-6. Thus, early low-dose and short-term administration of corticosteroids was associated in patients with acute COVID-19 pneumonia with faster progress of clinical symptoms.

In addition, methylprednisolone has been used in COVID19 patients, in association with antibiotics, oseltamivir and oxygen therapy (Huang et al., 2020; Rosa and Santos, 2020). However, a recent study has shown that prednisolone was not capable of suppressing viral SARS-CoV-2 growth in infected VeroE6/TMPRSS2 cells. Moreover, another corticosteroid called ciclesonide, which is an inactive prodrug and activated by esterase in the lung to the metabolite des-ciclesonide, was highly effective in treating SARS-CoV-2 infection.

These data strongly indicate that ciclesonide activity was specific to coronavirus; the authors of the aforementioned study have suggested that ciclesonide is a promising pharmaceutical to treat MERS or COVID-19 patients (Matsuyama et al., 2020).Actually, clinical trials are already in course[1] was able to prevent death in one over eight ventilated COVID-19 patients and one over of 25 patients receiving oxygen only. Over 11,500 patients have been enrolled from over 175 National Health Service (NHS) hospitals in the UK[2] [3]. This study showed that dexamethasone diminished deaths by one-third in ventilated patients and by one fifth in patients receiving only oxygen. The medical staff implied that based on these outcomes, one death could be avoided by treatment of about eight ventilated patients or near 25 patients requiring oxygen alone. Actually, there are several clinical trials in recruiting phase (NCT04325061Spain; NCT04347980-France; NCT04395105-Argentina; NCT 04344730-Fance; NCT04327401-Brazil).

RNA-Dependent RNA Polymerase

RNA-dependent RNA polymerase (RdRp) is another possible target against SARS-CoV-2. It is so, because SARS-CoV-2 is certainly a strand RNA virus, whose reproduction is based on a multiple subunit replication or/and transcription complex of viral unstructured proteins (nsp) (Ziebuhr, 2005). The main element of this structure is a subunit of catalytic activity (nsp12) of an RNA, which is RNA polymerase-dependent (RdRp) (Ahn et al., 2012; Te Velthus et al., 2010).

It was observed that nsp12 has insignificant activity and that its functions need supplementary factors such as nsp7 and nsp8 (Subissi et al., 2014; Kirchdoerfer and Ward, 2019), which lead to increased RdRp scaffold binding and treatability. Remdesivir is one of the best antiviral targeting RdRps (Wang et al., 2020c; Holshue et al., 2020; Warren et al., 2016); this pro-drug is transformed into an active product derivative (triphosphate) form (RTP) in cells (Siegelet al., 2017). Allstructures related to RdRp were ofrigorous structural biological achievements (Kirchdoerfer and Ward, 2019; Zhai et al., 2005; Peti et al., 2005; Johnson et al., 2010; Gao et al., 2020), make available the complete design of the RdRp complex (Yin et al., 2020). In order to understand the actual and in course antiviral activity against COVID-19 it will be an analysis of the actual pharmaceutics using on this disease.

Remdesivir

Remdesivir was effective against SARS and MERS in murine models (Holshue et al., 2020). It is an RNA polymerase-dependent RNA antagonist that leads to early viral RNA termination (Sheahan et al., 2017); this prodrug must undergo metabolization to enable its active form of GS-441524-triphospahate. Remdesivir presented excellent outcome during the West African Ebola virus epidemic (2013–2016) and the Kivu Ebola epidemic (2018) (Warren et al., 2015), a fact that also made this drug tested against COVID-19 (Wang et al., 2020b). Remdesivir (RDV) and IFN-β have higher antiviral activity than lopinavir (LPV) and ritonavir (RTV) *in vitro*. Both prophylactic and therapeutic remdesivir applications have improved the pulmonary function, as well as reduced lung viral loads and severe lung pathology in mice.

On the other hand, prophylactic LPV/RTV-IFN-β treatment has slightly reduced viral loads, although without affecting other disease parameters in the investigated model. Therapeutic

---

[1] (Clinical trial.gov NCT04323592Italy; NCT04343729-Brazil. Recently, a clinical trial (randomized) has demonstrated that a low-price steroid named dexamethasone (low-dose)

[2] (https://www.recoverytrial.net/files/recovery_dexamethasone_statement_ 160620_v2final.pdf)

[3] (Clinical trial gov.: NCT04381936)

LPV/RTV-IFN-β has enhanced the pulmonary function but it did not diminish virus replication or severe lung pathology in mice. This outcome provided evidence *in vivo* of remdesivir potential to treat MERS-CoV infections (Sheahan et a., 2020).SARS-CoV-2 replication needs viral RNA-dependent RNA polymerase (RdRp), which is a target of the antiviral drug called remdesivir.

The cryo-EM structure of the SARS-CoV-2 RdRp was reported either in its apo-form or in the complex with 50-base template-primer RNA and remdesivir can be a good solution under these conditions. This complex structure shows that the partial double-stranded RNA template is introduced in the central channel of the RdRp, where remdesivir is covalently added to the primer strand at the first replicated base pair and terminates the chain elongation. This structure provides critical insights about the viral RNA replication mechanism and a rational model for drug design to treat viral infections (Yin et al., 2020).

A clinical trial with double-blind, placebo-controlled and randomized of intravenous remdesivir was recently conducted with adult COVID-19 patients hospitalized with confirm of lower respiratory tract implication. All patients were randomly assigned to accept either remdesivir or placebo for up to 10 days. The total of 1,063 patients underwent randomization (ClinicalTrials.gov: NCT04280705-USA). Data and safety monitoring board advised early unblinding the results based on analysis findings that showed shortened recovery time in the remdesivir group. Initial results of 1,059 patients (538 treated with remdesivir and 521 with placebo) based on data available after randomization have indicated that individuals who received remdesivir recorded median recovery time of 11 days, whereas those who received placebo recorded median recovery time of 15 days. Based on Kaplan Meier's estimates for 14 days, remdesivir and placebo recorded 7.1% and 11.9% patient mortality, respectively. Severe adverse events were reported in the remdesivir (21.1%) and placebo (27.0%) groups subjected to randomization.

Thus, remdesivir was more effective than placebo in shortening the recovery time in adult COVID-19 individuals hospitalized with evidence of lower respiratory tract involvement. However, given the high mortality rate observed despite remdesivir use, it is clear that treatments with antiviral drug alone are not likely to be sufficient against COVID-19 (Wang et al., 2020; Beigel et al., 2020).

A randomized, double-blind, placebo-controlled, multicentre trial conducted in China with 237 patients with laboratory-confirmed SARS-CoV-2 infection (ClinicalTrials.gov.: NCT04257656China) has observed faster clinical improvement; however, adverse events were also reported in 102 (66%) of 155 remdesivir recipients and in 50 (64%) of 78 placebo recipients. Remdesivir treatment was interrupted early in 18 (12%) patients because of adverse events versus four (5%) patients who stopped placebo treatment early. The authors of the aforementioned study inferred that remdesivir was not related to statistically significant clinical benefits. However, further studies should be conducted in order to confirm the shorter time necessary for individuals subjected to early remdesivir treatment to present clinical improvement (Wang et al., 2020c).Actually, clinical trials are already in course (ClinicalTrials.gov Identifier: NCT04365725-France; NCT04280705-USA; NCT04302766-USA).

Avifavir (Favipiravir)

Favipiravir (Fig.1) has been authorized as therapy to treat influenza in Japan. But, only suggested for new influenza (strains causing acute disease) instead than seasonal influenza (Shiraki and Daikoku, 2020).The action´s mechanism is believe to be associated to the selective suppress of viral RNA-dependent RNA polymerase (Jin et al., 2013).

Baranovivh et al. (2013) suggested that favipiravir caused lethal RNA transversion mutations, causing a no-viable viral phenotype (Baranovich et al., 2013). Favipiravir is a pro-drug which is metabolized to its reactive form, favipiravir-ribofuranosyl-5'-triphosphate (favipiravir-RTP), usable in both intravenous and oral formulations (Guedj et al., 2028). HGPRT (human hypoxanthine guanine phosphoribosyl-transferase) is presumed to play a crucial role in this activation activity. Interesting, that favipiravir acts as non-inhibitor of RNA or DNA synthesis in mammalian cells and is non-toxic to them. From 2014 is used in Japan, but, favipiravir has not been demonstrated to be efficient in primary human airway cells, causing doubt on its efficiency in influenza therapy (Yoon et al., 2018) In 2020, favipiravir was used as treatment in China in emergent COVID-19 (Li and De Clercq, 2020) [1]

A study on 80 patients comparing the use of lopinavir/ritonavir demonstrated that it diminished viral clearance period, and that 91% of patients had enhanced CT scans with almost no side effects. Unfortunately, this was not randomized double-blinded and placebo-controlled trial (Cai et al., 2020; Dong et al., 2020). Recently, the favipiravir has been approved for use in clinical trials of coronavirus disease in China.[2]Italy, in March 2020,Italy authorized favipiravir for research use against COVID19 and has initiated trials in three locals most involved in the contamination.[3] There are in progress to initiate in three hospitals in Massachusetts, USA , trials with favipiravir[4].

In a first week of May 2020, a trial is initiating in London, UK.[5] The favipiravir was also approved for the therapy of COVID-19 in the hospital installations in Russia on May 29, 2020, after taking place open-label randomized clinical trial had recruited 60 patients on.

As claimed by the government clinical trial registry as COVID-FPR-01 is predicted to enroll 390 patients overall and end by December 31, 2020. On May 30, 2020, the Russian Health Ministry authorized a generic form of favipiravir called Avifavir.Russian Direct Investment Fund (RDIF) supported the exploration of Avifavir and established it high efficiency in the first stage of clinical trials [6][7] Then, avifavir or favipiravir appears as a potential to treat COVID-19 in Russia and probably soon in England, Italy and USA.

Nucleocytoplasmic Trafficking of Viral Proteins Ivermectin

Protein signal-dependent targeting inside and outside the nucleus is regulated by components belonging to the importin (IMP) family of transport receptors, which are capable of identifying targeting signals in a load protein and of mediating transit over the complexes of nuclear pores in nuclear wrapping. This process is essential to activate cell division and differentiation; however, it is also crucial for viral reproduction and disease development. The phosphorylation process plays a key role in regulating viral protein nucleocytoplasmic trafficking and other post-translational transformations. Nucleocytoplasmic trafficking mechanisms are modulated by IMPs/EXPs (export members of the IMPβ superfamily) levels and distribution, as well as by the number and/or

---

[1] (https://www.fujifilmamericas.com.br/press/news/display_news? newsID=881796).

[2] (https://global.chinadaily.com.cn/a/202002/17/ WS5e49efc2a310128217277fa3.html)

[3] (https://www.ilfattoquotidiano.it/2020/03/22/coronavirus-il-veneto-sperimentalantivirale-giapponese-favipiravir-ma-laifa-ci-sono-scarse-evidenze-scientifiche-suefficacia/5745426/).

[4] (https://advances.massgeneral.org/research-and-innovation/article.aspx?id= 1171)

[5] (https://www.standard.co.uk/news/uk/uk-coronavirus-patients-trialjapanese-covid19-drug-a4429731.html)

[6] (https://www.bnnbloomberg.ca/russian-health-ministry-approves-anti-coronavirus-drugavifavir-1.1443601);

[7] https://www.reuters.com/article/ us-health-coronavirus-russiacases/russia-plans-coronavirus-vaccine-clinical-trials-in-two-weeks-reportidUSKBN2360BJ).

components of nuclear pore complexes (NPCs). One of the most investigated nuclear transport modulation mechanisms refers to the phosphorylation process near the NLS/NES (nuclear localization signal/nuclear export signal) and to change identification through IMP/EXP; however, transformations such as esterification (e.g., acetylation, ubiquitinoylation, among others) have also been reported to modulate the nucleocytoplasmic trafficking of cellular proteins (e.g., p53) and tumoUr suppressors (p110[Rb]), survivin, PTEN (phosphatase and tensin homolog on chromosome 10), nuclear factor NF-κB and MEMO (NF-κB essential modulator).

It is clear that viral proteins are often post-translationally transformed, and fully incorporate the action of cyclindependent kinases(CDKs), which account for the cell cycle-dependent regulation of nucleocytoplasmic trafficking (Fulcher and Jans, 2011; and references therein). Ivermectin was the central point of a phase-III clinical trial conducted to investigate dengue virus (DENV) infection in Thailand in 2014–2017;results have shown that a single oral dose a day was safe and significantly reduced serum viral NS1 protein levels, although it did not lead to changes in viremia or presented clinical benefits (Yamasmith et al., 2018).

A study has demonstrated that ivermectin was capable of dissociating the preformed IMPα/β1 heterodimer, beside avoiding its generation by linking to the IMPα armadillo (ARM) repeat domain to enable IMPα thermal stability and α-helicity. Ivermectin has also inhibited a non-structured protein 5 deriving from dengue virus (NS5)-IMPα association in cell context (Yang et al., 2020). Caly et al. (2020) have shown that ivermectin had antiviral action against SARS-CoV-2 clinical isolate *in vitro*; a single dose was capable of controlling viral replication within 24–48 h under that condition. It was hypothesized that it may have happened due to the inhibition of IMPα/β1-mediated nuclear import of viral proteins, as demonstrated in other RNA viruses. The confirmation of this mechanism in the case of SARS-CoV-2, and the identification of the specific SARS-CoV-2 and/or affected host constituent(s), is relevant topics to be investigated in future studies in this field (Figure 4).

According to Patel et al. (2020), the application of 150 μg/kg of ivermectin to patients after mechanical ventilation application has potential to diminish hospitalization time and to improve survival rates in comparison to conventional treatments. Unfortunately, this report did not take into consideration comorbidities that could lead to these results. Thus, if ivermectin really provided these clinical findings, it would suggest that the study *in vitro* conducted by Caly et al. (2020) did not correlate to low amounts of the drug at the action site in humans.

A clinical study with ivermectin must follow well controlled clinical dose-response at low dose (dose approved) and at dose higher than that of placebo in COVID-19 patients (Schmith et al, 2020). Ivermectin doses up to 120 mg have only been applied to a small number of patients (Guzzo et al., 2002). Daily ivermectin applications at the approved dose (200 μg/kg) for longer periods (e.g., 14 days) have only been investigated in case of severe infections where non-approved subcutaneous formulation was applied (Turner et al., 2005). Thus, if higher doses are applied on a weekly basis, or other administration method is adopted, patients should be closely monitored. Therefore, an interesting solution would lie on investigating whether ivermectin-inhaled therapy is realistic. Unfortunately, only one non-clinical research on inhaled ivermectin has been reported and presented NOAEL (no-observed-adverse-effect level) equal to 380 mg/m³ after 1 month of treatment(Ji et al., 2016).

The literature lacks studies focused on investigating this administration route in humans. Experts must evaluate whether ivermectin has the ideal properties for inhalation treatments and whether it does not present any risk that might limit this application route. Therefore, Schmith et al. (2020) suggested that the outcomes observed in the study by Caly et al. (2020) stablished the opportunity for an interdisciplinary collaboration to help better understand the best likelihood of achievement in ivermectin-based therapy, before the application of a less-than-ideal dose in clinical studies. Actually, clinical trials are already in Couse (ClinicalTrials.gov Identifier: NCT04381884-Argentina; NCT04390022-Spain; NCT04392713-Pakistan; NCT04373824-India).

Final Remarks

Based on data analysed in the current study, it is clear that despite tremendous efforts to access a new and effective antiviral drug against SARS-CoV-2 in clinical trials conducted during the COVID-19 pandemic, an efficient antiviral drug has not yet been found. The problem observed in clinical trials carried out to research potential therapies against COVID-19 hampers both the requirement and ability to generate high-quality prove, even in the middle of the COVID-19 pandemic. Although there are different mechanisms capable of inhibiting or killing SARS-CoV-2 virus, it is possible believing that the scientific community will be able to find a successful pharmaceutical capable of finishing this pandemic. Once we get to fully know the pathogenesis of COVID-19, we will be able to select a compound capable of presenting efficient results *in vivo*, rather than *in vitro*. This, it is due to the projection of the activity from culture cells is negligible to animal and then worse to human. Thus, it is necessary developing a well-stablished protocol for clinical trials in order to find a new and safe antiviral drug.It is important emphasizing that,in march 2020, WHO made public plans to initiate a global "megatrial" named SOLIDARITY, based on a practice trial design, for to randomize attested cases into either basic care or 1 of 4 active therapy arms (chloroquines, lopinavir/ritonavir alone, or lopinavir/ ritonavir plus IFN-β) based on regional medicone availability (Kupferschmidt and Cohen, 2020).
It was a really interesting proposal at that time; however, unfortunately, all priorities have changed from March to June 2020 and it is necessary re-evaluating all these possibilities.

Acknowledgments

The authors would like to thank the São Paulo Research Council (FAPESP grant 2014/11154-1; 2018/10052-1), the Brazilian National Council for Scientific and Technological Development (CNPq grant 552120/2011-1) and Hospital Municipal de Paulínia, Paulínia-SP.

Financial Support: São Paulo Research Council (FAPESP grant 2014/11154-1; 2018/10052-1) and the Brazilian National Council for Scientific and Technological Development (CNPq grant 552120/2011-1).

Individual Collaboration: Nelson Durán: study design, bibliographic search, data analysis, interpretation of results, writing, review and approval of the final version of the manuscript.

Wagner J. Fávaro: study design, bibliographic search, data analysis, interpretation of results, writing, review and approval of the final version of the manuscript.

REFERENCES

Ahn. D.G, Choi, J.K., Taylor, D.R, *et al.* (2012).Biochemical characterization of a recombinant SARS coronavirus nsp12 RNA-dependent RNA polymerase capable of copying viral RNA templates. *Arch Virol* 2012; **157**: 2095-2104.

Antony, F., Vashi, Y., Morla, S. (2020). Therapeutic potential of Nitazoxanide against Newcastle disease virus: A possible modulation of host cytokines. *Cytokine* 2020;**131**: 155115.

Baranovich, T., Wong, S,S., Armstrong, J, et al.(2013).T-705 (favipiravir) induces lethal mutagenesis in influenza A H1N1 viruses *in vitro*. *J Virol* 2013; **87**: 3741–51

Barnes, P.J. (2010). Inhaled corticosteroids. *Pharmaceuticals* 2010; **3**: 514-540.

Beigel, J.H, Tomashek, K.M, Dodd, Ç.L.E, *et al.* (2020).Remdesivir for the treatment of COVID-19. *Preliminary report* May 22, 2020. Doi: 10.1056/NEJMoa2007764.

Borba, M.G.D,, Val, F.F.A, Sampaio, V.S., *et al.* (2020). Effect of high vs low doses of chloroquine diphosphate as adjunctive therapy for patients hospitalized with severe acute respiratory syndrome coronavirus 2 (SARS-CoV-2) infection: A randomized clinical trial. *JAMA Network Open* 2020; **3**: e208857.

Caly, L., Druce, J.D, Catton, M.G., *et al.* (2020).The FDA-approved drug ivermectin inhibits the replication of SARS-CoV-2 in vitro. *Antiviral Res* 2020; **178**: 1047872.

Chang, D., Lin, M., Wei, L, *et al.* (2020).Epidemiologic and clinical characteristics of novel coronavirus infections involving 13 patients outside Wuhan, China. *JAMA* 2020; **323**: 1092-1093.

Cai, Q., Yang, M., Liu, D., et al. (2020).Experimental treatment with favipiravir for COVID-19: An open-label control study. *Engineering* 2020; doi:10.1016/j.eng.2020.03.007.

Chen, S.X, Wang, N., Zhu, Y. *et al.* (2020). The antimalarial chloroquine suppresses LPS-induced NLRP3 inflammasome activation and confers protection against murine endotoxic. *Mediat Inflamm* 2017; **2017**: Article ID 6543237.

Chen, C., Qi, F., Shi, K., *et al.*(2020). Thalidomide combined with low-dose glucocorticoid in the treatment of COVID-19 Pneumonia. *Preprints* 2020b; **2020:** 2020020395 .

Chen, N., Zhou, M., Dong, X., *et al.* (2020). Epidemiological and clinical characteristics of 99 cases of 2019 novel coronavirus pneumonia in Wuhan, China: A descriptive study. *Lancet* 2020a; **395**: 507-513.

da Silva, J.C. Mariz. H.A, da Rocha Júnior, L.F. *et al.*(2013).Hydroxychloroquine decreases Th17- related cytokines in systemic lupus erythematosus and rheumatoid arthritis patients. *Clinics* 2013; **68**:766-771.

Dastan, F., Tabarsi., P. Marjani, M. *et al.* (2020).Thalidomide against Coronavirus Disease 2019 (COVID-19): A medicine with a thousand faces.*Iran J Pharm Res* 2020; **19**: 1-2.

Dong, L., Hu, S., Gao, J. (2020).Discovering drugs to treat coronavirus disease 2019 (COVID19). *Drug Discov Ther* 2020; **14:** 58–60.

Durán, N., Fávaro, W.J. (2020) Pyroptosis in cancer cells and its perspectives in nanomedicine: A mini review. *Inter J Med Rev* 2020a; Submitted.

Durán, N., Fávaro, W.J.(2020). Pyroptosis: Physiological roles in viral infection. *medRxiv Preprint* 2020b; Submitted.

Fulcher, A.J. Jans, D.A. (2020).Regulation of nucleocytoplasmic trafficking of viral proteins: An integral role in pathogenesis? *Biochim Biophys Acta* 2011; **1813**: 2176-2190.

Geleris. J, Sun, Y., Platt. J. *et al.* (2020). Observational study of hydroxychloroquine in hospitalized patients with COVID-19. *N Engl J Med* 2020; DOI: 10.1056/NEJMoa2012410

Gao, Y., Yan, L., Huang, Y. *et al.* (2020).Structure of the RNA-dependent RNA polymerase from COVID-19 virus. *Science* 2020. Doi: 10.1126/science.abb7498.

Guedj, J., Piorkowski, G., Jacquot, F., et al. (2018). Antiviral efficacy of favipiravir against Ebola virus: A translational study in cynomolgus macaques. *PLOS Med* 2018; **15**: e1002535.

Guzzo, C.A., Furtek, C.I, Porras, A.G., *et al.* (2020).Safety, tolerability, and pharmacokinetics of escalating high doses of ivermectin in healthy adult subjects. *J Clin Pharmacol*. 2020; **42**: 1122-1133.

Henry, B.M, de Oliveira, M.H.S, Benoit, S., *et al.* (2020). Hematologic, biochemical and immune biomarker abnormalities associated with severe illness and mortality in coronavirus disease 2019 (COVID-19): A meta-analysis. *Clin Chem Lab Med* 2020; https://doi.org/10.1515/cclm-2020-0369.

Hickson, S.E., Margineantua, D., Hockenbery, D.N., *et al.* (2018).Inhibition of vaccinia virus replication by nitazoxanide. *Virology* 2018; **518**: 398-405.

Holshue, M.L., DeBolt, C., Lindquist, S, *et al.* (2020).First case of 2019 novel coronavirus in the United States. *N Engl J Med* 2020; **382:** 929-936.

Jin. Z., Smith, LK., Rajwanshi, V.K., et al. (2013). The ambiguous base-pairing and high substrate efficiency of T-705 (Favipiravir) Ribofuranosyl 5'-triphosphate towards influenza A virus polymerase. *PLOS One* 2013; **8**: e68347.

Johnson, M.A., Jaudzems, K., Wüthrich, K. N.M.R Structure of the SARS-CoV Nonstructural Protein 7 in Solution at pH 6.5. *J Mol. Biol*2010; **402**, 619-628.

Huang, C., Wang, Y.,Li X, *et al.* (2020). Clinical features of patients infected with 2019 novel coronavirus in Wuhan, China. *Lancet* 2020; **395**: 497-506.

Jakobsen, M.R., Bak, R.O., Andersen, A, *et al.*(2013).IFI16 senses DNA forms of the lentiviral replication cycle and controls HIV-1 replication. *Proc Nat Acad Sci USA*. 2013; **110**: E4571-4580.

Ji L, Cen J, Lin, S, *et al.*(2016).Study on the subacute inhalation toxicity of ivermectin TC in rats. *Chin J Comparative Med* 2016; **26**: 70-74.

Keller, M., Sollberger, G., Beer H-C. (2009). Thalidomide inhibits activation of caspase-1. *JImmunol* 2009; **183**: 5593-5599.

Kirchdoerfer, R.N, Ward, A.B. (2019). Structure of the SARS-CoV nsp12 polymerase bound to nsp7 and nsp8 co-factors. *Nat Commun* 2019; **10**: 2342.

Kupferschmidt, K., Cohen, J. (2020). WHO launches global megatrial of the four most promising coronavirus treatments. *Science*. Published March 22, 2020. Accessed March 23, 2020. https://www. sciencemag.org/news/2020/03/who-launchesglobal-megatrial-four-mostpromising-coronavirustreatments#. https://www.who.int/emergencies/diseases/novelcoronavirus-2019/global-research-on-novel-coronavirus-2019-ncov/solidarity-clinicaltrial-for-COVID-19-treatments

Lam, M.F, Ooi, G.C, Lam, B., *et al.* (2004). An indolent case of severe acute respiratory syndrome. *Am J Respir Crit Care Med* 2004; **169**:125-128

Li, G., De Clercq, E. (2020). Therapeutic options for the 2019 novel coronavirus (2019-nCoV). *Nat Rev Drug Discov* 2020; Doi:10.1038/d41573-020-00016-0

Liang, F., Zhang, F., Zhang, L., *et al.* (2020). The advances in pyroptosis initiated by infammasome in infammatory and immune diseases. *Inflamm Res* 2020; **69**:159-166.

Lippi,G.,Plebani, M. Laboratory abnormalities in patients with COVID-2019 infection. *Clin Chem Lab Med* 2020; https://doi.org/10.1515/cclm-2020-0198.

Ma, Y.Z., Jiang, J.X, Gao, Y., *et al.* (2018).Research progress of the relationship between pyroptosis and disease. *Am J Transl Res* 2018; **10**: 2213-2219.

Mali, S.N, Pratap, A.P., Thorat, B.R. (2020). The rise of new coronavirus infection (COVID-19): A recent update and potential therapeutic candidates. *Eurasian J Med Oncol* (EJMO)2020; **4**: 35-41.

Matsuyama, S., Kawase, M., Nao, N., *et al.* (2020). The inhaled corticosteroid ciclesonide blocks coronavirus RNA replication by targeting viral NSP15. *bioRxiv preprint* Doi: https://doi.org/10.1101/2020.03.11.987016.

Patel, A., Desai, S. (2020). Ivermectin in COVID-19 Related Critical Illness.. 2020; *SSRN* 2020; https://ssrncom/abstract=3570270 or http://dxdoiorg/102139/ssrn3570270.

Peti, E.W., Johnson, M.A., Herrmann, T, *et al.* (2005). Structural genomics of the severe acute respiratory syndrome coronavirus: Nuclear magnetic resonance structure of the protein nsP7. *J Virol* 2005; **79**: 12905-12913.

Qin Y-Y, Zhou Y-H, Lu Y-Q, *et al.* (2020). Effectiveness of glucocorticoid therapy in patients with severe coronavirus disease 2019: Protocol of a randomized controlled trial. *Chin Med J* 2020; Doi: 10.1097/CM9.0000000000000791.

Rosa, S.G.V, Santos, W.C. (2020). Clinical trials on drug repositioning for COVID-19 treatment. *Rev Panam Salud Publica*. 2020; **44**:e40. https://doi.org/10.26633/RPSP.2020.40

Rosenberg, E.S., Dufort, E.M., Udo, T., *et al.*(2020). Association of treatment with hydroxychloroquine or azithromycin with in-hospital mortality in patients with COVID19 in New York State. *JAMA* 2020; Doi:10.1001/jama.2020.8630

Rossignol, J.F. (2020). Nitazoxanide, a new drug candidate for the treatment of Middle East respiratory syndrome coronavirus. *J Infect Public Heal* 2016; **9**: 227-230.

Sanders, J.M., Monogue, M.L, Tomasz, Z., *et al.* (2020).Pharmacologic treatments for coronavirus disease 2019 (COVID-19): A review. *JAMA* 2020; **323**:1824-1836.

Schmith. V.D,Zhou, J.,Lohmer, L.RL. (2020).The Approved dose of ivermectin alone is not the ideal dose for the treatment of COVID-19. *medRxiv Preprint* doi: https://doi.org/10.1101/2020.04.21.20073262

Siegel, D., Hui, H.C, Doerffler E, *et al.* (2020).Discovery and synthesis of a phosphoramidate prodrug of a pyrrolo[2,1-f][triazin-4-amino] adenine Cnucleoside (GS-5734) for the treatment of Ebola and emerging viruses. *J Med Chem* 2017; **60**:1648-1661.

Sheahan, T.P., Sims, A. C, Leist, S.R, *et al.* (2020).Comparative therapeutic efficacy of remdesivir and combination lopinavir, ritonavir, and interferon beta against MERSCoV. *Nat Commun* 2020; **11**: 222.

Shiraki. K., Daikoku, T. (2020). Favipiravir, an anti-influenza drug against life-threatening RNA virus infections. *Pharmacol Ther* 2020; **209**:107512.

Sollberger, G., Strittmatter, G.E, Garstkiewicz, M. *et al.* (2014).Caspase-1: the inflammasome and beyond. *Innate Immun* 2014; **20**:115-125.

Subissi, L, Posthuma, C.C., Collet, A., *et al.* (2014). One severe acute respiratory syndrome coronavirus protein complex integrates processive RNA polymerase and exonuclease activities. *Proc Nat. Acad Sci USA* 2014; **111**: E3900-E3909.

Tabata, C., Tabata, R., Takahashi, Y., et al. (2015). Thalidomide prevents cigarette smoke extractinduced lung damage in mice. *Inter Immunopharmacol* 2015; 25: 511-517.

Tay, M.Z., Poh, C.M., Rénia, L., *et al.* (2020). The trinity of COVID-19: immunity, inflammation and intervention. *Nat Rev Innmunol*2020; https://doi.org/10.1038/s41577-020-0311-8.

Te Velthuis, A.J.W., Arnold, J.J., Cameron, C.E., *et al.* (2010). The RNA polymerase activity of SARScoronavirus nsp12 is primer dependent. *Nucleic Acids Res* 2010; **38**: 203-214 (2010).

Thi HTH, Hong., S. (2017). Inflammasome as a therapeutic target for cancer prevention and treatment review. *J Cancer Prev* 2017; **22**: 62-63.

Turner, S.A., Maclean, J.D., Fleckenstein, L, *et al.* (2005). Parenteral administration of ivermectin in a patient with disseminated strongyloidiasis. *Am J Trop Med Hyg* 2005; **73**: 911-914.

Wang, M, Cao, R., L. Zhang, L, *et al.* (2020). Remdesivir and chloroquine effectively inhibit the recently emerged novel coronavirus (2019-nCoV) in vitro. *Cell Res* 2020; **30**: 269-271.

Wang, M., Cao, R., Zhang ,L, *et al.* (2020).Remdesivir and chloroquine effectively inhibit the recently emerged novel coronavirus (2019-nCoV) *in vitro*. *Cell Res* 2020a; **30**: 269-271

Wang, Y., Jiang, W., He, Q, *et al.* (2020). A retrospective cohort study of methylprednisolone therapy in severe patients with COVID-19 pneumonia. *Signal Transduc Target Ther* 2020b; **5**: 57

Wang, Y., Zhang, D., Du, G. *et al.* (2020). Remdesivir in adults with severe COVID-19: a randomised, double-blind, placebo-controlled, multicentre trial. *Lancet* 2020c; **395**: 1569-1578.

Warren, T., Jordan, R., Lo, M., *et al.* (2015).Nucleotide prodrug GS-5734 is a broad-spectrum filovirus inhibitor that provides complete therapeutic protection against the development of Ebola virus disease (EVD) in infected non-human primates. *Open Forum Infect Dis 2* (Suppl. 1). 2015; LB-2. https://doi.org/10.1093/ofid/ofv130.02.

Warren, T.K., Jordan, R., Lo, M.K., *et al.* (2016).Therapeutic efficacy of the small molecule GS-5734 against Ebola virus in rhesus monkeys. *Nature* 2016; **531**: 381-385.

Yamasnith, E, Saleh-arong, F.A, Aviruntan, P, *et al.* (2018). Efficacy and safety ofivermectin against dengue infection: a phase III, randomized, double-blind, placebo-controlled trial, In: *The 34th Annual Meeting The Royal College of Physicians of Thailand*, Internal Medicine and One Health. 2018, Pattaya, Chonburi, Thailand.

Yang, M. Cell(2020). Pyroptosis, a potential pathogenic mechanism of 2019-nCoV Infection *SSRN,* 2020 ;https://ssrn.com/abstract=3527420; http://dx.doi.org/10.2139/ssrn. 3527420.

Yang, Y., Peng, F., Wang, R., *et al.* (2020). The deadly coronaviruses: The 2003 SARS pandemic and the 2020 novel coronavirus epidemic in China. *J Autoimmun* 2020a; **109**: 102434.

Yang, S.N.Y, Atkinson, C., Wang, C.,*et al.* (2020). The broad spectrum antiviral ivermectin targets the host nuclear transport importin $\alpha/\beta1$ heterodimer. *Antiviral Res* 2020b; **177**: 104760.

Yin, W., Mao, C., Luan, X., *et al.* (2020).Structural basis for inhibition of the RNA-dependent RNA polymerase from SARS-CoV-2 by remdesivir. *Science* 2020; Doi: 10.1126/science.abc1560.

Yoon, J.J. Toots M, Lee S, et al. (2018).Orally efficacious broad-spectrum ribonucleoside analog inhibitor of influenza and respiratory syncytial viruses. *Antimicrob AgentsChemother* 2018; **62**: e00766–18.

Zeng, C., Wang, R., Tan, H. (2019). Role of pyroptosis in cardiovascular diseases and its therapeutic implications. *Inter J Biol Sci* 2019; **15**:1345-1357.

Ziebuhr, J. (2005). The coronavirus replicase. *Curr Top Microbiol Immunol*2005; **287**: 57-94.

Zhai, Y., Sun, F., Li X, *et al.* (2005).Insights into SARS-CoV transcription and replication from the structure of the nsp7-nsp8 hexadecamer. *Nat Struct Mol Biol*2005; **12**: 980-986.

Zhang, R., Wang, X., Ni, L, *et al.* (2020). COVID-19: Melatonin as a potential adjuvant treatment. *Life Sci.* 2020a; **250**: 117583.

Zhao, C. Zhao, W. (2020).NLRP3 Inflammasome: A key player in antiviral responses. *Front Immunol* 2020; **11**:211 (and reference therein).

FIGURES

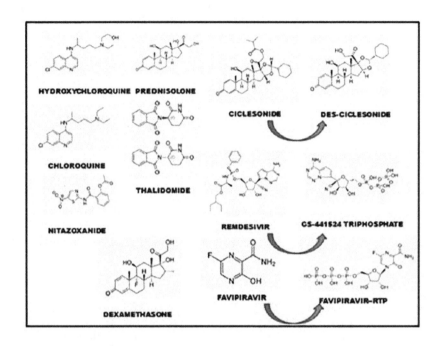

Figure 1. Potential antiviral pharmaceutics.

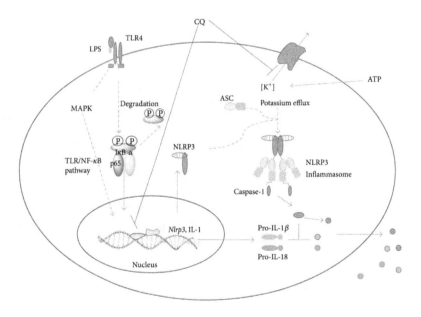

Figure 2. The proposed mechanism of Chloroquine for the inhibition of NLRP3 inflammasome activation (extracted from ref. Chen et al., 2017 and under Creative Commons Attribution Licenseapproved by Hindawi).

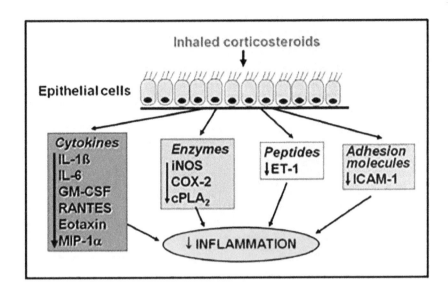

Figure 3. Inhaled corticosteroids may inhibit the transcription of several inflammatory genes in airway epithelial cells and thus reduce inflammation in the airway wall. GMCSF = granulocyte-macrophage colony stimulating factor; IL-1 = interleukin-1; RANTES = regulated on activation, normal T cell expressed and secreted; Eotaxin = potent and selective chemoattractant for eosinophils; MIP-1α = macrophage inflammatory protein; iNOS = inducible nitric oxide synthase; COX-2 = inducible cyclooxygenase; cPLA2 = cytoplasmic phospholipase A2; ET = endothelin; ICAM = intercellular adhesion molecule (extracted from ref. Barnes, 2010; authorized by MDPI (Basel, Switzerland- underCreative Commons Attribution license) .

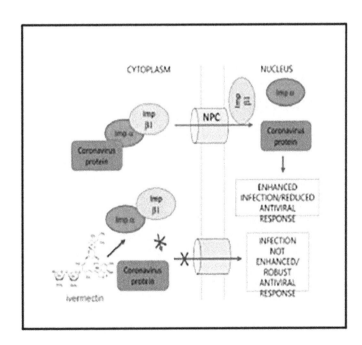

Figure 4. Ivermectin is a potent inhibitor of the SARS-CoV-2 clinical isolate Australia/VIC01/2020. Vero/hSLAM cells were in infected with SARS-CoV-2 clinical isolate Australia/VIC01/2020 (MOI = 0.1) for 2 h prior to addition of vehicle (DMSO) or Ivermectin at the indicated concentrations. Samples were taken at 0–3 days post infection for quantitation of viral load using real-time PCR of cell associated virus (A) or supernatant (B). IC50 values were determined in subsequent experiments at 48 h post infection using the indicated concentrations of Ivermectin (treated at 2 h post infection as per A/B). Triplicate real-time PCR analysis was performed on cell associated virus (C/E) or supernatant (D/F) using probes against either the SARS-CoV-2 E (C/D) or RdRp (E/F) genes. Results represent mean ± SD (n = 3). 3 parameter dose response curves were fitted using GraphPad prism to determine IC50 values (indicated). G. Schematic of ivermectin's proposed antiviral action on coronavirus. IMPα/β1 binds to the coronavirus cargo protein in the cytoplasm (top) and translocates it through the nuclear pore complex (NPC) into the nucleus where the complex falls apart and the viral cargo can reduce the host cell's antiviral response, leading to enhanced infection. Ivermectin binds to and destabilises the Impα/β1 heterodimer thereby preventing Impα/β1 from binding to the viral protein (bottom) and preventing it from entering the nucleus. This likely results in reduced inhibition of the antiviral responses, leading to a normal, more efficient antiviral response (extracted from ref. Caly et al., 2020; authorized by Elsevier B.V.).

5.Teach, And Teach And Teach: Does The Average Citizen Use Masks Correctly During Daily Activities?

[1]Evaldo Stanislau Affonso de Araújo [1,2]; Fatima Maria Bernardes Henriques Amaral [1]; Dongmin Park [1]; Ana Paola Ceraldi Cameira [1]; Murilo Augustinho Muniz da Cunha [1]; Evelyn Gutierrez Karl [1]; Sheila J. Henderson [3].

1.Sao Judas Tadeu University, Medical School
2.Hospital das Clinicas, University of Sao Paulo Medical School
3. Alliant International University

ABSTRACT

COVID-19 is a new disease with no treatment and no vaccine so far. The pandemic is still growing in many areas. Among the core measures to prevent disease spread is the use of face masks. We observed 12,588 people in five Brazilian cities within the Baixada Santista metropolitan area. Even though this is densely populated region and heavily impacted by COVID-19 with a high-risk population, only 45.1% of the observed population wore in face masks in a correct way, and another 15.5% simply did not use masks at all. The remainder used masks incorrectly, which is evidence of the worst scenario of people believing that they are protected when they are not. This is among the first studies, to the best of our knowledge, that measures real life compliance with face masks during this COVID-19 pandemic. It is our conclusion that it is paramount to first control the virus before allowing people back in the streets. We should not assume that people will wear masks properly. Equally important is to instruct and sensitize people on how to use face masks and why it is important.

INTRODUCTION

The impact of COVID-19 has been enormous; everyone has had to change their social and health behaviours. Nonetheless, with every new day, COVID-19 becomes an easier and less frightening subject for the less informed. Especially with the need for daily income, the lack of social support for the stay at home policy, and in some countries like Brazil, the political misguidance contrary to the recommendations of the Science and Health Authorities [1], public pressure has mounted to end the quarantine. Some Brazilian cities are arranging the progressive reopening of commercial areas and allowing people to move freely about town. As the quarantine ends, with the numbers of cases and deaths on the rise, it has now become obligatory to wear a face mask.

[1] Correspondent author: Evaldo Stanislau Affonso de Araújo. E-mail: evaldo.araujo@hc.fm.usp.br
Hospital das Clinicas HC-FMUSP
Av.Dr.Eneas de Carvalho Aguiar 255, Sao Paulo
Brazil ZIP 05403-000 Tel: +55 11 2661-6397

The Baixada Santista metropolitan area is an immense harbour region (the largest in Latin America), providing an oil and industrial area close to São Paulo, with a large retired population of 60+ years in age. COVID-19 is highly prevalent with rising deaths (1,706 cases/100,000 inhabitants and 65.3 deaths/100,000, as of June 20, 2020, for the city of Santos) [2]. Although a population-based serologic survey conducted in the region every two weeks in the last two months (since June 11, 2020) showed a variation in anti-SARS-CoV-2 antibodies from 1.4 to 6.6%, the region still eased on the Social Distancing Rules. Due to the strategic nature of the region, its aging population, and the growing numbers of cases, and antibodies prevalence, the impact of COVID-19 is growing rapidly and perilously. For a proper risk assessment, it is critical to understand the degree of public compliance with protective measures. The face mask is a cornerstone measure to protect against the COVID-19 infection [3]. To evaluate if, how often, and in what way people wear their face masks, we conducted an observational study in five major cities in the Baixada Santista metropolitan area with a sample of over 12,000 observations.

MATERIAL AND METHODS

From June 17th to 19th, 2020, medical student researchers went to large commercial streets in the cities of Santos, São Vicente, Cubatão, Guarujá, and Praia Grande. For three consecutive days, for a period of one hour, the same researcher occupied the same spot on the same street, at the same time, and observed and recorded if, how many, and in what way, people were wearing their face masks. The sample size was based on the numbers of people at streets seen and recorded during the specified hours of observation at the specified place, which reflected the real-life scenario for an average weekday. To guard against observer bias, the researchers were included in determining the categories of face mask use, and we ensured consensus about these categories before the study began. The following categories were observed: people wearing masks covering mouth and nose, firmly adjusted; or individuals wearing a mask with their nose and/or mouth exposed; people not wearing masks; others were wearing a poorly fitting mask; and, finally, people who touch their masks during use. Results were plotted and analysed in total and by city.

RESULTS

Table 1 (by number and percentage) and Figure 1 (by percentage) display the research results by city and in total. Overall, an average of 45.1% of the people observed wore their masks properly, within a city by city range of 39.1% to 63.5%. Within the remaining 54.9%, 15.5% wore no mask (ranging from 12.7% to 18.8%), 12.9% wore masks but exposed their mouth and nose (range: 9.9% to 17.6%), 12.0% exposed their nose only (7.9% to 16.6%), 17.8% touched their mask during use (0.0% to 14.0%), and 6.5% wore poorly fitted masks (1.2% to 10.7%). The number of observations across the five cities was similar from 2,270 people (18.0%) in São Vicente to 3055 (24.6%) in Santos.

Table 1: Observations of face mask compliance by city and region

City	Date in June 2020	Correct Use	No mask	Exposed Mouth and Nose	Exposed Nose	Touching Face During Use	Poorly Fitted Mask	City Total	%
CUBATAO	17th	640	130	104	62	0	14		
	18th	604	120	68	50	0	10		
	19th	266	152	76	76	0	5		
TOTAL CUBATAO		1,510	402	248	188	0	29	2,377	18.8%
%		63.5%	16.9%	10.4%	7.9%	0%	1.2%	100%	
PRAIA GRANDE	17th	360	108	76	66	38	46		
	18th	318	170	194	108	40	92		
	19th	411	188	96	62	53	42		
TOTAL PRAIA GRANDE		1,089	466	366	236	131	180	2,468	19.6%
%		44.1%	18.8%	14.8%	9.5%	5.3%	7.3%	100%	
SANTOS	17th	321	145	66	174	179	146		
	18th	351	130	161	103	116	73		
	19th	349	172	141	228	135	65		
TOTAL SANTOS		1,021	447	368	505	430	284	3,055	24.6%
%		33.4%	14.6%	12.0%	16.6%	14.0%	9.3%	100%	
GUARUJA	17th	198	107	138	114	80	101		
	18th	295	71	161	103	65	61		
	19th	304	170	128	126	98	98		
TOTAL GUARUJA		797	348	427	343	243	260	2,418	19.2%
%		32.9%	14.3%	17.6%	14.1%	10.0%	10.7%	100%	
SAO VICENTE	17	447	97	79	79	58	27		
	18	384	96	78	78	50	23		
	19	436	96	68	82	71	21		
TOTAL SAO VICENTE		1,267	289	225	239	179	71	2,270	18.0%
%		55.8%	12.7%	9.9%	10.5%	7.8%	3.1%	100%	
Region TOTAL		5,684	1,952	1,634	1,511	983	824	12,588	100%
%		45.1%	15.5%	12.9%	12.0%	7.8%	6.5%	100%	

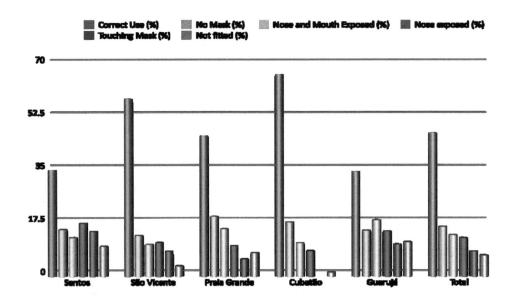

Figure 1. Relative use of face masks by city and region (%)

DISCUSSION

At the present time, there is little, if any, research data on face mask compliance worn to prevent the spread of COVID-19. In this study, over three consecutive days, we observed 12,588 people in the streets wearing, or not, masks in their routine lives. Overall, only 45.1% of the people observed wore their masks properly, 39.4% wore their masks improperly, and 15.5% did not wear masks at all. The 39.4% who were wearing masks improperly were likely to be as dangerous as those not wearing a mask. This suggests that many mask-wearing people were feeling safe, but in reality, were not, and therefore risking presence in the streets in an inadvisable fashion.

Non-pharmacological measures are the main line of defence against COVID-19 [3]. Several barriers, such as physical or behavioural, should exist between the susceptible host and SARS-CoV-2. Face masks have grown in relevance during this pandemic, particularly going from health care facilities to the average people daily activities. Face masks are now a cornerstone in prevention, no matter who or where the need exists. Nevertheless, face masks are new for the public. Face masks are not comfortable to wear, and they require a new routine for how to wear, how to remove, how to preserve and clean, and so forth. Many people complain of a lack of oxygen while wearing masks. Therefore, it may be overly optimistic to count on public compliance with face masks as a tool to prevent infection and as a measure to make it safe to relax hard social distancing.

Our results are quite disturbing. We found that only 45.1% of people wore face masks properly and safely in a research sample observed in a region with significant prevalence of COVID-19, among people at high risk of infection (because of poverty and high prevalence) and complications (due to age and pre-existing health conditions). According some mathematical models, more than 80% of people must wear a face mask properly for efficacy in COVID-19 spread prevention [4]. As a public health measure and the successful defence against the spread of COVID-19, the use of masks to protect the public, in lieu of quarantine, depends on each individual adhering to proper use [5]. We must ask ourselves: who are we deceiving with the false belief of high compliance? Before we move to some plan of further relaxing control measures, it's clear that safe social distancing is still a critical target to be achieved in order to reduce circulation of the virus. These research results from Baixada Santista, revealing inadequate public compliance, suggest that we are playing with fire and jeopardizing people lives, and quite literally, offering them over to the virus. Prevention of COVID-19, like some other infectious diseases, (so far) lacks an effective vaccine and therefore requires a change in public behaviour. HIV taught us how hard is to avoid risk with a single behavioural change, such as using a condom. So, before we move ahead with peace of mind, and erroneously assume that people will wear masks routinely and properly, it is paramount that we teach, and teach, and teach use of face masks, and explain why one's life depends on proper use.

To the best of our knowledge, this study is the first to observe COVID-19 prevention from the perspective of actual observed compliance. This was an observational study, in a single region with no intervention. The generalizability of this study is unknown; however, this study can be easily replicated at low cost in other regions around the world. Observational studies are useful as preliminary but rapid research to raise significant red flags in current efforts against COVID-19.

Author Contributions

Evaldo Stanislau Affonso de Araújo [a] Fatima Maria Bernardes Henriques Amaral [b] Dongmin Park [b] Ana Paola Ceraldi Cameira [b]Murilo Augustinho Muniz da Cunha [b] Evelyn Gutierrez Karl [b]Sheila J. Henderson [c]

[a] concept of the study, wrote manuscript, prepared dataset

[b] field observation

[c] reviewed and prepared manuscript

REFERENCES

1. Editorial. COVID-19 in Brazil: "So what?". Lancet, 2020, 339: 1461, May 9, 2020. https://doi.org/10.1016/S0140-6736(20)31095-3
2. ESPECIAL COVID-19 – Dados por Município, 2020. https://www.brasil.io/covid19/ Accessed 20th June 2020
3. DK Chu, EA Akl, S Duda, K Solo, S Yaacoub, et al. Physical distancing, face masks, and eye protection to prevent person-to-person transmission of SARS-CoV-2 and COVID-19: a systematic review and meta-analysis. Lancet, In press. https://doi.org/10.1016/S01406736(20)31142-9.
4. SE Eikenberry, M Mancuso, E Iboi, T Phan, K Eikenberry, et al. (2020). To mask or not to mask: Modeling the potential for face mask use by the general public to curtail the COVID19 pandemic. Infectious Disease Modelling, 5: 293-306, 2020. https://doi.org/10.1016/j.idm.2020.04.001
5. WHO. Advice on the use of masks in the context of COVID-19. Interim guidance. 5 June 2020. https://www.who.int/publications/i/item/advice-on-the-use-of-masks-in-thecommunity-during-home-care-and-in-healthcare-settings-in-the-context-of-the-novelcoronavirus-(2019-ncov)-outbreak Accessed 20th June 2020

6.How Brazil Can Hold Back COVID-19?

Wanderson Kleber de Oliveira, Elisete Duarte,
Giovanny Vinícius Araújo de[1] França Leila Posenato Garcia

ABSTRACT

This article presents the strategies and actions adopted by the Brazilian Ministry of Health to hold back COVID-19. The response to the disease was immediate and occurred prior to the first case being detected in Brazil. Provision of information and communication to the population and the press was adopted as a fundamental strategy for addressing the epidemic. Guidance provided to the population has been clear, stressing the importance of coronavirus transmission prevention measures. Efforts have been directed towards strengthening health surveillance and health care, as well as boosting research, development and innovation. Actions have targeted human resource training and expanding coverage afforded by the Brazilian National Health System (SUS). Protecting health workers is a priority. All SUS health workers, managers and directors are dedicated to preserving the health and life of each and every Brazilian citizen.

INTRODUCTION

COVID-19, a disease caused by the novel coronavirus named SARS-CoV-2, was identified for the first time in China, in December 2019. [1] On January 30th 2020, the World Health Organization (WHO) declared the event to be a Public Health Emergency of International Concern, [2] and on March 11th 2020 declared it to be a pandemic. In Brazil, the Ministry of Health (MoH) acted immediately as soon as news began to be broadcast about the emerging disease. [3] On January 22nd the Ministry's Emergency Operations Centre was deployed. The Centre is coordinated by the Health Surveillance Secretariat to harmonize, plan and organize activities with the stakeholders involved and to monitor the epidemiological situation. Several government sectors were mobilized, and a variety of actions were implemented, including the preparation of a contingency plan. [4] On February 3rd 2020, human infection by the novel coronavirus was declared a Public Health Emergency of National Concern (PHENC). [5]Right from the start the MoH has turned to information and communication with the population and the press as fundamental strategies for withstanding the epidemic. The numbers of confirmed cases and deaths have been publicized daily. Epidemiological bulletins have been published, containing guidance on surveillance actions within the context of the PHENC. [6] In addition, press conferences have been held almost daily, emphasizing MoH commitment to transparent information and rapid communication about the epidemiological situation and actions to address it. [3]

The MoH has also provided new forms of service provision to the population, such as the Coronavírus - SUS application and a specific WhatsApp channel. [9] The MoH Press Office has been working shifts, including at weekends. [10] Recognizing that fake news promotes disinformation and can contribute to making the situation worse, the MoH has acted to provide the population and the press

[1] Special article • Epidemiol. Serv. Saúde 29 (2) 27 Apr 20202020

with reliable information. Guidance provided by the MoH to the population has been clear, right from the beginning, in the sense of reinforcing the importance of measures to prevent coronavirus transmission, which include: (i) washing hands with soap and water or sanitizing them with alcohol-based gel; (ii) "respiratory etiquette", which consists of covering one's nose and mouth when sneezing or coughing; (iii) social distancing; (iv) not sharing objects intended for individual use, such as glasses and cutlery; and (v) keeping rooms well ventilated.

With effect from April 2020, the MoH began advising the population to use cloth facemasks as a barrier against the spread of SARS-CoV-2. [11] Brazil's first COVID-19 case was confirmed on February 26 th 2020. The case was that of an elderly man living in São Paulo/SP who had returned from a trip to Italy. The disease spread rapidly. In less than one month after the first case was confirmed, community transmission was already happening in some cities. Brazil's first COVID-19 death occurred on March 17 th 2020. This case was also that of an elderly man living in São Paulo/SP who had diabetes and hypertension but had no record of having travelled abroad recently. On March 20 th 2020, community transmission of COVID-19 was recognized throughout the national territory. [13] Figure 1 shows the daily number of new cases, from February 26 th to April 6 th 2020. Figure 2 shows the daily number of deaths, from March 17 th to April 6 th 2020.

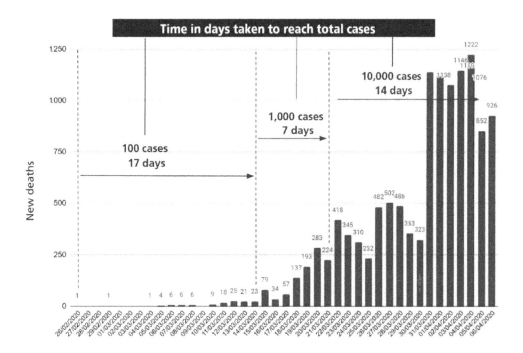

**Figure 1:– Number of new COVID-19 cases notified in Brazil,
from February 26th to April 6th 2020**

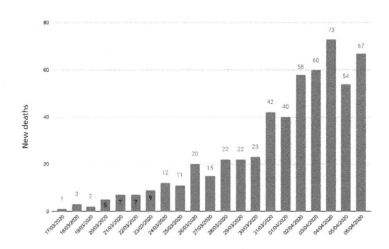

Figure 2:– Number of COVID-19 deaths in Brazil, from March 17th to April 6th 2020

At the time the disease was introduced into the country, the majority of cases were imported and the strategy to contain it was based on tracing and isolating cases and contacts, in order to avoid sustained person-to-person transmission of the virus. With the growth in the number of COVID-19 cases and the occurrence of community transmission, mitigation strategies were introduced with the aim of avoiding the occurrence of severe cases and deaths from the disease. These strategies include hospital care measures for severe cases, as well as isolation measures for mild cases and contacts. [15] In this sense, MoH actions have also been based on strengthening health care.

Actions have targeted human resource training and increasing National Health System (SUS) coverage, by hiring more health workers, especially physicians. A total of 5,811 additional job positions have been made available for doctors to work in Primary Health Care Centres in 1,864 municipalities, as well as in 19 Special Indigenous Health Districts, nationwide. State capital cities and large urban centres have been benefited, since they have higher population density and are places more propitious to coronavirus spreading. Another highlight is the strategic action called " *O Brasil conta comigo* " (Brazil can count on me), involving registration and training of health workers to join the fight against COVID-19. Students in the final year of medicine, nursing, physiotherapy and pharmacology courses at both public and private higher education institutions can also become part of this effort. [18]

Moreover, ensuring protection of health workers is a priority, as they form the front line in the battle against COVID-19, fulfilling their role as protagonists in case diagnosis and treatment. The MoH has paid special attention to producing, purchasing and distributing personal protective equipment for health workers throughout the entire country. Infection prevention measures must be implemented in all health services and their vehicles. [19] Scaling up structure to care for severe cases that require hospitalization and/or intensive care is being done by purchasing equipment and supplies, building hospital units, increasing the capacity of existing units, renting beds in private or supplemental health sector hospitals, as well as providing support for field hospitals to be set up. Priority has also been given to encouraging production and purchasing of ventilators, the availability and distribution of which are essential for meeting the needs of severe cases.

In March 2020, the federal administration transferred over BRL 1 billion to state and municipal governments to fund actions to combat COVID-19. [20]

The MoH has made efforts to fulfill the WHO recommendations for testing suspected cases, detecting positive cases and advising isolation of people with the disease and their household contacts, so as to reduce dissemination. However, once COVID-19 began to spread via community transmission, there was not sufficient SUS health centre capacity to test everyone suspected of having the disease. The MoH rapidly increased the number of tests for COVID-19 diagnosis, including two types of tests: (i) RT-PCR, which detects virus present in the sample; and (ii) the rapid serologic test, which detects coronavirus antibodies. Initially, priority was given to testing health workers and the police, as well as severe cases and deaths. [21]In order to guarantee an adequate response to the emergency, the MoH is working to expand the Influenza-Like Syndrome Sentinel Network. The number of establishments that collect samples for surveillance of this condition is expected to increase from 168 to 500 within three months. [21] Logistics will be enhanced, and testing capacity will be increased through partnerships with the private sector.

The TeleSUS initiative uses artificial intelligence for active tracing of suspected COVID-19 cases by means of telephone calls. People with signs and symptoms of SARS-CoV-2 infection can get guidance at home without needing to go to a health service. [22] Moreover, by means of cellular telephones, the Chronic Disease Risk and Protective Factor Surveillance Telephone Survey (Vigitel COVID-19) will obtain information from people aged 18 or over, living in all the Brazilian state capitals and Federal District, about COVID-19 prevention practices, as well as information about their state of health. [23] Use of telemedicine is another strategy. The Federal Council of Medicine CFM) [24] has produced regulations for on-line medical consultations, as well as telesurgery and telediagnosis, among other forms of remote medical care, which will be important for ensuring care not only for people affected by COVID-19, but for all people who need medical assistance.

Another area focused by MoH actions is the promotion of research, innovation and development. The MoH Science, Technology and Strategic Supplies Secretariat is leading the production of evidence summaries to guide the decisions of the MoH Emergency Operations centre. Support for research projects on COVID-19 and other severe acute respiratory diseases will be provided by the MoH in partnership with the National Scientific and Technological Development Council, by means of a call for proposals. [25] Priority will be given to projects following different research tracks capable of contributing to the production of evidence about the natural history of the disease, diagnosis, health care organization, effectiveness of surveillance, prevention and control measures, treatment alternatives, as well as support for development and evaluation of diagnostic test accuracy. Research considered to be priority is being supported in a more agile manner through the collaboration of research institutions and charitable hospitals that take part in the National Health System Institutional Development Program, by means of the initiative called the Brazil Covid Coalition. National multicentre clinical trials to evaluate the efficacy and safety of medication and combination treatment have been prioritized. The Oswaldo Cruz Foundation (Fiocruz) is taking part in the global SOLIDARITY trial, launched by WHO to test promising treatment for COVID-19. The Ministry of Science, Technology, Innovation and Communication is also collaborating with these initiatives and has created a Virus Network Specialists Committee with the aim of promoting integration of scientific research and technological development efforts. Notwithstanding the efforts made by the MoH, the characteristics of COVID-19 make it difficult to control. Its high transmissibility, including through asymptomatic cases, and its tendency to lead to severe complications, hospitalizations and deaths, together with the absence of prior immunity (as it is a virus unknown to the human species), inexistence of vaccine or treatment known to be efficacious and the vulnerability of the Brazilian population (living and health conditions), mean it can assumed that infection incidence will be high and that the number of severe cases, needing hospitalization and/or intensive care, may exceed health service capacity. [26]In this context it is recommendable to adopt measures that contribute to flattening the COVID-19 epidemic curve, preventing an abrupt increase in the number of cases and reducing the peak in demand for health services. The aim is to avoid the health system from becoming overloaded and collapsing, which could lead to increased mortality owing to lack of hospital beds and intensive care. In view of the disease's characteristics, finding the balance between COVID-19 incidence and availability of medium and high complexity health care will be fundamental for avoiding deaths among severe cases. [27]

In order to stand up to a disease that spreads very quickly, and which not only attacks people, but also compromises the health system and society as a whole, individual prevention measures are not sufficient and community measures must also be adopted. Such measures include restricting access to schools, universities, community gathering places, public transport, as well as other places where large numbers of people gather, such as social and sports events, theatres, cinemas and commercial establishments, which are not characterized as providing essential services. [28] Adoption of such measures is recommended based on the experience of countries affected by COVID-19 before Brazil, WHO recommendations and evidence available so far about effective interventions for controlling the disease, based on studies conducted in other nations.

The time at which these measures are adopted and how long they last for are fundamental for their success. It is a considerable challenge to determine the best time to start community restriction measures, as if they are implemented too soon this can result in social and economic hardships with limited benefit for public health and, over time, can result in fatigue and the population ceasing to commit to the measures. On the other hand, late implementation, after the disease has become widespread, can limit their benefits. In other words, the intervention needs to start soon enough to prevent the initial sharp rise in the number of cases, and last long enough to cover the peak of the expected epidemic curve. [14]

In Brazil, a country of continental dimensions and very diverse local realities, it is not appropriate to adopt from the outset a uniform procedure for all states and municipalities. The need exists to have knowledge of and assess local data in order to inform decision making. A plan also needs to be built to make feasible actions that can and must continue, especially those considered to be essential and which guarantee production, storage and distribution of equipment, materials and supplies needed to address the pandemic. [14] As such, the Brazilian National Health System (SUS) needs to be fully mobilized in an articulated manner, with the indivisible participation of the municipalities, the states and the Union, as well as involvement of all governments at all three levels of administration, the National Congress, the Judiciary and Brazilian society. Hard times are ahead, and the course of the epidemic will demand that strategies be constantly reviewed. The work of epidemiological surveillance services is therefore crucial. Timely and correct case and death notification will help to inform sounder decision making.

The COVID-19 pandemic is exposing SUS structural weaknesses and bottlenecks, in particular the lack – or unequal distribution –, in the territory, of health workers and medium and high complexity care infrastructure, as well as limited capacity to produce and perform diagnostic tests. It does, however, also bring to light the strengths of the world's largest public and universal health system, which plays a paramount role in health surveillance and health care, as well as in organizing and articulating actions to address the pandemic, at all three levels of administration, in all the Brazilian Federative units. The challenges that are looming are huge and made worse by our social situation, which imposes precarious living and health conditions, especially for people who live on the poor outskirts of large urban centres. Escalation of mental health conditions is expected, as a consequence of fears caused by the pandemic and isolation. The fact that COVID-19 will overlap in space and time with other diseases – such as arboviruses transmitted by *Aedes aegypti*, seasonal influenza, tuberculosis, AIDS, noncommunicable diseases and conditions, among others – is an further challenge

The country not only faces a new disease, but also an unprecedented situation, which requires radical changes in behaviour at both individual and community level. Collaboration by society in standing up to COVID-19 will be a determining factor for the epidemic's progression. Everyone without fail should follow the guidance of health authorities, based on available scientific evidence and in line with WHO recommendations, respecting isolation, quarantine and restrictions on movement and social contact, as indicated in each situation. Common sense and solidarity need to guide the actions of all Brazilians, in order for it to be possible to reduce the impact of COVID-19 on the population's health and on the economy. Protecting the elderly is a priority strategy, given that they form a group at greater risk of complications and death due to COVID-19. Because they are more vulnerable, people aged over 60 should stay at home whenever possible, restrict their movements to doing only strictly necessary activities, avoid using public transport and not frequent places where people are gathered. People in other age groups should also do their part, since reducing transmission in the community is necessary for everyone's protection. Children and those who develop asymptomatic infection can contribute to spreading the disease and infecting the elderly and other groups more prone to suffering complications, such as people with diabetes, hypertension and cancer. [29] SUS performance will be a determining factor. The SUS is a national heritage, a State policy that guarantees access to health actions and services to the more than 210 million people who live in Brazil. Since it was created in 1988, the SUS has become ever more present in people's lives. SUS workers, including community health agents and professionals who work on the front line, SUS managers and MoH directors will do their utmost to preserve the health and life of each and every Brazilian. Through SUS strength and the contribution of society, Brazil can hold back COVID-19. Before long the country will be able to return to normal, with more strength, more solidarity, more empathy, and with new habits and values that will enable social development and economic growth to be resumed, in a more sustainable and equitable manner, towards a better future.

REFERENCES

1. Zhu N, Zhang D, Wang W, Li X, Yang B, Song J, et al. A novel coronavirus from patients with pneumonia in China, 2019. N Engl J Med [Internet]. 2020 Feb [cited 2020 Apr 7];382:727-33. Available from: http://doi.org/10.1056/NEJMoa2001017
   » http://doi.org/10.1056/NEJMoa2001017
2. World Health Organization. Statement on the second meeting of the international health regulations (2005) emergency committee regarding the outbreak of novel coronavirus (2019-nCoV) [Internet]. Geneva: World Health Organization; 2020 [cited 2020 Apr 7]. Available from: https://www.who.int/news-room/detail/30-01-2020-statement-on-the-second-meeting-of-the-international-health-regulations-(2005)-emergency-committee-regarding-the-outbreak-of-novel-coronavirus-(2019-ncov)
   » https://www.who.int/news-room/detail/30-01-2020-statement-on-the-second-meeting-of-the-international-health-regulations-(2005)-emergency-committee-regarding-the-outbreak-of-novel-coronavirus-(2019-ncov)
3. Croda JHR, Garcia LP. Resposta imediata da Vigilância em Saúde à epidemia da COVID-19. Epidemiol Serv Saúde [Internet]. 2020 mar [citado 2020 abr 7];29(1):e2020002. Disponível em: https://doi.org/10.5123/s1679-49742020000100021
   » https://doi.org/10.5123/s1679-49742020000100021
4. Ministério da Saúde (BR). Centro de Operações de Emergências em Saúde Pública COE-COVID-19. Plano de contingência nacional para infecção humana pelo novo coronavírus COVID-19 [Internet]. Brasília: Ministério da

Saúde; 2020 [citado 2020 abr 7]. 24 p. Disponível em: https://portalarquivos2.saude.gov.br/images/pdf/2020/fevereiro/13/plano-contingencia-coronavirus-COVID19.pdf
» https://portalarquivos2.saude.gov.br/images/pdf/2020/fevereiro/13/plano-contingencia-coronavirus-COVID19.pdf

5. Brasil. Ministério da Saúde. Portaria MS/GM nº 188, de 3 de fevereiro de 2020. Declara Emergência em Saúde Pública de importância Nacional (ESPIN) em decorrência da Infecção Humana pelo novo Coronavírus (2019-nCoV) [Internet]. Diário Oficial da União, Brasília (DF), 2020 fev 4 [citado 2020 abr 7]; Seção Extra:1. Disponível em: http://www.in.gov.br/web/dou/-/portaria-n-188-de-3-de-fevereiro-de-2020-241408388
» http://www.in.gov.br/web/dou/-/portaria-n-188-de-3-de-fevereiro-de-2020-241408388

6. Ministério da Saúde (BR). Secretaria de Vigilância em Saúde. Infecção humana pelo novo coronavírus (2019-nCoV). Bol Epidemiol [Internet]. 2020 jan [citado 2020 abr 7];COE 1:1-17. Disponível em: https://www.saude.gov.br/images/pdf/2020/fevereiro/04/Boletim-epidemiologico-SVS-04fev20.pdf
» https://www.saude.gov.br/images/pdf/2020/fevereiro/04/Boletim-epidemiologico-SVS-04fev20.pdf

7. Ministério da Saúde (BR). Secretaria de Vigilância em Saúde. Infecção humana pelo novo coronavírus (2019-nCoV): errata. Bol Epidemiol [Internet]. 2020 fev [citado 2020 mar 30];COE 2:1-23. Disponível em: https://www.saude.gov.br/images/pdf/2020/marco/24/03--ERRATA---Boletim-Epidemiologico-05.pdf
» https://www.saude.gov.br/images/pdf/2020/marco/24/03--ERRATA---Boletim-Epidemiologico-05.pdf

8. Ministério da Saúde (BR). Secretaria de Vigilância em Saúde. Doença pelo coronavírus 2019: ampliação da vigilância, medidas não farmacológicas e descentralização do diagnóstico laboratorial. Bol Epidemiol [Internet]. 2020 [citado 2020 abr 7];5:1-11. Disponível em: https://portalarquivos2.saude.gov.br/images/pdf/2020/fevereiro/13/Boletim-epidemiologico-COEcorona-SVS-13fev20.pdf
» https://portalarquivos2.saude.gov.br/images/pdf/2020/fevereiro/13/Boletim-epidemiologico-COEcorona-SVS-13fev20.pdf

9. Ministério da Saúde (BR). Ministério da Saúde lança canal para atender população no WhatsApp [Internet]. Brasília: Ministério da Saúde; 2020 [citado 2020 abr 7]. Disponível em: https://www.saude.gov.br/noticias/agencia-saude/46607-ministerio-da-saude-lanca-canal-para-atender-populacao-no-whatsapp
» https://www.saude.gov.br/noticias/agencia-saude/46607-ministerio-da-saude-lanca-canal-para-atender-populacao-no-whatsapp

10. Ministério da Saúde (BR). Assessoria de imprensa atende em regime de plantão [Internet]. Brasília: Ministério da Saúde; 2020 [citado 2020 abr 7]. Disponível em: https://www.saude.gov.br/noticias/agencia-saude/46564-assessoria-de-imprensa-atende-em-regime-de-plantao-70
» https://www.saude.gov.br/noticias/agencia-saude/46564-assessoria-de-imprensa-atende-em-regime-de-plantao-70

11. Ministério da Saúde (BR). Máscaras caseiras podem ajudar na prevenção contra o coronavírus [Internet]. Brasília: Ministério da Saúde; 2020 [citado 2020 abr 7]. Disponível em: https://www.saude.gov.br/noticias/agencia-saude/46645-mascaras-caseiras-podem-ajudar-na-prevencao-contra-o-coronavirus
» https://www.saude.gov.br/noticias/agencia-saude/46645-mascaras-caseiras-podem-ajudar-na-prevencao-contra-o-coronavirus

12. Garcia LP. Uso de máscara facial para limitar a transmissão da COVID-19. Epidemiol Serv Saúde. No prelo. 2020.

13. Ministério da Saúde (BR). Ministério da Saúde declara transmissão comunitária nacional [Internet]. Brasília: Ministério da Saúde; 2020 [citado 2020 abr 7]. Disponível em: https://www.saude.gov.br/noticias/agencia-saude/46568-ministerio-da-saude-declara-transmissao-comunitaria-nacional
» https://www.saude.gov.br/noticias/agencia-saude/46568-ministerio-da-saude-declara-transmissao-comunitaria-nacional

14. Ministério da Saúde (BR). Secretaria de Vigilância em Saúde. Especial: doença pelo coronavírus 2019. Bol Epidemiol [Internet]. 2020 abr [citado 2020 abr 7];7(spe):1-28. Disponível em: https://portalarquivos.saude.gov.br/images/pdf/2020/April/06/2020-04-06-BE7-Boletim-Especial-do-COE-Atualizacao-da-Avaliacao-de-Risco.pdf
» https://portalarquivos.saude.gov.br/images/pdf/2020/April/06/2020-04-06-BE7-Boletim-Especial-do-COE-Atualizacao-da-Avaliacao-de-Risco.pdf

15. Brasil. Ministério da Saúde. Portaria MS/GM n. 356, de 11 de março de 2020. Dispõe sobre a regulamentação e operacionalização do disposto na Lei nº 13.979, de 6 de fevereiro de 2020, que estabelece as medidas para enfrentamento da emergência de saúde pública de importância internacional decorrente do coronavírus (COVID-19) [Internet]. Diário Oficial da União, Brasília (DF), 2020 mar 12 [citado 2020 abr 7];Seção 1:185. Disponível

em: http://www.in.gov.br/web/dou/-/portaria-n-356-de-11-de-marco-de-2020-247538346
» http://www.in.gov.br/web/dou/-/portaria-n-356-de-11-de-marco-de-2020-247538346

16. Ministério da Saúde (BR). Coronavírus, COVID-19: fast-track para a atenção primária em locais com transmissão comunitária, fluxo rápido [Internet]. Brasília: Ministério da Saúde; 2020 [citado 2020 abr 7]. Disponível em: https://portalarquivos.saude.gov.br/images/pdf/2020/marco/30/20200330-FAST-TRACK-ver06-verFinal.pdf» https://portalarquivos.saude.gov.br/images/pdf/2020/marco/30/20200330-FAST-TRACK-ver06-verFinal.pdf

17. Ministério da Saúde (BR). Projeto Lean nas emergências: plano de resposta hospitalar ao COVID-19 [Internet]. Brasília: Ministério da Saúde; 2020 [citado 2020 abr 7]. 44 p. Disponível em: https://portalar-quivos.saude.gov.br/images/pdf/2020/April/03/Ebook-SirioLibanes-PlanodeCriseCOVID19-LeannasEmerg--ncias-0304-espelhadas.pdf » https://portalarquivos.saude.gov.br/images/pdf/2020/April/03/Ebook-Sirio-oLibanes-PlanodeCriseCOVID19-LeannasEmerg--ncias-0304-espelhadas.pdf

18. Ministério da Saúde (BR). Alunos da área de saúde poderão ajudar no combate ao coronavírus [Internet]. Brasília: Ministério da Saúde; 2020 [citado 2020 abr 7]. Disponível em: https://www.saude.gov.br/noticias/46636-alunos-da-area-de-saude-poderao-ajudar-no-combate-ao-coronavirus
» https://www.saude.gov.br/noticias/46636-alunos-da-area-de-saude-poderao-ajudar-no-combate-ao-corona-virus

19. Nacoti M, Ciocca A, Giupponi A, Brambillasca P, Lussara F, Pisano M, et al. At the epicentre of the COVID-19 pandemic and humanitarian crises in Italy: changing perspectives on preparation and mitigation: in a Bergamo hospital deeply strained by the COVID-19 pandemic, exhausted clinicians reflect on how to prepare for the next outbreak. NEJM Catalyst [Internet]. 2020 Mar [cited 2020 Apr 7]. Available from: https://cata-lyst.nejm.org/doi/full/10.1056/CAT.20.0080?query=CON&cid=DM88964_Catalyst_Non_Sub-scriber&bid=172148390
» https://catalyst.nejm.org/doi/full/10.1056/CAT.20.0080?query=CON&cid=DM88964_Catalyst_Non_Sub-scriber&bid=172148390

20. Ministério da Saúde (BR). Saúde destina mais R$ 600 mi para ações de combate à pandemia [Internet]. Brasília: Ministério da Saúde; 2020 [citado 2020 abr 7]. Disponível em: https://www.saude.gov.br/noticias/agencia-saude/46602-saude-destina-mais-r-600-mi-para-acoes-de-combate-a-pandemia
» https://www.saude.gov.br/noticias/agencia-saude/46602-saude-destina-mais-r-600-mi-para-acoes-de-combate-a-pandemia

21. Ministério da Saúde (BR). Saúde amplia testes para profissionais de saúde e segurança [Internet]. Brasília: Ministério da Saúde; 2020 [citado 2020 abr 7]. Disponível em: https://www.saude.gov.br/noticias/agencia-saude/46596-saude-amplia-testes-para-profissionais-de-saude-e-seguranca
» https://www.saude.gov.br/noticias/agencia-saude/46596-saude-amplia-testes-para-profissionais-de-saude-e-seguranca

22. Ministério da Saúde (BR). TeleSUS fará busca ativa de informações sobre coronavírus [Internet]. Brasília: Ministério da Saúde; 2020 [citado 2020 abr 7]. Disponível em: https://www.saude.gov.br/noticias/agencia-saude/46633-ministerio-da-saude-fara-busca-ativa-de-informacoes-sobre-coronavirus
» https://www.saude.gov.br/noticias/agencia-saude/46633-ministerio-da-saude-fara-busca-ativa-de-infor-macoes-sobre-coronavirus

23. Ministério da Saúde (BR). Saúde avalia comportamento dos brasileiros no combate à COVID-19 [Internet]. Brasília: Ministério da Saúde; 2020 [citado 2020 abr 7]. Disponível em: https://www.saude.gov.br/noticias/agencia-saude/46639-saude-avalia-comportamento-dos-brasileiros-no-combate-a-COVID-19
» https://www.saude.gov.br/noticias/agencia-saude/46639-saude-avalia-comportamento-dos-brasileiros-no-combate-a-COVID-19

24. Conselho Federal de Medicina (BR). Resolução CFM n. 2.227, de 26 de fevereiro de 2019. Define e disciplina a telemedicina como forma de prestação de serviços médicos mediados por tecnologias [Internet]. Diário Oficial da União, Brasília (DF), 2019 mar 6 [citado 2020 abr 7];Seção 1. Disponível em: https://portal.cfm.org.br/im-ages/PDF/resolucao222718.pdf
» https://portal.cfm.org.br/images/PDF/resolucao222718.pdf

25. Ministério da Ciência, Tecnologia, Inovações e Comunicações (BR). Conselho Nacional de Desenvolvimento Científico e Tecnológico – CNPq. Ministério da Saúde (BR). Chamada MCTIC/CNPq/FNDCT/MS/SCTIE/Decit nº 07/2020: pesquisas para enfrentamento da COVID-19, suas consequências e outras síndromes respiratórias agudas graves [Internet]. Brasília: Ministério da Ciência, Tecnologia, Inovações e Comunicações; 2020 [citado 2020 br 15]. Disponível em: http://resultado.cnpq.br/6022243470135030
» http://resultado.cnpq.br/6022243470135030

26. Castro MC, Carvalho LR, Chin T, Kahn R, Franca GVA, Macario EMM, et al. Demand for hospitalization services for COVID-19 patients in Brazil. MedRxiv [Internet]. 2020 Apr [cited 2020 Apr 7]. Available from: https://www.medrxiv.org/content/10.1101/2020.03.30.20047662v1
   » https://www.medrxiv.org/content/10.1101/2020.03.30.20047662v1

27. Garcia LP, Duarte E. Intervenções não farmacológicas para o enfrentamento à epidemia da COVID-19 no Brasil. Epidemiol Serv Saúde [Internet]. 2020 abr [citado 2020 abr 7];29(2). Disponível em: https://doi.org/10.5123/s1679-49742020000200009» https://doi.org/10.5123/s1679-49742020000200009

28. Qualls N, Levitt A, Kanade N, Wright-Jegede N, Dopson S, Biggerstaff M, et al. Community mitigation guidelines to prevent pandemic influenza — United States, 2017. MMWR Recomm Rep [Internet]. 2017 Apr [cited 2020 Apr 7];66(1):1-34. Available from: https://doi.org/10.15585/mmwr.rr6601a1
   » https://doi.org/10.15585/mmwr.rr6601a1

29. Weiss P, Murdoch D. Clinical course and mortality risk of severe COVID-19. Lancet [Internet]. 2020 Mar [cited 2020 Apr 8];395(10229):1014-5. Available from: https://doi.org/10.1016/S0140-6736(20)30633-4
   » https://doi.org/10.1016/S0140-6736(20)30633-4

30. CDC COVID-19 Response Team. Severe outcomes among patients with coronavirus disease 2019 (COVID-19) — United States, February 12–March 16, 2020. MMWR Morb Mortal Wkly Rep [Internet]. 2020 Mar [cited 2020 Apr 7];69(12):343-6. Available from: http://dx.doi.org/10.15585/mmwr.mm6912e2
   » http://dx.doi.org/10.15585/mmwr.mm6912e2

7. What Has The COVID-19 Pandemic Taught Us About Adopting Preventive Measures?[1]

Adriana Cristina de Oliveira[1]
[1]Universidade Federal de Minas Gerais, Escola de Enfermagem,
Programa de Pós-graduação em Enfermagem. Belo Horizonte, Minas Gerais, Brasil.

Thabata Coaglio Lucas[2]
[2]Universidade Federal dos Vales do Jequitinhonha e Mucuri, Departamento de Enfermagem,
Programa de Pós-graduação em Ensino em Saúde. Diamantina, Minas Gerais, Brasil.

Robert Aldo Iquiapaza[3]
Universidade Federal de Minas Gerais, Faculdade de Ciências Econômicas,
Departamento de Ciências Administrativas. Belo Horizonte, Minas Gerais, Brasil.

ABSTRACT

Objective: to analyze the COVID-19 pandemic and what we have (re)learned from the world experience of adopting prevention measures recommended by the World Health Organization as well as the epidemiological overview in the world, in Latin America and in Brazil. **Results:** the World Health Organization has pointed out that the path to reduce the speed of circulation of the virus, control and decrease in the number of cases and deaths resulting from this pandemic can only be accomplished with mass adoption of fundamental measures that include hand hygiene, alcohol gel use, cough etiquette, cleaning surfaces, avoiding agglomerations and social distancing. The epidemiological curve of the disease clearly shows the devastating proportions in Italy, Spain and the United States, surpassing China in death records, due to the delay in adopting the aforementioned measures. In Brazil, the rapid progression in relation to the world and Latin America points to an important increase in the number of cases. **Conclusion:** this is possibly the most serious pandemic in recent human history, and its course can be influenced by the rigor in adopting individual and collective behavioural measures.

INTRODUCTION

On the world stage, although distant from our daily lives, the beginning of 2020 was characterized by an outbreak of a mysterious pneumonia caused by a variation of coronavirus, whose first case was reported in December 2019 in the city of Wuhan, China.[1] The increase in the number of cases quickly characterized the infection as an outbreak, so that, at the end of January 2020, the World Health Organization (WHO) declared the situation as a public health emergency of international interest.[1] This is a virus isolated for the first time in 1937, and in 1965 was described as coronavirus, due to its profile under microscopy, similar to a crown.[2] Between 2002 and 2003, the WHO reported

[1] Texto & Contexto Enfermagem 2020, v. 29: e20200106   2/14
ISSN 1980-265X DOI https://doi.org/10.1590/1980-265X-TCE-2020-0106

774 deaths due to Severe Acute Respiratory Syndrome (SARS-CoV). In 2012, 858 deaths from Middle East Respiratory Syndrome (Mers-CoV) were confirmed in Saudi Arabia, both complications caused by members of the coronavirus family.[2]

Eight years later, 2019-2020, the world found the mutating RNA virus expanding, especially asymptomatically, as an emerging infection, with milder symptoms than SARS-CoV and Mers-CoV, but with greater transmissibility, thus generating considerable impacts on health systems.[1] Most people are infected with coronavirus throughout their lives, especially children, in which case α-coronavirus 229E and NL63, β-coronavirus OC43 and HKU1 are recognized.[2]

However, they can occasionally cause serious respiratory diseases in the elderly and the immunocompromised.[2-3]From virus isolation in initial cases, researchers identified genetic mutation in a spike surface protein, which the virus uses to attack the human organism and multiply.[3] Little by little, information about its incubation period, between two and ten days, and of propagation through contaminated droplets, hands and surfaces were described in the literature.[4-5] Immediately, the news reports recorded increase in infected people, deaths, and high rate of contamination in Wuhan, where the first control measures included suspension of public transport, closure of entertainment venues, prohibition of public meetings, cleaning of buildings, streets and compulsory home restrictions on all citizens.[6] Spread of cases to other geographic areas has been greatly accelerated due to globalization and lack of knowledge to adopt restrictive measures for travellers. There were many questions and few answers at first, a direct and active mobilization by WHO to monitor cases and virus spread to all continents. Then, by the results of the first researches, the picture was outlined with human-human transmission of n-COVID-19.[7]

In this setting, WHO declared COVID-19 a pandemic on March 11, 2020, and instituted essential measures for prevention and confrontation. They included hand washing with soap and water whenever possible and alcohol gel use in situations where access to water and soap is not possible. They also recommended avoiding touching the eyes, nose and mouth, and protecting people around them when sneezing or coughing, with the adoption of a cough etiquette, by using a flexed elbow or disposable handkerchief.[8] Moreover, the WHO indicated maintaining social distancing (minimum of one meter), avoiding crowding and using a mask in case of flu or infection by COVID-19, or if a health professional in caring for suspected/infected patients.[8]

In Brazil, on February 3, 2020, it was declared, through Ordinance 188 from the Ministry of Health, a public health emergency of national importance, corresponding to a risk classification at level 3, due to human infection with the new coronavirus (SARS-CoV-2). This action aimed to favour that administrative measures were taken with greater agility so that the country began to prepare itself to face the pandemic, although at the time there was still no record of a confirmed case.[9] The first case of infection in Brazil was notified by the Ministry of Health on February 26, in the city of São Paulo, and the entire country from that moment on went on alert. Hand hygiene measures and cough etiquette were reinforced.[10]

However, the advance of the disease has been rapid, evolving in less than thirty days of cases imported for community or sustainable transmission. Imported cases are those in which it is possible to identify the origin of the virus, in general, when a person acquires it on trips abroad, at first, coming from countries like China and Italy.[10] In community transmission, the origin of the disease can no longer be identified, in addition to asymptomatic cases that come to represent a greater risk, considering that they spread the virus effectively.[10] In this new context of transmission at the national level, we witnessed, in parallel, estimates based on mathematical models proposed by researchers, and progression of COVID-19 cases in countries whose entry of the virus occurred in the period prior to notification in Brazil. In this perspective, this paper set out to analyse the COVID-19 pandemic, what we have (re) learned from the world experience of adopting prevention measures recommended by the WHO, as well as the epidemiological overview in the world, in Latin America and in Brazil.

TRANSMISSION OF COVID-19 AND MEASURES TO PREVENT ITS SPREAD

The term "virus" comes from Latin, understood as "poison" or "toxin". They are mostly 20-300 nm in diameter, have a genome consisting of one or more nucleic acid molecules (DNA or RNA), covered by a protein wrapper formed by one or more proteins, and by a complex envelope in a lipid bilayer.[2] Coronaviruses are enveloped positive-RNA viruses, and have a unique replication strategy, which makes it possible to vary their pathogenicity and ease of adaptation in different environments.[2] SARS-CoV-2 comes from a new strain identified in 2019 and, because it has not yet been isolated in humans, the measures to be implemented to face the pandemic are aimed at destroying the virus, preventing rapid transmission from person to person.[1-3]

SARS-CoV-2 transmission from person to person occurs through autoinoculation in mucous membranes (nose, eyes or mouth) and contact with contaminated inanimate surfaces, which has increasingly called attention to the need for rapid and preventive adoption of human protection measures to prevent contamination of persons.[5] For this reason, one of the most important measures for preventing transmission refers to hand hygiene, considered a low-cost and high-effectiveness measure, since hands are the main vehicle of cross-contamination. Countless studies point to inadequate adoption of this practice among professionals during care for patients in health services.[5,11-13]Admittedly, the practice of hand hygiene by rubbing with water and soap reduces the occurrence of preventable infections, reducing morbidity and mortality in health services.[14-18] However, the complexity involved in complying with this measure is great, and can often be related to factors such as human behaviour, including false perceptions of an invisible risk, underestimation of individual responsibility and lack of knowledge, behaviours that can interfere with compliance with preventive measures.[16-18]

People have emphasized compliance with this measure and its importance, but, in addition to the difficulties mentioned, some barriers that should not exist are still part of institutional realities, such as lack of sinks and supplies such as soap and water or even paper in public places that are characterized by high handling and contact of people, transit of escalators, toilets, buses, subways etc., as well as in communities without regular water and sewage supply. Due to the potential of the virus to survive in the environment for several days, facilities and areas potentially contaminated with SARS-CoV-2 must be cleaned before being reused, with products containing antimicrobial agents known to be effective against coronaviruses.[13,17] Although there is a lack of specific evidence of its effectiveness against SARS-CoV-2, cleaning with water and household detergents and common disinfectant product use are considered sufficient for general household cleaning.[19-20]

In hospital, several antimicrobial agents have been tested against different coronaviruses such as isopropanol, povidone-iodine, ethanol, and sodium hypochlorite.[5,14] Some of the active ingredients, for instance, sodium hypochlorite and ethanol, are widely available in non-medical and non-laboratory environments, which contributes to population access.[5,14] Evidence points out that surfaces that were cleaned with 70% alcohol had an expected disinfecting effect for two types of coronaviruses (mouse hepatitis virus and transmissible gastroenteritis virus) after one minute of contact, compared to 0.06% of sodium hypochlorite.[19] Tests carried out with SARS-CoV showed that sodium hypochlorite is effective at a concentration of 0.05% to 0.1% after five minutes when it is mixed with a solution containing SARS-CoV.[5,14] A study analysed surface stability of SARS-CoV-2, compared to SARS-CoV-1, the closest related human coronavirus.[5] The result of the experimental study is illustrated in Chart 1.

Chart 1 – Persistence of coronaviruses on inanimate surfaces.
Belo Horizonte, Minas Gerais, Brazil, 2020.

Type of surface	Persistence
Steel	48 hours
Metal	5 days
Paper	4-5 days
Glass	4 days
Plastic	< 5 days
Silicone rubber	5 days
Latex Glove	< 8 hours

Source: Adapted from Kampf et al.[5]

The results indicated that the virus can remain viable and infectious on surfaces from hours to days (depending on the inoculum), reinforcing the importance of hand hygiene after contact with inanimate environments and surfaces. This is most likely because the droplets of viruses that cause respiratory infections are expelled by coughing and sneezing, and a single droplet can easily contain an infectious dose. Furthermore, social distancing is also among the priorities of institutions to decrease transmission of SARS-CoV-2. Separation minimizes contact between potentially infected and healthy individuals, or between groups with high rates of transmission and or those with no or low levels, in order to delay the peak of the epidemic and lessen the magnitude of its effects, to protect assistance capacity clinic.[8] Isolation effectiveness depends on some epidemiological parameters, such as the number of secondary infections generated by each new infection and the proportion of transmissions that occur before the onset of symptoms.[14-15]

These measures are justified due to the risk that asymptomatic people who remain in the community may infect others until their isolation, which makes it a challenge to control the pandemic. Based on this premise, Figure 1 shows the main public health measures to be adopted early to reduce the impact of the pandemic.

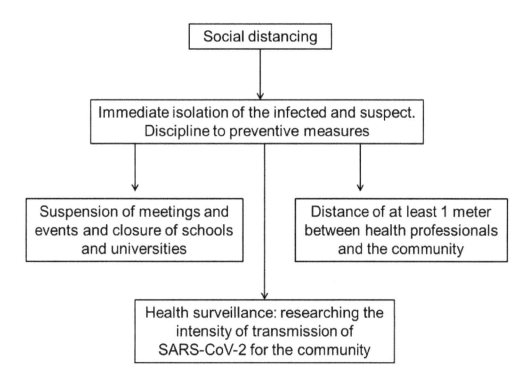

Figure 1 - Flowchart of measures to contain the circulation of the new coronavirus aiming at reducing the impact of the pandemic by COVID-19.[13] Belo Horizonte, Minas Gerais, Brazil, 2020.

A study that evaluated the case isolation effectiveness concerning COVID-19 control showed that isolation control over a period of three months, is more effective when there was low transmission, before the onset of symptoms.[21] However, isolation, without adequate preventive measures, may be considered insufficient to control the outbreak. Thus, community, at this moment, is alerted to the importance of correct hand hygiene technique, mask use and surface hygiene measures that jointly prevent spread of the virus.[8,22] Surgical mask use by patients reduces aerosol transmission, when in contact with suspected people of COVID-19 and with mild respiratory symptoms, since arrival at the health service, at the isolation site and during circulation within the service (transport from one area/sector to another), avoiding touching the mask, eyes, mouth and face as much as possible.[22-23] This measure can limit the spread of respiratory diseases, including the new coronavirus. However, only mask use is insufficient to provide safe level of protection in isolation and should always be associated with those already referred to as hand hygiene, especially before and after using masks. It should also be remembered that wearing masks when not indicated can generate unnecessary costs and create a false sense of security,
inducing negligence to other measures, such as hand hygiene and cleaning of inanimate surfaces potentially contaminated with SARS-CoV -2.[22-23] For performing procedures

in patients with suspected or confirmed infection with coronavirus (SARS-CoV-2), which can generate aerosols, such as procedures that induce cough, intubation or tracheal aspiration, invasive and non-invasive ventilation, cardiopulmonary resuscitation, manual ventilation before intubation, sputum induction, nasotracheal sample collections), healthcare professionals must use respiratory protection masks with minimum efficiency in the filtration of 95% of particles up to 0.3 μ (type N95, N99, N100, PFF2 or PFF3).8,23.

Procedures that can generate aerosols should preferably be performed in a respiratory isolation unit with negative pressure and a Hepa filter (high efficiency particulate arrestance).

In the absence of this type of unit, patients should be placed in a room with closed doors (and open windows) and restrict the number of professionals during these procedures.[23] To use respirators or mask N95 or PFF2, it must be considered that the equipment must be properly adjusted to the face. How they are uses, handled and stored must follow the manufacturer's recommendations, also the accessory must never be shared among professionals. The following checks of the components must be made before use, including strips and material of the nasal bridge, to ensure its fit and sealing: visually inspect the N95 mask to determine if its integrity has been compromised (damp, dirty, torn, dented or creased masks cannot be used). It is also important to note that the surgical mask should not be superimposed on the N95 mask or equivalent, as, in addition to not guaranteeing protection from filtration or contamination, it can also lead to the waste of another Personal Protective Equipment (PPE), which can be very damaging in this pandemic setting.[23]

Another relevant aspect is that exceptionally, in situations of lack of supplies and to meet the demand of the COVID-19 epidemic, the N95 mask or equivalent can be reused by the same professional, provided that mandatory steps are taken to remove the mask without contamination. inside. To minimize the contamination of the N95 mask or equivalent, if available, a face shield can be used. Also, if the mask is intact, clean and dry, it can be used several times during the same shift by the same professional (up to 12 hours or as defined by the Hospital Infection Control Commission - HICC - of the health service).[23] To remove the mask, the side elastics must first be removed, and the inner surface must not be touched. After removal, the mask must be packed in a paper bag or envelope with the elastics out, to facilitate the removal of the mask for new use.

Plastic bag use, however, may contribute to the mask remaining moist and potentially contaminated. Another aspect to be highlighted is about its cleaning, after use, these cannot be cleaned or disinfected for later use and when wet they lose their filtration capacity.[23] On the other hand, with the indication of mask use for health professionals, there was a rush to pharmacies to acquire these by the general population, which has generated a shortage for health services, in the care of patients with COVID-19. On April 2, 2020, the Ministry of Health of Brazil began to recommend the use of masks made of cotton, non-woven-textiles, among others, for the population in contact with suspects at home and that needs to go out to perform activities that may require contact with other people, so that masks act as a mechanical barrier.[24] However, attention must be paid to the other preventive measures already recommended, such as social distancing and keeping hands away from the eyes, nose and mouth, in addition to proper hand hygiene.

This indication is justified by the fact that the tissue mask can reduce the spread of the virus by asymptomatic or pre-symptomatic people who may be transmitting the virus without knowing it, but it does not protect the individual who is using it, as it has no filtering capacity of microorganisms. It should be noted that its use must be individual, and cannot be shared, and that, in health services, fabric masks should not be used under any circumstances, considering the provisions of Technical Note 4/2020, of the Brazilian National Surveillance Sanitary Agency (ANVISA – correspondent to US' FDA).[24] This measure favours the potential for contagion of people to happen, gradually, without the occurrence of a peak in the curve. Therefore, it contributes for the health system to be able to effectively care for those who are contaminated, with availability of equipment and personnel, without the overload found in the experience of other countries, due to the high number of infected in a short period of time.[4,11]

The other preventive and professional protection components must be aligned to the type of contact and procedure to be performed and to the vestment for assistance to the suspected patient/ carrier of COVID-19 and include the use of gloves, cloak/apron, goggles or protection facial, hat and apron. The cloak or apron (minimum weight of 30 g/m²) must be used to avoid contamination of the skin and clothing of professionals, who, after removal, needs to wash their hands.[23] Waterproof apron should be used to care for people suspected or infected by SARS-Cov-2.[23] Professionals should assess the need for the use of a waterproof coat or apron (minimum weight 50 g/m²) depending on the patient's clinical condition (vomiting, diarrhoea, orotracheal hypersecretion, bleeding, etc.).

The cloak or apron must have long sleeves, a mesh or elastic cuff and a rear opening. In addition, it must be made of good quality material, non-toxic.[23] It is recommended that the impermeable cloak or apron, after use, be considered contaminated, and should be removed and discarded as an infectious residue after performing the patient's procedure with COVID-19 before leaving the isolation room.[8,23] However, in a considerable part of places far from large centres in Brazil, the aprons available at the institutions are made of fabric, not disposable.

In these cases, however, at this time of the pandemic, it is necessary that after use, it is sent immediately to the laundry, and its reuse is not recommended during new appointments. Contamination risk and spread may increase in the case of apron reuse, increasing the demand for beds destined to more serious cases and even removal of health professionals due to their contamination. As for the use of procedure gloves, they must also be discarded before professionals leave the isolation room of patients. In addition, long-barrelled rubber glove use should be implemented for support personnel, such as cleaning professionals.[23] Care and attention of all professionals is essential for the premise that glove use does not replace hand hygiene and that the areas around patients, infected or not, such as tables and bedside rails, are considered contaminated. The areas should not be touched with gloves, in order not to favour spread of the virus in the environment. Thus, glove use inappropriately, especially in isolation sites with more than one patient with COVID-19, may cause cross-contamination among patients, favouring increased morbidity.

SPREAD OF COVID-19 WORLDWIDE

Experiences of affected countries, as well as evolution of the disease and the number of deaths in the world show an association between preventive measures that were implemented by the State and Government through health authorities and rigor with which they were incorporated by the population, as well as their impact on coping and progressing cases of the disease (Figure 2).

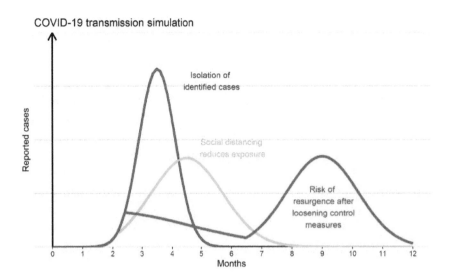

Figure 2 – Illustration of the COVID-19 transmission curve and its relationship with the population's adoption of hygiene, social restriction and non-agglomeration measures.[25] Belo Horizonte, Minas Gerais, Brazil, 2020.

What we have observed, however, is that even though the Ministry of Health reinforces the relevance of adopting such measures on a daily basis, its compliance at first showed a new learning for the population, above all, regarding the restriction or social distancing, threatened in part by the risk of increased unemployment, drop in income and/or often by minimizing the potential risk of the pandemic. These behaviours could decrease effectiveness of measures and increase the risk of resurgence of cases,[25] as shown in Figure 2. Efforts by health and political authorities in the states to encourage the population to stay at home to achieve a flattening of the curve and less circulation of the virus have been verified, as well as review of some recommendations.

In this setting of daily learning and monitoring of each case in the states and in the country, until April 18, 2020, by following the growth curve of cases in Brazil compared to other countries, it is possible to verify that the growth line shows itself differently from the devastating situation recorded in Italy, Spain, and the United States (Figure 3, left panel).[11-12] However, in the initial phase, a similar evolution can be seen in such countries, but which over time has distanced, possibly due to the impact of greater population compliance and strengthening of state policies for social restriction. The evolution of COVID-19 cases in Brazil in relation to some countries in Latin America (Figure 3, right panel) shows a prominent progression curve, followed by Peru, Chile and Ecuador. This figure shows the daily evolution of the infection, after each country has notified at least ten cases.[26] From the rapid evolution, world statistics consolidated by John Hopkins University, in the United States, until April 18, 2020, point out that after 39 days of recognition by WHO of the outbreak as a pandemic. The world registered 2,317,758 cases and 159,509 deaths, affecting 185 countries and regions worldwide.[26] The total number of confirmed cases increased from 100 thousand to 200 thousand, with an interval of twelve days.

Six days later, it exceeded 400 thousand cases, reaching more than 800 thousand seven days later; and, went from 500 thousand to 1 million in seven days, and passed the 2 million infected people 13 days later, showing a high speed in the doubling of the number of cases worldwide.[26] On the other hand, it is necessary to consider a certain difference in spread of infections in each country in a particular way, worldwide. The evolution of the doubling time of cases of the new coronavirus is shown in Figure 4, prepared considering information dated April 18, 2020.[27]

Therefore, it appears that, for instance, the estimated speed of duplication of cases, until March 24, for Canada and the United States (US), should occur every two and a half days. However, on April 7, this time increased to around seven days, showing a reduction in the speed of the spread, although it keeps these countries on alert for the total number of cases.[27] Colombia and Brazil, in the same interval, behaved differently, increasing the doubling time, that is, decreasing the speed of spread of the infection, until March 29 and 30, respectively. However, until April 3, this speed was higher for Brazil, reaching a doubling interval slightly higher than four days, showing the need to reinforce measures to contain the epidemic, seeking effective arrest of its advance. Until the end of the interval, on April 18, in general the times for doubling cases increased, showing a reduction in the speed of infections dissemination; in Mexico, Bolivia, Peru and Brazil the cases would be duplicated in up to 8 days, and the other countries in figure 4 showed duplication intervals of more than eleven days, up to eighteen days in the case of Colombia.

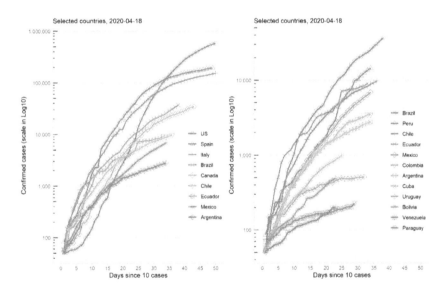

Figure 3 – Daily evolution curve for notified COVID-19 cases in Brazil, compared to other countries, from ten confirmed cases.[26] Belo Horizonte, Minas Gerais, Brazil, 2020.

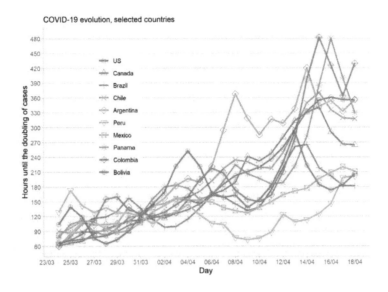

Figure 4 – Time distribution of doubling the number of COVID-19 cases in Brazil, compared to other countries.27 Belo Horizonte, Minas Gerais, Brazil, 2020.

EPIDEMIC CONTROL

The COVID-19 outbreak is still new and its duration uncertain. Thus, reducing exposure to the virus is necessary to control/delay spread of the disease and negative impacts, such as increased mortality and degradation of the economic and social situation.

Experiences from countries that adopted measures such as social distancing and early suspension of classes, Singapore, South Korea and Japan, point out that immediate implementation of these measures as well as rigorous management of cases and mass diagnoses influenced the course of transmissibility, resulting in a lower number of deaths. Singapore, for instance, on February 17, 2020, recorded the largest number of confirmed cases outside mainland China.

However, it immediately implemented control measures such as isolating all suspected or confirmed cases in rooms with negative pressure; training and re-education of health professionals to use personal protective equipment; use of respirators and air purifiers; monitoring of isolation teams for COVID-19 symptoms with thermal scanners to track fever; and investment in single-use equipment such as disposable bronchoscopes for bronchoscopy and percutaneous tracheostomy.[28] And even though there was an increase in cases in the last week, until April 18, Singapore recorded eleven deaths and 5,992 confirmed infections.[26]South Korea, had its first case registered on January 20, 2020, adopted contact management between suspects and infected people for epidemiological investigation. It also implemented a system for assessing the risk of exposure among people in all places where they were confirmed cases (after the onset of symptoms) and classified the contact persons based on that risk.

In addition, to eliminate the possibility of exposure to infection in the places visited by the confirmed patient, it performed appropriate disinfection of areas that could harbour environmental contamination.[29] Thus, systematic investigations were successful due to a rigorous control process based on scientific principles and continuous feedback assessment cycles to contain the outbreak.

Although there were more than 10,600 patients as of April 18, new infections have been abruptly reduced in recent weeks.[26] Japan carried out a rigorous surveillance between the time from the onset of the disease in a primary (suspected) case to its manifestation in a secondary (infected) case to understand the transmissibility of the disease.[30-31] With the mapping of suspect/infected data, it was initially possible to control spread and transmissibility from substantial pre-symptomatic transmissions and early isolation of people with COVID-19 in a population of 120 million.

As a result, as of April 18, 2020, cases reached 10,300, with a total of 222 deaths.[26] The Chinese special administrative region of Hong Kong, where 7.5 million people live, which shares a land border with the rest of China, recorded 1,024 cases and four deaths on April 18, 2020.[26] In this setting, WHO and experts agree that early detection of cases is a fundamental factor to contain the spread of a virus.

CONCLUSION

The involvement of the whole society in the conscious adoption of preventive measures against COVID-19 requires a change in individual and collective behaviour at that moment, immediately and rigorously. In this pandemic setting, it is possible to learn that its course and impacts in Brazil depend on the collaborative effort of all, government, families, and citizens. The world reality still points to a situation of great attention and can support choices of the path to be followed to face this critical moment, in order to allow interference in the rapid evolution of COVID-19.

REFERENCES

1. Word Health Organization. Considerations for quarantine of individuals in the context of containment for coronavirus disease (COVID-19): Interim guidance [Internet]. Geneva (CH); 2020 [cited 2020 Mar 24]. Available from: https://apps.who.int/iris/handle/10665/331299

2. Chang Le, Yan Y, Wang L. (2020).Coronavirus disease 2019: Coronaviruses and blood safety. Transfus Med Rev [Internet]. 2020 Feb 21 [cited 2020 Mar 23]. Available from: https://dx.doi.org/10.1016/j.tmrv.2020.02.003

3. Shang, J., Wan, Y., Liu, C., Yount, B., Gully, K., Yang. Y., et al(2020). Structure of mouse coronavirus spike protein complexed with receptor reveals mechanism for viral entry. PLoS Pathog [Internet]. 2020 [cited 2020 Mar 23];16(3):e1008392. Available from: https://dx.doi.org/10.1371/journal.ppat.1008392

4. Li R, Pei S, Chen, B., Song, Y., Zhang, T., Yang W, et al. (2020). Substantial undocumented infection facilitates the rapid dissemination of novel coronavirus (SARS-CoV2). Science [Internet]. 2020 Mar 16 [cited 2020 Mar 21]. Available from: https://www.ncbi.nlm.nih.gov/pubmed/32179701

5. Kampf G, Todt T, Pfaender S, Steinmann E. (2020).Persistence of coronaviruses on inanimate surfaces and their inactivation with biocidal agents. J Hosp Infect [Internet]. 2020 [cited 2020 Mar 22];104(3):246-

6. Available from: https://dx.doi.org/10.1016/j.jhin.2020.01.022

7. Tian, H., Liu, Y., Li, Y., Wu, C.H, Chen, B., Kraemer, M.U.G, et al. (2020).The impact of transmission control measures during the first 50 days of the COVID-19 2 epidemic in China. MedRxiv [Internet]. 2020 Mar 10 [cited 2020 Mar 23]. Available from: https://dx.doi.org/10.1101/2020.01.30.20019844

8. Kim, J.Y., Choe PG, Oh Y, Oh KJ, Kim J, Park SJ, et al. (2020).The first case of 2019 novel coronavirus pneumonia imported into Korea from Wuhan, China: implication for infection prevention and control measures. J Korean Med Sci [Internet]. 2020 [cited 2020 Mar 21];10;35(5):e61. Available from: https://dx.doi.org/10.3346/jkms.2020.35.e61

9. World Health Organization. Rational use of personal protective equipment (PPE) for coronavirus disease (COVID-19): interim guidance [Internet]. Geneva (CH); 2020 [cited 2020 Mar 23]. Available from: https://apps.who.int/iris/handle/10665/331498

10. Ministério da Saúde (BR). Portaria nº 454, de 20 de março de 2020: declara, em todo o território nacional, o estado de transmissão comunitária do coronavírus (COVID-19). Diário Oficial da União [Internet]. 2020 Mar 20 [cited 2020 Mar 26]; 1:1. Available from: http://www.in.gov.br/en/web/ dou/-/portaria-n-454-de-20-de-marco-de-2020-249091587

11. Valente, J. (2020).COVID-19: governo declara transmissão comunitária em todo o país. Agência Brasil [Internet]. 2020 Mar 20 [cited 2020 Mar 21]. Available from: https://agenciabrasil.ebc.com.br/ saude/noticia/2020-03/COVID-19-governo-declara-transmissao-comunitaria-em-todo-o-pais

12. Vetter, P., Guitart C, Lotfinejad N, Pittet D(2020).. Understanding the emerging coronavirus: what it means for health security and infection prevention. J Hosp Infect [Internet]. 2020 Mar 4 [cited 2020 Mar 17];104(4):440-8. Available from: https://dx.doi.org/10.1016/j.jhin.2020.02.023

13. Remuzzi A; Remuzzi, G. (2020). COVID-19 and Italy: what next? Lancet [Internet]. 2020 Mar 13 [cited 2020 Mar 24];395:1225-8 Available from: https://doi.org/10.1016/S0140-6736(20)30627-9

14. European Centre for Disease Prevention and Control. Considerations relating to social distancing measures in response to the COVID-19 epidemic [Internet]. Stockholm (SW); 2020 Mar 23 [cited 2020 Mar 23]. Available from: https://www.ecdc.europa.eu/en/publications-data/considerationsrelating-social-distancing-measures-response-COVID-19-second

15. World Health Organization. Critical preparedness, readiness and response actions for COVID-19 [Internet]. Geneva (CH); 2020 [cited 2020 Mar 18]. Available from: https://www.who.int/emergencies/ diseases/novel-coronavirus-2019/technical-guidance/critical-preparedness-readiness-andresponse-actions-for-COVID-19

16. World Health Organization. 2019 Novel coronavirus (2019-nCoV): strategic preparedness and response plan [Internet]. Geneva (CH); 2020 [cited 2020 Mar 17]. Available from: https://reliefweb. int/report/world/2019-novel-coronavirus-2019-ncov-strategic-preparedness-and-response-plandraft-3

17. European Centre for Disease Prevention and Control Rapid risk assessment: Novel coronavirus disease 2019 (COVID-19) pandemic: increased transmission in the EU/EEA and the UK: sixth update [Internet]. Stockholm (SW); 2020 Mar 12 [cited 2020 Mar 17]. Available from: https:// www.ecdc.europa.eu/en/publications-data/rapid-risk-assessment-novel-coronavirus-disease2019-COVID-19-pandemic-increased

18. Oliveira, A., De Paula, A., Souza, M., Silva, A. (2020).. Adesão à higiene de mãos entre profissionais de um serviço de pronto atendimento. Rev Med [Internet]. 2016 [cited 2020 Mar 20];95(4):162-7. Available from: https://dx.doi.org/10.11606/issn.1679-9836.v95i4p162-167

19. Amorim, C..S..V, Pinheiro, I.F., Vieira, V.G., Guimarães, R.A., Nunes, O.S., Marinho, T.A. (2020). Hand hygiene and influenza prevention: knowledge of health students. Texto Contexto Enferm [Internet]. 2018 [cited 2020 Apr 3];27(4):e4570017. Available from: https://dx.doi.org/10.1590/0104-070720180004570017

20. European Centre for Disease Prevention and Control. Interim guidance for environmental cleaning in non-healthcare facilities exposed to SARS-CoV-2 [Internet]. Stockholm (SW); 2020 Feb 18 [cited 2020 Apr 2]. Available from: https://www.ecdc.europa.eu/en/publications-data/interimguidance-environmental-cleaning-non-healthcare-facilities-exposed-2019

21. Van Doremalen, N, Bushmaker, T., Morris, D.H., Holbrook, M.G., Gamble, A., Williamson, B.N. Aerosol and surface stability of SARS-CoV-2 as compared with SARS-CoV-1. N Engl J Med [Internet]. 2020 Mar 17 [cited 2020 Mar 23];382:1564-7. Available from: https://dx.doi.org/10.1056/NEJMc2004973

22. Gostic, K., Gomez, A.C, Mummah, R.O., Kuchars. (2020). ki AJ, Lloyd-Smith JO. Estimated effectiveness of symptom and risk screening to prevent the spread of COVID-19. Elife [Internet]. 2020 Feb 24 [cited 2020 Mar 18];2020;9:e55570 Available from: https://dx.doi.org/10.7554/eLife.55570

23. Hellewell, J., Abbott, Gimma, A., Bosse, N.I., Jarvis ,C.I, Russel, T.W., et al. Feasibility of controlling COVID-19 outbreaks by isolation of cases and contacts. Lancet Glob Health [Internet]. 2020 [cited 2020 Mar 15];8(4):e486. Available from: https://www.thelancet.com/journals/langlo/article/ piis2214-109x(20)30074-7/fulltext

24. Agência Nacional de V.(2020). igilância Sanitária (BR). Nota técnica GVIMS/GGTES/ANVISA nº 04/2020: orientações para serviços de saúde: medidas de prevenção e controle que devem ser adotadas durante a assistência aos casos suspeitos ou confirmados de infecção pelo novo coronavírus (SARS-CoV-2) [Internet]. Brasília, DF(BR); 2020 [cited 2020 Mar 23]. Available from: http://portal. anvisa.gov.br/documents/33852/271858/nota+t%c3%a9cnica+n+04-2020+gvims-ggtes-anvisa/ ab598660-3de4-4f14-8e6f-b9341c196b28

25. Ministério da Saúde (BR). Máscaras caseiras podem ajudar na prevenção contra o Coronavírus [Internet]. Brasília, DF(BR);2020 [cited 2020 Apr 3]. Available from: https://www.saude.gov. br/noticias/agencia-saude/46645-mascaras-caseiras-podem-ajudar-na-prevencao-contra-ocoronavirus

26. Anderson, R.M., Heesterbeek, H., Klinkenberg, D., Hollingsworth, T.D. (2020).How will country-based mitigation measures influence the course of the COVID-19 epidemic? Lancet [Internet]. 2020 [cited 2020 Apr 4];395(10228):931-34. Available from: https://www.thelancet.com/journals/lancet/article/ piis0140-6736(20)30567-5/fulltext

27. Dong, E, Du, H, Gardner, L. An interactive web-based dashboard to track COVID-19 in real time. Lancet Infect Dis [Internet]. 2020 Feb 27 [cited 2020 Apr 3].

28. Abbott, S., Hellewell, J., Munday, J.D., Chun, J.Y., Thompson, R.N. Bosse., NI, et al. (2020).Temporal variation in transmission during the COVID-19 outbreak. CMMID Repository [Internet]. 2020 Mar 2 [cited 2020 Apr 2]. Available from: https://cmmid.github.io/topics/covid19/current-patterns-transmission/ global-time-varying-transmission.html

29. Liew, M.F, Siow, W.T., MacLaren, G,, See KC. Preparing for COVID 19: early experience from an intensive care unit in Singapore. Crit Care [Internet]. 2020 [cited 2020 Mar 26];24(1):83. Available from: https://dx.doi.org/10.1186/s13054-020-2814-x

30. COVID-19 National Emergency Response Centre, Epidemiology & Case Management Team, Korea Centres for Disease Control & Prevention. Contact Transmission of COVID-19 in South Korea: novel investigation techniques for tracing contacts. Osong Public Health Res Perspect [Internet]. 2020 [cited 2020 Mar 25];11(1):60-3. Available from: https://dx.doi.org/10.24171/j. phrp.2020.11.1.09

31. Kakimoto, K, Kamiya, H., Yamagishi, T., Matsui, T., Suzuki, M., Wakita, T (2020).. Initial investigation of transmission of COVID-19 among crew members during quarantine of a cruise ship: Yokohama, Japan, February 2020. MMWR Surveill Summ. [Internet]. 2020 [cited 2020 Mar 18];69(11):312-3. Available from: https://dx.doi.org/10.15585/mmwr.mm6911e2

32. Nakazawa, E., Ino H, Akabayashi, A. (2020). Chronology of COVID-19 cases on the Diamond Princess cruise ship and ethical considerations: a report from Japan. Disaster Med Public Health Prep [Internet]. 2020 Mar 24 [cited 2020 Mar 20]. Available from: https://dx.doi.org/10.1017/dmp.2020.50

8.Dark Future For Brazil In The Fight Against Coronavirus

Fernando Alcoforado*

Many rulers in the world regard the fight against Coronavirus as a war against an invisible enemy. The indispensable condition for a nation to win the war is to be united against the common enemy, the Coronavirus. In Brazil, this condition is not respected because whoever should lead the fight against Coronavirus, the President of the Republic, Jair Bolsonaro, is opposing it by systematically disrespecting all restrictive measures on the gathering of people under the pretext that it is necessary to save, also, the Brazilian economy from debacle. In his action to compromise the fight against Coronavirus, Bolsonaro says that people must go back to work because Chloroquine cures the disease that is not proven by the WHO - World Health Organization and by scientists around the world. The fact that Bolsonaro assumes this attitude is encouraging a large number of people to leave the isolation in which they find themselves and return to the street as is already happening in several cities in Brazil. The end of many people's social isolation is also related to the fact that they need to work to survive, given that the Bolsonaro government does not offer all Brazilians the necessary conditions for their survival.

In addition to acting to destroy the effort of governors and mayors to fight the Coronavirus, the Bolsonaro government does not act with the necessary urgency in the economic plan with the use of the financial resources it has to help vulnerable populations to fight hunger, companies in general not to be bankrupt and states and municipal governments to avoid their insolvency. All economic initiatives adopted to date have come from the National Congress. Brazil urgently needs strategic alignment in health actions with those of an economic nature, in order to facilitate the isolation of people to fight the Coronavirus. Total social isolation should only be replaced by partial isolation, as Bolsonaro suggests, in a second stage after which everything would return to normal in a third stage. This process should be implemented based on data that indicate a downward trend in the number of contaminated and killed by Coronavirus. As these numbers regress, the least affected areas should move to partial isolation followed by total clearance. In the third stage, to reactivate the Brazilian economy, massive public investments in public works and private investments facilitated by the government with the reduction of bank interest and tax burden should occur. This should be the rational process that would make health and economics compatible. The need for total social isolation is imperative in order not to collapse the health system in Brazil. At least 2.8 billion people - representing more than a third of the world's population - currently live under some kind of restriction of circulation to contain the rapid advance of Covid-19, a disease caused by the new coronavirus (Sars-Cov -2), points out a balance sheet by the agency France Presse (AFP). At a time when the pandemic is accelerating at an exponential rate, WHO advocates the physical isolation of people, despite its significant social and economic cost.

Without aggressive action in all countries, millions could die, said the organization's director general, Tedros Ghebreyesus. The rules of social isolation, which vary from country to country, aim to reduce the transmission time of the virus from person to person, giving governments time to equip and strengthen their health systems with equipment, expansion of beds, construction of hospitals and hiring health professionals and, above all, avoiding the collapse of health systems as occurred in Italy and Spain and may occur in the United States. The countries that have adopted social isolation are the following: China, South Korea, Taiwan, United States, Singapore, Hong Kong, France, Germany, Italy, India, United Kingdom, Spain, Brazil, Chile, Argentina and Peru. In general , the restriction model depends on the degree of spread of the disease, the political context and the alignment with WHO recommendations. It usually starts with limitations of agglomerations, suspension of classes, advances with restrictions on circulation and, in the most extreme cases, even provides for a curfew and a fine for those who leave home.

Bolsonaro's attitude in opposition to the total social isolation policy adopted in the vast majority of countries in the world and against the will of 76% of the Brazilian population in favour of this measure in a recent Data Folha survey, does not collaborate in overcoming the common enemy of Brazilian people, which is the Coronavirus. The fight against Coronavirus should be led by Bolsonaro, as President of the Republic, who, on the contrary, sabotages all necessary actions. In practice, the true commander in the war against the Coronavirus should follow the teachings of Sun Tzu, a great military strategist, who in his work The Art of War states that: 1) A leader leads by example, not by force. This is not the case with Bolsonaro because he does not set an example by exposing himself in public and the people he contacts, in addition to wanting to forcefully impose his will to end total social isolation through a decree that is prevented by the National Congress and the Judicial power; and, 2) The enlightened ruler establishes plans to follow, and the good general cultivates his resources. This is not the case with Bolsonaro who, as a ruler, does not establish plans to fight the Coronavirus and, on the contrary, acts to torpedo the plans of the Ministry of Health and of the governors and mayors.

In the article "How and when will this pandemic end? published on the website[1]

Belgian virologist Guido Vanham, former head of virology at the Antwerp Institute of Tropical Medicine in Belgium, answered the following questions: how will this pandemic end? and what factors might it depend on? In this article there is synthetically the following:

5. It will probably never end, in the sense that this virus is clearly here to stay, unless we eradicate it. And the only way to eradicate this virus would be with a very effective vaccine that is delivered to every human being. We did this with smallpox, but that is the only example - and it took many years. So, it will probably stay. It belongs to a family of viruses that we know - the coronaviruses - and one of the questions now is whether it will behave like other viruses.

6. We know that people develop antibodies. This has been clearly demonstrated in China, but we are still not sure how protective these antibodies are. There is still no convincing evidence that people who have recovered will fall ill again after a few days or weeks - so antibodies are probably at least partially protective. But how long will this protection last - is it a matter of months or years? Epidemiology in the future will depend on that - the level of protective immunity you get at the population level after this wave of infections, which we really cannot stop. We can mitigate it, we can flatten the curve, but we can't really stop it, because at some point we will have to leave our homes again and go to work and study. Nobody really knows when that will be.

7. What are some of the factors at play? What do we know and what do we not know? The first thing we know is that it is a very infectious virus. But what is not known is the infectious dose - how many viruses you need to produce an infection - and that will be very difficult to know, unless we carry out

---

[1] <https://www.weforum.org/agenda/2020/04/how-and-when-will-this-pandemic-end-we- asked-a-virologist />,

experimental infections. The virus will run its course and there will be a certain level of immunity - but the answer to how long it will take will determine the periodicity and extent of the epidemics to come. Unless, of course, we find a way to block it in a year or more from now with an effective vaccine.

On the vaccine against Coronavirus, researchers from the United States and Germany are ahead in this race and with about 20 groups dedicated to finding an immunization against the disease. China has developed its first prototype and the Ministry of Defence has announced that the country is ready to start clinical trials on humans. Volunteers between 18 and 60 are being called in to test the vaccine. The United States, which started the first phase of its clinical trials the day before the Chinese announcement, is also pursuing a quick, effective and safe solution. The vaccine problem, however, does not end with the discovery. It is necessary to produce it on a large scale and distribute it to millions of people. No government believes that this can happen in less than twelve months. Another promising news comes from Japan, where a drug called Favipiravir, also known as Avigan, has been recommended by Chinese health officials because it speeds up the recovery of infected people. Those who received Favipiravir were negative for the virus after an average of four days after becoming positive, while those who did not use the drug needed an average of eleven days to recover. Other drugs, chloroquine and hydroxychloroquine, drugs that regulate the immune system in the face of infections, are considered harmful to health in the treatment of Coronavirus according to the opinion of highly qualified professors at Oxford University and Birmingham University. The widespread use of hydroxychloroquine exposes some patients to rare but potentially fatal damage, including severe skin reactions, fulminant liver failure and ventricular arrhythmias (especially when prescribed with azithromycin), says the article signed by Professor Robin Ferner of the Institute of Clinical Sciences from the University of Birmingham, and Jeffrey Aronson, from the Department of Health Sciences at the University of Oxford, UK. Vaccines and medicines can be the antidote to the pandemic. But that will not come anytime soon and what we have left for now, if we want to collaborate with society, is total social isolation. At this time, individual conduct may be more important in containing the plague than government actions. From the above, it can be concluded that total social isolation is absolutely necessary at the moment in Brazil, that chloroquine is not yet proven as a drug capable of beating Coronavirus, that there is no vaccine capable of preventing people from the disease and that Brazil will not win the war against the virus if Bolsonaro's will prevails. The future of Brazil is gloomy with the increase in people infected with Coronavirus and deaths of people from any type of disease and by the Coronavirus itself that will not be attended to due to the collapse of the Brazilian health system.

CHAPTER 21

ADHERANCE AND RESISTANCE TO COVID-19 INTERVENTION STRATEGIES

1.Is Social Distancing And Movement Constraints Responsible For The COVID-19 Outbreak Brazil?

Matheus Tenório Baumgartner[a][*][¶], Fernando Miranda Lansac-Tôha[a][*][¶],Marco Túlio Pacheco Coelho[b], Ricardo Dobrovolski[c] & José Alexandre Felizola Diniz-Filho[b][1]

ABSTRACT

As thousands of new cases of COVID-19 have been confirmed, there is an increasing demand to understand the factors underlying the spread of this disease. Using country level data, we modelled the early growth in the number of cases for over 480 cities in all Brazilian states. As the main findings, we found that the percentage of people respecting social distancing protocols was the main explanatory factor for the observed growth rate of COVID-19. Those cities that presented the highest spread of the new coronavirus were also those that had lower averages of social distancing. We also underline that total population of cities and connectivity, represented by the city-level importance to the air transportation of people across the country, plays important roles in the dissemination of SARS-CoV-2. Climate and socioeconomic predictors had little contribution to the big-picture scenario. Our results show that different States had high variability in their growth rates, mostly due to quite different public health strategies to retain the outbreak of COVID-19. In spite of all limitations of such a large-scale approach, our results underline that climatic conditions are likely weak limiting factors for the spread of the new coronavirus, and the circulation of people in the city- and country-level are the most responsible factors for the early outbreak of COVID-19 in Brazil. Moreover, we reinforce that social distancing protocols are fundamental to avoid critical scenarios and the collapse of healthcare systems. We also predict that economic induced decisions for relaxing social distancing might have catastrophic consequences, especially in large cities.

INTRODUCTION

In late December 2019, the novel Coronavirus Disease 2019 (COVID-19) emerged in Wuhan, the capital city of Hubei Province in great China (Zhu et al., 2020). At the beginning of the infection outbreak, the disease caused by the SARS-CoV-2 virus has been suggested to be of bat origin (Cheng et al., 2007; Guo et al., 2020; Zhou et al., 2020), and might have been transmitted to humans through intermediate mammals (Andersen et al., 2020; Li et al., 2020; Zhang et al., 2020). The initial diffusion of the virus suddenly became exponential, increasing the number of infected cases and deaths in Wuhan (Kraemer et al., 2020). In the next few weeks, it has become clear that the high

---

[1] aDepartamento de Biologia, Centro de Ciências Biológicas, Universidade Estadual de Maringá, Maringá, PR, Brasil
bDepartamento de Ecologia, Universidade Federal de Goiás, Goiânia, GO, Brazil cInstituto de Biologia, Universidade Federal da Bahia, Salvador, BA, Brazil

virulence of the new coronavirus posed a considerable health threat on a global scale, quickly spreading to Asia, Europe, North America, and, more recently, South America and Africa.

On March 11, 2020, the World Health Organization (WHO) declared the coronavirus as a global pandemic. The declaration reflected the concern by WHO that countries were unable to control the dissemination of the virus (Li et al., 2020). The novel coronavirus is still spreading rapidly worldwide, with millions of infections and hundreds of thousands of deaths addressed to COVID-19, most of them concentrated in the United States and Europe. Common symptoms of COVID-19 infections include fever, dry cough, and dyspnoea but the most serious clinical case is lung failure associated with severe acute respiratory syndrome (SARS) (Yang et al., 2020). From all infected patients, about 30% require mechanical ventilation and 2-5% die, with higher death rates in elderly people and those with comorbidities (Rothan and Byrareddy, 2020). Fortunately, most people have very mild symptoms or are even asymptomatic (Yang et al., 2020).

Conventionally, laboratory testing by real-time polymerase chain reaction (RT-PCR) and quick antigen tests have been conducted prioritizing symptomatic or high-risk groups (Mizumoto et al., 2020). However, a recent study showed that substantial undocumented infection facilitates the rapid dissemination of the novel coronavirus (R. Li et al., 2020), which forced the WHO to recommend that policymakers should mobilize mass testing in an attempt to retain initial local outbreaks effectively (Balilla, 2020). With clinical symptoms that are indicative of many ordinary conditions, the new coronavirus is the largest concern for human populations because it may cause severe clinical conditions that can readily overcome the carrying capacity of healthcare facilities. Although vaccines and immunotherapy protocols have been conducted in a rate never seen before, there is no effective treatment for COVID-19 yet (Lurie et al., 2020).

The available interventions include rapid diagnosis and isolation of confirmed cases, and restrictions on mobility (Kraemer et al., 2020). Especially for in-development countries, social isolation has been listed as the most effective strategy to deal with COVID-19 and mitigate the risk for public health and economy (Coelho et al., 2020). However, understanding how other environmental and social factors are associated with human-to-human transmissions of SARS-CoV-2 are fundamental for the decision-making process at a country-level. Building on evidence about the role of environmental factors such as temperature and humidity on the survival of viruses, some studies forecasted the near future of the current outbreak (Sajadi et al., 2020; Wang et al., 2020). For instance, Araújo and Naimi (2020) built a global ensemble to model the monthly spread of COVID-19 under the prediction of temperature and humidity, although with some later criticism (Chipperfield, 2020). While these variables are known to interfere with the spread and survival of other coronaviruses (e.g., SARS-CoV and MERS-CoV; Gaunt *et al.*, 2010; Chan *et al.*, 2011; Cauchemez *et al.*, 2014), considering only the environment and ignoring social and behavioural factors might be inadequate to determine effective restraint strategies in the near future (Pybus et al., 2015).

Considering socioeconomic aspects, countries and regions across the world have a very skewed distribution of income and wealth (Dabla-Norris et al., 2015; Davies et al., 2017). Even within countries, there are clear spatial distribution patterns of economic development, as it is explicit within Brazil (Skidmore, 2004). In terms of healthcare, socioeconomic indicators can be considered as a proxy for the ability of each city to identify and treat people with COVID-19 effectively (Coelho et al., 2020). Additionally, the dispersal of viruses among hosts follows a geographic pattern (Holmes, 2004).

Thus, the physical distance among cities (and people) is certainly crucial for how the actual pandemic state will evolve (Chipperfield, 2020). In an attempt to investigate these factors, Coelho et al. (2020) found evidence that the air transportation of people across the word overcame environmental and socioeconomic factors, posing a strong argument towards social distancing and traveling restraint. Thus, here we extended the investigation on which factors could be related to the spread of the new coronavirus in Brazil, considering all cities on a nation-wide scale. We studied the exponential growth of time series data for over 460 cities with reported cases of infections by the new coronavirus, considering the effect of the environment, socioeconomic indicators, movement of people across the country, and social distancing. We demonstrate that the growth of COVID-19 in different cities is mostly determined by population size, transportation among cities, and the percentage of people respecting social distancing protocols. This evidence points towards social distancing and mobility restriction as the main actions necessary to reduce the spreading of the pandemic and avoid its worst consequences.

MATERIAL AND METHODS

Dataset and Exponential Growth Model

We obtained data on the daily number of people manifesting the COVID-19 in Brazil, available at the digital panel from the Ministry of Health [1] This dataset comprises real-time information on disease cases that were confirmed through laboratory analysis and quick tests for every city. Our most recent data retrieval was conducted on April 20, 2020, which comprised information of 40,581 cases and time series data for 1,456 cities with at least one confirmed case, since the first recorded case in Brazil on February, 25, 2020. We chose April 20 as the last day because several cities have gradually relaxed their quarantine protocols and allowed many working activities to restore their functioning since then. In our analyses, we used only the exponential part of each time series by excluding previous days before the first confirmed cases in each city, and no time series had reached stabilization or decrease in the total number of confirmed records yet. We fitted exponential growth models to the time series of each city and calculated the intrinsic growth rate (r), as well as the slope coefficient (b) of the log growth model. Because our focus was on the overall growth of the number of confirmed cases, these two parameters were candidates to be used as response variables in our approach. However, some convergence failures for exponential models applied on short time series and the high goodness-of-fit of log-transformed models (average R^2 = 0.84) led us to use the log-growth slope in our subsequent analysis.

Predictor Variables

In order to explore potential correlates of the early increase in the number of cases, we used climatic and socioeconomic data. Climatic variables included average temperature (ºC) and precipitation (mm), retrieved from the most recent year available at the WorldClim online database [2] This database comprises monthly information on these climatic variables. We downloaded temperature and precipitation values between February and April, which coincided

---

[1] (http://www.covid.saude.gov.br).
[2] (http://www.worldclim.org; Fick & Hijmans, 2017).

with the time series of COVID-19 cases in Brazil and with the late summer season of the Southern Hemisphere, matching the world outbreak of the virus.

From these data, we extracted values for each city according to their geographic coordinates, using the QGIS 3.12.1 software (QGIS Development Team, 2020).

For each city, we also extracted information on total population, Human Development Index (HDI), and average income. These demographic data were obtained from the digital platform maintained by the Institute of Applied Economic Research, under the '*Atlas do Desenvolvimento Humano no Brasil*' project This initiative encompasses data[1] about more than 5,500 municipalities in all 27 Brazilian federal units, with several socioeconomic descriptors derived from the 2010 national census. As an additional correlate to the increase of the infestation by the new virus, we also considered information on transportation of people across the country. First, we obtained data on air transportation available at the Open Flights database [2]which included information on 122 airports within Brazil, and whether there is a direct flight connecting each pair of them (1,193 flights). To match the information on the spread of the virus across cities, we filtered these airport records to consider only those cities that had at least one confirmed infection, which yielded us a database containing 100 cities with 1,164 registered flights (Fig 1).

We then used these cities and flights to construct an oriented graph with cities assigned as notes and flight routes as edges (West, 2001). From this network, we extracted a variable that weighted the importance of each city to the country-level network: the Eigenvector Centrality (Bonacich, 1987). This metric quantifies both how surrounding cities are connected to a focal city and its connection to the whole network, directly and indirectly. Second, many cities with confirmed cases are not large enough to carry airports with commercial flights. In these cases, we used the geographic coordinates to calculate the proximity to the nearest airport (1 - standardized Euclidean distances), which was then multiplied by the centrality of their respective nearest airport. These two procedures yielded connectivity, a variable that represented the direct and indirect movement of people among large cities, based on their centrality, as well as their potential exchange of people with smaller municipalities nearby, described by the proximity-weighted centrality.

---

[1] (http://www.atlasbrasil.org.br/).

[2] (http://openflights.org/data.html),

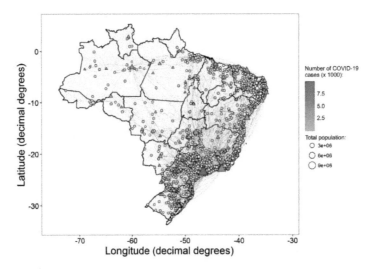

Fig. 1: Geographic distribution of 1,456 cities with at least one confirmed case of COVID-19 in Brazil by April 20, 2020. Blue circles represent cities with less than five confirmed cases, which were not included in our analyses. Yellow, orange, and red symbols depict cities that had at least five confirmed cases, with (82 cities; triangles) and without (383 cities; circles) airports. Flying routes are depicted by grey traces and State borders are in black. See Fig. S1 for more details on the names and locations of each Brazilian state.

In order to assess the effectiveness of social distancing on the early spread of the new coronavirus in Brazilian cities, we used State-level data on mobility of citizens[1] which comes from a monitoring program that was exclusively implemented to be useful against the new coronavirus. This database comprises the percentage of people performing social distancing for each state on a daily basis. The index is based on information provided by telephone companies about the location of electronic devices (e.g., cell phones and tablets), which are tracked through their physical displacement under Wi-Fi, Bluetooth, and GPS connections. In practice, whenever an electronic device leaves a radius of ~200 m from what it is considered as 'home', the system records the event as a movement. Therefore, this protocol ensures the privacy and preserves the identity of citizens by focusing on the binary record of movement, rather than on the destination or specific routes of each citizen. This information yielded us a database with the time series of social distancing for each state.

To obtain city-level data, we averaged the percentages between the first day of COVID-19 record in Brazil and the day where the thresholds of the minimum number of cases was achieved at each city (see below).See Supplementary Material Fig. S1 for more details on the names and locations of each Brazilian state. Time series of percentages of people respecting social distancing protocols at each Brazilian state are given in Fig. S2.

Data Analysis

We investigated whether the city-level growth rate of COVID-19 was related to the climatic, socioeconomic, connectivity, and social distancing predictors using multiple linear regression models. Models were fitted using sequential subsets of the 465 cities considering increasing thresholds of the minimum number of confirmed cases: 5, 10, 20, 40, 80, and 160.This sequential sub-modelling approach intended to assess whether and how the COVID-19 outbreak across Brazil was related to each one of our predictors along the early spread of the disease, considering cities at

---

[1] (https://mapabrasileirodacovid.inloco.com.br/),

different stages of the dissemination wave. All predictors were checked, and only total population required log transformation to approximate a normal distribution. Before statistical analyses, we checked the multicollinearity of predictors, by computing the variance inflation factors (VIF), and removed those that the variance of a regression coefficient was inflated in the presence of other explanatory variables (i.e. VIF > 5; (Borcard et al., 2018)). In this case, HDI and average income showed collinearity, so we kept the later in our analyses because of its larger variation. In addition, we used Moran's I correlograms (Legendre and Legendre, 2012) to check if the control for spatial autocorrelation bias was required, which could somehow inflate the significance of each predictor. A summary of all the predictors used to fit the regression models is provided in Fig 2.

Finally, we fitted independent linear models to each State to investigate potential regional trends in the COVID-19 growth, using the most important predictors identified in the previous steps, separately. For this procedure, we used only those states that had at least five cities with at least five confirmed cases. For inference, we then plotted the log-transformed total number of confirmed cases against the standardized slopes of the models, which portrays the state-dependent context of growth in COVID-19 cases. All analyses were performed in the R Environment (R Core Team, 2019) using packages *ape* (Paradis and Schliep, 2019), *car* (Fox and Weisberg., 2019), and *igraph* (Csardi and Nepusz, 2006).

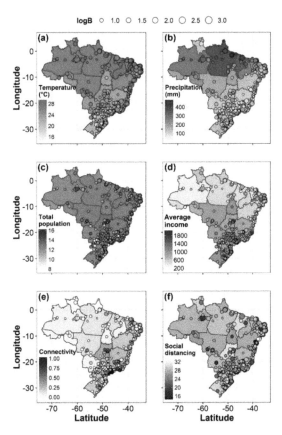

Fig. 2: Brazilian maps showing the geographic patterns of all predictors considered in the regression models: temperature (a), precipitation (b), log-total population (c), average income (d), connectivity (e), and social distancing (f). States borders are depicted by black traces and colours of each State represents the mean value considering all cities. Circles depict cities that had at least five confirmed cases. The colours within circles represent the values of each predictor, whereas the circle size depicts the b log growth rate (logB) for each city.

RESULTS

The overall performance of models fitted to the exponential growth of COVID19 in each city was particularly good. The average variance explained by our predictors (R^2) were 0.51 (>= 5 cases; 465 cities), 0.60 (>= 10 cases; 252 cities), 0.61 (>= 20 cases; 158 cities), 0.64 (>= 40 cases; 104 cities), 0.56 (>= 80 cases; 62 cities), and 0.67 (>= 160 cases; 33 cities). Considering the effect of each predictor on the exponential growth across all sub-models, social distancing had significant relationships in all cases, with an average standardized coefficient of -0.15 (Table 1, Fig 3). This variable was also the only with negative significant slope coefficients. Most importantly, social distancing had an intensifying trend in its negative coefficient across sub-models, showing an enhanced effect as the number of confirmed cases evolved. In addition, total population and connectivity of each city had significant relationships in five out of six sub-models, with average standardized coefficients of 0.14 and 0.07, respectively. Another predictor that played a secondary role was precipitation, which was significant in the first four sub-models, although with a considerably weak average standardized coefficients (0.05). Average income was only significant for the first sub-model, whereas temperature was not significant in any sub-model. None of the six sub-models presented bias related to spatial autocorrelation structures according to Moran's I correlograms.

Table 1. Parameter estimates (standardized β's) for all variables used as predictors of the slope coefficient (b) of the log-growth models, fitted for the number of confirmed cases of infection by Coronavirus Disease (COVID-19). Significant estimates (at $\alpha = 0.05$) are in bold; see Table S1 for full results.

	Number of cases					
	>= 5 (df=458)	>= 10 (df=245)	>= 20 (df=151)	>= 40 (df=97)	>=80 (df=58)	>=160 (df=26)
Intercept	0.93	1.17	1.38	1.55	1.71	1.93
Temperature (°C)	0.02	0.02	0.04	0.04	0.00	-0.03
Precipitation (mm)	**0.08**	**0.09**	**0.07**	**0.06**	0.07	0.09
Total population	**0.13**	**0.17**	**0.18**	**0.11**	**0.11**	0.09
Average income	**0.05**	0.03	0.01	0.00	0.00	-0.01
Connectivity	**0.07**	**0.07**	**0.07**	**0.06**	**0.08**	0.04
Social distancing	**-0.13**	**-0.13**	**-0.11**	**-0.17**	**-0.15**	**-0.19**

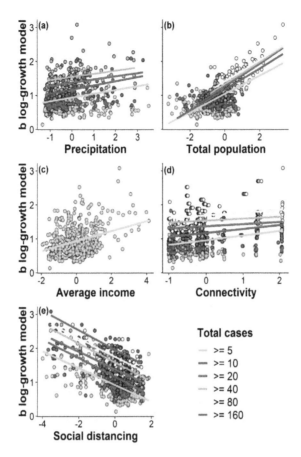

Fig. 3: Relationships between the slopes of log-growth models fitted to time series of confirmed COVID-19 cases for every city. Only significant regression models are shown.

Comparatively, the variable with the clearest effect on the exponential growth during the COVID-19 early outbreak was social distancing (Table 1; Fig 3e). In practice, this result suggest that the more frequent people circulated within cities (lower social distancing), the faster the early spread of the new coronavirus (a result that was consistent across all sub-models). The results also reveal that the log-growth of the disease caused by the SARS-CoV-2 virus increased with the total population of cities (Fig 3). Thus, larger population sizes led to faster spread of the new coronavirus. The third most important variable, connectivity (Fig 3d), had a similar trend but with considerably lower standardized coefficients (at least two times lower than total population, Table 1). In contrast, we observed that precipitation (Fig 3a) showed trends that were more important during the initial days in each city, with positive but very low coefficients (Table 1).

When we built one independent model for each State, considering total population, connectivity, and social distancing (i.e., the three most important predictors), there was a high variation in the results depending on the focal State (Fig 4). Notably, the rate of increase in the number of COVID-19 cases was mostly determined by respecting social distancing protocols (i.e., higher R^2; Fig 4c), followed by population size (Fig 4a). Although not with the same intensity, connectivity also had an important role on the observed growth patterns (Figure 4b).

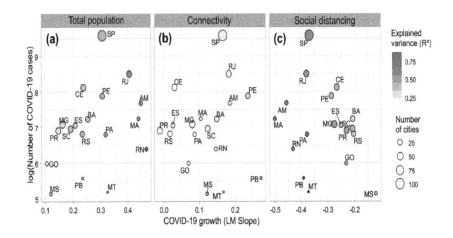

Fig. 4: Relationship between the log-transformed total number of confirmed cases against the standardized slopes of the models. (a) total population, (b) connectivity, and (c) social distancing for 18 Brazilian states. See Fig. S1 for more details on the names and locations of each Brazilian state.

The overall trend was that those states where people were performing social distancing less effectively (leftward circles in Fig 4c) coincided with those states under the most positive effect of total population and connectivity (rightward circles in Figures 4a,b, respectively) on the spread of COVID-19. These examples include Amazonas (AM), Maranhão (MA), Rio Grande do Norte (RN), and Rio de Janeiro (RJ). Moreover, total population and social distancing shared similar slices of explained variance (i.e., similar colour in Figures 4a,c), such as in Amazonas (AM) and Maranhão (MA). Where the number of cases were the highest in Brazil, such as São Paulo (SP), Rio de Janeiro (RJ), Ceará (CE), and Pernambuco (PE), both population size and social distancing shared nearly similar contributions for their observed condition of the spread of COVID-19. Particularly, the situation of Pernambuco (PE) can be considered as the fairest trade-off between population size and distance of citizens (i.e., similar circle colours). By contrast, those states where the social distancing and the effect of total population were combined to produce the mildest scenarios of COVID-19 spread were Espírito Santo (ES), Goiás (GO), Mato Grosso do Sul (MS), Paraná (PR), and Santa Catarina (SC), compared to other federal units.

DISCUSSION

In addition to the pandemic state and the thousands of deaths caused by COVID19 worldwide, some government boards and leaders manifest that their foremost concern regards the economic retraction, which is expected to last longer than the harmful effects of the COVID-19 outbreak themselves. In fact, they are not completely controversial from their perspective. While in-development countries' systems depend on economic income (e.g., sales of commodities), further projections are certainly contingent upon the creation and offer of jobs to remain sustainable. However, the transmission of the virus and the complications arising from severe illness conditions may never rest on the bottom of the country-level priorities of one's management actions. By contrast, decision-makers should provide raw information to fuel research and development of effective containment and treatment of diseases. Hereafter we discuss our results in light of the situations that other countries and cities around the world have experienced.

Our results show that the early spread of the new coronavirus in Brazil was mitigated by social distancing in some regions but was also positively related to the size of the population of cities and how people moved across them. These outcomes underline that the direct and indirect contact among individuals was the most responsible for the rapid spread of the disease caused by the SARS-CoV-2 virus in Brazil. Contrary to initial perspectives, the ability of COVID-19 to spread, estimated by the basic reproduction number (R0) statistic, seems to be higher than the WHO estimated (Liu et al., 2020). Moreover, substantial transmission before symptom onset facilitates the rapid dissemination of the novel coronavirus (Hellewell et al., 2020). As diseases transmitted by respiratory droplets require a certain proximity of people, social distancing certainly reduce transmission rates (Anderson et al., 2020). For this reason, keeping people apart from each other, whenever feasible, should be the primary goal of public health programs to prevent human-to-human transmission. We found evidences that the tools adopted by states and municipalities, including the closure of schools and commercial buildings, lock down of restaurants and malls, and prohibitions of mass gatherings had a negative impact on the expansion of COVID-19 in Brazil. Most importantly, this result somehow evidences that the combination of ignoring social distance especially in large and well-connected cities will have catastrophic consequences.

In Great China, the ongoing COVID-19 outbreak expanded fast throughout the country and the majority of early cases reported outside of its origin had admitted recent travels to Wuhan, the core of the disease spread (Chinazzi et al., 2020). Because of the association between both international and domestic air travel and the dissemination of COVID-19 (Bogoch et al., 2020; Zhao et al., 2020), one of the initial plans for the contagious control was to prevent people from flying around when the outbreak emerged (Kraemer et al., 2020).

Actions such as reducing human mobility by restricting travels and declaring quarantine were fundamental to reduce the dissemination of SARS-CoV-2 within and outside Wuhan, highlighting the importance of mobility restrictions in cities where there is a clear potential for spread of the new coronavirus (Fang et al., 2020). Fortunately, in China, the government-level positions were declared when contagious boundaries were relatively discrete (Kraemer et al., 2020).

Comparatively, this was not the case in Brazil, where the number of confirmed cases of COVID-19 are still growing exponentially (Crokidakis, 2020). The first case in Brazil was registered on February 25, 2020, in São Paulo City (Rodriguez-Morales et al., 2020). It was a man with recent travel to the Italy, precisely for the Lombardy region. Contrary to China, Italy did not conduct a fast protocol of social isolation and already had a high number of cases and deaths. Similarly, to the observed in the United States, until the establishment of local transmission in Brazil, all reported cases had returned from recent travels abroad. Among them, it is noteworthy that 23 members of the delegation that accompanied the Brazilian President on a visit to the United States in March had since tested positive for COVID-19. Indeed, the proportion of estimated imported cases by airport of destination is highly correlated with the proportion of detected imported cases (Candido et al., 2020). For this reason, the Brazilian government announced a temporary ban on foreign air travellers by March 31, 2020.

Moreover, most State governors have imposed quarantines to contain the spread of the virus, but with no support from the federal government. A recent study suggests that more than 40% of social isolation in Brazil is necessary to flatten the epidemic curve of the new coronavirus and to prevent the collapse of the healthcare system (Croda et al., 2020). We defend that the only feasible way to achieve this target is to keep on with social distancing and avoid gatherings of people. Despite the aforementioned efforts, most of them being contemporaneous among many countries, the effective containment of COVID-19 is still a delicate task because of the characteristic mild symptoms and the transmission before the full onset of the disease (Fraser et al., 2004; R. Li et al., 2020). However, the example of the sanitary action conducted in Great China was fundamental when the contagious boundaries were discrete. In Brazil's context, there are cities such as São Paulo, Rio de Janeiro, and other capitals such as Fortaleza and Manaus that likely act as super spreaders of SARS-CoV-2. In a network context, these cities maximize their influence on COVID-19 spread by exporting many cases to cities nearby (Madotto and Liu, 2016).

This fact highlights that these centres should be of foremost concern, especially because some of them are near (e.g. Ceará and Rio de Janeiro) or have already saturated (e.g., Manaus) their health system carrying capacity, given that the number of cases is growing very fast (Crokidakis, 2020). Therefore, the multiple potential Wuhan-alike regions in Brazil require government-level actions towards the necessity of multiplicative movement restrictions and social distancing. Moreover, there are speculations that the number of documented Brazilian cases is likely more than ten times lower than the real number (Bastos and Cajueiro, 2020), considering that tests are being conducted mostly only in cases of severe acute respiratory syndrome (SARS). As an alternative to contour this situation, especially in those countries where several undocumented cases are expected (e.g., in Brazil), decision-makers could base their actions on the recent increase in number of SARS-related hospital records as a surrogate to the real amount of COVID-19 cases.

In addition to social distancing and restrictions on mobility, interventions available include rapid diagnosis and isolation of confirmed cases (Kraemer et al., 2020). However, in Brazil, the diagnosis is completely biased towards people already at advanced clinical stages, in contrast to other countries such as China, Singapore, Germany, and the United States. Clearly, the growth rates of infections by the new coronavirus differ across countries (Coelho et al., 2020; Ficetola and Rubolini, 2020).

As the rate differs, the factors determining the expansion of the infection within populations inevitably result from the policies adopted by each country. Our results reveal that this variation also occurs within Brazil. We believe that the reasons for this can be addressed to the continental-wide nature of our country, or the non-uniform demographic distribution across regions (Reis-Santos et al., 2013). Thus, the responsibility for the local spread of COVID-19 is directly dependent on Mayors' and Governors' positions. Several studies have shown that environmental factors such as local temperature and precipitation may affect the SARS-CoV-2 virus survival and transmission, with significant consequences for the seasonal and geographic patterns of outbreaks (Bukhari and Jameel, 2020; Ficetola and Rubolini, 2020; Ma et al., 2020). The mechanism underlying these patterns of climate determination is likely linked with the ability of the virus to survive external environmental conditions prior to reaching a host (Harmooshi et al., n.d.).

A recent study showed that COVID-19 is more viable at lower temperatures (5-11°C) and was inversely related to humidity (Sajadi et al., 2020). However, our results indicate that climate variables had secondary roles in explaining the COVID-19 growth rate in Brazil. This weak relationship suggests that seasonal climatic variation plays a minor role in the spatial spread and severity of COVID-19 outbreaks, as observed in recent studies on other regions (Baker et al., 2020; Coelho et al., 2020).

For instance, Manaus, the largest metropolitan city in North Brazil, is located at the core world's largest rainforest, the Amazon, and is characterized by extremely high rainfall and temperatures throughout all over the year. This city registered more than one thousand confirmed cases and, recently, the state health department is suffering from the collapse of the health network due to the excessive cases of COVID-19. Among these, over 85 cases have been recorded in indigenous peoples and four deaths have been confirmed, including young people.

Historically, due to the absence of antibodies, indigenous people are likely more susceptible to diseases such as flu, measles, rubella, and tuberculosis, which caused dramatic epidemic cases with the arrival of Europeans on the South American continent (Montenegro and Stephens, 2006). According to the latest census, more than 300 thousand of indigenous people currently live in the Amazon region, which is home to more than 100 tribes that are still isolated. The advance of illegal mining is a major threat to these peoples. Furthermore, instead of allowing religious missionaries to get in contact with isolated Indigenous groups, all means of transportation to these areas should be restricted (Ferrante and Fearnside, 2020).

Therefore, the thoughtlessness by the federal government about COVID-19 potentially leads to a dramatic scenario for indigenous people. It is important to highlight that the low predictability of climatic variables in explaining the virus outbreaks patterns may be explained by the climatic peculiarities of Brazil during the summer that matched with the arrival and spread of the virus. Among all cities with confirmed cases, the average temperature was 24°C and the lowest temperature was 18°C, which is still far from what was indicated as ideal for the survival of the virus (Sajadi et al., 2020; Wang et al., 2020). We found a positive relationship between temperature and precipitation variables and the growth in the number of COVID-19 cases, which is in line with previous findings in Brazil (Auler et al., 2020), but contrary to a global tendency. Although the coefficients were quite weak, this suggests that high temperatures and precipitation are not limiting factors for the spread of the virus.

Conversely, a scenario of extreme concern is emerging, since the Winter season approaches, so temperatures will drop dramatically across many areas, especially in the South region. Therefore, at this early outbreak, any generalization is hasty and results have to be considered with extreme caution. Most importantly, the climate must not be used as an easing argument as particularly declared by the Brazilian President. The actual emergence of the novel infectious agent has revealed the vulnerability of societies to new health threats (Morse et al., 2012). Brazil has recently experienced other public health emergencies under polio, smallpox, cholera, H1N1 (Influenza A), avian flu, yellow fever, dengue and zika (Croda et al., 2020).Along with the current COVID-19 outbreak, we judge that all these examples constitute an important legacy on the role of scientific research on dealing with epidemics. Thus, we may now face the most important event, in the recent decades, to learn on how to respond to emergencies effectively (Croda et al., 2020).

We need to assume that this study does not intend to serve as specific guidelines for any decision-making process within any specific administrative council. Nevertheless, at a country-scale, we disapprove any government declaration or exposure that confronts the statements and protocols from the World Health Organization (WHO) or the United Nations (UN), which are international institutions that are presumed to be sovereign in their actions and recommendations since their utmost concern is the health and human wellbeing on a global scale. If eventually confronted, the arguments for doing so should be based on clear and strong scientific evidence, although it is very unlikely that these organizations have ignored such information while developing their protocols. It is now clear that the most likely determinant of the virus spread is the vicinity of infected peoples and cities. While evacuating cities is not reasonable at this point, the easiest and the most feasible way to decelerate the COVID-19 spread is to avoid people transportation among them.

This is fundamental within cities. While the virulence of the SARS-CoV-2 virus is remarkably high and we are not able to tear houses or buildings apart, the only way to allow for the healthcare systems to treat ill people effectively is performing social distancing. In the absence of any effective treatment and vaccine, we support that social distancing is still the only feasible way to avoid the collapse of our national health system. Specially in Brazil, a '3rd world country', we have few hospitals and clinics with beds and respirators that are autonomous for treating SARS, which means that if we allow it to grow fast by not maintaining restrictions in movement between cities/states and social distancing within cities, we may certainly hope for the best but expect for the worst. We assume that the indicator for the efficiency of social distancing is a conundrum because the response about its effectiveness might come only weeks after the execution of any plans. In fact, people tend to underrate social isolation because the more effective it is, the less needed it seems to be. We also admit that any delayed action can be catastrophic, both for the health and economy of any country. Nevertheless, the expeditious suspension of social distancing under the coating of restoring the economic trades and jobs likely has even more dangerous side effects than COVID-19 itself.

Acknowledgements

This study was developed as a contribution to the Brazilian Ministry of Health about the overall evaluation of collected data on COVID-19. Most of the merit of this study belongs to all those individuals involved in collecting epidemiologic data and working in favour of health, directly or indirectly, inside or outside the healthcare facilities. They deserve sincere acknowledgements for their daily work.

Author contribution

MTB conceived the study with extensive suggestions from FMLT. MTB gathered and organized information and FMLT analysed data. Visual results were produced by FMLT. MTB and FMLT wrote the first draft, which was thoroughly reviewed and approved by all authors.

REFERENCES

Andersen, K.G., Rambaut, A., Lipkin, W.I., Holmes, E.C., Garry, R.F., (2020). The proximal origin of SARS-CoV-2. Nat. Med. 26, 450–452. https://doi.org/10.1038/s41591-020-0820-9

Anderson, R.M., Heesterbeek, H., Klinkenberg, D., Hollingsworth, T.D., (2020). How will country-based mitigation measures influence the course of the COVID-19 epidemic? Lancet 395, 931–934. https://doi.org/10.1016/S0140-6736(20)30567-5

Araujo, M.B., Naimi, B., (2020). Spread of SARS-CoV-2 Coronavirus likely to be constrained by climate. medRxiv 2020.03.12.20034728. https://doi.org/10.1101/2020.03.12.20034728

Auler, A.C., Cássaro, F.A.M., Silva, V.O. da, L.F. Pires, A., (2020). Evidence that high temperatures and intermediate relative humidity might favor the spread of COVID19 in tropical climate: A case study for the most affected Brazilian cities. Sci. Total Environ. 1–5. https://doi.org/10.1016/j.bbamem.2019.183135

Baker, R.E., Yang, W., Vecchi, G.A., Metcalf, C.J.E., Grenfell, B.T., (2020). Susceptible supply limits the role of climate in the COVID-19 pandemic. medRxiv 2020.04.03.20052787. https://doi.org/10.1101/2020.04.03.20052787

Balilla, J., (2020). Assessment of COVID-19 Mass Testing: The Case of South Korea. SSRN Electron. J. 6. https://doi.org/10.2139/ssrn.3556346

Bastos, S.B., Cajueiro, D.O., (2020). Modeling and forecasting the early evolution of the COVID-19 pandemic in Brazil 1–15.

Bogoch, I.I., Watts, A., Thomas-Bachli, A., Huber, C., Kraemer, M.U.G., Khan, K., (2020). Pneumonia of unknown aetiology in Wuhan, China: potential for international spread via commercial air travel. J. Travel Med. 27, 1–3. https://doi.org/10.1093/jtm/taaa008

Bonacich, P., (1987). Power and Centrality: A Family of Measures. Am. J. Sociol. 92, 1170–1182. https://doi.org/10.1086/228631

Borcard, D., Gillet, F., Legendre, P., (2018). Numerical ecology with R. Springer, New York.

Bukhari, Q., Jameel, Y., 2020. Will Coronavirus Pandemic Diminish by Summer? SSRN Electron. J. https://doi.org/10.2139/ssrn.3556998

Candido, D.D.S., Watts, A., Abade, L., Kraemer, M.U.G., Pybus, O.G., Croda, J., Oliveira, W., Khan, K., Sabino, E.C., Faria, N.R., (2020). Routes for COVID-19 importation in Brazil. J. Travel Med. https://doi.org/10.1093/jtm/taaa042

Cauchemez, S., Fraser, C., Van Kerkhove, M.D., Donnelly, C.A., Riley, S., Rambaut, A., Enouf, V., van der Werf, S., Ferguson, N.M., (2014). Middle East respiratory syndrome coronavirus: quantification of the extent of the epidemic, surveillance biases, and transmissibility. Lancet Infect. Dis. 14, 50–56. https://doi.org/10.1016/S1473-3099(13)70304-9

Chan, K.H., Peiris, J.S.M., Lam, S.Y., Poon, L.L.M., Yuen, K.Y., Seto, W.H., (2011).The Effects of Temperature and Relative Humidity on the Viability of the SARS Coronavirus. Adv. Virol. 2011, 1–7. https://doi.org/10.1155/2011/734690

Cheng, V.C.C., Lau, S.K.P., Woo, P.C.Y., Yuen, K.Y., (2007). Severe Acute Respiratory Syndrome Coronavirus as an Agent of Emerging and Reemerging Infection. Clin. Microbiol. Rev. 20, 660–694. https://doi.org/10.1128/CMR.00023-07

Chinazzi, M., Davis, J.T., Ajelli, M., Gioannini, C., Litvinova, M., Merler, S., Pastore y Piontti, A., Mu, K., Rossi, L., Sun, K., Viboud, C., Xiong, X., Yu, H., Halloran, M.E., Longini, I.M., Vespignani, A., (2020). The effect of travel restrictions on the spread of the 2019 novel coronavirus (COVID-19) outbreak. Science (80-.). 9757, eaba9757. https://doi.org/10.1126/science.aba9757

Chipperfield, J.D., (2020). On the inadequacy of species distribution models for modelling the spread of SARS-CoV-2 : response to Araújo and Naimi. medRxiv.

Coelho, M.T.P., Rodrigues, F.J.M., Medina, A.M., Scalco, P., Terribile, L.C., Vilela, B., Diniz-filho, A.F., Dobrovolski, R., (2020). Exponential phase of covid19 expansion is not driven by climate at global scale. medRxiv.

Croda, J., Oliveira, W.K. De, Frutuoso, R.L., Mandetta, L.H., Baia-da-Silva, D.C., Brito-Sousa, J.D., Monteiro, W.M., Lacerda, M.V.G., (2020). COVID-19 in Brazil: advantages of a socialized unified health system and preparation to contain cases. Rev. Soc. Bras. Med. Trop. 53, 2–7. https://doi.org/10.1590/0037-8682-0167-2020

Crokidakis, N., (2020). Data analysis and modeling of the evolution of COVID-19 in Brazil.

Csardi, G., Nepusz, T., (2006). The igraph software package for complex network research.

Dabla-Norris, E., Kochhar, K., Suphaphiphat, N., Ricka, F., Tsounta, E., (2015). Causes and Consequences of Income Inequality: A Global Perspective. Staff Discuss. Notes 15, 1. https://doi.org/10.5089/9781513555188.006

Davies, J.B., Lluberas, R., Shorrocks, A.F., (2017). Estimating the Level and Distribution of Global Wealth, 2000-2014. Rev. Income Wealth 63, 731–759. https://doi.org/10.1111/roiw.12318

Fang, H., Wang, L., Yang, Y., (2020). Human Mobility Restrictions and the Spread of the Novel Coronavirus (2019-nCoV) in China. Cambridge, MA. https://doi.org/10.3386/w26906

Ferrante, L., Fearnside, P.M., (2020). Protect Indigenous peoples from COVID-19.Science (80-.). 368, 251.1-251. https://doi.org/10.1126/science.abc0073

Ficetola, G.F., Rubolini, D., (2020). Climate affects global patterns of COVID-19 early outbreak dynamics. medRxiv 2020.03.23.20040501. https://doi.org/10.1101/2020.03.23.20040501

Fick, S.E., Hijmans, R.J., (2017). WorldClim 2: new 1-km spatial resolution climate surfaces for global land areas. Int. J. Climatol. 37, 4302–4315. https://doi.org/10.1002/joc.5086

Fox, J., Weisberg., S., (2019). An R companion to applied regression., 3rd ed. Sage publications.

Fraser, C., Riley, S., Anderson, R.M., Ferguson, N.M., (2004). Factors that make an infectious disease outbreak controllable. Proc. Natl. Acad. Sci. 101, 6146–6151. https://doi.org/10.1073/pnas.0307506101

Gaunt, E.R., Hardie, A., Claas, E.C.J., Simmonds, P., Templeton, K.E., (2010). Epidemiology and Clinical Presentations of the Four Human Coronaviruses 229E, HKU1, NL63, and OC43 Detected over 3 Years Using a Novel Multiplex Real-Time PCR Method. J. Clin. Microbiol. 48, 2940–2947. https://doi.org/10.1128/JCM.00636-10

Guo, Y.-R., Cao, Q.-D., Hong, Z.-S., Tan, Y.-Y., Chen, S.-D., Jin, H.-J., Tan, K.-S., Wang, D.-Y., Yan, Y., (2020). The origin, transmission and clinical therapies on coronavirus disease 2019 (COVID-19) outbreak – an update on the status. Mil. Med. Res. 7, 11. https://doi.org/10.1186/s40779-020-00240-0

Harmooshi, N.N., Shirbandi, K., Rahim, F., n.d. Environmental concern regarding the effect of humidity and temperature on SARS-COV-2 (COVID-19) survival : Fact or Fiction 2.

Hellewell, J., Abbott, S., Gimma, A., Bosse, N.I., Jarvis, C.I., Russell, T.W., Munday, J.D., Kucharski, A.J., Edmunds, W.J., Funk, S., Eggo, R.M., Sun, F., Flasche, S.,Quilty, B.J., Davies, N., Liu, Y., Clifford, S., Klepac, P., Jit, M., Diamond, C., Gibbs, H., van Zandvoort, K., (2020). Feasibility of controlling COVID-19 outbreaks by isolation of cases and contacts. Lancet Glob. Heal. 8, e488–e496. https://doi.org/10.1016/S2214-109X(20)30074-7 #

Holmes, E.C., (2004). The phylogeography of human viruses. Mol. Ecol. 13, 745–756. https://doi.org/10.1046/j.1365-294X.2003.02051.x

Kraemer, M.U.G., Yang, C.-H., Gutierrez, B., Wu, C.-H., Klein, B., Pigott, D.M., du Plessis, L., Faria, N.R., Li, R., Hanage, W.P., Brownstein, J.S., Layan, M., Vespignani, A., Tian, H., Dye, C., Pybus, O.G., Scarpino, S. V., (2020). The effect of human mobility and control measures on the COVID-19 epidemic in China. Science (80-.). eabb4218. https://doi.org/10.1126/science.abb4218

Legendre, P., Legendre, L.F., (2012). Numerical ecology. Elsevier, New York.

Li, R., Pei, S., Chen, B., Song, Y., Zhang, T., Yang, W., Shaman, J., (2020). Substantial undocumented infection facilitates the rapid dissemination of novel coronavirus (SARS-CoV2). Science (80-.). 3221, eabb3221. https://doi.org/10.1126/science.abb3221

Li, X., Zai, J., Zhao, Q., Nie, Q., Li, Y., Foley, B.T., Chaillon, A., (2020). Evolutionary history, potential intermediate animal host, and cross-species analyses of SARS-CoV-2. J. Med. Virol. 92, 602–611. https://doi.org/10.1002/jmv.25731

Liu, Y., Gayle, A.A., Wilder-Smith, A., Rocklöv, J., (2020). The reproductive number of COVID-19 is higher compared to SARS coronavirus. J. Travel Med. 27, 1–4. https://doi.org/10.1093/jtm/taaa021

Lurie, N., Saville, M., Hatchett, R., Halton, J., (2020). Developing COVID-19 Vaccines at Pandemic Speed. N. Engl. J. Med. NEJMp2005630. https://doi.org/10.1056/NEJMp2005630

Ma, Y., Zhao, Y., Liu, J., He, X., Wang, B., Fu, S., Yan, J., Niu, J., Zhou, J., Luo, B., (2020). Effects of temperature variation and humidity on the death of COVID-19 in Wuhan, China. Sci. Total Environ. 724, 138226. https://doi.org/10.1016/j.scitotenv.2020.138226

Madotto, A., Liu, J., 2016. Super-Spreader Identification Using Meta-Centrality. Sci Rep. 6, 1–10. https://doi.org/10.1038/srep38994

Mizumoto, K., Kagaya, K., Zarebski, A., Chowell, G., (2020). Estimating the asymptomatic proportion of coronavirus disease 2019 (COVID-19) cases on board the Diamond Princess cruise ship, Yokohama, Japan, 2020. Eurosurveillance 25, 1–5. https://doi.org/10.2807/1560-7917.ES.2020.25.10.2000180

Montenegro, R.A., Stephens, C., (2006). Indigenous health in Latin America and the Caribbean. Lancet 367, 1859–1869. https://doi.org/10.1016/S0140-6736(06)68808-9

Openflights.org database. http://openflights.org/data.html. [WWW Document], n.d. URL http://openflights.org/data.html.(accessed 4.7.20).

Paradis, E., Schliep, K., (2019). ape 5.0: an environment for modern phylogenetics and evolutionary analyses in R. Bioinformatics 35, 526–528. https://doi.org/10.1093/bioinformatics/bty633

Pybus, O.G., Tatem, A.J., Lemey, P., (2015). Virus evolution and transmission in an ever more connected world. Proc. R. Soc. B Biol. Sci. 282, 20142878. https://doi.org/10.1098/rspb.2014.2878QGIS Development Team, 2020. QGIS Geographic Information System.

R Core Team, (2019). R: A language and environment for statistical computing.Reis-Santos, B., Locatelli, R., Horta, B.L., Faerstein, E., Sanchez, M.N., Riley, L.W., Maciel, E.L., 2013. Socio-Demographic and Clinical Differences in Subjects with Tuberculosis with and without Diabetes Mellitus in Brazil – A Multivariate Analysis. PLoS One 8, e62604. https://doi.org/10.1371/journal.pone.0062604

Rodriguez-Morales, A.J., Gallego, V., Escalera-Antezana, J.P., Méndez, C.A., Zambrano, L.I., Franco-Paredes, C., Suárez, J.A., Rodriguez-Enciso, H.D., Balbin-Ramon, G.J., Savio-Larriera, E., Risquez, A., Cimerman, S., (2020). COVID-19 in Latin America: The implications of the first confirmed case in Brazil. Travel Med. Infect. Dis. 101613. https://doi.org/10.1016/j.tmaid.2020.101613

Rothan, H.A., Byrareddy, S.N., (2020). The epidemiology and pathogenesis of coronavirus disease (COVID-19) outbreak. J. Autoimmun. 109, 102433. https://doi.org/10.1016/j.jaut.2020.102433

Sajadi, M.M., Habibzadeh, P., Vintzileos, A., Shokouhi, S., Miralles-Wilhelm, F., Amoroso, A., (2020). Temperature and Latitude Analysis to Predict Potential Spread and Seasonality for COVID-19. SSRN Electron. J. https://doi.org/10.2139/ssrn.3550308

Skidmore, T.E., (2004). Policy Issues Brazil's Persistent Income Inequality: Lessons from History. Lat. Am. Polit. Soc. 46, 133–150. https://doi.org/10.1111/j.1548-2456.2004.tb00278.x

Wang, J., Tang, K., Feng, K., Lv, W., (2020). High Temperature and High Humidity Reduce the Transmission of COVID-19. SSRN Electron. J. https://doi.org/10.2139/ssrn.3551767

West, D.B., (2001). Introduction to graph theory, 2nd ed. Prentice hall, Upper Saddle

River. Yang, J., Zheng, Y., Gou, X., Pu, K., Chen, Z., Guo, Q., Ji, R., Wang, H., Wang, Y., Zhou, Y., (2020). Prevalence of comorbidities in the novel Wuhan coronavirus (COVID-19) infection: a systematic review and meta-analysis. Int. J. Infect. Dis. https://doi.org/10.1016/j.ijid.2020.03.017

Zhang, T., Wu, Q., Zhang, Z., (2020). Probable Pangolin Origin of SARS-CoV-2 Associated with the COVID-19 Outbreak. Curr. Biol. 30, 1346-1351.e2. https://doi.org/10.1016/j.cub.2020.03.022

Zhao, S., Zhuang, Z., Cao, P., Ran, J., Gao, D., Lou, Y., Yang, L., Cai, Y., Wang, W., He, D., Wang, M.H., (2020). Quantifying the association between domestic travel and the exportation of novel coronavirus (2019-nCoV) cases from Wuhan, China in 2020: a correlational analysis. J. Travel Med. 27, 1–3. https://doi.org/10.1093/jtm/taaa022

Zhou, P., Yang, X. Lou, Wang, X.G., Hu, B., Zhang, L., Zhang, W., Si, H.R., Zhu, Y., Li, B., Huang, C.L., Chen, H.D., Chen, J., Luo, Y., Guo, H., Jiang, R. Di, Liu, M.Q., Chen, Y., Shen, X.R., Wang, X., Zheng, X.S., Zhao, K., Chen, Q.J., Deng, F., Liu, L.L., Yan, B., Zhan, F.X., Wang, Y.Y., Xiao, G.F., Shi, Z.L., (2020). A pneumonia outbreak associated with a new coronavirus of probable bat origin. Nature 579, 270–273. https://doi.org/10.1038/s41586-020-2012-7

Zhu, N., Zhang, D., Wang, W., Li, X., Yang, B., Song, J., Zhao, X., Huang, B., Shi, W., Lu, R., Niu, P., Zhan, F., Ma, X., Wang, D., Xu, W., Wu, G., Gao, G.F., Tan, W., (2020). A Novel Coronavirus from Patients with Pneumonia in China, 2019. N. Engl. J. Med. 382, 727–733. https://doi.org/10.1056/NEJMoa2001017

2. Monitoring Social Distancing And SARS-Cov-2 Transmission
In Brazil Using Cell Phone Mobility Data

[1]Silvano Barbosa de Oliveira†[1,2], Victor Bertollo Gomes Pôrto†[1],

Fabiana Ganem[1,3],Fabio Macedo Mendes,[2] Maria Almiron[4], Wanderson Kleber de Oliveira[1], Francieli Fontana Sutile Tardetti Fantinato[1], Walquiria Aparecida Ferreira de Almeida[1], Abel Pereira de Macedo Borges Junior[5], Hector Natan Batista Pinheiro[5], Raíza dos Santos Oliveira[5], Jason R. Andrews[6], Nuno R Faria[7,8], Marcelo Barreto Lopes[9], Wildo Navegantes de Araújo[2], Fredi A. DiazQuijano[10], Helder I. Nakaya[11,12], Julio Croda[13,14,15]*.

ABSTRACT

Social distancing measures have emerged as the predominant intervention for containing the spread of COVID-19, but evaluating adherence and effectiveness remains a challenge. We assessed the relationship between aggregated mobility data collected from mobile phone users and the time-dependent reproduction number R(t), using severe acute respiratory illness (SARI) cases reported by São Paulo and Rio de Janeiro. We found that the proportion of individuals staying home all day (isolation index) had a strong inverse correlation with R(t) (rho<-0.7) and was predictive of COVID-19 transmissibility (p<0.0001). Furthermore, indexes of 46.7% had the highest accuracy (93.9%) to predict R(t) below one. This metric can be monitored in real time to assess adherence to social distancing measures and predict their effectiveness for controlling SARS-CoV-2 transmission.

INTRODUCTION

The coronavirus diseases 2019 (COVID-19) pandemic has caused more than 2,900,000 cases and 200,000 deaths worldwide as of April 26, 2020(1). In the absence of vaccines and effective pharmacological interventions, social distancing measures are critical to mitigate the impact on healthcare systems and allow time for a public health response around the globe (2, 3).

There is growing evidence that a significant reduction in new locally-transmitted cases have been achieved in Asia and Europe following restrictions on urban mobility and travel (2–6). To reduce the peak of transmission, starting in March of 2020, the Brazilian states of São Paulo and Rio de Janeiro in Brazil, with a population of 63 million people, implemented non-pharmacological interventions and recommended social distancing measures. This implied reductions in public gatherings; the closure of schools, universities, and businesses such as restaurants, bars and gyms; and the institution of remote or virtual work for older adults and individuals with underlying

---

[1] *Correspondence to: julio.croda@fiocruz.br

medical conditions. In light of these public health interventions only essential services (i.e., grocery stores, emergency health service) remained open. To prevent the expansion of COVID-19 epidemic, the non-pharmacological measures have to bring the time-dependent reproduction number (R(t)) to less than 1. This requires a 50-60% reduction of a baseline R(t) between 2 and 2.5(2).

Using data from hospitalization due to severe acute respiratory illness (SARI) as a proxy for severe cases of COVID-19, we recently reported an important decline in the R(t) in the metropolitan area of São Paulo after the implementation of social distancing measures (7). Although R(t) is a useful tool to monitor the epidemic, it is subject to significant delays in notification. In Brazil, a time lag of 8 days exists between the date of onset of symptoms and the date of notification of a SARI case (8). Given this time, relying solely on the measurement of R(t) bears a likely risk of introducing significant delays in detecting changes in the epidemic dynamics. In an epidemic with cases doubling in 5.2 days (9), a delay of 1-2 weeks in the implementation of effective social distancing would overwhelm the capacity of the healthcare system, resulting in a growing number of excess deaths (10–13). Thus, a timelier metric for COVID-19 transmission potential is required to evaluate social distancing interventions.

The wide-ranging usage of mobile phone provides a unique opportunity to monitor and control the spread of infectious diseases (14–17). Mobile phones with geolocation enablement can track movement in a timely and precise manner. To our knowledge, no study thus far has assessed the use of mobile phones for this purpose in Brazil. Monitoring human activity through mobile aggregated data can permit measurement of the effectiveness of social distancing measures in reducing transmissibility of the SARS-CoV2 virus (18). Nonetheless, the association between urban mobility and COVID-19 transmissibility has not yet been established.

In this study, we assessed the relationship between social isolation measures, by using human urban movement data and the transmissibility of COVID-19. From February 1st to April 10th, 2020 a total of 21,426 hospitalizations in 853 hospitals (58%) due to SARI were reported in the São Paulo (SP) state. A clinical diagnosis of COVID-19 was confirmed by molecular testing for 4,111 (19% of total SARI cases), 16,892 (79%) remained as suspected COVID-19 cases and 423 (2%) were confirmed for other respiratory virus diseases in SP state. During the same period the RJ state had reported 2,540 hospitalizations in 320 hospitals (62%) due to SARI, 402 (16%) were confirmed by molecular testing for COVID-19, 2,090 (82%) remained as suspected and 48 (2%) have been confirmed for other respiratory viruses (Fig. 1A and 1D). Most SARI cases in SP and RJ have not been tested due to the shortage of SARS-CoV2 real-time polymerase cycle reaction (RT-PCR) diagnostic screening. In 2019, during the same period, 1,550 and 220 SARI cases were reported in SP and RJ, respectively. This corresponds to 1,282% and 1,054% increase in SARI cases in SP and RJ respectively between the same periods in 2019 and 2020.

Implemented Social Distancing Measures

Starting on March 13, 2020, two days after the World Health Organization declared COVID-19 as a pandemic, the states of São Paulo and Rio de Janeiro implemented a series of nonpharmacological interventions. These measures were implemented gradually in both states, some of these interventions are described on **Figure 1**. To investigate the impact of social distancing measures in SARS-CoV-2 transmission, we compared daily aggregated mobility data for São Paulo and Rio de Janeiro with R estimates obtained from SARI data. Here, we calculate an "isolation index" as a ratio between the number of people staying at home on a given day divided by the number of cell-phone users living in the state or city (see **Material and Methods**). First, we find that the mean isolation index from February 1st to April 10th was 40.2%, ranging from 18.5% to 69.4%. In São Paulo state, mean isolation index ranged from 13.5% to 67.9% and in the Rio de Janeiro State from 16.6% to 69.4%, with no significant difference observed between the two states (p-value = 0.210). Second, after the start of interventions we observe a sharp and significant increase in the isolation index and a corresponding decrease in the R(t) (**Figs. 1B** and **1E**). Overall, we find that temporal periods with R(t) ≥1 had a mean isolation index below 29.3% (SD = 8.2%) while those with R(t) <1 had a mean isolation index above 53.4% (SD = 3.0%) (**Figs. 1C** and **1F**).

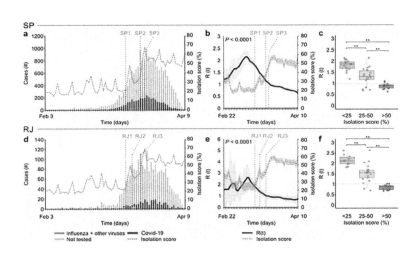

Fig. 1. Impact of interventions in the reduction of severe acute respiratory transmission São Paulo and Rio de Janeiro states, Brazil.

A and D: epidemic curve of SARI cases by date of onset of symptoms for São Paulo and Rio de Janeiro, respectively; B and E: Daily Time dependent reproductive number (R(t)) (grey) and isolation index (orange) (curves smoothed by Kalman Filtering method), SP and RJ respectively; C and F: boxplot showing the median, interquartile range and range of the association between of R(t) and isolation index categories. SP1: March 13, 2020, SP recommended reduction in public gatherings events and closure of schools; SP2: March 20, 2020, SP declares Public Calamity and prohibits religious ceremonies; SP3: March 22, SP establishes quarantine in the entire state, closure of night clubs, shopping centres, gyms, bars, restaurants and bakeries; RJ1: March 13, 2020, RJ recommended remote work, suspended public gathering events, closed schools, and entertainment establishments, prohibited the access of visitors to prisons and to COVID-19 hospitalized patients; RJ2: March 16, 2020, RJ prohibited the access to tourist places, including beaches and public pools, restricted public transport such as bus lines, airlines and cruise ships coming from states or countries with COVID-19 circulation, closed bars and restaurants, closed gyms, shopping centres and similar establishments and set restrictions on public transportation; RJ3:March 20, 2020, RJ declared Public Calamity due to the COVID-19 pandemic

Mobility Data Predicted the Time-Dependent Reproduction Number R(T)

We next conducted cross-correlation analyses with different lag days and the Granger test to investigate if the isolation index measure obtained from mobility data is able to predict R(t). After the intervention began, it was also observed a gradual decrease in R(t) (Fig. 1B and 1E). Furthermore, using SARI cases, cross-correlation analyses showed that isolation was highly correlated with R(t) (rho<-0.7) in a lag period of up to five days in SP and RJ. Considering only COVID-19 confirmed cases, the R(t) and isolation index were moderately correlated (rho >-0.7) using a lag period from -2 to 0 (Fig. 2A and B).

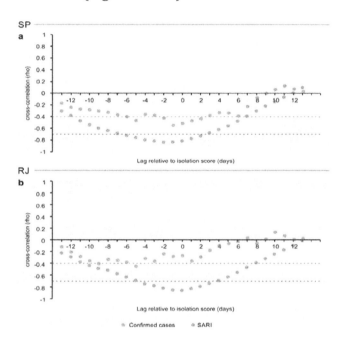

Fig. 2. Cross-correlation (rho) between isolation index and reproductive number (R(t) estimated using SARI (purple circles)and confirmed COVID-19 (red circles) cases in São Paulo (A) and Rio de Janeiro (B).

The isolation score exhibited an area under the ROC curve 93.8% (95% CI: 88% - 99.5%) to predict *R* values under 1.0 (**Fig. 3A**). We obtained the best accuracy with score values close to 50%. Particularly, we observed the highest accuracy (93.9%) with the cut-off of 46.7%, and cut-offs higher than 50% exhibited specificity greater than 93% (**Fig. 3B**). Furthermore, 88.9% of the areas with at least 50% isolation score had an *R* <1. In contrast, 90.3% of the observations with an isolation score <50% had an *R* ≥1. The isolation scores, for both states combined, when greater than 50%, were associated with a mean *R* of 0.9 (ranging from 0.6 to 1.1) (**Fig. 1C and 1F**). Scores between 25-50% had a mean *R* of 1.4 *R* (ranging from 0.7 to 2.6). On the other hand, isolation scores lower than 25% exhibited a mean *R* of 1.9 (ranging from 1.2 to 2.6).

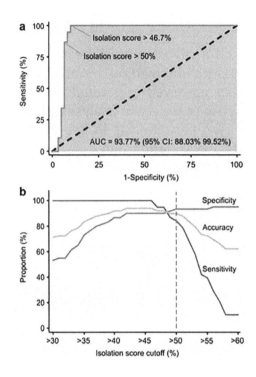

Fig. 3. A. Receiver operating characteristic curve of isolation index for prediction of R(t)<1. B. Sensitivity, Specificity and Accuracy of isolation index cut-offs to predict R(t)<1.

To investigate the effectiveness of interventions in areas with different human development indexes (HDI), we analyzed the isolation score time series for the 10 largest cities in the states of São Paulo and Rio de Janeiro stratified by HDI(*19*). We found no significant difference between the groups). To validate the findings, we aggregated 20 cities in two groups stratified by HDI (lower and higher values). We observed the same trend and strong correlation, regardless of the group (higher and lower HDI) (**Fig. S1A**). Interestingly, we found an identical cut-off point of isolation index (50%) which was correlated with R(t) values below 1 (**Fig. S1B**).

Simulation Of Different Interventions Scenarios With Isolation Index's Above 50%

Assuming the R(t) values associated with isolation indexes above 50% we next simulated different lengths of social distancing interventions, 30, 60 and 90 days (see **Materials and Methods**). An intervention of only 30 days was able to revert the intensive care units (ICU) demand curve only in those scenarios with the lowest values of R(t) and was also associated with a quick rebound of the ICU demand curve far above the existing capacity (Figure 5). Prolonging the intervention to 60 days managed to revert the curve in most scenarios and delayed the second epidemic wave. An intervention of 90 days substantially delayed the second epidemic wave in all scenarios, although it had minimal impact on the height of both curves. According to our simulation, Rio de Janeiro state is able to stay below the ICU bed capacity threshold in the first epidemic wave in all scenarios. Conversely, São Paulo state needs to steadily increase its capacity in order to manage the first epidemic curve. Lower values of R(t) were associated with smaller epidemic waves during the intervention but higher second epidemic waves (Figure 4).

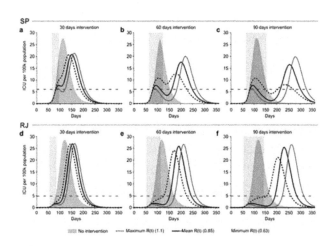

Fig. 4.Simulations of intensive care unit (ICU) demand according to different lengths of social distancing interventions for the states of São Paulo (top row) and Rio de Janeiro (bottom row).

A, B and C: simulations for the São Paulo state assuming *R* values associated 5 with isolation scores above 50% during30, 60 and 90 days of intervention respectively; D, E and F: simulations for the Rio de Janeiro state assuming R(t)values associated with isolation scores above 50% during t 30, 60 and 90 days of intervention respectively. For each scenario we plotted the mean, minimum and maximum R(t) values in the >50% isolation score category. The red horizontal line corresponds to ICU capacity for each state.

DISCUSSION

Individual-based control efforts of COVID-19 can be challenging to implement due to the high infectiousness, relatively mild and moderate symptoms and pre symptomatic transmission[23-25]. Consequently, social distancing measures are required to control COVID-19 in most scenarios. Here, we demonstrated that the initial social distancing measures adopted by the states of São Paulo and Rio de Janeiro successfully reduced R(t) < 1 by decreasing mobility across populations with lower and higher development index. We further demonstrated a strong correlation between the social isolation index and R(t) and showed that isolation indexes above 50% lead to R(t)<1 in most cases (89%). Our findings suggest that the isolation index can be used to monitor the effectiveness of social distancing measures and guide further interventions. By using aggregated mobility data, public health officials and policymakers can monitor in real time regional differences in social distancing intervention effectiveness and propose specific actions to reduce the transmission in specific locations (*20*). Individual-based control efforts for COVID-19 can be challenging to implement due to the high infectiousness, relatively mild and moderate symptoms and pre-symptomatic transmission (*21– 23*). Consequently, social distancing measures are required to control COVID-19 in most scenarios.

The structural impacts of social distancing should also be considered while managing its impact on disease transmission and, consequently, the healthcare systems' capacity. A previous analysis demonstrated that social distancing adopted during the Spanish flu pandemic was associated with better economic outcomes (*24*).However, society dynamics have changed dramatically during the past 102 years, and a continued monitorization of the COVID-19 socioeconomic impact is urgently needed. Suboptimal interventions for COVID-19 could be potentially catastrophic to public health and lead to a significant number of deaths.

Thus, finding the optimal "therapeutic dosage" of such interventions is crucial, and requires a reliable and timely tool to monitor its effects. R(t) depends on the contact-rate among individuals; but the frequency of these contacts is difficult to quantify in real time through conventional approaches (*25*). We observed an inverse relationship between R(t) and the isolation index for São Paulo and Rio de Janeiro States, the two mostly affected by the epidemic. We find that increases in the isolation index from lower than 25% to greater than 50% have led to a reduction of R(t) from approximately 2 to values less than 1, such as we observed. Highly effective social distancing could reduce COVID-19 transmission enough to make a strategy based on contact tracing feasible, as is taking place in South Korea and Singapore (*26, 27*).

By using the R(t) values associated with isolation indexes above 50%, we simulated social distancing interventions with varying time extensions. In most scenarios, interventions lasting between 30 to 60 days would blunt the first epidemic wave, although a shorter intervention led to a quick rebound and was not enough in scenarios with higher values of R(t) during the intervention. Lower values of R(t) resulted in a more effective control during the first wave, but with a caveat that the second epidemic wave was became significantly larger (albeit smaller than the initial peak that would have been otherwise seen in the absence of interventions).

Furthermore, the delay in this peak allows the preparation of healthcare systems to mitigate health impacts by securing equipment and supplies, bolstering ICU capacity, planning for personnel needs and implementing infection control policies. Higher values of R(t) during the intervention led to more evenly distributed epidemic waves, which would make it possible to implement less stringent interventions during following waves.

Although it is tempting to propose that social distancing interventions that would lead to an R(t) value of 1.1, such a strategy could have potentially catastrophic consequences. The reason for this is that values of social indexes below 50% are associated with a mean R(t) value of 1.4 (ranging from 0.7 to 2.6), which was not significantly different from no intervention. Aiming at achieving a R(t) value of 1.1 by lowering the social isolation index could therefore lead to a scenario similar to the natural history of COVID-19. It is thus more effective and probably safer to set a goal of R(t) below 1 and implement social distancing interventions that lead to social isolation indexes above 50%. This will require close monitoring after the intervention is relaxed, since it is very likely that a second intervention will be needed to flatten a second epidemic wave.

The findings of our simulations need to be interpreted cautiously. We did not aim to precisely replicate the epidemic in both states but merely to simulate hypothetical scenarios, exploring different strategies. Also, our simulations are heavily influenced by the assumptions and parameters that were built into the model. A key assumption in our model is that infection leads to persistent immunity after recovery. Data on SARS-CoV-2 immunity is scarce, preliminary data on rhesus macaques have demonstrated immunity after an initial infection (28, 29) and plasma from recovered individuals was tested to neutralize the virus *in vitro* and *in vivo* (30–33). On the other hand, antigenic drifts (34) as well as waning immunity might lead to the loss of herd immunity. If immunity is not long lasting, as has been estimated for other coronaviruses such as HCoV-OC43 and HCoV-HKU1, COVID-19 will likely enter a regular transmission cycle and become endemic (35).

Another aspect that needs to be taken in consideration is that we simulated epidemics in entire states, assuming homogeneous transmission within the state. However, it is possible that different cities will have non synchronized COVID-19 epidemics, hence interventions will need to be tailored for each city or metropolitan area individually. Moreover, our assumption that only 50% of the established ICU capacity could be used for COVID-19 might be an underestimation of the total capacity, given that during the epidemic efforts have been made to increase hospital capacity in both states, which could lead to the need of less stringent interventions. Another potential source of bias is that we assumed that the reporting rates were stable during the epidemic. If reporting rates of SARI cases increased during the initial stages of the epidemic our initial R(t) estimates would have been overestimated.

Further, if the reporting rates are decreasing, it could mean that the decrease in R(t) that was observed would be partially a result of a reporting bias. Although Brazil has had changes in the reporting systems for COVID-19 during the epidemic, the dataset which was used is based solely on hospitalized SARI cases which required hospitalizations. However, we used SIVEP-GRIPE data, a stable and a well-established system and recommendations for its use have not changed during the epidemic, we believe that this is the most reliable and consistent source of data for severe cases of COVID-19 in Brazil. We also accounted for potential bias related to reporting delays, which affect the end of a time series, by applying a correction factor which corresponds to the inverse of the probability of being reported up to the last date of data being collected.

Another limitation of our approach is that mobility data from mobile phones are a coarse measure of physical distancing, which does not directly capture changes in the number, duration or character of human interactions. Additionally, this approach does not account for other behavioural changes in the population (such as hand washing, respiratory etiquette and universal mask usage) that could also alter transmission patterns and lead to changes in R(t). Our findings underscore the importance of early implementation of social distancing measures to reduce SARS-CoV-2 transmission. The strong association observed here indicates that urban mobile phone-derived isolation scores can track temporal fluctuations in *R* during social distancing interventions in Brazil. If additional behavioural changes are undertaken and sustained, the isolation score could provide a real-time metric to assess effectiveness of interventions. A major contribution of our approach is that the social isolation index data is readily available on a daily basis, in contrast with the R(t) measurement, which is subject to delays (up to two weeks). Using this index will allow for a more timely assessment of the epidemic dynamics and for planning of public health mitigation strategies.

Affiliations:

1National Immunization Program, Department of Immunization and Communicable Diseases, Secretariat of Health Surveillance, Ministry of Health, Brasília, Brazil.

2 University of Brasilia, Brasília, Brazil.

3Programa de Doctorado en Metodología de la Investigación Biomédica y Salud Pública, Universidad Autónoma de Barcelona, Barcelona, Spain.

4Panamerican Health Organization, Brasilia, Brazil.

5 Inloco Company, Recife, Brazil.

6 Division of Infectious Diseases and Geographic Medicine, Stanford University School of Medicine, Stanford, CA, USA.

7 Department of Zoology, University of Oxford, United Kingdom.

8 Instituto Medicina Tropical, University of São Paulo, Brazil.

9Arbor Research Collaborative for Health, Ann Arbor, USA.

10 University of São Paulo, School of Public Health, Department of Epidemiology, Laboratório de Inferência Causal em Epidemiologia, São Paulo, SP, Brazil.

11 Department of Clinical and Toxicological Analyses, School of Pharmaceutical Sciences, 25 University of São Paulo, São Paulo, Brazil

12Scientific Platform Pasteur USP, São Paulo, Brazil.

13 School of Medicine, Federal University of Mato Grosso do Sul, Campo Grande, MS, Brazil.

14 Department of Epidemiology of Microbial Diseases, Yale University School of Public Health, New Haven, United States of America.

15Oswaldo Cruz Foundation, Mato Grosso do Sul, Campo Grande, MS, Brazil.

REFERENCES AND NOTES

1. WHO, Coronavirus disease (COVID-2019) situation reports (2020), (available at https://www.who.int/emergencies/diseases/novel-coronavirus-2019/situation-reports).

2. Anderson, R.M.,Heesterbeek, H., Klinkenberg, D., Hollingsworth, T.D. (2020) How will country based mitigation measures influence the course of the COVID-19 epidemic? *The Lancet.* **395**, 931–934.

3. Maier, B.F &Brockmann, D. (2020) Effective containment explains subexponential growth in recent confirmed COVID-19 cases in China. *Science*, eabb4557.

4. M. Chinazzi, J. T. Davis, M. Ajelli, C. Gioannini, M. Litvinova, S. Merler, A. P. y Piontti, K. Mu, L. Rossi, K. Sun, The effect of travel restrictions on the spread of the 2019 novel coronavirus (COVID-19) outbreak. *Science* (2020).

5. H. Tian, Y. Liu, Y. Li, C.-H. Wu, B. Chen, M. U. G. Kraemer, B. Li, J. Cai, B. Xu, Q. Yang, B. Wang, P. Yang, Y. Cui, Y. Song, P. Zheng, Q. Wang, O. N. Bjornstad, R. Yang, B. T. Grenfell, O. G. Pybus, C. Dye, An investigation of transmission control measures during the first 50 days of the. *Science* (2020), doi:10.1126/science.abb6105.

6. K. E. C. Ainslie, C. Walters, H. Fu, S. Bhatia, H. Wang, M. Baguelin, S. Bhatt, A. Boonyasiri, O. Boyd, L. Cattarino, C. Ciavarella, Z. Cucunubá, G. Cuomo, A. Dighe, I. Dorigatti, S. L. van Elsland, R. FitzJohn, K. Gaythorpe, L. Geidelberg, A. C. Ghani, G. Nedjati-Gilani, L. C. Okell, I. Siveroni, H. Thompson, J. Unwin, R. Verity, M. Vollmer, P. G. Walker, Y. Wang, O. Watson, C. Whittaker, P. Winskill, C. A. Donnelly, N. M. Ferguson, S. Riley, Report 11: Evidence of initial success for China exiting COVID-19 social distancing policy after achieving containment, 8 (2020).

7. The impact of early social distancing at COVID-19 Outbreak in the largest Metropolitan Area of Brazil. | medRxiv, (available at https://www.medrxiv.org/content/10.1101/2020.04.06.20055103v1).

8. Fiocruz, FGV/EmaP, InfoGripe: Monitoramento de casos reportados de síndrome respiratória aguda grave (SRAG) hospitalizado (2020), (available at http://info.gripe.fiocruz.br/).

9. J. T. Wu, K. Leung, M. Bushman, N. Kishore, R. Niehus, P. M. de Salazar, B. J. Cowling, M. Lipsitch, G. M. Leung, Estimating clinical severity of COVID-19 from the transmission dynamics in Wuhan, China. *Nat. Med.*, 1–5 (2020).

10. D. Nogee, A. Tomassoni, Concise Communication: COVID-19 and the N95 Respirator Shortage: Closing the Gap. *Infect. Control Hosp. Epidemiol.*, 1–4 (2020).

11. S. M. Moghadas, A. Shoukat, M. C. Fitzpatrick, C. R. Wells, P. Sah, A. Pandey, J. D. Sachs, Z. Wang, L. A. Meyers, B. H. Singer, A. P. Galvani, Projecting hospital utilization during the COVID-19 outbreaks in the United States. *Proc. Natl. Acad. Sci. U. S. A.* (2020), doi:10.1073/pnas.2004064117.

12. R. J. Hatchett, C. E. Mecher, M. Lipsitch, Public health interventions and epidemic intensity during the 1918 influenza pandemic. *Proc. Natl. Acad. Sci. U. S. A.* **104**, 7582– 7587 (2007).

13. R. Li, C. Rivers, Q. Tan, M. B. Murray, E. Toner, M. Lipsitch, *medRxiv*, in press, doi:10.1101/2020.03.09.20033241.

14. A. Wesolowski, N. Eagle, A. J. Tatem, D. L. Smith, A. M. Noor, R. W. Snow, C. O. Buckee, Quantifying the Impact of Human Mobility on Malaria. *Science*. **338**, 267–270 (2012).

15. A. Wesolowski, C. J. E. Metcalf, N. Eagle, J. Kombich, B. T. Grenfell, O. N. Bjørnstad, J. Lessler, A. J. Tatem, C. O. Buckee, Quantifying seasonal population fluxes driving rubella transmission dynamics using mobile phone data. *Proc. Natl. Acad. Sci.* **112**, 11114–11119 (2015).

16. A. Wesolowski, T. Qureshi, M. F. Boni, P. R. Sundsøy, M. A. Johansson, S. B. Rasheed, K. Engø-Monsen, C. O. Buckee, Impact of human mobility on the emergence of dengue epidemics in Pakistan. *Proc. Natl. Acad. Sci.* **112**, 11887–11892 (2015).

17. C. M. Peak, A. Wesolowski, E. zu Erbach-Schoenberg, A. J. Tatem, E. Wetter, X. Lu, D. Power, E. Weidman-Grunewald, S. Ramos, S. Moritz, C. O. Buckee, L. Bengtsson, Population mobility reductions associated with travel restrictions during the Ebola epidemic in Sierra Leone: use of mobile phone data. *Int. J. Epidemiol.* **47**, 1562–1570 (2018).

18. C. O. Buckee, S. Balsari, J. Chan, M. Crosas, F. Dominici, U. Gasser, Y. H. Grad, B. Grenfell, M. E. Halloran, M. U. G. Kraemer, M. Lipsitch, C. J. E. Metcalf, L. A. Meyers, T. A. Perkins, M. Santillana, S. V. Scarpino, C. Viboud, A. Wesolowski, A. Schroeder, Aggregated mobility data could help fight COVID-19. *Science* (2020), doi:10.1126/science.abb8021.

19. S. A. da Silva, Regional Inequalities in Brazil: Divergent Readings on Their Origin and Public Policy Design. *EchoGéo* (2017), doi:10.4000/echogeo.15060.

20. S. V. Leavitt, R. S. Lee, P. Sebastiani, C. R. Horsburgh, H. E. Jenkins, L. F. White, Estimating the relative probability of direct transmission between infectious disease patients. *Int. J. Epidemiol.*, dyaa031 (2020).

21. M. Day, COVID-19: identifying and isolating asymptomatic people helped eliminate virus inItalian village. *BMJ*. **368**, m1165 (2020).

22. M. Day, COVID-19: four fifths of cases are asymptomatic, China figures indicate. *BMJ*. **369**, m1375 (2020).

23. Y. Bai, L. Yao, T. Wei, F. Tian, D.-Y. Jin, L. Chen, M. Wang, Presumed asymptomatic carrier transmission of COVID-19. *Jama* (2020) (available at https://jamanetwork.com/journals/jama/article-abstract/2762028).

24. S. Correia, S. Luck, E. Verner, "Fight the Pandemic, Save the Economy: Lessons from the 5 1918 Flu" (Federal Reserve Bank of New York, 2020).

25. F. A. Diaz-Quijano, A. J. Rodriguez-Morales, E. A. Waldman, Translating transmissibility measures into recommendations for coronavirus prevention. *Rev. Saude Publica*. **54**, 43 (2020).

26. J. R. Koo, A. R. Cook, M. Park, Y. Sun, H. Sun, J. T. Lim, C. Tam, B. L. Dickens, 10 Interventions to mitigate early spread of SARS-CoV-2 in Singapore: a modelling study. *Lancet Infect. Dis.* (2020), doi:10.1016/S1473-3099(20)30162-6.

27. B. Tang, F. Xia, N. L. Bragazzi, X. Wang, S. He, X. Sun, S. Tang, Y. Xiao, J. Wu, *medRxiv*, in press, doi:10.1101/2020.03.09.20033464.

28. L. Bao, W. Deng, H. Gao, C. Xiao, J. Liu, J. Xue, Q. Lv, J. Liu, P. Yu, Y. Xu, F. Qi, Y. Qu, 15 F. Li, Z. Xiang, H. Yu, S. Gong, M. Liu, G. Wang, S. Wang, Z. Song, W. Zhao, Y. Han, L. Zhao, X. Liu, Q. Wei, C. Qin, "Reinfection could not occur in SARS-CoV-2 infected rhesus macaques" (preprint, Microbiology, 2020), , doi:10.1101/2020.03.13.990226.

29. M. Ota, Will we see protection or reinfection in COVID-19? *Nat. Rev. Immunol.* (2020), doi:10.1038/s41577-020-0316-3.

30. L. Chen, J. Xiong, L. Bao, Y. Shi, Convalescent plasma as a potential therapy for COVID19. *Lancet Infect. Dis.*, S1473309920301419 (2020).

31. K. Duan, B. Liu, C. Li, H. Zhang, T. Yu, J. Qu, M. Zhou, L. Chen, S. Meng, Y. Hu, C. Peng, M. Yuan, J. Huang, Z. Wang, J. Yu, X. Gao, D. Wang, X. Yu, L. Li, J. Zhang, X. Wu, B. Li, Y. Xu, W. Chen, Y. Peng, Y. Hu, L. Lin, X. Liu, S. Huang, Z. Zhou, L. Zhang, 25 Y. Wang, Z. Zhang, K. Deng, Z. Xia, Q. Gong, W. Zhang, X. Zheng, Y. Liu, H. Yang, D. Zhou, D. Yu, J. Hou, Z. Shi, S. Chen, Z. Chen, X. Zhang, X. Yang, Effectiveness of convalescent plasma therapy in severe COVID-19 patients. *Proc. Natl. Acad. Sci. U. S. A.* (2020), doi:10.1073/pnas.2004168117.

32. J. D. Roback, J. Guarner, Convalescent Plasma to Treat COVID-19: Possibilities and 30 Challenges. *JAMA* (2020), doi:10.1001/jama.2020.4940.

33. C. Shen, Z. Wang, F. Zhao, Y. Yang, J. Li, J. Yuan, F. Wang, D. Li, M. Yang, L. Xing, J. Wei, H. Xiao, Y. Yang, J. Qu, L. Qing, L. Chen, Z. Xu, L. Peng, Y. Li, H. Zheng, F. Chen, K. Huang, Y. Jiang, D. Liu, Z. Zhang, Y. Liu, L. Liu, Treatment of 5 Critically Ill Patients With COVID-19 With Convalescent Plasma. *JAMA* (2020), doi:10.1001/jama.2020.4783.

34. T. Koyama, D. Weeraratne, J. L. Snowdon, L. Parida, "Emergence of Drift Variants That May Affect COVID-19 Vaccine Development and Antibody Treatment" (preprint, LIFE SCIENCES, 2020), , doi:10.20944/preprints202004.0024.v1. S. M. Kissler, C. Tedijanto, E. Goldstein, Y. H. Grad, M. Lipsitch, Projecting the transmission dynamics of SARS-CoV-2 through the postpandemic period. *Science* (2020), doi:10.1126/science.abb5793.

35. R. Li, S. Pei, B. Chen, Y. Song, T. Zhang, W. Yang, J. Shaman, Substantial undocumented infection facilitates the rapid dissemination of novelcoronavirus (SARS-CoV2). *Science* (2020), doi:10.1126/science.abb3221.

36. R. Verity, L. C. Okell, I. Dorigatti, P. Winskill, C. Whittaker, N. Imai, G. CuomoDannenburg, H. Thompson, P. G. T. Walker, H. Fu, A. Dighe, J. T. Griffin, M. Baguelin, S. Bhatia, A. Boonyasiri, A. Cori, Z. Cucunubá, R. FitzJohn, K. Gay-thorpe, W. Green, A. Hamlet, W. Hinsley, D. Laydon, G. Nedjati-Gilani, S. Riley, S. van Elsland, E. Volz, H. Wang, Y. Wang, X. Xi, C. A. Donnelly, A. C. Ghani, N. M. Ferguson, Estimates of the severity of coronavirus disease 2019: a model-based analysis. *Lancet Infect. Dis.*, doi:10.1016/S1473-3099(20)30243-7.

37. Novel Coronavirus Pneumonia Emergency Response Epidemiology Team, [The epidemiological characteristics of an outbreak of 2019 novel coronavirus diseases (COVID19) in China]. *Zhonghua Liu Xing Bing Xue Za Zhi Zhonghua Liuxingbingxue Zazhi.* **41**, 145–151 (2020).

38. D. Wang, B. Hu, C. Hu, F. Zhu, X. Liu, J. Zhang, B. Wang, H. Xiang, Z. Cheng, Y. Xiong, Y. Zhao, Y. Li, X. Wang, Z. Peng, Clinical Characteristics of 138 Hospitalized Patients With 2019 Novel Coronavirus–Infected Pneumonia in Wuhan, China. *JAMA* (2020), doi:10.1001/jama.2020.1585.

3. Viral Surveillance: Governing Social Isolation In São Paulo, Brazil, During The COVID-19 Pandemic[1]

Dr. Alcides Eduardo dos Reis Peron
Dr. Daniel Edler Duarte
Ma. Letícia Simões-Gomes
Dr. Marcelo Batista Nery
Prof. Almeida Prado,

INTRODUCTION

The COVID-19 pandemic imposes extraordinary challenges to governments and societies. At the time of writing, it has killed nearly5 Million people worldwide and paralysed most of China, India, Europe, the US and Latin American countries, causing an upsurge in unemployment rates and still incalculable economic losses. Before it is over, the pandemic will kill thousands more and most likely it will be followed by a period of global recession and social unrest. In response to the virus, most epidemiologists and policy-makers seem to agree on the need to restrict freedom of movement, to invest in personal protective equipment (PPEs) and hospital resources (tests, drugs and ventilators), and, finally, to build up virus-tracing capacities to identify clusters of infections, anticipate contagion, and contain further outbreaks.

In this context, while robust public policies have been said to be vital to tackle the pandemic, boosting claims for universal healthcare systems and basic income programs, travel restrictions, strict quarantine rules, and surveillance measures also become increasingly popular solutions. Indeed, the World Health Organisation (WHO) issued a flattering report on China's ability to contain initial outbreaks, exhorting other governments to adopt similar actions and, particularly, to ramp up their monitoring capacities to "expand surveillance to detect COVID-19 transmission chains" (WHO, 2020a, p. 21). Interestingly, the pandemic has elicited both solidarity networks and widespread suspicion, combining practices of care, calculations of risk, and disciplinary techniques of population control.

initial approaches to the matter have emphasized the ambiguous aspects of current policy responses. Many scholars expressed fears of "surveillance creep" (Lyon, 2007), which could end up inducing techno-totalitarian states, in which authorities keep powers and techniques to snoop on people indefinitely (Morozov, 2020). Others advanced revolutionary readings of the current crisis claiming neoliberal dogmas might be witnessing their last days (Zizzed, 2020). Accordingly, the coronavirus "laid bare the exploitative structures that govern our social and political lives" (Goldenfein et al, 2020), opening gaps for solidarity-based systems in which markets are fettered and the common good, including green economy, become mainstream politics (Latour, 2020).

---

[1] Corresponding Author. Department of Sociology, University of São Paulo, Av. Prof. Luciano Gualberto, 315, Butantã, São Paulo, 05508-010, Brazil. E-mail address: dudperon@gmail.com

In this paper, we engage with such debates, but advance a different perspective to contemporary security practices and disciplinary politics of health and care. Looking into local responses to COVID-19 in São Paulo, Brazil, we trace the adoption and reconfiguration of surveillance technology as multiple devices are developed or repurposed to enhance pandemic control.

Specifically, we put our lenses over two main projects, the Smart Monitoring System (SIMI-SP) and the Social Isolation Index (SII). SIMI-SP entails the collection of cell-phones positioning data to feed maps of mass gatherings, indicating where authorities need to enhance patrols and social isolation recommendations.

SII was designed by InLoco, a data-savvy media/advertising company, to measure aggregate data on people's movement and issue daily rates of social distancing across the urban landscape. Both tools comprise a digital platform used by the state to better assess and efficiently manage local responses to the health crisis. Hence, the article raises evidence of the rearticulating of surveillant assemblages in São Paulo. The monitoring techniques and social sorting algorithms used to tackle the pandemic are not exactly new. Similar devices were already deployed by the police, media and health professionals. We argue that the changing composition of the assemblage produces relevant effects. Emerging technologies comprise of public and private actors, biometrics, commercial databases, digital infrastructures, mathematical models, epidemiologists, and data scientists which were previously dispersed. In this process, practices of body surveillance and urban monitoring effectively coalesce, juxtaposing notions of disciplinary power, governmentality, and self-care (Foucault, 2015).

In this article, we investigate the biopolitics of local responses to the virus, stressing the cross contamination of medical, political, security, and technological knowledge and practices. The production of data of contagion patterns is inherently connected both to the deployment of population monitoring systems and police repression. Thus, São Paulo is arguably going through a "medicalization of security" (Elbe, 2011), as epidemiologists, physicians, and sanitary authorities become relevant voices in the making of deviant profiles, in designing monitoring techniques and enforcing practices of control. Public health measures are arguably undissociated from public security measures, while virology discourses support arrests of those who break the lockdown and justify stricter surveillance of urban flows (Wright, 2020).

To develop this analysis, the first section presents a brief overview of current debates on security practices during the pandemic, also depicting the surveillance apparatus in the interstices of control and care. In the second part, we describe how monitoring tools have been developed and deployed in São Paulol, and, most importantly, how they articulate with disciplinary practices (including heavy fines and summary arrests) to enforce social isolation recommendations. The third section explores social and political impacts of emerging surveillant assemblages, analysing dilemmas of data privacy, human rights, and the managing of mobility during the pandemic. Technologies might mitigate the spread of the virus but, as we argue in the conclusion, there needs to be more transparency about their implementation, use and effects. Promises of techno-solutions to the pandemic must be balanced with public awareness about their accuracy, biases, and limits.

The Apparatus of Social Isolation and Self Care

São Paulo registered its first COVID-19 infection on February 26th, roughly three months after the disease was identified in Wuhan, China. The subject was immediately isolated while authorities attempted to track his previous contacts and monitor potential contagions. Initial efforts, however, proved insufficient to hold local spread of the virus. Four weeks after "patient zero", the state already recorded about fourteen thousand cases, in 228 cities, and more than a thousand deaths. São Paulo's capital alone – a 12-million-people metropolis – is responsible for 68% of infections, which makes it the pandemic epicentre in Brazil (Governo do Estado de São Paulo, 2020).[1] In response to the widespread disease, João Dória, the state's governor, issued a decree of public calamity, expanding executive powers over the state's budget and centralizing public information and decisions in a crisis cabinet under his authority.

Local pandemic control measures encompassed redirecting emergency funds to the purchase of PPEs, assembling three makeshift hospitals for COVID-19 patients, importing tests, and suspending every non-essential service, effectively closing most of commerce, parks, schools, etc. In parallel, public authorities also invested in massive public health campaigns which advised people to avoid social activities, stay at home, and adopt meticulous personal hygiene routines. Such measures are in accordance with WHO's list of best practices of health emergency preparedness, which advocates for physical isolation to disrupt the chain of infection and halt communitarian transmission. As Michael Ryan, WHO's director to the Health Emergencies Programme, explains:

"[T]ere are a toolkit of measures that can be taken to deal with this virus when the disease has reached a certain level, especially in community transmission, and it's no longer possible to identify all the cases or all of the contacts then you move to separating everybody from everybody else. You create physical distance between everybody because you don't know exactly who might have the virus" (WHO, 2020b). Multiple countries have since adopted these recommendations on social distancing and contact-tracing, imposing emergency social isolation laws and developing a myriad of digital devices to monitor people's interactions. In São Paulo and elsewhere health authorities have turned to private companies and experts to collect data and establish virus transmission chains, to trace individuals who might have been infected, to identify mass gatherings, and, finally, to design predictive models of future outbreaks.

Unsurprisingly, controversies on privacy rights and bio surveillance followed governments' attempts to scale up social control amid the pandemic. Agamben (2020), for one, alerted to the perils of authoritarian oppression stemming from "frantic, irrational, and absolutely unwarranted emergency measures adopted for a supposed epidemic of coronavirus". Byung-Chul Han (2020) resonated this criticism, pointing out that decisions to close borders and ramp up digital surveillance are based in disproportionate fears of the virus. Naomi Klein (2020) also addressed the issue through the prism of exception and rupture. For her, we are currently living in a "pandemic shock doctrine", which will catalyse radical free market policies.

David Harvey (2020) contributed with a similar note, raising awareness to the risk of sitting leaders to declare "imperial presidenc[ies] to save capital". In short, many authors set states' responses to COVID-19 as attempts to frame health emergencies as existential threats, thus gathering support for draconian reactions. As different as they might be, these standpoints share a perception that liberty and freedom are at risk since "wartime" responses to the pandemic jeopardize well-being and democracy (Mudde, 2020). Against the "state of exception" argument, many commentators

---

[1] Data of infections in Brazil vary on a daily basis. The numbers presented here were collected at the end of April 2020.

have contextualized initially feeble responses to the virus, especially in the US, Brazil and the UK, as enactments of neoliberal necropolitics, claiming economically vulnerable populations, those on the fringes of capitalism and deemed surplus or disposable, would also be the most affected by the disease (Purnell, 2020; Diniz & Carino, 2020). In this perspective, to act normally and avoid extreme reactions are not real options, at least not for those willing to flatten the curve of infections.

As Panagiotis Sotiris (2020) puts it, *bare life* is "closer to the pensioner on a waiting list for a respirator or an ICU bed, because of a collapsed health system, than the intellectual having to do with the practicalities of quarantine measures". Although critical scholars have been prolific in raising awareness to the biopolitics of pandemics, contemporary practices of population control are much more ambivalent and entangled than the above debates might indicate. State responses are not limited to lockdowns and mobility control; they also comprise massive investments in public health infrastructure and prophylactic attempts at disrupting the infection chain. As we will see in the next section, self-care conducts and preventive social control policies coalesce, assembling a hybrid pandemic-response apparatus which articulates health professionals, security agents, surveillance devices, private companies, international institutions, local policy-makers, etc.

As (Foucault, 2015; Murphy & Whitty, 2009; Elbe, 2011),and others have shown this heterogeneous apparatus is hardly exceptional. Early modern medicine in the 19th Century already encompassed articulations between police, sanitary and demographic registers and statistics. Hence public health policies and security practices were intertwined in the politico-scientific control of growing urban populations. Also, "health emergency preparedness", as promoted by the WHO for decades, already articulated techniques of body examination and surveillance with collective forms of intervention and regulatory controls (Sanford, Polzer & McDonough, 2016).

However, while many commentators have taken up Foucault's much cited analysis on leprosy and the plague to discuss present responses to the virus in terms of powers to exclude or to confine and discipline,[1] we argue that social isolation policies in São Paulo do not equate to the "biopolitical dream" in which "governments, advised by physicians, impose pandemic dictatorship on entire populations" (Sarasin, 2020). Following the executive decree on public calamity, non-essential services were obliged to shut doors and major gatherings have been prohibited (i.e. music concerts and sports events), but social distancing, despite being closely monitored, is mostly voluntary.

There have been very few cases of police repression and, to this moment, local authorities seem to prefer media campaigns about preventive care and healthy behaviours.

In this sense, São Paulo witnesses an unstable, hence, contingent juxtaposition of different social control techniques, which might be better described as a governmentality of pandemics in which the police take part, but the main "instruments of government, become diverse tactics rather than laws" (Foucault, 2007, p. 99). In other words, in parallel to repression and actual surveillance, responses to the COVID-19 aim at developing self-care awareness and collective solidarity, also educating people to identify symptoms of infection and to make responsible decisions about whether to leave their homes or not. For Foucault, governmentality is a form of population management based on statistical, economic and health knowledge. It targets people's interactions and mobilities. In this sense, governmentality acts in the interstices of self-government and the government of others, in which the technologies of the self (knowledge about the human body and

---

[1] Foucault (2001) describes disciplinary medical measures for social control, differentiating the isolation against leprosy (a preventive form based on total exclusion) from the confinement practices during the plague (when even if restrictive circulation is mandatory, he portrays it as an inclusion, meaning that it allows a permanent monitoring of individual health, and relationships among residents).

self-preventive care) are mobilized as techniques for population's control (general preventive care). As Foucault points out:

"[...] the principle of care of oneself became rather general in scope. The precept according to which one must give attention to oneself was in any case an imperative that circulated among a number of different doctrines. It also took the form of an attitude, a mode of behaviour; it became instilled in ways of living; it evolved into procedures, practices, and formulas that people reflected on, developed, perfected, and taught. It thus came to constitute a social practice, giving rise to relationships between individuals, to exchanges and communications, and at times even to institutions. And it gave rise, finally, to a certain mode of knowledge and to the elaboration of a science" (Foucault, 1986, pp. 44/45). Self-care as prevention is generalized as a technology of the self (self-conduct) in the security device of governmentality, as Lemke points out (2012, p. 21): "[they are] techniques that permit individuals to affect a certain number of operations on their bodies, souls, thoughts, and so on, to transform themselves in order to attain a certain desired state". These technologies of the self-allow an exercise of control and of driving people in a more palatable way and without resistance.

Thus, the notion of government resides precisely in the interaction between control and care (prevention). It aims to tutor and organize large contingents of people, to modulate their behaviours from the introduction of a mentality in the social body that relates prevention (the management of risks), selfcare and environment, and the production of quality of life. Thus, we analyse social isolation policies as governmental techniques that introduce precautionary rationalities in which self-care is generalized as a safety device within the social body. Specifically, health professionals, deeply articulated within the pandemic-response apparatus (Elbe, 2011), propose that physical interactions are the cause of contagion. So, individual practices of reduced mobility and cautious hygiene routines produce collective effects on public health security. The above measures target the population. They configure a non-individualized technique of power informed by statistics and generalized surveillance. However, they do not exclude other forms of social control. Hence, the governmentality of pandemics overlaps and juxtaposes disciplinary practices – those based on minute details of individualized bodies – with the biopolitics of the population.[1] In the next section, we debate two techniques of control that have been central to São Paulo's governmentality of pandemics: the making of a social isolation index and the sociotechnical surveillance devices used by state authorities to monitor people's adherence to lockdown recommendations.

These techniques bring together public and private actors and mobilize medical and security knowledge in the governing of conducts and mobilities. As we will see, the governmentality of pandemic encompasses threats of repressive actions, campaigns of persuasion, political disputes, and controversies on privacy and intrusiveness. In this context, we argue that the social isolation index mediates between disciplinary and biopolitical practices.

---

[1] About this, Foucault (2015, pp. 295-296) pointed out that in governmentality, disciplinary techniques are not necessarily canceled, but overlapped and often act simultaneously. Similarly, Klauser (2017), when looking from a spatial logic of surveillance practices, admits the possibilities of overlapping and simultaneity of securitarian (crowd management) and disciplinary (individualizing and normative) logics of monitoring and exercise of power.

In pursuit of a metrics: The public-private assemblages for monitoring the isolation

Local authorities had been monitoring risks of COVID-19 infections in São Paulo since January, but contingency plans were only made public in late February, when initial outbreaks were confirmed. The state government then imposed lockdown and assembled a crisis cabinet, composed by multiple secretariats, technical bodies, security agencies and municipal authorities. The cabinet occupies a well-appointed control room close to the governor's office and has since become the main source of information for both state officials and the media. Equipped with scanning software, multiple communication devices, and digital platforms, the cabinet gathers data from public and private institutions in order to build situational awareness about the pandemic.

Projected in a line-up of screens, several dashboards aggregate information on the toll of infections, ICU's occupation rate, PPEs demands, distribution of tests, critical infrastructure, real-time camera feeds, and contagion forecasts (Ghirotto, 2020). In this multi-stakeholder operational environment, authorities aim at breaking the chain of contagions with a more efficient management of resources. In practice, this means monitoring social adherence to social isolation measures. In this context, state and municipal officials approached private companies to develop social distancing indicators and maps of urban mobilities and variations in demographic densities. These partnerships resulted in two main surveillance tools, the Smart Monitoring System (SIMI-SP) and Inloco's Social Isolation Index (SII).[1] Both tools allow taskforces to check whether risk groups follow lockdown policies and to flag hotspots of disease potential outbreaks.

As such, they are valuable tools to assess government's actions on a daily basis. Most importantly, they guide the allocation of resources, indicating where the police and sanitary authorities need to focus next. SIMI-SP was designed by local cell-phone providers and relies on regular collection of data by telecom antennas to produce structured databases of urban flows and heat maps of mass gatherings. As people move around the city, their cell-phones connect to various broadcast spots, leaving registers of data transmission in different neighbourhoods. Specifically, the system geo-references every cell phone position between 10pm and 2am to infer where individuals spent the night. In the next day, if any data is captured by antennas more than 200 meters away from the initial site, SIMI-SP will consider the individual did not follow lockdown rules (Gomes, 2020).

The government says that it only accesses anonymized data and cannot visualize heat maps in real-time. Telecoms aggregate information collected on the previous day and erases time frames of movements before feeding the system.

So, digital maps only display average rates of flows and isolation in different neighbourhoods. Inloco's solution has a different architecture.[2] The SII collects data through a Software Development Kit (SDK - i.e. code) embedded in smartphone applications of partner companies, which mostly consist of banks, retail stores, telecoms, and fintechs.[3] By accepting the apps' terms of service, clients agree to have their geolocation information used for other purposes, such as digital address validation, target advertisement, and population mobility indexes. According to InLoco, its database comprises about 60 million smartphones (four million in the city of São Paulo alone) (InLoco, 2020).

---

[1] InLoco is a Recife-based technology company focused on location data analysis, as means of targeted advertisement and consumer profiling.

[2] Although the company individually provides "tech solutions" for the pandemic, their development is also related to academia research, as evidenced by its partnership with the Pasteur Institute and the Pharmaceutical Sciences Faculty at University of São Paulo. In this case, InLoco shared its database to an ongoing epidemiological research based on smartphone patient tracking.

[3] It is highly probable that their sample is biased; InLoco's database of the city of São Paulo comprehends approximately 4 million devices, in a population of 12 million inhabitants (Queiroz et al., 2020). Moreover, their data is mostly derived from apps' whose public are middle and high income consumers.

In order to build its mapping service, data is extracted by different sensors, including GPS, Wi-Fi connections, Bluetooth-LE, cell-phone signals, and activity recognition. Whereas other companies stick to GPS signals or cell-phone antennas, Inloco's myriad of sources allegedly enables them to provide more precise geolocation. The social isolation index is calculated by tracking individual users' mobility data, which is later anonymised and aggregated, so public authorities are only presented a percentage of lockdown abiders in different neighbourhoods.[1]

Health authorities are still struggling to convince citizens on the need to respect social distancing, so SIMI-SP's and Inloco's heat maps not only guide their responses but help in performing the pandemic to the public (Lynch, 1985). Digital interfaces provide valuable illustrations of risks of infections. Maps, diagrams, and graphs make the hitherto invisible virus easily accessible, so the palpable consequences of the disease become suitable for state intervention.

Furthermore, indexes, as social processes of measurement and commensuration, have the attribute of simplifying observed facts by transforming qualities into quantities, and differences into comparable magnitudes (Espeland and Stevens, 1998: 316). In short, these representations are objects as well as tools of power relations. By abstracting and reducing complexities, both heat maps and indexes turn social isolation into a continuum, which contributes to depict mass gatherings and spatial mobility as unwelcome/undesirable behaviours to be socially (and potentially normatively) sanctioned.

While these technologies indicate the effectiveness of social isolation and the possibility of loosening lockdown rules, they also act upon the population's fear, stimulating self-care as means of collective care and solidarity. As Porter notes: "Numbers alone never provide enough information to make detailed decisions [...]. Their highest purpose is to instil an ethic. Measures of [...] achievement in general succeed to the degree they become, in Nikolas Rose's phrase, "technologies of the soul." They provide legitimacy for administrative actions, in large part because they provide standards against which people judge themselves" (Porter, 1998, p. 45).

Also, practices around technologies do not necessarily follow their strict purposes, they are creatively and situationally resignified. In this sense, they comprise a contingent and heterogeneous governmentality of pandemics which consists of three emerging and overlapping techniques of control: educational campaigns for improved personal hygiene, incentives for individuals to inform authorities on others' undesirable behaviour, and straightforward police repression. In spatializing and communicating threats, the government expects to educate the population on the need to change everyday habits. Beyond media campaigns, local authorities send SMS messages on potential outbreaks to residents of neighbourhoods where people are not upholding social distancing.

Those who inhabit risky areas (where infections concentrate) also receive customized messages about hygiene precautions. State and municipal authorities have even used cars with sound systems to inform on personal safety precautions in the urban outskirts. As Patrícia Ellen, state secretary for economic development, science, and technology, declared, government strategies of containment are ineffective without people's cooperation, so SIMI-SP and SII are key political tools of persuasion. In her words, "we must have at least 60% of isolation rate so we can control the curve [of the spread] of the virus.

---

[1] It is not yet clear whether the data analysed is compared on a longitudinal basis (such as patterns of user mobility before and after the lockdown), or just relative signal immobility. Regarding its pandemic-specific products, InLoco offers the public sector a wide range of mapping and tracking programs: a) integrating its SDK to office services apps', as to generate input for social isolation metrics, monitor "risk areas", and provide a direct communication channel with its users; b) mobility analysis through health and essential services; c) Mobility index by neighbourhood/state; d) Social isolation index par residence (clustered by neighbourhood); e) Social isolation and mobility indexes for academic research; f) Journey analysis; g) Mass gathering heatmaps (Moura and Ferraz, 2020).

The government cannot cope with it alone, and we have lives on the line. This technology is at people's service. The data that we have is also accessible for you [the media] to follow the results and evaluate our actions" (Balanço Geral, 2020). The normalizing apparatus is also manifested by how citizens inform authorities on lockdown disengagement in their neighbourhoods. In 2017, the municipal department of public safety developed a platform so people could notify public services of urban disorder incidents that might require intervention. SP+Segura, as the system is named, registers multiple cases, ranging from safety measures to fallen trees.[1]

During the pandemic, however, the platform became a mediator for horizontal surveillance on undesirable/unhealthy behaviours. In other words, citizens have been exercising their normalizing gaze through SP+Segura. We observed that it has been used to warn authorities about public gatherings, markets that do not follow hygiene recommendations (i.e. employees without masks and gloves), non-essential commerce that insists to keep doors open, bars that deceive sanitary authorities by claiming to be markets, private parties, and all sorts of unwelcome behaviours that might put society in risk. The juxtaposition of self-care and government, or discipline and control, is also seen in this platform-mediated contact between municipal agencies and local citizens. Finally, the third technique of control is the state resort to police repression. After experiencing high isolation rates in the first weeks of the lockdown, the SII and SIMI-SP began to alert on increasing mobilities and gatherings. In response, the state government performed another aspect of the governmentality of the pandemics and threatened that severe measures would be taken against those who break the rules, which meant heavy fines and up to 18-month prison sentences. In the governor's words:

"If we don't take isolation rates from 50% to more than 60%, and move towards 70% in the next week, [...] [public authorities] will take more rigid measures. I wanted to avoid that, because it means people will receive official warnings, fines, and may even be arrested. People must be conscious about the situation we're in. [...] People must be responsible and we're monitoring that with the cell-phones. [..] I hope we don't need to reach that level [of repression], but, if we have to do it, we'll do it in defence of life" (Pauluze & Trindade, 2020). These disciplinary measures are provided by the state decree of calamity, which lists a few instruments to enforce social isolation. Indeed, the police were already being used to disperse parties in public places and to close non-essential commerce, but arrests were few and sparse. It is not yet clear, however, what the governor's threats will entail. Although data on lockdown-related police operations is not available, the media has not reported on an upsurge in arrests and the news are limited to occasional altercations between police officers and individuals who resist requests to leave public parks or to close local bars (Chagas, 2020).

As we will see below, the governor's statement was also met with scepticism by the police. Despite claims that the pandemic surveillance apparatus is essential to better manage public resources and effectively control the virus, ultimately saving lives, local authorities and private companies have been criticised for stepping up their monitoring capacities. Anticipating controversies about client's privacy, the cell-phone companies that designed SIMI-SP argued that their database is "non-intrusive" since it cannot be used to identify and track individuals. According to Sinditelebrasil, a syndicate of private media companies, public authorities cannot reverse the anonymization process, so they have no access to clients' gender, name, or phone number: "It's only statistics. It's like you go to a metro turnstile. People will see you passing through and the turnstile will only register the

---

[1] Its name can be roughly translated as São Paulo+Safe. For a longer description of its functionalities and a debate on its impacts in São Paulo's security assemblage, see: Peron and Alvarez (2019).

number of people. At the end of each day, station managers check the turnstile and know how many people passed through. […] It's impossible to reverse [i.e. deanonymize], There's no way to see who passed the turnstile, you only know that someone did it" (Gomes, 2020a). Furthermore, the databases offered to local authorities on a pro-bono agreement are not unprecedented, on the contrary. The companies already collected aggregate data on cell-phone positions in order to improve their services and make profit selling in the data market. As the vice president for data and AI in one of the telecoms confirmed: "In the past five years we have invested in big data and artificial intelligence to improve clients' experience. So, when the pandemic came, we built applications to help in the fight" (Mello, 2020).

In Loco also dismissed accusations of privacy breaches and emphasized that we are going through a crisis, which requests coordination between public and private actors so health professionals may have the best technology and information at their disposal. Also, Raísa Moura, InLoco's head of data privacy, stressed that the company can protect individuals' identity while also providing public authorities with statistics, maps and other helpful representations of mobility and concentration. As she explained, the company adopts a "privacy by design" approach, which means that neither their programmers nor public officials have access to identifiable personal information. Identifiers in each smartphone (IMEI and MAC codes) and client's accounts or documents (e-mail, phone number, ID registers, etc) are not collected. She also ensures that, even during the pandemics, the company has not integrated different databases, nor triangulated information to identify individual users. So, there is no need to be caught in the privacy vs. security trade-off. In her words: "During a calamity, many rights are relativized, norms become more flexible and all the efforts must be directed to saving as many lives as we can. However, the "Sophie's choice" should not be about "pandemic control vs. privacy", with the risk of inducting arbitrary governments.

More than ever, discussions about privacy, so much debated before the pandemic, should stay under the spotlight" (Moura and Ferraz, 2020, p. 5). Despite the above justifications and government's claims about the relevance of surveillance platforms for the virus containment strategy, privacy watchdogs insist that companies should have asked users whether they were willing to surrender personal data to the government before implementing the systems (Bioni et al, 2020). We did not find judicial claims mentioning InLoco, but many clients opened litigations against the telecoms and managed to get their numbers out of SIMISP's monitoring list (Gomes, 2020b). At least one lawyer had a request for collective *habeas corpus*, which would stall monitoring and prevent private companies from further transferring personal data to public authorities, denied by federal courts (UOL, 2020). Others developed and shared on social media inventive ways to elude surveillance and avoid tracking. A similar solution for monitoring social isolation rates on a national level was blocked by the president, who criticized São Paulo's attempts to reduce individual freedom and claimed privacy risks should be better assessed before setting such systems up.

The president of Brazil and São Paulo's governor have adopted radically different stances towards the pandemic. While the governor blames the president for "politicizing the virus" (Dória, 2020), Bolsonaro has taken sides with local businessmen who claim lockdowns will cause severe economic damages.

Despite the growing toll of deaths, the president has repeatedly downplayed the consequences of the COVID-19, which he calls "just a minor flu", and advised Dória and other governors that "the treatment should not be worse than the disease" (Bolsonaro, 2020). His position resonates within São Paulo's police. The Association of Military Police Officers of São Paulo (Defenda PM), for example, has publicly antagonised the governor. In their perspective, social isolation is a suggestion, not an order, so the police should not be deployed to arrest citizens who choose not to follow the lockdown. Furthermore, the retired police colonel Elias Miler, Defenda PM's president, declared state attempts to prevent people's mobility are against the constitution. For him, the governor's threats were "truculent, arbitrary and configure misfeasance" (Miler, 2020). As the reduced number of arrests might indicate, these disputes have jeopardized the state's capacity to enforce social isolation and seems to have contributed to undermine further disciplinary measures.

While the governor maintains that current monitoring practices are in accordance with national laws on telecommunications, the Civil Rights Framework for the Internet, and the criminal law, there are at least three issues to be raised. The first concern is transparency. São Paulo follows the spread of the virus in the crisis cabinet, which has straight contact with the media to broadcast relevant information. However, to the moment, transparency has been synonym to official statistics and not much more. Scholars have limited access to control rooms and struggle to understand its surveillance architecture.

Since most devices were designed by private companies, even members of public security institutions have restricted access to digital platforms and limited knowledge about how infection rates and other statistics are produced. We tried contact with many professionals placed in public institutions with experience in digital technologies and georeferencing (including the police), but none of them could tell us much about what happens inside the crisis cabinet. The second concern refers to practices of anonymization. Cyber security specialists often argue that there is no anonymous data per se, only a successful or unsuccessful process of anonymization in which specific information is generalized and a few data entries are discarded.

Although anonymization is hardly an irreversible process, public and private data holders can make this a lengthy and costly endeavour for those trying to identify individuals in a database. So, it is not enough to erase names and phone numbers, as InLoco seems to suggest. Data analysts must ensure that other data sources cannot be used to triangulate personal information and deanonymize individuals. This is exactly what an investigative reporter did with the supposedly anonymous data collected by telecoms (Dias, 2020). Using information from social media, the reporter managed to identify a few names in a database that is similar to the one used in SIMI-SP. Interestingly, none of them knew their data was collected and used for purposes other than the telecom service.

The last issue is that monitoring capabilities recently introduced are not built upon a blank slate but articulate with previous surveillance practices and rationales.

In 2014, for example, state authorities launched a digital platform aimed at mapping crimes in São Paulo in order to improve police patrols and investigations, and to inform crime control strategies in general.

The platform was named "intelligent monitoring system" and offered security professionals detailed representations of aggregate crime data, so police officers could identify crime patterns in specific neighbourhoods and react accordingly. This system was later connected to video-monitoring devices which allowed operators to trace suspects and produce real-time alerts on potential crimes. Despite claims that SIMISP and the SII will be discontinued after the pandemic, recent history of surveillance teaches us that society should be alert to future articulations between data on urban fluxes and peoples' gatherings and other security monitoring systems. The governmentality of pandemic might have durable effects on surveillant assemblages.

Equating Privacy and Proportionality Under the Pandemic

These surveillance and monitoring technologies, in parallel with restrictive measures, seem to produce a great amount of knowledge about patterns of population mobility. The Institute for Applied Economic Research (IPEA), a public think tank that provides technical support to the federal government, produced a report discussing the benefits of social isolation measures to control COVID19 outbreaks and evaluating different social isolation indexes, including InLoco's platform. In their perspective, while public campaigns have positive effects, restrictive policies are essential for maintaining social distancing in Brazilian cities. Hence, governments are advised to uphold monitoring practices throughout the pandemic (Moraes, 2020). However, state surveillance and policies of restrictive mobility should be closely followed. Civil society organisations have alerted the risks of excesses and, most importantly, to the fact that surveillance devices designed for pandemic control might be deployed for general security purposes once the crisis is over (Bioni et al, 2020). In this regard, Han (2020) warns that extensive use of forms of surveillance seem to have been essential to contain the pandemic in China. In sustaining that the halt of the disease does not operate only through doctors, but also through data scientists, Han (2020) states:

"Critical awareness of digital surveillance is practically non-existent in Asia. There is almost no talk regarding data protection, including liberal states like Japan and Korea. No one is irritated by the authorities' frenzy to compile data (...) The entire infrastructure for digital surveillance has now proved to be extremely effective in containing the epidemic. (...) Digitization directly intoxicates them. This is also due to a cultural motive. In Asia, collectivism prevails.

There is no strong individualism. Individualism is not the same as selfishness, which of course is also widespread in Asia". In other words, the absence of a critical culture about surveillance, of trust in the State, and a peculiar perception of collectivism, facilitate the adoption of more intrusive surveillance measures, and greater exposure of people to massive data collection. Paradoxically, these same measures seem to be most effective in tackling the pandemic. To Han (2020), their spread would reinforce the evolution of police states in Western societies.

Also, it would undermine legal safeguards that limit surveillance practices, which draws his argument closer to Agamben's (2020).Nonetheless, the availability of these surveillance and monitoring technologies in the "West" encouraged debates on discriminatory and authoritarian practices, such as facial recognition systems (Ajana, 2013; Garvie, et. al, 2016; Peron and Alvarez, 2019), algorithmic surveillance instruments and risk classification (Amoore, 2013).

In São Paulo, both the SII and SIMI may perpetuate disciplinary policing practices in post-pandemic techniques of control.

However, there are alternatives to mitigate surveillance creep and even prevent intrusive monitoring practices from taking hold after the crises. A joint statement of several civil society organisations notes that "The COVID-19 pandemic is a global public health emergency that requires a coordinated and large-scale response by governments worldwide. However, States' efforts to contain the virus must not be used as a cover to usher in a new era of greatly expanded systems of invasive digital surveillance" (7amleh, et al, 2020). Thus, how should we balance its use and limit the pervasiveness of these technologies? Is it possible to employ them to manage the spreading of COVID-19, while reconciling it to Human Rights demands?

Controversies about emergency (intrusive) measures during pandemics and the preservation of human rights often derived from past experiences (O'Malley et al., 2009; Murphy and Whitty, 2009;

Elbe, 2011; Carney and Bennett, 2012; Ventura, 2016). Many authors have shown that pandemic crisis management often bring medical-sanitary knowledge to the security apparatus[1], conforming a policy of permanent care as "health security" that will inform decisions (Elbe, 2011). However, pandemic management goes beyond ordinary monitoring, and, once declared, often requires rapid and exceptional measures, and demands wit from political elites (Prescott, 2007: 02). They elude the traditional democratic process of decision-making. Thus, an epidemic deflagration should be met with public health emergency legal preparedness, which "is all about having the right laws in place and then using them in the right way in a time of public health emergency (...)

it is both proactive and reactive" (Murphy and Whitty, 2009, p. 220). Medical-sanitary knowledge gains prominence in the context of a pandemic, informing conducts of care and safety based on its own ethical principles. As public health has its focus on promoting collective well-being (Gilbert, 2012), commensuration and monitoring could offer smarter and less intrusive mechanisms for pandemic management. The underlying assumption is that all humans are potential victims and vectors of contagion[2]; therefore, measures taken must comprehend the social group in its totality, and should not be directed at specific groups[3], i.e., "maximize the minimum" of well-being or expand to all its benefits as a form of solidarity (Gilbert, 2012, p. 129). Still, adopting public health ethics for halting contagion does not preclude human rights observation. To make use of restraining technologies, authorities must comply with the criteria of "necessity" and "proportionality" posed by International Humanitarian Law (IHL) and International Health Regulation (IHR). In this respect, the IHR is complementary regarding the IHL, as it promotes the latter's standards of dignity, personal freedoms, transparency, non-discrimination, and consent (Murphy and Whitty, 2009, pp. 226-228). As article 43(1) of the International Health Regulations states: pandemic control measures should not be "more invasive or intrusive to persons than reasonably available alternatives that would achieve the appropriate level of health protection" (WHO, 2005, p. 29). Murphy and Whitty (2009) reject the "sceptical" view that confers legitimacy to exceptional measures that incur in Human Rights violations. In their analysis, there should not be a trade-off between political objectives (with intrusive measures) and Human Rights protection, as that draw principles and objectives to the same level (Murphy and Whitty, 2009, p. 236).

For them, proportionality is the key to deal with rights and their relationship to invasive policies, by acknowledging that rights can indeed restrict public and collectivist interests, but also contributing to set legitimate goals and practices: "Rights outweigh goals that are not legitimate and, where goals are legitimate, any measures giving effect to them must be suitable, the least restrictive possible, and proportionate between the effects of the measures and the objective to be achieved. (...) if risk evidence is to be used to justify limitations on rights, the evidence of threats to security must be disclosed and scrutinized according to identifiable legal norms" (Murphy and Whitty, 2009, pp. 236237).Albeit respecting human rights might seem counterproductive in economic and political terms, they are essential for assessing risk and proportionality in technological solutions to the pandemic. Social isolation policies in São Paulo, for instance, have been proportional. To the moment, public authorities kept police repression to a minimum, investing instead in massive educational campaigns to convince local citizens of the need to stay at home and adopt hygienic

---

[1] Others, in Global Health Studies, argue the other way around: seeing pandemic situations as processes of securitization of global health, under the banner of right to health implementation and/or preservation (see Ventura, 2016).

[2] Such a stance is also known as the Rawsilian veil of ignorance, in which every individual is taken as free, rational, and morally equal.

[3] Targeting groups during pandemics has historically been a source of discrimination and abuse, such as during the 1980s AIDS outbreak, against LGBT communities (Murphy and Whitty, 2009).

routines. Likewise, the lockdown can be considered necessary and proportional inasmuch as mobility restrictions aim at a greater good, i.e., halting the spread of the disease and protecting the right to life. At the same time, technologies such as Simi and SII call for greater attention. Besides supporting the lockdown in the terms, we discussed above, their enactment depends on individual data collection for state monitoring purposes, without explicit consent, jeopardising people's privacy.

Afterwards, these tools have the potential to be redirected to crime control, making them both disproportionate and unnecessary.

As the United Nations Human Rights office poses, "(...) we are aware of growing use of tools of surveillance technology to track the spread of the coronavirus. While we understand and support the need for active efforts to confront the pandemic, it is also crucial that such tools be limited in use, both in terms of purpose and time, and that individual rights to privacy, non-discrimination, the protection of journalistic sources and other freedoms be rigorously protected" (UNHR, 2020). Hence, proportionality meets a clear need for information production. Notwithstanding, their employment ought to be subjected to criteria guiding data collection, processing, and storage. In this spirit, Data Privacy Brasil developed 18 guidelines comprising implicit notions and fundamental values for orienting data collection during the pandemic. Compliance with these guidelines, in a way, would ensure proportionality in data collection.

As widely discussed in digital surveillance studies (Murphy and Whitty, 2009; O'Neil, 2016; Zuboff, 2019), transparency is a core element of technologies in general - not to mention in pandemics - since it allows identifying and circumscribing uses, preventing pandemic measures from being as harmful as the disease itself: "If the recommended data protection principles and best practices are internalized and well implemented, the likelihood of efficiency of these measures will increase while ensuring their legitimacy, in addition to enjoying greater trust on the part of society. The use of personal data is just one of the measures to contain the pandemic of COVID-19, which must be conceived as such so that it is, in fact, a measure of containment and not of increasing the damage experienced by such an epidemic. The set of recommendations above makes it clear that data protection does not rival this purpose, but rather allows the State to be efficient in combating the epidemic and to do so with respect to the fundamental rights and guarantees of the population" (Bioni, et al; 2020, p. 27). SIMI's deployment, for one, presented several difficulties and loopholes, failing to follow the proportionality criterion. First, it appears that there is no detailed deadline for its cessation - although it is assumed that they may cease along with the pandemic, this is not clearly stated, raising doubts as to whether it would be directed to other uses. Moreover, *The Intercept Brasil* argued that although telephone companies and the state affirm that geolocation data cannot be individualized, numerous loopholes that allow the identification of users were registered, exposing them to prosecution risks in a hypothetical case of (disciplinary) hardening of the insulation (Dias, 2020).

Finally, Data Privacy alerted to the fact that SIMI's software is not designed with open source code, which could facilitate the understanding of third parties and consultants regarding the collection, processing and disposal of data (Gomes, 2020a). Lack of transparency was also remarkable when conducting this study, as few actors from either the public and private sectors were interested in providing explanations about the technologies' implementation.

FINAL REMARKS

Pandemics are extraordinary and multifaceted events, calling for intricate human intervention to their mitigation. Coronavirus' propagation happened in an age of massive data collection, with widespread availability of sensors and other informational devices, which constantly interact with our social life. Thus, it is no surprise that these informational systems were to be put into action to address the pandemic and enhance policy making efficiency.

As discussed above, those technologies draw similarities with security/surveillance tools, and present potential to be redirected to monitoring and managing populations. From a human rights perspective, that could violate people's privacy and hurt the proportionality principle. Concerning São Paulo's security landscape, those urban management systems also interplay public and private interests. They produce indexes that commensurate and hence perform social isolation through individual "self-care". Notwithstanding, international experiences show us that privacy violations may lead to discriminatory outcomes. In this sense, Brazilian General Law for Data Protection, yet to be put forth, offers a starting point to conciliate privacy and technology use. Yet some questions remain open, how to guarantee that much needed data will not be used for other purposes than to assist health authorities in providing better care?

How do we disentangle security and public health articulations once the pandemic is over? If, on the one hand, governments do need large swaths of data on patients, urban flows, and sites of agglomeration to track recent outbreaks, understand mobility patterns, and, hopefully, limit contagion in new areas, on the other hand, technology corporations have been found breaking public trust before. Personal data collected for one purpose has been used for commercial and security initiatives without clear consent, and supposedly anonymized data has been found to be easily deanonymized again and again. In this sense, considering that Human Rights provides enough tools to equate social isolation control and preservation of rights by limiting arbitrary and disproportionate practices, it's possible to consider that the privacy versus pandemics' management dilemma is false. Thus, remitting its principles might be particularly damaging to countries that still lack robust legal frameworks on data protection, and which carry a long history of police and military abuse, such as Brazil. In this context, surveillance technologies could be indiscriminately used by security agencies to reduce political freedom. Hence, it is paramount that the implementation of these technologies be evaluated and audited, considering its effects and results in society.

Acknowledgements

This work was supported by the São Paulo Research Foundation (Fapesp) under the Grants No. 2016/24525-3, No. 2019/02612-0, and No. 2013/07923-7; and Capes Research Foundation, Grant No. 88887.368551/2019-00.

7amleh, Access Now, African Declaration on Internet Rights and Freedoms Coalition, AI Now, Algorithm Watch, Alternatif Bilisim, Amnesty International … et al (2020) *Joint statement:States use of digital surveillance technologies to fight pandemic must respect human rights*. Available at: <https://www.amnesty.org/en/documents/pol30/2081/2020/en/>(accessed 29 April 2020).

REFERENCES

Agamben, G. (2020). The state of Exception provoked by an unmotivated emergency.*Positions Politics*. Available at: http://positionswebsite.org/giorgio-agamben-the-state-of-exception-provokedby-an-unmotivated-emergency/ (accessed 29 April 2020).

Amoore, L (2013). *The Politics of Possibility: Risk and Security Beyond Probability*. Durham, ed. Duke University Press.

Ajana, B. (2013). *Governing through Biometrics: The Biopolitics of Identity*. London: Palgrave Macmillan.

Balanço Geral (2020, April 10). *Governo de SP usa dados do GPS do celular para monitorar aglomerações*. https://www.youtube.com/watch?v=lBgv7AEERLk (accessed 29 April 2020).

Bioni, B., Zanatta, R., Monteiro, R.L., Rielli, M. (2020). Privacidade e Pandemia: Recomendações para o uso legítimo de dados no combate à COVID-19. *Data Privacy Brasil*. https://www.dataprivacybr.org/wpcontent/uploads/2020/04/relatorio_privacidade_e_pandemia_final.pdf (accessed 29 April 2020).

Bolsonaro, J. (2020, April 6). *Pronunciamento do presidente da República, Jair Bolsonaro (08/04/2020)*. https://www.youtube.com/watch?v=x04OKkxT2Tc (accessed 29 April 2020).

Carney, T., Bennett, B. (2012). Governance, Rights and Pandemics: Science, Public Health or Individual Rights? In: Selgelid, M.J; Enemark, C. (eds*.*) *Ethics and Security Aspects of Infectious Disease Control: Interdisciplinary Perspectives* (201-217). Oxon: Routledge.

Chagas, G. (2020). Mulher Morde guarda e é detida após abordagem por descumprir decreto em Araraquara*. Portal G1*. Available at: https://g1.globo.com/sp/sao-carlos-regiao/noticia/2020/04/13/mulher-morde-guarda-municipal-ao-ser-detida-por-caminhar-em-pracade-araraquara.ghtml (accessed 29 April 2020).

Dias, T. (2020). Vigiar e Lucrar. *The Intercept Brasil*. Available at: https://theintercept.com/2020/04/13/vivo-venda-localizacao-anonima/ (accessed 29 April 2020).

Dória, J. (2020). O maior desafio da história de São Paulo. *Folha de São Paulo*. Available at: https://www1.folha.uol.com.br/opiniao/2020/04/o-maior-desafio-da-historia-de-sao-paulo.shtml (accessed 29 April 2020).

Diniz, D., Carino, G. (2020) A necropolítica das pandemias. *El País*. available at: https://brasil.elpais.com/opiniao/2020-03-09/a-necropolitica-das-epidemias.html (accessed 29 April 2020).

Elbe, S. (2011). Pandemics on the Radar Screen: Health Security, Infectious Disease and the Medicalisation of Insecurity. *Political Studies*, 59(4), 848-866. https://doi.org/10.1111/j.14679248.2011.00921.x

Espeland, W.N., Stevens, M.L. (1998). Commensuration as a social process. *Annual Review of Sociology, 24,* 313–343. https://doi.org/10.1146/annurev.soc.24.1.313

Foucault, M. (2015). *Ditos e Escritos. Volume IV: Estratégia Poder-Saber*. Rio de Janeiro: Forense Universitária.

Foucault, M. (2007) Security, Territory, Population: Lectures at the Collège de France, 1977-78. Basingstoke, UK: Palgrave Macmillan.

Foucault, M. (1986). *The History of Sexuality: The Care of the Self.* New York: Pantheon Books.

Garvie, C., Bedoya, A,. Frankle, J. (2016). The Perpetual Line-up: Unregulated Police Face Recognition in America. *Centre of Privacy & Technology*, Georgetown University.

Gilbert, G.L. (2012). Electronic Surveillance for Communicable Disease Prevention and Control: Health Protection or a Threat to Privacy and Autonomy? In: Selgelid, M.J; Enemark, C. (eds.) *Ethics and Security Aspects of Infectious Disease Control: Interdisciplinary Perspectives* (127-144). Oxon: Routledge.

Ghirotto, E. (2020). Os bastidores do comitê de emergência montado por SP devido ao coronavírus. *Revista Veja*. https://veja.abril.com.br/brasil/os-bastidores-do-comite-de-emergencia-montado-porsp-devido-ao-coronavirus/ (accessed 29 April 2020).

Goldenfein, J., Green, B., Viljoen, S. (2020). Privacy Versus Health Is a False Trade-Off. *Jacobin*. https://jacobinmag.com/2020/04/privacy-health-surveillance-coronavirus-pandemic-technology (accessed 29 April 2020).

Gomes, H.S. (2020a). Monitoramento de celular para combate a COVID-19 escorrega feio em 5 pontos.*Tilt Uol*. https://www.uol.com.br/tilt/noticias/redacao/2020/04/17/sem-data-para-acabar-e-maismonitoramento-no-brasil-escorrega-em-5-pontos.htm (accessed 29 April 2020).

Gomes, H.S. (2020b). 'Invasão de privacidade', diz advogado que barrou monitoramento na Justiça. *Tilt Uol*. https://www.uol.com.br/tilt/noticias/redacao/2020/04/18/invasao-de-privacidade-dizadvogado-que-barrou-monitoramento-na-justica.htm (accessed 29 April 2020).

Governo do Estado de São Paulo. (2020). *Coronavírus: Casos em São Paulo*. https://www.seade.gov.br/coronavirus/ (accessed 29 April 2020).

Han, B.C. (2020). O Coronavírus de hoje e o mundo de amanhã. *El País* [online]. https://brasil.elpais.com/ideas/2020-03-22/o-coronavirus-de-hoje-e-o-mundo-de-amanha-segundoo-filosofo-byung-chul-han.html (accessed 29 April 2020).

Harvey, D. (2020). Anti-Capitalist Politics in the Time of COVID-19. Jacobin [online]. https://jacobinmag.com/2020/03/david-harvey-coronavirus-political-economy-disruptions? (accessed 29 April 2020).

InLoco (2020). Privacy policy. https://public.inloco.ai/en/privacy-policy#covid (accessed 23 April 2020).

Klauser, F.R. (2017). *Surveillance & Space*. London: Sage.

Klein, N. (2020). Coronavirus Capitalism: Naomi Klein's Case for Transformative Change Amid Coronavirus Pandemic. *Democracy Now*. https://www.democracynow.org/2020/3/19/naomi_klein_coronavirus_capitalism (accessed 29 April 2020).

Latour, B. (2020).La crise sanitaire incite à se préparer à la mutation climatique. *Le Monde*. https://www.lemonde.fr/idees/article/2020/03/25/la-crise-sanitaire-incite-a-se-preparer-a-lamutation-climatique_6034312_3232.html (accessed 29 April 2020).

Lemke T. (2017). *Foucault, Governmentality, and Critique.* London and New York: Routledge.

Lynch, M. (1985) Discipline and the Material Form of Images: An Analysis of Scientific Visibility. *Social Studies of Science*, 15(1), pp. 37–66. doi: 10.1177/030631285015001002.

Lyon, D. (2007). *Surveillance Studies: An Overview*. Cambridge: Polity Press.

Miller, E. (2020) Liberdades Individuais e direitos Fundamentais em Tempos de Quarentena. *DEFENDA PM*. Available at: https://defendapm.org.br/liberdades-individuais-e-direitos-fundamentais-emtempos-de-quarentena/ (accessed 29 April 2020).

Moraes, R. F. (2020). Medidas Legais de Incentivo ao Distanciamento Social: Comparação das Políticas de Governos Estaduais e Prefeituras das Capitais no Brasil. *Nota Técnica n. 16 IPEA* . https://www.ipea.gov.br/portal/images/stories/PDFs/nota_tecnica/200415_dinte_n_16.pdf (accessed 28 April 2020).

Moura, R; Ferraz, L. (2020). Meios de Controle à Pandemia da COVID-19 e a Inviolabilidade da Privacidade. InLoco Report. https://bit.ly/2Ybwxca (accessed 29 April 2020).

Mozorov, E. (2020). The tech 'solutions' for coronavirus take the surveillance state to the next level. *The Guardian*. https://www.theguardian.com/commentisfree/2020/apr/15/tech-coronavirussurveilance-state-digital-disrupt (accessed 29 April 2020).

Mudde, C. (2020). Wartime' coronavirus powers could hurt our democracy – without keeping us safe. *The Guardian*.https://www.theguardian.com/commentisfree/2020/mar/24/wartime-coronaviruspowers-state-of-emergency (accessed 29 April 2020).

Murphy, T., Whitty, N. (2009). Is Human Rights Prepared? Risk, Rights and Public Health Emergencies. *Medical Law Review*, 17, 219-244. https://doi.org/10.1093/medlaw/fwp007

O'Malley, P., Rainford, J., Thompson, A. (2009). Transparency during public health emergencies: from rhetoric to reality. *Bulletin of the World Health Organization*, 87, 614-18.

O'Neil, C. (2016) *Weapons of Math Destruction*. New York: Crown Books.

Pauluze, T., Trindade, L. (2020). João Doria Ameaça Prender quem violar regras de quarentena em São Paulo. *Folha de São Paulo*. https://www1.folha.uol.com.br/cotidiano/2020/04/doria-diz-na-televisaoque-mandara-prender-quem-se-aglomerar-nas-ruas.shtml (accessed 29 April 2020).

Peron, A., Alvarez, M.C. (2019). Governing the City: The Detecta Surveillance System in São Paulo and the Role of Private Vigilantism in the Public Security. *Sciences et actions sociales*, 12, p. 1-36.

Porter, T. M. (1998.) *Trust in numbers: the pursuit of objectivity in science and public life.* Princeton, N.J: Princeton Univ. Press.

Prescott, E.M. (2007). The politics of disease: governance and emerging infections. *Global Health*, 1(1), p. 1-8.

Purnell, K. (2020) The Body Politics of COVID-19. *The Disorder of Things*. Available at: https://thedisorderofthings.com/2020/04/06/the-body-politics-of-COVID-19/ (accessed 29 April 2020).

Queiroz, L., Ferraz, A., Melo, J. L., Barboza, G., Urbanski, A., Nicolau, A., Oliva, Sergio, Nakaya, H. (2020, March 26). Large-scale assessment of human mobility during COVID-19 outbreak. https://doi.org/10.31219/osf.io/nqxrd

R7 (2020) Isolamento é mais respeitado na periferia de São Paulo, diz estudo. *R7*, Available at:

https://noticias.r7.com/sao-paulo/isolamento-e-mais-respeitado-na-periferia-de-sao-paulo-dizestudo-03042020?fbclid=IwAR0DRVQmXPAOCTbbZMh5PRLPjRD69oPUsaaTUyeVVG9uJInhoLJKGxEdRM (accessed 29 April 2020).

Sanford, S., Polzer, J., McDonough, P. (2016). Preparedness as a technology of (in)security: Pandemic influenza planning and the global biopolitics of emerging infectious disease. *Social Theory Health*, 14, p. 18–43. https://doi.org/10.1057/sth.2015.8.

Sarasin, P. (2020). Understanding the Coronavirus Pandemic with Foucault? Foucaultblog. DOI: 10.13095/uzh.fsw.fb.254

Sotiris, P. (2020) Against Agamben: Is a Democratic Biopolitics Possible? *Critical Legal Thinking*. Available at: https://criticallegalthinking.com/2020/03/14/against-agamben-is-a-democraticbiopolitics-possible/(accessed 29 April 2020).

Tunes, S. (2020) Inteligência artificial contra a COVID-19. *FAPESP*, Available at: https://revistapesquisa.fapesp.br/2020/04/14/inteligencia-artificial-contra-a-COVID-19/ (accessed 29 April 2020).

UNHR. (2020). COVID-19: Governments must promote and protect access to and free flow of information during pandemic – International experts. https://www.ohchr.org/EN/NewsEvents/Pages/DisplayNews.aspx?NewsID=25729&LangID=Eccess (accessed 29 April 2020).

Ventura, D (2016). From Ebola to Zika: international emergencies and the securitization of global health. *Cad. Saúde Pública*, 32(4), p. 1-32. https://doi.org/10.1590/0102-311X00033316

World Health Organization. (2020a). *Report of the WHO-China Joint Mission on Coronavirus Disease 2019 (COVID-19)*. https://www.who.int/docs/default-source/coronaviruse/who-china-joint-missionon-COVID-19-final-report.pdf (accessed 29 April 2020).

World Health Organization. (2020b). *WHO Emergencies Press Conference on Coronavirus Disease outbreak – 20 March*. https://www.who.int/emergencies/diseases/novel-coronavirus-2019/mediaresources/press-briefings (accessed 29 April 2020).

World Health Organization. (2005 [2016]). International Health Regulations. 3rd ed. https://www.who.int/ihr/publications/9789241580496/en/ (accessed 28 April 2020).

Wright, R. (2020). Coronavirus and the Future of Surveillance: Democracies Must Offer an Alternative to Authoritarian Solutions. *Foreign Affairs* [online]. https://www.foreignaffairs.com/articles/2020-0406/coronavirus-and-future-surveillance (accessed 29 April 2020).

Zizek, S. (2020). Zizek vê o poder subversivo do Coronavírus. *Outras Palavras*. https://outraspalavras.net/crise-civilizatoria/zizek-ve-o-poder-subversivo-do-coronavirus/ (accessed 29 April 2020).

Zuboff, S. (2019). *The Age of Surveillance Capitalism: The fight for a Human Future at the New Frontier of Power*. London: Profile Books.

4. Personality Differences And COVID-19: Are Extroversion and Conscientiousness Personality Traits Associated with Engagement with Containment Measures?[1]

Lucas de F. Carvalho,[1] Giselle Pianowski,[1] André P. Gonçalves[1]

ABSTRACT

Introduction: In December 2019, an outbreak of the novel coronavirus, the coronavirus disease 2019 (COVID-19) probably occurred in Wuhan, China. By March 2020, the World Health Organization (WHO) had declared a pandemic. Containment measures such as social distancing and hand hygiene were recommended. In this study, we start from the hypothesis that engaging with containment measures in a pandemic situation should be more comfortable for some people than for other people. Thus, individual differences should be associated with engagement with containment measures. **Objective:** To investigate the extent two personality traits, extroversion and conscientiousness, are associated with engagement with two containment measures (social distancing and handwashing). **Methods:** The sample consisted of 715 Brazilian adults aged 18-78 years, who answered the Big Five Inventory 2 Short (BFI-2-S) and factors from the Dimensional Clinical Personality Inventory 2 (IDCP-2) **Results:** Higher scores for extroversion were associated with lower means for social distancing ($p < 0.001$) and higher scores for conscientiousness were associated with higher means for social distancing and handwashing ($p < 0.05$). **Conclusion:** The findings indicate the importance of acknowledging extroversion and conscientiousness traits as relevant to people's engagement with the measures recommended for COVID-19 containment.

INTRODUCTION

In December 2019, cases of life-threatening pneumonia were reported in Wuhan, China, catching the attention of the international audience. The number of reported cases increased rapidly in Wuhan and other Chinese cities. Cases were also diagnosed in other parts of the world. The source of the outbreak of this novel coronavirus, the coronavirus disease 2019 (COVID-19), is believed to be related to live animal markets selling wild and domestic animals in proximity to large cities with high levels of human density. On January 30, 2020, the World Health Organization (WHO) declared that COVID-19 constituted a Public Health Emergency of International Concern. By March 19, 2020, within a matter of 3 months since the beginning of the outbreak and about one week after the WHO had officially declared a pandemic, more than 240,000 confirmed cases of COVID 19 had been announced and almost 10,000 deaths had been registered, mostly in Italy and China. Outside of

[1] 1 Universidade São Francisco, Campinas, SP, Brazil.
Suggested citation: Carvalho LF, Pianowski G, Gonçalvez AP. Personality differences and COVID-19: are extroversion and conscientiousness personality traits associated with engagement with containment measures? Trends Psychiatry Psychother. 2020;00(0):000-000.
Http://dx.doi.org/10.1590/2237-6089-2020-0029

these, 176 countries had reported more than 130,000 cases. Unfortunately, as we write this paper, the COVID-19 emergency is evolving rapidly.[1-3]Similar to other coronaviruses (e.g., MERS-COV),[4] the negative impact of COVID-19 and its consequences are vast, including negative outcomes in mental health, with increased depressive and anxiety symptoms, stress disorders, insomnia, anger, and fear.[5-10] Pandemics are known to provoke social disruptions.[1,2] Several publications warned of the need for containment measures,[11-15] Such social distancing [16] and hand hygiene. Although lacking empirical evidence, previous publications have argued that habits and behavioural trends have impacts on containment measures,[17,18] stressing that individual behaviour is crucial to controlling the spread of COVID-19.Li et al.[19] conducted a study in China (n = 4,607)

investigating the impact of people's behaviour on COVID-19 containment measures. The authors focused on social participation, precautionary behaviour, and perceived severity, among other behaviours. Findings indicated that people are tending to avoid social events since the outbreak of COVID-19, to exhibit precautionary behaviours such as wearing a facemask and washing hands, and to perceive the impacts of COVID-19 as highly negative (e.g., high mortality and negative influence on social order and economics). We can therefore observe some initial results indicating that people are inclined to adhere to containment measures in extreme situations.

A necessary further step is to investigate the role of individual differences in the propensity to adhere to containment measures, which is the scope of our study. In this study, we start from the assumption that engaging with containment measures in a pandemic situation should be easier for some people than others. Individual differences are expected to be associated with the disposition to engage in these measures. We aimed to investigate associations between two personality traits, extroversion and conscientiousness, and engagement with two containment measures (social distancing and handwashing). Therefore, we used the Five-Factor Model (FFM) as the framework for personality traits, since it is the model closest to the scientific consensus.[20] The FFM proposes that personality is best described in five broad traits: extroversion (or extraversion), agreeableness, conscientiousness, neuroticism, and openness. A personality trait is a stable psychological characteristic that contributes to determining how people experience the world as well as to the impact of these experiences.[21]

Our focus is on the extroversion trait, since people who score high for this trait are outgoing and generally prone to closeness and social contact; and on conscientiousness, since people who score high for this trait are organized, meticulous, and tend to respect norms and social rules. We hypothesize that extroverted people are less likely to engage with the COVID-19 pandemic containment measures than highly conscientious people.

METHODS

This is a cross-sectional study, nested within a larger mental health project in Brazil, with research ethics committee approval (CAAE: 09112419.7.0000.5514). All participants signed an informed consent form before participating.

Participants

The study sample consisted of 715 Brazilian adults, recruited by convenience between March 18 and 19 of 2020. The sole eligibility criterion was age ≥ 18 years.

Measures
Questionnaire On COVID-19-Related Behaviour

We developed a questionnaire to measure general information and behaviour-related to the COVID-19 pandemic situation. Focusing on our objective, we selected two variables associated with containment measures, specifically, social distancing and handwashing behaviours. We presented participants with "yes or no" response format questions, "Do you think it is necessary to avoid approaching people as much as possible until the coronavirus situation is controlled?" and "Do you think it is necessary to wash your hands and/or use alcohol gel as many times a day as possible until the coronavirus situation is controlled?".

Big Five Inventory-2 Short (BFI-2-S)[22]

The BFI-2-S is a self-report measure of personality traits based on the FFM, evaluating extroversion, agreeableness, conscientiousness, neuroticism, and openness. This measure is composed of 30 items that are answered on a 5-point Likert scale. Psychometric investigations of the BFI-2-S in Brazil have not yet been published, although the Ayrton Senna Institute has published documents regarding the previous version of the BFI-2-S.[23] Prior evidence suggests the BFI-2-S has good psychometric properties and indicates strong correlations between the BFI-2 and the BFI.[22]

Dimensional Clinical Personality Inventory 2 (IDCP-2)[24]

The IDCP-2 was developed in Brazil and is a self-report measure that assesses pathological traits, i.e., extreme maladaptive variants of personality traits. It is composed of 206 items answered on a 4-point Likert scale. The IDCP-2 encompasses 47 factors. In this study, we administered four factors, two related to extroversion, Need for attention and Intimacy avoidance (negatively related), and two related to conscientiousness, Thoroughness and Concern with details. Studies support the psychometric properties of this measure, including studies focused on the factors we administered (e.g., Carvalho et al.[25,26]).

PROCEDURE

After approval by the São Francisco University research ethics committee, data collection was performed online via Google Forms. We shared the research link on the social media website Facebook and via the WhatsApp app, inviting individuals to participate and relying on the snowball strategy to reach a larger number of participants. For both Extroversion and Conscientiousness dimensions, we administered measures on healthy and maladaptive variant levels of personality, using the BFI-2-S and IDCP-2 respectively; and administered a questionnaire focusing on COVID19-related behaviour.

Data Analysis

We divided participants into four groups: None = people who think that containment measures are not important (n = 6); Social distancing = people who think social distancing is important, but handwashing is not (n = 17); Handwashing = people who think handwashing is important, but social distancing is not (n = 23); and All = people who think that all containment measures are important (n = 669). We conducted analysis of variance (ANOVA) with a post hoc test (Tukey method) to compare groups by personality measures. We applied the bootstrapping procedure because the groups' sizes varied widely. We used 0.05 as the significance level, and partial eta squared was used as an indicator of effect size. We performed the analysis using SPSS version 23.

RESULTS

The descriptive statistics for basic sociodemographic data and specific information related to COVID-19. The total number of participants was 715 adults, mostly female (77.3%), single (52.2%), Caucasian (69.5%), and holding post-graduate degrees (40%).All pre-existing medical conditions related to increased risk of death from COVID-19 were reported by at least one participant. Two participants from the Southwest region reported being positive for COVID-19, and 25 (14 from the Southwest, six from the Mid-west, and five from the Northeast) reported knowing someone positive for COVID-19.The results of the ANOVA, show a trend towards lower extroversion scores in the social distance group (p < 0.001), indicating that people who are more concerned with social distance tend to be less extroverted. We also observe a trend to lower conscientiousness scores for the groups that considered neither of the containment measures were essential in the current pandemic situation (p = 0.011). When compared to extroversion, we observe higher means for conscientiousness in the groups of people who reported adhering to both or one of the containment measures. Factors related to maladaptive variants of personality traits (i.e., Need for attention [p = 0.003], Intimacy avoidance [p = 0.010], Concern with details [p < 0.016], and Thoroughness [p = 0.018]) presented larger group differences in comparison to factors related to healthy personality traits.

DISCUSSION

We are living with a pandemic caused by a coronavirus that spreads the COVID-19. Containment measures have been recommended,[11-15]including social distancing and handwashing. However, several factors can increase or decrease people's engagement with these measures. We aimed to investigate to what extent two personality traits, extroversion and conscientiousness, are associated with engagement with two containment measures (social distancing and handwashing). To achieve this, we collected data from a Brazilian sample. The findings corroborate our hypothesis, indicating that extroverted functioning seems to lack engagement with the COVID-19 containment measures. At the same time, a conscientiousness pattern is more cautious in following all the recommendations. Although preliminary, these findings add empirical data to the critical debate on individual behavioural responsibility in co-operating with containment measures to prevent even worse outcomes from this pandemic.[17,18]

The lower scores for extroversion observed in the social distancing group, indicate the challenging task of reducing the social proximity typical of extroverted people, which seemed not to greatly impact their readiness to engage with hand hygiene recommendations. The difficulty in reducing social proximity is coherent with the typical characteristics of extroversion.[20,22] Moreover, the factors evaluating maladaptive variations of extroversion,[21] Need for attention and (negatively) Intimacy avoidance, highlighted the trend of extroverted people to avoid social distancing.

These results suggest that pathological levels may bring even more difficulty with engagement with pandemic containment measures.

In a manner that differs from what was observed for the extroversion trait, low conscientiousness scores were presented by people reporting that they did not engage with any of the containment measures. We can hypothesize that an increase in conscientiousness scores is associated with a decrease in the propensity to break safety recommendations for containment of the pandemic. Moreover, engaging with social distancing does not seems to be a problem for people who score high for this trait. These trends are consistent with the conceptualization of the conscientiousness trait.[20,22]

The Concern with details and Thoroughness factors corroborated this trend, even though they relate to maladaptive variations of conscientiousness. Our results comprise initial evidence on the association between personality traits and engagement with measures for containment of the COVID-19 pandemic. People who score high for extroversion are probably experiencing more difficulty in following the global recommendations to slow down the spread of the COVID-19, especially the social distancing containment measures. In contrast, people who score high for conscientiousness are more likely to find it easy to adhere to the proposed containment measures. The impact of these different experiences in mental health is yet to be known. However, our findings indicate the importance of acknowledging extroversion and conscientiousness traits as relevant to people's engagement with the recommended actions.

They are an alert to the need for strategies that promote adherence to containment measures by people high in extroversion, since their difficulty in maintaining social distance can put them at a higher risk of contamination and of acting as transmission vectors. Our results provide data for psychological assessment and intervention during the COVID-19 pandemic. The methodological limitations of our study must be acknowledged. First, this is a cross-sectional study with a restricted convenience sample, and potential uncontrolled confounding variables, which introduce biases to the findings. Second, we only administered self-report scales and did not employ a multimethod approach. Third, we focused on two containment measures and not on all possible measures recommended in the present pandemic situation.

We hope our findings can contribute to dealing with this gruelling time for humanity. Many efforts to minimize the damage of the COVID-19 pandemic are underway. We can only agree with the closing words of Wang et al.[3]: "Every effort should be given to understand and control the disease, and the time to act is now."

REFERENCES

1. Higemura J, Nakamoto K, Ursano, R.J. (2009). Responses to the outbreak of novel influenza A (H1N1) in Japan: risk communication and shimaguni konjo. Am J Disaster Med. 2009;4:133-4.
2. Shigemura, J., Tanigawa, T., Saito, I., Nomura, S. (2012). Psychological distress in workers at the Fukushima nuclear power plants. JAMA. 2012;308:667-9.
3. Wang C, Horby PW, Hayden FG, Gao GF. A novel coronavirus outbreak of global health concern. Lancet. 2020;395:470-3.
4. Kim, J.S., Choi, J.S..(2016). Factors influencing emergency nurses' burnout during an outbreak of Middle East respiratory syndrome coronavirus in Korea. Asian Nurs Res. 2016;10:295-9.
5. Bao, Y., Sun, Y., Meng, S., Shi, J., Lu, L. (2019) COVID-19 epidemic: address mental health care to empower society. Lancet. 2020;395:e37-8.
6. Duan, L, Zhu, G. (2020).Psychological interventions for people affected by the COVID-19 epidemic. Lancet Psychiatry. 2020;7:300-2.
7. Kang, L, Li Y, Hu, S, Chen, M., Yang, C., Yang, B.X., et al. (2020). The mental health of medical workers in Wuhan, China dealing with the 2019 novel coronavirus. Lancet Psychiatry. 2020;7:e14.
8. Shigemura, J., Ursano, R.J., Morganstein, J.C., Kurosawa, M., Benedek, D.M. (2020). Public responses to the novel 2019 coronavirus (2019-nCoV) in Japan: mental health consequences and target populations. Psychiatry Clin Neurosci. 2020;74:281-2.

9. Yang, Y, Li, W., Zhang, Q, Zhang, L., Cheung, T., Xiang, Y.T. (2020). Mental health services for older adults in China during the COVID-19 outbreak. Lancet Psychiatry. 2020;7:e19.

10. Wang G, Zhang Y, Zhao J, Zhang J, Jiang F. Mitigate the effects of home confinement on children during the COVID-19 outbreak. Lancet. 2020;395:45-7.

11. Kickbusch, I, Leung, G. (2020). Response to the emerging novel coronavirus outbreak. BMJ. 2020;368:m406.

12. Mahase E. China coronavirus: WHO declares international emergency as death toll exceeds 200. BMJ. 2020;368:m408.

13. Wilder-Smith A, Chiew C.J., Lee, V.J. (2020). Can we contain the COVID-19 outbreak with the same measures as for SARS? Lancet Infect Dis. 3099(20)30129-8. [Epub ahead of print]

14. Wilder-Smith A, Freedman, D.O. (2020).Isolation, quarantine, social distancing and community containment: pivotal role for old-style public health measures in the novel coronavirus (2019-nCoV) outbreak. J Travel Med. 2020;13:23-7.

15. Xiang, Y.T, Zhao, Y.J., Liu, Z.H., Li, X.H., Zhao, N., Cheung, T., et al. (2020). The COVID-19 outbreak and psychiatric hospitals in China: managing challenges through mental health service reform. Int J Biol Sci. 2020;16:1741-4.

16. World Health Organization. "COVID-19". WHO. 2020 [cited 25 March 2020]. http:// https://www.who.int/docs/default-source/ coronaviruse/transcripts/who-audio-emergencies-coronaviruspress-conference-full-20mar2020.pdf

17. Lunn, P., Belton, C., Lavin, C., McGowan, F., Timmons, S., Robertson, D. (2020). Using behavioural science to help fight the coronavirus. ESRI. 2020. [cited 25 March 2020]. https://www.esri.ie/system/files/ publications/WP656.pdf

18. Anderson, R.M., Heesterbeek, H., Klinkenberg, D., Hollingsworth, T.D. (2020). How will country-based mitigation measures influence the course of the COVID-19 epidemic?. Lancet. 2020;395:931-4.

19. Li, JB, Yang, A., Dou, K., Wang, L.X., Zhang, M.C., Lin, X., (2020). Chinese public's knowledge, perceived severity, and perceived controllability of the COVID-19 and their associations with emotional and behavioural reactions, social participation, and precautionary behaviour: a national survey. PsyArXiv. 2020. [cited 25 March 2020]. https:// doi.org/10.31234/osf.io/5tmsh

20. Saulsman, L.M., Page, A.C. (2004). The five-factor model and personality disorder empirical literature: a meta-analytic review. Clin Psychol Rev. 2004;23:1055-85.

21. Allik. J, Realo, A., McCrae, R.R., Universality of the five-factor model of personality.

22. Soto, C.J., John. O.P. (2017).The next Big Five Inventory (BFI-2): developing and assessing a hierarchical model with 15 facets to enhance bandwidth, fidelity, and predictive power. J Pers Soc Psychol. 2017;1:113-7.

23. Santos D, Primi R. Desenvolvimento socioemocional e aprendizado escolar: uma proposta de mensuração para apoiar políticas públicas. Relatório sobre resultados 929reliminaries do projeto de medição de competências socioemocionais no Rio de Janeiro. São Paulo: OCDE, SEEDUC, Instituto Ayrton Senna; 2014.

24. Carvalho, L.F., Primi, R. (2020).Technical manual of the Dimensional Clinical Personality Inventory 2 (IDCP-2) and Dimensional Clinical Personality Inventory screening version (IDCP-triagem). São Paulo: Pearson. Forthcoming 2020.

25. Carvalho, L.F, Sette, C.P., Capitão, C.G., (2014). Primi R. Propriedades psicométricas da versão revisada da dimensão necessidade de atenção do inventário dimensional clínico da personalidade. Temas Psicol. 2014;22:147:60.

26. Carvalho, L.D., Souza, B.D., (2014).Primi R. Psychometric properties of the revised conscientiousness dimension of Inventário Dimensional Clínico da Personalidade (IDCP). Trends Psychiatry Psychother. 2014;36:23-31.

5. Between Behavioural and Psychosocial Factors Among Brazilians Quarantined Due To COVID-19

Alberto Filgueiras[1]
Universidade do Estado do Rio de Janeiro (UERJ)

Matthew Stults-Kolehmainen
Yale University - Yale New Haven Hospital (YNHH)

ABSTRACT

Background: During quarantine, both physical and mental health are a concern. To the same extent that physicians are a scarce resource during this crisis, psychiatrists and psychologists are also limited in number. In order to help practitioners and public managers to decide where to put their mental health resources, the present research investigated the relationship between stress, depression and state anxiety levels with sociodemographic and behavioural variables. **Methods:** Data were collected in Brazil between March 18 and 22, 2020 in 1,468 volunteers during quarantine. Participants with history or current mental health illnesses were excluded leaving 1,460 individuals in the final sample.

The online assessment included instruments for psychological stress, depression and state anxiety; whereas, a sociodemographic and behavioural questionnaire with 15 items was used to assess other factors. A multiple linear regression was performed for each psychological dimension so a hierarchy of independent variables could be developed.

Findings: Stress, depression and state anxiety levels were all predicted by gender (women higher than men), quality of nutrition, attendance in tele-psychotherapy, exercise frequency, presence of elderly persons in quarantine with the person, obligation to work outside, level of education (more educated, lesser risk for mental illness) and age (younger age, greater risk). Having a perceived risk factor for COVID-19 predicted depression and state anxiety, but not stress. Finally, the presence of children in quarantine with the participant was a protective factor for depression. **Interpretation:** Even though this research is limited by its cross-sectional design, it is possible to infer that mental health varies by demographic attributes, obligations and health behaviours. Those who report higher distress must work outside during quarantine, live with an elderly person and carry a risk factor for COVID-19, among other factors. Identifying those who are most vulnerable would help to prioritize those who may need the greatest psychological aid and assist public health practitioners in developing support strategies.

---

[1] For Supplementary chart table and data contact: julio.croda@fiocruz.br

INTRODUCTION

Mental health can be defined as an internal state of well-being, balance and cognitive and coping abilities used in harmony with the universal values of society which allows individuals to work, cope and solve problems in everyday tasks [1,2]. According to the World Health Organization (WHO), 14% of the global burden of disease can be attributed to mental health disorders [3, 4]. Consequently, the WHO developed the Mental Health Gap Action Programme (mhGAP), which is a project that aims to raise awareness about the deficit between physical and mental health. Moreover, the programme aims to provide evidence-based practices and guidelines to help mental health practitioners in their everyday work [4]. Of particular emphasis in this report is the urgent need to "scale up" mental health interventions, which requires acute knowledge of situational factors, the needs of population and identifying those most at risk.

Due to the outbreak of the Corona Virus Disease 2019 (COVID-19), quarantine was adopted as a strategy to avoid its spread in several countries in the first quarter of 2020 [5, 6]. Although it became clear that public policies to prohibit people from going outside their homes were necessary [6], physicians, nurses, physical therapists and other healthcare providers remained working to protect the physical health of COVID-19 (SARS-CoV-2) and other inpatients [7]. However, other members of the workforce, such as supermarket employees, public servants and police, are also on the streets to maintain a functioning society, exposing them to a greater risk of contracting COVID-19 than those in quarantine [5-8].

Social isolation poses an additional big challenge to workers both inside and outside of the home [7-11]. Some research has been conducted in quarantined samples [9]; however, the current condition is one of the few times when a large amount of the global population has been confined to their own homes. Therefore, those in quarantine are facing stressful living conditions confronted without any previous training and little time for preparations [7]. For example, in 2016 Jeong, Yim, Song and colleagues investigated anxiety and anger in participants confined for two weeks due to Middle East Respiratory Syndrome (MERS). The results showed that both psychological variables were higher during confinement. Anxiety measured during confinement had a prevalence of 7.6% and 3.0% out of isolation; whereas, anger was reported among 16.6% of confined participants decreasing to 6.4% six months after the end of isolation [12]. This is the only Longitudinal quantitative study of psychological symptoms in participants obliged to social isolation thus far in the literature [10].

However, similar studies with cross-sectional sampling have been conducted to assess different psychological conditions and states among participants in quarantine. Hawryluck, Gold, Robinson et al. collected post-traumatic stress and depression symptom-like data from 129 participants supposedly exposed to SARS and prohibited to leave quarantine for an average of ten days. Results showed a greater amount of symptoms when compared to normative data [13]. Other papers presented similar results for: stress [12-17], depression [12, 16], anxiety [12, 13] and hopelessness [16]. Although the present paper does no compare its results to normative data due to the lack of norms in some of the measures, it is important to highlight the need to understand the role of behavioural and psychosocial factors to predict mental health in people going through confinement and social isolation. Even though people in quarantined conditions seem to have higher levels of stress, anxiety and depression-like symptoms [10], mental health practitioners are not a limitless resource.

In fact, the current availability of resources may be only a small fraction of what is needed at the peak of a crisis. Consequently, public policies and strategies should be adopted to appropriately match psychology and psychiatry professionals with those most vulnerable. Regarding mental health, or more specifically distress, anxiety and depression, some demographics (e.g., gender [18-20], age [21], education, number of people in confinement with the person [11], other variables [15, 22]) and behavioural (balanced nutrition [23], regular exercise [24, 25], psychotherapy [26], and telepsychology [27, 28]) outcomes seem to be associated with or directly reduce or increase its levels. However, the vast majority of this evidence was gathered with people who were not in confinement at home. Altogether, this evidence leads to the question: which demographic and behavioural variables predict stress, anxiety and depression levels among people in quarantine?

METHOD

Participants

Participants of the present study were 1,468 volunteers in different levels of government-mandated confinement at home. Inclusion criteria were adults (two volunteers were not included due to this criterion), Brazilian Portuguese speakers who were in quarantine or who lived with another person in quarantine for at least 3 days due to COVID-19 outbreak. Included participants signed a consent form (two individuals refused and were not included). The exclusion criteria were volunteers under psychiatric treatment or any history of previous treatment (four volunteers were excluded based on these criteria) which lead to the final number of 1,460 participants.

Procedure

The project of the present research was approved by the institution's Ethics Committee before data collection. All procedures follow the Brazilian Legislation (i.e., Resolution #196/96 of the Brazilian National Health Council [29]) and the Declaration of Helsinki.

After the approval, a website in Google Forms presented the following instruments in the same order for all participants: (i) Consent form, (ii) stress measure (Perceived Stress Scale-10), (iii) depression measure (Filgueiras Depression Inventory), state anxiety measure (State and Trait Anxiety Inventory: state subscale), (iv) sociodemographic information. After beginning, no answer could be left blank, so the entire form had to be filled in order to complete and send it to the server. The recruitment for volunteers occurred through the first author's and his laboratory's social media, which consequently lead to a convenience sample. Data collection happened between March 18th and March 22nd of 2020, from 3 to 7 days after the COVID-19 quarantine Lockdown declared by the Brazilian States Governors on National Television. The spreadsheet generated by the Google Drive was saved in Microsoft Excel format for further analysis.

Instruments

Four instruments were adopted: three psychometric assessment measures and one sociodemographic questionnaire.

The characteristics of those instruments are presented below:

Perceived Stress Scale-10 items version (PSS-10)[30]:

The PSS-10 is a 10-item self-reporting scale with questions regarding the frequency which one perceives stressful variables in daily activities in the last month. The participant answers to those questions in a 5-point Likert-type scale that ranges from "0-never" to "4-very often". Sample of questions are: "In the last month, how often have you been able to control irritations in your life?" and "In the last month, how often have you felt that you were unable to control the important things in your life?". Items 4, 5, 7 and 8 are reverse-scored before summing the 10 items to generate the total score.

Filgueiras Depression Inventory (FDI)[31]:

The FDI is a 20-item inventory of words that are related to depression-like symptoms according to the DSM-V. The participant associates each one of these twenty words to his own feelings in the last fortnight through a Likert-type scale of six categories of endorsement ranging from "0-not related to me at all" to "5-totally related to me". Sample of the 20-item words list are: "Melancholy", "Sadness", "Disgust", "Displeasure" and "Death". The total score is simply the sum of all items.

The Spielberg State and Trait Anxiety Inventory – State Subscale (SSTAI)[32]:

The SSTAI is one in a set of two subscales developed to assess two dimensions of anxiety: trait and state. The trait anxiety refers to personality characteristics of an individual that facilitates the occurrence of anxiety-like symptoms and behaviours. On the other hand, state anxiety comprises how one feels in the moment the inventory is completed rather than enduring aspects of personality. The state anxiety subscale has a 20-item structure that is answered in a 4category Likert scale. Specifically, the SSTAI, responses range from "1-not at all" to "4-very much so". Sample of items are: "I feel calm", "I feel nervous" and "I am presently worrying over possible misfortunes". Items 1, 2, 5, 8, 10, 11, 15, 16, 19 and 20 are reverse-scored before summing the answers of all items to provide the total score.

Sociodemographic questionnaire:

Due to potential social and demographic characteristics found in the literature linked to stress, anxiety and depression among diverse samples, including recent studies about COVID-19 [7-12]. A simple "yes" or "no" dichotomous response was provided for the following questions: "Is an elderly person in quarantine with you?", "Are children in quarantine with you?" and "Do you have any risk factors for COVID19?". A question about quarantine status at home was asked with two possible responses: either "Yes (I am not going outside)" or "No (I do go outside, even if rarely)". A 3-category response("yes", "sometimes" and "no") was used for two questions: "Does your job require you to go outside?" and "Have you used telemedicine services yet?". Another three questions provided the participant a 3-category response options, although they were presented differently. The item called "Nutrition" offered the following options: "Balanced meals every time", "Balanced meals sometimes" and "Meals that are not balanced". The item called "Exercise" provided these possible responses: "At least 4 times a week", "Between 1 and 3 times a week" and "No exercise". The question "Do you attend psychotherapy (online)?" had these options for responding: "Regularly", "Only for emergencies" and "No psychotherapy at all". Gender was also collected with three possible categories: "men", "women" and "other". Education had five response levels: "Elementary school", "High school", "Bachelor's degree", "Master's degree" and "Doctoral degree". Finally, there were four items of the sociodemographic questionnaire that required a numeric response: "Age", "Total number of members in the nuclear family" (not necessarily with the participant at home), "Number of family members in quarantine with you" and "Number of days in quarantine".

Data Analysis

Descriptive statistics for stress, anxiety and depression levels were calculated for each categorical variable: mean and standard deviation (S.D.). Continuous demographic variables (i.e., age, total number of members in the nuclear family, number of family members in quarantine with you and number of days in quarantine) and total scores of psychometric measures were also described in terms of average and S.D. Null-hypothesis tests were performed to compare means of PSS-10, FDI and SSTAI for different categories in demographic variables. Specifically, for independent variables with two categories the t-test was used and effect-size was measured by Cohen's d; for independent variables with more than two categories, a one-way ANOVA was chosen to compare groups and Cohen's f was used for effect-size. Significant differences were considered when the $p$value was below 0.05; whereas effect-size interpretation followed the cut-offs from Cohen [33]: for Cohen's d, the values indicate a small effect-size between 0.20 and 0.50, between 0.50 and 0.80 is interpreted as a moderate size and above 0.80 depicts a large effect-size; for Cohen's f, the values are considered a small effect-size between 0.10 and 0.25, between 0.25 and 0.40 is understand as a moderate size and above 0.40 entails a large effect-size.

Three multiple linear regressions were performed to identify which sociodemographic and behavioural variables predict stress, state anxiety and depression independently. The stepwise method was adopted to retain variables if they contributed significantly to predict the dependent variable (i.e., improve the statistical linearity of the function in comparison to the constant). Inclusion and exclusion of variables was based on t-test p-values; whereas, the level of contribution of the sociodemographic or behavioural variables was assessed through Beta. Because most of variables used in the regression were categorical, Positive Beta does not necessarily mean positive association and *vice-versa*; it applies only when variables were continuous. The coefficient of determination (r^2) was also calculated to reveal the amount of variance explained by the independent variables. Acceptable values of r^2 for social sciences and clinical studies with humans may vary between 0.20 and 0.40, although the closer to 1.0, the better [34]. Three dispersion graphs with the line of tendency were plotted with the total score of PSS-10, FDI and SSTAI in the axis y and the results of the linear function in the axis x.

RESULTS

Participants reported an average of 4.09 (S.D. = 0.97) days in quarantine. The sample's mean for age was 32.9 (S.D. = 12.1), number of members in the nuclear family was 3.9 (S.D. = 3.3) and for family members in quarantine with the person was 3.1 (S.D. = 1.7). PSS-10, FDI and SSTAI descriptive statistics stratified for each categorical independent variable, along with null-hypothesis tests.

Two information are important to depict: (i) even though "other" was an option for gender, it was not checked in this data collection, (ii)Five factors had effect sizes above 0.2 for all 3 indicators of mental health: gender, nutrition, exercise frequency, being quarantined with an elder and having perceived risk factors for COVID-19. Multiple Linear regression revealed that several variables were predicted mental health variables. Specifically, stress was predicted by gender, nutrition, quarantine along with an elderly person, exercise frequency, level of education, a job requirement to work outside, the use of tele-psychotherapy and age, in order by strength of standardized betas. The coefficient of determination (r^2) was 0.23.

The protective factors based on the strength of standardized betas were: being man, having a balanced diet, attending to tele-psychotherapy (or telepsychological counselling), having children at home during quarantine and higher levels of education. On the opposite side, risk factors for mental illness during quarantine were being a woman, living with elders, job requirement to go outside, caring any risk factor for COVID-19 and being younger. In terms of depression, gender, nutrition, presence of children in quarantine with the participant, use of tele-psychotherapy, whether the person carries a perceived risk factor for COVID-19, exercise frequency, level of education, presence of an elderly person in quarantine with the participant, the need to go outside the home due to job commitments and age, respectively. The coefficient of determination (r^2) for the depression model was 0.24. Finally, state anxiety was significantly linked to the same variables of Depression with exception of the presence of children or elderly in quarantine with the participant. The coefficient of determination (r^2) for the SSTAI model was 0.21.

DISCUSSION

The current study helps to identify factors associated with poorer mental health among people in quarantine. First, women scored significantly higher for stress, depression and state anxiety levels when compared to men. Indeed, there is ample evidence that gender and gender have a relationship with mental health [18-20]. Such a finding may suggest that psychological care be tailored by gender. The second most relevant variable based on the strength of standardized betas to predict all three psychological variables was nutrition. A balanced diet and regular feeding habits are linked to better mental health indices [23]. Although exercise appeared as an important factor to predict stress, depression and state anxiety levels [24], it was not as relevant according to betas as other sociodemographic and behavioural variables, such as characteristics of people in quarantine or the use of telepsychology. Evidence from epidemiological research on COVID-19 suggests that elderly individuals are more susceptible to the virus than other age groups [6, 11]. The findings depicted here reveal that stress and depression levels are associated with the presence of older people in quarantine with participants. In fact, this variable had the third strongest beta in the PSS-10 multiple regression model.

Probably two main factors are to be considered: leaving an elder at home and coming back later is stressful due to the risk of contagion, so, people who lives with elders tend to feel more stressed because they can contaminate those who have greater risk of health problems due to COVID-19 [6]. In addition, taking care of elderly implicates more time dedicated to cleaning and organizing the house to avoid contamination [11]. Also, regarding age-related variables, the presence of children in quarantine with volunteers was, interestingly, a protective whether than a depressive factor.

People who had children among them in confinement reported less depression levels than those without children. It is a surprising finding, since it is a stressful condition to take care of children in quarantine [22]; however, in this sense, perhaps parents perceive that the condition of their offspring is safer so it might decrease worry or increase happiness. Age itself is also a demographic variable that predicts psychological outcomes; however, it is negative associated, and it has the smallest correlation in the regression when compared to other variables.

The Younger people are a little bit more stressed, depressed and anxious with the quarantine situation than those who are older, which actually contradicts the literature [21]. On the other hand, the economic impact of COVID-19 and the growing trend of hopelessness among young adults [11] may explain the present findings. Interestingly, higher levels of education appears to be protective for psychological distress, depression and state anxiety. The current results showed significant differences between participants with post-graduate education (Master's and Ph.D. degrees) and those who completed lower levels (bachelor's and high school). Accordingly, Steele, Dewa, Lin and colleagues [35] found evidence that those completing higher levels of education were more likely to seek psychological or psychiatric help.

It corroborates with another finding of the present study: the efficacy of tele-psychotherapy. All three dependent variables were partially predicted by the attendance of the participant in tele-psychotherapy (or online psychotherapy). Previous studies have shown the relevance of this kind of practice [26-28]; however, the results depicted here highlight the importance of psychological interventions during quarantine and isolation. In fact, telepsychology seems to be more associated with depression and anxiety levels than exercise, age and education. Finally, factors relevant for one's personal exposure to the novel coronavirus predicted all 3 indicators of mental health. There is already evidence in the scientific literature that COVID-19 raises levels of distress among people in quarantine also due to the lethal threat it poses to the population and to the person himself [11]. Two pertinent risk variables were predictive of stress, depression and anxiety: job obligation to leave the home and having perceived risk factors for SARS-CoV-2. Participants whose jobs obliged them to go outside the home to work showed higher stress, depression and state anxiety levels when compared to those who were not required to leave home. Worse mental health was also reported for those who perceived themselves as having risk factors for COVID-19.

Recent evidence implicates several physical factors that render a person more vulnerable to a viral infection: age, obesity, diabetes, heart diseases, asthma, bronchitis and other breathing disorders, chronic and autoimmune diseases [5-6]. Consequently, participants who classified themselves as having one or more of these illnesses also reported more depression and anxiety than those volunteers who categorized themselves without these vulnerabilities. It is understandable that a disease that is newly emerging, not fully understood by science and poses a real and lethal threat to people is perceived as very stressful - even more to those who have greater infection risk and have to face death [11]. Unfortunately, PSS-10 and SSTAI do not have any normative data to Brazilian population, so, neither prevalence nor comparison to norms were possible in the present study.

Regardless, the number of participants who presented values above FDI's cut-off point for depression was 4.1% [31], similar number to the prevalence of major depression among Brazilians [36]. Although this research provides a step further to understand psychological needs during quarantine of COVID-19, it also has several limitations. All data were self-report and not verifiable from other sources. Furthermore, no other psychological and environmental variables were considered, such as personality traits, economic conditions, size of the city and proximity of contamination that could provide more information regarding possible relationships between psychological, physical, behavioural and demographic dimensions [5, 6-10].

Another problem is the design of the study: data were cross-sectional (no comparison group) and the analysis was composed of a linear regression technique, which limits inferences about causality. Thus, everything that this paper can state is the level of association between variables. Future studies may benefit from longitudinal designs. Differently from previous studies with people in quarantine [10-17], the present study aimed to identify and quantify the strength of associations of various risk factors with mental health outcomes. Based on the findings here depicted, mental health services, either public or private, may be able to prioritize their services to those in greater danger to developing mental illness.

The results suggest that less educated women who have unbalanced diets, do not exercise, have no psychological aid, work outside, are in quarantine with older people, have perceived physical risk factors for COVID-19 contamination and are at young age are more likely to report higher levels of distress, depression and state anxiety. Effect sizes observed suggests that several factors were of a moderate magnitude: levels of education, nutrition, practicing exercise regularly, the presence of elders in quarantine living with participants and caring any risk factor for COVID-19. Those factors may need special consideration. Regardless, the sociodemographic and behavioural variables identified in the current study should be carefully considered when establishing strategies to provide psychological help to those at greater risk for developing mental illness.

Contributors

AF designed the method, collected data, performed statistical analyses and wrote the manuscript. MSK performed analyses and wrote the manuscript.

Role of the funding source

The funders of the study had no role in study design, data collection, data analysis, data interpretation, or writing of the report. The corresponding author had full access to all the data in the study and had final responsibility for the decision to submit for publication.

Acknowledgements

This study was supported by the Fundação Carlos Chagas de Amparo à Pesquisa do Estado do Rio de Janeiro (FAPERJ) and the Coordenação de Aperfeiçoamento de Pessoal de Nível Superior (CAPES) through the Brazilian Government Programm PROAP.

REFERENCES

1. World Health Organization. *Promoting mental health: concepts, emerging evidence, practice (Summary Report)*. Geneva: World Health Organization, **2004**.
2. Galderisi, S, Heinz, A., Kastrup, M., et al. (2015).Toward a new definition of mental health. *World Psychiatry* **2015**; **14**: 231-33.
3. Prince, M., Patel, V., Saxena, S., et al. (2007). No health without mental health. *The Lancet* **2007**; **370**: 859-77.
4. World Health Organization. *mhGAP: Mental Health Gap Action Programme: Scaling up care for mental, neurological, and substance use disorders*. Geneva: World Health Organization, **2008**.
5. Wilder-Smith A, Freedman, D. (2020).Isolation, quarantine, social distancing and community containment: pivotal role for old-style public health measures in the novel coronavirus (2019-nCoV) outbreak. *Journal of travel medicine* **2020**; **27:** taaa020.
6. World Health Organization. *Considerations for quarantine of individuals in the context of containment for coronavirus disease (COVID-19): interim guidance, 19 March 2020* (WHO/2019-nCoV/IHR_Quarantine/2020.2). Geneva: World Health Organization, **2020**.
7. Rubin, G., Wessely, S. (2020).The psychological effects of quarantining a city. *Bmj* **2020**; **368**.
8. Webster R, Brooks S, Smith L, et al. (2020).How to improve adherence with quarantine: Rapid review of the evidence. *medRxiv* **2020**; **23**.
9. Xiao, C. (2020). A Novel Approach of Consultation on 2019 Novel Coronavirus (COVID-19)Related Psychological and Mental Problems: Structured Letter Therapy. *Psychiatry investigation* **2020**; **17**: 175.
10. Brooks, S., Webster, R., Smith L., et al. The psychological impact of quarantine and how to reduce it: rapid review of the evidence. *The Lancet* **2020**; **395**: 14-20.
11. Qiu J, Shen, B., Zhao, M., et al. (2020). A nationwide survey of psychological distress among Chinese people in the COVID-19 epidemic: implications and policy recommendations. *Bmj* **2020**; **33**: e100213.
12. Jeong, H., Yim, H.W., Song Y-J, et al. (2016). Mental health status of people isolated due to Middle East respiratory syndrome. *Epidemiol Health* 2016; 38: e2016048.
13. Hawryluck, L., Gold, W., Robinson, S, et al. (2004). SARS control and psychological effects of quarantine, Toronto, Canada. *Emerg Infect Dis* **2004**; **10**: 1206-12.
14. Reynolds, D., Garay, J., Deamond, S.L, et al.(2007). Understanding, compliance and psychological impact of the SARS quarantine experience. *Epidemiol Infect* **2008**; **136**: 997-1007.
15. Taylor, M., Agho, K., Stevens, G., et al. (2008). Factors influencing psychological distress during a disease epidemic: data from Australia's first outbreak of equine influenza. *BMC Public Health* **2008**; **8**: 347.
16. Wu, P., Fang, Y., Guan, Z., et al.(2009). The psychological impact of the SARS epidemic on hospital employees in China: exposure, risk perception, and altruistic acceptance of risk. *Can J Psychiatry* **2009**, **54**: 302-11.
17. Wang, Y., Xu, B,, Zhao, G. et al. (2011). Is quarantine related to immediate negative psychological consequences during the 2009 H1N1 epidemic? *Gen Hosp Psychiatry* **2011**; **33**: 75-7.
18. Nolen-Hoeksema S. (2011).Gender differences in depression. *Current directions in psychological science* **2001**; **10**: 173-76.
19. Almeida, D., Kessler, R.(1998). Everyday stressors and gender differences in daily distress. *Journal of personality and social psychology* **75**: 670-80.
20. McLean, C.P. (2009). Anderson ER. Brave men and timid women? A review of the gender differences in fear and anxiety. *Clinical psychology review* **29**: 496-505.
21. Christensen, H., Jorm, A., Mackinnon, A. et al.(1999). Age differences in depression and anxiety symptoms: a structural equation modelling analysis of data from a general population sample. *Psychological medicine* . **29**: 325-39.
22. Timmer, S.G., Ho, L.K., Urquiza, A.J., et al. (2011). The effectiveness of parent–child interaction therapy with depressive mothers: The changing relationship as the agent of individual change. *Child Psychiatry & Human Development*. **42**: 406-23.
23. Lim S, Kim, E. Kim, A. et al. (2016). Nutritional factors affecting mental health. *Clinical nutrition research* **25**: 143-52.
24. Paluska, S.A., Schwenk, T.L.(2000). Physical activity and mental health. *Sports medicine* **29**: 167-80.
25. Stults-Kolehmainen M, Sinha, R. (2014). The effects of stress on physical activity and exercise. *Sports medicine* **44**: 81-121.

26. Lambert, M.J., Bergin, A.E., Garfield, S.L. (1994). *The effectiveness of psychotherapy: Encyclopedia of Psychotherapy.* New York, NY: Elsevier Science.
27. Bolton, A.J., Dorstyn, D.S. (2015). Telepsychology for posttraumatic stress disorder: A systematic review. *Journal of telemedicine and telecare***21**: 254-67.
28. Varker, T., Brand, R.M., Ward, J. et al. (2019).Efficacy of synchronous telepsychology interventions for people with anxiety, depression, posttraumatic stress disorder, and adjustment disorder: A rapid evidence assessment. *Psychological services***16**: 621-35.
29. National Council of Health. *Resolução nº 196, de 10 de Outubro de 1996.* Brasilia: Ministry of Health of Brazil, **1996**.
30. Cohen, S. Williamson, G.M. (1988). Perceived stress in a probability sample of the United States. In: Spacapan S, Oskamp S. *The social psychology of health: Claremont Symposium on Applied Social Psychology* (pp. 31–67). Newbury Park: Sage.
31. Filgueiras, A., Hora, G., Fioravanti-Bastos AC, et al. (2014). Development and psychometric properties of a novel depression measure. *Trends in Psychology***22**: 249-69.
32. Spielberger, C.D., Gorsuch, R.L., Lushene, R.D. (1970). *STAI: manual for the State-Trait Anxiety Inventory.* Palo Alto, CA: Consulting Psychologists Press.
33. Cohen, J. (1988). *Statistical Power Analysis for the Behavioural Sciences.* New York, NY: Lawrence Erlbaum Associates.
34. Hamilton, D.F., Ghert. M, Simpson, A.H.R.W. (2015). Interpreting regression models in clinical outcome studies. *Bone Joint Res***4**: 152-3.
35. Steele, L.S, Dewa, C.S, Lin, E, et al (n.d). Education level, income level and mental health services use in Canada: Associations and policy implications. *Healthcare Policy* , **3**: 96.
36. Barros, B.A.B., Lima, G.L, De Azevedo, C.S.A, et al. (2017). Depression and health behaviours in Brazilian adults – PNS 2013. *Rev Saude Publica* **51**: 8s.

Contributors

AF designed the method, collected data, performed statistical analyses and wrote the manuscript. MSK performed analyses and wrote the manuscript.

Role of the funding source

The funders of the study had no role in study design, data collection, data analysis, data interpretation, or writing of the report. The corresponding author had full access to all the data in the study and had final responsibility for the decision to submit for publication.

Acknowledgements

This study was supported by the Fundação Carlos Chagas de Amparo à Pesquisa do Estado do Rio de Janeiro (FAPERJ) and the Coordenação de Aperfeiçoamento de Pessoal de Nível Superior (CAPES) through the Brazilian Government Programm PROAP.

6. Mayoral Party Identity and Social Distancing in Brazil

Jeff Chan*and Ridwan Karim†

Wilfrid Laurier University

ABSTRACT

Does the political affiliation of local policymakers determine the citizens' compliance to social distancing behaviours? We provide causal estimates of the effect of political party affiliation of municipal mayors on regional differences in engaging in preventive behaviours in the context of Brazil. We employ a sharp regression discontinuity design based on close mayoral elections in 2016 to examine the effects of having a mayor from one of three political parties that President Jair Bolsonaro is closely associated with, by combining Facebook mobility data that tracks regional movement relative to February levels with electoral data from the 2016 mayoral municipal elections. Our methodology compares municipalities that are similar along a wide array of predetermined and observable correlates of the spread of the coronavirus, and where the incumbent mayor was selected as-if randomly.

We find that residents of Bolsonaro-affiliated municipalities exhibit 60% smaller relative declines in regional movement and are 13% more likely to cross regional boundaries over the months of March, April, and May. The findings hold for each of the three political parties, for each of the three months since the onset of the pandemic, and after controlling for anti-lockdown measures of March 15 in Brazil. We also provide evidence consistent with the notion that Bolsonaro-affiliated municipalities systematically under-report COVID-related cases and deaths on any given day, relative to comparable municipalities within close geographical proximity but with an incumbent mayor from a different political party.

---

* Assistant Professor, Department of Economics, Lazaridis School of Business & Economics, Wilfrid Laurier University, email: jchan@wlu.ca, phone: 519.884.0710 x3197, mailing address: Wilfrid Laurier University, 75 University Avenue W., Waterloo, Ontario, Canada N2L 3C5, Office: LH3016

† Assistant Professor, Department of Economics, Lazaridis School of Business & Economics, Wilfrid Laurier University, email: rkarim@wlu.ca, phone: 519.884.0710 x2820, mailing address: Wilfrid Laurier University, 75 University Avenue W., Waterloo, Ontario, Canada N2L 3C5, Office: LH3084

• INTRODUCTION

Does the political affiliation of local policymakers determine the response of citizens to the COVID19 pandemic in terms of adhering to social distancing behaviours? Studies examining the broad correlates of the spread of the coronavirus disease have reported differences along partisan lines in regional policies to tackle the global pandemic (Adolph et al. (2020), Allcott et al. (2020), Gupta et al. (2020)), as well as the variation in individual compliance to social distancing measures that are associated with political beliefs and party identity (Barrios and Hochberg (2020), Painter and Qiu (2020), Desmet and Wacziarg (2020)).

While these correlations are suggestive, it is often difficult to identify the underlying mechanisms due to the potentially endogenous relationship between responses by policymakers and citizen behaviours. We provide causal estimates of the effect of political party affiliation of municipal mayors on regional differences in engaging in social distancing behaviours in the context of Brazil. President Jair Bolsonaro's response to the COVID pandemic, and, his stringent opposition to the imposition of state-mandated social distancing measures, has exposed political fault lines over the desirability of lockdown policies in Brazil.

We examine the effects of having a mayor from one of three political parties that President Jair Bolsonaro is closely associated with on citizen behaviours at the level of local municipalities. The difficulties in identifying the causal effects of partisan policies on COVID-relate outcomes arise from both joint determination and reverse causality, both of which bias OLS estimates in directions that are ambiguous ex ante. Demographic variables (e.g. population density, extent of urbanization, average age of citizens) can jointly determine both local political outcomes and regional prevalence of the pandemic. On the other hand, growth in COVID cases due to ineffective policy response to the pandemic could induce a change in the party in power. We circumvent these endogeneity concerns by employing a sharp regression discontinuity design based on close mayoral elections in 2016, where the eventual mayor was selected as-if randomly and provides a source of plausibly exogenous variation in the party in power[1].

We combine electoral data from the 2016 mayoral municipal elections with Facebook mobility data that tracks regional movement relative to February levels, and data on daily incidences of new cases and COVID-related deaths at the local municipality level. We examine close elections where the eventual winner belonged to one of three political parties: Social Christian Party (PSC), Brazil Labour Renewal Party (PRTB), and Social Liberal Party (PSL). All three of these parties are closely affiliated with President Bolsonaro, with party platforms that closely align with his.

We find that residents of municipalities where the winning mayoral candidate in 2016 belonged to one of these three parties exhibited smaller relative declines in regional movement and are more likely to cross regional boundaries over the months of March, April, and May. Specifically, the decline in regional movement relative to February levels is approximately 60% less compared to municipalities where the mayoral candidates from one of these three parties barely lost. Moreover, the proportion of residents of these municipalities who cross regional boundaries from March to May are 13% higher relative to the average of the comparison municipalities.

The findings hold for each of the three political parties separately, for each of the three months since the onset of the pandemic separately as well as in regressions combining the three parties together and are robust to a wide variety of specification choices. We demonstrate that 'treatment' municipalities are similar to municipalities along a wide array of predetermined and observable characteristics that have been identified in the literature as broad correlates of the spread of the coronavirus. We also provide evidence consistent with the notion that Bolosonaro-affiliated municipalities systematically under-report COVID-related cases and deaths on any given day, relative to comparable municipalities within close geographical proximity but with an incumbent mayor from a different political party.

---

[1] Cornelson et al. (2020) employ a similar methodology to investigate in USA the effect of the political identity of state governors on the extent to which individuals engage in preventive behaviors.

With more than a million cases of the coronavirus, Brazil has emerged as the new epicenter of the outbreak in Latin America[1]. The response to the pandemic has been a particularly contentious political flashpoint between Brazil's populist president Jair Bolsonaro and his political rivals and has divided public opinion along partisan lines[2]. Among his public pronouncements, President Bolsonaro underplayed the seriousness of the coronavirus[3], blamed the media for creating a panic surrounding the pandemic[4], and has criticized the protocols recommended by public health officials[6].

His public actions include joining demonstrations against stay-at-home order[7] and firing Health Minister Luiz Henrique Mandetta who advocated for social distancing[8]. These positions have led to well-documented instances of verbal clashes with municipal mayors from rival political parties[9]. Given the potential persuasive effect of political messaging on social distancing compliance (Simonov et al. (2020)), we examine the consequences of the political rhetoric and actions of the president of Brazil on COVID-related outcomes in Brazil. We study this at the local municipality level and focus on mayors that belong to one of three political parties: PSC, PSL, and PRTB. These three parties have been consistently classified as far-right parties by political scientists, and all three of them are closely associated with the President. President Bolsonaro is a former member of both the PSL and PSC and is credited with substantially altering the party platform of both parties. For the Brazilian general election of 2018, PRTB formed coalition with PSL to support then candidate Bolsonaro. His pick for Vice President is also a member of PRTB. We find sharp discontinuities in various COVID-related outcomes in our comparison of municipalities where a mayoral candidate from one of these three parties won in a close election in 2016, as opposed to municipalities where a mayoral candidate from one of the same three parties lost in a close election. In particular, residents of municipalities with a mayor from one of these three parties reduce their movement relative to levels in February to a lower extent and are more likely to cross regional boundaries. Our identification strategy overcomes the effect other confounding factors may have on our key variables of interest. We demonstrate balance in important predetermined covariates that are known to be correlated with COVID prevalence, which include variables such as population density, proportion of rural population, proportion of population above the age of 65, geographical location of particular municipalities, and per capita public health expenditures.

mayors-media-for-covid-19-crisis-1.4953827
6 Sims, Shannon. "Bolsonaro Criticizes Lockdown Measures as Brazil Becomes Hotspot".May 10. 2020. BNNBllomberg.ca, https://www.bnnbloomberg.ca/bolsonaro-criticizes-lockdown-measures-as-brazil-becomeshotspot-1.1434280 7 "Brazil's Bolsonaro joins protest against coronavirus restrictions".20 Apr. 2020.AlJazeera.com. https://www.aljazeera.com/news/2020/04/brazil-bolsonaro-joins-protest-coronavirus-curbs-200420042616860.html
8 Philips, Dom. "Bolsonaro fires popular health minister after dispute over coronavirus response". 16 Apr. 2020. TheGuardian.com https://www.theguardian.com/world/2020/apr/16/bolsonaro-brazil-president-luizmandetta-health-minister 9 Walsh, Nick. Shelley, Jo. Duwe, Eduardo. Picheta, Rob. "Brazilian mayor launches attack on 'stupid' Bolsonaro over coronavirus response". 25 May. 2020. CTVNews.ca, https://www.ctvnews.ca/world/brazilian-mayor-launchesattack-on-stupid-bolsonaro-over-coronavirus-response-1.4952996

1 The data are updated daily and available at https://www.nytimes.com/interactive/2020/world/americas/brazilcoronavirus-cases.html and https://github.com/wcota/covid19br/blob/master/cases-brazil-cities-time.csv.
2 Encarnacion, Omar. "Brazil Is Suffering. Bolsonaro Isn't." Foreign Policy. 28 May. 2020. ForeignPolicy.com https://foreignpolicy.com/2020/05/28/brazil-is-suffering-bolsonaro-isnt/
3 Fearnow, Benjamin. "Brazilian President Bolsonaro Rejects Calls for Coronavirus Lockdown, Says 'We're All Going to Die One Day'" 30 Mar. 2020. Newsweek.com, https://www.newsweek.com/brazilian-president-bolsonarorejects-calls-coronavirus-lockdown-says-were-all-going-die-one-1495020
4 Biller, David. "Brazilian president blames health minister, mayors, media for COVID-19 crisis". 25 May. 2020. CTVnews.ca, https://www.ctvnews.ca/health/coronavirus/brazilian-president-blames-health-minister-

Since there are no pre-existing differences between our 'treatment' and 'control' municipalities along these dimensions, the observed divergence in citizen behaviours and COVID cases can be attributed to as-if randomly assigned political identity of local mayors. Our preferred specifications include both state and date fixed effects, in order to control for the timing of the onset of the disease and lockdown measures initiated by particular state governors. Our results hold for each of the three political parties, as well as regressions combing the three parties together. Our analysis examines the role party affiliation of local mayors at various points in time, starting on March 01, 2020 and ending on May 31, 2020. The patterns observed hold for each month of March, April, and May, and after controlling for March 15 demonstrations against lockdown measures that President Bolsonaro participated in.

There are several mechanisms that could help explain the link between local political affiliation and citizens' observance of social distancing behaviours. There may be important and systematic differences across political lines in declaring and/or enforcing (in the case of state-mandated social distancing policies that apply to all its constituent municipalities) various lockdown measures. Local mayors may also control the flow of information available in local media platforms regarding recommended social distancing practices. Thus, our results may also be capturing the effects of differential messaging by politicians across municipalities. We then employ a similar methodology to see the effects of party identity on COVID cases and deaths.

However, there are important caveats to keep in mind when analyzing the officially released data. It is widely considered that the official number of cases and COVID-related deaths provided by the Ministry of Health are unreliable, due to a number of reasons. These include underreporting and comparatively very low levels of testing in Brazil, as well as the substantial variation in testing frequency across states, municipalities, and days that are likely correlated with, among other factors, local political conditions (Ajzenman, Cavalcanti, and Da Mata, 2020).

Curiously, the regression discontinuity estimates show that Bolsonaro-affiliated municipalities on average experience 1.4 fewer new cases, and 0.14 fewer deaths per one hundred thousand residents relative to comparison municipalities.

Further exploration shows that non-Bolsonaro municipalities that are in close geographical proximity of a Bolsonaro municipality and belong to the same state report more cases and deaths on any given day, holding constant unobservable factors common to all municipalities belonging the same state. We also do not find any evidence of higher prevalence of COVID cases induced by the low levels of compliance with social distancing behaviours by residents in Bolsonaro municipalities. These two results combined point towards Bolsonaro municipalities experiencing systematically fewer cases and deaths due to either less testing or less reporting. We would require information on testing frequency to formally test this hypothesis, data for which is not yet available.

Our paper is closely related to various literatures. Firstly, this paper is related to other work that report differences along partisan lines in regional policies to tackle the global pandemic (Adolph et al. (2020), Allcott et al. (2020), Gupta et al. (2020)). Adolph et al. (2020) employ an event study methodology to study differences in state-level social distancing policy responses in USA. They find that political partisanship is a key determinant of timing of lockdown policies. In particular, Republican governors with a stronger mandate delayed the adoption of social distancing policies. Gupta et al. (2020) document differences across political lines in declaring and enforcing various lockdown measures, e.g. emergency declarations, and school closures, across state and local governments in USA. There is a related strand of the literature that examines individual compliance to social distancing measures that are associated with political beliefs and party identity (Barrios et al. (2020) Barrios and Hochberg (2020), Painter and Qiu (2020), Desmet and Wacziarg (2020)). Galasso et al. (2020) report results that suggest that political leanings, among other factors, influence COVID-19 Related Attitudes and Behaviour.

Barrios and Hochberg (2020) use data on internet searches and county-level average daily travel distance from a large sample of U.S. smartphones at the daily level and show that political preferences of residents affect perceptions of risk associated with the COVID-19 virus and as well as levels of social distancing behaviour. Painter and Qiu (2020) report that Democrats are more likely to switch to e-commerce ad more likely to completely stay at home after state orders on lockdown are implemented. Desmet and Wacziarg (2020) document the growing political divide among individual citizens in USA over policies to ease stay-at-home orders; as well as the difference in the political willingness to suspend social distancing measures between Republican-leaning locations as compared to Democratic-leaning locations. Fan et al. (2020) documents substantial differences in behaviours, beliefs, and risk preferences across partisanship lines (among other observable covariates) from a nationally representative survey covering 5,500 adult respondents in the U.S.

Another literature utilizes various social connectedness measures gleaned from social media platforms and its association with COVID-related behaviours. For example, Kuchler et al. (2020) use anonymized and aggregated data from Facebook to show that areas with stronger social ties to two early COVID-19 "hotspots" (Westchester County, NY, in the U.S. and Lodi province in Italy) generally have more confirmed COVID-19 cases as of March 30, 2020. These relationships hold after controlling for geographic distance to the hotspots as well as for the income and population density of the regions. Barrios and Hochberg (2020) use data on internet searches and travel distance gleaned from U.S. smartphones and find that counties with higher percentage of Trump voters consider COVID-19 virus to be less risky, and also engage in lower levels of social distancing behaviour. Painter and Qiu (2020) use geolocation data to track and estimate differences across party lines in compliance with social distancing measures in USA. Allcott et al. (2020) utilize location data from smartphones to show that regions within USA with more Republicans engage in less social distancing, controlling for other factors. Finally, our paper contributes to the literature looking at the political economy determinants of COVID-related outcomes in Brazil. Mariani et al. (2020) employ a differences-in-differences strategy to estimate the effects of president's Bolosonaro's decision to ignore health ministry recommendations on March 15. Ajzenman et al. (2020) employ an event study methodology to show pro-Bolsonaro municipalities reduce social distancing compliance post-March 15 relative to non Bolsonaro municipalities. Calvo and Ventura (2020) employ a social media framing experiment to show how public perceptions are differentially affected along party identities by social media messages from politicians. The rest of the paper is structured as follows. In Section 2, we describe the identification strategy; Section 3 describes the data sources; Section 4 presents the results and their interpretation; and section 5 concludes.

(2) EMPIRICAL METHODOLOGY

Estimating the effects of political identity of local mayors on the response of citizens to the COVID19 pandemic can be frustrated by classic endogeneity concerns. For example, various demographic and geographical variables known to exert an influence on the spread of the coronavirus - population density, extent of urbanization, average age of citizens are also well-documented determinants of local electoral outcomes. The direction of causality could also flow in the opposite direction, as perceived ineffectual policy response to the pandemic could induce a change in the party in power. Moreover, selection bias can overpower estimates, or even change the direction of the effect.

We overcome these endogeneity concerns by using a regression discontinuity design based on close mayoral election in Brazil in 2016, where the treatment is the electoral victory of one of the three parties (PSC, PSL, PRTB) affiliated with President Bolsonaro[1]. This methodology allows us to quantify the effects in a transparent manner of the partisan identity of local mayors on citizens' decisions regarding their social mobility patterns. In this section, we explain the regression discontinuity design that we employ as the main identification strategy. We also detail the tests of the key assumptions embedded in this strategy.

2.1 Regression Discontinuity

The identification of local average treatment effects through regression discontinuity analysis is now well established in the literature (Angrist and Lavy (1999), Lee (2008)). We use local linear regressions, dropping observations outside a set bandwidth of the cut-off (Lee and Lemieux (2010)) in order to reduce bias from including observations far away from the cut-off where the assumptions underlying the identification is likely to not hold. The treatment in this context is winning an election under plurality rules, and the forcing variable is the margin of victory of a particular party (PSC, PRTB, or PSL) in the 2016 mayoral elections. The margin of victory for a given party is defined as the vote share obtained by the mayoral candidate from that party minus the vote share obtained by its closest electoral opponent in the 2016 mayoral elections.

This regression discontinuity design is referred to as the Multi-Cutoff Regression Discontinuity Design (Cattaneo et al. (2016)), and we follow the standard practice of normalizing the forcing variable so that the cutoff is zero percent for all observations. If the margin of victory crosses zero percent, it acts as an exogenous trigger for the mayoral candidate from a particular party to assume power. The multi-cutoff RD design has been used widely in many contexts to study causal mechanisms.

For example, Brollo et al. (2013) utilizes a series of cut offs to study the effects of federal transfers on political corruption in Brazil. Cattaneo et al. (2016) analyzes the properties of such a design by exploring the effects of a party winning in a local election on the probability of the same party winning the following election. The formal equation describing the RD design is as follows, using only observations that satisfy the requirement that the margin of victory $\in (0.8 - h, 0.8 + h)$, where h is the choice bandwidth around the zero percent threshold:

$$Y_i = \alpha + \beta_1 D_i + \beta_2 [Margin\ of\ Victory]$$

$$+ \beta_3 D_i X [Margin\ of\ Victory] + \epsilon_i \tag{1}$$

Here, Y_i is the relevant outcome variable (e.g. social mobility measures) in municipality i, D_i is a dummy variable that takes on the value of 1 if the municipality crosses the threshold of zero percent, i.e. if either PSC, PRTB, or PSL wins.

---

[1] RD designs based on close elections have a long tradition in the political economy literature. Although the identifying assumptions do not always hold, as is the case with US House election (Caughey and Sekhon (2011)), the validity of this identification strategy is generally accepted in other contexts (Eggers et al. (2015), De la Cuesta and Imai (2016))

This specification allows for a linear relationship between the outcome and the forcing variable to be estimated separately on each side of the discontinuity within the bandwidth window.

The regressor of interest is D_i, which provides the reduced form estimate for the existence of any discontinuity at the threshold. We include state and date fixed effects in all our specifications. Therefore, the identifying variation comes from comparing municipalities on either side of the zero-percent threshold within a given state and on a given day.

The zero-percent trigger leads to exogenous variation in the party identity of the winning mayoral candidate. Undergoing the treatment is a deterministic function of the margin of victory for the party in question. As such, we report sharp regression discontinuity results using the Calonico, Cattaneo and Titiunik's "rdrobust" package (Calonico et al. (2015b) with a triangular kernel. A key decision is h, the kernel bandwidth, and the trade-off between precision and bias. We report estimates based on Imbens and Kalyanaraman (2012) optimal bandwidth choice (IKBW), which is itself a function of the data and hence different for each outcome variable.

For the RD strategy to be valid, agents cannot have precise control over the forcing variable (Lee, 2008). This condition should hold in the setting that we study, since close victories are often determined by forces outside of a candidate's precise control, including deaths of voters, cancellations, new voter registrations, outflows of voters etc. Moreover, the setting passes the McCrary Density test. Figure A1 shows that there is no precise sorting around the cut-off. To check if municipalities above and below the cut-off are comparable, we present estimates of the effects of the treatment on a wide array of predetermined covariates at the municipality level in Table A2. These are per capita health expenditures, municipality population, population density, distance to state capital, geographical location, media presence, life expectancy, infant mortality, literacy rates, Gini coefficient, proportion of population aged above 65, and proportion of rural population. All effects are close to zero in magnitude and statistically insignificant, with the exception of regional identifiers, which will be controlled for with state fixed effects in our regressions.

We calculate the margin of victory and conduct analyses for each party separately. We also combine all observations to carry out a pooled regression discontinuity design. In these pooled regressions, we combine the margin of victory of all three parties to form a common forcing variable. The total number of mayoral elections held in 2016 exceed five thousand. Out of these elections, there are only 8 elections where a mayoral candidate from one of these three parties ran against a candidate from one of the other two parties. In computing the common forcing variable, we drop a particular party's margin of victory from a given election, if one of the three other parties won in that election. We show in the results section that our results hold individually for each of these three political parties, as well as in the combined regressions.

3. DATA DESCRIPTION

3.1 Facebook Mobility Data

The data for mobility during the COVID-19 pandemic come from Facebook at the GADM level 2 region level for Brazil starting from March 1, 2020 to May 31, 2020. The regional aggregation chosen by Facebook mostly corresponds with municipalities in Brazil, although there are some differences in boundaries. We use GIS to construct a crosswalk between the GADM regions used by Facebook and official Brazilian municipality boundaries.[1] The Facebook mobility data are drawn from Facebook users who use the mobile version of the application and enable location tracking. Movement in each day from March 1 onwards is calculated relative to February levels. Specifically, Facebook takes tiles of roughly several hundred square meters each and calculates the mean number of tiles visited per day by users in a GADM region.

It then, for each day, compares that average number of tiles visited to a baseline from February (based on all the February days on that same day of the week) and calculates the percentage change in the average tiles visited. Similarly, Facebook also produces a measure of staying put. This is calculated as the share of users in an area who remain in the same tile for that day without moving to another.

The Facebook data are not available for all GADM regions. In addition, not all GADM regions that have data have it for all the days in the sample period examined. Whenever a municipality is missing data from at least one of the GADM regions that it consists of, we treat that municipality as missing for that day. We ultimately have an unbalanced panel of 2846 municipalities with data. Despite these issues, the Facebook data represent the most disaggregated, freely accessible mobility based information on movement reductions during COVID-19 in Brazil. In addition, Facebook is very popular in Brazil. From 2018 data collected by Statistica,[2] there were 75.6 million users in Brazil that logged in at least once a month, relative to an overall population of just under 210 million. In addition, according to Statistica, Facebook had the highest penetration rate in Brazil of all social media platforms as of the fourth quarter of 2015. While these statistics cannot guarantee that Facebook users in the mobility data are representative of the Brazilian population, they reassure us that they are a non-trivial proportion of that population.

3.2 Elections Data

Municipal elections are held every four years in Brazil. The electoral data related to the municipal elections in 2016 are obtained from the Superior Electoral Court (TSE). These include data on turnout, votes for different candidates, party affiliations of candidates, and other voting statistics for locations within each municipality. We use this data to construct measures of margin of victory and number of candidates in each election at the municipality level.

3.3 COVID-19 Cases and Deaths Data

We use municipality-day level data on COVID-19 confirmed cases and deaths at the municipality level from Cota (2020). The data are collected from numerous official sources and updated regularly in an accessible format for researchers and policymakers.[3] The Cota (2020) data have been used by the New York Times in its COVID-19 case tracker for Brazil, amongst others.[4]

We report summary statistics for our main variables in Table A1. Mayoral candidates belonging to PSC, PRTB, and PSL took part in 310, 78, and 128 municipal elections respectively in 2016. We also have observations at the municipal-day level from March to May on social mobility variables, and

---

[1] For more information on this crosswalk construction, see the Appendix.

[2] https://www.statista.com/statistics/244936/number-of-facebook-users-in-brazil/

[3] The data can be downloaded from https://github.com/wcota/covid19br (As of June 19, 2020).

[4] https://www.nytimes.com/interactive/2020/world/americas/brazil-coronavirus-cases.html

daily incidences of COVID cases and deaths. As can be seen, mobility relative February levels declined on average across Brazilian municipalities during these months. Moreover, 29% of the population on average do not cross regional boundaries on a given day during this time-period. Municipalities in Brail report 2.3 new cases and 0.08 deaths per one hundred thousand inhabitants daily on average, based on the officially released figures.

4. RESULTS

4.1. Main Results: Social Mobility

We begin by providing graphical evidence of the effects of the party barely winning a municipal election in 2016 on social mobility patters of its residents from March - May of 2020. Figures 1 and 2 presents RD plots in the pooled sample, where we combine the margin of victory of each of the three parties to combine one common forcing variable, as described in section 2. Figures A2 and A3 presents the RD plots for each of the three parties separately. These figures plot social mobility patters on the y-axis against the party's margin of victory in the 2016 elections within a threshold of 10% around the cut-off of 80%. The patterns presented are robust to different selections of the bandwidth around the threshold. Each marker represents a local average: the mean of the outcome in a bin of 20 municipalities.

A straight line is fitted on the original (i.e., "unbinned") data at each side of the vertical threshold, so that the point where the lines are not connected is where the discontinuity in outcomes could be visible. All observations to the right of the cut off correspond to municipalities ("treatment" group) where the party (or parties) won in the 2016 elections, and all observations to the left correspond to municipalities ("control" group) where the party faced an electoral defeat.

As can be seen, there are visible and statistically significant discontinuities in the patterns of social mobility for two different measures, although the treatment municipalities are similar to the control municipalities along a wide array of predetermined and observable characteristics. Municipalities where the incumbent mayor belongs to one of PSC, PRTB, or PSL, and won in a close election in 2016 are also municipalities where the decline in residents' change in movement across regional boundaries during the time period relative to February levels are the smallest.

These residents are also less likely to remain within their regional boundaries during the three months of March - May, relative to residents where a mayoral candidate from PSC, PRTB, or PSL, lost in a close election in 2016. Figures A2 and A3 demonstrate that the exact same patterns hold for each of the three parties separately.

Table 1 presents the local linear regression estimates of the treatment effects on these social mobility variables. We report the sharp RD estimates, using the methods in Calonico et al. (2015a), estimated using the optimal Imbens and Kalyanaraman bandwidth. We include state fixed effects, to control for state specific patterns of the spread of corona virus and/or directives issued by state governors. We also include date fixed-effects, to control for any sources of temporal variation across municipalities that may be correlated with our main outcomes.

Therefore, the discontinuities are being estimated by comparing treatment municipalities against control municipalities from the same state on a given day.

Confirming the graphical analysis, the table shows that, although residents across all municipalities reduce their movement relative to February levels; a close PSC, PRTB, or PSL victory leads to residents in these municipalities reducing their movement by 60% less relative to the average decline in movement, compared to residents where one of those three parties lost by a close margin (Column 1). Moreover, the residents of these municipalities are 13% less likely to remain within their regional boundaries relative to the mean for Brazilian municipalities within the estimation sample, compared to residents of the control municipalities. These results are statistically significant at the 1% level. Table 2 shows that the results are statistically significant for each of the three parties separately using the same estimation framework.

We estimate sharp discontinuities that are significant and point towards the same effects on social mobility patterns across all three parties. A PRTB victory leads to the biggest estimated effects, while the effects of a PSC or PSL victory are comparable to each other and the main results in magnitude. Residents of treatment municipalities are less likely to exhibit behaviours consistent with observing recommended social distancing patterns, and the magnitudes of the deviations are both statistically and economically significant.

4.2 Main Results with Different Sample Selection Criteria and Alternate Specifications

We now conduct additional analyses by employing certain sample selection criteria and exploring alternate specifications. In table A3, we restrict the sample of municipalities to a balanced panel. Therefore, we only retain those municipalities for which we have data on social mobility for each of the 92 days spanning the months of March, April, and May. As can be seen from the table, the number of observations drop by around 4% relative to our main results, but our RD estimates are identical in magnitudes, direction, and significance to the ones presented in Table 1.

Table A4 reports the results for each month of March, April, and May, employing the common forcing variable calculated by combining the margins of victory of all three parties. Once again, we estimate sharp discontinuities that are consistently significant across all three months. The RD estimate on change in relative movement grows bigger in magnitude in each subsequent month, while the RD estimate for staying within regional boundaries increase in April and remain stable for May. In Table A5, we take the mean of social mobility patterns for each municipality from our balanced panel sample (i.e. municipalities for which we observe measures of social mobility across all 92 days in the three months of March, April, and May). We collapse the data at the municipality level such that each municipality appears once in our regression discontinuity design. We can only add state-fixed effects in these regressions by design. We find that the results remain robust and significant with almost identical magnitudes even in this reduced sample. Finally, Table A6 shows that our results are robust to controlling for March 15 demonstrations against lockdown measures that President Bolsonaro participated in.

4.3 Results: COVID-Related Cases and Deaths

We now employ a similar methodology to investigate whether treatment municipalities experience higher levels of coronavirus cases and deaths, due to lower levels of observance of social distancing behaviours. At the onset, it is important to clarify that the official number of cases and COVID related deaths provided by the Ministry of Health is widely considered to be unreliable.

Ajzenman, Cavalcanti, and Da Mata (2020) describe some of the issues plaguing case reporting data in Brazil, including underreporting and disproportionately low levels of testing in Brazil relative to other nations.

Moreover, the little testing that is carried out varies in its frequency substantially across states, municipalities, and days, and are very likely to be correlated to local political determinations, among other factors. This is best exemplified by the Brazilian government decision to stop releasing its total numbers of Covid-19 cases and deaths from the official website as ordered by President Jair Bolsonaro himself a decision that the Ministry of Health back tracked. Therefore, the data we have on daily frequencies of cases and deaths is likely to have systematic measurement errors. Table A7 reports the results for new cases and deaths, alongside our main results on social mobility, for comparison. Curiously, the patterns observed are exactly opposite to those that might be expected based on our results on social mobility patterns. Treatment municipalities on average experience 1.4 fewer new cases, and 0.14 fewer deaths per one hundred thousand residents, relative to control municipalities, and this difference is statistically significant. One possibility is that the relationship between movement and cases/deaths is likely to be heavily endogenous, (eg. municipalities with high rates of infection may also observe reduced movement).

Another possibility is that COVID-cases are systematically under-reported (due to lower levels of testing) in Bolosonaro affiliated municipalities. To test this possibility, we would need access to testing data as well as some form of data capturing excess mortality, either of which is not publicly available as of now. We explore further, employing two different specifications, to examine whether Bolosonaro affiliated municipalities have systematically lower number of cases and deaths.

To do this, we compute geographical distances between each pair of municipalities. We then run regressions to compare municipalities where the mayor is affiliated to one of our three Bolosonaro affiliated parties, to municipalities that are within close proximity of these municipalities but have an incumbent mayor that belongs to a different political party.

Table A8 reports the results for deaths and cases. All specifications employ state and date fixed effects. As can be seen, municipalities that are within 20 kilometres of a treatment municipality but did not receive the treatment themselves (i.e. a mayoral candidates from PSC, PRTB, or PSL did not win in elections in these municipalities), report more cases and deaths on a given day, holding constant other confounding factors common to all municipalities belonging the same state.

The systematic results holds for distance of 30 kilometres, 40 kilometres, as well as 50 kilometres, and becomes statistically significant in the last two specifications. There are two possible reasons for this finding that we consider: a) the higher relative social mobility in treatment municipalities lead to the spread of the infection to other municipalities, or b) treatment municipalities are systematically under-reporting cases and deaths relative to others that are within the same state and in close proximity on any given day. We test the first possibility by comparing control municipalities that are in close geographical proximity to treatment ones, relative to other control municipalities farther away in the same state on any given day.

The thought experiment is as follows: within a given state and on a given day, do control municipalities that are closer to treatment ones exhibit more cases and deaths relative to other control municipalities in the same state that are farther away? This test assumes that there are no systematic reporting and testing differences across control municipalities.

We report the results in Table A9 and find no significant differences in the occurrences of cases and deaths per capita between these two sets of municipalities. In fact, closer municipalities are likely to experience fewer cases in one of our specifications. The results run counter to the idea that residents from treatment municipalities are spreading the disease to nearby municipalities and is more consistent with the second possibility: treatment municipalities have systematically fewer cases and deaths due to either less testing or less reporting. Of course, a formal test of this hypothesis can only be conducted once we have access to testing and reporting data across municipalities on any given day. However, this data is not yet available

.

5. CONCLUSION

In this paper, we explored the effect of political party affiliation of municipal mayors on regional differences in engaging in preventive behaviours in the context of Brazil. We employ a sharp regression discontinuity design based on close mayoral elections in 2016 to examine the effects of having a mayor from one of three political parties that President Jair Bolsonaro is closely associated with, by combining Facebook mobility data that tracks regional movement relative to February levels with electoral data from the 2016 mayoral municipal elections.

Our methodology circumvents the endogeneity concerns by comparing municipalities that are similar along a wide array of predetermined and observable correlates of the spread of the coronavirus, and where the incumbent mayor was selected as-if randomly. We find that residents of Bolsonaro-affiliated municipalities exhibit 60% smaller relative declines in regional movement and are 13% more likely to cross regional boundaries over the months of March, April, and May.

The findings hold for each of the three political parties, for each of the three months since the onset of the pandemic, and after controlling for anti-lockdown measures of March 15 in Brazil. The results are robust to a wide array of alternate specifications and sample selection criteria. We then explore the effects of party identity of local mayors on incidences of COVID-19 cases and deaths.

We document that, counter-intuitively, Bolsonaro municipalities experience fewer cases and deaths on any given day. We then explore further, and report that non-Bolsonaro municipalities that are in close geographical proximity of a Bolsonaro municipality and belong to the same state report more cases and deaths on any given day, holding constant unobservable determinants of the spread of the infection. We also do not find any evidence of higher prevalence of COVID cases induced by the low levels of compliance with social distancing behaviours by residents in Bolsonaro municipalities. Thus, the evidence we provide is consistent with the notion that Bolsonaro-affiliated municipalities systematically under-report COVID-related cases and deaths on any given day, relative to comparable municipalities within close geographical proximity but with an incumbent mayor from a different political party. We plan to collect data on testing frequency and variations in policy across Brazilian municipalities to formally test this hypothesis, data for which is not yet available.

REFERENCES

Adolph, Christopher, Kenya Amano, Bree Bang-Jensen, Nancy Fullman, and John Wilkerson, "Pandemic politics: Timing state-level social distancing responses to COVID-19," *medRxiv*, 2020.

Ajzenman, Nicolas, Tiago Cavalcanti, and Daniel Da Mata, "More than words: Leaders' speech and risky behavior during a pandemic," *Available at SSRN 3582908*, 2020.

Allcott, Hunt, Levi Boxell, Jacob Conway, Matthew Gentzkow, Michael Thaler, and David Y Yang, "Polarization and public health: Partisan differences in social distancing during the Coronavirus pandemic," *NBER Working Paper*, 2020, (w26946).

Angrist, Joshua D and Victor Lavy, "Using Maimonides' rule to estimate the effect of class size on scholastic achievement," *The Quarterly journal of economics*, 1999, *114* (2), 533–575.

Barrios, John M and Yael Hochberg, "Risk perception through the lens of politics in the time of the covid-19 pandemic," Technical Report, National Bureau of Economic Research 2020.

_ , Efraim Benmelech, Yael V Hochberg, Paola Sapienza, and Luigi Zingales, "Civic capital and social distancing during the covid-19 pandemic," Technical Report, National Bureau of Economic Research 2020.

Brollo, Fernanda, Tommaso Nannicini, Roberto Perotti, and Guido Tabellini, "The political resource curse," *American Economic Review*, 2013, *103* (5), 1759–96.

Calonico, Sebastian, Matias D Cattaneo, and Rocio Titiunik, "Optimal data-driven regression discontinuity plots," *Journal of the American Statistical Association*, 2015, *110* (512), 1753–1769.

, and , "rdrobust: An R Package for Robust Nonparametric Inference in RegressionDiscontinuity Designs.," *R J.*, 2015, *7* (1), 38.

Calvo, Ernesto and Tiago Ventura, "Will I get COVID-19? Partisanship, Social Media Frames, and Perceptions of Health Risk in Brazil," 2020.

Cattaneo, Matias D, Roc´ıo Titiunik, Gonzalo Vazquez-Bare, and Luke Keele, "Interpreting regression discontinuity designs with multiple cutoffs," *The Journal of Politics*, 2016, *78* (4), 1229–1248.

Caughey, Devin and Jasjeet S Sekhon, "Elections and the regression discontinuity design: Lessons from close US house races, 1942–2008," *Political Analysis*, 2011, *19* (4), 385–408.

Cornelson, Kirsten, Boriana Miloucheva et al., "Political polarization, social fragmentation, and cooperation during a pandemic," Technical Report 2020.

Cota, Wesley, "Monitoring the number of COVID-19 cases and deaths in Brazil at municipal and federative units level," 2020.

Desmet, Klaus and Romain Wacziarg, "Understanding Spatial Variation in COVID-19 across the United States," Technical Report, National Bureau of Economic Research 2020.

Eggers, Andrew C, Anthony Fowler, Jens Hainmueller, Andrew B Hall, and James M Snyder Jr, "On the validity of the regression discontinuity design for estimating electoral effects: New evidence from over 40,000 close races," *American Journal of Political Science*, 2015, *59* (1), 259–274.

Fan, Ying, A Ye,sim Orhun, and Dana Turjeman, "Heterogeneous Actions, Beliefs, Constraints and Risk Tolerance During the COVID-19 Pandemic," Technical Report, National Bureau of Economic Research 2020.

Galasso, Vincenzo, Vincent Pons, Paola Profeta, Michael Becher, Sylvain Brouard, and Martial Foucault, "Gender Differences in COVID-19 Related Attitudes and Behavior: Evidence from a Panel Survey in Eight OECD Countries," Technical Report, National Bureau of Economic Research 2020.

Gupta, Sumedha, Thuy D Nguyen, Felipe Lozano Rojas, Shyam Raman, Byungkyu Lee, Ana Bento, Kosali I Simon, and Coady Wing, "Tracking public and private response to the covid-19 epidemic: Evidence from state and local government actions," Technical Report, National Bureau of Economic Research 2020.

Imbens, Guido and Karthik Kalyanaraman, "Optimal bandwidth choice for the regression discontinuity estimator," *The Review of economic studies*, 2012, *79* (3), 933–959.

Kuchler, Theresa, Dominic Russel, and Johannes Stroebel, "The geographic spread of COVID-19 correlates with structure of social networks as measured by Facebook," Technical Report, National Bureau of Economic Research 2020.

la Cuesta, Brandon De and Kosuke Imai, "Misunderstandings about the regression discontinuity design in the study of close elections," *Annual Review of Political Science*, 2016, *19*, 375–396.

Lee, David S, "Randomized experiments from non-random selection in US House elections," *Journal of Econometrics*, 2008, *142* (2), 675–697.

_ and Thomas Lemieux, "Regression discontinuity designs in economics," *Journal of economic literature*, 2010, *48* (2), 281–355.

Mariani, L, Jessica Gagete-Miranda, and P Retti, "Words can hurt: How political communication can change the pace of an epidemic," DOI: https://doi. org/10.31235/osf. io/a32r7, 2020

Painter, Marcus and Tian Qiu, "Political beliefs affect compliance with covid-19 social distancing orders," *Available at SSRN 3569098*, 2020. Simonov, Andrey, Szymon K Sacher, Jean-Pierre H Dub´e, and Shirsho Biswas, "The persuasive effect of fox news: non-compliance with social distancing during the covid-19 pandemic," Technical Report, National Bureau of Economic Research 2020.

7.Impact of Socioeconomic Vulnerability On Covid-19 Outcomes And Social Distancing In Brazil

[1]Paulo Cardoso Lins-Filho[1], Millena Mirella Silva de Araújo[1], Thuanny Silva de Macêdo[1], Maria Cecília Freire de Melo[1], Andressa Kelly Alves Ferreira[1], Elizabeth Louisy Marques Soares da Silva[1], Jaciel Leandro de Melo Freitas[1], Arnaldo de França Caldas Jr[1,2].

[1] Universidade Federal de Pernambuco, Recife, Pernambuco, Brazil
[2] Universidade de Pernambuco, Camaragibe, Pernambuco, Brazil

ABSTRACT

Objective: To assess the impact and correlation of socioeconomic vulnerability on COVID-19 outcomes and social distancing in Brazil. **Methods:** The Gini Coefficient (GC), the Social Vulnerability Index (SVI), epidemiological data on COVID-19 epidemic in Brazil, and the Social Distancing Index (SDI) were retrieved from online databases and assessed for each Brazilian state. Data was statistically analyzed through non-parametric tests and multiple linear regressions. **Results:** The mean values for the GC and SVI were 0.495 and 0.261, respectively. A positive statistically significant correlation between the socioeconomic indicators and the three variables related to the COVID-19 outbreak was found. States with very low social vulnerability presented fewer deaths per 100 thousand inhabitants due to COVID-19 than states with moderate social vulnerability. SVI was a predictor of accumulated cases, confirmed deaths, and social distancing in Brazilian states during COVID-19. **Conclusions:** The COVID-19 outcomes and SDI in Brazilian states are correlated to the socioeconomic condition. The pandemic impacts are more severe in less favoured communities.

INTRODUCTION

Less than four months after the first confirmed case of the 2019 novel coronavirus disease (COVID-19) in Brazil, the country reaches the mark of more than one million accumulated cases, and over 50.000 confirmed deaths [1]. These numbers are estimated to be even greater, considering the likely occurrence of underreporting as the country is testing only severe cases [2]. During the pandemic, the country has been facing a political crisis, which has been misleading the efforts to mitigate COVID-19 spread and its socioeconomic impacts [3]. Brazil is the largest and most populous Latin-American country; its continental dimension favours to diversity in socioeconomic and geographical aspects [4].

---

[1] Corresponding Author: E-mail: caldasjr@alldeia.com.br

Each Brazilian region is different, based on social behaviour, genetics, and economic backgrounds raising the need for different measures and health policies to direct medical resources, and to manage social issues, respecting each area's particularities [2]. All regions in Brazil have confirmed cases of COVID-19 [1]. There is a socioeconomic disparity among regions corroborating several issues related with COVID-19 pandemic such as access and understanding of information about the disease, availability of diagnostic tests, health human resources, and intensive care units, besides the political decisions to control the pandemic [2,3]. Despite statements like "COVID-19 virus does not discriminate", made by some politicians and part of the media, COVID-19 is not a socially neutral disease [5]. Special attention must be paid to vulnerable populations, since recent reports indicate that incidence and deaths are disproportionately affecting less favoured communities [6,7,8]. Scientific evidence and broader surveillance are in urgent need to improve response and planning, such as resources allocation, to tackle health inequities in the current COVID19 pandemic [9]. Thus, the present study aims to assess the impact and correlation of socioeconomic vulnerability on COVID-19 outcomes and social distancing in Brazil.

METHODS

The Gini Coefficient (GC) and Social Vulnerability Index (SVI) were adopted as socioeconomic indicators. The values scored in these indicators for each Brazilian state were retrieved from the online database of the Brazilian Institute of Geography and Statistics [10] and the Institute of Applied Economic Research [11], respectively. In addition to socioeconomic indicators epidemiological data on COVID-19 epidemic in Brazil and the Social Distancing Index (SDI) were assessed for each Brazilian state.

The GC is a measure of statistical dispersion used in economics intended to represent the income or wealth distribution among residents of a certain area and is the most used measurement of inequality. This indicator has been applied in the health field to measure disparities. The GC value ranges from 0 (perfect equality, where every household earns the same income) to 1.0 (perfect inequality, where households earn a diverse range of incomes) [12]. The SVI is an index that seeks to highlight different indicatives of exclusion and social vulnerability in a perspective that goes further the comprehension of poverty only as insufficient monetary resources. Thus, the SVI intends to signal the access, absence, or insufficiency of some "assets" in areas of the Brazilian territory, which should be available to every citizen, by virtue of State action. The three sub-indices that comprise it are urban infrastructure, human capital, and income and labour.

Those sub-indices represent three large sets of assets, whose possession or deprivation determines the conditions of well-being of populations in contemporary societies. The index value ranges from 0 to 1, the closer to 1, the greater the social vulnerability of a region. Values between 0 and 0.200, indicate very low social vulnerability; between 0.201 and 0.300 indicate low social vulnerability; between 0.301 and 0.400 indicate moderate social vulnerability; between 0.401 and 0.500 indicate high social vulnerability; and between 0.501 and 1 indicate very high social vulnerability [13]. Epidemiological data concerning accumulated cases and confirmed deaths (per 100 thousand inhabitants) due to COVID-19 in each state were collected from the Brazilian government Health Ministry database, available online [1]. The data used in this research comprises information from February 25, 2020 (first case recorded in Brazil) to June 20, 2020.

The SDI was created to help mitigate the spread of COVID-19, since its launch, it has been improved with the sole objective of providing increasingly accurate data for public authorities and research institutes.

To achieve the index, highly accurate geolocation data was treated with a distance algorithm. Polygons from all regions of the IBGE were adopted to ensure a more accurate categorization and more reliable data [14].

Data is available on the Inloco website[1] displayed as a map and chart. SDI values are represented in percentual of social distancing, ranging from 0 to 100%. Data were submitted to statistical analysis, all tests were applied considering an error of 5% and the confidence interval of 95%, and the analyzes were carried out using SPSS software version 23.0 (SPSS Inc. Chicago, IL, USA). As the hypothesis of normal distribution of data was not confirmed by the Kolmogorov-Smirnov test, the statistical analysis was performed through the application of nonparametric tests. The strength of the association between distinct measures was tested with Spearman rank correlation. States in different groups according with SVI categorization were compared by KruskalWallis test and post-hoc Dunn test. Multiple linear regressions were performed to verify whether GC or SVI were predictors of accumulated cases, confirmed deaths, and social distancing index in Brazilian states during COVID-19 outbreak.

RESULTS

For the period evaluated, the mean of accumulated cases and confirmed deaths per 100 thousand inhabitants in the Brazilian states was approximately 697 and 24, respectively. The states mean SDI score was 38.77%. Regarding the socioeconomic indicators, the mean values for the GC and SVI were, respectively, 0.495 and 0.261, as shown in table 1. The SVI values ranged from 0.134 to 0.374, thus none of the states presented high or very high social vulnerability. The comparison among states with different social vulnerability indices found statistically significant differences in the number of deaths. States with very low social vulnerability presented fewer deaths per 100 thousand inhabitants due to COVID-19 than states with moderate social vulnerability, as shown in table 2.

The Spearman correlation test found a positive statistically significant correlation between the socioeconomic indicators and the three variables related to the COVID-19 outbreak in Brazil, except for the correlation between the GC and confirmed deaths (table 3). The analysis of multiple linear regressions resulted in statistically significant models where the SVI was a predictor of accumulated cases, confirmed deaths, and social distancing index in Brazil during COVID-19 epidemic. Higher SVI, indicative of greater social vulnerability, was associated with higher accumulated cases (β = 0.409; t=2.243; p=0.034), confirmed deaths (β = 0.498; t=2.874; p=0.008), and social distancing index (β = 0.544; t=3.242; p=0.003). The values that describe these relationships are shown in table 4.

DISCUSSION

Health inequities are a worldwide issue [5]. The COVID-19 pandemic can affect the whole of society, however, its repercussions will be experienced in different ways, depending on the level of equity that exists in each social reality [15]. The findings of the present study support this statement since areas with different socioeconomic conditions are not being proportionally affected in Brazil. The number of confirmed deaths due to COVID-19 presented a positive correlation with GC and SVI

---

[1] (https://mapabrasileirodacovid.inloco.com.br/pt/)

(table 3). In addition, states with moderate social vulnerability presented an average of 30 deaths per 100 thousand inhabitants more than states with very low social vulnerability (table 2).

Furthermore, greater social vulnerability was a predictor of increase in deaths (table 4). These findings demonstrate the impact of socioeconomic vulnerability on COVID-19 mortality. Vulnerable communities are also disproportionately affected by pre-existing chronic conditions. Studies carried out in Brazilian populations found that in areas with more marked poverty or inequality a higher prevalence of hypertension [16], diabetes [17], cancer [18], asthma [19], and multiple comorbidities[20] were observed, those conditions represent an increased risk for severe COVID-19 health outcomes [21, 22]. In addition, the availability of resources such as diagnostic tests, intensive care units, and health human resources are not equally distributed in the Brazilian territory [2]. Risk communication is an integral element of any public health emergency response [23], however, vulnerable populations may not have the necessary language and literacy skills to understand and appropriately respond to pandemic messaging [15] because low health literacy is more prevalent among vulnerable populations [24].

This may be associated with the difficulty to control the spread of COVID-19, particularly in regions of greater social vulnerability. In addition, lower sanitary standards, and the inability to maintain social distancing due to the need to leave home in search of work and income increase the exposure risk of people in social vulnerability. In the present study income inequality and social vulnerability showed a positive correlation with the cumulative cases of COVID-19 (table 3). SVI was a predictor of increased cases per 100 thousand inhabitants in Brazilian states (table 4).

These findings support studies that alert to health inequalities during COVID-19 pandemic [5, 25].

Social distancing measures to control the spread of COVID-19 are likely to have large effects on health and health inequalities[26]. Countries worldwide implemented rigorous isolation measures in response to the pandemic. The aim of social distancing is to mitigate transmission by reducing close contact, however, the measures have profound socioeconomic and health consequences [26].

In Brazil, according to the present investigation, the SDI is correlated to the socioeconomic status, as shown in table 3. In addition, greater social vulnerability was predictor of increased SDI in Brazilian states. Since socioeconomic disparities are an aggravating factor in the course of the health crisis, it is expected that, in response to higher rates of cases and deaths, as shown by the findings of the present study, more stricter measures of social distancing are implemented in more vulnerable areas. Social distancing has led to a reduced workforce in all economic sectors and has caused job losses, resulting in income losses for workers unable to work and increased long-term unemployment if companies fail [26, 27].

Isolation measures should be thoughtfully planned and executed, policymakers must consider its broader effects on health and health equity, otherwise, the decrease in income will exacerbate the pre-existing socioeconomic disparities, deepening the problems of local health inequity in epidemic areas [9, 28]. Besides the immediate health effects for the vulnerable populations, the pandemic will certainly have long-term socioeconomic impacts on less favoured communities [9]. The public health policy responses must ensure that considerations of health equity and social justice principles remain at the forefront of pandemic responses to ensure that the COVID-19 pandemic does not increase health inequalities for future generations [5].

CONCLUSIONS

The COVID-19 outcomes and SDI in Brazilian states are correlated to the socioeconomic condition. States with moderate social vulnerability presented more deaths per 100 thousand inhabitants than states with very low social vulnerability. SVI was a predictor of accumulated cases, confirmed deaths, and social distancing index in Brazilian states during COVID-19. Health authorities might apply these data on disease control efforts, guiding interventions and resource allocations to improve outcomes in vulnerable communities.

ACKNOWLEDGMENTS

The authors would like to thank the Coordenação de Aperfeiçoamento de Pessoal de Nível Superior (CAPES) for scholarship granting.

REFERENCES

1. Brazilian Health Ministry. *Painel Coronavírus (2020)* [accessed 20/06/2020]. Available at: https://covid.saude.gov.br/.
2. Marson FL, Ortega M. COVID-19 in Brazil. *Pulmonology* 2020; 26(4):241-244.
3. The Lancet. COVID-19 in Brazil: "So What?". *Lancet* 2020; 395(1): 1461.
4. The Brazilian EPIGEN Project Consortium. Origin and dynamics of admixture in Brazilians and its effect on the pattern of deleterious mutations. *PNAS* 2015; 112 (28): 8696-8701.
5. Bambra C, Riordan R, Ford J, Matthews F. The COVID-19 pandemic and health inequalities. *J Epidemiol Community Health* 2020; 0: 1-5.
6. Dorn A, Cooney RE, Sabin ML. COVID-19 exacerbating inequalities in the US. *Lancet* 2020; 395(10232):1243-1244.
7. Turner-Musa J, Ajayi O, Kemp L. Examining Social Determinants of Health, Stigma, and COVID-19 Disparities. *Healthcare* 2020; 8: 1-7.
8. Dyer O. Covid-19: Black People and Other Minorities Are Hardest Hit in US. *BMJ* 2020; 369: 1-2.
9. Wang Z, Tang K. Combating COVID-19: Health Equity Matters. *Nature* 2020; 26: 458–464.
10. Brazilian Institute of Geography and Statistics (IBGE). *Continuous National Household Sample Survey - Continuous PNAD*. Brasília: 2019.
11. Institute of Applied Economic Research (IPEA). *Atlas of Social Vulnerability*. Brasília: 2017.
12. Pabayo R, Chiavegatto Filho ADP, Lebrão ML, Kawachi I. Income Inequality and Mortality: Results From a Longitudinal Study of Older Residents of São Paulo, Brazil. *Am J Public Health* 2013; 103(9):43-49.
13. Institute of Applied Economic Research (IPEA). *Atlas of social vulnerability in Brazilian municipalities*. Brasília: 2015.
14. Inloco. *Mapa brasileiro da COVID-19* [accessed 23/05/2020]. Available at: https://mapabrasileirodacovid.inloco.com.br/pt/.
15. Smith JA, Judd J. COVID-19: Vulnerability and the power of privilege in a pandemic. *Health Promot J Austr* 2020; 31:158-160.
16. Santos DMS, Prado BS, Oliveira CCC, Almeida-Santos MA. Prevalence of Systemic Arterial Hypertension in Quilombola Communities, State of Sergipe, Brazil. *Arq Bras Cardiol* 2019; 113(3):383-390.
17. Meiners M et al, Tavares NUL, Guimarães LSP, Bertoldi AD, Dal Pizzol TS, Luiza VL, Mengue SS, Merchan-Hamann E. Access and Adherence to Medication Among People with Diabetes in Brazil: Evidences from PNAUM. *Rev Bras Epidemiol* 2017; 20(3):445-459.
18. Barbosa IR, Souza DL, Bernal MM, Costa ICC. Cancer mortality in Brazil: Temporal Trends and Predictions for the Year 2030. *Medicine (Baltimore)* 2015; 94(16): 1-6.

19. Cunha SS, Pujades-Rodriguez M, Barreto ML, Genser B, Rodrigues LC. Ecological study of socio-economic indicators and prevalence of asthma in schoolchildren in urban Brazil. *BMC Public Health* 2007; 7(1): 1-6.

20. Cabral JF, Silva AMC, Mattos IE, Neves AQ, Luz LL, Ferreira DB, Santiago LM, Carmo CN. Vulnerability and Associated Factors Among Older People Using the Family Health Strategy. *Cien Saude Colet* 2019; 24(9): 3227-3236.

21. Xu PP, Luo S, Tian RH, Zu ZY. Risk Factors for Adverse Clinical Outcomes with COVID-19 in China: A Multicenter, Retrospective, Observational Study. *Theranostics* 2020; 10(14):6372-6383.

22. China Medical Treatment Expert Group for COVID-19. Comorbidity and its impact on 1590 patients with COVID-19 in China: a nationwide analysis. *Eur Respir J* 2020; 55(5): 1-14.

23. Shrivastava SR, Shrivastava PS, Ramasamy J. Risk Communication: An Integral Element in Public Health Emergencies. *Int J Prev Med* 2016; 7(1): 1-2.

24. Lynch M, Franklin G. Strategies to Reduce Hospital Mortality in Lower and Middle Income Countries (LMICs) and Resource-Limited Settings. *IntechOpen* 2020.

25. Ramírez I, Lee J. COVID-19 Emergence and Social and Health Determinants in Colorado: A Rapid Spatial Analysis. *Int J Environl Res Public Health* 2020; 17(11): 1-15.

26. Douglas M, Katikireddi SV, Taulbut M, McKee M, McCartney G. Mitigating the Wider Health Effects of covid-19 Pandemic Response. *BMJ* 2020; 369: 1-6.

27. Nicola M, Alsafi Z, Sohrabi C, Kerwan A, Al-Jabir A, Iosifidis C, Agha M, Agha R. The socio-economic implications of the coronavirus pandemic (COVID-19): A review. Int J Surg 2020; 78:185-193.

28. Ioannidis JPA. Coronavirus disease 2019: The harms of exaggerated information and non-evidence-based

29. measures. Eur J Clin Invest 2020; 50: 1-5.

Table 1. Descriptive Statistics of Socioeconomic Vulnerability Indicators And COVID-19 Outcomes in Brazilian States

Variables	Mean (SD)	Median	Minimum	Maximum
Gini Coefficient	0.495 (0.039)	0.495	0.398	0.548
Social Vulnerability Index	0.261 (0.056)	0.258	0.134	0.374
COVID-19 cases[†]	697.48 (510)	541.00	113	2353
COVID-19 deaths[†]	23.76 (18.537)	19.76	1.44	63.31
Social Distancing Index	38.76 (2.68)	39.65	30.70	42.65

per 100 thousand inhabitants

Table 2.. Descriptive statistics of different Brazilian states groups according with degree of social vulnerability.

	Very low social vulnerability (n=4)	Low social vulnerability (n=18)	Moderate social vulnerability (n=5)
COVID-19 cases[†]			
Mean (SD)	329.2 (322.6)	693.7 (534.9)	1005.6 (376.6)
Median	198	523.5	968
Minimum	113	123	520
Maximum	808	2356	1488
COVID-19 deaths[†]			
Mean (SD)	7.6 (9.6)*	23.5 (18.1)	37.6 (16.3)*
Median	3.5	18.2	33.1
Minimum	1.4	2.8	23.2
Maximum	22	60.1	63.3
Social Distancing Index			
Mean (SD)	36 (4.2)	38.9 (2.1)	40.2 (1.6)
Median	36.2	39.1	40.1
Minimum	30.7	34.3	38.1
Maximum	40.1	42.9	42.6

†per 100 thousand inhabitants

* Significant statistical differences between the groups (Kruskal-Wallis test and post-hoc Dunn test)

Table 3 Correlation between socioeconomic disparities indicators measures and COVID-19 outcomes in Brazilian states.

	Gini coefficient	Social Vulnerability Index
COVID-19 cases†	0.490*	0.504**
COVID-19 deaths†	0.356*	0.544**
Social Distancing Index	0.394*	0.520**

Spearman's correlation test

†per 100 thousand inhabitants

* p≤0.05; ** p≤0.01

Table 4. Multiple linear regression according to the Social Vulnerability Index.

Variables in the equation

	F	df	R²	β	t	95% Confidence Interval		p-value
						Lower bound	Upper bound	
)VID-19 cases†	5.031	1	0.168	0.409	2.243	46.387	280.860	0.034
OVID-19 deaths†	8.262	1	0.248	0.498	2.874	302.223	7091.379	0.008
Social stancing Index	10.513	1	0.296	0.544	3.242	9.426	42.251	0.003

†per 100 thousand inhabitants

8. Determinants of Physical Distancing During The Covid-19 Epidemic In Brazil: Effects From Mandatory Rules, Numbers of Cases And Duration Of Rules

Rodrigo Fracalossi de Moraes

ABSTRACT

During the covid-19 pandemic, physical distancing is being promoted to reduce the disease transmission and pressure on health systems. Yet, what determines physical distancing? Through a panel data analysis, this article identifies some of its determinants.

Using a specifically built index that measures the strictness of physical distancing rules in the 27 Brazilian states, this paper isolates the effect of mandatory physical distancing rules from other potential determinants of physical distancing. The article concludes that physical distancing is influenced by at least three variables: the strictness of mandatory physical distancing rules, the number of confirmed cases of covid-19, and the duration of rules. Evidence also indicates that the effect of physical distancing measures is relatively stronger than that of the number of cases physical distancing is determined proportionally more by mandatory policies than people's awareness about the severity of the epidemic. These results have at least two policy implications. First, governments should adopt mandatory measures in order to increase physical distancing – rather than expect people to adopt them on their own. Second, the timing of adopting them is important, since people are unlikely to comply with them for long periods of time.

What Determines Physical Distancing?

In the context of an epidemic in which there are no better alternatives to reduce the transmission of a disease and no effective treatment, the answer to this question might determine government policies to contain an epidemic. If people practice physical distancing voluntarily, based on the severity of the epidemic or out of a sense of social responsibility, strict physical distancing measures would be largely unnecessary.

However, if people respond mainly to mandatory restrictions (closing non-essential shops, suspending classes, suspending mass gatherings, etc), governments should adopt these non-pharmaceutical interventions (NPIs) in order to contain an epidemic. **Maloney and Taskin (2020)**[1] argued that the covid-19 pandemic *per se* led to voluntary demobilization and that this effect is stronger than that of NPIs, what was observed in all but the poorest countries.

This finding was reinforced by case studies on the US and Sweden, where evidence indicates that physical distancing increased *before* mandatory measures were adopted. The causal mechanism could be not only the fear of getting infected but also empathy for those most vulnerable to the virus[2] or people's belief in science[3]. If this is true, lifting restrictive measures during the epidemic would not have a great impact, as people would practice physical distancing anyway. From a different angle, Engle et al.[4], **Brzezinski et al. (2020)**[5]**, Painter and Qiu**[6] **and Anderson et al**

(2020).[7]demonstrated that mandatory physical distancing measures in the United States significantly increased the probability of someone staying at home.

In addition, physical distancing levels may depend on the length of restrictions on people's mobility: the longer they last the higher the costs for people to stay at home, reducing their probability of complying with physical distancing rules. Frequent extensions may also create confusion and frustration, leading people to reduce levels of compliance, something that was observed in Italy[8]. Through a panel data analysis, this paper seeks to answer the question of what influences physical distancing during the covid-19 pandemic. It looks at the effects of mandatory physical distancing rules, numbers of covid-19 cases, and the duration of mandatory rules on the levels of physical distancing in Brazil. As physical distancing policies in Brazil were implemented mainly by states (27 in total, including the Federal District), comparing their policies and respective outcomes might indicate the extent to what mandatory policies are necessary to increase physical distancing in the context of an epidemic. Evidence presented in this article suggests that levels of physical distancing are positively correlated with the strictness of mandatory restrictions and the severity of the epidemic, as well as negatively correlated with the number of days since the first mandatory measures were adopted.

METHOD AND DATA

In order to identify some of the potential determinants of physical distancing levels during the covid-19 pandemic in Brazil I conducted a panel data analysis (using a balanced panel) covering the period 22 Mar – 24 May 2020. I created a daily series for all variables starting from 22 Mar, when all Brazilian states had reported at least one case of covid-19. The model has the following variables and uses the following data sources.

Dependent Variable: Physical Distancing

The Brazilian geolocation company In Loco generates data on daily levels of physical distancing discriminated by state, using data collected through apps in over 60 million smartphones in Brazil. The company monitors movement trends, producing data similar to those of Google Mobility Reports. In Loco uses various apps, including those of the main telecommunication companies, retailer stores, banks, etc. in Brazil[9]. Data is aggregated into the 'social distancing index', which is used here as a proxy for physical distancing, a method used in previous research[10,11]. The index has values expressed in percentages (in a scale of 0% to 100%), in which 100% is a hypothetical situation in which the whole population stays at home for a whole day. In the model, I use rolling averages (7 days) to minimize the effect of short-term variations.

Independent Variables: Strictness of Mandatory Physical Distancing Rules

I created an index that measures the strictness of physical distancing rules, which I have called the *physical distancing rules index* (PDI). This index is composed of six variables, measuring: whether mass gatherings, as well as cultural, sport or religious activities are suspended; whether bars, pubs, restaurants and similar places are closed; whether non-essential shops are closed; whether non-essential industries are closed; whether classes are suspended; and whether there are restrictions on passenger transportation. Each of these variables represents a type of agglomeration of people that may be restricted by NPIs: if these activities were all suspended, the aggregate effect should be a broad reduction in the number of agglomerations. For each of these variables, values o f 2, 1 or 0 were assigned depending on whether suspension or restriction was full, partial or non-existent (details are in Table 1 and Chart 1). As the sum of the values would vary between 0 and 12 (there are six variables), the index's values w ere adjusted to be between 0 and 10 (a more intuitive scale), in which 10 is the greatest level of restriction. This index has at least one caveat: its values are a non-weighted sum of the variables, regardless of how much the activities they measure produce in terms of agglomerations. This could be corrected by an index with weighted variables, but this would require data about how much different activities produce agglomerations of people (not available) or arbitrary assumptions.

Number of Cases of Covid-19

A high number of cases should make people more aware of the epidemic or more afraid of getting infected, which is likely to influence their behaviour. In the model, I use rolling averages (7 days) to compensate for random factors affecting the number of reported cases in a given day. For example, cases during weekends and bank holidays take longer to be reported to the Ministry of Health. which consolidates data from all Brazilian states. Underreporting is of course a problem, but the high correlation between the number of cases and the number of deaths (0.80) indicates that underreporting rates did not vary substantially over time. Number of deaths were not used in the model due to a high number of observations with a value of zero: in a log scale these observations would either be discarded or have arbitrary values, which is likely to bias results. Data for this variable come from Brazil's Ministry of Health.

Duration of physical distancing rules

Levels of physical distancing should be negatively correlated with the number of days since mandatory physical distancing rules were introduced. The longer the rules last the less likely people are to comply with them (holding everything else constant), which should occur for a few reasons: their savings (in case they have them) were all spent; people are looking for jobs or need to increase their income; social isolation produces stress; or people may seek to escape from domestic abuse. In the model, this variable is measured by the number of days since the first mandatory physical distancing rule was introduced in a given state.

Levels of Development

In poorer places people should be less likely to practice physical distancing as they are less likely to have savings and more likely to have informal jobs, reducing incentives for them to stay at home. This variable is measured through GDP per capita, which has a substantial variation in Brazil: between R$ 12,800 a year in the poorest state (Maranhão) and R$ 80,500 in the richest one (Distrito Federal). The interpretation of results for this variable should be cautious though as it is likely to capture the effect of others: lower levels of GDP per capita are associated with a lower number of ICU beds, a lower percentage of people living in urban areas, a lower population density, less access to reliable information and a lower educational level, which might all influence levels of physical distancing. Data for this variable come from the Brazilian Institute of Geography and Statistics (IBGE)

# of the variable	Description of the variable	Values
1	Mass gatherings and cultural, sport or religious activities	2 = Full suspension
2	Bars, pubs, restaurants and similar places	1 = Partial suspension or restriction
3	Non-essential shops	0 = No suspension or restriction
4	Non-essential industries	
5	Classes	
6	Public transportation	

- Information used to code the values of these variables come from open sources, especially legal documents from state governments, complemented by news from local media. Details are in the Chart 1 and in Moraes[12,13]. The original dataset is in Moraes[14].

Chart 1. Variables And Values Of The Physical Distancing Rules Index (PDI).

Variable 1 (mass gatherings and cultural, sport or religious activities)
Full (2):
The following activities or places are suspended or closed: gatherings with more than 20 people, gyms, religious temples, concert halls, cinemas, theatres, cultural centres, etc. Partial (1):
At least one of the abovementioned activities or places is suspended or closed (even if only in part of the territory).
No suspension (0):
None of the abovementioned activities or places is suspended or closed.

Variable 2 (bars, pubs, restaurants, etc.)
Full (2):
The following places must remain closed: bars, pubs, restaurants, cafés, etc. (except for takeaway or delivery) Partial (1):
At least one of the abovementioned places' activities is suspended or there are strict rules for those that remain open (even if only in part of the territory), including the use of no more than 50% of their capacity.
No suspension (0):
None of the abovementioned places has to suspend or reduce activities.

Variable 3 (non-essential shops)
Full (2):
Only essential shops and services can remain open
Partial (1):
Some non-essential shops or services can remain open (for example: electronic stores, clothing shops or beauty salons) or they can remain open but limited to up to 50% of their capacity (even if only in part of the territory).
No suspension (0):
None of the abovementioned places has to suspend or reduce activities.

Variable 4 (non-essential industry)
Full (2):
Only essential industries can remain open.
Partial (1):
Some non-essential industries can remain open or they can operate at a maximum of 50% of their capacity (even if only in part of the territory).
No suspension (0):
There are no restrictions.

Variable 5 (classes)
Full (2):
All classes are suspended.
Partial (1):
Some classes are authorized,or schools can open with a maximum of 50% of their capacity (even if only in part of the territory).
No suspension (0):
There are no restrictions.

Variable 6 (public transportation)
Full (2):
Both intermunicipal and interstate public transportation are suspended.
Partial (1):
Only intermunicipal or interstate public transportation is suspended, or they can operate with a maximum of 50% of their capacity (even if only in part of the territory).
No suspension (0):
There are no restrictions.

Health infrastructure

In places with limited health infrastructure, people should have more incentives to practice physical distancing as they would be less likely to have healthcare available. In the model, this is measured by the number of ICU beds per 100,000 people. Data for this variable come from Brazil's Ministry of Health (DATASUS).

Political party or coalition in power

The ideology of a government in power might indicate people's willingness to practice physical distancing. A stronger sense of social responsibility might be more common among leftwing people, so that voters who elected left-wing candidates would be more likely to practice physical distancing. In contrast, people who elected right-wing candidates might put more emphasis on their freedom of going and coming, making them less likely to practice physical distancing. In the model there are three values for this variable: 0 for a left-wing party or coalition; 1 for a centrist party or coalition; or 2 for a right-wing party or coalition.

Population density

People living in places with a high population density have a greater risk of getting infected and infecting others, creating more incentives for people to stay at home. In the model, this is measured by the log of the population density. Data for this variable come from the Brazilian Institute of Geography and Statistics (IBGE).

RESULTS AND DISCUSSION

As observed in Figure 1, values of the PDI are highly and positively correlated with values of the social distancing index, suggesting that these two phenomena are associated.

Yet, there is substantial variation across states, suggesting that other variables also determine levels of physical distancing. Moreover, physical distancing's decrease over time was on average higher than the decrease in the strictness of mandatory physical distancing rules. This is puzzling because it coincided with rising numbers of cases and deaths due to covid-19, which should make people comply more – rather than less with physical distancing rules. This indicates that the length of legal rules of physical distancing may be negatively correlated with levels of physical distancing.

Results from a panel data analysis indicate that levels of physical distancing depend on the strictness of mandatory physical distancing rules, on the number of confirmed cases of covid-19 and on the number of days since the first mandatory measures were introduced. As observed in Table 2, the coefficients of these three variables were similar across different models. An increase of one additional unit in the PDI (which has a scale of 0 to 10) is expected to increase physical distancing by about 0.8 percentage point. The effect of an increase in the number of cases is also significant: one additional unit increases physical distancing by about 0.9 percentage point.

Yet, it is important to consider that one unit in the log scale represents an increase of about 3 times in the number of cases per 100,000 people. Consequently, an increase of 3 times in the number of cases have an effect only slightly stronger than the effect of increasing one additional unit in the strictness of mandatory physical distancing rules. The duration of mandatory physical distancing measures is also statistically significant: holding everything else constant, an additional day of physical distancing mandatory rules decreases physical distancing by about 0.2 percentage point. This implies that keeping physical distancing levels constant over time requires an increase in the strictness of physical distancing rules or other measures that increase physical distancing (Table 2).Data indicates that GDP per capita might have an influence but it does not add predictive power to the model. Due to a high or medium correlation of GDP per capita with the number of ICUs per 100,000 people (correl = 0.82), the ideology of the political party/coalition in power (correl = -0.50), and population density (correl = 0.34), separate models with each of these variables were built. The number of ICU beds and population density were significant but did not increase the predictive power of the models, and the political party (or coalition) in power was not statistically significant. The R^2 values for models with state dummies should be interpreted with caution as they are inflated by the use of these dummies. The R^2 of 0.54 in model 2 indicates a good predictive power of the model, suggesting that more than 50% of the variation in physical distancing levels is caused by the strictness of physical distancing rules, the number of confirmed covid-19 cases, and the length of mandatory physical distancing measures.

There are at least three limitations in these models. First, the physical distancing rules index captures only the suspension or restriction of activities, not including measures that are also essential to contain an epidemic, such as awareness campaigns, mandatory use of PPE, cash transfers (which encourages people to stay at home), or the enforcement of legal rules. Second, the models do not capture overall social norms, which may lead people to stay at home more in certain states than in others. Third, there is variation over time for the independent variables of interest (strictness of physical distancing rules, number of covid-19 cases, and number of days since mandatory measures were introduced), but not for the other covariates, either because there was no daily data available or because they only change substantially over larger periods of time. Therefore, the results for population density, GDP per capita, ideology and ICU beds should be interpreted with caution.

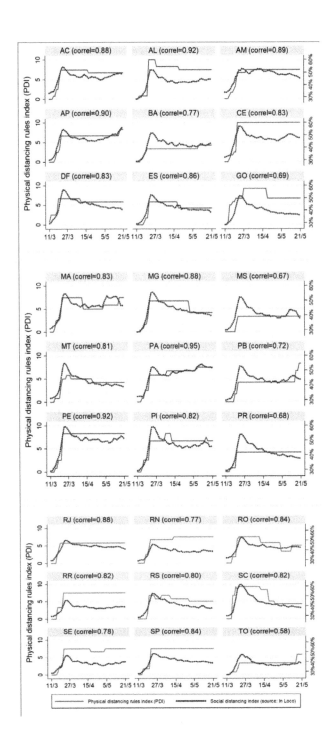

Figure 1. Physical Distancing Rules Index (PDI) And Social Distancing Index, 11 Mar-21-May (Only Business Days).

- Centred-moving averages (3 days) for values of the social distancing index.
- AC: Acre, AL: Alagoas, AM: Amazonas, AP: Amapá, BA: Bahia, CE: Ceará, DF: Distrito Federal, ES: Espírito Santo, GO: Goiás, MA: Maranhão, MG: Minas Gerais, MS: Mato Grosso do Sul, MT: Mato Grosso, PA: Pará, PB: Paraíba, PE: Pernambuco, PI: Piauí, PR: Paraná, RJ: Rio de Janeiro, RN: Rio Grande do Norte, RO: Rondônia, RR: Roraima, RS: Rio Grande do Sul, SC: Santa Catarina, SE: Sergipe, SP: São Paulo, TO: Tocantins.

Table 2. Determinants Of Physical Distancing In Brazil (22 March – 24 May 2020).4

Social distancing index (0-100%)	(1)	(2)	(3)	(4)	(5)	(6)
Physical distancing rules index (PDI)	0.799*** (0.055)	0.788*** (0.054)	0.799*** (0.055)	0.799*** (0.055)	0.799*** (0.055)	0.799*** (0.055)
Number of days	-0.194*** (0.007)	-0.195*** (0.006)	-0.194*** (0.007)	-0.194*** (0.007)	-0.194*** (0.007)	-0.194*** (0.007)
Log cases	0.926*** (0.075)	0.945*** (0.074)	0.926*** (0.075)	0.926*** (0.075)	0.926*** (0.075)	0.926*** (0.075)
Log GDP per capita			1.008** (0.298)			
ICU beds				0.048** (0.014)		
Ideology					0.048 (0.445)	
Log population density						0.287** (0.085)
Constant	49.287*** (0.533)	49.166*** (0.600)	39.118*** (3.239)	48.362*** (0.682)	49.287*** (0.533)	49.370*** (0.524)
State dummies	Yes	No	Yes	Yes	Yes	Yes
# of observations	1.725	1.725	1.725	1.725	1.725	1.725
R^2	0.772	0.544	0.772	0.772	0.772	0.772

*** $p < 0.001$, ** $p < 0.01$, *< 0.05.
- The numbers of the models are indicated at the top row.
- Physical distancing rules index (PDI): strictness of mandatory physical distancing rules; number of days: days since the first mandatory physical distancing rules was adopted; log cases: log of the number of new confirmed cases; Log GDP per capita: log of the GDP per capita; ICU beds: number of ICU beds per 100,000 people; ideology: ideology of the political party or coalition in power (left-wing, centre or right-wing); log population density: log of the population density.

These findings do not imply that similar results should be found in other countries, as there might be specific determinants in Brazil not captured in this model. Among others, the federal government encouraged people not to respect physical distancing and sought to undermine states' policies of physical distancing, which is likely to have influenced people's behaviour[15].

CONCLUSIONS

This paper was an attempt to estimate the determinants of physical distancing levels. Results show that mandatory physical distancing rules and the number of confirmed covid-19 cases are positively correlated with physical distancing levels, while the duration of rules are negatively correlated with them. It also shows that the effect of physical distancing mandatory rules is relatively stronger than the effect of the number of cases, suggesting that people respond more to mandatory rules of physical distancing than to the severity of the epidemic. These findings have at least two policy implications. First, increasing physical distancing to high levels requires governments to adopt mandatory measures, especially when numbers of cases and deaths are not high. For a variety of reasons, a substantial part of the population seems to have a risk-taking behaviour, which might result from economic needs, cultural or psychological traits, or influence from pandemic-negationists. Second, evidence indicates that mandatory physical distancing rules have an 'expiry date': for a variety of reasons people's compliance with mandatory rules decrease over time, even if the number of cases and deaths from covid-19 increases.

This implies that the 'timing' for adopting mandatory measures is important, as compliance with rules might decrease when it is most needed. This also implies that keeping levels of physical distancing constant over time are likely to require additional mandatory restrictions, a greater enforcement or non-mandatory measures (awareness campaigns or cash transfers to people, for example). This problem might be minimized by an on-off lockdown policy, as suggested by Scherbina[16], which may not be the best solution from an epidemiological point of view, but necessary in some cases for practical reasons.

Acknowledgements
I would like to thank Acir dos Santos Almeida, Amanda Reis Montenegro, Flávia de Holanda Schmidt, Paulo de Tarso Linhares and an anonymous reviewer for comments and suggestions on drafts of this paper or the research project as a whole.

REFERENCES

1. Maloney WF, Taskin T. Determinants of social distancing and economic activity during COVID-19: A global view. *World Bank Policy Res Work Pap* 2020. [cited 2020 Jun 9]. Available from: http://documents. worldbank.org/curated/en/325021589288466494/ Determinants-of-Social-Distancing-and-Economic-Activity-during-COVID-19-A-Global-View.

2. Pfattheicher S, Nockur L, Böhm R, Sassenrath C, Petersen MB. The emotional path to action: Empathy promotes physical distancing during the COVID-19 pandemic. [Preprint] 2020. [cited 2020 Jun 9]. Available from: https://psyarxiv.com/y2cg5.

3. Brzezinski A, Kecht V, Van Dijcke D, Wright AL. Belief in science influences physical distancing in response to covid-19 lockdown policies. *Univ Chic Becker Friedman Inst Econ Work Pap.* 2020. [cited 2020 Jun 9]. Available from: https://bfi.uchicago.edu/working-paper/belief-in-science-influences-physical-distancing-in-response-to-covid-19-lockdown-policies

4. Engle S, Stromme J, Zhou A. Staying at home: mobility effects of covid-19. *Covid Economics* 2020; 4:86102.

5. Brzezinski A, Deiana G, Kecht V, Van Dijcke D. The covid-19 pandemic: government vs. community action across the United States. *INET Oxford Work Pap* 2020; 06. [cited 2020 Jun 9]. Available from: https://

www.inet.ox.ac.uk/publications/no-2020-06-thecovid-19-pandemic-government-vs-communityaction-across-the-united-states.

6. Painter M, Qiu T. Political beliefs affect compliance with covid-19 social distancing orders. [Preprint] 2020. [cited 2020 Jun 9]. Available from: SSRN 3569098.

7. Anderson RM, Heesterbeek H, Klinkenberg D, Hollingsworth TD. How will country-based mitigation measures influence the course of the COVID-19 epidemic? *Lancet* 2020; 395(10228):931-934.

8. Briscese G, Lacetera N, Macis M, Tonin M. Compliance with covid-19 social-distancing measures in Italy: the role of expectations and duration. *IZA - Institute of Labor Economics Discussion Paper Series* 2020. [cited 2020 Jun 9]. Available from: http://ftp.iza.org/ dp13092.pdf.

9. In Loco. Mapa brasileiro da COVID-19 [Internet]. In Loco; 2020. [cited 2020 Jun 9]. Available from: https:// mapabrasileirodacovid.inloco.com.br/pt.

10. Ajzenman N, Cavalcanti T, Da Mata D. *More than words: Leaders' speech and risky behavior during a pandemic.* [Preprint] 2020. [cited 2020 Jun 9]. Available from: SSRN 3582908.

11. Peixoto PS, Marcondes DR, Peixoto CM, Queiroz L, Gouveia R, Delgado A, Oliva SM. *Potential dissemination of epidemics based on Brazilian mobile geolocation data. Part I: Population dynamics and future spreading of infection in the states of São Paulo and Rio de Janeiro during the pandemic of COVID-19.* [Preprint] 2020. [cited 2020 Jun 9].

12. Moraes RF. Medidas legais de incentivo ao distanciamento social: comparação das políticas de governos estaduais e prefeituras das capitais no Brasil. *Nota Téc - Ipea.* 2020; 16. [cited 2020 Jun 9]. Available from: https://www.ipea.gov.br/portal/images/stories/PDFs/ nota_tecnica/200415_dinte_n_16.pdf.

13. Moraes RF. Covid-19 e medidas legais de distanciamento social: tipologia de políticas estaduais e análise do período de 13 a 26 de abril de 2020. *Nota Téc - Ipea.* 2020; 18. [cited 2020 Jun 9]. Available from: http://www.ipea.gov.br/portal/images/stories/PDFs/ nota_tecnica/200429_nt18_covid-19.pdf.

14. Moraes RF. Índice de medidas legais de distanciamento social. Brasília: Ipea; 2020.

15. Ajzenman N, Cavalcanti T, Da Mata D. *More than words: Leaders' speech and risky behavior during a pandemic.* [Preprint] 2020. [cited 2020 Jun 9]. Available from: SSRN 3582908.

16. Scherbina A. *Determining the optimal duration of the COVID-19 suppression policy: A cost-benefit analysis.* [Preprint] 2020. [cited 2020 Jun 9]. Available from: SSRN 3562053.

CHAPTER 22

MANAGING DEATHS BY COVID-19

1. Deaths Due To COVID-19 In Brazil: How Many Are There And Which Are Being Identified?

Elisabeth Barboza Franç[I,II] , Lenice HarumiIshitani II ,
Renato Azeredo Teixeira[II] ,Daisy Maria Xavier de Abreu[II] ,
Paulo Roberto Lopes Corrêa[I,III] Fatima Marinho[II,IV]
Ana Maria Nogales Vasconcelos[V]

ABSTRACT

COVID-19 was initially notified in February, 2020, in Brazil, and the first death was reported on March 17[1]. Since then, national spread has been rapid, with over 9,000 deaths reported less than two months later[2]. These deaths refer to people who tested positive for the polymerase chain reaction test (PCR), which detects the genetic material of SARS-CoV-2 and establishes the presence of the virus. This figure, however, represents only the tip of the iceberg, because the PCR test has been performed with priority on hospitalized patients under suspicion of having the disease and, in some states, as a *post-mortem* exam[3]. It can be deduced that there are certainly many deaths from suspected cases without a confirmed diagnosis. Thus, two major challenges are how to estimate the degree of underreported deaths due to COVID-19 and what the actual number is.

DEATH CERTIFICATE, INFORMATION SYSTEMS AND COVID-19

Cause of death information is gathered from the death certificate (DC), a standard international document that should be filled out by doctors in Brazil. In a DC, the cause(s) of death is(are) declared in Part I (immediate, intervening, and underlying cause). For mortality statistics purposes, the underlying cause of death (COD) is selected, which should be the cause stated on the lowest used line of the DC, if the causal sequence leading to death was filled in correctly. The underlying COD is the disease or circumstances of injuries that initiated the chain of events leading to death[4]. In the case of disease due to SARS-CoV-2, the COD must be reported as COVID-19, and clinical suspicion without laboratory results, as suspected COVID-19. Pre-existing comorbidities responsible for worsening the disease should not be considered the underlying COD [5].The DC form is issued in three copies, the first (white) copy for the municipal, state and federal health services, responsible for monitoring causes of death with the Mortality Information System (*Sistema de Informações Sobre Mortalidade* – SIM).

The second copy (yellow) is destined to the Civil Registry (CR) notary offices for the registration of the death and the drawing up of a copy of the DC to the family, which are essential to proceed with the burial. The third copy (pink) must be retained by the issuing institution[4].For the insertion of deaths in the SIM, the death surveillance service of the health municipal department performs an active search for the DC in hospitals and other establishments, and/or notary offices, and uses international standardized rules for selecting the underlying COD. In the case of deaths that have not yet been confirmed as COVID-19, an attempt is made to streamline the routine process of investigating unspecified causes with an active search in medical records of hospitals and laboratories for the qualification and confirmation of the disease. Deaths captured at the municipal department are transferred to the state and to the federal level, to consolidate the national base[6]. Because of qualification processes in the mortality information system, there is a delay in the final registration in the system, which may vary according to different municipalities and causes.

Deaths registered in notary offices across the country make up the CR statistics system, coordinated by the Brazilian Institute of Geography and Statistics (*Instituto Brasileiro de Geografia e Estatística* – IBGE). This system, based on data from notary registrations, does not have the function of monitoring vital events occurring in the territory, but it contributes for the timely detection by municipal, state and federal health services of atypical occurrences in the various locations throughout the country. Over the last 10 years, it is estimated that the two systems, CR and SIM, have captured almost the total number of deaths that occur in large urban centres where the epidemic is concentrated. However, for a substantial proportion the cause of death is still ill-defined or imprecise (35% of deaths investigated in 60 cities in 2017)[7].

In the case of COVID-19, it is most likely that there is an expressive underreporting of deaths due to the difficulty in identifying the cases, considering that many did not have material collection for the PCR test. Even with samples collected, countless individuals evolve to death before having their results released. In addition, collection quality problems, since collecting specimens late or very early in the infection period as well as not handling and shipping them appropriately, may be responsible for false negative results[8]. Therefore, the timely inclusion of confirmed cases of COVID-19 in the SIM depends on the physician having adequate results of the PCR test available when filling in the DC. The major problem, however, concerns the criterion of suspected COVID-19 cases.

Given the delay in the release of a national protocol by the Brazilian Ministry of Health to standardize the adequate completion of DCs due to the disease, some institutions[3] have issued guidelines that differ from those recommended by the World Health Organization (WHO). The WHO proposes to consider as suspected case of COVID-19 all cases with clinically compatible disease even without confirmatory laboratory results.[5] In the epidemic, the poor completion of the DC is reinforced by the limited or non-existent medical care during the terminal illness and by the precarious working conditions of physicians in urgent and emergency settings. Thus, a high proportion of deaths from COVID-19 stated as other causes could compromise the understanding of the real magnitude of mortality from this specific cause.

DEATHS FROM PNEUMONIA, SEVERE ACUTE RESPIRATORY SYNDROME, RESPIRATORY FAILURE, SEPTICEMIA AND ILL-DEFINED CAUSES CAN ALSO OCCUR DUE TO THE NEW CORONAVIRUS

The disease caused by the new coronavirus was initially detected in China with the investigation of seven cases of pneumonia of unknown aetiology that occurred in late December 2019 in hospitalized patients, and which evolved into a severe acute respiratory syndrome (SARS)[9]. Therefore, pneumonia and SARS are causes that are part of the causal sequence of severe cases of COVID-19 which progress to death, and sepsis is also a possible complication[10]. Deaths classified as respiratory failure or ill-defined/undetermined causes conceal other causes, and the underlying COD can be any other specific cause. Research results for investigation of respiratory failure performed in 2017 on medical records, indicate that this diagnosis is the result of different underlying CODs, from chronic diseases, such as cardiovascular diseases (24% of 518 reclassified cases) to external causes[11] (Table 1). Ill-defined causes and sepsis had a similar pattern in previous investigations, indicating that they also hide a huge variety of underlying CODs[12,13].

The CR data on death in the recent Covid Registral panel, made available by the National Association of Natural Persons Registers (*Associação Nacional dos Registradores de Pessoas Naturais* – ARPEN Brasil)[14], come from the country's notary offices. A single cause of death was selected according to hierarchical criteria for the causes stated in the certificate. Endeavouring to measure mortality from coronavirus, deaths that had COVID-19 mentioned in the DC were identified, followed by deaths with mention of acute respiratory syndrome and those with pneumonia mentioned with no mention of SARS; finally, those with respiratory failure (with or without mentioned sepsis), and sepsis and ill-defined causes when they were the unique stated causes[14]. It appears that SARS increased in capital cities where there was an increase in confirmed cases of COVID-19 (data not shown) in 2020. When analysing three capital cities with a higher increase in cases of COVID-19 (Figure 1), an important rise in respiratory failure is observed as cause of death in São Paulo and Rio de Janeiro, whereas there was also an increase in mentioned pneumonia deaths in Manaus. The CR data, despite having some limitations, indicate that deaths from coronavirus are probably included among deaths registered as other causes, with different behaviour patterns in the municipalities. It then becomes urgent and necessary to face the challenge of building a picture closer to reality about the epidemic, which heavily impacts the life of the

Table 1 Deaths according to underlying causes after investigation of causes registered as respiratory failure. Brazil, 2017.

Underlying cause of death	< 20	20–39	40–49	50–59	60–69	70–79	80 and+	Total	%
Ischemic heart disease, hypertensive heart disease, cerebrovascular and other cardiovascular diseases	0	3	3	9	13	28	70	126	24.3
Neoplasms	0	2	6	8	13	15	7	51	9.8
Pneumonia and other respiratory infections	5	0	0	5	6	7	25	48	9.3
Chronic obstructive pulmonary disease	0	1	0	3	9	11	12	36	6.9
Diabetes and chronic kidney disease	0	2	3	2	3	9	17	36	6.9
Falls and other external causes	6	3	0	0	3	7	16	35	6.8
Tuberculosis, diarrhea and other communicable diseases	1	3	3	4	5	5	10	31	6.0
Alzheimer's disease and other dementias	0	0	0	1	0	2	24	27	5.2
Urinary tract disease and other natural causes	12	9	5	5	8	7	19	65	12.5
Ill-defined causes and other garbage codes	6	5	6	3	11	11	21	63	12.2
Reclassified causes after investigation (total)	30	28	26	40	71	102	221	518	53.8
Maintained respiratory failure	34	28	43	31	41	79	189	445	46.2
Total	64	56	69	71	112	181	410	963	100.0

Source: raw data from the Mortality Information System[11].

Epidemiological

Rio de
Cit

Numberofdeaths

1 2 3 4 5 6 7 8 9 1 1 1 1 1 1 1 1 1

Epidemiological

São
Cit

Numberofdeaths

1 2 3 4 5 6 7 8 9 1 1 1 1 1 1 1 1 1

Epidemiological week

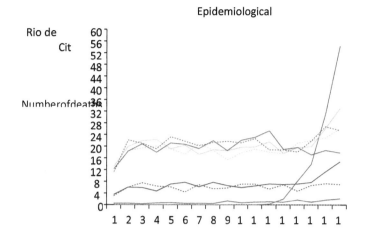

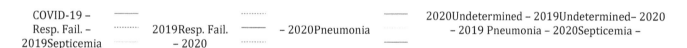

COVID-19 –				2020Undetermined – 2019Undetermined– 2020
Resp. Fail. –		2019Resp. Fail.	– 2020Pneumonia	– 2019 Pneumonia – 2020Septicemia –
2019Septicemia		– 2020		

*For COVID-19 and pneumonia, deaths were considered with mention of the cause in the death certificate.
Source: Covid Registral panel, made available by the National Association of Natural Persons Registers (*Associação Nacional dos Registradores de Pessoas Naturais* – ARPEN Brasil)[14].

Figure 1 Number of deaths due to COVID-19, pneumonia, respiratory failure and septicaemia per epidemiological week. Manaus, Rio de Janeiro and São Paulo Cities, 2019 and 2020*. Brazilian population. In addition to expanding laboratory tests of suspected cases and deaths with a higher quality control of performance[15], two additional approaches are recommended to enable a rapid assessment and better knowledge of the situation of deaths from COVID-19 in the country's municipalities:

- Consider as a suspected death of COVID-19 all deaths registered as SARS as from March 2020;
- Consider municipalities with probable underreporting of deaths from COVID-19 those with a number of deaths due to pneumonia, respiratory failure, septicaemia or ill-defined causes higher than the expected maximum limit for the number of weekly occurrences of each cause, based on a control diagram for deaths from these causes.

These two approaches will allow health municipal departments to conduct investigations of deaths due to Covid-related causes and, thus, have a better estimation of the real number of deaths from the disease. In a study in cooperation with Universidade Federal de Minas Gerais and Vital Strategies, health departments of three municipalities in the country started, with priority, an investigation process based on these guidelines last March. The results of this study should provide the degree of probable underreporting of deaths due to COVID-19 with greater precision. In an epidemic such as COVID-19, reliable and timely cause-of-death data are essential to define measures to control the spread of the disease and better manage health services. It is estimated that when a single death occurs in one place, hundreds of cases are probably present in the population[16]. Hence, we suggest that the protocols for investigating causes of death already found in the routine of the municipal health departments include the proposal presented in this article. It is essential that federal, state and municipal governments and society have a greater understanding of the risks involved and take the necessary effective measures to prevent them.

REFERENCES

1. Brasil. Ministério da Saúde. Secretaria de Vigilância em Saúde. Boletim Epidemiológico Especial. COE-COVID19. 26 abr. 2020. [Links]

2. Coronavírus Brasil. Painel Coronavírus [Internet]. [acessado em 7 maio 2020]. Disponível em: Disponível em: https://covid.saude.gov.br/ [Links]

3. Estado de São Paulo. Resolução SS-32. Diário Oficial. 20 mar. 2020. [Links]

4. Brasil. Ministério da Saúde. Conselho Federal de Medicina. Centro Brasileiro de Classificação de Doenças. A declaração de óbito: documento necessário e importante. Brasília: Ministério da Saúde; 2009. 38 p. (Série A. Normas e Manuais Técnicos.) [Links]

5. World Health Organization. International Guidelines for Certification and Classification (Coding) of COVID-19 as cause of death. Genebra: World Health Organization; 20 abr. 2020. [Links]

6. Brasil. Ministério da Saúde. Secretaria de Vigilância em Saúde. Portaria n° 116, 11 de fevereiro de 2009. Brasil: Ministério da Saúde; 2009. [Links]

7. Marinho MF, França EB, Teixeira RA, Ishitani LH, Cunha CC, Santos MR, et al. Dados para a saúde: impacto na melhoria da qualidade da informação sobre causas de óbito no Brasil. Rev Bras Epidemiol [Internet] 2019 [acessado em 7 maio 2020]; 22(Supl. 3): e19005.supl.3. Disponível em: Disponível em: http://www.scielo.br/scielo.php?script=sci_arttext&pid=S1415-790X2019000400403&lng=en https://doi.org/10.1590/1980-549720190005.supl.3 [Links]

8. Xie X, Zhong Z, Zhao W, Zheng C, Wang F, Liu J. Chest CT for Typical 2019-nCoV Pneumonia: Relationship to Negative RT-PCR Testing. Radiology 2020. https://doi.org/10.1148/radiol.2020200343 [Links]

9. Zhou P, Yang X-L, Wang XG, Hu B, Zhang L, Zhang W, et al. A pneumonia outbreak associated with a new coronavirus of probable bat origin. Nature 2020; 579: 270-3. https://doi.org/10.1038/s41586-020-2012-7 [Links]

10. Alhazzani W, Møller MH, Arabi YM, Loeb M, Gong M, Fan E, et al. Surviving Sepsis Campaign: Guidelines on the Management of Critically Ill Adults with Coronavirus Disease 2019 (COVID-19). Crit Care Med 2020. https://doi.org/10.1097/CCM.0000000000004363 [Links]

11. Brasil. Ministério da Saúde. Informações de saúde (Tabnet): estatísticas vitais: mortalidade geral [Internet]. Brasília: Ministério da Saúde ; 2019 [acessado em set. 2019]. Disponível em: Disponível em: http://www2.datasus.gov.br/DATASUS/index.php?area=0901&item=1&acao=26 [Links]

12. França EB, Ishitani LH, Teixeira RA, Cunha CC, Marinho MF. Improving the usefulness of mortality data: reclassification of ill-defined causes based on medical records and home interviews in Brazil. Rev Bras Epidemiol 2019; 22(Supl. 3). http://dx.doi.org/10.1590/1980-549720190010.supl.3 [Links]

13. Santos MR, Cunha CC, Ishitani LH, França EB. Mortes por sepse: causas básicas do óbito após investigação em 60 municípios do Brasil em 2017. Rev Bras Epidemiol 2019; 22(Supl. 3). https://doi.org/10.1590/1980-549720190012.supl.3 [Links]

14. Associação Nacional dos Registradores de Pessoas Naturais (ARPEN Brasil). Painel Covid Registral [Internet] [acessado em 11 maio 2020]. Disponível em: Disponível em: https://transparencia.registrocivil.org.br/registral-covid [Links]

15. Barreto ML, Barros AJD, Carvalho MS, Codeço CT, Hallal PRC, Medronho RA, et al. O que é urgente e necessário para subsidiar as políticas de enfrentamento da pandemia de COVID-19 no Brasil? Rev Bras Epidemiol [Internet] 2020 [acessado em 5 maio 2020; 23: e200032. Disponível em: Disponível em: http://www.scielo.br/scielo.php?script=sci_arttext&pid=S1415-790X2020000100101&lng=en https://doi.org/10.1590/1980-549720200032 [Links]

16. Jombart T, Zandvoort K, Russell T, Jarvis C, Gimma A, Abbott S, et al. Inferring the number of COVID-19 cases from recently reported deaths. medRxiv 2020. https://doi.org/10.1101/2020.03.10.20033761 [Links]

Financial support: Vital Strategies, as part of the Bloomberg Philanthropies Data for Health Initiative.

2. Considerations of Coronavirus (COVID-19) Impact and The Management of The Dead in Brazil

Melina Calmon[520]

ABSTRACT

During a pandemic such as COVID-19, the forensic community plays a key role in the management of the crisis, both nationally and internationally. Much has been written and disseminated regarding protocols for death investigation, infection mitigation and risks, and management of dead. However, in many contexts, the ability of forensic practitioners to follow best-practice procedures is limited by the resources available to them. This article examines some of the impact of the novel coronavirus[521] (COVID-19) in Brazil, with emphasis on management of the dead and challenges faced by medicolegal services.

INTRODUCTION

Forensic practitioners are important professionals whose work have legal, social, and economic consequences for communities, deceased individuals, and families of the deceased. During a pandemic such as COVID-19, the forensic community plays a key role in the management of the crisis, both nationally and internationally. The challenge for forensic practitioners has been twofold: first, to minimize the spread of the virus and, second, to advise authorities, hospitals, and funerary workers on proper protocols when deaths risk exceeding the capacities of local medicolegal services. Much has been written and disseminated regarding protocols for death investigation, infection mitigation and risks, and management of dead [[1], [2], [3], [4], [5]]. However, in many contexts, the ability of forensic practitioners to follow best-practice procedures is limited by the resources available to them. The capacity of forensic experts often depends on a large bureaucratic chain of events and many existing guidelines are predicated on a fully functioning laboratory or necropsy area and the availability of personal protective equipment[522] (PPE) and other materials. The reality for some countries, or regions within a country, is much different. Particularly, for Brazil, the current pandemic is likely to intensify the country's political and socioeconomic disparities. The goal of this article is to examine the impact of the novel coronavirus (COVID-19) in Brazil, with emphasis on management of the dead and challenges faced by medicolegal services.

---

[520] https://doi.org/10.1016/j.fsir.2020.100110
[521] https://www.sciencedirect.com/topics/medicine-and-dentistry/coronavirinae
[522] https://www.sciencedirect.com/topics/medicine-and-dentistry/personal-protective-equipment

Coronavirus and Politics

COVID-19 has been spreading rapidly across Brazil, prompting concerns over the potential collapse of the healthcare system. From February 27th to May 18th 2020, there were 241,080[523] confirmed cases of COVID-19 with 16,118 deaths [6]. On April 8th 2020, the state of Amazonas was the first to declare that the collapse of its healthcare system was imminent, with its capital, Manaus, having 95 % of the 293 ICU beds occupied at both private and public hospitals [7]. Bruno Covas, mayor of São Paulo, the capital of the state with the same name, declared on May 17th that the city's public hospitals had reached 90 % capacity and can potentially run out of space in two weeks [8].

São Paulo is the country's epicentre with almost 3000 deaths [8]. Concurrent with these potentially devastating impacts of the pandemic, federal government officials have downplayed the public health threat posed by the virus, with the current President Jair Bolsonaro calling COVID-19 a "little flu" and encouraging both the reopening of the country for the sake of the economy and the use of hydroxychloroquine[524] as a medicine to treat COVID-19 [9,10].

Although the federal government introduced measures such as a welfare stimulus package to contain the imminent financial fallout of the crisis [9], more rigorous health measures, such as a "stay at home" or social distancing order, were held back. Rather, local officials, such as governors and mayors, are at the forefront of holding the population accountable for staying at home and engaging in social distancing.

These officials have been publicly denounced as taking "extreme measures" by the President. In addition, two officials left the post of the Minister of Health in Brazil, leaving the country now facing a pandemic without a person appointed for such post [8]. Brazil is one of the countries garnering international media attention for the repercussions resulted from the country's Presidential pressure for disregarding guidelines issued by international public health authorities and deviate from actions taken by most other nations. Other leaders, such as President Alexander Lukashenko from Belarus, President Andrés Manuel López Obrador from México, President John Magufuli from Tanzania, President Gurbanguly Berdymukhamedov from Turkmenistan, and Kim Jong-Un from North Korea have either denied the existence of the disease, or downplayed the effects of coronavirus[525] in their respective countries [11].

Coronavirus and The Management of The Dead

On March 25th 2020, the Brazilian Ministry of Health published a guideline on the management of the dead in the context of COVID-19 [12]. Many important points can be drawn from this document, including:-Transmission of infectious disease[526] can occur through the management of dead bodies, especially if workers are not in possession of adequate personal protective equipment[527] (PPE). Funerals of confirmed or suspected patients of COVID-19 are not recommended due to the agglomeration of people.

---

[523] https://www.sciencedirect.com/topics/medicine-and-dentistry/americium-241
[524] https://www.sciencedirect.com/topics/medicine-and-dentistry/hydroxychloroquine
[525] https://www.sciencedirect.com/topics/medicine-and-dentistry/coronavirinae
[526] https://www.sciencedirect.com/topics/medicine-and-dentistry/horizontal-disease-transmission
[527] https://www.sciencedirect.com/topics/medicine-and-dentistry/personal-protective-equipment

This recommendation is valid for the quarantine and social distancing period. Autopsies must not be performed, and it is unnecessary in case of a confirmed COVID-19 case.- It is necessary to provide information and explanation to the family of the deceased regarding the care of the body. The document details the PPE and procedures to be followed for cases of death in hospital facilities, domicile, and public spaces. For hospital facilities, the directions are straightforward, with a physician in charge of signing the death certificate in situ. The PPE recommended for those who manage bodies in hospitals are:

-

- Hair cover
- Goggles or face shield
- Fluid-resistant or impermeable gown with long sleeves
- Surgical mask (N95, PFF2, or equivalent)
- Nitrile[528] gloves
- Impermeable boots

The management of the body follows directives given by the World Health Organization (WHO) and the International Committee of the Red Cross (ICRC) [1,12,13]. This includes the non-recommendation of embalming, the correct use of PPE, and the use of sheets, impermeable body bags, and a second body bag cleaned with 70 % ethanol, bleach solution 0.5–1.0 %, or another type of sanitizer approved by ANVISA, the regulatory sanitary agency in Brazil. For domicile or public spaces deaths, the recommendation is that a health department team investigates the case, verifying the need to collect samples to attest for the cause of death (in case of suspected COVID-19).

In case autopsy is deemed necessary, the autopsy must be conducted in a room with an adequate air treatment system (negative pressure with a minimum of six air exchanges). The number of professionals must be limited to one technician and one forensic pathologist[529]. The use of regular autopsy equipment such as oscillating saws is discouraged, with manual methods being preferred. Practitioners must avoid the use of techniques that might produce residues or protect the space with a vacuum cover. If the collection of soft tissue is necessary, it must be done through a minimally invasive autopsy technique (image and percutaneous intervention). For autopsy staff, the PPE required is:

-

1. Double surgical gloves interposed with a layer of cut-proof synthetic mesh gloves
2. Fluid-resistant or impermeable gown, or aprons over gowns
3. Goggles or face shields
4. Shoe covers or impermeable boots
5. N95 masks or superior
6. For other body handlers the PPE recommended are:
7. Non-sterile nitrile gloves while handling infectious materials
8. In case cuts or perforations are a risk, wear heavy duty gloves over the nitrile ones.

---

[528] https://www.sciencedirect.com/topics/medicine-and-dentistry/nitrile
[529] https://www.sciencedirect.com/topics/medicine-and-dentistry/forensic-pathologist

It is clear that the measures disseminated through the Ministry of Health guidelines follow the information by the WHO and other health and international organizations [[1], [2], [3], [4], [5],[12], [13], [14]]. However, the reality of Brazil is threefold:

1. Brazil, and other nations in Latin America and Africa, are scrambling for supplies while countries such as the United States and European countries are buying most stocks or simply rerouting them.

2. The country lacks the volume of trained personnel needed to deal with bodies following an infectious disease outbreak.

3. There is a lack of a coordinated and standardized manner of investigating and managing the dead throughout the country.

Until the release of the guidelines by the Ministry of Health in Brazil on March 25th 2020, there were no protocols for the care of bodies during the novel coronavirus[530] outbreak. Furthermore, the guidelines presuppose that the materials and equipment needed are available, when in reality there is an acute lack and disproportionate distribution of PPE and healthcare equipment in the country [15,16]. For instance, the equipment necessary to perform a minimally invasive autopsy is not available in adequate numbers throughout Brazil, with some regions not having the equipment at all.

The result is that many cases that required autopsy or collection of biological material for the confirmation of death by COVID-19 will not be performed. Therefore, current numbers are not a reflection of the real number of cases. Ultimately, it means that the numbers of deceased persons by COVID-19 will probably be an epidemiological assessment based on overall numbers of deaths compared with the average for the same period in the past two to five years. The exceeding numbers can then be assumed to be related to COVID-19. T

Therefore, the crucial problem with post-mortem testing is the contribution to the underestimation of cases today, which also means that families are not properly informed, and opportunities to trace contact and help control the epidemic, are neglected. The Adolfo Lutz Institute, an analytical laboratory accredited as a National Laboratory of Public Health and Reference Laboratory Macroregional by the Brazilian Ministry of Health, and current reference in coronavirus testing in São Paulo, had allegedly a backlog of 16,000 tests waiting to be finalized by April 1st 2020 [17]. According to the unofficial platform worldometer, Brazil has 3462 coronavirus tests performed for every one million people [18].

Many forensic workers, especially those in funerary services, have been struggling to balance following correct procedures for victims of coronavirus while still handling deaths non-related to the virus. The Public Ministry of Rio de Janeiro, for instance, has received reports of improper management of the dead by funerary services, who are reportedly not following the WHO recommendations for the proper preparation of bodies for burial of deaths occurring the pandemic. [19]. One problem is that some bodies arrive with death certificates describing "respiratory disease" with an observation "awaiting results." Funerary service workers have reported being threatened

---

[530] https://www.sciencedirect.com/topics/medicine-and-dentistry/coronavirinae

by families who wish to pursue traditional burial services for deceased individuals who have no explicit confirmation of COVID-19 as their cause of death. Other cases might be documented as "cause of death undetermined," which results in the same problem for post-mortem examination and handling. The delay in exams and tests to confirm the infection, even after the death of someone possibly infected, has affected how forensic personnel follow the management of the dead procedures and leads to a probable underreporting of deaths by the new coronavirus.

Coronavirus and reporting procedures

The underreporting of COVID-19 cases in Brazil has been a cause for investigation in some states. A funeral home in Belo Horizonte, Minas Gerais received 41 bodies in 48 h, some with the cause of death stated as COVID-19. However, the state of Minas Gerais at that point had not yet reported any cases of death by coronavirus[531]. Another funeral home in the same state had 73 bodies during the days of 20 to 22nd of March. The State Secretary of Health explained that many of the bodies with notations of COVID-19 might not necessarily have died of the new coronavirus, but that the death occurred during the pandemic period, causing again confusion among forensic personnel [20].

The underreporting of COVID-19 deaths in Brazil is especially evident after the release of a more flexible way of certifying deaths during the pandemic. The Resolution SS 32, passed on March 20th, 2020 by the São Paulo state government, established that the cause of death by coronavirus cannot be attested by autopsies, due to risk of contamination. Therefore, many deaths due to COVID-19 will never be documented if they are not readily attested in a hospital prior to death. With the lack of tests and personnel to run the exams, it is possible that the real number of COVID-19 deaths will never be known [21,22].

The São Paulo government has determined that:

"(...) every cadaver, with or without the suspicion of coronavirus infection (COVID-19), in external or internal hospital environment, without any indication of violent death, are now the responsibility of the City Death Verification Services (SVOM). The Medical Legal Institutes, which in normal instances perform autopsies of natural deaths of unidentified persons, is now only performing investigations of bodies related to violent deaths" [22]. However, because the new guidelines in place do not recommend the autopsy of bodies, the SVOM has up to 24 h after an individual's death to collect swabs from the cadaver suspected of being infected. This would allow for the possible infection to be confirmed at a later time through post-mortem exams. Alternately, the death can be certified by a verbal questionnaire in which the family provides information about the deceased's health. One problem regarding the second certification of death is that sometimes the family will still not have a confirmation of a possible death by COVID-19, especially if no swab was collected to accompany the questionnaire.

---

[531] https://www.sciencedirect.com/topics/medicine-and-dentistry/coronavirinae

Coronavirus and Burials

The main problem with burial during this pandemic in Brazil is the lack of space in cemeteries and an insufficient number of body handlers. According to the mayor's office in São Paulo city, the number of daily burials increased around 30 % in the biggest cemetery of Latin America, the Vila Formosa. Since April 1st, 2020, cemetery workers have been digging approximately 100 new graves a day, doubling the amount in relation to pre-pandemic levels. Because any death caused by respiratory problems in São Paulo is being treated as a potential COVID-19 case, all cemetery staff needs to work with proper recommended PPE. However, cemetery staff and body handlers have been speaking out against the lack of proper PPE, with funeral staff refusing to perform burials due to fear of contamination. Cemetery staff are threatening to strike over the conditions they have been experiencing during this time [23,24]. Nevertheless, it is important to stress that there is a lack of evidence regarding the transmissibility of COVID-19 from bodies of deceased persons of confirmed or suspected cases [25].

Coronavirus and The New Missing Persons

Another risk is an emergence of a new type of missing persons, the "disappeared via the pandemic." The rise of these disappeared would be due to unintentional errors such as documentation being lost or misplaced, which may happen when services are in a crisis and operating above capacity. Such errors hinder the positive identification of the dead or cause bodies to be moved without following a proper chain of custody. Examples of such problems have already been found in Brazilian cities. During the pandemic crisis, two families received unsettling news regarding their loved ones after they were informed of their death. In one case, the body of the deceased could not be located in the hospital, and on the other case the family received the death certificate with the name of another deceased person [26]. Another case reports that two bodies were swapped in the hospital. Due to funerals and burials being done with closed and sealed coffins, the family of one of the deceased was only informed of the error once the procedures were finalized [27].

The Procuradoria Federal dos Direitos do Cidadão (Federal Prosecution for Citizen's Rights – free translation), in the capital Brasília, stated that the rights of families, descendants and heirs, as well as the correct identification of the dead during the pandemic, must be guaranteed.

The document[1] described that it is equally important to guarantee that unidentified bodies and unclaimed bodies can, in a reasonable time, be buried without the loss of any rights to the family. The family has the right to the death certificate, with clearly documented causes and circumstances, and information regarding the burial location of the remains. Such directives are to uphold dignity and respect of the deceased, and to allow the possibility of mourning to the families.

The document references internationally recognized organizations such as WHO, Pan-American Health Organization (PAHO) ICRC, International Federation of the Red Cross (IFRC), and Interpol, emphasizing guidelines such as the Management of Dead Bodies after Disasters and the Disaster Victim Identification Guide and the International Humanitarian Law.

The existence of such recommendations highlights the needs that are anticipated to emerge due to the coronavirus[532] pandemic, such as the need to exhume remains for future identification or

---

[532] https://www.sciencedirect.com/topics/medicine-and-dentistry/coronavirinae

proper post-mortem examination such as the recovery of projectiles. Some of the recommendations are:

- That bodies of unidentified or unclaimed remains are not cremated but buried

- Buried bodies must have water-proofed identification tags, following the guidelines by the ICRC, WHO, and IFRC, and Interpol manuals.

- The use of standardized forms for the identification of remains (making direct reference to forms provided by WHO and ICRC).

- That all the personal effects are buried together with the remains, in plastic bags matching the identification tag of the remains.

- That funeral services maintain a precise identification of the graves with an easy access for matching of data with the burial registry.

- That a unique database is used to insert the identification form data as well as the burial location of the remains.

- That the collection of fingerprints[533] or genetic material (via nasopharyngeal swabs) becomes mandatory and is accompanied by photographs.

- That professionals are trained in a standardized manner to perform procedures and that the data collected (swab, photographs, and fingerprints) are entered in the unified database.

- That in cases where exhumation is needed to free space in cemeteries, unidentified or unclaimed bodies are not destroyed but instead individually placed in ossuary's or equivalent places following guidelines for eventual retrieval (traceability).

Additional Considerations of The Brazilian Reality

Brazil is the world's fifth-largest country by area, and the sixth most populous (over 211 million people). According to the National Council of the Public Ministry (CNMP), in 2019 Brazil had 727,227 incarcerated persons [28]. Many prisons are operating at or over their capacity, with the overall system operating at 166 % capacity according to data released by the Public Ministry in 2019. Therefore, the prison environment, especially instances of overcrowding, makes individuals susceptible for the transmission of diseases such as tuberculosis, HIV, measles, and other bacterial and viral illnesses [29]. According to the National Penitentiary Department (DEPEN), 483 incarcerated persons have confirmed cases of coronavirus, 303 are suspected cases, and 22 persons have died due to the disease [30]. The overburdened Brazilian healthcare system, aggravated by the deep inequality in the country, will also disproportionally affect the population of the favelas. Favelas are informal, unregulated settlements of low to middle-income people. Favela neighbourhoods and communities have historically been neglected by government, and have

---

[533] https://www.sciencedirect.com/topics/medicine-and-dentistry/finger-dermatoglyphics

limited access to security, water, sanitation, health care, public education, and formal employment, making the coping mechanism of the residents regarding COVID-19 worrisome. According to the 2010 census, 14 million Brazilians were estimated to live in favelas across the country [31]. Many of these individuals do not have the luxury of quarantine.

They are informal employers, street vendors, delivery drivers or domestic workers, all still working while living in a highly dense environment. To monitor the real situation of the pandemic in the favelas of Rio de Janeiro, inhabitants of the favelas have collected data that indicate that the number of deaths caused by coronavirus in the favelas is 41 % higher than the number reported by the Mayor's Office [32]. The underreporting of cases and deaths have brought NGOs that act on those communities to launch initiatives to collect data inside the favelas [33]. The community newspaper of the Complexo do Alemão, one of the most famous favelas in Rio de Janeiro, organized a database panel with the data collected from 13 communities [34]. The data is collected from the family clinics and Rapid Appointment Units (UPAs), of the regions, providing a better precision for the area where the patient came from. The numbers are discrepant to the ones released by the Mayor's Office because the latter only releases it by neighbourhoods, and many favelas intersect between multiple neighbourhoods of the city. As of May 19th 2020, 504 cases of coronavirus have been confirmed in the favelas of Rio de Janeiro, with 172 deaths, a death rate of 34.1 % [34]. Another population who needs to be highlighted are the Native Brazilians. The coordinator of the Xingu Project, at the Federal University of São Paulo, states that the COVID-19 might have an impact comparable to previous epidemics, such as measles [35]. Many practices disseminated to prevent the spread of coronavirus, such as the cleaning of hands with 70 % alcohol, are impracticable in many Native Brazilian villages. Moreover, PPEs are not distributed throughout different rural or remote communities. According to the FUNAI, the national foundation for the Native Brazilians, 107 indigenous groups in the Brazilian Amazon are still deprived of contact with the modern society [36]. According with the Special Secretary of Indigenous Health (SESAI) and the Brazil's Indigenous People Articulation (APIB), around 81,000 indigenous people from 230 territories are threatened by the coronavirus pandemic. Many of the territories occupied by native groups are targeted by missionaries, hunters, and people who want to extract wood.

This creates risk for native individuals who travel out of indigenous villages to gather resources (food, supplies, etc.) and may come into contact with outsiders who might carry the virus. In addition, many villages are isolated from governmental health systems. Until May 12th, APIB reported that 308 indigenous people were infected by the disease, and 77 individuals died from it. A death rate of 25 % [37]. It is important that in addition to knowledge regarding public health measures to mitigate the coronavirus spread, we also take into consideration the reality of many of |novel coronavirus reaches these vulnerable populations or others such as displaced communities, migration camps, or prison environments in different parts of the world the result will be a humanitarian crisis. The containment of the spread will be impossible, and the death toll caused by the disease will be unprecedented for modern times.

Last Comments

While other countries face or will face some or many of the challenges detailed above, Brazil illustrates a constellation of factors that create unique problems and exceptional risk. The country is in a current political crisis, with acute socioeconomical disparities[534], it has a large territory and voluminous population, and unequal availability of basic services.. It is imperative for professionals across disciplines to work together to share and disseminate accurate and precise information to the public and each other. For the forensic community, these partnerships include but are not limited to the fields of health, public health, medico legal, public policy, law enforcement, and scientific institutions. Special attention must be paid to vulnerable populations who are on the verge of being disproportionately impacted by the spread of COVID-19.

The rights of families and the deceased must be upheld to the extent that these rights do not jeopardize public health or the safety of forensic staff. Professionals involved with management of the dead must provide families with information regarding their deceased relatives, including death certificates and any protocols that must be followed for the care and handling of the body. Effectively and ethically managing large numbers of dead from COVID-19 requires an increase of human and material resources, including building local capacity and supporting and/or carrying out recovery and identification processes. It is imperative that authorities anticipate and prepare for the grave challenges they might encounter regarding managing those who died during the pandemic.

REFERENCES

1. Management of the Dead After Disasters. A Field Manual for First Responders, 2nd edition, International Committee of the Red Cross (ICRC), the World Health Organization (WHO), the Pan American Health Organization (PAHO) and the
International Federation of Red Cross and Red Crescent Societies (IFRC), Geneva, 2016. (Accessed 18 April 2020) https://shop.icrc.org/gestion-des-depouillesmortelles-lors-de-catastrophes-manuel-pratique-a-l-usage-des-premiersintervenants-669.html.

2. Briefing on COVID-19: Autopsy Practice Relating to Possible Cases of COVID-19
(2019-nCov, Novel Coronavirus From China 2019/2020), Royal College of Pathologists, London, 2020. (Accessed 18 April 2020 https://www.rcpath.org/ uploads/assets/d5e28baf-5789-4b0f-acecfe370eee6223/fe8fa85a-f004-4a0c81ee4b2b9cd12cbf/Briefing-on-COVID-19-autopsy-Feb-2020.pdf.

3. World Health Organization, 19 March 2020. Infection Prevention and Control During Health Care When Novel Coronavirus (nCoV) Infection Is Suspected (Interim Guidance), (2020) . (Accessed 17 May 2020) https://www.who.int/publicationsdetail/infection-prevention-and-control-during-health-care-when-novelcoronavirus-(ncov)-infection-is-suspected-20200125.

4. Centres for Disease Control and Prevention. Interim Health Recommendations for Workers Who Handle Human Remains After a Disaster, (2020) . (Accessed 17 May 2020) https://www.cdc.gov/disasters/handleremains.html.

5. Centres for Disease Control and Prevention, February 2020. Guidance for Collection and Submission of Postmortem Specimens From Deceased Persons Under Investigation (PUI) for COVID-19, (2020) . (Accessed 17 May 2020) https://www.cdc. gov/coronavirus/2019-ncov/hcp/guidance-postmortem-specimens.html.

6. World Health Organization Data by Country, Brazil, (2020) . (Accessed 19 May 2020) https://covid19.who.int/region/amro/country/br.

---

[534] https://www.sciencedirect.com/topics/medicine-and-dentistry/disparity

7. Brasil.io. Bolentins informativos e casos do coronavírus por município por dia, (2020) .

8. BBC News, Coronavirus: Hospitals in Brazil's São Paulo 'near collapse', (2020) . (Accessed 18 May 2020) https://www.bbc.com/news/world-latin-america52701524.

9. President Jair Bolsonaro Official Statement Transcript. March 24th 2020, (2020) . (Accessed 18 April 2020) https://www.gov.br/planalto/pt-br/acompanhe-oplanalto/pronunciamentos/pronunciamento-em-cadeia-de-radio-e-televisao-dosenhor-presidente-da-republica-jair-bolsonaro.

10. President Jair Bolsorano Official Statement Transcript. April 8th 2020, (2020) . (Accessed 18 April 2020) https://www.gov.br/planalto/pt-br/acompanhe-oplanalto/pronunciamentos/pronunciamentos-do-presidente-da-republica/ pronunciamento-do-senhor-presidente-da-republica-jair-bolsonaro-em-cadeia-deradio-e-televisao-4.

11. The Globe and Mail. The Notorious Nine: These World Leaders Responded to the Coronavirus With Denial, Duplicity and Ineptitude, (2020) . (Accessed 17 May 2020) https://www.theglobeandmail.com/world/article-the-notorious-nine-these-worldleaders-responded-to-the-coronavirus/.

12. Ministério da Saúde, March 25th 2020. Version 1. Manejo De Corpos No Contexto Do Novo Coronavirus COVID-19. Brasília/DF, (2020) https://www.saude.gov.br/ images/pdf/2020/marco/25/manejo-corpos-coronavirus-versao1-25mar20-rev5. pdf.

13. World Health Organization Website, (2020) . (Accessed 18 May 2020) https://www. who.int/emergencies/diseases/novel-coronavirus-2019/technical-guidance/ infection-prevention-and-control.

14. World Health Organization, Infection Prevention and Control for the Safe Management of a Dead Body in the Context of COVID-19, (2020.

15. NY Times, J. Bradley, Scramble for Coronavirus Supplies, Rich Countries Push Poor Aside, (2020) . (Accessed 10 April 2020) https://www.nytimes.com/2020/04/09/ world/coronavirus-equipment-rich-poor.html.

16. C.S. Alves, M.M.F. Gomes, L.M. Brasil, Project management for clinical engineeringconsiderations in the evaluation and acquisition of medical equipment for health services in Brazil, World Congress on Medical Physics and Biomedical Engineering, June 7-12, 2015, Toronto, Canada, 2015, pp. 1497–1500 Springer, Cham.

17. G1. April 1st 2020. Instituto Adolfo Lutz libera 0.4% dos testes de coronavirus; 16 mil aguardam análise, (2020) . (Accessed 15 April 2020) https://g1.globo.com/sp/saopaulo/noticia/2020/04/01/instituto-adolfo-lutz-liberou-apenas-04percent-dostestes-para-coronavirus-recebidos-na-semana-passada.ghtml.

18. Worldometer https://www.worldometers.info/coronavirus/? utm_campaign=CSauthorbio? (Accessed 20 May 2020).

19. O. Globo, C. Otávio, Coronavírus: MP recebe denúncia de que manejo de corpos por funerárias não estaria seguindo recomendação da OMS, (2020) https://oglobo.globo. com/rio/coronavirus-mp-recebe-denuncia-de-que-manejo-de-corpos-por-funerariasnao-estaria-seguindo-recomendacao-da-oms-24347322.

20. O. Estado de São Paulo, P. Camporez, Minas investiga excesso de corpos em funerária e cogita exumação para testar coronavírus, (2020) https://brasil.estadao.com.br/ noticias/geral,minas-investiga-excesso-de-corpos-em-funeraria-e-cogita-exumacaopara-testar-coronavirus,70003251680.

21. El País M. Rossi, Mortes sem diagnóstico reforçam suspeitas de que estatísticas de coronavírus em São Paulo estão defasadas, (2020) https://brasil.elpais.com/politica/ 2020-03-31/mortes-sem-diagnostico-levantam-suspeita-de-subnotificacao-de-casosdo-coronavirus-em-sao-paulo.html.

22. S.S. Resolução, 32. São Paulo. March 20th 2020, (2020) . (Accessed 10 April 2020) http://www.co-semssp.org.br/noticias/resolucao-ss-32-20-03-2020-dispoe-sobre-asdiretrizes-para-manejo-e-seguimento-dos-casos-de-obito-no-contexto-da-pandemiaCOVID-19-no-estado-de-sao-paulo/.

23. Veja, M. Zylberkan, Coronavírus leva prefeitura de São Paulo a dobrar número de coveiros, (2020) . (Accessed 17 April 2020) https://veja.abril.com.br/brasil/ coronavirus-leva-prefeitura-de-sao-paulo-a-dobrar-numero-de-coveiros/.

24. Medium, M. Tegon, Profissão em alta: coveiro, (2020) . (Accessed 17 April 2020) https://medium.com/@maritegon/profissão-em-alta-coveiro-bd9037b0b4d9.

25. S. Yaacoub, H.J. Schünemann, J. Khabsa, A. El-Harakeh, A.M. Khamis, F. Chamseddine, R. El Khoury, Z. Saad, L. Hneiny, C.C. Garcia, G.E.U. Muti-Schünemann, Safe management of bodies of deceased persons with suspected or confirmed COVID19: a rapid systematic review, BMJ Glob. Health 5 (5) (2020) p.e002650.

26. G1 Rio de Janeiro, R. Coutinho, A. Prado, E. Maria, Famílias de pacientes mortos com coronavírus têm dificuldade para localizar corpos em hospitais do RJ, (2020) . corpos-em-hospitais-do-rj.ghtml.

27. G1 São Paulo, Corpo de isoda é trocado em hospital de Santo André durante pandemia de coronavírus, (2020) . (Accessed 17 May 2020 https://g1.globo.com/sp/sao-paulo/ noticia/2020/04/09/corpo-de-idosa-e-trocado-em-funeraria-de-santo-andredurante-pandemia-de-coronavirus.ghtml.

28. Conselho Nacional do Ministério Público. Relatório do Sistema Prisional, (2019) . (Accessed 16th April 2020 https://www.cnmp.mp.br/portal/relatoriosbi/sistemaprisional-em-numeros.

29. R. Sánchez, A.A.M. Maria, Tuberculose em População Carcerária do Estado do Rio de Janeiro: prevalência e subsídios para formulação de estratégias de controle Doctoral dissertation, (2008) .

30. Departamento Penitenciário Nacional. Painel Mundial, (2020) . (Accessed 17 May 2020) http://depen.gov.br/DE-PEN/Covid19PainelMundial08MAIO20.pdf.

31. Intsituto Brasileiro de Geografia e Estatística. Censo Demográfico, (2010) . (Accessed 17 April 2020)

32. Exame. Favelas do Rio têm mortes por vocid-19 for a de boletim oficial, (2020) . (Accessed on 17 May 2020) https://exame.abril.com.br/brasil/favelas-no-rio-temmortes-por-COVID-19-fora-de-boletim-oficial/.

33. Agência Brasil. Nitaha, A. May 16th 2020. https://agenciabrasil.ebc.com.br/saude/ noticia/2020-05/organizac-oes-monitoram-situacao-da-COVID-19-nas-favelas-do-rio (Accessed 17 May 2020).

34. COVID-19 nas Favelas, (2020) . (Accessed 20 May 2020 https://painel. vozdascomunidades.com.br/.

35. Universidade Federal de São Paulo. Projeto Xingu, (2020) . (Accessed 20 May 2020) https://www.unifesp.br/reitoria/dci/index.php? option=com_k2&view=item&id=1913:ha-50-anos-cuidando-da-saude-dos-povosindigenas.

36. Fundação Nacional do Índio (FUNAI). Povos Indígenas Isolados e de Recente Contato, (2020) . (Accessed 20 May 2020) http://www.funai.gov.br/index.php/nossas-acoes/ povos-indigenas-isolados-e-de-recente-contato.

Articulação dos Povos Indígenas do Brasil (APIB), (2020) . (Accessed 20 May 2020) http://apib.info/2020/05/14/01-indigenous-lives-and-COVID-19/?lang=en

3. How To Reduce And Paralyze The Climb Of Contamination And Deaths By The New Coronavirus In Brazil

Fernando Alcoforado*

ABSTRACT

This article aims to present what and how to do to reduce and halt the advance of the new Coronavirus in Brazil, which accounted for 10,627 deaths with 155,939 confirmed cases until 05/10/2020 and 730 deaths in the last 24 hours. It is demonstrated by these figures that the policies adopted so far by the federal, state and municipal governments of Brazil are insufficient to contain the progress of the new Coronavirus and that more effective measures urgently need to be put in place to reduce the number of contaminated and killed by the viruses without which more than 1 million deaths from the new Coronavirus in Brazil may occur. Imperial College London report about the new New Coronavirus in Brazil, prepared by Thomas A Mellan, Henrique H Hoeltgebaum, Swapnil Mishra et al., Is entitled "Report 21: Estimating COVID-19 cases and reproduction number in Brazil". In this report, there is information that Brazil is an epicentre of the COVID-19 in Latin America where the most affected states correspond to São Paulo, Rio de Janeiro, Ceará, Pernambuco and Amazonas, which account for 81% of the deaths reported until now. In Brazil, the number of infections continues to grow with the record of almost twice as many deaths by covid19 as in China and more than 100,000 confirmed cases.

INTRODUCTION

This report predicts that, in the worst-case scenario, if no one is quarantined and the tests are not multiplied, there would be up to 188 million people infected (the equivalent of 88% of the entire Brazilian population) and 1.1 million people killed. More than 6.2 million people would pass through hospitals in the country because of the coronavirus collapsing the health system. In a quarantine scenario only for the elderly, the number of deaths would vary between 322 thousand and 530 thousand, depending on the transmission rate and public health measures. In the best scenario calculated with 75% of the entire population in quarantine, with tests for all suspected patients, the number of deaths from COVID-19 in the country would not exceed 44,300. In these conditions, at the peak of the pandemic, there would be a demand for 72 thousand beds at the same time. Therefore, with the best quarantine scenario for 75% of the entire population, it can save up to 1 million people in Brazil, calculates Imperial College.

In this report from Imperial College there is information that the interventions employed in Brazil to combat COVID-19 so far are insufficient because they fall short of the generalized and mandatory blockages implemented in parts of Asia and Europe that have proven to be highly effective in containing the spread of the virus. It also informs that the results of the study on Brazil show that until now the changes in mobility adopted have not been rigorous enough. The epidemic is expected to continue to grow throughout Brazil and to increase the associated number of cases and deaths, unless other more vigorous actions are taken. There is a suggestion of the need to break the chain of transmission of the virus as essential to control it and prevent its exponential growth. The study concludes that "the rapid adoption of proven public health measures, including testing, case isolation and greater social distancing" are essential to contain the impact of the pandemic.

This is what would "flatten" the contaminated curve, which would reduce the burden on hospitals and consequently reduce the proportion of deaths per week - one of the variables calculated by Imperial College. After breaking the record for the daily increase in deaths (610 new deaths) and cases of the new Coronavirus (9,888 cases of the disease) this week, Brazil has 9,146 deaths and 135,106 infected by COVID-19. Faced with this situation, lockdown, that is, confinement or total closure as the most radical method imposed by governments for people to fulfill the period of social distancing, begins to spread throughout the country, reaching 18 cities in five states. First state in the Southeast to enact the strictest isolation regime, Rio de Janeiro announced yesterday the measure in Niterói and Bangu. Salvador decreed the lockdown in some neighbourhoods of the city. Most states that have already decreed lockdown are on the list of 12 federal units that exceed 100 deaths from the disease. The group includes São Paulo (3,206), Rio de Janeiro (1,394), Ceará (903), Pernambuco (845), Amazonas (806), Pará (410), Maranhão (305), Bahia (165), Espírito Santo (155), Minas Gerais (106), Paraná (104) and Paraíba (101). Together, these states account for 8,500 deaths, that is, 92% of deaths in Brazil.

Considering the reports from Imperial College, which states that the actions taken to date in Brazil were not rigorous enough to contain the spread of the new Coronavirus, there is no other solution to prevent the spread of the virus that could catastrophically affect the entire population with its deadly effects with over 1 million deaths except by breaking its transmission chain. This disruption of the virus transmission chain would have to be radical like the one adopted by China, which, by adopting the lockdown with the isolation of Wuhan (epicentre of the virus) from the rest of the country, was successful in controlling the spread of the new Coronavirus by the rest of the country. In Brazil, there is no other way but to adopt the lockdown of the cities and regions most affected for an indefinite period. In each city and region most affected by the new Coronavirus and isolated from the rest of the state and country, mass tests should be adopted along the same lines as those adopted in China to identify who should be quarantined and who should be released for social coexistence. There should be strict control on the movement of people at the entrance and exit of cities and regions in lockdown, with tests to verify whether or not they are contaminated by the new Coronavirus. This would be one of the measures to prevent the collapse of economic activities by eliminating the conflict between the need to prevent the spread of the virus with the collapse of the health system and the resumption of economic activity.

Lockdown cities and regions should only be released gradually in the same way as in China with the population wearing a facemask, being subjected to constant temperature measurements, in addition to being controlled by means of a QR code (Quick Response code) of health that works as an immunity passport. In several Chinese cities, there is a QR for each inhabitant, informing their health condition based on both their own statements and data available to the government. Thus, citizens receive codes marked in green, yellow or red. Only residents with a green code can move freely around the city. Yellow and red code holders must keep quarantine and register daily on an internet platform to provide information, until they obtain the green code.

In addition to these measures that must be adopted by states and municipalities, income should be distributed by the federal government to the populations, especially the vulnerable ones, to avoid that, due to the need for survival, they are forced to leave their homes to work in offices or in streets. In other words, the federal government should pay people not to take to the streets to avoid contaminating or being contaminated by the virus. Measures should also be adopted by the federal government to help companies, especially micro, small and medium-sized companies, to survive at this time of falling revenues, as well as states and municipalities to avoid their insolvency due to the drop in tax collection. Only the federal government has the capacity to implement these measures.

For these measures to be successful and result in the successful fight against the new Coronavirus in Brazil, coordinating action by the federal government is urgent. The indispensable condition for Brazil to win the war against the new Coronavirus is the government at all levels and the population being united against the common enemy.

Unfortunately, in Brazil, this situation does not exist because the President of the Republic Jair Bolsonaro is against the social isolation of the population, systematically disrespecting all restrictive measures to the gathering of people under the pretext that it is also necessary to save the Brazilian economy from debacle. In his compromising action in the fight against the new Coronavirus, Bolsonaro says that people should go back to work. The fact that Bolsonaro takes this attitude is encouraging a large number of people to leave the isolation in which they find themselves and return to the street as is already happening in several cities in Brazil, contributing to the increase in the number of contaminated and killed by the new Coronavirus. The end of the social isolation of many people is also related to the fact that they need to work to survive, given that the Bolsonaro government does not offer people and companies the conditions necessary for their survival.

In addition to acting to destroy the effort of governors and mayors to fight the new Coronavirus, the Bolsonaro government does not act with the necessary urgency in the economic plan with the release of the financial resources it has approved by the National Congress to help vulnerable populations to fight hunger, companies in general to avoid bankruptcy and states and municipal governments to avoid their insolvency. This is one more reason why Jair Bolsonaro's removal from the Presidency of the Republic is necessary with his replacement by Vice President Hamilton Mourão who, in addition to being more qualified to play the role of general commander in the fight against the new Coronavirus for being general Army, would be better able to unite the nation against the common enemy. The political leaders of all parties need to act as soon as possible to remove Bolsonaro from power to avoid the catastrophe that is envisaged with the dizzying advance of the number of contaminated and killed by the new Coronavirus in Brazil. n the article "How and when will this pandemic end? [535] Belgian virologist Guido Vanham, former head of virology at the Antwerp Institute of Tropical Medicine in Belgium, replied that it will probably never end, in the sense that this virus is clearly here to stay, unless we eradicate it . In addition, the only way to eradicate this virus would be with a very effective vaccine that be delivered to every human being. We did this with smallpox, but that is the only example - and it took many years. Therefore, it will probably stay. It belongs to a family of viruses that we know - the coronaviruses - and one of the questions now is whether it will behave like other viruses.

---

[535] Published on the website <https://www.weforum.org/agenda/2020/04/how-and-when-will-this-pandemic-end-weasked-a-virologist/>

Therefore, the vaccine is the only weapon we have to use to eradicate the new Coranavirus. Throughout history, vaccines have helped to significantly reduce the incidence of flu, chicken pox or chickenpox, mumps, dengue, yellow fever, hepatitis, rubella, measles, smallpox, herpes simplex, rabies, polio, measles and tetanus. Today, vaccines are considered the most cost-effective treatment in public health. The reality now is that the world needs a vaccine against the new Coronavirus that causes COVID-19. It will probably not be ready in the next few months. Maybe this will only happen in 12 or 18 months. More than 90 vaccines are being developed against COVID-19 by research teams at companies and universities around the world. The researchers are testing different technologies, some of which have never been used in a licensed vaccine before. At least six groups have already started to inject formulations into volunteers in safety tests; others started testing on animals. It is through the vaccine that what is called "herd immunity" is rationally obtained, ie the immunization of the virus of the entire population. The other way to obtain "herd immunity" is to allow the entire population to be infected by the virus. This was the idea developed by Donald Trump, President of the United States, and Boris Johnson, British Prime Minister, who considered only crossing their arms while the population of their respective countries was infected with the new Coronavirus. This idea, put into practice initially and abandoned later, was based on the premise that only the most vulnerable should be protected. This was the proposal defended by Bolsonaro to be applied in Brazil.

The idea was to create what they understood to be "herd immunity", that is, the greater the number of infected with COVID-19, the more people would become resistant to the virus due to the acquired immune memory. Thus, there would come a time when the pathogen would stop spreading due to the lack of susceptible hosts. The problem with this reasoning is that the new Coronavirus is a new infectious agent and it is not known how many people it is able to infect and kill if no action is taken. If too many people are allowed to become infected in a short period, health systems will not be able to handle the cases that will get worse. In addition, herd immunity is only performed in a rational manner, obtaining excellent results when it is done in a controlled manner, using vaccines.

From the above, it can be said that without the total isolation or lockdown of cities and regions affected by the new Coronavirus, without the effective help of the federal government to populations, especially the most vulnerable, to companies, especially micro, small and medium companies, and to states and municipalities and without the coordinating action of the federal government to combat the common enemy, there will be no success in the war against the virus. Without the adoption of these measures, Brazil will be subjected to the greatest humanitarian disaster in its history. In addition, these measures are essential because in the absence of a vaccine that will immunize the population against the new Coronavirus, the humanitarian disaster that is envisaged will turn into the collective murder of the Brazilian population whose biggest responsibility will be the Bolsonaro government if nothing is done to avoid it. To avoid the foreseeable humanitarian disaster that is envisaged in Brazil, it is necessary to remove Jair Bolsonaro from the Presidency of the Republic with his replacement by Vice President Hamilton Mourão who, in addition to being more qualified to play the role of general commander in the fight against new Coronavirus because he is an army general, he would be better able to unite the nation against the common enemy.

REFERENCES

Cann, A. J.(2005). Principles Of Molecular Virology. 4. Ed. Massachusetts: Elsevier Academic Press.

Carter, J.; Saunders, V. (2007) Virology: Principles And Applications. Chichester: Wiley, 2007.

Mahy, B. W. J. (2001). Dictionary of Virology. 3. Ed. London: Academic Press, 2001.

Imperial College. Report 21: Estimating COVID-19 Cases And Reproduction Number In Brazil. Disponível No Website <Https://Www.Imperial.Ac.Uk/Media/Imperialcollege/Medicine/Mrc-Gida/2020-05-08-Covid19-Report-21.Pdf>.

Pasternak, Natalia E Almeida, Luiz Gustavo De.Coronavírus: Quase Todo Mundo Tem Que Pegar Para A Pandemia Passar? Disponível No Website <Https://Saude.Abril.Com.Br/Blog/Cientistas-Explicam/Coronavirus-Quase-Todo-Mundotem-Que-Pegar-Para-A-Pandemia-Passar/>.

Piffero, Luiza. Em Busca Da "Imunização De Rebanho": O Contra-Ataque Da Ciência Diante Do Coronavírus. Disponível No Website < Https://Gauchazh.Clicrbs.Com.Br/Saude/Noticia/2020/04/Em-Busca-Da-Imunizacao-Derebanho-O-Contra-Ataque-Da-Ciencia-Diante-Do-Coronavirusck8u9z90e01pv01qw6vod7kx9.Html>.

Ribeiro, Krukemberghe Divino Kirk Da Fonseca. Vírus. Brasil Escola. Disponível No Website <Https://Brasilescola.Uol.Com.Br/Biologia/Virus.Htm>.

* Fernando Alcoforado, 80, awarded the medal of Engineering Merit of the CONFEA / CREA System, member of the Bahia Academy of Education, engineer and doctor in Territorial Planning and Regional Development by the University of Barcelona, university professor and consultant in the areas of strategicplanning, business planning, regional planning and planning of energy systems, is author of the books Globalização (Editora Nobel, São Paulo, 1997), De Collor a FHC-O Brasil e a Nova (Des)ordem Mundial (Editora Nobel, São Paulo, 1998), Um Projeto para o Brasil (Editora Nobel, São Paulo, 2000), Os condicionantes do desenvolvimento do Estado da Bahia (Tese de doutorado.

Universidade de Barcelona,http://www.tesisenred.net/handle/10803/1944, 2003), Globalização e Desenvolvimento (Editora Nobel, São Paulo, 2006), Bahia- Desenvolvimento do Século XVI ao Século XX e Objetivos Estratégicos na Era Contemporânea (EGBA, Salvador, 2008), The Necessary Conditions of the Economic and Social Development- The Case of the State of Bahia (VDM Verlag Dr. Müller Aktiengesellschaft & Co. KG, Saarbrücken, Germany, 2010), Aquecimento Global e Catástrofe Planetária (Viena- Editora e Gráfica, Santa Cruz do Rio Pardo, São Paulo, 2010), Amazônia Sustentável- Para o progresso do Brasil e combate ao aquecimento global (Viena- Editora e Gráfica, Santa Cruz do Rio Pardo, São Paulo, 2011), Os Fatores Condicionantes do Desenvolvimento Econômico e Social (Editora CRV, Curitiba, 2012), Energia no Mundo e no Brasil- Energia e Mudança Climática Catastrófica no Século XXI (Editora CRV, Curitiba, 2015), As Grandes Revoluções Científicas, Econômicas e Sociais que Mudaram o Mundo (Editora CRV, Curitiba, 2016), A Invenção de um novo Brasil (Editora CRV, Curitiba, 2017),Esquerda x Direita e a sua convergência (Associação Baiana de Imprensa, Salvador, 2018, em co-autoria) and Como inventar o futuro para mudar o mundo (Editora CRV, Curitiba, 2019).

4. Struggling To Cope Up With Surge In Dead Bodies Due To COVID-19[536]

Brazil is struggling to handle the rising number of dead bodies due to the coronavirus pandemic. The country which is the hardest-hit country in Latin America, registered a daily record of 13,944 new cases on Thursday, bringing its total to 202,918 confirmed cases of the virus and 13,933 deaths since the outbreak began, according to health ministry data. Brazil's failure to provide enough hospital beds for the surging number of critical coronavirus patients is yielding increasingly grim results across the country, but particularly in Manaus, a city of 2 million people on the Amazon River deep in the rainforest. More than 2,000 people died in Manaus in April, more than four times the monthly average. Now, the city is running out of coffins. Hundreds are dying at home, either because they can't get treatment at the hospitals or because they fear they won't.

Brazil's Sao Paulo state is building thousands of vertical funeral plots in order to meet the demand caused by the surge in coronavirus victims. Heber Vila, director of Evolution Technology Funderaria, the company that manufactures these vertical cemeteries, said the plots being constructed of recyclable materials are safe as it prevents any type of contact between cemetery visitors in the form of liquids or gases from the body. An estimated 13,000 vertical plots are being built in three cemeteries in Sao Paulo state, one of the areas in Brazil hardest-hit by the COVID-19 outbreak. The impact of the virus on Sao Paulo prompted Gov. Joao Doria to repeat his stance of gradually easing lockdown restrictions, although President Jair Bolsonaro has complained that the lockdown measures to contain the spread of the virus have hurt the economy.

Meanwhile, Brazilian President Jair Bolsonaro has frequently swum against the tide of scientific opinion since the crisis broke out, first by playing down the threat of the virus and by focusing on the country's economies despite rising cases.

---

[536] WION Web Team Sao Paolo, Brazil May 15, 2020, 04.57 PM(IST)

5. Yanomami Mothers Fight For The Right To Bury Their Children During The COVID-19 Pandemic In Brazil

Written by **Amazônia Real**
Translated by **Liam Anderson**

On July 1, a mother of Yanomami[537] ethnicity, and member of the Sanöma subgroup, received her daughter's body in Onkopiu village, in Brazil, after a two-month wait.

The baby died of hydranencephaly and septicaemia in a state hospital at Boa Vista, the capital of Roraima state. According to the state's Medical Legal Institute, the body was kept all this time in a cold storage facility. The reason for the delay, according to a document by Brazil's Indigenous Health Secretariat (Sesai), to which Amazônia Real had access, was that the mother had contracted COVID-19 and been hospitalized. The mother recovered from the illness. The child, though, was not infected, which would make the transfer to the village for the funeral ritual safe.

In another part of the document, Sesai informed that it could not make the transfer because there was no "flight scheduled to enter the territory of the relatives of the deceased".

The situation is similar to that of other Yanomami mothers seeking the right to bury their children according to their traditions, faced with the funeral restrictions in place all over Brazil due to the new coronavirus pandemic.

Another three[538] Yanomami babies, who died between April and May as a result of COVID-19, were buried in a private cemetery in Boa Vista without the consent of their mothers. For them, their children's bodies were missing they were located during Amazonia Real's[539] investigations for this report. Junior Hekurari Yanomami, president of the Yanomami District Health Council, an agency attached to Sesai, said the Sanöma mother was aware that the child's body was in the Medical Legal Institute and had asked to have the funeral ritual in their village.

"Even the communities are questioning it, calling, asking us to send [the body] as soon as possible," he told Amazônia Real the day before the body was taken to the mother's land.

Amazônia Real asked Sesai for an explanation of why the child's body had remained at the IML for two months, but received no answer. The head of the agency, Robson Silva, visited the Yanomami land on July 1 with General Fernando de Azevedo Silva, the defense minister in Jair Bolsonaro's government, and representatives of the National Indigenous Foundation (Funai). On Brazilian Air Force planes, they brought medical care, medicines, supplies, as well as teams of international journalists to the Yanomami communities. On the same day, the child's body was taken to the Onkopiu village, at 11 a.m., by plane — the journey took less than 2 hours from Boa Vista. The

---

[537] https://www.indios.org.br/pt/Povo:Yanomami

[538] https://brasil.elpais.com/brasil/2020-06-24/maes-yanomami-imploram-pelos-corpos-de-seus-bebes.html

[539] https://amazoniareal.com.br/criancas-yanomami-tres-corpos-de-bebes-estao-em-cemiterio-e-um-no-iml-de-boa-vista-rr/

transfer only happened because the child did not have COVID-19, according to the Yanomami District Health Council.

Asked about the community's reaction to receiving the body of the Sanöma child, Junior Yanomami said it brought them some comfort, but the whole community was in mourning.

Other Cases

This is not the first time health authorities have failed to inform Yanomami parents about their children's burials in Boa Vista's cemeteries. The first case of the new coronavirus in the ethnic group was a 15-year-old boy in the town of Alto Alegre, also in Roraima, a region where there are a lot of rogue miners around the Uraricoera River.

Although he had symptoms since March 18, he was only tested on April 6. Three days later, the young man died in a hospital in Boa Vista. At the time, Dario Kopenawa Yanomami, director of the Hutukara Yanomami Association, said[540] officials lacked respect and knowledge of traditional ceremonies of indigenous culture.

The case was denounced at the Federal Prosecutor's Office.

"The parents [even though they were in Boa Vista] were not informed of the funeral, this is wrong and we are questioning it," he said. For the French anthropologist[541] Bruce Albert, burying a Yanomami victim without the consent of relatives shows a lack of ethics and empathy from the authorities. "Moreover, dealing with a dead person without traditional funeral rituals constitutes, for the Yanomami, as for any other people, an inhuman and therefore ignominious act". The Federal Prosecution opened a procedure to ensure the identification of the Yanomami bodies and subsequent return to their indigenous lands when it is sanitarily safe and if desired by their community of origin. Speaking with Amazônia Real, the office said it has been holding meetings with indigenous leaders and health representatives to discuss the burial of indigenous victims of COVID-19. The objective, it said, is "to align protocols with the objective of having greater communication, information and follow-up with indigenous people, but respecting the communities' health to avoid risks".

On June 30, Dario Kopenawa Yanomami said that the mothers were only informed where the babies' bodies were "after a lot of criticism" and that "they were notified very late".

On July 2, he travelled to Brasilia and me[542]t with Brazil's Vice President, General Hamilton Mourão, and the indigenous legislator Joênia Wapichana[543]. As well as talking about the Yanomami peoples' fight against the pandemic, they also discussed the invasion[544] of their territory by 20,000 miners. As well as the baby who was at the Medical Legal Institute, the report found[545] the graves of three other Yanomami children for whom the mothers were searching. They are at the private cemetery Campo da Saudade in Boa Vista.

These three Yanomami mothers are still waiting for answers about when they will receive their babies' bodies, so as to perform their funeral rituals in their villages. The babies died with suspected

---

[540] https://amazoniareal.com.br/coronavirus-povo-yanomami-ira-questionar-na-justica-enterro-de-jovem-sem-autorizacao-dos-pais-em-roraima/
[541] https://amazoniareal.com.br/sepultamento-de-yanomami-vitima-da-covid-19/
[542] https://www.socioambiental.org/pt-br/noticias-socioambientais/em-encontro-com-dario-yanomami-mourao-promete-combater-o-garimpo-ilegal-e-promover-a-desintrusao-da-terra-indigena
[543] https://pt.globalvoices.org/2019/03/10/pela-primeira-vez-na-historia-do-brasil-uma-indigena-ocupa-cadeira-no-congresso-nacional/
[544] https://g1.globo.com/rr/roraima/noticia/2020/07/03/trf-1-determina-que-governo-federal-retire-garimpeiros-da-terra-yanomami-em-roraima.ghtml
[545] https://amazoniareal.com.br/criancas-yanomami-tres-corpos-de-bebes-estao-em-cemiterio-e-um-no-iml-de-boa-vista-rr/

infection by the new coronavirus. Sesai confirmed the cause of the deaths. One of the babies, a boy, died on April 29 in a hospital under the management of Roraima's government. The mother also tested positive for COVID-19. The baby's body was not buried until three weeks after his death, on May 20, according to documents accessed by this report. The other two babies, two boys from the Sanöma subgroup, died on May 25 and were buried next to each other. One of them was two months old and died of acute renal failure and suspected COVID-19 infection in a hospital managed by Boa Vista city. The other was three days old and died after contracting an infection.

The risk of contamination because of the pandemic prevents the bodies from being removed from the cemetery at the moment. "It's only possible to retrieve buried bodies by judicial means or by waiting for the minimum period before exhumation, which is three years for adults and two years for children and newborns," said Anselmo Martinez, the manager of the cemetery where the children's bodies are. Since the first case of COVID-19 appeared among the Yanomami people, in April, more than 200 others have been contaminated in their territory, which lies in the Brazilian states of Roraima and Amazonas. Sesai's most recent epidemiological report[546], dated July 15, reported that 262 Yanomami have been infected by the virus. Four deaths have been confirmed: the three babies and the 15-year-old.

---

[546] https://saudeindigena.saude.gov.br/corona

6. Explosion In Mortality In The Amazonian Epicentre Of The COVID-19 Epidemic 19

Jesem Douglas, Yamall Orellana, Geraldo Marcelo da Cunha, Lihsieh Marrero, Bernardo Lessa Horta, Luri da Costa Leite

ABSTRACT

Manaus, the capital of the Brazilian State of Amazonas, is the current epicentre of the COVID-19 epidemic in Amazonia. The sharp increase in deaths is a huge concern for health system administrators and society. The study aimed to analyse excess overall mortality according to Epidemiological Week (EW) in order to identify changes potentially associated with the epidemic in Manaus. Overall and cause-specific mortality data were obtained from the Central Database of the National Civil Registry and the Mortality Information System for 2018, 2019, and 2020. The study analysed age bracket, sex, place of death, EW, calendar year, and causes of death. Ratios were calculated between deaths in 2019/2018 and 2020/2019 to estimate excess deaths, with 5% confidence intervals. No significant excess overall mortality was seen in the ratios for 2019/2018, independently of EW. Meanwhile, the ratios for 2020/2019 increased from 1.0 (95%CI: 0.9-1.3) in EW 11 to 4.6 (95%CI: 3.9-5.3) in EW 17. Excess overall mortality was observed with increasing age, especially in individuals 60 years or older, who accounted for 69.1% (95%CI: 66.8-71.4) of the deaths. The ratios for 2020/2019 for deaths at home or on public byways were 1.1 (95%CI: 0.7-1.8) in EW 12 and 7.8 (95%CI: 5.4-11.2) in EW 17. The explosion in overall mortality in Manaus and the high proportion of deaths at home or on public byways reveals the epidemic's severity in contexts of heavy social inequality and weak effectiveness of government policies, especially policies meant to deal with social inequalities and strengthen the Unified Health System.

INTRODUCTION

As of May 20, 2020, two months after the World Health Organization (WHO) declared COVID-19 a pandemic, some five million cases and approximately 320,000 deaths had been reported in 216 countries/areas/territories. Even with strong evidence of underestimation of its official statistics [1], Brazil is now the third most heavily affected country, with 280,000 cases and 18,000 deaths[547]. Distribution of COVID-19 mortality reflects Brazil's social and geographic heterogeneity, with five states accounting for 81% of the deaths: São Paulo, Rio de Janeiro, Ceará, Pernambuco, and Amazonas, the latter having the highest proportion of infected individuals, with 10.6% (95%CI: 8.8-12.1) [2].

---

[547] (World Health Organization. WHO coronavirus disease (COVID-19) dashboard. https://covid19.who.int/, accessed on 20/May/2020)

The State of Amazonas is located in the Brazilian Amazonia, a region occupying approximately 60% of Brazil's territory and whose population has been exposed historically to poverty and social inequality [3].

A study on the Greater Metropolitan Area of Manaus identified extensive inequality in access to health services [4]. This is a common reality for populations living in remote areas and on indigenous lands [5], whose social and economic vulnerability limits their mobility in the territory, making them more susceptible to the dramatic spread of COVID-19, especially in the more serious forms of the disease. For more than four weeks, Manaus has shown signs of exhaustion of the public hospital network due to the rapid increase in COVID-19 cases. In the first two weeks of May alone, there were nearly 7,000 new cases, double the number identified until then. In addition, from April 19 to 28, the average daily number of burials in Manaus was 123, four times more than the daily average in the same period in 2019 [6]. The average daily number of COVID-19 deaths confirmed by health services during the same period was only 14, suggesting extensive underreporting, a problem seen elsewhere in the world, especially in places with precarious testing and deficient health services [7,8]. Despite uncertainties on COVID-19-specific mortality [9], indicators of excess deaths are one of the most objective and comparable parameters to assess the epidemic's impact on mortality [10]. This study thus aimed to analyse excess overall mortality according to Epidemiological Week (EW) in order to identify changes in the risk of death potentially associated with the epidemic.

METHODS

Study design and data sources. This was a cross-sectional study with mortality data from the Central Database of the National Civil Registry[548]. Due to the pandemic scenario, the National CRC assembled a COVID-19 Registration Panel (Portal da Transparência[549] accessed on 10/May/2020), aimed at furnishing data on causes of death from Death Certificates recorded at notary public offices, which represents the totality of natural deaths, treated here as a proxy for general mortality. The data are updated daily and comply with legal guidelines and deadlines. The time between recording of the death and its transfer to the COVID-19 Registration Panel is 14 days or less, after which the data become public.

Working Definitions

According to the National CRC criteria, a suspected or confirmed death from COVID-19 is one in which the death certificate mentions the terms COVID-19, coronavirus, or novel coronavirus in sections I (lines a, b, c, d) or II (other pre-existing disease conditions not directly related to the death and not recorded in the causal sequence listed in part I). Besides COVID-19, other possible causes were considered based on the National CRC: severe acute respiratory syndrome (SARS); pneumonia; septicaemia; and respiratory failure. Deaths not classified in any of the above-mentioned conditions were included in the category "other causes". Finally, "indeterminate" deaths

---

[548] (National CRC. https://sistema.registrocivil.org.br) and the Mortality Information System (SIM. http://www2.datasus.gov.br)

[549] . https://transparencia.registrocivil.org.br/registral-COVID,

(causes of deaths related to respiratory causes, but inconclusive) accounted for fewer than 1% of the sample and were not presented separately. The National CRC data were updated on May 19, 2020, 66 days after the start of EW 12 and 24 days after the last day of EW 17. The start of EW 12 corresponds to the two days after confirmation of the first case of COVID-19 and to the 15 days prior to the first death from COVID-19 in Manaus. For purposes of comparison, we also used data on overall mortality from the SIM, furnished for the EW in question in 2018 in the city of Manaus.

Study Variables

The study variables were age bracket, sex, death at home or on public byways, EW, calendar year, and causes of death. Deaths from SARS, pneumonia (PNM), and respiratory failure (RF) were aggregated in a variable called "SARS+PNM+RF", which excludes the group of deaths suspected or confirmed by COVID-19 and according to the criteria of the National CRC.

Data Analysis

We calculated the ratios between deaths in 2019 and 2018 (2019/2018) and in 2020 and 2019 (2020/2019), in EW 12 to 17 in Manaus. We also calculated the ratios between deaths in 2020/2019 in EW 14 to 17, stratified by sex, age bracket, and cause of death. For the mortality ratios, we calculated confidence intervals with 5% significance. The analyses were performed in the R program, version 3.6.1 (http://www.r-project.org).

RESULTS

In 2018, according to the SIM, the mean weekly number of deaths in Manaus was 230, close to the weekly number observed in the first 70 days of 2019 and 2020 according to data from the National CRC, or 225 and 218 deaths, respectively. As shown in Figure 1, the overall mortality ratio for 2019/2018 is very close to one, independently of EW, while the ratio 2020/2019 only showed a similar pattern (close to one) from EW 12 to 14, with a major increase in the subsequent weeks. In other words, the ratio increased from 1.0 (95%CI: 0.9-1.3) in EW 12 to 4.6 (95%CI: 3.9-5.3) in EW 17.Overall mortality ratios for the years 2019/2018 and 2020/2019 by Epidemiological Week (EW). Manaus, Amazonas State, Brazil. The overall mortality ratios for 2020/2019 according to age bracket were not statistically significant in males under 40 years of age or females under 30 years of age, revealing the excess mortality from those age brackets upwards in 2020, especially in males (Table 1).

Overall mortality and respective ratios and confidence intervals for Epidemiological Weeks (EW) 14 to 17, according to age bracket and sex. Manaus, Amazonas State, Brazil. When comparing the 2020/2019 mortality ratio according to groups of causes of death, the data showed a gradual increase over the weeks, especially starting in EW 15, for deaths from "SARS+PNM+RF" (Figure 2). In the group of "other causes", the mortality ratio remained close to one until EW 14, when it increased, reaching a ratio of 3 by EW 17.
Mortality ratios by specific groups of causes for the years 2020/2019 by Epidemiological Week (EW). Manaus, Amazonas State, Brazil. As for the distribution of deaths across age brackets, 69.1% of the deaths occurred in individuals 60 years or older (95%CI: 66.8-71.4). The ratio of deaths

occurring at home or on public byways (43/38) in EW 12 was 1.1 (95%CI: 0.7-1.8). This same ratio (268/33) reached 8.1 (95%CI: 5.7-11.7) in EW 17 (data not shown).

Figure 1

Overall mortality ratios for the years 2019/2018 and 2020/2019 by Epidemiological Week (EW). Manaus, Amazonas State, Brazil.

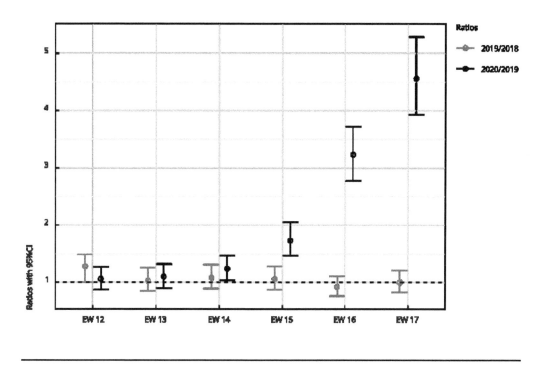

Sources: Civil Registry National Database (National CRC. https://sistema.registrocivil.org.br) and Mortality Information System (SIM. http://www2.datasus.gov.br).

Table 1

Overall mortality and respective ratios and confidence intervals for Epidemiological Weeks (EW) 14 to 17, according to age bracket and sex. Manaus, Amazonas State, Brazil.

Sex/Age bracket (years)	2020 (n)	2019 (n)	Ratio	95%CI
Male				
0-9	51	61	0.84	0.58-1.21
10-19	9	6	1.50	0.53-4.21
20-29	35	27	1.30	0.78-2.14
30-39	54	37	1.46	0.96-2.22
40-49	110	38	2.89	2.00-4.19
50-59	195	42	4.64	3.33-6.48
60-69	315	87	3.62	2.86-4.59
70-79	332	91	3.65	2.89-4.60
80 and over	317	89	3.56	2.82-4.50
All	1,418	478	2.97	2.67-3.29

(continues)

Sex/Age bracket (years)	2020 (n)	2019 (n)	Ratio	95%CI
Female				
0-9				
10-19	48	48	1.00	0.67-1.49
20-29	3	8	0.38	0.10-1.41
30-39	15	11	1.36	0.63-2.97
40-49	30	12	2.50	1.28-4.89
50-59	65	28	2.32	1.50-3.62
60-69	94	38	2.47	1.69-3.61
70-79	175	47	3.72	2.70-5.14
80 and over	185	79	2.34	1.80-3.05
All	263	108	2.44	1.95-3.04
Both sexes	878	379	2.32	2.05-2.61
0-9				
10-19	99	109	0.91	0.69-1.19
20-29	12	14	0.86	0.40-1.85
30-39	50	38	1.32	0.86-2.01
40-49	84	49	1.71	1.21-2.43
50-59	175	66	2.65	1.99-3.50
60-69	289	80	3.61	2.82-4.63
70-79	490	134	3.66	3.02-4.43
80 and over	517	170	3.04	2.56-3.62
All	580	197	2.94	2.50-3.46
	2,296	857	2.68	2.48-2.90

Source: Civil Registry National Database (National CRC. https://sistema.registrocivil.org.br) .Figure 2

DISCUSSION

According to the results, total deaths reported in 2019 were similar to 2018, comparing EW 12 through 17 in those two years. However, the comparison between total deaths in 2020 and 2019 revealed excess mortality starting in the 15th EW of 2020, with the ratio exploding in EW 17, when the number of deaths was 200% higher than in 2019.The increase in deaths started in EW 15, approximately 15 days after confirmation of the first 30 cases of COVID-19 in Manaus. In EW 17, the anomalous number of deaths coincided with the collapse in the public hospital system. During this period, the mean number of burials per day tripled. Deaths at home or on public byways also increased, as did COVID-19 cases in neighbouring municipalities.

This set of events probably resulted from a major acceleration in the epidemic in Manaus [11] in the previous weeks.

The fragility of the healthcare network in Manaus and in neighbouring municipalities [4], combined with extensive social inequality [3], help explain the critical situation with the COVID-19 epidemic. Excess mortality in the pandemic is not limited to low- and middle-income countries, but has also appeared in New York City, United States, and in the provinces of Bergamo and Brescia in northern Italy [9,12,13]. In relation to age, nearly 70% of the deaths occurred in persons 60 years or older, consistent with studies in other countries [9,12,13,14]. In this age bracket, comorbidities are more prevalent and have been associated with worse prognosis in cases of hospitalization for COVID-19 [15] Another key aspect involves gender differences, with a higher risk of mortality among men, corroborating findings from other studies [16,17].

Lower case-fatality may be associated with women's heightened perception of the symptoms and search for health services, whereas men would only tend to turn to health services in the more serious stages of COVID-19, when therapeutic possibilities are more limited. However, Zeng et al. [18] argued that higher IgG antibody levels in women could partially explain the relatively higher case-fatality in men. There was an explosive increase in mortality from respiratory problems (SARS+PNM+RF), common complications of COVID-19 [14], during the COVID-19 pandemic. There was also a significant increase in mortality from other causes, possibly resulting from factors such as: the patient's postponement of treatment in order to avoid exposure to the virus in hospitals, health services' prioritization of care for COVID-19 [19].One strength of this study was the use of the overall mortality indicator to estimate excess deaths, which appears to be a useful resource for rapid and low-cost evaluations, besides serving as a more robust and comparable indicator in a pandemic scenario [10]. Unlike COVID-19-specific mortality, overall mortality does not depend on testing strategies, health systems' organization and financing, demographic structure, or the choice of denominator, which can make the case-fatality estimates vary widely [9].

However, the interpretation of this study's results should take some limitations into account, such as the lack of standardization or review of the causes of death on the death certificates and a possible under-recording of deaths on the digital platform of the National CRC, especially in 2019, which could overestimate the ratios between total deaths in 2020 and 2019, for example. However, judging by the comparisons between total deaths in 2019 and 2018, where the ratios were always close to one, this distortion may possibly be small. The analytical strategy adopted in this study unequivocally reveals the high excess mortality in Manaus and the epidemic's severity in contexts of great social inequality, weak effectiveness of public policies, and fragility in health services. Efforts must be stepped up by administrators at the municipal, state, and federal levels to contain or mitigate the harmful effects of COVID-19, especially in more vulnerable areas where the pandemic tends to have a heavier impact on mortality.

REFERENCES

The Lancet. COVID-19 in Brazil: "so what?". Lancet 2020; 395:1461.

Mellan TA, Hoeltgebaum HH, Mishra S, Whittaker C, Schnekenberg RP, Gandy A, et al. Estimating COVID-19 cases and reproduction number in Brazil. London: Imperial College London; 2020. (Report 21).

Waisbich LT, Shankland A, Bloom G, Coelho VSP. Introduction. The accountability politics of reducing health inequalities: learning from Brazil and Mozambique. Novos Estudos CEBRAP 2019; 38:271-89.

Galvão TF, Tiguman GMB, Caicedo RM, Silva MT. Inequity in utilizing health services in the Brazilian Amazon: a population-based survey, 2015. Int J Health Plann Manage 2019; 34:e1846-53.

Ferrante L, Fearnside PM. Protect indigenous peoples from COVID-19. Science 2020; 368:251.

Prefeitura de Manaus. Manaus registra quase 2,5 mil sepultamentos em abril. http://www.manaus.am.gov.br/noticia/manaus-registra-quase-25-mil-sepultamentos-em-abril/ (acessadoem10/Mai/2020).
» http://www.manaus.am.gov.br/noticia/manaus-registra-quase-25-mil-sepultamentos-em-abril/

Ji Y, Ma Z, Peppelenbosch MP, Pan Q. Potential association between COVID-19 mortality and health-care resource availability. Lancet Glob Health 2020; 8:e480.

Castro MC, Carvalho LR, Chin T, Kahn R, Franca GV, Macario EM, et al. Demand for hospitalization services for COVID-19 patients in Brazil. medRxiv 2020; 1 abr. https://www.medrxiv.org/content/10.1101/2020.03.30.20047662v1
» https://www.medrxiv.org/content/10.1101/2020.03.30.20047662v1

Onder G, Rezza G, Brusaferro S. Case-fatality rate and characteristics of patients dying in relation to COVID-19 in Italy. JAMA 2020; [Online ahead of print].

Leon DA, Shkolnikov VM, Smeeth L, Magnus P, Pechholdová M, Jarvis CI. COVID-19: a need for real-time monitoring of weekly excess deaths. Lancet 2020; 395:e81.

Programa de Pós-graduação em Ciências do Ambiente e Sustentabilidade na Amazônia, Universidade Federal do Amazonas. Atlas dos objetivos de desenvolvimento sustentável no Amazonas. (Especial COVID-19, 2). https://edoc.ufam.edu.br/handle/123456789/3198/ (acessado em 03/Mai/2020).
» https://edoc.ufam.edu.br/handle/123456789/3198/

Weinberger D, Cohen T, Crawford F, Mostashari F, Olson D, Pitzer VE, et al. Estimating the early death toll of COVID-19 in the United States. medRxiv 2020; 29 abr. https://www.medrxiv.org/content/10.1101/2020.04.15.20066431v2
» https://www.medrxiv.org/content/10.1101/2020.04.15.20066431v2

Ghislandi S, Muttarak R, Sauerberg M, Scotti B. News from the front: excess mortality and life expectancy in two major epicentres of the COVID-19 pandemic in Italy. medRxiv 2020; 13 mai. https://www.medrxiv.org/content/10.1101/2020.04.29.20084335v2
» https://www.medrxiv.org/content/10.1101/2020.04.29.20084335v2

Shi S, Qin M, Shen B, Cai Y, Liu T, Yang F, et al. Association of cardiac injury with mortality in hospitalized patients with COVID-19 in Wuhan, China. JAMA Cardiol 2020; e200950.

Dietz W, Santos-Burgoa C. Obesity and its implications for COVID-19 mortality. Obesity (Silver Spring) 2020; 28:1005.

Ciminelli G, Garcia-Mandicó S. COVID-19 in Italy: an analysis of death registry data. VOX 2020; 22 abr. https://voxeu.org/article/COVID-19-italy-analysis-death-registry-data
» https://voxeu.org/article/COVID-19-italy-analysis-death-registry-data

Huang C, Wang Y, Li X, Ren L, Zhao J, Hu Y, et al. Clinical features of patients infected with 2019 novel coronavirus in Wuhan, China. Lancet 2020; 395:497-506.

Zeng F, Dai C, Cai P, Wang J, Xu L, Li J, et al. A comparison study of SARS-COV-2 IgG antibody between male and female COVID-19 patients: a possible reason underlying difference outcome between gender. medRxiv 2020; 27 mar.

Vandoros S. Excess mortality during the COVID-19 pandemic: early evidence from England and Wales. medRxiv 2020; 17 mai. https://www.medrxiv.org/content/10.1101/2020.04.14.20065706v6
» https://www.medrxiv.org/content/10.1101/2020.04.14.20065706v6

J. D. Y. Orellana Instituto Leônidas e Maria Deane, Fundação Oswaldo Cruz. Rua Teresina 476, 2º andar, sala 203, Manaus, AM 69057-070, Brasil. jesem.orellana@fiocruz.br

Contributors

J. D. Y. Orellana, G. M. Cunha and I. C. Leite participated in the study's conception, interpretation, and final drafting of the manuscript. L. Marrero and B. L. Horta participated in the interpretation and final drafting of the manuscript.

Authors Details

Jesem Douglas Yamall Orellana
Instituto Leônidas e Maria Deane, Fundação Oswaldo Cruz, Manaus, Brasil.
http://orcid.org/0000-0002-5607-2615
Geraldo Marcelo da Cunha
Escola Nacional de Saúde Pública Sergio Arouca, Fundação Oswaldo Cruz, Rio de Janeiro, Brasil.
http://orcid.org/0000-0001-7128-933X
Lihsieh Marrero
Universidade do Estado do Amazonas, Manaus, Brasil.
http://orcid.org/0000-0002-2856-5682
Bernardo Lessa Horta
Centro de Pesquisas Epidemiológicas, Universidade Federal de Pelotas, Pelotas, Brasil.
http://orcid.org/0000-0001-9843-412X
Iuri da Costa Leite
Escola Nacional de Saúde Pública Sergio Arouca, Fundação Oswaldo Cruz, Rio de Janeiro, Brasil.
http://orcid.org/0000-0002-9136-8948

CHAPTER 23

HOW THE PANDEMIC EXACERBATES SOCIAL DISPARITIES

1. Just Like Trump, Brazil's Bolsonaro Puts The Economy Ahead Of His People During Coronavirus

Bruno Dupeyron,
Professor, Johnson Shoyama
Graduate School of Public Policy, University of Regina

Catarina Segatto
Visiting Professor, Universidade Federal do ABC

The COVID-19 coronavirus has infected more than two million people and killed more than 150,000 in almost 200 countries — figures that will be outdated by the time you read this article[550]. Different countries have responded to the crisis by imposing national strategies that include the shutdown of non-essential places, home confinement and physical distancing. We now know that many countries were late in imposing social distancing measures, often because the leaders of those countries failed to acknowledge[551] the seriousness of the problem. China and the United States have been criticized for their lax response. Brazil should also be lumped into the same category. Official figures from the Brazilian health ministry have shown a relatively small number of deaths from COVID-19, about 2,000 people killed by the disease in a country with a population of more than 200 million. But researchers have shown Brazil is under-reporting COVID-19 infections and deaths, and that the country likely has 12 times more coronavirus cases than the official numbers.[552] Like the leaders of China and the United States did in the early stages of the outbreak, Brazilian President Jair Bolsonaro has downplayed the risks of the coronavirus. In late March, he argued[553]: "Life must go on, employments should be kept, people's income should be preserved, so all Brazilians should go back to normal." The elderly were the most susceptible to infection, he said, so "why should schools be closed?"[554]

Health Minister Was Fired

Bolsonaro has opposed his own Ministry of Health's policies regarding social isolation — so much so that he fired Minister of Health Luiz Henrique Mandetta on April 16[555]. The final straw came after Mandetta criticized Bolsonaro when the president visited a hospital near Brasilia, but then went

---

[550] https://gisanddata.maps.arcgis.com/apps/opsdashboard/index.html#/bda7594740fd40299423467b48e9ecf6
[551] https://www.nytimes.com/2020/04/11/us/politics/coronavirus-trump-response.html
[552] https://nationalpost.com/pmn/health-pmn/brazil-likely-has-12-times-more-coronavirus-cases-than-official-count-study-finds
[553] https://www.reuters.com/article/us-health-coronavirus-brazil/bolsonaro-urges-brazilians-back-to-work-dismisses-coronavirus-hysteria-idUSKBN21B2H2
[554] https://www1.folha.uol.com.br/internacional/en/brazil/2020/03/bolsonaro-criticizes-the-closure-of-schools-attacks-governors-and-blames-the-media-in-televised-statement.shtml
[555] https://www.washingtonpost.com/world/the_americas/coronavirus-brazil-bolsonaro-luiz-henrique-mandetta-health-minister/2020/04/16/c143a8b0-7fe0-11ea-84c2-0792d8591911_story.html

outside, walked among a crowd without his mask, shook hands and signed autographs. Bolsonaro, 65, said if he were infected, he would not feel anything, or he would feel symptoms similar to "a little flu.[556]" He has played up the fact that people under the age 40 are less likely to die from COVID-19, telling Brazilians that 90 per cent of "us" would not have any symptoms even if "we" were infected. Brazilians should be careful not to spread the virus to "our" parents and grandparents, he conceded. If some people die, such as his mother, who is more than 90 years old, then he would say: "I'm sorry … that's life[557]."The main reason why Bolsonaro thinks the elderly and people with high-risk conditions can be sacrificed for the sake of the economy is that Brazil cannot afford an increase in unemployment, poverty and hunger[558]. Being suddenly concerned about Brazilians' poor and unemployed is something new for the neoliberal populist president. He has been more concerned about the conservatives who support his government including conservative Catholics and evangelicals. Bolsonaro has promised to increase Brazil's GDP, but has also backed policies favoured by his conservatives base, such as opposing gender recognition and the legalization of abortion.

Why Are Some Considered Disposable?

If we follow Bolsonaro's rationale, some groups should be considered disposable, particularly the very old and unhealthy people with high-risk conditions. But this eugenic view is absurd: emerging data from affected countries show that healthy young and middle-aged people are not spared by COVID-19[559], and many end up in intensive care. While Bolsonaro strongly opposes abortion, old people's deaths from COVID-19 seem to be quite acceptable. Bolsonaro, a former army captain, was elected in 2018 with a strong majority[560] after campaigning as a "defender of freedom." He has often been described as the South American version of Donald Trump[561], but his anti-democracy views[562] have made him a political outcast. In the midst of the COVID-19 crisis, he appeared at a public rally where right-wing protesters were calling for an end to stay-at-home orders and a return to military rule[563] for the country that was a military dictatorship from 1964-85.

Anti-China Theories

Bolsonaro has been guided by Trump's anti-China theories about the coronavirus, presented in Washington, D.C., and Mar-a-Lago, where the two presidents met in March[564]. Relations between China and Brazil have been strained — especially after one of Bolsonaro's cabinet ministers said in a tweet the coronavirus pandemic was part of Beijing's "plan for world domination." Bolsonaro's contrarian views about the pandemic have been questioned by Brazil's governors and municipal leaders, as well as physicians and other experts. The vast majority of Brazilians have been following the World Health Organization's recommendations of physical distancing — even criminal

---

[556] https://youtu.be/Vl_DYb-XaAE

[557] https://www.reuters.com/article/us-health-coronavirus-brazil/brazils-bolsonaro-questions-coronavirus-deaths-says-sorry-some-will-die-idUSKBN21E3IZ

[558] https://g1.globo.com/fantastico/noticia/2020/03/29/bolsonaro-passeia-por-brasilia-um-dia-apos-ministro-da-saude-defender-isolamento-social.ghtml

[559] https://www.washingtonpost.com/health/2020/04/08/young-people-coronavirus-deaths/

[560] https://www.cnn.com/2018/10/28/americas/brazil-election/index.html

[561] https://www.nytimes.com/2019/03/19/us/politics/bolsonaro-trump.html

[562] https://www.theguardian.com/commentisfree/2019/nov/21/bolsonaro-brazil-military-dictatorship-violence#maincontent

[563] https://www.aljazeera.com/news/2020/04/brazil-bolsonaro-joins-protest-coronavirus-curbs-200420042616860.html

[564] https://www.usatoday.com/story/news/politics/2020/03/12/trump-florida-meeting-brazil-official-now-has-coronavirus/5031802002/

organizations in favelas[565]. A coalition against Bolsonaro has been coming together, made up of ministers, governors, judges, senior civil servants, experts, journalists and citizens. This show of solidarity indicates most Brazilians are willing to pay a heavy socio-economic price for the protection of people's lives. But when this moment ends, what will Brazilians do?

More than 55 per cent of voters backed him in 2018, but his popularity was dropping[566] even before the coronavirus outbreak. Will they approve of Bolsonaro's example of trying to conduct "business as usual" during the pandemic for the sake of the economy, or will a new movement emerge that tries to address the country's abject inequality? The crisis facing Brazil may be the perfect time to rethink and rebuild the country.

---

[565] https://www.occrp.org/en/daily/11930-organized-crime-enforcing-quarantine-in-brazilian-favelas
[566] https://www.americasquarterly.org/content/bolsonaro-faces-his-biggest-crisis-and-struggling

5. Social Disparity in Magnifying Glass: The Inequality Among the Vulnerable People During COVID-19 Pandemic[567]

Andre Luis Ribeiro Ribeiro,
Naama Waleria Alves Sousa,
Vitor Oliveira Carvalho,

The editorial written by Stein and Ometa, (2020) [1] about the dilemma between health system and socioeconomic conditions created by the COVID-19 pandemic has called our attention as a very appropriated topic. Indeed, there are different repercussion in all aspects in unequal societies, which goes from financial issues to the chances to adhere of the current recommended measures of the WHO. For instance, social distancing and basic personal hygiene without proper social, economic and healthcare support may contribute to exacerbate disparity in fragile societies. In Brazil, the virus SARS-COV-2 is spreading fast and crashing our healthcare system and economy. The government is struggling to pay the financial supporting defined by the congress of 600 Brazilian real per month (about 100USD) for all the living costs and only reached around 15% of the population.

Demographic data show that 48% of Brazilians live in places without sewage and 35 million do not have access to running water in their homes [2]. Furthermore, 5-10% live in slum-like areas known as "favelas" [3], where most residences accommodate an average of 5 individuals per room with a housing density 10x higher than the rest of the city [4]. Finally, 40.6% of the Brazilian working-age population are in the informal economy, living without social protection [5]. Keeping these in mind, how can these vulnerable people protect themselves in times of COVD-19? How can they keep basic hygiene without regular running water and sewage? How to accomplish social distancing living in over-crowded places?

If the COVID-19 wasn´t challenging enough, Brazil still struggles with other important infectious diseases, such as Dengue fever, Zika e Chikungunya. These viral mosquito-borne infections (Aedes aegypti mosquito) are endemic in Brazil and can show initial similar signs and symptoms to COVID-19. The rainy season is the most favourable time for mosquito proliferation and disease spread [6], which this year the seasonality (usually peaks in April) is coinciding with the spread of SARS-COV-2 in Brazil [7]. Socially vulnerable people are more prone to acquire Aedes aegypti-related infections due to poor housing, poor sanitation and high-density population housing in "favelas" [8] [9].

Current recommendations for people with COVID-19 mild illness is to stay at home. However, the panic-state created by the COVID-19 pandemic is taking these vulnerable people, which may be suffering of mosquito-borne infections, to health units and exposing them to SARS-COV-2. Thus, the

[567] Am. J. Trop. Med. Hyg., 00(0), 2020, pp. 1–4

overlapping of infections is overburdening even more the health system and increasing the transmission rate of COVID-19 in Brazil. Furthermore, many people in the informal market don't have bank accounts and are agglomerating in huge lines in bank branches to get the financial aid. While many developed countries have struggled to give assistance to COVID-19 patients, Brazil must battle against two powerful enemies. So, the hard question to answer is: how many extra souls will be lost due to Brazil's chronic problems?

Brazil was used as an example we know well, but many other non-developed countries, especially the African ones may be struggling with some of these problems as well.

REFERERENCES

1. Stein, R.A. and Ometa, O. (2020)."When Public Health Crises Collide: Social Disparities and COVID-19," *Int. J. Clin. Pract.* , pp. 0–2, May 2020. doi:10.1111/IJCP.13524

2. Federal, S.(2020). "Brasil tem 48% da população sem coleta de esgoto, diz Instituto Trata Brasil — Senado Notícias," 2020. [Online]. Available: https://www12.senado.leg.br/noticias/materias/2019/09/25/brasil-tem-48-da-populacao-sem-coleta-de-esgoto-diz-instituto-trata-brasil.

3. Boehm, C. (2020). "Moradores de favelas movimentam R$ 119,8 bilhões por ano," *Empresa Brasil de Comunicação* , 2020. [Online]. Available: https://agenciabrasil.ebc.com.br/geral/noticia/2020-01/moradores-de-favelas-movimentam-r-1198-bilhoes-por-ano. [Accessed: 19-May-2020].

4. Souza, B, (2020). "Junto e misturado – Data Labe," *data_labe* . [Online]. Available: https://datalabe.org/junto-e-misturado-isolamento-e-quarentena-sao-possiveis-nas-favelas/. [Accessed: 25-May-2020].

5. Nitahara, A. (2020). "Informalidade cai , mas atinge 38 milhões de trabalhadores," *Empresa Brasil de Comunicação* , 2020. [Online]. Available: https://agenciabrasil.ebc.com.br/economia/noticia/2020-03/informalidade-cai-mas-atinge-38-milhoes-de-trabalhadores. [Accessed: 19-May-2020].

6. Ministério da Saúde, "Combate ao Aedes Aegypti: prevenção e controle da Dengue, Chikungunya e Zika," *Ministério da Saúde* , 2020. [Online]. Available: https://www.saude.gov.br/saude-de-a-z/combate-ao-aedes. [Accessed: 20-May-2020].

7. Viana, D,V, and Ignotti, E. (2020)."The ocurrence of dengue and systematic review," *Rev Bras Epidemiol* , vol. 16, no. 2, pp. 240–256, 2013.

8. Heukelbach, F. A., Sales De Oliveira, L., Kerr-Pontes,R. S.andFeldmeier, H. (2001). "Risk factors associated with an outbreak of dengue fever in a favela in Fortaleza, north-east Brazil," *Trop. Med. Int. Heal.* , vol. 6, no. 8, pp. 635–642, 2001.

9. Maciel-de-Freitas,R., Souza-Santos, R.,Codeço, C.T., and LourençO-De-Oliveira, R. (2010) "Influence of the spatial distribution of human hosts and large size containers on the dispersal of the mosquito Aedes aegypti within the first gonotrophic cycle," *Med. Vet. Entomol.* , vol. 24, no. 1, pp. 74–82, 2010.

3. The Impacts Of COVID-19 On Brazil's Precarious Labour Market: Informality, Citizenship and The Universal Basic Income[4]

Mara Nogueira[1]
Birkbeck, University of London, A-id

Aiko Ikemura Amaral[2]
London School of Economics and Political Science

Gareth A. Jones[3]
London School of Economics and Political Science

The first case of COVID-19 in Brazil was announced by the Ministry of Health[568] on 26 February 2020. Two weeks earlier, the Brazilian Institute of Geography and Statistics (IBGE) had published data from the National Household Survey (PNAD) showing supposedly secure jobs. that around 38 million people[569] in Brazil work in the informal sector. In eleven out of 27 states, more than 50 per cent of workers were in the informal sector and therefore fell outside the bounds of protective labour laws. Beyond informal work, a recent report by researchers from Rede de Pesquisa Solidária[570] estimated that the pandemic would impact up to 81 per cent of the country's labour force[571], thereby jeopardising even their livelihoods or taking risks[572] to keep working in order to survive day-to-day.

The pandemic exposes the dismantling of welfare regimes in the Global North and their historical limitations in the Global South, where a citizenship regime mediated by formal waged labour has always been exclusionary. All around the world, various countries have adopted emergency transfer programmes that target vulnerable groups, rekindling debates around universal basic income as a mechanism that can redistribute wealth and expand access to citizenship. Globally, the pandemic has highlighted the sheer level of precarity engendered by global restructuring of labour markets. Without access to protective safety nets, many workers in the so-called "informal economy[573]" and "gig economy[574]" face a choice between losing

---

[568] https://www.saude.gov.br/noticias/agencia-saude/46435-brasil-confirma-primeiro-caso-de-novo-coronavirus

[569] https://www.saude.gov.br/noticias/agencia-saude/46435-brasil-confirma-primeiro-caso-de-novo-coronavirus

[570] http://oic.nap.usp.br/wp-content/uploads/2020/04/Boletim_1_Covid19__revisadov2.pdf

[571] http://oic.nap.usp.br/wp-content/uploads/2020/04/Boletim-n%C2%BA2_22Covid1922pdf.pdf

[572] https://noticias.uol.com.br/saude/ultimas-noticias/redacao/2020/03/24/sem-banheiro-e-alcool-gel-entregadores-de-app-ignoram-corona-por-sustento.htm

[573] https://6minutos.com.br/economia/covid-19-o-virus-sem-fronteiras-ameaca-2-bilhoes-que-vivem-na-informalidade/

[574] https://equitablegrowth.org/the-coronavirus-recession-exposes-how-u-s-labor-laws-fail-gig-workers-and-independent-contractors/?mkt_tok=eyJpIjoiTURFd01qUmpZVGMyWXpVeiIsInQiOiJ1SHNDSmJSN2txSGN5dit3XC9PNlU2U2xFSUpiTmU3TVl6RkZwXC84cWU3SDRzN2t3SlBDaVcwQ2ZoTjYOdVwvTlpjZUdLYjVYclZSSWRSeG5jZXhlT2pPdHg2dHJ4R2Rodmp3a2hzeXBUaUHHcGFjeFV4V0VrK0ZlSGtWVU1VUFM2ZyJ9

Percentage of informal workers by state, 2019

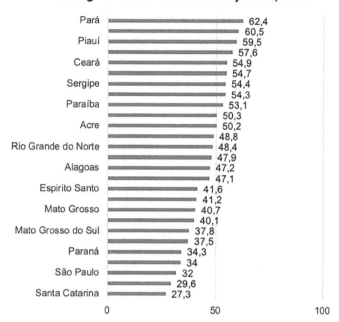

Note: Informal workers include: employees without formal contracts, domestic workers without formal contracts, employers without a business register, self-employed workers without a business register, and auxiliary household workers. Source: IBGE.

Life and Death in Brazil's "Racial Democracy"

Brazil is the seventh most unequal country in the world[575] in terms of income distribution. The same inequality is manifest in the country's heterogeneous labour market, which is stratified by race and gender[576], amongst other categories. Only in 2018 did black and brown students become a majority[577] amongst public university undergraduate students. Yet, data for the same year also showed that black and brown workers with a university degree were paid 45 per cent less than their white counterparts. Across the labour force, the average monthly income of the white population (£386/$486) was 74 per cent higher than that of the black and brown population (£222/$279). Accordingly, vulnerability is higher amongst black and brown people[578], who make up just 29 per cent of managers but constitute a clear majority amongst the poor[579] and informal workers[580].

[575] http://hdr.undp.org/sites/default/files/hdr_2019_pt.pdf
[576] https://agenciadenoticias.ibge.gov.br/agencia-noticias/2012-agencia-de-noticias/noticias/25223-mercado-de-trabalho-reflete-desigualdades-de-genero
[577] https://www.nexojornal.com.br/expresso/2019/11/13/A-desigualdade-racial-do-mercado-de-trabalho-em-6-gr%C3%A1ficos
[578] http://oic.nap.usp.br/wp-content/uploads/2020/04/Boletim-n%C2%BA3_PPS_24abril.pdf
[579] https://biblioteca.ibge.gov.br/visualizacao/livros/liv101681_informativo.pdf
[580] https://www.nexojornal.com.br/expresso/2019/11/13/A-desigualdade-racial-do-mercado-de-trabalho-em-6-gr%C3%A1ficos

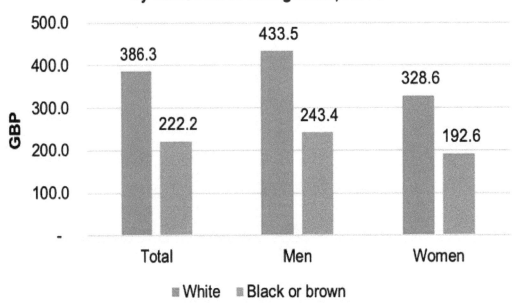

Average monthly salary (GBP) in main job, by race/colour and gender, 2018

■ White ■ Black or brown

Notes: People aged 14 or over. GBP values calculated using the exchange rate on 13 May 2020 (1 GBP = BRL 7.24). Based on socioeconomic similarities between black (*preto*) and brown (*pardo*) categories, analyses using census data commonly pool the two together into a single non-white (*negro*) category. Source: IBGE. Brazil's longstanding structural inequalities have only been exacerbated by the pandemic, which has further undermined Brazil's so-called "racial democracy". In Brazil, the black and brown population is more reliant on the overstretched and underfunded public health system and more prone to diseases such as diabetes, tuberculosis, and hypertension – comorbidities likely to aggravate COVID-19. The data clearly show the racial undertones of the pandemic: amongst victims who are severely affected or ultimately die, the majority are black or brown[581].The disproportionate effects of the disease and its ensuing economic impact on vulnerable groups – migrants, black and brown people, the indigenous, informal workers, and the poor – reveal the intersectional historical inequalities that mediate access to basic rights and citizenship in the country.

Waiting For The "Coronavoucher"

On 30 March, the Brazilian Senate approved a bill to implement a three-month emergency income for informal workers[582] of £83 (BRL $600) per month, with double that amount for female heads of household. The bill was sanctioned by President Jair Bolsonaro[583] and is widely referred to as the "coronavoucher". The benefit, currently being rolled out through the state bank Caixa

---

[581] https://g1.globo.com/bemestar/coronavirus/noticia/2020/04/11/coronavirus-e-mais-letal-entre-negros-no-brasil-apontam-dados-do-ministerio-da-saude.ghtml

[582] https://www12.senado.leg.br/noticias/materias/2020/03/30/coronavirus-senado-aprova-auxilio-emergencial-de-r-600

[583] https://g1.globo.com/politica/noticia/2020/04/01/bolsonaro-sanciona-lei-que-preve-auxilio-de-r-600-mensais-a-trabalhadores-informais-diz-planalto.ghtml

Econômica Federal[584], is anxiously anticipated around the country. The WhatsApp group "Dignidade Ambulante" ("Street Trader's Dignity"), which brings together street vendors and social activists in the city of Belo Horizonte, has seen intense information exchange and discussion about this benefit. The vote, broadcast live on 30 April, was widely publicised in the group and was compared to a "World Cup final" that would bring in the channel's largest-ever audience. Such high expectations can be explained by the precarious situation of non-waged workers unprotected by labour laws, for whom everyday subsistence and housing[585] depend on daily work in the streets. Moreover, the life strategies of the urban poor often combine several kinds of informal practices, as demonstrated by Mara Nogueira in the article "Displacing Informality[586]". For this group, confinement represents an extreme decrease in their quality of life and carries the real threat of hunger. In this context, many workers resist social isolation, echoing the president's argument that "Brazil cannot stop[587]".

Informality and Citizenship

Bolzano's disastrous handling of the pandemic has been widely condemned inside and outside Brazil. The president, however, finds supporters amongst workers in the popular economy[588]. Historically excluded from a citizenship regime mediated by formal waged labour[589], street vendors' lives are pervaded by uncertainty and a persistent struggle against state repression.
As a result, they tend to hold negative views of the state and of politicians, linking both to corruption. In Brazil, with some regional variations, municipal governments also handle workers in the popular economy punitively by applying hygienist policies[590] that seek to remove street vendors from urban centres.
Paradoxically, the emergency income already approved represents an almost unprecedented degree of recognition for a group of citizens whose relationship with the state has never been mediated by a logic of rights. The reality, however, is that many of these people face technological difficulties in accessing the new benefit because eligibility is linked to digital records. Uncertainty was compounded after the federal government excluded certain categories[591] (e.g. street vendors and gig-economy workers) from the so-called "corona voucher".

This label itself, which the media has echoed, has been criticised by specialists[592] for stigmatising its recipients, as it could associate them with the disease and thereby reproduce a kind of hygienist rhetoric. The corona voucher label thus reinforces the idea of abnormality, denying logics of citizenship and rights while conveying an idea of impermanence. Through these semantic acrobatics, the government attempts to move away from historical debates on universal basic income, which have recently been rekindled amidst forecasts of an imminent economic crisis.

---

[584] https://agora.folha.uol.com.br/grana/2020/04/caixa-tem-fila-de-espera-de-mais-de-5-horas-para-saque-do-auxilio-emergencial.shtml
[585] https://www.ijurr.org/article/displacing-informality-rights-and-legitimacy-in-belo-horizonte-brazil/
[586] https://www.ijurr.org/article/displacing-informality-rights-and-legitimacy-in-belo-horizonte-brazil/
[587] https://www.theguardian.com/commentisfree/2020/apr/02/brazil-message-world-our-president-wrong-coronavirus-jair-bolsonaro
[588] http://www.a-id.org/wp-content/uploads/2020/03/MN_COMMENTARY_.pdf
[589] https://onlinelibrary.wiley.com/doi/abs/10.1111/dech.12115
[590] https://onlinelibrary.wiley.com/doi/full/10.1111/anti.12584
[591] https://agenciabrasil.ebc.com.br/politica/noticia/2020-05/bolsonaro-sanciona-com-11-vetos-lei-que-altera-auxilio-emergencial
[592] https://www.uol.com.br/ecoa/ultimas-noticias/2020/04/03/por-que-voce-nao-deve-falar-coronavoucher-e-estigmatizar-mais-as-pessoas.htm

Universal Basic Income Under Debate

In Brazil, the first mentions of the idea of a minimum income date back to the 1970s, but the first bill proposing such a measure dates back to 1991[593]. The author was the then senator Eduardo Suplicy (Workers' Party, São Paulo), perhaps the most famous advocate of the policy in the country[594]. Approved by the Senate, the proposal to implement a negative income tax[595] was never voted on in Congress. It was eventually abandoned, as the national anti-poverty strategy took a different path. In Latin America, the rise[596] of unemployment, poverty, and informality in the aftermath of structural adjustment programmes [597]created the need for "social adjustment[598]" policies, often in the form of conditional cash transfers[599]. Bolsa Família, the largest and most successful income transfer programme in the country, was implemented in 2004, during the first term of President Lula (Workers' Party). The programme currently reaches 13.4 million families[600], but despite much international recognition, it continues to attract a wide range of detractors and supporters. From the right, it is criticised as a handout[601] that discourages hard work[602], and from the left as a policy that fails to tackle the structural roots of inequality[603].

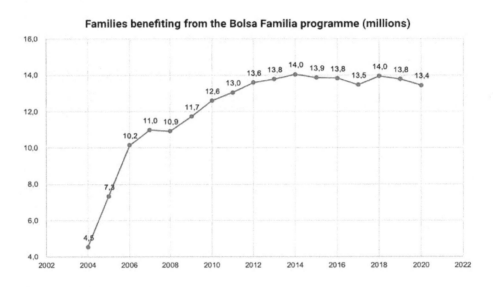

Source: Ministry of Social Development

[593] https://www.camara.leg.br/proposicoesWeb/fichadetramitacao?idProposicao=18311

[594] https://www.camara.leg.br/proposicoesWeb/fichadetramitacao?idProposicao=18311

[595] http://www.scielo.br/scielo.php?script=sci_arttext&pid=S0101-41612008000300006

[596] https://revistas.uniandes.edu.co/doi/pdf/10.7440/colombiaint9.1990.01

[597] http://www.scielo.br/scielo.php?script=sci_arttext&pid=S1413-81232018000702187

[598] https://journals.sagepub.com/doi/abs/10.1177/1468018108090638?casa_token=72xDwT8w1BkAAAAA:UJMiTIbt88_zdusfoYygET8pLHm3iviav_94-rz81hsW1bPT7tgwd_UKccwGFThPEUCBmIN74Q

[599] https://www.academia.edu/download/42938153/The_Nuts_and_Bolts_of_Brazils_Bolsa_Fam20160222-1046-se130n.pdf

[600] http://mds.gov.br/area-de-imprensa/noticias/2019/setembro/bolsa-familia-atende-mais-de-13-5-milhoes-de-beneficiarios-em-setembro

[601] https://politica.estadao.com.br/noticias/geral,bolsa-familia-e-um-programa-que-vicia-afirma-cnbb,20061117p59474

[602] https://oglobo.globo.com/brasil/apos-criticar-bolsonaro-agora-defende-bolsa-familia-22753361

[603] https://passapalavra.info/2010/04/21315/

Similar criticisms have been levelled against universal basic income. But even if they might seem similar at first sight, universal basic income differs from conditional cash transfers in that it grants all citizens the right to an unconditional and individual (rather than family) income.

This policy would increase coverage of the target population by avoiding exclusion errors, remove the stigma experienced by beneficiaries, eliminate the bureaucratic apparatus required to monitor conditionalities, and reduce the disincentive to work by delinking benefits from family income.

In the past, universal basic income has been derided as fanciful and fiscally infeasible.

Yet today it has resurfaced in several countries, including the US[604] and the UK[605]. as a policy option with real potential[606] to counter the effects of the pandemic. Even with social distancing, a global economic recession[607] is widely expected. For Brazil in particular, the IMF has estimated a 5.2 per cent fall in GDP[608] for 2020, with the economy's structural characteristics then leading to a slow recovery.

The world in which the COVID-19 crisis unfolded was one in which labour markets were already weakened by decades of restructuring, with growing levels of informalisation and precarity; stability had long since become a privilege rather than a right. Inequalities and hardship were already a reality in normal times, and they were only deepened and exacerbated by the pandemic. We urgently need to recover the logic of rights and expand it beyond a weakened welfare state with limited coverage that still revolves around labour relations. Universal basic income represents a real alternative that can extend citizenship beyond formal labour relations, granting a minimum of stability to those whose daily goal is simply to sustain their livelihoods.

---

[604] https://www1.folha.uol.com.br/mercado/2020/03/governo-trump-quer-mandar-dinheiro-as-familias-para-enfrentar-coronavirus.shtml
[605] https://www.ft.com/content/6b00fa50-d811-41cd-975b-6a8382ca6e91
[606] https://www1.folha.uol.com.br/ilustrissima/2020/03/renda-basica-antes-folclorica-vira-medida-essencial-para-enfrentar-crise-do-coronavirus.shtml
[607] https://news.un.org/pt/story/2020/04/1710372
[608] https://valorinveste.globo.com/mercados/brasil-e-politica/noticia/2020/04/17/brasil-deve-ter-ritmo-menor-de-recuperacao-pos-covid-do-que-paises-vizinhos-diz-fmi.ghtml

4. Brazil's So-Called 'Invisibles' Will Need More Than Resilience To Redress The Unequal Impacts Of COVID-19

Aiko Ikemura Amaral[609]
LSE Latin America and Caribbean Centre

Gareth A. Jones[610]
LSE Latin America and Caribbean Centre

Mara Nogueira[611]
(Birkbeck, University of London

Brazil's 13 million favela dwellers have often been asked to show resilience in the face of the country's sharp inequalities. Getting through the coronavirus crisis, however, will require more than the ability to make ends meet. Community-based initiatives have done much to protect local people from the most damaging impacts of the Bolsonaro government's deficient response and toxic rhetoric. But now as in the long term, the deep inequalities revealed by coronavirus must be kept visible and properly addressed, In Brazil, the COVID-19 pandemic has become an integral part of a political struggle involving politicians across the board[612].

But even though "the war against coronavirus" has become a means of gaining political capital, concrete responses from the government have been both lagging and lacking. The first week of April saw some measures begin to be implemented, not least the distribution of monthly vouchers worth R$600 (less than £100) to those financially affected by the coronavirus. Appealing to Brazilians' sense of kindness, Minister of Finance Paulo Guedes asked the population to help those he called "the invisibles" to register for the voucher via smartphone apps. Guedes' misplaced insinuation was that this population either lacked smartphones or were not themselves smart enough to follow the guidelines issued by the government. But who are "the invisibles"? According to Guedes[613], these are the people who "never asked for anything, [who] never needed the government ... a cleaner, a cab driver, a street vendor." This rhetorical acknowledgement of informal workers is revealing of his disconnect with the working classes in Brazil, whose contributions are central to the country's economy and society.

---

[609] https://blogs.lse.ac.uk/latamcaribbean/2020/05/14/brazils-so-called-invisibles-will-need-more-than-resilience-to-redress-the-unequal-impacts-of-covid-19/#author-info
[610] https://blogs.lse.ac.uk/latamcaribbean/2020/05/14/brazils-so-called-invisibles-will-need-more-than-resilience-to-redress-the-unequal-impacts-of-covid-19/#author-info
[611] https://blogs.lse.ac.uk/latamcaribbean/2020/05/14/brazils-so-called-invisibles-will-need-more-than-resilience-to-redress-the-unequal-impacts-of-covid-19/#author-info
[612] https://blogs.lse.ac.uk/latamcaribbean/2020/03/27/bolsonaros-brazil-and-coronavirus-contesting-the-incontestable/
[613] https://valor.globo.com/brasil/noticia/2020/04/03/guedes-pede-que-ajudem-a-informar-os-invisiveis-sobre-auxilio-de-r-600.ghtml

Yet in favelas, where the eyes of the state have rarely fallen, a number of collaborative, community-based initiatives to counteract the impacts of the disease have emerged and flourished. For those who were already struggling to get by without coronavirus, however, invisibility before the state is not just a cause for resilience and resourcefulness but also a product of deeper socioeconomic inequalities and restricted access to rights. The virulence of COVID-19 does not make it more democratic in highly unequal societies: collective action is required, and fast. But getting through the pandemic will need more than just bottom-up solutions from low-income Brazilians and the few limited measures already adopted by the government.

Lives and Livelihoods in Favelas

Stark socioeconomic inequalities have a direct impact on health and wellbeing[614], and these socioeconomic disparities are most graphically revealed by Brazil's classic *asfalto–morro* divide: that is, between the formal, tarmacked city (*asfalto*) and the improvised favelas climbing the hillsides (*morro*). Even before COVID-19, the higher prevalence of other infectious conditions like tuberculosis (TB) in favelas has been an underlying cause of public health concern. Rocinha, the biggest favela in Rio de Janeiro, for instance, has an annual TB notification rate five times higher than the citywide average[615]. Sadly, but perhaps unsurprisingly, existing data on COVID-19's death toll indicates that the mortality rate is considerably higher[616] in low-income areas of Brazil's largest cities. Yet, favelas are not homogeneously destitute spaces, and broader inequalities are also reproduced across and within favelas.

This becomes evident in the very architecture of houses.

While some homes are built of brick-and-mortar and can cost tens of thousands of Brazilian reais, more recent constructions are usually made of less-durable materials and located in more hazardous areas considered "at risk", such as floodplains or steep slopes. For some favela residents, *lajes* [617] concrete slabs serving as rooftops – provide much-needed respite[618] from the lockdown, with residents able to socialise, go about their everyday chores, or live-stream funk concerts[619] via social media. For those who do not own a *laje*, the streets – usually bustling with commerce, services, and people – are still the place to go out and get some fresh air. The centrality of the street in peoples' everyday lives goes beyond its economic importance: streets are spaces of conviviality, community-building, and organising.

Indeed, social media posts with the hashtag #COVID19nasFavelas[620] suggest that these spaces remain very lively[621], despite growing awareness of the virus. But busy streets also suggest that the "stay at home" guidelines issued by city mayors and state governors also present other serious threats to people's subsistence. In favelas, the majority of self-employed and informal employees

---

[614] https://blogs.lse.ac.uk/latamcaribbean/2020/04/14/brazils-urban-inequalities-will-exacerbate-the-impacts-of-covid-19/
[615] https://www.ingentaconnect.com/content/iuatld/ijtld/2013/00000017/00000012/art00014
[616] https://oglobo.globo.com/sociedade/covid-19-mais-letal-em-regioes-de-periferia-no-brasil-1-24407520
[617] http://www.scielo.br/pdf/ts/v31n1/1809-4554-ts-31-01-0153.pdf
[618] https://www.rioonwatch.org/?p=58809
[619] https://revistaforum.com.br/cultura/em-meio-ao-isolamento-dj-de-funk-faz-live-em-laje-na-favela-em-sp-e-explode-nas-redes/
[620] https://twitter.com/hashtag/covid19nasfavelas?src=hash
[621] https://agora.folha.uol.com.br/sao-paulo/2020/04/lider-em-mortes-brasilandia-tem-rua-cheia-e-comercio-aberto.shtml

(respectively 47% and 8% of favela residents[622]) rarely have the option of working from home. While some continue to risk infection on public transport and at work, others have no choice but to close their businesses or lose their jobs. The connection between these two dimensions sociability and liveability is thrown into ever starker relief as small entrepreneurs and workers see their incomes threatened by COVID-19's looming socioeconomic effects. The pervasiveness of so-called *viração*[623] making ends meet through a variety of precarious jobs despite the difficulties – can be taken as a sign of Brazilian inventiveness and resilience, but it is also a clear indication that material resources and economic opportunities do not trickle down to the poorest.

A month into quarantine measures in a number of states, 72 per cent of favela residents[624] had already experienced a deterioration in their living standards. The same research[625] also indicated that 92 per cent of mothers[626] living in favelas believed they would not be able to access staples, including food, if they were to lose their incomes for another month. In the absence of more comprehensive social security programmes, favela residents are left with a false and yet all too real – choice between their lives and their livelihoods.

Bottom-Up Initiatives in The Favela

Official responses to the COVID-19 crisis have been contradictory, slow, and insufficient, leading many favelas across Brazil to take things into their own hands. Local initiatives have often relied on dense, pre-existing networks of social organisations, collectives, and projects. Some focus on raising awareness[627] and fighting the spread of fake news. Loudspeakers, banners[628], and signs reinforce the message that residents should, as best as they can, follow the World Health Organization guidelines. Online, social media initiatives such as Favelas Contra o Coronavirus[629] disseminate the latest information about the virus, its spread, and how to prevent it.

Meanwhile, crowdfunding websites like the national civil society network Central Única das Favelas[630] (CUFA, have been able to finance a variety of local projects. In Rio's Complexo da Maré, meanwhile, the community NGO Redes da Maré[631] has organised the distribution of food baskets and hygiene kits with items purchased from local shops; this effort simultaneously addresses people's immediate needs and the survival of local businesses.

In Paraisópolis[632], in São Paulo, the neighbourhood association has used its own initiative and a crowdfunding campaign[633] to hire three ambulances, distribute free meals to the homeless, and create a decentralised network that monitors the wellbeing of over 100,000 residents. This new structure was implemented both to contain the spread of the virus and to locate those who are most

---

[622] https://brasil.elpais.com/sociedade/2020-03-28/sem-acoes-especificas-86-dos-moradores-de-favelas-vao-passar-fome-por-causa-do-coronavirus.html

[623] https://periodicos.fclar.unesp.br/estudos/article/view/89/85

[624] https://www1.folha.uol.com.br/equilibrioesaude/2020/03/em-quarentena-72-dos-moradores-de-favelas-tem-padrao-de-vida-rebaixado.shtml?origin=folha&sfns=mo

[625] https://www1.folha.uol.com.br/equilibrioesaude/2020/03/em-quarentena-72-dos-moradores-de-favelas-tem-padrao-de-vida-rebaixado.shtml?origin=folha&sfns=mo

[626] https://www.bbc.com/portuguese/brasil-52131989

[627] https://www.rioonwatch.org/?p=58575

[628] https://twitter.com/pisbihis/status/1248236059038814208

[629] https://www.facebook.com/favelascontraocoronavirus/

[630] https://www.vakinha.com.br/vaquinha/ajude-a-cufa-a-ampliar-seu-combate-ao-coronavirus

[631] http://redesdamare.org.br/br/artigo/86/coronavirus-entenda-como-voce-pode-ajudar-a-mare

[632] https://g1.globo.com/jornal-nacional/noticia/2020/04/11/favela-de-sao-paulo-vira-exemplo-em-acoes-contra-o-coronavirus.ghtml

[633] https://www.esolidar.com/br/crowdfunding/detail/3-g10-apoie-paraisopolis-a-combater-o-corona-virus?lang=br

vulnerable to sharp losses in income. Between making ends meet, entrepreneurship, and strong grassroots organisations, favela residents continue to demonstrate their capacity to forge strong alliances and find creative solutions to deadly circumstances that just weeks ago seemed inconceivable. That said, their actions cannot and should not have to make up for decades of state negligence and poorly planned, unsustainable interventions. Resilience is often required from those who are not able to enjoy even basic citizenship, let alone full human rights.

But surviving the pandemic is not a matter of patience and painstaking dedication from those "who never asked for anything". The inequalities and issues exposed by the pandemic have long been present and will not disappear as a result of the measures recently adopted by the government. The momentum generated by increased awareness of such inequalities, however, might serve as a strong push towards substantive change. Guaranteeing better and stable income, as well as higher living standards for favela residents, is not only important during COVID-19. It is an issue of basic social justice and a vitally important goal in and of itself.

Notes:
• The views expressed here are of the authors rather than the Centre or the LSE
• This article is part of an ongoing project entitled 'Engineering Food: infrastructure exclusion and 'last mile' delivery in Brazilian favelas', which is funded by The British Academy under its Urban Infrastructure and Well-Being programme.
• Please read our Comments Policy before commenting

About the author

Dr Aiko Ikemura Amaral is post-doctoral research officer at LSE Latin America and Caribbean Centre for the British Academy project "Engineering food: infrastructure exclusion and 'last mile' delivery in Brazilian favelas". She holds a PhD in Sociology from the University of Essex and is also a teaching associate at the Centre of Latin American Studies, University of Cambridge.

Gareth Jones is Director of the Latin America and Caribbean Centre, as well as Professor of Urban Geography in the Department of Geography and Environment at LSE and an Associate Member of the International Inequalities Institute. He has an interdisciplinary academic background, having studied economics, geography, and urban sociology. He holds an undergraduate degree from University College London and a doctorate from the University of Cambridge. He has held numerous visiting positions, including at the University of California San Diego, the University of Texas at Austin, and the Universidad Iberoamericana.

Mara Nogueira is a lecturer in geography at Birkbeck, University of London and a visiting fellow at the LSE Latin America and Caribbean Centre. She is an urban geographer whose research focuses on socio-spatial inequality and the urban politics of urban space production in Brazil. She completed a PhD in Human Geography and Urban Studies at LSE. She also holds a BSc and a MSc in Economics from the Federal University of Minas Gerais, Brazil.

5. Who's Going to Pay the Price of COVID 19? : Reflection About an Unequal Brazil[634]

Fabiana Ribeiro
University of Luxemburg

ABSTRACT

The COVID-19 pandemic has caused high mortality rates among older people, and in order to avoid a healthcare system crisis, almost all countries worldwide have adopted social isolation measures to prevent the spread of the disease. However, in Brazil, a country demarcated by economic inequalities, in which approximately 25% of the population live below the poverty line, these measures will cost severe economic losses and accentuated starvation. For this reason, the underprivileged population should be immediately prioritized and well informed through good practice to avoid the virus. Since, government discrepancies in dealing with the COVID-19 outbreak leaves the population without congruent guidelines on how to react or what to believe, allowing the spread of fake news and political crises. Here, we discuss who will pay the price of the Brazilian government denying the impact of COVID19 pandemic and suggest some measures to ensure that clear information and protection reach this population.

INTRODUCTION

We've been facing a pandemic crisis caused by COVID-19, which has produced high hospitalization rates after infection and an elevated mortality rate among the elderly aged over 60. To partially decrease public health problems, interventions relying on travel bans, social distancing, quarantine, and self-isolation have been implemented in almost all countries worldwide. These practices prevent the spread of potential infection to other individuals; nevertheless, it will cost, in the short term, severe economic damage. The situation in Brazil is rapidly evolving as in all countries over the last months. Almost three months ago, on 25th February, Brazil confirmed the first case of COVID19 in the state of São Paulo, brought by a wealthy patient coming from Italy, who spread the virus to other people, including her domestic servant with an age of over 60 years who would die a few days later. In the face of this scenario, several experts have already argued that COVID19 affects people differently, in other words, according to their social class: the marginalized populations will suffer the most significant consequences [1–3]. At this moment, Brazil is considered the new global centre of the pandemics, with substantial increases in daily deaths, and mounting to more than 19,000 deaths due to COVID-19 in total. These are the possible results of late measures of quarantine

---

[634] Correspondence: fabiana.ribeiro@uni.lu
1Institute for Research on Socio-Economic Inequality (IRSEI), University ofLuxembourg, Esch-sur-Alzette, Luxembourg
2Centro de Matemática, Computação e Cognição, Universidade Federal do

implementation by governors, strongly criticized by the president. Furthermore, these numbers seem to be underestimated since testing has been carried out in approximately 3462 people per 1 million, which represents one of the lowest testing numbers in the world. It is essential to highlight that since the outbreak of the COVID-19 pandemic, the situation in Brazil can be characterized as official communication not adhering to the WHO guidelines and a series of measures that ignored the danger of the COVID-9 crisis for public health, leading to a spread of the epidemic across the country. Brazil is characterized by increased inequalities, such as a large number of low-income people and a small elite that controls economic and political powers [4].

Poverty in Brazil affects mainly blacks and browns who compose 72.7% of low-income people, of which over half are women.

These people live in crowded living conditions and with limited possibilities to follow hygiene and social distancing related recommendations in many urban communities, which makes a significant, hardly containable spread of the disease very likely to happen. Allied to this, a large part of the people over 60 years old, cannot follow the quarantine recommendations since they have to work to, with their income, still help a large number of family members as a consequence of the weak system of pensions which favours the nonpoor [5]. Moreover, 6.9% of the Brazilian population is illiterate, 30% of the Brazilians between the age of 15 to 64 years old are functionally illiterate people [6], 26.9% have 11 years of formal education, and only 16.5% have completed undergraduate education [7], which means that a large part of the population is unable to interpret information related to COVID-19, especially when conflicting messages are disseminated.

Another important point regarding inequality in Brazil is related to the public health system that covers healthcare of approximately 80% of the population [7], of which many people who cannot afford to pay for private healthcare. In other words, Brazil has a public health system that can rapidly collapse if measures to prevent the spread of the virus are not followed. It has been shown in Brazil that low schooling and consequently low purchasing power combined with a weak health system is aggravating the development of chronic health problems in the population: Beltrán-Sánchez and Andrade [8] noticed that Brazilians without formal education had higher levels of diabetes, hypertension, and heart disease as a result of higher prevalence of obesity compared to those with some formal education, especially among women. Congruently, with a higher number of adults presenting chronic diseases, the impact of COVID-19, which has caused a high number of deaths among older people in developed countries, in a developing country like Brazil, the possible victims will also be younger ones. This trend has already been observed, as 30% of the reported deaths were from patients under the age of 60 [9]. Who is going to pay the price of COVID-19 in Brazil? The marginalized groups that support the elite of Brazilian society will be the potential victims of COVID-19, which represent informal workers or those in essential services [10].

Although more men are dying at this moment from COVID-19 around the world, outcomes of COVID-19 seem to be associated with health comorbidities and also by social inequalities [11].

Given that women in Brazil are those who integrate the most significant numbers of informal jobs [7] it is possible to suppose that more women will be affected by COVID-19 when compared to countries with greater gender equality. Furthermore, the numbers of the Ministry of Health [9] have been showing that, when considering hospital admissions, the percentage of white persons hospitalized for COVID-19 is higher than the rates of black and brown persons. However, about 54.8% of deaths are of the latter, which are overwhelmingly users of the public health system.

As urgent measures to ensure that the situation does not get even worse, the government must promote, with information based on scientific evidence, public health campaigns with congruent and clear guidelines across the country using easy language (e.g. distributing flyers and providing masks), so its population can understand how to act. Furthermore, the population of Brazil needs to be tested, and contacts of cases need to be traced, to provide precise data on the pandemic and stop further spread. Without testing and tracing, there can be no effective healthcare response.

REFERENCES

1. Ahmed. F., Ahmed,N.E, Pissarides C, Stiglitz J. (2020).Why inequality could spread COVID-19. Lancet Public Health. 2020. https://doi.org/10.1016/S24682667(20)30085-2.
2. Chiriboga, D., Garay, J., Buss, P., Madrigal, R., Rispel, L. (2020). Health inequity during the COVID-19 pandemic: a cry for ethical global leadership. Lancet Public Health. 2020. https://doi.org/10.1016/S0140-6736(20)31145-4.
3. Dorn, A.V., Cooney, R.E., Sabin, M.L. (2020). COVID-19 exacerbating inequalities in the US. Lancet. 2020;395(10232):1243–4. https://doi.org/10.1016/S0140-6736(20)30893-X.
4. Medeiros, M. (2020). Income inequality in Brazil: new evidence from combined tax and survey data: World Social Science Report. Paris: UNESCO. 2016. https:// unesdoc.unesco.org/ark:/48223/pf0000245949. Accessed 07 May 2020.
5. Gasparini, L, Alejo, J., Haimovich, F., Olivieri, S., Tornarolli, L. (2020).Poverty among the elderly in Latin America and the Caribbean. Background paper for the World Economic and Social Survey2007. http://www.ced-las.econo.unlp.edu. ar/wp/wp-content/uploads/doc_cedlas55.pdf. Accessed 5 May 2020.
6. Lima, A., Catelli, R. Indicador de Alfabetismo funcional - INAF Brasil 2018: resultados preliminares. São Paulo, Ação Educativa & Ação Social do IBOPE; 2018. https://ipm.org.br/relatorios. Accessed 12 May 2020.
7. Brazilian Institute of Geography and Statistics: IBGE. (2019) http://www.ibge. gov.br. Accessed 13 May 2020.
8. Beltrán-Sánchez, H., Andrade, F.C.D. (2020).Time trends in adult chronic disease inequalities by education in Brazil: 1998–2013. Int J Equity Health. 2016. https://doi.org/10.1186/s12939-016-0426-5.
9. Ministry of Health of Brazil. Boletins epidemiológicos. (2020) https://www. saude.gov.br/boletins-epidemiologicos. Accessed 16 May 2020.
10. Loayza, N.V., Pennings, S. (2020). Macroeconomic Policy in the Time of COVID-19:A Primer for Developing Countries. World Bank, Washington, DC. (2020) https:// openknowledge.worldbank.org/handle/10986/33540. Accessed 21 May 2020.
11. The Lancet. The gendered dimensions of COVID-19. Lancet (London, England). 2020;395:10231. https://doi.org/10.1016/S0140-6736(20)30823-0.

6. Vulnerability, Poverty and COVID-19: Risk Factors and Deprivations in Brazil[635]

Fernando Flores Tavares[*] and Gianni Betti[*]

*Department of Economics and Statistics, University of Siena, Italy..

INTRODUCTION

The COVID-19 outbreak exposes to a greater extent the inequalities and the lack of basic human needs in developing countries. Planning an efficient response to the pandemic requires a comprehension of the increased risk of exposure experienced by people, especially those on unsafe conditions. This briefing aims to show how much and in which way people in Brazil are deprived in living standards indicators directly related to the capacity to prevent and heal COVID-19. In this manner, we hope to contribute with information, supporting actions to guarantee that all the population could follow international health recommendations.

The first confirmed case in Brazil was diagnosed on February 26. Currently there are 25,262 confirmed cases in a rapid contamination path (DATASUS, 2020)[636]. The potential threats of the pandemic are worsening the quality of life of entire communities. There are at least[637] two sets of additional risk factors faced by families under multidimensional vulnerability condition.

First, people may not be able to follow the essential prevention recommendations.

Sheltering at home may be currently infeasible, both because many people do not have a fixed monthly payment salary, and also because the house structure is not adequate to keep them safe and comfortable during the quarantine. Moreover, due to inadequate access to clean water and poor sanitation condition, it is not always possible to properly wash hands, and clean and disinfect the home. Also, in case of necessity, keeping a safe distance from others is not practicable in an overcrowded household. **Second**, poor living standards may increase the risk of contamination to COVID-19 and reduce the capacity to recover from it. Drinking unsafe water and being exposed to improper sewage disposal is highly correlated to preventable diseases (WHO, 2019; WHO, 2018b), which can compromise the immune systems. Families cooking with polluting fuels may be a group of risk to COVID-19 as indoor air pollution is associated with respiratory diseases (WHO, 2018a). Moreover, food security is now under threat for families that have schoolchildren dependent on daily school meals.In order to capture these aspects, we use the Alkire-Foster (AF) method to measure multidimensional vulnerability (Alkire and Foster, 2011). AF method is an appropriate tool to provide clear evidence of overlapping deprivations.

---

[635] This is a preliminary brief. Further details and analysis will be presented in future work.
[636] Last updated on 14/04/2020.
[637] For example, other publications also discuss: access to public health, gender issues, employment, and others (Coelho et al. (2020); UNFPA (2020); ILO (2020); Alkire et al. (2020), Pires et al. (2020)).

Using the Brazilian Consumer Expenditure Survey (POF-IBGE) for 2017-18, we selected eight interlinked vulnerability indicators in the dimensions of hygiene, shelter, physical distance, and health recovery capacity (see Table 1). Five of these indicators are also part of the ten global Multidimensional Poverty Index (MPI)[638] (OPHI and UNDP, 2019).

2. Vulnerability to COVID-19 and Poverty
2.1 Deprivations in Brazil

By first looking into the living standards data in Brazil is possible to see that, independently of the pandemic context, a large proportion of Brazilians do not have access to basic human needs. The main results are:

- **81 million people (39.1% of the • population)** are deprived in sanitation, and **61.5 million (30%)** may have inadequate access to safe drinking water.

- **45.5 (21.9%) million** may have indoor pollution, **26.3 million (12.7%)** live in an over-crowd house, **22.2 million (10.7%)** have poor material housing condition, and **22 million (10.6%)** have children relying on daily school meal.
  9.8 million people (4.7%) have a high number of older adults or children per working-age people at home, and **457.7 thousand (0.2%)** do not have access to electricity.

---

[638] The Global MPI indicators are: nutrition, child mortality, years of schooling, school attendance, cooking fuel, sanitation, drinking water, electricity, housing, and assets.

Table 1 - Vulnerability indicators and its association to COVID-19
Source: Elaborated by the authors.

Dimension	Variable	Description	Association to COVID-19
Hygiene	Drinking water	The household does not have daily indoor access to water from the public network.	Clean water is crucial to prevent COVID-19 by washing hands, and unsafe drinking water is associated with weakened immune systems (WHO, 2019).
	Sanitation	The household's sanitation facility is not improved, or it is shared with other families, or the sewage disposal is not connected to the public system.	Improper sanitation is a major cause of infectious diseases (WHO, 2018b), which can affect the immune system compromising recovery from COVID-19.
Staying at Home	Electricity	The household does not have electricity available.	Electricity is a basic human need to guarantee well-being and safe food storage.
	Housing	The household's housing materials for at least one of floor, wall and roof, walls are inadequate.	An inadequate house structure makes it difficult to stay an extended period at home due to excessive indoor heat, exposure to natural disasters and other factors.
Physical Distance	Overcrowded housing	The household has three or more residents per permanent bedrooms.	Having adequate space is not related only to being comfortable at home, but also crowded homes are more exposed to infectious diseases (WHO, 2018c), and people cannot maintain safe physical distance in case of necessity.
	Dependency Ratio	The household has four or more non-working-age per workingage residents.	There is a higher need for caution because there may be older adults at home which is a group of risk. A highdependency ratio is also associated with bigger household vulnerability to shocks (Naudé et al., 2009).
Recovery Capacity	Cooking fuel	The household cooking fuel is wood, oil, kerosene, or other chemical fuel.	Inadequate cooking fuel is associated with indoor pollution that harms the respiratory systems (WHO, 2018a).
	School meals	The household has one or more children at home that daily have breakfast, or lunch, or dinner for free at school.	It is an indication that the household food security may be compromised. Families will have to spend more to feed their children during the quarantine.

2.2

Table 2 - Number and proportion of people deprived in each indicator

	Freq.	% of Total population
Drinking Water	61,478,436	29.68%
Sanitation	80,970,486	39.1%
Electricity	457,742	0.22%
Housing	22,155,805	10.7%
Cooking Fuel	45,478,041	21.96%
Crowded Housing	26,313,116	12.71%
Dependency Ratio	98,12,883	4.74%
School meals	21,959,815	10.6%
Total Pop.	207,103,790	100%

Source: POF 2017/2018. Calculated and elaborated by the authors.

Overlapping Deprivations and Poverty

We consider a person as vulnerable to COVID19 when she or he is deprived in at least two of the eight indicators. People under severe risk are those deprived in half of the eight vulnerability indicators. Poverty is calculated based on household consumption expenditure per capita with a poverty line at $3.20 a day (2018 PPP), which is equivalent to R$298.86 per capita. The main messages are:

- **78.7 million people (38% of the population)** are deprived in at least one of the indicators.
- More than **2.3 million people (1.1% of the population)** are deprived in at least half of the indicators, which is considered a severe risk to COVID-19.
- **10.17 million people (4.9% of the population)** are simultaneously vulnerable to COVID-19 and poor.
- **1.19 million people (0.6% of the population)** are simultaneously at severe risk to COVID-19 and poor.

This outcome shows that not all the people vulnerable and at severe risk to COVID-19 are monetarily poor, and vice-versa. Of course, money is essential for families to fight the pandemic, but what this result implies is that policy responses also need to involve the basic human necessities to prevent and recover from COVID-19.

Table 3 – Incidence and number of people under vulnerability, severe risk, and poverty conditions

	Vulnerable	At Severe Risk	Poor	Vulnerable and Poor	At Severe Risk and Poor
Incidence (%)	18.20%	1.13%	9.96%	4.91%	0.58%
Pop.(in thousands)	37,672	2,340	20,636	10,169	1,193

Source: POF 2017/2018. Calculated and elaborated by the authors.

2.3 Overlapping Deprivations Disaggregated by Region and Area

As an indication of regional inequalities, Figure 1 shows the number and proportion of vulnerable people and the current number of COVID-19 cases by State. The key outcomes are:

- The percentage of people that are deprived in at least one of the indicators ranges from **15.8%** in Rio de Janeiro state to **80.6%** in Rondônia state.

- The states with the highest proportion of vulnerable people are Acre, Maranhão e Pará, with **26.9%, 22.8%** and **18.7%,** respectively. The regions with the lowest ratios are São Paulo, Distrito Federal and Paraná, with **1.5%, 1.5%** and **2.1%,** respectively.

- São Paulo is the region with the highest number of COVID-19 cases (**9371 people**). Acre, Maranhão and Pará together account to **900** cases.

- In terms of COVID-19 cases per million people, states of the north region present the highest number: Amazonas, Amapá and Roraima have **381, 377** and **223 cases per million**, respectively.

- **20.4 million people in rural areas (66.9% of the rural population)** are vulnerable to

- COVID-19.

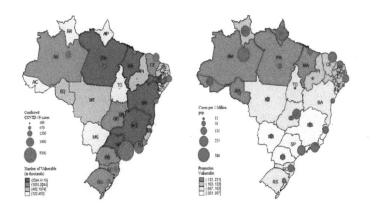

(a) Number of COVID-19 cases and number of vulnerable and proportion

(b) COVID-19 cases per 1 million population of vulnerable

Figure 1 –COVID-19 and vulnerability by state
Source: DATASUS (2020) and POF 2017/2018. Calculated and elaborated by the authors

2.4 Overlapping Deprivations Disaggregated by Ethnicity

The risks to COVID-19 are also very different among ethnicities. Figure 2 depicts the incidence of vulnerability for each group. The main outcome is:

- Indigenous people have the highest population proportion vulnerable to COVID-19 (**28.5%**), followed by brown (**23.8%**), black (**19.2%**), white (**12.5%**), and yellow7.5%.

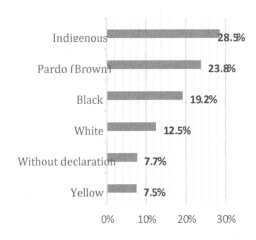

Figure 2 - Incidence of vulnerability by ethnicity

Source: POF2017/2018. Calculated and elaborated by the authors.

This information means that more than a quarter of the indigenous population is deprived in at least two indicators. The fact that the virus is spreading quickly towards the north region is an additional concern. North is the region with the highest proportion of the population under vulnerability and severe risk to COVID-19 and concentrates 22.7% of the Brazilian indigenous population. This evidence reinforces the urgent need to act to avoid the virus to achieve the most vulnerable groups and be prepared in advance in case of necessity.

3.CONCLUSIONS

This briefing intended to call attention to the number of people vulnerable to COVID-19 in Brazil. In the short run, we need rapid actions preventing to spread the virus in vulnerable regions and to alleviate the risks involved. To achieve these results, it is essential also to promote prevention in low-risk areas. Policy response must ensure that people with multiple deprivations can follow as much international prevention recommendations as they can and have quality public health services available. A priority action is to guarantee a basic income for all people in vulnerable conditions. Another crucial complementary response is to massively distribute masks, hand sanitizers, basic supplies, mineral water, cooking gas, and non-perishable food prioritizing people under vulnerability. Moreover, an evident plan is to follow examples of international responses. For instance, increasing the number of available beds for COVID-19 in public hospitals; suspending rents, taxes and public services bills to people under unsafe conditions; bringing doctors from other countries to help on the pandemic. In the long run, the hope is that these pandemic crisis responses turn, as written by Alkire et al. (2020), an inflexion point in ending poverty in all its forms.

REFERENCES

Alkire, S., And J. Foster (2011). Counting and multidimensional poverty measurement. Journal of Public Economics 95: 476–487.

Alkire, S. Et Al. (2020). Multidimensional Poverty and COVID-19 Risk Factors: A Rapid Overview of Interlinked Deprivations across 5.7 Billion People. Oxford Poverty & Human Development Initiative, Briefing 53.

COELHO Et Al. (2020). Assessing the potential impact of COVID-19 in Brazil: Mobility, Morbidity and the burden on the Health Care System.

Datasus (2020), Painel de casos de doença pelo coronavírus 2019 (COVID-19) no Brasil pelo Ministério da Saúde.

Ilo (2020). COVID-19 and the world of work: Impact and policy responses. International Labour Organization Monitor 2nd Ed. https://www.ilo.org/wcmsp5/groups/public/@dgreports/@dcomm/documents/briefingnote/wcms_740877.pdf.

Naudé, W. et al. (2009). Vulnerability in developing Countries. UNUWIDER. United Nations University Press.

OPHI and UNDP (2019). Global multidimensional poverty index 2019: illuminating inequalities.

Pires, Et Al.(2020). COVID-19 e desigualdade: a distribuição dos fatores de risco no Brasil.

UNFPA (2020). COVID-19: A Gender Lens: Protecting Sexual And Reproductive Health And Rights, And Promoting Gender Equality. Technical Brief. https://www.unfpa.org/resources/COVID-19-gender-lens.

WHO (2019). Drinking-water Key Facts. World Health Organization

WHO (2018a). Household air pollution and health. World Health Organization. https://www.who.int/news-room/factsheets/detail/household-air-pollution-and-health.

WHO (2018b). Water sanitation hygiene. World Health Organization. https://www.researchgate.net/community/COVID-19.

WHO (2018c). WHO housing and health guidelines. World Health Organization. https://apps.who.int/iris/bitstream/handle/10665/276001/9 789241550376-eng.pdf.

CHAPTER 24

FOOD SUPPLY AND SCARCITY

1. Challenges Facing The COVID-19 Pandemic In Brazil: Lessons From Short Food Supply Systems

Potira V. Preiss[1]

During the first months of the quarantine in Brazil, the official numbers indicated that 40,000 people were infected and 2500 died from COVID-19. However, given the rationalized testing policy, specialists alert there is a high number of underreported cases, and the official numbers might account for nearly 10% of cases. We are in the deep dark and there is no indication of when we will be out of the woods. The challenging situation began in a fragile political moment in Brazil.

The Brazilian president has been completely despicable, disregarding the gravity of the situation, acting against mitigation strategies, and disseminating false news. There is no cohesive political leadership, governors and mayors are acting without a coordinated plan. Unemployment is growing faster and the population that was already in a precarious condition is becoming an easy prey.

We do not know what will kill them first, hunger or COVID-19.

Overall, activities in the country are restricted to essential services, such as health care and food supply. In this field, the main protagonists are farmer families who account for about 80% of the country's food production. This group is mostly in a context of social vulnerability due to their depravation of public policies because lawmakers prioritise the production of commodities and exportation. Currently, the profile of a Brazilian family farming is aging and in poverty, making them twice as victims of COVID-19. They should be supported and protected.

Supermarkets are recognised internationally for the low prices they pay to farmers and for offering ultra-processed foods, which are less healthy. Thus, prioritizing farmers' direct marketing channels is essential. Street farmers markets are the Brazilians second favourite place to buy food, and most of them remain open during the outbreak with a series of security measures in place such as: bigger distance between stands, stronger asepsis, supply of cleaning material, usage of masks and advertising how to prevent contamination. The indoor farmers markets have been suspended and in some cases the producers have organised home delivery schemes. The remaining challenge is the ability to quickly adapt to a completely different form of trading. For instance, the lack of a free e-commerce platform that could help advertise and facilitate ordering is an obstacle because it makes the job more work intensive.

Besides, it takes experience to become efficient in a new trading channel.

In the case of existing Solidarity Purchasing Groups (GAS), Community Supported Agriculture (CSA) and delivery system, there is a huge explosion in demand. Some producers report twice as many orders, overloading the capacity to cope. The above systems offer a simple buying experience for consumers and a stable demand for producers that guarantees continuous income and helps with production planning. Brazilian researches on agroecological markets, GAS and CSA systems demonstrate that those channels work mostly with family farmers that produce local organic or agroecological fresh food and can be up to 400 times cheaper than the organics commercialized by supermarkets. It generates higher revenue to farmers and more accessible quality products for costumers, breaking the myth 'clean food is expensive'. New consumers and new groups of farmers experiencing those channels offer an interesting potential for widening such strategies in size and number after the quarantine period. For those who cannot afford to buy food, the hope is also in family farming that can supply the vulnerable population with basic food—especially if the State inject emergency resources in the existing institutional programs. This is a strong demand from social movements in Brazil, however without action by the State yet. There are many civil society donation campaigns, but they do not meet the demand. It is hard to set any conclusion, but some lessons have been already learned. The agroecological farmers network experience and cooperative articulations stand out of the crowd with their resilience capacity. The disruption in recent years of a series of food policies in progress in the country aggravates the situation and demonstrates that the State's role is imperative for safeguarding food producers and ensuring food security. We urgently need to re-territorialise food systems by embedding them to social needs and ecological process. Consumers have a key role to play in this transformation by supporting economically and politically the type of food systems they want to foster. Finally, despite all, this crisis may be the wakeup call we all need to redirect society priorities and encourage us to endeavour the necessary changes.

Potira V. Preiss Post-Doctoral Researcher at Graduate Program in
Regional Development at University of Santa Cruz do Sul – PPGDR/
UNISC, PNPD/CAPES Fellow and researcher at Group of Studies and Research in Agriculture, Food and Development – GEPAD/UFRGS.

2. How COVID-19 Exposed Inequalities In Brazil's Food Supply Chain

Gareth A. Jones [639]

(LSE Latin America and Caribbean Centre),

Aiko Ikemura Amaral[640]

(LSE Latin America and Caribbean Centre),

The impact of the coronavirus crisis on livelihoods and prices has limited access to food in Brazil, particularly for those on lower incomes. Supply chains that fail to cover the "last mile" into poor urban communities are a significant part of the problem, and impressive community initiatives to meet nutritional needs are not enough to bridge that gap. So far the issue of food security has been used by the current government mainly for political point-scoring, but there are real steps that it could take to achieve a more resilient, fairer, and healthier food system.

(LSE Latin America and Caribbean Centre), and Mara Nogueira (Birkbeck, University of London) as part of a series of blogs[641] linked to their British Academy-funded project Engineering Food: infrastructure exclusion and "last mile" delivery in Brazilian favelas[642].

On April Fools' Day, Brazil's president Jair Bolsonaro tweeted a video of a near-deserted regional supply centre in Belo Horizonte. "Take a look at this", said the man in the video. "This is what we call a *food short–age!*". Bolsonaro's own caption[643] added that "[This is not about] a disagreement between the president and SOME state governors and SOME mayors", claiming that the video showed "some facts and truths that must be revealed".

This video[644] depicting supposed food shortages in Belo Horizonte was shared by President Jair Bolsonaro, but it was later found to be false

Bolsonaro's brief encounter with the "truth", however, ended only hours later when journalists visited the supply centre and found it operating as usual.[645] It later emerged that the video had deliberately been shot while the market was being cleaned and therefore empty. Bolsonaro later

---

[639] https://blogs.lse.ac.uk/latamcaribbean/2020/06/19/mixing-food-with-politics-how-covid-19-exposed-inequalities-in-brazils-food-supply-chain/#author-info

[640] https://blogs.lse.ac.uk/latamcaribbean/2020/06/19/mixing-food-with-politics-how-covid-19-exposed-inequalities-in-brazils-food-supply-chain/#author-info

[641] https://blogs.lse.ac.uk/latamcaribbean/tag/engineering-food/

[642] https://blogs.lse.ac.uk/latamcaribbean/tag/engineering-food/

[643] https://piaui.folha.uol.com.br/lupa/2020/04/01/twitter-bolsonaro-video-desabastecimento-ceasa-minas-gerais/

[644] https://www.youtube.com/watch?v=rZd_XQFIxI4&feature=emb_logo

[645] https://g1.globo.com/mg/minas-gerais/noticia/2020/04/01/policia-investiga-video-postado-por-bolsonaro-que-mostrava-ceasa-da-grande-bh-vazia.ghtml

apologised and deleted the tweet[646], but its message had gone out loud and clear. The food supply chain had become politicised, and was now one more issues like promoting treatment with chloroquine[647] or rejecting social distancing[648] that he could use to fire up his ardent supporters. Beyond Brazil, steps to control the pandemic[649] have led to a renewed focus on the resilience of food supply chains, raising important questions about availability and accessibility of food. Complex, time-sensitive supply chains, like those providing fresh fruit and vegetables[650], suddenly begin to look too long and too fragile[651]. Policy advice has highlighted logistical solutions that ensure future supply chains are more resilient and efficient[652]. But missing from this discussion, and from controversy around Bolsonaro's "shortages" has been a consideration of the actual politics of food insecurity and its far-reaching effects on health and wellbeing.

COVID-19, Food Security, And A Health Syndemic

Even before the pandemic, the impact of extreme weather events, conflicts, and persistent poverty on global food systems had led UN agencies to highlight the growing problem of food insecurity. But COVID-19 threatens to make the problem even worse, especially for the poor and vulnerable, including the elderly and lower-income households with children[653]. Widespread job losses[654] and rising prices during the crisis put pressure on people's ability to acquire food of sufficient quantity and variety. And when healthy foods are substituted with high-calorie, ultra-processed options, rates of undernutrition and obesity are exacerbated, which effectively serves to store up negative public health outcomes[655]. COVID-19 has highlighted how vulnerable populations[656] are negatively impacted by the complex interaction of socio-economic exclusion, low-nutrition diets, diagnostic markers indicating compromised immune systems, and policy decisions that provide uneven access to underfunded health services[657]. This situation can be viewed as a syndemic[658]: a complex web of illnesses, social factors, and environmental influences that promotes the negative effects of disease interaction. Leading up to the coronavirus crisis, data for Brazil showed that high levels of undernutrition and obesity[659] were co-present with associated diseases[660] such as diabetes, cardio-respiratory conditions, and some cancers[661]. These conditions have persisted despite numerous public policy interventions. During the 2000s, a combination of economic growth, decreasing

---

[646] https://www.correiobraziliense.com.br/app/noticia/brasil/2020/04/01/interna-brasil,841679/ceasa-de-minas-gerais-desmente-bolsonaro-apaga-video-de-rede-social.shtml

[647] https://brasil.elpais.com/brasil/2020-05-20/bolsonaro-amplia-uso-da-cloroquina-admitindo-que-pode-nao-ter-eficacia-e-trazer-efeitos-colaterais-graves.html

[648] https://oglobo.globo.com/brasil/bolsonaro-volta-criticar-isolamento-social-contra-coronavirus-24430964

[649] https://www.ifpri.org/blog/how-covid-19-may-disrupt-food-supply-chains-developing-countries

[650] https://doi.org/10.4060/ca8388en

[651] https://www.nytimes.com/2020/03/31/opinion/coronavirus-food-supply.html

[652] https://doi.org/10.4060/ca8466en

[653] https://www.brookings.edu/blog/up-front/2020/05/06/the-covid-19-crisis-has-already-left-too-many-children-hungry-in-america/

[654] https://blogs.lse.ac.uk/latamcaribbean/2020/06/03/the-impact-of-covid-19-on-brazils-precarious-labour-market-calls-for-far-reaching-policies-like-universal-basic-income/

[655] https://www.ids.ac.uk/opinions/will-the-covid-19-pandemic-increase-obesity-rates/?utm_campaign=News%20at%20IDS%208%20April%202020&utm_source=emailCampaign&utm_content=&utm_medium=email

[656] https://blogs.bmj.com/bmj/2020/05/01/covid-19-an-opportunity-or-risk-to-addressing-health-inequalities/

[657] https://www.thelancet.com/journals/lanplh/article/PIIS2542-5196(19)30244-X/fulltext

[658] https://www.thelancet.com/pdfs/journals/lancet/PIIS0140-6736(17)30602-5.pdf

[659] https://www.scielosp.org/article/csp/2017.v33n7/e00006016/pt/

[660] https://www.scielo.br/scielo.php?pid=S0034-75902018000300337&script=sci_arttext

[661] https://doi.org/10.1590/S0102-311X2008001400018

inequality, and targeted public policy (particularly the Zero Hunger programme) led to improved nutrition but also rising obesity. Once economic growth slowed, indicators for both nutrition and obesity worsened[662]. The 2020 Global Nutrition Report[663] showed Brazil was on track to miss all of its nutrition targets for 2025. While the process of nutritional transition has been extensively analysed, only recently have discussions focused on food security in cities, especially for low-income residents.

Our ongoing research project[664] examines the availability, accessibility, and consumption of fresh food in favela neighbourhoods in Belo Horizonte and São Paulo. In both cities, business models have produced supply chains that do not close the "last mile", failing to provide sufficient fresh food to favelas. Instead, residents buy food from street markets and "mom and pop stores", or from supermarkets outside the favela, often during long return journeys from work.

It is common to observe people, and especially women, carrying heavy loads, sometimes at night, on uneven pathways or up steep slopes. Acquiring food is a daily struggle for the urban poor.

The food burden is also an economic one, as budgetary constraints and limited storage options only allow for shopping in small quantities at higher unit prices. According to data from the Brazilian Institute of Geography and Statistics, families in the lowest income bracket spend almost four times more of their monthly income on food than those in the highest income bracket. This spending does not translate into a more balanced diet, however, as the proportional consumption of fruit and vegetables for people in lower-income brackets is far lower than for those with high incomes (as illustrated below).

[662] http://www.fao.org/state-of-food-security-nutrition/en/
[663] https://globalnutritionreport.org/reports/2020-global-nutrition-report/
[664] http://www.lse.ac.uk/lacc/research/engineering-food-infrastructure-exclusion-and-last-mile-delivery-in-Brazilian-favelas

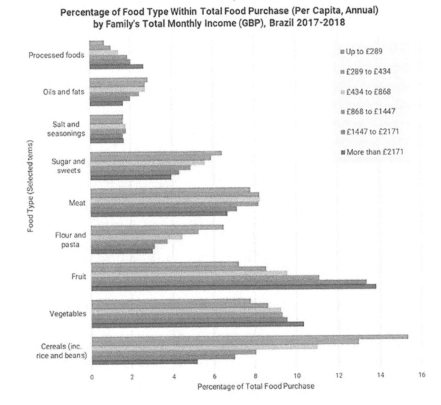

Percentage of Food Type Within Total Food Purchase (Per Capita, Annual) by Family's Total Monthly Income (GBP), Brazil 2017-2018

Source: Avaliação Nutricional da Disponibilidade Domiciliar de Alimentos no Brasil, IBGE. Notes: Income values in GBP calculated 28 May 2020 (GBP 1 = BRL 6.59) ; percentages based on annual purchases in kilograms; family units are defined as people sharing housing and food.

Adopting the idea of "people as infrastructure[665]"we find that social networks provide opportunities for people to borrow food, to look after each other during sickness, or to mind children and other relatives. A diverse array of actors, civic organisations, religious groups, political activists, trade unions, social entrepreneurs, and criminal networks operate, collaborate, and improvise to "engineer" food availability for vulnerable households. This dense network has set up community kitchens, urban gardens, food banks, savings schemes, and waste recycling projects, with many also seeking to raise awareness of nutritional issues and organic food[666].

These interventions are inherently, and sometimes explicitly, political actions. They respond to supply-chain models that perceive favela communities as "economically inviable" or excessively violent. This common disconnect from favela realities has tended to reinforce other inequalities, such as unequal economic power, limited state services, and citizenship rights[667].

[665] https://muse.jhu.edu/article/173743
[666] https://mst.org.br/2019/09/05/armazem-do-campo-sp-completa-tres-anos-de-luta-e-resistencia/
[667] https://blogs.lse.ac.uk/latamcaribbean/2020/04/14/brazils-urban-inequalities-will-exacerbate-the-impacts-of-covid-19/

Tackling the food crisis under COVID-19

The unfolding COVID-19 food crisis has highlighted cleavages of economic, social, and political power, and their intersections with gender, race, and class. Poor households have struggled to make ends meet, with further pressure on already precarious livelihoods leading to lower food consumption[668]. Without refrigerators or the money to pay for electricity, households are unable to store food or plan meals. School closures during lockdown, meanwhile, have made it harder for parents to go out to work, deprived children of free meals, and increased domestic food bills. Supply chains for processed foods have been less affected than for fresher and healthier foods, especially where more vulnerable urban households are concerned. Crowded streets and wholesale markets have become vectors for COVID-19, with nearly 80 per cent of vendors[669] in some Latin American markets becoming infected. Politicians have found themselves in a bind: leave markets open to protect livelihoods and food supply, hoping to dodge awkward questions about why sanitation conditions are often inadequate, or enforce lockdown measures and take the political hit. Instead, food supply has been supported by a series of extraordinary measures.

 Civil society organisations, church groups, unions, universities, private companies, and individuals have mobilised to deliver food parcels[670] to needy households. Community kitchens in neighbourhoods across Brazil have been supplied by social movements[671] and farm cooperatives, supporting the provision of basic meals and delivering lunch boxes for takeaway[672]. Even criminal groups[673] have become involved, sometimes forcing shops to remain open[674] or distributing food parcels. These responses are short-term interventions in an urgent situation.

They tackle the immediate threat of hunger, but they neither solve inadequate and disrupted supply chains nor combat widespread undernutrition and obesity. Most food parcels consist of items that are easy to transport, distribute, and store. But long-life milk, biscuits, and "dry goods" like rice, pasta, and noodles provide a particularly carbohydrate-heavy diet[675]. These interventions could also undermine the social infrastructure upon which local people generally rely, not least by jeopardising the livelihoods of "mom and pop stores" and market traders.

Building sustainable food systems after COVID-19

So what would a more resilient, more equitable, and healthier food system look like in the long term? First, there are innovative ways to make supply chains shorter[676] and more diverse. Low-friction farm-to-fork chains, already heralded as a viable response in the US[677], can deliver benefits like adaptability to sudden shocks and lower carbon footprints.

---

[668] https://www1.folha.uol.com.br/cotidiano/2020/04/quarentena-em-sao-paulo-reduz-dieta-de-criancas-na-periferia-a-arroz.shtml
[669] https://www.theguardian.com/world/2020/may/17/coronavirus-latin-america-markets-mexico-brazil-peru
[670] https://www.theguardian.com/global-development/2020/apr/14/were-abandoned-to-our-own-luck-coronavirus-menaces-brazils-favelas
[671] https://mst.org.br/2019/09/05/armazem-do-campo-sp-completa-tres-anos-de-luta-e-resistencia/
[672] https://doi.org/10.4060/ca8600en
[673] https://blogs.lse.ac.uk/latamcaribbean/2020/05/28/covid-19-is-increasing-the-power-of-brazils-criminal-groups/
[674] https://www1.folha.uol.com.br/amp/cotidiano/2020/05/cidade-da-baixada-fluminense-tem-saude-a-beira-do-colapso-e-comercio-aberto-a-mando-da-milicia.shtml?_twitter_impression=true
[675] https://theconversation.com/food-aid-parcels-in-south-africa-could-do-with-a-better-nutritional-balance-136417
[676] https://doi.org/10.4060/ca8600en
[677] https://now.tufts.edu/articles/how-covid-19-affects-farmers-and-food-supply-chain

In São Paulo, our co-researchers are working in collaboration[678] with a social enterprise called Frexco in an effort to use logistical solutions to enhance the circular economy between peri-urban small producers and urban consumers. The dual purpose of this initiative is to improve the provision of fresh food while strengthening livelihoods along the supply chain. Second, we will have to gain greater insight into how people engineer their access to food, especially under conditions of extreme precarity. How do people move across different networks, set preferences, improvise practices, and share knowledge around food? Lacking this information, interventions that aim to improve access in favelas and increase the involvement of private supply chains will fail to meet people's needs.

Third, we need to raise awareness of balanced diets and identify the barriers that poorer people especially face in acquiring and consuming fresh food. While budget constraints matter, data show low levels of interest in fruit and vegetables across all social groups[679] in Brazil. Wider public policy should also consider and integrate the Food-Based Dietary Guidelines[680] set out by the Ministry of Health and Pan American Health Organization. More specifically, past experiences of food awareness programmes (as once used in Belo Horizonte, for example) should be revisited, with local practices and preferences incorporated into their development and implementation.

Fundamentally, building sustainable food systems involves contentious political decisions: as the coordinator of a São Paulo organic food shop maintained by the Landless Movement recently noted, promoting good dietary practice is a political act[681]. The threat of food shortages, as symbolised by the supposedly empty supply centre in Bolsonaro's tweet, highlights the gap between the haves and the have-nots. Bolsonaro and his economy minister Paulo Guedes exploited this politics of food and subsequent "social disorder" to raise the pressure on state governors[682] to lift lockdown measures. But although a focus on supply chains is overdue, for now the Brazilian government continues to dodge the thornier underlying issue: that the social inequalities revealed by COVID-19 must be addressed if people's need for affordable, reliable, and health-appropriate food is to be met in the years ahead.

Notes:
* *The views expressed here are of the authors rather than the Centre or the LSE*
* *This article is part of an ongoing project entitled 'Engineering Food: infrastructure exclusion and 'last mile' delivery in Brazilian favelas', which is funded by The British Academy under its Urban Infrastructure and Well-Being programme*

•

---

[678] http://www.campofavela.ong.br/
[679] https://www.statista.com/statistics/919107/share-consumers-healthy-fresh-food-region-brazil/
[680] http://bvsms.saude.gov.br/bvs/publicacoes/dietary_guidelines_brazilian_population.pdf
[681] https://mst.org.br/2019/09/05/armazem-do-campo-sp-completa-tres-anos-de-luta-e-resistencia/
[682] https://uk.reuters.com/article/uk-health-coronavirus-brazil/brazils-guedes-warns-of-virus-control-measures-economic-toll-idUKKBN22J3KP

3. The Worst Time for A Pandemic – How Coronavirus and Seasonal Floods Are Causing Hunger in The Remote Amazon

Daniel Tregidgo

Instituto de Desenvolvimento Sustentável Mamirauá

Luke Parry

Associate Professor of Geography, Lancaster University

Patricia Carignano Torres

Postdoctoral Researcher in Food Security and Conservation,
Universidade de São Paulo

To slow the spread of COVID-19, a third of the global population is in lockdown[683]. While major cities are swamped with case[684]s, isolated ocean islands are among the last places on the planet free from the disease. Isolation, it seems, helps during a pandemic. Or does it? Millions of people live in isolated Amazonian towns and villages[685] that are only accessible by boat or plane. Many of these towns are a few days' boat ride from the nearest major city, and some of the villages are another few days' boat ride from the nearest town. And despite surviving the early part of the pandemic without many cases, the Brazilian Amazon is now experiencing a major COVID-19 outbreak[686]. The healthcare system of its largest city, Manaus collapsed just three weeks after its first confirmed case, and the city is now being forced to bury many of its victims in mass graves. By now, even some of the most isolated Amazonians[687] are being infected.

Stay Home or Feed Your Family

Amazonia's intensive care units are only found in its major cities, which can be well over 1,000km from some towns – about the same distance as London to Barcelona. To prevent the further spread of COVID-19, many Amazonians are trying to increase their isolation. Some indigenous groups are making camps deeper in the forest[688]. Other villages and whole cities have declared themselves closed to the world. Rural Amazonians still rely on visiting local towns to buy food, trade and receive salaries and welfare payments. This presents a wicked problem, stay home to avoid COVID-19 or feed your family[689]. The effect in poorer regions, where hunger/ malnutrition are already common,

---

[683] https://www.businessinsider.com/countries-on-lockdown-coronavirus-italy-2020-3?r=US&IR=T
[684] https://www.bbc.co.uk/news/world-asia-india-52306225
[685] https://www.tandfonline.com/doi/full/10.1080/24694452.2017.1325726
[686] https://www.theguardian.com/world/2020/apr/30/brazil-manaus-coronavirus-mass-graves?CMP=Share_iOSApp_Other
[687] https://edition.cnn.com/2020/04/10/world/yanomami-amazon-coronavirus-brazil-trnd/index.html
[688] https://time.com/5826188/amazons-indigenous-people-coronavirus/
[689] https://www.theguardian.com/world/2020/apr/21/latin-america-coronavirus-lockdowns-low-income

is predicted to be catastrophic[690]. Experts predict that malnutrition caused by the pandemic will leave an extra seven million children stunted[691]. Our research shows that remote Amazonian municipalities tend to have poor public services, deep poverty and high food prices[692] already. Traditional river-dwelling populations face much of this alone, largely invisible in Brazilian society[693]. In normal times, most households in remote Amazonian communities have trouble feeding themselves[694], and most children under five are anaemic[695].

Can Nature Provide?

Amazonia is exceptionally rich in natural resources. Rivers and forests[696] are likely to be providing some natural insurance[697] against hunger. The availability of natural resources varies throughout the year. Seasonal floods[698] allow fish to disperse across the flooded forest for months every year, peaking around April to July which coincides with the pandemic. Our latest research[699] showed this makes fish much harder to catch, meaning many families struggle to eat enough food during the highwater season. A third of rural households skip meals, and the chance of not eating for a whole day increases four-fold when compared with the low water season. People living on the floodplain can't easily switch from fishing to farming because the swollen rivers flood virtually all land in many areas, sometimes for hundreds of kilometres. Rural households rely on supplementing what they can catch or grow with food they buy in local towns.

That means queuing at the bank, stopping by the market on the way home, potentially bringing the virus with you. COVID-19 and the subsequent lockdown has arrived at a really bad time, as rising river levels exacerbate existing hunger, forcing many people to choose between limiting their exposure and that of their community to the virus, and eating. The Brazilian government's emergency stipend[700] aims to protect vulnerable citizens, such as informal workers, from the impacts of the pandemic, but its benefits could be offset by rising food prices in remote areas, which our contacts across the Amazon.. There are no obvious solutions, but they must involve helping people have a nutritious diet while being able to avoid neighbouring towns and cities. Acting quickly[701] will be vital for the health and wellbeing of Amazonian river-dwellers.

[690] https://www.theguardian.com/global-development/2020/apr/21/millions-hang-by-a-thread-extreme-global-hunger-compounded-by-covid-19-coronavirus

[691] https://www.ifpri.org/blog/biblical-steroids-and-across-generations-coming-food-and-nutrition-crash-can-be-averted-if-we

[692] https://doi.org/10.1080/24694452.2017.1325726

[693] https://doi.org/10.1016/j.socscimed.2019.112448

[694] http://wp.lancs.ac.uk/rede-cidada-am/files/2018/04/Seguranca-alimentar-divulgacao.pdf

[695] http://wp.lancs.ac.uk/rede-cidada-am/files/2018/04/Seguranca-nutricional-divulgacao.pdf

[696] https://onlinelibrary.wiley.com/doi/abs/10.1002/ajhb.21192

[697] https://doi.org/10.1111/j.1365-2400.2010.00750.x

[698] https://rainforests.mongabay.com/0604.htm

[699] https://doi.org/10.1002/pan3.10086

[700] https://auxilio.caixa.gov.br/#/inicio

[701] https://www.ifpri.org/blog/biblical-steroids-and-across-generations-coming-food-and-nutrition-crash-can-be-averted-if-we

Childhood Malnutrition Has Lifelong Consequences[702].

After the pandemic has passed, there must be significant investment in reducing poverty. That will enable people to better weather shocks like COVID-19. But poverty must be tackled not just in terms of income. Improving sanitation and access to clean water and healthcare is also vital. With intestinal infections and preventable diseases such as malaria so common in rural areas, even the most nutritious diet might not stop malnourishment.

---

[702] https://www.sciencedirect.com/science/article/pii/S0140673616316786

4. COVID-19 And Food Security In Brazil, Will Emergency Aid Be Enough To Guarantee Access To Food For The Country's Poor?

Stéphane Guéneau,
CIRAD Public Policy Specialist
&
Catia Grisa,
Researcher At The University Of Rio Grande Do Sul.

In Brazil, the COVID-19 health crisis has triggered a standoff between the President and local government. The rapid spread of the disease through the country has led many state governments and city mayors to take strict lockdown measures.

Conversely, the country's President, Jair Bolsonaro, continues to call for a return to economic activity, with selective isolation of "at-risk" citizens. Initially, the Brazilian judiciary supported the blanket lockdown strategy adopted by local authorities. However, certain state governors have already given in to pressure, for instance in Santa Catarina state, where non-essential businesses were authorized to reopen as of 22 April 2020.

The measures imposed have meant that a substantial proportion of Brazilians, and often the poorest, have lost their means of subsistence, particularly in terms of casual jobs, which concern 40% of the workforce. In a country where 13.5 million people are classed as extremely poor (less than 1 dollar per day), any sudden fall in casual income rapidly triggers hunger issues. Certain rural casual workers in the fishing and agricultural sectors have also seen a sudden loss of subsistence income following the closure of urban markets. The authorities, mainly on a federal level, have responded slowly, if at all, and the country's poorest people have rapidly found themselves caught between a rock and a hard place. Should they stay on lockdown and face misery and hunger, or continue to work and risk contamination, in a country where few people have satisfactory access to healthcare?

To compensate for the sudden fall in incomes among the poor, many local authorities rapidly introduced emergency programmes. They organized the distribution of food parcels containing staple goods (rice, beans, etc). However, although vital, these steps have fallen short of solving the growing food shortfalls. Moreover, the centralized distribution of large numbers of parcels has led to large gatherings of people and increased the risk of virus transmission. The question of introducing emergency income support for casual workers is therefore now on the political agenda. A law voted on 2 April 2020 allows for a monthly payment of BRL 600 (around 110 euros) per person (BRL 1200 per family) for casual workers and micro-entrepreneurs with the lowest individual incomes. However, the President did not sign the necessary decree until 7 April 2020. With the delay in implementing the measure, as of 9 April 2020, the country's poor had no choice but to take to the streets to look for sources of income to meet their basic requirements, hence increasing the risks of contamination. Moreover, that emergency income support is not universally guaranteed, particularly for people in rural areas.

Applications must be registered in a databank, accessible via an app, a dedicated website, state bank branches, or businesses specializing in payment services ("loterias"). Ironically, it is the most severely economically disadvantaged people who have the least chance of accessing such services, particularly since social services are currently at a virtual standstill. Additional emergency measures could be taken on a federal level, along the lines of those take successfully by the Maranhão state government: state purchasing of products from family farms to make up food parcels for direct distribution to local people, the poor, and restaurants, to ensure easy access for the homeless. In addition to the above measures, the current crisis could prove to be an opportunity to tackle the structural problem of inequality in Brazil.

5. High Prevalence of Food Insecurity, The Adverse Impact Of COVID-19 In Brazilian Favela

Catarina Vezetiv Manfrinato[1], Aluízio Marino[2],

Vitória Ferreira Condé[3],

Maria do Carmo Pinho Franco[1,4], Elke Stedefeldt[1],

Luciana Yuki Tomita[1*703 704]

ABSTRACT

Objective: To investigate food insecurity prevalence in two favelas in Brazil in the early weeks from physical distancing policy, between March 27, 2020 to June 1, 2020. **Design:** A cross-sectional study by means of an online questionnaire to elicit information on socioeconomic and demographic characteristics, the types of stores visited to buy food including food insecurity screening. Experience of food insecurity data was collected according to the Brazilian Food Insecurity Scale. Factors associated with moderate or severe food insecurity (EBIA≥3) were investigated using the logistic regression model. **Setting:** São Paulo city, Brazil. **Participants:** 909 householders. **Results:** 88% of the households included young women working as cleaners or kitchen assistants and in sales services. One-fifth of the participants were receiving federal cash transfer programme, called Bolsa Família. There were 92% households with children.

The most frequent experience reported was uncertainty about food acquisition or receiving more (89%), to eat less than one should (64%), not being able to eat healthy and nutritious food (46%) and skipping a meal (39%). 47% of the participants experienced moderate or severe food insecurity.

Factors associated with moderate and severe food insecurity were low income, being Bolsa Família recipient, a low level of education, and households without children. **Conclusions:** Half of the participants experienced moderate or severe food insecurity, and close to ten per cent was hungry. Our data suggest that families with children were at lower risk of moderate to severe food insecurity. It is possible that nationally established social programs like Bolsa Família were protecting those families.

[703] *Corresponding author: e-mail: luciana.tomita@unifesp.br phone: 55 11 55764876

[704] 1Universidade Federal de São Paulo, Escola Paulista de Medicina, Department of Preventive Medicine, São Paulo, SP, Brazil
2Universidade Federal do ABC, São Paulo, SP, Brazil
3Universidade Federal de São Paulo, Escola Paulista de Enfermagem, São Paulo, SP, Brazil
4Universidade Federal de São Paulo, Escola Paulista de Medicina, Medicine Department, São Paulo, SP, Brazil
5Instituto Estudos Avançados, Universidade de São Paulo, SP, Brazil

INTRODUCTION

The (COVID-19) pandemic has led to the tragic loss of human life with deep social and economic consequences, including on food insecurity and nutrition. Disproportionate burdens of infections, hospitalisations, and deaths from COVID-19 among already vulnerable communities were observed[1].Inequities in food and health access exacerbate inequalities in nutrition outcomes in the form of undernutrition and overweight individuals, obesity, and diet-related chronic diseases[2].

The lack of regular access to nutritious and sufficient food experienced by such people puts them at greater risk of malnutrition, hidden hunger, or micronutrient deficiencies. The ability to eat a healthy diet is determined by the person's access to affordable healthy food, the environment in which they live, and knowledge about the importance of those food groups for health[3].

People experiencing food insecurity may live in food deserts and may predominantly have access to low-cost, energy dense processed foods[3]. Those calorie-dense processed foods are risk factors for obesity and obesity-related chronic diseases, such as diabetes, hypertension, and cardiovascular disease, and are strongly associated with severe COVID-19 outcomes. Obesity, hidden hunger, and coronavirus could face the triple burden of disease[4].

In the COVID-19 pandemic, physical distancing or quarantine is impossible in regions such as the Brazilian favelas that house approximately 13 million individuals, which is crowded and has limited access to clean water or hygiene supplies[5]. Those people work in informal or less flexible jobs and are at a higher risk of losing their jobs completely or partially. On 25 February 2020, the first COVID-19 case was confirmed in São Paulo city, Brazil. Twenty days later, community transmission was announced. One month after the first COVID-19 case, a physical distancing policy was adopted with the closing of schools and non-essential services. The objective of the present study was to investigate food insecurity prevalence in two favelas in São Paulo city in the early weeks of the physical distancing policy.

METHODS

A cross-sectional study was conducted in two favelas in São Paulo city, Brazil, between 27th March 2020 and 1st June 2020.

The inclusion criteria were those living in those communities and householders. Heliopolis Favela is the biggest and most densely populated shantytown located close to the downtown area of São Paulo city. The population size is not precise. The last Brazilian census in 2010 estimated that 65 thousand people live in an area of approximately 1.2 km², but local public health services indicate that they attend 140 thousand patients; the local non-profit organisation, the UNAS, estimated that 220 thousand people live there. Vila São José is a favela located in the south of São Paulo city.

A projection of the local population from the Public Health Service is that 203 thousand people live in a 134 km² area. On 24 May 2020, newspapers published reports that the peripheral regions of the city of São Paulo are where most people died from COVID-19 [6]. The Vila São José community is located in a peripheral region.

Data Collection

A standardised online questionnaire was employed to elicit information on socioeconomic and demographic characteristics, the frequency of food purchases, the types of stores visited to buy food, finances, and food insecurity screening after the physical distancing policy came into effect. Data on the experience of food insecurity were collected according to the Brazilian Food Insecurity Scale[7].An online questionnaire was collected in Heliopolis Favela by the observatory 'De Olho na Quebrada' (Eyes in the Broken). Each questionnaire was available for one week.

The household level of food insecurity was assessed using the short version of the Brazilian Food Insecurity Scale (EBIA), adapted from the US Household Food Security Survey Measure (HPSSM) and validated for the Brazilian population[7].

The short version is comprised of five questions and presents high sensibility and specificity compared to the original food insecurity scale[8]. The householder should answer the scale. A family that reported any experience of food insecurity, by answering "yes", was scored as 1 point and 0 points for "no", with a maximum of five points in the questionnaire. The five questions were based on assessing the perception or experience of food intake in the household since the beginning of social distancing: 1) anxiety and worry about the ability to obtain food; 2) too poor to buy more food; 3) whether the quality and variety of food has been compromised, including nutritious food; 4) quantity reduction and 5) skipping meals[7]. The total score classifications of the food insecurity grade were: (0) no insecurity, (1–2) mild insecurity, (3–4) moderate insecurity, and (5) severe insecurity. The income per person was converted from Brazilian Real to U.S. Dollars using the currency conversion rate during the period. Ethical approval was obtained from the Institutional Review Board of the Universidade Federal de São Paulo and the Medical Ethical Committees of the participating hospitals (CAAE 30805520.7.0000.5505). Online consent was obtained from all participants. The present study complies with the Strengthening the Reporting of Observational Studies in Epidemiology guidelines.

Statistical Analysis

Crude and relative distributions and median and interquartile ranges were calculated for the descriptive statistics. Factors associated with moderate or severe food insecurity (EBIA≥3) were investigated using the logistic regression model. The reference category for exposure of interest was the lowest risk for food insecurity. For income, the first quartile among households with no food insecurity was the reference category. A level of significance of 5% was adopted. Statistical analysis was performed using STATA 14.0. (Texas, USA).

RESULTS

In the present study, 1 172 participants answered the online survey. Of these, 123 (10%) did not live in those communities, 86 (7.3%) were not householders, and 54 (4.6%) answers were repeated. In Heliopolis, a questionnaire was administered twice. The first was administered on 27 March, four days after the social distancing policy came into effect, collecting 653 responses.

The second was administered after one month, on 30 April, at which time 756 participants assessed their experience of food insecurity. For the present study, only participants who answered both questionnaires were considered. Of these, 909 (78%) were considered eligible participants; 697 lived in Heliopolis Favela and 212 in Vila São José. The majority of the households included young women working as cleaners or kitchen assistants and in sales services. One-fifth were Bolsa Família recipients, a federal cash transfer programme for families with children that attend school. There were many overcrowded households with children. The majority of participants purchased food in a local supermarket (55%) or a local market close to home (43%), and only 2% reported buying food in *feira*, an outdoor public market that sells fresh vegetables and fruits; 98% observed an increase in food prices. Foods were purchased monthly (66%), twice a month (23%), and weekly (8%). More than half of the participants were in moderate and severe food insecurity (56%). The most frequent experience reported was uncertainty about food acquisition or receiving more, to eat less than one should, not being able to eat healthy and nutritious food, and skipping a meal. A quarter reported that food was consumed before buying or receiving more (Table 1). Factors associated with moderate and severe food insecurity were low income, being a Bolsa Família recipient, a low level of education, and households without children (Table 2).

DISCUSSION

Our study presents the impact on food access immediately following the COVID-19-related physical distancing measure and school closure in two favelas in São Paulo city, Brazil. More than half of the participants experienced moderate or severe food insecurity, and close to ten per cent were hungry. Half were unable to eat healthy and nutritious food, while families with children were at a lower risk for insecurity. Almost all participants reported that food prices increased and the majority purchased food from supermarkets, but not from local outdoor markets where fresh vegetables and fruits are available. Unfortunately, a downward trend in food insecurity observed in Brazil from 2004 to 2013, 17% to 7.9% respectively, has been diverted[9]. At that time, the associated factors of moderate and severe food insecurity were living in the Northeast and Northern regions, being among the poorest and living in an urban area with inadequate sanitation, a household density of more than two persons per bedroom, less than four household material goods, and households headed by females, individuals younger than 60, non-whites, having less than four years of schooling, and being unemployed. These associated factors remained in the ten years covered by the National Survey[9].

Early effects of the COVID-19 pandemic were also observed among low income Americans, where 44% of households were food insecure[10]. However, among Americans, an increase in household food insecurity was observed in previous years, from 11% in 2018 to 38% in March 2020. People who were non-Hispanic, Black, or Hispanic, had children in the home, and had less than a college education were more likely to be at risk of food insecurity. According to the United Nations Department of Economic and Social Affairs (2020), the COVID-19 pandemic has affected all segments of the population, but it was reinforced among the poorest and most vulnerable people. Many of these people are workers in the informal economy, as observed in our study[11].

In the Heliopolis Observatory, collected in the first week after COVID-19 physical distancing measures were enacted, 65% reported that they were not working due to social distancing, 68% reported considerable income reduction, and 17% reported no wages, with higher impacts occurring among the poorest people[12]. A Brazilian Federal cash transfer of USD 110 was offered for informal workers after a social appeal, one month after the social distancing policy came into effect. However, according to the observatory, among the 83% who asked for emergency cash, only one-third received it.

As a result of the economic impact of COVID-19, the number of people around the world facing acute food insecurity is 265 million in 2020, an increase of 130 million from 135 million in 2019 according to the World Food Programme projection (WFP)[11]. The WFP recommended measures, including pre-positioning food closest to those most in need while supply chains are still working, providing double food rations per person to reduce the number of distributions, providing take home food rations to replace school meals, and launching health-education campaigns[12]. For many students around the world, school feeding is the only meal they receive during the day. To protect students from food insecurity, the São Paulo state government offered an additional cash payment of USD 10 per month for Bolsa Família recipients for 27% of students.

However, in our study, only 15% received it[12]. The distribution of food kits, called *cesta básica* in Portuguese, from the São Paulo city prefecture, comprised of 25 kg minimally processed food such as rice and beans, processed foods such as pasta, salt, sugar, tomato pasta, green beans, corn, maize flour, and vegetable oil, as well as ultra-processed food such as biscuits. This food kit was also offered to student recipients of Bolsa Família. The Brazilian public agenda has an intersectorial and participatory approach called Food and Nutrition Security, that aims to develop public policies to guaranty food and nutrition security. This concept is to ensure human rights for a healthy, accessible, and adequate diet, without compromising access to other essential needs, such as respecting healthy eating practises and cultural diversity, and should be socioeconomically and agro-ecologically sustainable[13].

Through this program, family farming from settlements should be supported in terms of sales to benefit socially vulnerable and marginalised populations, such as quilombolas (AfroBrazilian ancestry), indigenous people, and for school feeding, entitled Programa de Aquisição de Alimentos (PAA) or Program for Food Acquisition in English[14]. In the present situation of poor access to healthy food in a highly vulnerable community, this program should work.

However, in the actual government, financing for social programs has been reduced, including the PAA. Over the past fifteen years, the PAA has shown how a Brazilian public policy has importance in boosting local economies and short production/distribution circuits. In addition, the PAA also supports the structuring role and income provision for family farming and the guarantee of the human right to adequate food [15]. It would be essential in the context of the pandemic to offer logistical support so that farmers can directly market their products to consumers in urban centres, reducing the risk of COVID-19. At the same time, safe conditions must be offered for production to be acquired by the government for the distribution of food baskets. The strategic use of PAA in the crisis would also involve reactivating the modalities of direct purchases and stock formation.

Moreover, the program's institutional channels can serve federal resources and be transferred to states and municipalities to finance local strategies for responding to the effects of the pandemic [15]. Our data suggest that families with children were at lower risk of moderate to severe food insecurity. It is possible that nationally established social programs like Bolsa Família were protecting those families, as well as solidarity from non-profit organisations and private sectors that offer *cesta básica* instead of government defaults during the COVID-19 pandemic period.

A systematic review observed that female-headed households were 75% more likely to be food insecure than male-headed households. This could be because of the lower income earned by women compared to men due to the sex wage difference or reduced work time among women, the greater observation of household needs and food preparation among women than men[16] and the increased childcare burden shouldered by female household providers, such as feeding and education. The impact of COVID-19 among Brazilian families could be significant. Brazil was already experiencing food insecurity before the coronavirus pandemic: more than half of adults were excess weight and 19.8% were obese, 24.7% were diagnosed with hypertension, and 7.7% with diabetes, with a higher prevalence of morbidity among those with low levels of education; only 23% reported an intake of five or more portions of vegetables and fruits, with a lower frequency observed among those with lower levels of education[17]. Aadolescents, a cross-sectional national study showed that 3.3% were overweight, 21.3% were obese with a premature impact on their health was observed: 20% presented hypercholesterolaemia, 47% low HDL cholesterol, 7.8% hypertriglyceridaemia, 8% hypertension, 4% had high glucose levels, and 2.6% suffered from metabolic syndrome[18,19].

In the two editions of the National Adolescent School-based Health Survey, 2009 and 2012, the consumption of beans and fruits decreased; in the most recent survey, 60% reported bean intake and 29.8% fruits, 35.4% sweet beverages, and 42.6% reported to consuming sweets at least five days a week[20].

Together, the antagonistic health-related problems and double burden of malnutrition among Brazilian adolescents with a high body mass index (BMI) and low height for their age was observed at 0.3%[21]. The quality of food that was stocked up on before social distancing came into effect is a concern, as almost all participants reported buying food in supermarkets and only two per cent reported doing so in outdoor fresh vegetable and fruit stores. The increased consumption of ultra-processed food combined with reduced physical activity during the pandemic period could worsen or increase the number of overweight people and chronic diseases, risk factors that have been related to increasing the severity of COVID-19. An estimate obtained in a nationally representative Brazilian household-based health survey pointed out that 34% of adults present at least one risk factor for severe COVID-19[22]. In São Paulo city, the prevalence of one or more risk factors for severe COVID-19 was 56%, with a higher prevalence among less educated adults (86%) compared to those with a university education (49%); a similar distribution was seen according toincome or race[23].

The limitations of the present study should be considered. It is a cross sectional study, and no temporality and causality can be inferred. No statistical probabilistic sample was drawn since the population size of the communities in question is unknown. The web questionnaire was shared between both communities through local acting non-profit organisations and community leaders. It is possible that it reached many households due to their high capillarity and relevance to social policy. However, families that are going hungry could be under-represented since they may not have an internet plan or mobile phone. The present study showed the importance and swift impact of social distancing in São Paulo's favelas. These findings should be considered when designing and implementing social policy intended to act fast, closing family farming to socially vulnerable communities, as well as implementing assistance programs, especially for households without children, who are more likely to go hungry.

Acknowledgments: We thank members from the Observatory "De Olho na

Quebrada", André Luis Silva, Gabriel Feitosa, Gabrielle Souza, João Victor da Cruz,

Karoline Aparecida, Leonardo da Silva Pimentel, Letícia Avelino, Edgard Barki, Marina Lima, Isabela Lemos, Reginaldo José Gonçalves and Vila São José´s community leader Luiz Alberto F. Alves and CAPES (Coordenação de Aperfeiçoamento de Pessoal de Nível Superior) for CVZ scholarship and financial code 001.

REFERENCES

1. Chiriboga D, Garay J, Buss P, et al. (2020) Health inequity during the COVID19 pandemic: a cry for ethical global leadership. *Lancet* 395, 1690-1.

2. Mannar V, Micha R, Afshin A, et al. (2020) *The 2020 Global Nutrition Report in the context of COVID-19.* https://globalnutritionreport.org/reports/2020global-nutrition-report/2020-global-nutrition-report-context-COVID-19/ (Accessed July 2020).

3. Belanger MJ, Hill MA, Angelidi AM, et al. (2020) COVID-19 and Disparities in Nutrition and Obesity. *N. Engl. J. Med.* Published online: 27 July 2020. DOI:10.1056/NEJMp2021264

4. Cuevas A & Batz C (2020) Coronavirus, obesity and undernutrition: the triple burden for Latin America. *Plos Blogs Your Say.* May 2020. https://yoursay.plos.org/2020/05/26/coronavirus-obesity-and-undernutritionthe-triple-burden-for-latin-america/(Accessed July 2020).

5. Burki T (2020) COVID-19 in Latin America. *Lancet Infect Dis* 20: 547-8.

6. Souza C & Pessoa GS (2020) 20 bairros com mais mortes por COVID-19 estão nos extremos de São Paulo. São Paulo: https://noticias.uol.com.br/saude/ultimasnoticias/redacao/2020/05/24/coronavirus-avanca-mais-na-periferia-de-sp.htm (Accessed July 2020).

7. Pérez-Escamilla R, Segall-Corrêa AM, Kurdian Maranha L, et al. (2004) An Adapted Version of the U.S. Department of Agriculture Food Insecurity Module Is a Valid Tool for Assessing Household Food Insecurity in Campinas, Brazil. *J. Nutr* 134: 1923-8.

7. dos Santos LP, Lindemann IL, Motta JV dos S, et al. (2014) Proposal of a short-form version of the Brazilian Food Insecurity Scale. *Rev. Saude Publica* 48:783-9.

8. dos Santos TG, da Silveira JAC, Longo-Silva G, et al. (2018) Trends and factors associated with food insecurity in Brazil: The national household sample survey, 2004, 2009, and 2013. *Cad. Saude Publica* 34: e00066917.

9. Wolfson JA & Leung CW (2020) Food insecurity and COVID-19: Disparities in early effects for us adults. *Nutrients* 12: 1-13.

10. United Nations Population, Division of Economic andSocial Affairs (2020) Department of Economic and Social Affairs. *United Nations.* www. population.un.org. Accessed July 2020.

11. Silva AL, Feitosa G, Souza G, et al. (2020) *Heliópolis contra coronavírus: pesquisa sobre os impactos do coronavírus nas famílias de Heliópolis.* São Paulo.

12. Brasil. Presidência da República CC (2006) *Lei no. 11.346, de 15 de Setembro de 2006. Segurança Alimentar e Nutricional - SISAN.* Brasília: DF.

13. Marques PEM, Le Moal MF & Andrade AGF de (2014) Programa deAquisição de Alimentos (PAA) no estado de São Paulo. *RURIS* 8:63-89.

14. Jung NM, De Bairros FS, Pattussi MP, et al. (2017) Gender differences in the prevalence of household food insecurity: A systematic review and meta-analysis. *Public Health Nutr* 20:902-16.

15. Valadares AA (2020) *O desempenho recente das políticas de compras públicas da produção da agricultura familiar. Políticas Sociais: acompanhamento e análise.* Brasilia: DF.

16. Jung NM, De Bairros FS, Pattussi MP, et al. (2017) Gender differences in the prevalence of household food insecurity: A systematic review and metaanalysis. *Public Health Nutr* 20:902-16.

17. Ministério da Saúde. Secretaria de Vigilancia em Saúde. Departamento de Análise em Saúde e Vigilância de Doenças não Transmissíveis (2019) *VIGITEL Brasil 2018: Vigilância de fatores de risco e proteção para doenças crônicas por inquérito telefônico: estimativas sobre frequência e distribuição sociodemográfica de fatores de risco e proteção para doenças crônicas nas capitais dos 26 estados br. Vigitel* [Ministério da Saúde, editor]. Brasília: DF.

18. Kuschnir MCC, Bloch KV, Szklo M, et al. (2016) ERICA: prevalência de síndrome metabólica em adolescentes brasileiros. *Rev. Saude Publica* 50: S1S13.

19. Bloch KV, Klein CH, Szklo M, et al. (2016) ERICA: Prevalences of hypertension and obesity in Brazilian adolescents. *Rev. Saude Publica* 50, S1S12.

20. Malta DC, Iser BPM, Claro RM, et al. (2013) Prevalence of risk and protective factors for non-communicable chronic diseases among adults: cross-sectional study, Brazil, 2011. *Epidemiol.Serv.Saúde* 23: 609-22.

21. Uzêda JCO, Ribeiro-Silva RDC, Silva NDJ, et al. (2019) Factors associated with the double burden of malnutrition among adolescents, National Adolescent School-Based Health Survey (PENSE 2009 and 2015). *PLoS One* 14:e0218566

22. Rezende LFM, Thome B, Schveitzer MC, et al. (2020) Adults at high-risk of severe coronavirus disease-2019 (COVID-19) in Brazil. *Rev. Saude Publica* 54: 50-9.

23. Thomé B, de Rezende LFM, Schveitzer MC, et al. (2020) Differences in the prevalence of risk factors for severe COVID-19 across São Paulo city regions. DOI 10.1590/1980-579720200087.

Table 1. Brazilian´s favela household characteristics and COVID-19 impact after social distancing, Brazil, April, 2020 (n=909)

Brazilian´s favela	n (%) or P50 (P25, P75)
Householder characteristics	
Female (%)	796 (88%)
Age, years	33 (28, 39)
Monthly per capita income, USD	70.2 (46.6)
Bolsa família recipients	236 (26%)
Occupation	
Cleaner, kitchen assistant, driver, deliveryman	369 (40%)
Salesman, freelance, autonomous	290 (33%)
Unemployed, housewife, retired	211 (23%)
Graduated	39 (4%)
Household characteristics	
Number of dwellers	4 (3,5)
Household with child under 10y	836 (92%)
Food insecurity	
Score at risk of food insecurity*	3 (2, 4)
No insecurity	47 (5%)
Mild insecurity	353 (39%)
Moderate insecurity	426 (47%)
Severe insecurity	83 (9%)
Uncertainty about food acquisition or receiving more	807 (89%)
Ran out of food before buying or receiving more	208 (23%)
Unable to eat healthy and nutritious food	421 (46%)
Ate less than one should	584 (64%)
Skipped a meal	350 (39%)

* no insecurity (0), mild insecurity (1-2 points), moderate insecurity (3-4 points), severe insecurity (5points)

Table 2. Associated factors for moderate and severe insecurity after social distancing from COVID-19, Brazil, April, 2020

Characteristics	No food insecurity Or mild food insecurity n(%)	Moderate or severe food insecurity n(%)	OR (95%CI)
Income Per Person, USD			
≥62	223 (62)	200 (48)	1.00
≤61	134 (38)	217 (52)	1.81 (1.35-2.41)
Bolsa Família Recipient*			
No	309 (77)	364 (72)	1.00
Yes	91 (23)	145 (28)	1.35 (1.00-1.83)
Years Of Education			
≥9 Years	221 (56)	203 (40)	1.00
≤8 Years	176(44)	303 (60)	1.87 (1.44-2.44)
Household With Children			
Yes	383 (96)	453 (89)	1.00
No	17 (4)	56 (11)	2.77 (1.59-4.76)

* Federal Cash Transfer Program

CHAPTER 25

BRAZILIAN WORFORCE VULNERABITIES EXPOSED BY COVID-19

1. Brazilian Pandemic Exposure And Policy Response

Household Vulnerability

The 2020 pandemic hit Brazil at a time when the poorest 40 percent were still struggling to recover from the 2015–16 crisis. The economic crisis resulted in a significant increase in poverty and inequality. Between 2014 and 2016, nearly 5.6 million Brazilians fell into poverty (US$5.50 per day). Currently, 20.1 percent of the population live in poverty, while those living on less than US$1.90 grew by 2.5 million, and now exceed 8 million people. Inequality increased from a Gini index of 51.9 in 2015 to 53.3 in 2016—the largest single-year increase in Brazil since the early 1990s. The subsequent uneven recovery since 2017 has left the poorest 40 percent worse off than they were before the crisis. In real terms, the income of the poorest 40 percent was lower in 2018 than in 2014 in all but four states. Even before the pandemic, half of the Brazilians (52 percent) were economically vulnerable, being either already in poverty (living on less than US$5.50 per day in 2011 PPP) or at risk of falling into poverty (living on a per capita income between US$5.50 to US$13 per day). This is particularly true in the North and Northeast regions of Brazil, where in most states, between 70 percent and 80 percent of the population fall into this category. These people are mostly young (more than 7 out of every 10 Brazilian children and youth belong to this group), urban, and employed in precarious and unprotected jobs.[705] They belong to groups expected to suffer a higher income shock.

Figure 38 1: Half of the Brazilian population are Economically Vulnerable (reported COVID-19 cases and percentage of state population aged 65 and older who are poor or vulnerable, 2018)

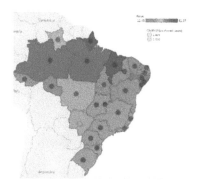

Source: World Bank (LAC TSD tabulations using SEDLAC) and Ministry of Health COVID-19 cases (as of May 31, 2020).

---

[705] The poor represent 20 percent of the Brazilian population, and include 36 percent of all Brazilian children (<15 years old) and 25 percent of the youth (15-24). Seventy-two percent of the poor live in urban areas, and 67 percent of those who work are in precarious jobs (informal or own-account), two groups likely to be particularly exposed to the COVID-19 crisis. This profile is very similar for the economically vulnerable (those living on US$5.50 to US$13 per day), who represent 32 percent of the country's population and 37 percent of all Brazilian children and youth. The proportion among those living in urban areas is even higher: 85 percent. Informal or own-account workers amount to 43 percent; and 67 percent are working in retail or services, which are expected to be the most affected sectors by the crisis.

The most vulnerable Brazilians were the urban poor; those in rural communities, including indigenous populations; women and children; and older people. About one in every five Brazilians live in slums or substandard housing, and another 32,000 are homeless. Epidemiological models find that COVID-1 was always going to spread in high-density areas, such as slums, making the urban poor particularly exposed. At the same time, rural populations, including indigenous peoples, forest and traditional communities, face additional risks arising from their difficult access to basic services, including health care. Children and youth face challenges from school closures and higher unemployment. Women and children, in particular also had to contend with increased risks of domestic violence. Quarantines and pandemics can increase widespread violence, as well as violence at home toward women and children.

Finally, while there is near-universal coverage of old-age benefits, either through pensions or social assistance schemes (such as the Continuous Cash Benefit program, or Benefício de Prestação Continuada BPC), a quarter of Brazil's population aged 65 and above live in vulnerable households, with higher proportions being found in the North and Northeast (figure 38 1).There is an important overlap between income vulnerability (ability to pay for food and rent) and vulnerability in living conditions (adequate housing and services). Poorer households have less access to improved sanitation, running water, and private bathrooms (figures 39 2 and 40 3)— all important services to reduce the spread of disease. hese critical deprivations affect the poorest 40 percent across all states in Brazil in similar proportions to other countries in Latin America (figure 41 4a, 41 4b, and 41 4c). e

Figure 39 2 : Lack of Access to Adequate Sanitation(percentage, 2018)   **Figure 40 3 : Water Supply Interruptions for Domestic Users (average hours per month, 2018)**

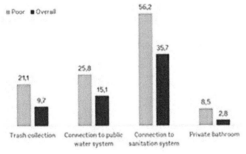

Figure 41 4 : Percentage of the Poorest 40 Percent Facing Deprivations in Housing and Related Services by State, 2018 a) Lacking Running Water b) Lacking Improved Sanitation c) Living in Overcrowded Housing

ercentage) (percentage) (percentage)

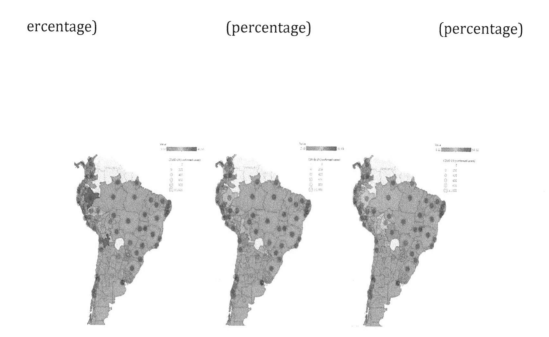

Source: LAC Team for Statistical Development tabulations of SEDLAC (CEDLAS and World Bank) for poverty data; and Public Health ministries for COVID-19 confirmed cases, circa May 31, 2020.

Transmission Channels

The key transmission channels through which the COVID-19 crisis will affect households are market demand and supply shocks, which are expected to translate into labour income losses. A large proportion of Brazilian households face a high risk of losing their income: two in every five Brazilians rely mostly on unprotected income sources (figure 425a). These are defined as the population for whom most of the household income derives from informal jobs, own-account work and formal employment with less than six months of wage protection in case of job loss.[706] Among the poorest 20 percent, the share of people relying on unprotected income increases to half the population. Another transmission channel through which the crisis may affect households is prices and, in particular, food security. Beyond the general equilibrium effects on prices, potential breakdowns in local logistics and labour availability could increase the cost of bringing food to market. This would especially affect lower-income net food buyers, consisting of both the urban population and a substantial number of rural dwellers. They would suffer a double hit—not only

---

[706] The analysis uses job and worker characteristics to simulate unemployment insurance eligibility, severance pay (multa) and employer-funded savings account (FGTS) balances. Based on these amounts, we calculate how many months of protected wages each formal private-sector wage worker will have in the case of a layoff.

are they more likely to experience income losses, but food is also a relatively larger part of their total consumption expenditure. The full impact of food price inflation on poverty depends on a range of factors, including the distribution of initial income/ expenditure across food producers and consumers, that is, whether net buyers have lower incomes than net sellers, or vice versa; whether households close to the poverty line are net sellers or net buyers; the concentration of households around the poverty line; the magnitude of price increases; and the extent to which medium-term adjustments in production and consumption—"second-round effects"—are able to reverse some of the short-term welfare losses. The food component of the IPC-C1 (a price index measured by FGV Ibre)[707] increased from 0.51 percent in February to 1.63 percent in March due to the initial run on supermarkets caused by the COVID-19 pandemic. However, while this initial pressure has receded a bit as the income shock compresses demand, supply constraints caused by lower labour availability and partial breakdown of supply chains still imply a danger of food price increases. Relatively few households can weather significant labour income shocks. It is particularly important to consider that Brazil's poorest were still recovering from the 2015–16 crisis, and the income of the poorest 40 percent is still below pre-crisis levels. Moreover, unemployment rates remain near crisis levels (figure 42 5b), with the youth facing particularly alarming levels of unemployment. In addition, household debt burden is high, at 45 percent of household income, reflecting increased non-mortgage debts since 2017 (figure 43 6). These factors suggest that many households have little room to absorb another shock.

---

[707] The IBGE suspended face-to-face data collection for the official national price indexes (IPCA, INPC) due to COVID-19, replacing it with phone and internet-based data collection. This may generate some discontinuity in the series.

Figure 42 5: Market Demand and Supply ShocksShare of Population by Majority Income Source
(percentage, 2018)

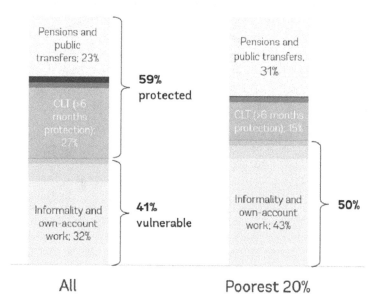

Source: World Bank.

(a) **Unemployment Rates (percentage of labor force, Q1 2012–Q1 2020)**

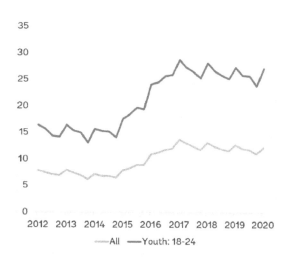

Figure 43: 6 Household Debt Burden
(percentage of household disposable income, 2007-20)

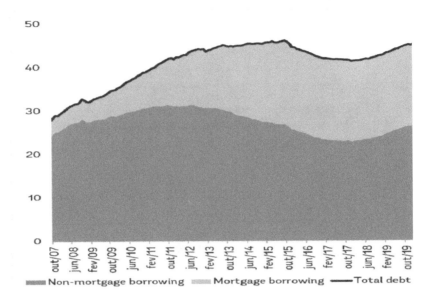

Source: World Bank.

Impact on Employment and Household Income

Vulnerability to pandemic-related unemployment or labour income shocks is heterogenous, affecting some types of workers more than others. As noted above, informal and own-account workers have no formal income protection mechanisms in place, whereas public sector workers and most formal private sector wage earners (CLT workers, that is, those covered by Brazil's labour law known as Consolidação das Leis do Trabalho) have employment protection and access to unemployment insurance, severance pay, and employer-funded savings accounts. Sectors are differently exposed as well. The risk of employment interruption is higher for sectors that rely more heavily on face to-face interactions. Low-wage workers and women are more likely to be in these sectors (figures 44 7a and 44 7b), and hence more prone to suffer the employment shock first.

Using subnational macroeconomic modelling techniques and crossing them with high-frequency data (such as credit card spending), estimates show that the most affected sector is that of services (export-crops benefit from the lower real exchange rate, but there is a risk of pressure on prices across food products, as reflected in early evidence of increasing food prices). This same model estimates the impact on real wages across sectors and across states, showing that they decrease across sectors, although there are some regional exceptions, especially in agriculture. In general, wages are "sticky", so adjustments from economic shocks, especially among formal workers, are more likely to take the form of reduced employment (including reduction in hours) than falling wages.

In order to understand how sectoral shocks will affect families, we have allocated them as employment interruptions to workers in a microsimulation model.[708] We estimate that these shocks will significantly reduce the earnings of 30 to 35 million workers, including as many as 70 percent of non-agriculture informal workers, and a third of CLTs. As a reference point, in February 2020, 12.3 million Brazilians were unemployed. More importantly, not all of these interruptions will necessarily become unemployment spells. The 2017 labour reform that regulated part-time work, and the recent Emergency Employment and Income Protection Benefit (BEm—Benefício Emergencial de Manutenção do Emprego e da Renda), which introduced flexibility for firms to suspend paid work, may help to reduce the amount of outright job destruction and mitigate workers' losses from cuts in paid hours, without forcing them to sever employment relations so as to activate unemployment insurance.

These unemployment shocks translate into significant reductions in family income and higher inequality. Simulations were run for two scenarios: a baseline and a downside scenario. The largest impact under both scenarios is in the middle of the income distribution. Under the baseline scenario, annualized per capita income is expected to fall by 7.6 percent overall, and 14.9 percent and 14 percent in the second and third quintiles, respectively (figure 44 7a). These are the quintiles hit the hardest by the crisis, and whose income depend less on government transfers. The first line of defence is Brazil's existing unemployment protection system for formal workers. Once unemployment benefits are considered, this effect is reduced to .3 percent nationally, and buffers 20 to 40 percent of the average income reduction in all but the poorest quintile.[709]

The effects are not expected to be income neutral—instead, they are likely to increase inequality, as informal workers and lower wage formal workers are more likely to suffer unemployment shocks. The disproportionate erosion of income for lower-income families would result in an increase of 3.1 percent in inequality—a significant one-year change, and larger than the 2.7 percent increase experienced between 2015 and 2016. The baseline scenario could lead to an increase in the population living on less than half a minimum wage (a proxy for poverty) by an estimated 8.4 million people in 2020. To assess the impact of the crisis on household welfare, we estimate the share of the population that will fall into poverty, defined in this analysis as living under the income threshold of half a minimum wage per capita. Because of the temporary nature of expected income shocks and of mitigation measures, results are based on annualized income.

We begin from a baseline poverty rate of 29.1 percent based on recently published 2019 PNAD-C data. For the baseline scenario, and after taking into account unemployment benefits received by formal workers who may be laid off, the result is a 13.4 percent increase in the share of people living on less than half a minimum wage. This translates into approximately 8.4 million people. Without unemployment benefits, this number would have been 11.5 million. These results are aligned with an increase in poverty (at the international poverty line of US$5.50 per day) for approximately 7.2 million Brazilians.[44]

---

[708] These estimates are based on results from the computable general equilibrium model and the BraSim microsimulation tool, assuming a baseline and a downside unemployment shock for affected workers. Unemployment shocks are allocated based on worker and household characteristics that are correlated with higher likelihood of non-employment.

[709] This analysis implicitly treats BEm, an emergency benefit which grants workers access to three months of unemployment benefits without a formal dismissal, as part of the unemployment insurance system.

The most affected quintiles are the second and the third—largely aligned with the economically vulnerable living on incomes that fall above the US$5.50-perday line, but below US$13 per day. Under the downside scenario, income reductions would be steeper, leading to higher increases in inequality and poverty. Overall, income would fall by 7.1 percent; and by 10.5 percent to 15.1 percent for the second and third quintiles (figure 45 8 c). Inequality would jump by 4.1 percent— an increase higher than what was seen in 2015–16. As a result, poverty would rise by 17.6 percent after taking into account formal workers' unemployment protection, pushing 11 million into poverty. Without unemployment protection measures, the increase in poverty would reach 24.5 percent, or over 15.4 million people.

[43]The value of half a minimum wage is an important poverty line proxy for Brazil, since it is the eligibility threshold for Cadastro Único, and it is close to the international poverty line for upper middle-income countries, US$5.50 per day (2011 PPP).[44]Due to methodological differences between the welfare aggregates used for the two poverty lines, the results are not directly comparable. The poverty change for the US$5.50 line is estimated based on historical elasticities of poverty to growth, but the selection of parameters is informed by the results of the microsimulation model.

Figure 44 7: Sectoral Distribution of Face-to-Face Interactions in the Formal Sector

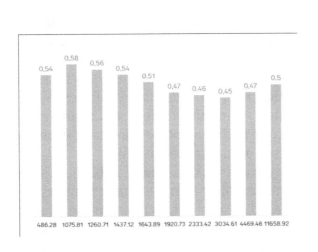
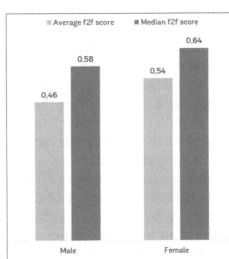

a) Average Score by Income Decileb) Average and Median Score by Gender

Source: World Bank tabulations based on RAIS. The results above highlight the importance of access to unemployment insurance benefits during this crisis, while also showing the magnitude of uncovered shocks among lower-income groups. Accessing unemployment insurance was initially slowed down by the closure of SINE offices, which traditionally process unemployment claims. These have now largely moved to online applications, which have allowed the continued processing of claims during the pandemic. Two particularly relevant policy responses announced by the government for alleviating the impact of the crisis on Brazilian households are (i) the expansion of the Bolsa Família Program (BFP) to include families that were already eligible; and (ii) Auxílio Emergencial, that is, an emergency aid program that grants three monthly transfers of R$600 to families with income levels below half a minimum wage per capita for informal and own-account workers (Microempreendedor Individual MEI, or self-employed), as well as the unemployed not receiving any unemployment insurance.

The expansion of the BFP is expected to add 1,225,000 families to the program, or approximately 3.3 million people. This increases the total coverage of the program by 8.6 percent to 14.26 million families at an estimated cost of R$3.1 billion. Although this expansion is expected to increase the income of these affected families, it should reduce poverty only marginally. The population living on less than R$178 per month (the BFP eligibility criteria, and a value close to US$1.90 per day) are expected to decrease by 0.1 percentage point. This is because of BFP's low generosity levels: 60 percent of families in the BFP receive less than R$200 per month. Moreover, an estimated 450,000 eligible families are still waiting to access the BFP, while it is possible that, in the coming months, new families will need assistance as a result of the pandemic. The Auxílio Emergencial program will have a significant impact on low-income households. Assuming

that the transfers are well disbursed to all eligible households, under the baseline scenario the benefit would more than offset the impact of the pandemic on the poorest quintiles, covering an estimated 54 to 68 million workers at a cost of R$106 billion to R$135 billion.[710] Relying only on the lower-bound estimates of coverage, the transfers would fully undo the annualized impact of the pandemic on income for the poorest 40 percent of the population. In annualized terms, the three months of transfers would increase the average income of the poorest quintile by 14 percent relative to 2019, when it was R$203.50 per capita, and of the second quintile by 3 percent. Auxílio Emergencial, if well implemented, would also significantly (though temporarily) mitigate the impact of the shock on inequality. Even with the resulting significant increase in income for the lowest income quintiles, inequality is expected to remain at a Gini index of 53.4, higher than its 2015 pre-crisis level.

The resulting increase in income for the poorest 40 percent has the potential to reverse the pandemic's impact on poverty. Using the annual average income for 2020, the poverty rate could fall by 2.3 percent relative to pre-shock poverty levels (figure 45 8b).[711]While the inclusion of all BFP families in this transfer means that a significant proportion of the poorest quintile will see their incomes increase (by an average of 14 percent), few BFP families are expected to exit poverty, as their income will remain below half a minimum wage. Rather, it is other households with higher incomes and who rely on informal and own-account work that are most likely to be pushed out of poverty. While the percent of families living on less than half one minimum salary is expected to fall as a result of the AE, it is important to note that, for about 1.2 million families who experience an income shock, the AE will not be sufficient to push them above this threshold. The median family in this category will see their monthly income fall to about R$420 per person. Figure 45d presents

---

[710] Lower-bound estimates are based on the application of income eligibility considering all informal income reported in the BraSim microsimulation model. Upper-bound estimates apply income eligibility, excluding income that is not reported by a third party (informal and self-employment income) and does not enforce the limit of 2 benefits per household. As of late May 2020, benefits had been approved for 60 million people.

[711] These results are based on the baseline and downside unemployment shock scenarios derived from CGE-based projections of sectoral income losses used above. This estimate takes into account unemployment benefits and the BFP expansion.

the impact of these transfers in the face of a more severe employment disruption scenario. In the downside scenario, the effects of the transfers are still positive and can offset most of the negative impact of the shock, but they are not able to reduce poverty below pre-shock levels.

Figure 458: Poverty and Income Impacts of Household Employment Shocks and Auxílio Emergencial: CGE—Microsimulation Household Analysis(a) Effects of the Pandemic on Household Income and (b) Effects of Expanded BFP and Auxílio Emergencial Poverty (before policies), Baseline Scenario on Household Income and Poverty, Baseline Scenario

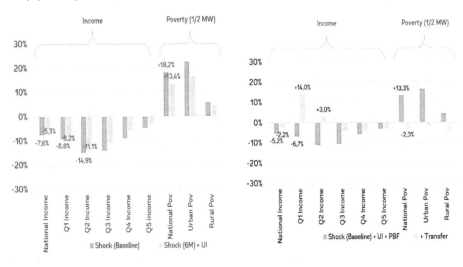

c) Effects of the Pandemic on Household Income and d) Effects of Expanded BFP and Auxílio Emergencial Poverty, Downside Scenario on Household Income and Poverty, Downside Scenario

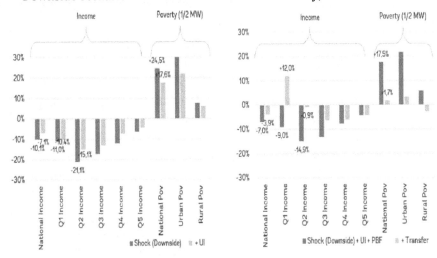

Source: World Bank.

The wage bill shock is based on the Brazil CGE model. Unemployment shocks are distributed based on worker and household characteristics using a fitted logit model. All figures are based on the lower-bound estimates of coverage for Auxílio Emergencial under each scenario. Successful implementation of Auxílio Emergencial requires a quick expansion of the national beneficiary registry (Cadastro Único) to include eligible workers that are not receiving benefits yet. This process has been hindered by a lack of identification numbers (known as CPF) for segments of the population, and the limited capacity of local social assistance offices (CRAS) to process new beneficiaries. A large segment of beneficiaries will be automatically covered— those who receive Bolsa Família. Under the lower-bound estimates of coverage, if we assume that only half of the eligible workers who do not receive Bolsa Família are able to access Auxílio Emergencial, 12.5 million fewer workers would receive it in the baseline scenario. The result would be 1.8 million people still entering poverty, instead of 1.4 million leaving it as a result of the transfers. Importantly, the results reported above, based on annualized income, obscure the severity of the short-term impact of these income shocks, assuming instead perfect income smoothing over the year. In reality, households in the lowest income groups will, on average, experience three months with higher-than-usual incomes during the onset of the pandemic (mostly April through July, depending on enrolment date) as a result of Auxílio Emergencial. Once these transfers end, and if employment remains weak, these same households will then experience a severe income reduction: relative to their pre-pandemic income, the income of the two bottom quintiles would fall by 26 percent on average—after taking into account unemployment insurance.

Beyond the two key policy responses explored above (expanded BFP and Auxílio Emergencial), policies are also being implemented to reduce unemployment shocks for formal workers, such as increased flexibility for remote working and leave policies, and bringing forward extra payments (such as the 13th salary and other wage subsidies). Other measures have also been adopted, such as expanding access to credit through increased lending, and steps to reduce food insecurity. Furthermore, there are also housing policies being implemented, such as the construction of subsidized housing; temporary suspension of mortgage payments for Minha Casa Minha Vida beneficiaries; and temporary resettlement of at-risk groups to government-managed facilities.

Brazil also has some notable sources of resilience, especially as compared to many other middle-income countries. Firstly, Brazil benefits from having a relatively large formal sector workforce with some unemployment protection and savings mechanisms in place. Secondly, Brazil has provided near-universal access to pensions and/or social security benefits to its older population, which is also among the most vulnerable to COVID-19. Thirdly, Brazil has robust infrastructure in place for the delivery of its emergency measures, such as Cadastro Único, with 76.4 million people registered, complemented by other tools, including an existing network of NGOs supporting government actions in the slums. While the country will still need to add a significant number of newly eligible informal, self-employed, and unemployed workers to the registry in order to effectively distribute Auxílio Emergencial, the rollout of this benefit to Bolsa Família beneficiaries provides a quick source of additional support to the poorest families in Brazil.

2. In Brazil's Raging Pandemic, Domestic Workers Fear For Their Lives – And Their Jobs

Mauricio Sellmann Oliveira
Visiting Scholar, Dartmouth College

Brazil has emerged as one of the worst-hit countries in the coronavirus crisis[712], with hundreds of thousands of cases affecting people from all backgrounds[713]. But in the early weeks of the pandemic, in March, many victims of the disease had a similar profile: a maid infected by her employer. The first confirmed COVID-19 patient in Brazil's north-eastern Bahia state was a woman recently returned from Italy. She infected her maid, who then infected her own 68-year-old mother[714]. On March 17, a 62-year-old live-in maid died[715] from the novel coronavirus in Rio de Janeiro. Her COVID-19 positive employer had also travelled to Italy. Domestic workers are central figures in Brazil[716], a hidden workforce that keeps society running. Most upper- and middle-class Brazilian households – and even many lower-middle class homes – employ an "empregada doméstica," or domestic employee. Brazil, with 209 million people, has 6 million maids, according to the government[717]. COVID-19 is bringing this enormous, often invisible workforce into sharp focus.

High Risk, No Safety Net

Brazilian domestic workers earn US$128 a month on average – less than minimum wage – though salary and working conditions vary greatly across social strata. Some domestic employees are live-in maids, who usually work their entire adult lives for one family. Others are paid monthly, and commute daily to work. Then there are daily maids who serve multiple households, akin to U.S. house cleaners. The tradition of domestic help can be traced back to the abolition of slavery in 1888, as I analyzed in my recent study on the evolution of Brazilian maids and their role in society.[718]After slavery ended in Brazil, the government left an estimated 1 million newly freed black people to survive with their own resources, which were usually none. Ninety-nine percent of black Brazilians were illiterate, according to Brazil's 1890 census. Most took menial jobs, with black women largely relegated to live-in domestic work serving mostly white homes. Black women still make up the majority of Brazil's "domésticas"[719] – 63% in 2018. Domestic work is so explicitly racialized in Brazil that, in 1994, soon-to-be Brazilian President Fernando Henrique Cardoso told reporters[720] he "had

[712] https://thehill.com/policy/international/americas/499460-brazil-has-worlds-highest-coronavirus-death-toll-for-first-time

[713] https://www.nytimes.com/interactive/2020/world/americas/brazil-coronavirus-cases.html

[714] https://www.correio24horas.com.br/noticia/nid/mae-de-domestica-infectada-e-terceiro-caso-confirmado-de-coronavirus-na-bahia/

[715] https://www.bbc.com/portuguese/brasil-51982465

[716] https://brazilian.report/society/2020/02/17/economy-minister-paulo-guedes-domestic-worker-brazil/

[717] https://www.ibge.gov.br/estatisticas/sociais/trabalho/9171-pesquisa-nacional-por-amostra-de-domicilios-continua-mensal.html?edicao=27527&t=quadro-sintetico

[718] https://www.springer.com/br/book/9783030332952

[719] https://www.ipea.gov.br/portal/images/stories/PDFs/TDs/td_2528.pdf

[720] https://www1.folha.uol.com.br/fsp/1994/5/31/brasil/18.html

one foot in the kitchen" to signal his mixed-race heritage. These days, having two feet in the kitchen signals a disproportionate COVID-19 risk. In April, the Health Ministry reported[721] that black Brazilians made up a quarter of those hospitalized with severe COVID-19 but about a third of COVID-19 fatalities. And officials in São Paulo, the epicentre of the pandemic in Brazil, recently reported that black residents were 62% more likely to die of COVID-19[722] than the general population. But Brazilian maids of all races are vulnerable in this crisis because most generally lack employment safeguards, commute long distances and are poor, with limited access to quality health care.All intensive care beds in public hospitals from five states[723] – Pará, Maranhão, Rio de Janeiro, Pernambuco and Ceará – are either occupied or soon will be, according to states reports. While wealthy COVID-19 patients can pay to be transported to top private hospitals in São Paulo or abroad[724], poorer Brazilians rely on the overwhelmed public health system.

Economic Devastation

Brazilian domestic workers' exposure to the pandemic is economic as well as physical. Approximately 4.3 million of Brazil's 6 million maids are employed informally[725], meaning they aren't registered with the government. As such, labour rights – which include the $178 national minimum monthly wage and 30-day paid vacations – do not apply. Since early March, 39% of daily maids in Brazil[726] have been let go. They are among the estimated 15 to 20 million Brazilians expected to be[727] unemployed by July, according to several projections[728]. Though the Office of the Federal Labour Attorney[729] officially recommends that maids receive paid leave to stay at home during the pandemic, only 39% of regular maids and 48% of daily maids have been given that benefit, according to the pollster Locomotiva[730]. Some states in Brazil have listed domestic work as an essential service, allowing them to continue working – assuming their employers will still pay them[731].

Solidarity Networks

The plight of domestic workers is one of many ways the pandemic is shining a hard light on inequality in Brazil. Brazil's Congress in March passed an aid bill authorizing a monthly $102 "emergency basic income" payment to the newly unemployed, including informal workers. So far, however, little more than half of the 55 million[732] people who've applied[733] have received funds,

---

[721] https://valor.globo.com/brasil/noticia/2020/04/11/coronavrus-mais-letal-entre-negros-no-brasil-apontam-dados-da-sade.ghtml

[722] https://saude.estadao.com.br/noticias/geral,em-sp-risco-de-morte-de-negros-por-covid-19-e-62-maior-em-relacao-aos-brancos,70003291431

[723] https://www1.folha.uol.com.br/cotidiano/2020/05/doze-capitais-tem-mais-de-80-de-leitos-publicos-de-uti-ocupados.shtml

[724] https://epoca.globo.com/sociedade/coronavirus-ricos-de-belem-escapam-em-uti-aerea-de-colapso-nos-hospitais-da-cidade-1-24412850

[725] https://www.ibge.gov.br/estatisticas/sociais/trabalho/9171-pesquisa-nacional-por-amostra-de-domicilios-continua-mensal.html?edicao=27527&t=quadro-sintetico

[726] https://noticias.uol.com.br/ultimas-noticias/bbc/2020/04/22/conoravirus-no-brasil-39-dos-patroes-dispensaram-diaristas-sem-pagamento-durante-pandemia-aponta-pesquisa.htm

[727] https://exame.com/economia/taxa-de-desemprego-no-brasil-pode-dobrar-por-covid-19-diz-salim-mattar/

[728] https://valorinveste.globo.com/mercados/brasil-e-politica/noticia/2020/03/27/desemprego-vai-explodir-no-brasil-com-coronavirus-a-duvida-e-o-tamanho-da-bomba.ghtml

[729] https://mpt.mp.br/pgt/noticias/nota-tecnica-no-4-coronavirus-1.pdf

[730] https://www.bbc.com/portuguese/brasil-52375292

[731] https://www.bbc.com/portuguese/brasil-52375292

[732] https://caixanoticias.caixa.gov.br/noticia/20795/auxilio-emergencial-clique-aqui-para-ver-os-ultimos-numeros

[733] https://caixanoticias.caixa.gov.br/noticia/20795/auxilio-emergencial-clique-aqui-para-ver-os-ultimos-numeros

due to faulty execution and bureaucratic delays. Lack of internet access and other poverty-related factors may prevent many millions more from even applying[734]. Brazilian maids are suffering in this pandemic, but not in silence. A federation of domestic workers unions called Fenatrad is challenging the state decrees that established domestic workers as essential service providers, pushing instead for this high-risk population to receive paid leave. In early May, the Brazilian Supreme Court ruled that COVID-19 qualifies as an occupational illness for the purposes of workers' compensation. This decision applies to maids. Communities have created their own grassroots initiatives to support domestic workers, too. An "Adopt a Daily Maid[735]" donation campaign is underway in São Paulo's Paraisópolis "favela" – a slum settlement that abuts an upper-class district – urging people with means to support house cleaners in the area. And in a sign of the remarkable social mobility Brazil fostered in the boom years of the early 21st century[736], the first-generation college-educated children of maids started a Change.org petition[737] asking employers to give domestic workers paid leave, advance vacation pay and isolate live-in maids who are at high COVID-19 risk. They latter added a donations option to support vulnerable maids[738]. "Maids belong to a group of workers that represents Brazil," reads the petition, which urges everyone raised by domestic workers to join their cause. So far, more than 90,000 people have signed on, "for the lives of all our mothers[739]."

---

[734] https://redepesquisasolidaria.org/wp-content/uploads/2020/05/boletim5.pdf

[735] https://www.esolidar.com/en/crowdfunding/detail/6-adote-uma-diarista-durante-o-coronavirus-covid19?lang=br

[736] https://theconversation.com/as-brazil-tilts-rightward-lulas-leftist-legacy-of-lifting-the-poor-is-at-risk-65939

[737] https://www.theguardian.com/global-development/2020/may/05/for-the-lives-of-our-mothers-covid-19-sparks-fight-for-maids-rights-in-brazil-coronavirus

[738] https://www.instagram.com/pelavidadenossasmaes/

[739] https://www.facebook.com/cartamanifesto/posts/103226661321138:0?_tn_=K-R

3. COVID-19 Among Health Workers In Brazil: The Silent Wave

Emanuelle Pessa Valente,[1] Lia Cruz Vaz da Costa Damásio,[2] Leonardo Sérvio Luz,[2] Marília Francisca da Silva Pereira,[2] and Marzia Lazzerini[1]

According to the most recent WHO estimates, Brazil has the highest number of diagnosed COVID-19 cases in the Americas Region after the United States [1]. Community transmission has been documented throughout all federal units (26 states and Federal district). Since the beginning of pandemic, many organizations have raised concerns with the lack of personal protective equipment (PPE), low observance of social distancing measures, and scarce availability of diagnostic tests in Brazil [2,3]. MoH recommended use of diagnostic swabs be reserved for severe cases with Acute Respiratory Distress Syndrome (ARDS) [4]. No specific federal recommendations on case finding among health workers (HW) currently exist. Data from other countries have clearly indicated that HW are disproportionally affected by COVID-19 and can be carriers of the disease. In Italy, 20 618 COVID-19 cases have been reported so far among HW (10.4% of total cases) [5]. The Italian National Federation of Medical Doctors and Odontologists has reported 151 deaths among doctors [6]. These data do not include other HW categories such as nurses or midwives. In US, the Centres for Disease Control and Prevention (CDC) reported 9282 COVID-19 cases confirmed among HW [7] among these 723 (8%-10%) were hospitalized and 184 (2%-5%) required intensive care unit (ICU) admission.

In defence of HW safety, the Brazilian Federal Council of Medicine (FCM) has taken several measures. HW safety guidelines have been widely circulated, with hospital inspections carried out to verify their implementation. An online platform has been established for professionals to report shortcomings of resources, such as lack of PPE in workplaces, either public or private. Finally, the FCM is advocating for expanding criteria for COVID-19 diagnostic tests to all symptomatic HW [8]. Yet frontline workers are dangerously ill-equipped due to decades of underinvestment in the public health sector and limited access to appropriate PPE and training [9,10]. The Brazilian Federal Council of Nursing highlighted around 4800 reports of lack of PPE made by associate members since the beginning of pandemic. In the same time period, there have been more than 4600 sick leaves for "influenza-like symptoms" and 32 deaths among nurses, numbers significantly higher than usual trends [10]. Brazilian media have claimed that the number of COVID-19 cases and related deaths among HW, in particular in selected states such as São Paulo and Maranhão, is rapidly increasing [11].

Open Knowledge Brazil (OKBR), a civil society organization that operates in support of open-access data of public interest, ranked Brazilian states with a "Transparency index", evaluating 13 criteria related to content, format and level of detail of information disclosed via official portals during COVID-19 pandemic [12]. Despite improvements in the last weeks, on 22 April only four (15.3%) Brazilian states published data on the availability of COVID-19 diagnostic tests, while 11 (42.3%)

provided data on incidence of new ARDS cases [12]. The "Transparency index" had a major impact on public opinion in Brazil, and civil public legal action was taken against San Paulo state using these data. However, the Transparency index does not include availability of data on COVID-19 among HW to evaluate states. We report here the results of a rapid review performed by systematically screening each of the 27 federal health department websites and COVID-19 dedicated portals in order to identify specific policies for HW health screening and testing, and related HW morbidity and mortality data. Data collection procedures were integrated by research on social networks. Data are updated on 27 April 2020. Results indicated that Pernambuco, a state in Northeast, was the first to develop a policy to perform diagnostic swabs among all symptomatic HW on 4 April 2020, giving priority to HW in ICUs and emergency departments. Policies in other states were less clear, with limited availability on official websites. Major investments were made in rapid tests for qualitative antibody detection whose accuracy is still unclear.

Information regarding COVID-19 confirmed cases among HWs was available in the official bulletins of only six (22.2%) Brazilian Federal states (**Figure 1**). As expected based on current policies, a significantly higher number of cases was detected in Pernambuco compared to other states, with a high prevalence in HW (30.8% of total cases). As many states are currently implementing massive rapid test programs, increased numbers of COVID-19 cases among HW are expected in coming weeks.

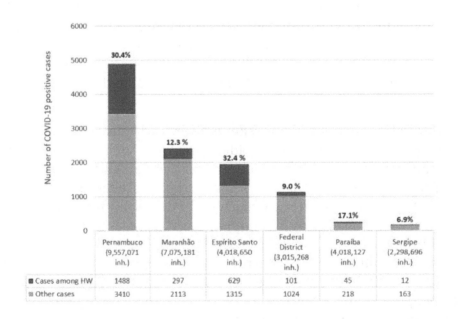

	Pernambuco (9,557,071 inh.)	Maranhão (7,075,181 inh.)	Espírito Santo (4,018,650 inh.)	Federal District (3,015,268 inh.)	Paraíba (4,018,127 inh.)	Sergipe (2,298,696 inh.)
■ Cases among HW	1488	297	629	101	45	12
▩ Other cases	3410	2113	1315	1024	218	163

Figure 1

COVID-19 positive cases among health workers by Brazilian federal state. HW – health worker. Note: only six states had data available on health worker infection; Pernambuco state has a policy for HW testing. Data sources: State epidemiological bulletins, accessed 27 April 2020 [13-19].

These data demonstrate a lack of a homogeneous, transparent, and comprehensive surveillance system for COVID-19 cases among Brazilian HW during the current pandemic. Coordinated policies are needed to increase HW protection, and availability of surveillance data, to protect both HW and the entire Brazilian population.

ACKNOWLEDGMENTS

The authors would like to thank Rebecca Lundin for the English language review.
Ethical statement: This article does not contain any studies involving human participants.

Notes.

Authorship contributions: EPV conceived the paper in discussion with LCVCD and ML. LSL, MFSP and EPV collected data. EPV drafted the initial manuscript and all authors reviewed/edited the manuscript for critically important intellectual content and approved the final version of the manuscript.

Conflict of interest: The authors completed the ICMJE Unified Competing Interest form (available upon request from the corresponding author) and declare no conflicts of interest.

REFERENCES

1. World Health Organization. Coronavirus disease (COVID-2019) situation reports. Available: https://www.who.int/emergencies/diseases/novel-coronavirus-2019/situation-reports. Accessed: 30 April 2020.
2. Conselho Nacional de Saúde – Brasil. NOTA PÚBLICA: CNS defende manutenção de distanciamento social conforme define OMS (08/04/2020). Available: https://conselho.saude.gov.br/ultimas-noticias-cns/1102-nota-publica-cns-defende-manutencao-de-distanciamento-social-conforme-define-oms. Accessed: 20 April 2020.
3. PAHO. COVID-19: PAHO Director calls for "extreme caution" when transitioning to more flexible social distancing measures. Available: https://www.paho.org/en/news/14-4-2020-COVID-19-paho-director-calls-extreme-caution-when-transitioning-more-flexible-social. Accessed: 20 April 2020.
4. BRASIL. Diretrizes para Diagnóstico e Tratamento da COVID-19. Versão 1. Secretaria de Ciência, Tecnologia, Inovação e Insumos Estratégicos em Saúde – SCTIE. Brasília – DF, 6 de abril de 2020.
5. Istituto Superiore di Sanità. Epidemia COVID-19. "Sorveglianza integrata COVID-19 in Italia". Aggiornamento 27 aprile 2020. Available: https://www.epicentro.iss.it/coronavirus/bollettino/Infografica_27aprile%20ITA.pdf. Accessed: 28 April 2020.
6. Federazione Nazionale degli Ordini dei Medici Chirurghi e degli Odontoiatri. Elenco dei Medici caduti nel corso dell'epidemia di COVID-19. Available: https://portale.fnomceo.it/elenco-dei-medici-caduti-nel-corso-dellepidemia-di-COVID-19/. Accessed: 27 April 2020.
7. Characteristics of Health Care Personnel with COVID-19 — United States February 12–April 9, 2020. MMWR Morb Mortal Wkly Rep. 2020;69:477-81. [PubMed] [Google Scholar]
8. Conselho Federal de Medicina. PANDEMIA COVID-19: Notas e esclarecimentos do CFM. Available: http://portal.cfm.org.br/index.php?option=com_content&view=article&id=28634 Accessed: 22 April 2020.
9. Confederação Nacional dos Trabalhadores na Saúde – Brasil. Profissionais de saúde estão expostos e sem proteção. Available: https://cnts.org.br/noticias/profissionais-de-saude-estao-expostos-e-sem-protecao/. Accessed: 20 April 2020.
10. COFEN. Conselho Federal de Enfermagem. "Mais de 4 mil profissionais foram contaminados pela COVID-19" (20/04/2020). Available: http://www.cofen.gov.br/mais-de-4-mil-profissionais-de-enfermagem-foram-contaminados-pela-COVID-19_79240.html. Accessed: 20 April 2020.
11. Atual RB. "Sindicato registra morte de 16 trabalhadores da saúde pela COVID-19 em São Paulo" (13/04/2020). Available: https://www.redebrasilatual.com.br/trabalho/2020/04/trabalhadores-saude-COVID-19/ Accessed: 20 April 2020.
12. Brasil OK. (OKBR). Índice de Transparência da COVID-19. Available: https://www.ok.org.br/projetos/indice-de-transparencia-da-COVID-19/. Accessed: 27 April 2020.
13. Epidemiológico B. COVID-19. Secretaria de Estado da Saúde do Maranhão (Boletim atualizado até às 18h – 26/04/2020. Portal da Saúde. Available: http://www.saude.ma.gov.br/boletins-COVID-19/. Accesses: 27 April 2020.

14. Governo do Estado do Espírito Santo. Painel COVID-19 do Espírito Santo. Available: https://coronavirus.es.gov.br/painel-COVID-19-es. Accessed: 27 April 2020.
15. Secretaria de Saúde de Pernambuco. ATUALIZAÇÕES EPIDEMIOLÓGICAS SES/PE. Informe Epidemiológico Coronavírus (COVID-19). Nº 56 – Pernambuco 26/04/2020. Available: https://www.cievspe.com/novo-coronavirus-2019-ncov. Accessed: 27 April 2020.
16. Secretaria de Saúde de Pernambuco. Secretaria-Executiva de Vigilância em Saúde. COVID-19: Nota orienta testagem de profissionais (04/04/2020). Available: http://portal.saude.pe.gov.br/noticias/secretaria-executiva-de-vigilancia-em-saude/COVID-19-nota-orienta-testagem-de-profissionais. Accessed: 20 April 2020.
17. Secretaria de Estado da Saúde. Gerência Executiva de Vigilância em Saúde. COVID-19 SES-PB, Boletim Epidemiológico n.10 (21/04/2020). Available: https://paraiba.pb.gov.br/diretas/saude/consultas/vigilancia-em-saude-1/boletins-epidemiologicos. Accessed 27 April 2020.
18. Governo do Estado de Sergipe. Secretaria de Estado da Saúde de Sergipe. Boletins. Availablet: https://todoscontraocorona.net.br/boletins/. Accessed: 27 April 2020.
19. Secretaria de Saúde do Distrito Federal. Boletins Informativos sobre Coronavirus (COVID-19) (SVS/DIVEP/CIEVES). Informe nº 55 – 26 abril 2020. Available: http://www.saude.df.gov.br/boletinsinformativos-divep-cieves/. Accessed: 28 April 2020.

4. Management of The Health Workforce In Facing COVID-19: Disinformation And Absences In Brazil's Public Policies.

Silvana Nair Leite

Universidade Federal de Santa Catarina. Departamento de Ciências Farmacêuticas. Programa de Pósgraduação em Farmácia. Florianópolis-Brasil

Mirelle Finkler

Universidade Federal de Santa Catarina. Departamento de Odontologia e Programa de Pós-graduação em Saúde Coletiva.Florianópolis-Brasil

Jussara Gue Martini

Universidade Federal de Santa Catarina. Departamento de Enfermagem. Programa de Pós-graduação em Enfermagem. Florianópolis-Brasil

Ivonete Heidemann

Universidade Federal de Santa Catarina. Departamento de Enfermagem. Programa de Pós-graduação em Enfermagem. Florianópolis-Brasil

Marta Verdi

Universidade Federal de Santa Catarina. Departamento de Saúde Pública. Programa de Pós-graduação em Saúde Coletiva Florianópolis-Brasil.

Fernando Hellmann

Universidade Federal de Santa Catarina. Departamento de Saúde Pública. Programa de Pós-graduação em Saúde Coletiva. Florianópolis-Brasil.

Maria Fernanda Vásquez-Autora

de correspondênciaUniversidade Federal de Santa Catarina. Bolsista PRINT-CAPES, Jovem Talento. Programa de Pósgraduação em Saúde Coletiva e Programa de Pós-graduação em Enfermagem.Florianópolis-Brasil.

ABSTRACT

How well a country manages the Covid-19 crisis depends largely on how effectively the health workforce is used. Much can be done to ensure that the workforce is prepared to deal with the pandemic. The objective of this research was to highlight the strategies implemented in Brazil in relation to the health workforce in the context of the Covid-19 pandemic and to analyse federal government interventions in crisis management and the consequences for health professionals. This is a documentary-type qualitative research project. Brazilian federal regulations referring to work and health education produced during the pandemic emergency of COVID-19, published from January 28 to June 2, 2020, were identified. Of the total of 845 documents, 62 were selected in accordance with the inclusion criteria and were then submitted to Thematic Content Analysis. The results and discussions were grouped into four categories: Workforce management, Workforce protection, Workforce training and Academic-Workforce relationship. An absence of a federal coordinating actions aimed at the governance of the health workforce facing the pandemic in Brazil was identified. It is considered that this lacking mechanisms for coordination contributed decisively to the tragic epidemiological situation still underway, especially in terms of the exposure of health workers to the risk of contamination, revealed in the extremely high rates of professionals infected or killed by Covid-19 in Brazil and the failure to control the pandemic in the population.

INTRODUCTION

Since the World Health Organisation (WHO) characterized the spread of Sars-CoV-2 as a pandemic on March 11, 2020, healthcare systems across high, lower and middle-income countries have been put under tremendous pressure to control the spread of the novel coronavirus[1]. The pandemic, together with a fragile and questionable economic model, has worsened global disparities by weakening the already precarious essential services (health and education) of the poorest countries, such as those in Latin America[2]. Issues related to lack of infrastructure, resources and the capacity to acquire equipment have been of crucial importance. The major responsibility of health systems is to maintain and support frontline health care workers, who are putting their lives on the line[1,3]. Government leaders and regulators need to help expand capacity and ensure the full use of the workforce under safe conditions throughout the pandemic[3,4].

In this sense, it is not only imperative to treat infected people and prevent new cases, but it is also of great importance to ensure that there are sufficient healthcare professionals (HCP) and a safe working environment[1,4,5]. Around the world, risks and harm to healthcare professionals have been reported. In the United States, a total of 9,282 health care professionals were confirmed with COVID-19 and reported to the CDC in April. This is likely an underestimate because HCP status was available for only 16% of reported cases nationwide[4]. In Wuhan, a total of 3.5% patients that presented with severe disease or death were health care workers[6]. In April 2020, Brazil already presented more than 50% of the deaths of nursing professionals from all over the planet[7]. In July 2020, the number of confirmed cases in HCP was 173,000 (about 10% of total cases). The nursing workforce was the most affected professional category with more than 37,680 professionals in the field infected by COVID-19, 396 of whom had died by 02/09/20[8]. The risk to healthcare workers is one of the greatest vulnerabilities of healthcare systems worldwide. To protect HCP is one of the major challenges and should be the crucial mission for health systems and institutions. The media and scientific publications have denounced the shortages in personal protective equipment for frontline health care workers. All the scientific recommendations agree that testing frontline health care staff is a priority[1,9,] together with ensuring conditions for self-isolation, social isolation and quarantine and utilization of training, knowledge and protocols[1,10] as well as developing an evidence-based menu of interventions from which careful selection may occur, and which are tailored to various workplace settings[11]. Effective strategies towards improving mental health should also be provided to the frontline professionals[12], because of high rates of reported symptoms of depression, anxiety, insomnia and distress[13,14].

Since late May 2020, three months after the first reported case of coronavirus in Brazil, an average of more than 1000 daily deaths has been recorded. Currently, Brazil has one of the fastest growing coronavirus epidemics in the world[15], with more than 3,950,931 confirmed cases - the second largest number in the world - and more than 122,596 deaths, according to official data[16]. Brazil has become one of the epicentres of the COVID-19 pandemic and is experiencing "a public health disaster"[17]. The vacuum of actions by the federal government to command the fight against the pandemic only aggravates the difficulty faced in the country, due to conditions in such an unequal society with a huge population of people in situations of extreme vulnerability[18]. The focus of this research was the policies implemented by the Brazilian government, specifically with regard to the health workforce tackling the Covid-19 pandemic. The health workforce concept adopted is the contingent of people engaged in actions whose primary intent is to enhance health, who are at many different stages of their working lives, work in many different organisations and under changing conditions and pressures[19]. The objective of the study was to highlight the strategies implemented in the management of the health workforce in Brazil and to analyse the way the federal government has dealt with the pandemic in terms of its consequences for health professionals.

METHODOLOGY

This research employed a qualitative approach, of the documentary type. Documentary research uses diverse sources such as statistical tables, newspapers, magazines, reports and official documents. It is a type of research that uses primary sources, that is, data and information that have not yet been treated scientifically or analytically [37].

A survey of all federal regulations and legislation produced during the pandemic emergency of COVID-19 in Brazil was carried out. The search included documents published between 28/01/2020 and 02/06/2020, on the two official websites that compile them: The National Council of Health Secretaries (CONASS)[20] and the Presidency of the Republic/ General Secretariat[21]. Both constantly update the publications and offer a direct link to their content, which is published in the Official Federal Gazette.

The selection had as inclusion criteria: regulations and laws related to the pandemic and to Education and/or Health; and that were federal in scope. 771 documents related to COVID-19 were found and organized in an Excel® spreadsheet to assist in the data collection stage. Of these, 706 were removed due to duplication or because they did not meet the inclusion criteria, resulting in a total of 65 documents. After a critical and thorough reading, it was possible to develop an overview of the published federal acts, according to a list of predetermined categories, namely:

Workforce Management; Workforce Protection; Teleworking; Workforce-Academia Relationship; and Workforce Training.

From this first analysis, we sought to identify the need to complement the investigation with documents that addressed the national combat of the pandemic within the scope of actions in Education and Health. Thus, a second stage of collecting directives was carried out, including technical notes, dispatches, technical reports and protocols published on the websites of the federal councils of Pharmacy (CFF), Medicine (CFM), Nursing (COFEN), Dentistry (CFO) as well as the Special Secretariat for Indigenous Health (SESAI), the Ministry of Education, the Brazilian Company and Hospital Services (EBSERH) and the Coordination for the Improvement of Higher Education Personnel (CAPES). In this second stage, 74 documents that met the study inclusion criteria were considered. The total number of documents was 139.

After reading and critically evaluating each of the documents, 77 were excluded because they did not meet the inclusion criteria, resulting in 62 documents that were actually analysed. These were synthesized and allocated to one or more of the previously defined categories. For the selection of documents, the recommendations of the Preferred Reporting Items for Systematic Reviews and Meta-Analyzes (PRISMA) were used, represented in figure 1.

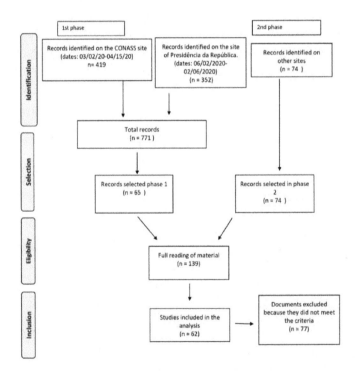

Figure 1. Flowchart of the document selection process.

Using the *tableu public* application, details of the characteristics of the included documents were obtained, such as temporal distribution, typology, grouping by categories and authoring institutions. For the evaluation of the documents, the steps of Thematic Content Analysis were followed, which provided methodological organisation and rigor to the study. In this process, it was noticed that the six previously defined categories formed four different thematic categories: Workforce Management, Workforce Protection, Workforce Training and Academia-Workforce Relationship.

RESULTS AND DISCUSSION

The arrival and spread of the coronavirus in Brazil required new regulations and laws in order to minimize the impact of COVID-19 on the lives and work of people, in particular HCP who are on the front line of resulting emergency public health measures. The two-stage review of various sites offered a total of 845 records. Of the total of official documents published in this period, the central theme of this study, federal governance of the health workforce, was present in a small portion (62 documents out of a total of 845), categorized into four different categories (Table 1).

Categories	Subcategories	Analysed Documents	
Workforce Management	Primary Care	Portaria nº 430[1]	
	Hospitals	Lei n. 13995[2]	Parecer normativo COFEN n.2[3]
	Material resources	Portarias 245[4], 488[5]	Nota Técnica n.4 SESAI[59]
	Professional resources	Portarias 55[9], 151[58], 188[6], 356[16], 639[7] Resolução RDC 356[8]	Edital EBSERH 1[10], 2[11] Editais 5[12],8[13],9[14],10[15]
	Protective measures	Portaria 356[17], 428[18]	Lei 13979[19] Resolução 682[20]
Workforce Protection	Organisation and dissemination of preventative and control measures	MS/SESAI Notas Informativas 2[21], 6[22] MS Protocolo de Manejo Clínico 3A[23]	MS Procedimento Operacional 3B[24] MS Fluxograma 3C [25] MS/SAPS Protocolo Específico[26]
	PPE:standardisation for commercialisation and use	Resolução RDC356[8] MS/ANVISA Nota Técnica 4[37] Portarias 337[36], 9471[38] MS Protocolo Manejo Clínico 3A[23] MS Procedimento Operacional 3B[24] MS Fluxograma 3C [25]	MS/SAPS Protocolo Específico[26] CFM despacho 193[27] MS/SAPS/CGSB Notas Técnicas 9[28], 16[29] MS/SESAI Plano de Contingência[35]
	Leave of absence for groups at risk	MS/SESAI Informes Técnicos 1[30], 2[31], 3[32], 4[33], 5[34]	CFM despacho 193[27]
	Teleworking	Portaria 397[39], 467[40] Despacho CFM 204[41]	Resoluções CFO 226[42] e COFEN 634[43] Recomendação CREMEPE 1[44]
	Alteration of working processes	MS Protocolo Manejo Clínico 3A[23] MS Fluxograma 3C[25] CFM despacho 193[27]	MS/SAPS/CGSB Notas Técnicas 9[28] e 16[29] MS/SESAI Informes 1[30], 2[31], 3[32], 4[33] 5[34]

			Portaria 337[36]
	Provision of tests	MS/SESAI Nota Técnica 21[45]	CFM despacho 193[27]
	Priority vaccination for influenza	CFM despacho 193[27]	
	Telephone service to inform professionals	MS/SESAI Notas Informativas 2[21] e 6[22] MS Protocolo Manejo Clínico3A [23]	MS Procedimento Operacional 3B [24] MS Fluxograma 3C[25]
	Guaranteed working conditions	Portaria 151[46]	
Workforce Training	Directions for training of healthcare professionals	MS/ANVISA Nota Técnica 4[37] MS/SESAI Informes Técnicos 2[31], 3[32], 4[33], 5[34]	Portarias 492[47], 639[7] Nota técnica 22 SESAI[60]
	Offer of lifelong learning courses by SUS educational institutions	OMS/OPAS escolavirtual.gov.br nasus.gov.br uvasus.ufrn.br	campusvirtual.fiocruz.br universus.saude.gov.br fiocruzbrasilia.fiocruz.br
AcademiaWorkforce Relationship	Flexibility of classes	Portarias 343[48], 376[49], 473[50], 544[51]	
	Inclusion of students	Portarias 356[47], 374[62], 492[47], 580[52]	Resoluções COFEN 637[53], 636[61]
	Education and research	Editais CAPES 9[54], 11[55], 12[56]	Edital CNPq 7[57]

*See additional material for references

How well a country manages the Covid-19 crisis depends largely on how effectively the health workforce is used. Much can be done to ensure that the workforce is prepared to deal with the pandemic. According to Fraher et al.[13], "government leaders and regulators will need to help expand capacity and ensure the full use of the workforce throughout the pandemic". The analysis of the standards and documents reported here identified how the Brazilian federal government has conducted the management of the health labour force in this period. From a bibliometric point of view, analysis of the temporal distribution of the documents showed greater publication in March 2020, when the first death from COVID-19 was registered in the country (12/03). Despite the exponential worsening of the pandemic in the following months, the number of published documents decreased sharply, instead of the expected and necessary expansion (Figure 2). Such data must be analysed in the political context of the country, in which the Minister of Health in office at the beginning of the pandemic, doctor Luis Henrique Mandetta, was replaced on April 17 by Nelson Teich, a doctor from the private sector, who remained in post for just a month. Since then, the health ministry has been replacing career civil servants with military personnel, including the current interim minister. This seems to be contributing to the near absence, in June, of regulations regarding the orientation of the workforce in combating Covid-19.

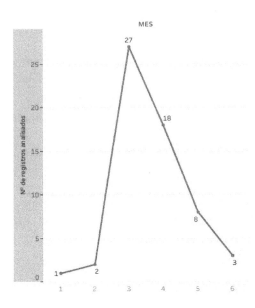

Figure 2. Records analysed by month

With respect to the type of records analysed, of the 62 documents included, 22 are decrees, being the most common legislative type for administration, regulation and application of laws and regulations, as well as general provisions, reporting on the acts carried out by public bodies. This trend is related to the type of institution that published such acts, mostly the Ministry of Health. From the analysed records, publications by the Special Secretariat for Indigenous Health (SESAI) predominate, it being responsible for 22.59% of the documents, followed by the regulations issued by the cabinet of the Minister of the Ministry of Health and the Secretariat of Primary Health Care (SAPS), with 19.35% and 11.29%, respectively. Despite the profusion of regulations in the area of indigenous health, systematizing regulations, guidelines and recommendations for management and specific care to be implemented in Special Indigenous Health Districts across the country, the level of contamination among more than 155 indigenous peoples reveals the social vulnerability to which they are subjected and the failure of the federal government to protect these native peoples. The underreporting of cases and deaths from COVID-19 in the indigenous context is evident, forcing indigenous leaders, with support from social organisations, to develop a registration system parallel to that of the government.

While the Ministry of Health counts 20,723 indigenous people infected and 348 deaths, the parallel survey has registered more than 29,381 infections and 775 deaths[22,23].

With regard to the other categories analysed, it is observed that more than half of the documents addressed some measure related to the Wworkforce Protection (64.29%). Themes related to the categories of Workforce Management and Academia-Worforce Relationship were less present (in 14.29%). The category of Workforce Training was the least identified among the documents analysed (7.14%). For the management and increase in the number of professionals in services to combat the pandemic, few regulations have been published. Only a few specific notices were issued, relating to hiring of additional professionals in university hospitals, which constitute a small portion of health services. The shortage of doctors in the public health system, especially in remote and poorer regions, is a longstanding problem. Globally, investment in the health workforce is lower than is often assumed, reducing the sustainability of the workforce and health systems[24]. In order to solve the persistent lack of doctors in poor areas of the country, in 2013, the Brazilian government launched the More Doctors Program (PMM). As a strategy to provide professionals, the PMM had more than 16,000 vacancies, mostly filled by foreigners, reaching

12,000 Cuban physicians hired through international cooperation between Brazil and Cuba, brokered by PAHO. Despite positive evaluations by the PMM, in November 2018, this cooperation was interrupted by the Cuban government after aggressive demonstrations by President-elect Bolsonaro disqualifying the training and performance of Cuban doctors [25]. In the urgency of the pandemic, state governments pushed for the reintroduction of these doctors, and some were contracted again. The Doctors Council did not agree. COFEN, on the other hand, authorized the professional registration of university leavers who had already completed the course, but were awaiting graduation, in an effort to expedite entry into the work front, of nurses who had already completed the degree program.

The fragility of workforce planning and actions for its resilience and sustainability that has been observed in Brazil resulted in the disastrous situation of facing a pandemic without having solved the basic demands for medical assistance that already existed. Analysis of the content of the documents revealed that to protect health workers, different specific actions were identified.

The most frequently encountered were the withdrawal of workers of the groups at greatest risk for Covid-19 (people aged 60 or over, people with comorbidities or pregnant women), the use of personal protective equipment (PPE), the possibility of teleworking, and the dissemination of infection prevention and pandemic control measures.

There were also recommendations for changes in work processes, especially those that generate aerosols or increase the risk for vulnerable populations, such as dental care and health worker visits to indigenous territories. Among the measures to prevent infection and control the pandemic, we highlight the control of the care environment and the movement of users between services by disinfecting surfaces and instruments, hand hygiene, respiratory etiquette, use of masks by patients, ventilation of the environments, use of barriers for interpersonal spacing, rotation in the work shifts to reduce the occupation of spaces, adequate management of waste and displaying information posters in health services. The PPE were addressed in the documents from two perspectives: the specification of characteristics for their commercialization and the establishment of usage protocols.

Although such recommendations have been included in several documents, guidelines for the adequate provision of PPE by the management of the services were rare, which suggests that the protection measures were envisaged more in the sense of maintaining the assistance services and controlling the pandemic itself rather than in the effective protection of workers' health and life.

Regarding the workforce and working conditions of HCP. it is identified that they live with potential sources of exposure to the virus and spread of the disease, stress and risk factors. In order to ensure working conditions that provide a reduction in virus transmission, it is essential to establish clear and robust strategies to face the pandemic[26]. However, the results of the present study indicate erratic and fragmented recommendations in different sectors of the Ministry of Health and other institutions. This understanding is supported by the lack of emphasis on important preventative, diagnostic and follow-up measures directed at HCP on a priority basis, and the transparent monitoring of infected workers and deaths. Added to this is the near absence of measures related to mental health and labour rights.

A report by Filho et al.[26] indicates that there has been little debate about the working conditions of professionals involved in the care of people with Covid-19 in Brazil. There is a predominance of protocols and recommendations for basic individual measures, but these are insufficient to control the spread of the virus. There are reports of professionals and unions denouncing precarious working conditions, inadequate hygiene, strenuous hours, lack of training and insufficient PPE .

A lack of protection for health workers was also found in an online survey of 1,456 public HCP in Brazil[17]. The study concluded that professionals are in a situation of extreme vulnerability, both due to the scarcity of PPE and the lack of information and government support. More than half of the interviewees affirm that they do not feel that the government supports them, this figure being higher when they evaluate the federal government (67%) than in relation to states governments (51%). These conditions have also been reported in other, especially low and middle-income, countries. This highlights the difficulty for health services in addressing the growing demands of COVID-19, and the need to reflect on the consequences of the pandemic. Since workers are overloaded, there are few resources to maintain the workforce and an inability to protect the well-being of HCP (Griffin 2020)[27].

Amnesty International[28] reports that despite the fundamental role of health and essential services workers during the pandemic, they have faced enormous challenges in doing their jobs and governments worldwide have not adequately protected them. On the contrary, many have been exposed, silenced and attacked: at least 3,000 health workers are known to have died after contracting COVID-19 in 79 countries around the world until June 2020; many others have worked in unsafe environments and unfair conditions; they have faced reprisals from the authorities and their employers for raising safety concerns, including arrests and dismissals; and in some cases have been subject to violence and stigma from members of the public. In Brazil, it is impossible to know the total number of HCP who are falling ill and dying from Covid-19, because there is no transparency in the publication of these data. Epidemiological bulletins released by the federal government show much lower numbers of infected workers than those recorded by professional organisations, such as COFEN (Federal Nursing Council), which implemented a digital Observation Platform for daily monitoring of contamination or death cases among nursing professionals. However, the Ministry of Health should "collect and publish data by occupation, including categories of health and other essential workers who have been infected by COVID-19, and how many have died as a result, in order to ensure effective protection in the future, as recommended by Amnesty

International. This data should be classified since prohibited grounds of discrimination, including but not limited to gender, race and workplace[28].

Teleworking or remote work was a proposed method for coping with the pandemic. It may be considered as another form of accessing health care while taking care to protect HCP by ensuring social distancing, as well as protecting users of the health system. Although legislation related to teleworking predates the Covid-19 pandemic, specific rules for the current moment were issued by the Ministry of Health and the professional councils of the categories directly involved with patient care, such as Nursing, Pharmacy, Medicine and Dentistry. The Ministry of Health also issued regulations regarding telemedicine, instituting, remote interaction. Telemedicine actions cover pre-clinical care, assistance support, consultation, monitoring and diagnosis, prescription of medicines through information and communication technology.

Published documents related to the management of the pandemic in Brazil provide, in general, guidelines for the organisation of some services, such as in Primary Health Care, in the dispensing of medicines, in hospital and dental services and protocols that can be understood as guidelines for the work of work teams, managers and health professionals. However, only a few documents guide or require the training of the workforce in the form of specific training for professionals.

The chronic under-investment in HCP education and training in some countries and the mismatch between education strategies in relation to health systems and population needs are resulting in continuous shortages and low resilience of the workforce[24].

Only a technical note from the National Health Surveillance Agency (ANVISA) instructs that all health professionals must be trained in the correct use of PPE, and that health services must ensure that all professionals are trained and make the appropriate PPE use. Among the specific areas or programs of the Ministry of Health, only the Special Secretariat for Indigenous Health (SESAI) advises, in its technical notes, that health professionals attend training courses on the topic offered by public institutions.

It also names the courses that should be completed by all professionals. Strengthening capacity of the national health workforce in emergency and disaster risk management for greater resilience and health-care response capacity is a general recommendation of the WHO, predating the current pandemic. The WHO has recommended that health systems develop and draw upon the capacities of the national health workforce in risk assessments, prevention, preparedness, response and recovery. This should encompass the provision of resources, training and equipment for the health workforce, who should be included in policy and implementation of operations for emergencies at local, national and international levels. Brazil has never experienced systematic preparation of its workforce for large-scale emergency situations. However, SUS (Unified Health System) has great experience and investment in "continuing education", such as the Open University of SUS (UNA-SUS), a network of public higher education institutions, which provides largescale courses in e-learning and blended methods[29].

The incongruity of guidelines for professional practices in facing the pandemic is a fact to be highlighted. The official federal government discourse, since the beginning of the pandemic, has been ambiguous, tending to deny scientific evidence. An emblematic example is the use of the drug hydroxychloroquine in the treatment (in early or advanced stages of the disease): even after the publication of studies that do not supply evidence of its efficacy in the management of the disease, the federal government continues (until September 2020) to encourage its prescription and use.

Since June 2020, the Ministry of Health has maintained a protocol of clinical practice to encourage the prescription of this drug.

Recurring official speeches also guide practices that are not scientifically based, such as denying the need for social distancing and biased use of epidemiological data. In this context, there is a lack of formal training for professionals in the management of the pandemic, plus the disinformation created by the federal government itself. Noteworthy is the total absence of regulations, technical notes or guidelines from Department of Labour Management and Health Education of the Ministry of Health (MS), which is the secretariat designed to coordinate professional education actions for SUS.

No document from the Ministry of Health explicitly addresses the need for training/ qualification of SUS workers. Furthermore, its website does not highlight initiatives to offer online courses by institutions that are maintained with resources from the Ministry itself (such as those of UNA-SUS). Several institutions and projects financed by MS have taken the initiative to create and offer a large number of places on online courses about Covid-19. However, there is no coordinated action for this offer and no general guidance for the entire SUS workforce, or for specific professional categories. This perhaps explains why only 14.2% of health professionals interviewed in an online survey[17] feel prepared to deal with Covid-19. The majority (64.97%) reported that they are not adequately prepared. Only 21.91%, most of whom are doctors, report having received training.

With regard to work relations within the academic sphere, one of the most influential actions was the suspension of face-to-face classes throughout the educational system. Ministry of Education issued directives that replace face-to-face classes with classes in digital media, at different levels of education, including technical, professional education. Initially this applied for 30 days, then another 30 and, finally, until Dec 31st 2020. In response to the need to increase the number of health professionals to serve to the growing number of infected and/ or hospitalized people, the Ministry of Health launched the public call "Brazil Counts On Me" (*Brasil Conta Comigo*) - in which those in the final year of courses in Medicine, Nursing, Physiotherapy and Pharmacy are encouraged to join the front line services in coping with the pandemic.

The practice of students must be preceded by a short preparatory course online via UNA-SUS. The public call fails to require the signature of an engagement agreement contract between the intern, health service, and educational institution. There is no assessment of the compatibility between the activities performed in the internship and those established in the syllabus of the undergraduate course. The public call only establishes that managers of the health units receiving students are responsible for nominating health professionals to supervise the interns. The interns have no health insurance of employment security. There is no detailed description of the activities in which they may or may not be involved. Such measures provoked reactions on the part of the main professional bodies, such as CFM, COFEN and Brazilian Nursing Association (ABEn) who pointed out the need for caution in relation to the risks arising from these students carrying out professional service during the pandemic. ABEn and COFEN expressed their opposition to the "Brazil Counts On Me" Program, considering the demand on and overload of health service professionals as an aspect that would make the supervision of students unfeasible.

Also because the shortage of Personal Protective Equipment (PPE) would put the students' health at risk[30]. COFEN argued that its opposition took into account that Nursing accounts for more than 60% of human resources in health and that this category is experiencing physical and mental exhaustion due to the immense demand generated by the pandemic. It is considered, therefore, inappropriate to expect nursing professionals to supervise trainees[31,32].

On the other hand, many discussions developed in the wider society point out that the pandemic could be considered a great opportunity for the development of competences by students, improving knowledge and skills essential to the fulfilment of what is specified in the National Curriculum Guidelines for undergraduate courses in the health field.

However, they emphasize that it is necessary to provide for the safety of service users, professionals and students, as well as to guarantee the quality of health care for the population[32]. The positions of ABEn and COFEN are like the decisions of the American Association of Medical Schools, which discouraged student participation in tackling the pandemic[32]. At the international level, reactions to the early entry of students in the health field into the job market has also provoked discussions[33].

Some countries prohibit healthcare students from having any interaction with COVID-19 patients, while others recruit students from the final years of the course to jobs in hospitals and, in some cases, accelerate the completion of undergraduate courses with the objective of increasing the active workforce. Some recent international publications claim that nursing and medical students and interns feel caught between the gratifying possibilities of contributing and learning from the pandemic and the concern of contracting the disease or contaminating their family members, or even causing damage to patients through malpractice.

Such contradictory feelings cause moral distress in students[34,35]. Reflections on students' difficult decisions lead us to think about the possibility that they could contribute in other, safer ways by developing, for example, health promotion and education actions in communities or creating and disseminating educational materials on social media[36]. Within the context of stimulating the development of research on COVID-19 and training postgraduate professionals in the areas of health, CNPq and CAPES (Brazilian agencies which promote and support research and postgraduate studies) announced, in recent months, public calls that aimed to contribute to the advancement of knowledge, training of human resources, generation of products, formulation, implementation and evaluation of public actions aimed at improving conditions to deal with the pandemic.

The education system and support for scientific activities in general, however, are under constant threat, with budget cuts and lack of planning for the sector during and post-pandemic. The lack of coordination by the authorities together with a succession of errors made by the federal government seems to be related to the multiplication of deaths caused by Covid-19 in the country, including deaths of health professionals. Coping with the pandemic in Brazil has required creativity and the ability to mobilize HCPs and health care institutions individually, far beyond the official directives and protocols, as a possibility to transform the work process of health professionals and encourage an interprofessional context. When examining recent legislation, it is evident that there is no leadership dedicated to formulating comprehensive policies and strategies that can deal with the fragmentation that prevails in all governmental bodies in the country. A committee to tackle the pandemic, interested in developing long-term strategic understanding, based on science, could increase cooperation and define the priorities of each region of the country. A coordinated approach to actions, involving all those dealing with the Covid-19 pandemic, is necessary to define priorities, especially in a scenario with challenges as complex and diverse as the Brazilian reality.

FINAL CONSIDERATIONS

The absence of a federal policy coordinating actions aimed at the governance of the health workforce to face the pandemic in Brazil has been noted. The opposing position of Federal Councils of health professions to federal regulations corroborates this perception.

This absence contributes decisively to the tragic epidemiological situation, both in terms of the general population and in terms of infection and mortality of HCP from Covid-19. The published regulations include isolated, superficial, repetitive and insufficient aspects as a set of measures to resize the workforce and enable it to properly manage the pandemic, as well as to protect it in terms of working conditions, physical and mental health, and labour rights by recognizing Covid-19 as an occupational disease.

These findings, added to the lack of transparency regarding the illness and death of health workers, reveal the immense carelessness in relation to professionals in the area and, consequently, the population itself. This neglect was evidenced by other recent actions of the federal government, widely disseminated by the media: the presidential veto of laws that provided compensation to disabled professionals after contracting SARS-CoV2 while working; vetoes on proposals that defined measures to combat the spread of the disease among indigenous, quilombola and traditional communities; vetoes of bills that required the use of masks in places such as churches, shops, schools and prisons. By July 2020, when the country had already accounted for almost 100,000 deaths from Covid-19, the federal government had invested only 29% of the financial resources that had been earmarked to combat the pandemic, and the Ministry of Health remained without an appointed Minister. In this context, the initiatives of the states and municipalities, as well as those of the professional health councils end up assuming a leading role in dealing with some of the gaps left by the federal executive without, however, being able to replace it in the strategic management of Covid- 19. The conclusions of this research need to be considered in the context of the serious Brazilian political crisis, which further intensifies the health crisis triggered by the pandemic, and vice versa. After the official figure of 3 million contaminated and 122 thousand Brazilians killed by Covid-19, such conclusions reinforce a dramatic appeal for the immediate organisation of a national response on a scale that the ongoing tragedy demands, in order to mitigate its irreversible consequences to Brazilian society and its health workers. This is a duty of the Brazilian State and a right of its citizens and workers.

REFERENCES

1. Nagesh S, Chakraborty S. Saving the frontline health workforce amidst the COVID-19 crisis:
2. Challenges and recommendations. *J Glob Health*. 2020;10(1). doi:10.7189/jogh.10.010345
   Litewka SG, Heitman E. Latin American healthcare systems in times of pandemic. *Dev World Bioeth*. 2020;20(2):69-73. doi:10.1111/dewb.12262
3. Fraher EP, Pittman P, Frogner B, et al. Ensuring and Sustaining a Pandemic Workforce. *N Engl J Med*. 2020;382(23):2181-2183. doi:10.1056/NEJMp2006376
4. CDC. Characteristics of Health Care Personnel with COVID-19 —. *Morb Mortal Wkly Rep*. 2020;69(15):477-481.

5   Black JRM, Bailey C, Przewrocka J, Dijkstra KK, Swanton C. COVID-19: the case for health-care worker screening to prevent hospital transmission. *Lancet*. 2020;395(10234):1418-1420. doi:10.1016/S0140-6736(20)30917-X

6   Guan W, Ni Z, Hu Y, et al. Clinical characteristics of coronavirus disease 2019 in China. *N Engl J Med*. 2020;382(18):1708-1720. doi:10.1056/NEJMoa2002032

7   Fundação Getulio Vargas. Nucléo de estudos da burocracia (NEB). *Nota Técnica. A Pandemia de Covid-19 e Os Profissionais de Saúde Pública No Brasil.*; 2020. https://bit.ly/3aTlmZX

8   Brasil. Conselho Federal de Enfermagem (COFEN). Profissionais infetados com Covid-19 informado pelo serviço de saúde. Accessed August 24, 2020. http://observatoriodaenfermagem.cofen.gov.br/

9   Heinzerling A, Stuckey MJ, Scheuer T, et al. *Morbidity and Mortality Weekly Report Transmission of COVID-19 to Health Care Personnel During Exposures to a Hospitalized Patient-Solano County, California, February 2020.*.

10 Tanne JH, Hayasaki E, Zastrow M, Pulla P, Smith P, Rada AG. Covid-19: How doctors and healthcare systems are tackling coronavirus worldwide. *BMJ*. 2020;368(March):1-5. doi:10.1136/bmj.m1090

11 Dewey C, Hingle S, Goelz E, Linzer M. Supporting clinicians during the COVID-19 pandemic. *Ann Intern Med*. 2020;172(11):752-753. doi:10.7326/M20-1033

12 Luo M, Guo L, Yu M, Jiang W, Wang H. The psychological and mental impact of coronavirus disease 2019 (COVID-19) on medical staff and general public- A systematic review and metaanalysis. *Psychiatry Res*. 2020;291(113190). doi:10.1016/j.psychres.2020.113190

13 Lai J, Ma S, Wang Y, et al. Factors associated with mental health outcomes among health care workers exposed to coronavirus disease 2019. *JAMA Netw Open*. 2020;3(3):203976. doi:10.1001/jamanetworkopen.2020.3976

14 Ersoy A. The frontline of the COVID-19 pandemic: Healthcare workers. *Turkish J Intern Med*. 2020;2(2):31-32. doi:10.46310/tjim.726917

15 Johns S. COVID-19 in Brazil : Research reveals how epidemic spread around country. Imperial College London. Published 2020. Accessed August 19, 2020. https://bit.ly/31qPMzv

16 Brasil. Covid-19. Painel coronavirus. SUS. Published 2020. Accessed August 24, 2020. https://covid.saude.gov.br/

17 Lotta G, Wenham C, Nunes J, Pimenta DN. Community health workers reveal COVID-19 disaster in Brazil. *Lancet*. 2020;396(10248):365-366. doi:10.1016/S0140-6736(20)31521-X

18 The Lancet. COVID-19 in Brazil: "So what?" *Lancet*. 2020;395(10235):1461. doi:10.1016/S0140-6736(20)31095-3

19 OMS. *The World Health Report 2006 - Working Together for Health*. OMS; 2006. Brasil. Conselho Nacional de Secretários de Saúde (CONASS). Published 2020. Accessed April 6, 2020. https://www.conass.org.br/

20 Brasil. Presidência da République. Secretaria geral. Sub-chefia para assuntos jurídicos. Published 2020. Accessed April 6, 2020. http://www.planalto.gov.br/CCIVIL_03/Portaria/quadro_portaria.htm

21 Brasil. Ministério da Saúde. Secretaria Especial de Saúde Indigena. Boletin epidemiológico da SESAI. Published 2020. Accessed August 20, 2020. https://saudeindigena.saude.gov.br/corona

22 Instituto Socioambiental (ISA). Covid-19 e os povos indígenas. Plataforma de monitoramento da situação indígena na pandemia do novo coronavírus (Covid-19) no Brasil. Published 2020. Accessed August 20, 2020. https://covid19.socioambiental.org/

23 OMS. *Working for Health and Growth: Investing in the Health Workforce. Report of the High-Level Commission on Health Employment and Economic Growth*. OMS; 2016.

24 Pacheco Santos LM, Millett C, Rasella D, Hone T. The end of Brazil's More Doctors programme? *BMJ*. 2018;363:12-13. doi:10.1136/bmj.k5247

25 Fiho JMJ, Assunção AÁ, Algranti E, Garcia EG, Saito CA, Maeno M. A saúde do trabalhador e o enfrentamento da COVID-19. *Rev Bras Saúde Ocup*. 2020;45(e14):10-12. doi:10.1590/2317-6369ed0000120

26 Griffin MF. An invited commentary: international surgical guidance for COVID-19: validation using an international Delphi process. *Int J Surg*. 2020;80:41-42. doi:https://doi.org/10.1016/j.ijsu.2020.06.040

27 Amnesty International. *Exposed, Silenced, Attacked: Failures to Protect Health and Essential Workers during the Covid-19 Pandemic.* Amnesty International Ltd.; 2020.

28 Oliveira AEF, FERREIRA EB, SOUZA RR, JUNIOR EF de C, MOURA M de FL. Educação a

29 Distância e Formação Continuada: em Busca de Progressos para a Saúde Distance Learning and Continuing Education: Searching for Progress in Health. *Rev Bras Educ Med.* 2013;37(4):578-583. http://www.scielo.br/pdf/rbem/v37n4/a14v37n4.pdf

30 Associação Brasileira de Enfermagem. Nota da ABEN Nacional em relação à ação estratégica "O Brasil conta comigo." Published 2020. Accessed July 5, 2020. https://bit.ly/3aZqdJd

31 Brasil. Conselho Federal de Enfermagem (COFEN). Cofen se manifesta sobre Portaria n° 356 do MEC. Published 2020. Accessed July 14, 2020. http://www.cofen.gov.br/cofen-se-manifesta-sobrea-portaria-356-do-mec_78941.html

32 Miller DG, Pierson L, Doernberg S. The Role of Medical Students During the COVID-19 Pandemic. *Ann Intern Med.* 2020;173(2):145-146. doi:10.7326/M20-1281

33 Choi B, Jegatheeswaran L, Minocha A, Alhilani M, Nakhoul M, Mutengesa E. The impact of the COVID-19 pandemic on final year medical students in the United Kingdom: a national survey. *BMC Med Educ.* 2020;20(1):206. doi:10.1186/s12909-020-02117-1

34 Swift A, Banks L, Baleswaran A, et al. COVID-19 and student nurses: A view from England. *J Clin Nurs.* 2020;29(17-18):3111-3114. doi:10.1111/jocn.15298

35 Gallagher T, Schleyer A. "We Signed Up for This!"-Student and Trainee responses to the Covid-19 pandemic. *N Engl J Med.* 2020;96(1):1-2. doi:DOI: 10.1056/NEJMp2009027

36 Rose S. Medical student education in the time of Covid-19. *JAMA Netw Open.* 2020;323(2131-2132). doi:doi:10.1001/jama.2020.5227.

37 Kripka R, Scheller M, De Lara Bonotto D. La investigación documental sobre la investigación cualitativa: conceptos y caracterización. Revista de Investigaciones UNAD. 2015;14(2): 55-73. doi.org/10.22490/25391887.1455

CHAPTER 26

DISASTER LOOMS LARGE FOR INDIGENOUS AMAZONIANS

1.COVID-19, Isolated Indigenous Peoples and The History of The Amazon

François-Michel Le Tourneau

Géographe, directeur de recherche au CNRS, École normale supérieure – PSL

William Milliken

Research leader, Royal Botanic Gardens, Kew

The current situation of a global pandemic invites reconsideration of similar situations that happened in the past, such as the great plague in Europe in the 14th century, or the successive and devastating influenza and measles epidemics (amongst others) which decimated indigenous populations in the post-Columbian era in Latin America, and especially in the Amazon.

There, in indigenous villages, people got sick and quickly died, and subsistence activities were disrupted because crippled people were too weak to gather food or tend their agricultural plots. This story unfortunately played out until a few decades ago. Among many indigenous groups, the Parakanã experienced it when opening the Transamazonian highway (see John Hemming's book *Die If You Must: The Brazilian Indians in the 20th Century*). After contact with Brazilian society in the 1970s, more than half the population of the Yanomami, and the Matis (Vale do Javari) died from epidemics .Most of them witnessed lethality rates equal or superior to 30% – an incredible toll on any society (COVID-19 lethality is approximately 2%, and perhaps lower)[740]. Despite recent, better-organised contacts, hepatitis B and D epidemics continue to afflict recently contacted populations such as the Korubo in the Javari valley, adding the toll of malaria and influenza.

With Each Contact, An Epidemic

Given the disruption of economic and social activities in our lives today, it is difficult to overstate the impact of the epidemics on indigenous populations after Europeans came to the shores of the Amazon. Like us, indigenous peoples were caught by an invisible enemy and had to choose between severing social and economic ties between villages and families or confront infection and death. In the case of the Yanomami, epidemics appeared during each of their initial contacts: in 1959 with the Brazilian Border Commission; in 1967 with the New Tribes Mission; in 1973-74 with the Perimetral Norte road construction and in 1987-1990 with the illegal gold miners. They soon suspected that the incomers were the source of the problem and attributed the disease to the smell of the grease that wrapped the metal tools they were given: their word for disease is *xarawa* which also means fume or smoke[741]. The desirable and useful metal tools were a source of mortal danger, in what may be an early tale about epidemics and globalisation. Previous experiences by indigenous peoples in the Amazon might assist a critical look at what is happening now in Brazil. Recently the Brazilian

---

[740] https://smw.ch/article/doi/smw.2020.20203
[741] https://www.persee.fr/doc/hom_0439-4216_1988_num_28_106_368972

National Indian Foundation (FUNAI) banned external entries to indigenous territories to prevent transmission of the COVID-19 disease, which might wreak havoc in populations with low resistance to any kind of respiratory illness.

But at the same time, President Jair Bolsonaro is aiming to alter the law so that mining companies could enter indigenous territories[742] and, with his tacit approval, thousands of illegal gold miners are currently extracting gold in many of them, especially the Yanomami territory[743], which FUNAI will not be able to prevent. Bolsonaro also appointed Ricardo Lopes Dias[744], a former missionary of an evangelical church known for aggressively seeking contact and evangelising indigenous peoples, as head of FUNAI's department for isolated and recently contacted tribes. It is feared that the FUNAI's policy of "leave them alone unless there is a good reason" in relation to isolated groups may be changed, leading to further potentially disastrous contacts.

A "Pristine" Jungle That Never Was

What happened to indigenous peoples in the Amazon during the 20th century[745] also sheds light to the colonial period. Epidemics were frequent[746], sometimes deliberately sowed by Europeans (see *Os Indios e a civilização*, by Brazilian anthropologist Darcy Ribeiro). Regrouping Indians around missions turned out to be a source of dissemination for diseases, and interethnic conflicts incited by the colonists wiped out an unknown number of people and tribes. Father Acuña, who was on the Pedro Teixeira expedition in 1637-38[747], describes numerous villages and thriving life along the banks of the Amazon, but a few decades later this region will be seen only as the realm of nature: a "pristine" forest. The disappearance of the indigenous populations of the Amazon explains, in part, assertions by anthropologist Betty Meggers in her 1954 article "Environmental Limitation on the Development of Culture[748]", that the rainforest does not allow for large villages due to resource scarcity. Today, however, naturalists, ethnobotanists and archaeologists are compiling more and more data that proves that the Amazon was probably relatively densely populated[749].

The rainforest has been heavily transformed by indigenous peoples[750], and it is only the untrained Western eye that cannot accept human influence can be present – and lasting – in the apparent disorder of the forest. Uncovering big earth structures, heavily modified soils[751] innumerable traces of villages and plant domestication,[752] we are now able to see how a whole world of thriving civilisations disappeared. The disappearance probably occurred in two ways. The first one by the collapse of villages/networks, such as the Marajoara civilisation of the Amazon estuary. Only a few items, especially funerary urns, earth mounds and canals, yet once a thriving and complex

[742] https://www.sciencedirect.com/science/article/pii/S1462901119309864

[743] https://www.survivalinternational.org/news/12158

[744] https://www.reuters.com/article/us-brazil-indigenous/brazil-prosecutors-seek-to-remove-ex-missionary-from-indigenous-post-idUSKBN2052KY

[745] https://acervo.socioambiental.org/acervo/publicacoes-isa/cercos-e-resistencias-povos-indigenas-isolados-na-amazonia-brasileira

[746] https://www.ncbi.nlm.nih.gov/pmc/articles/PMC4564847/

[747] https://bdor.sibi.ufrj.br/bitstream/doc/287/1/203 PDF - OCR - RED.pdf

[748] https://www.jstor.org/stable/663814

749 https://www.jstor.org/stable/24395921

750 https://www.sciencedirect.com/science/article/abs/pii/S2213305414000241

751 https://www.springer.com/gp/book/9781402018398

752 https://royalsocietypublishing.org/doi/full/10.1098/rspb.2015.0813

civilization existed[753]. The second may have been adaptation and the simplification of lifestyles to escape both the epidemics and the predation by slavers or missionaries (See A. Roosevelt's book *Moundbuilders of the Amazon: Geophysical Archaeology on Marajó Island*[754], 1991).

Current hunter-gatherer groups may in fact be remnants of older civilisations that adapted and chose to be mobile in order to escape destruction. The vision of the Amazon as a relatively densely populated region, and a centre of dissemination of cultivars and civilisations is now recognised among the scientific community and has recently been passed to a wider audience[755], as the recent communication around archaeological discoveries in the Mamiraua reserve, the Tefé National Forest or in the Llanos de Moxos (Bolivia) show. However, a great number of people continue to perpetuate old images of "the world's last virgin forest" each time the Amazon is threatened by fires or deforestation. Maybe now that we are faced with the consequences of a global pandemic, we can start rethinking, and accept that its population was wiped out principally by disease and predation. Likewise, how indigenous peoples of the Amazon transformed the forest and adapted it to their needs without destroying it.[756]

Pulling Back From The "Tipping Point"

When the COVID-19 pandemic is over and the world starts thinking again about our impact on the environment, such an example might prove inspiring, especially at a time when the Amazon forest is at the "tipping point"[757] and repeatedly faces giant fires[758]. We might also want to reflect on the fact that advances of Western-style consumption of remaining forests can be the sources of new diseases, especially of viruses passing from animals to humans[759] like Ebola[760]. Like a boomerang, such diseases currently strike us in the same way that indigenous peoples across the world were struck by germs that were disseminated at the time of the colonial conquest.

753 https://link.springer.com/chapter/10.1007/978-0-387-74907-5_19

754 https://www.researchgate.net/publication/230492523_Moundbuilders_of_the_Amazon_Geophysical_Archaeology_on_Marajo_Island_Brazil

755 https://www.nationalgeographic.com/news/2018/03/amazon-jungle-ancient-population-satellite-computer-model/

756 https://www.pnas.org/content/117/6/3015

757 https://advances.sciencemag.org/content/5/12/eaba2949

758 https://advances.sciencemag.org/content/6/2/eaay1632

759 https://royalsocietypublishing.org/doi/10.1098/rsif.2014.0950

760 https://www.sciencemag.org/news/2019/01/bat-species-may-be-source-ebola-epidemic-killed-more-11000-people-west-africa

2. COVID-19 And Brazilian Indigenous Populations[761]

[1]Graziela Almeida Cupertino,[1] Marli do Carmo Cupertino,[1,2] Andreia Patricia Gomes,[2] Luciene Muniz Braga,[2]
Rodrigo Siqueira-Batista[1,2]*

2 School of Medicine, Faculdade Dinamica do Vale do Piranga, Ponte Nova, Minas Gerais, Brazil;^
Department of Medicine and Nursing, Universidade Federal de Viçosa, Viçosa, Minas Gerais, Brazil

ABSTRACT

The newly discovered SARS-CoV-2 is the cause of COVID-19, including severe respiratory symptoms with an important lethality rate and high dissemination capacity. Considering the indigenous people of Brazil, it is feared that COVID-19 will spread to these communities, causing another stage of decimation. Despite advances in indigenous health care in the country, there are still many challenges due to the social vulnerability of this population, whose lands continue to be illegally exploited. Based on these considerations, this article discusses challenges in caring for the indigenous population in the context of the COVID-19 pandemic in Brazil.

INTRODUCTION

The indigenous population that inhabited Brazil in 1500 was, according to estimates, around 3 million people strong, distributed throughout the national territory in more than a thousand different ethnic groups. Of these, 2 million occupied the Brazilian coast and the rest the interior. Seventy years after the discovery of Brazilian lands and contact with the indigenous peoples by Europeans, this population was drastically reduced, estimated at 1,200,000 Indians distributed in the country, 200,000 of them on the coast and one million in the interior.[1,2] For centuries, the indigenous ethnic groups continued to suffer from the decimation of their peoples and, in 1957, reached their lowest number of inhabitants in the country, about 70,000 (5,000 along the coast and 65,000 in the interior). Diseases, wars, persecutions, and socioeconomic ruptures were mainly responsible for this reduction. Various epidemics of infectious and parasitic diseases were most likely the greatest cause of the demographic decline of these peoples.[1,2] Among the many illnesses that have affected the indigenous Brazilians, from the arrival of the Portuguese to the present day, are helminthiasis, syphilis, gonorrhoea, rickettsiosis, tuberculosis, pneumonia, whooping cough, malaria, yellow fever, smallpox, measles, chicken pox, and respiratory viruses.[1] Pandemic influenza, the Spanish flu, raged during 1918–1919 and was responsible for the deaths of 20 million people around the world. In Brazil, this disease was responsible for the extinction of countless indigenous ethnic groups.

[761] Am. J. Trop. Med. Hyg., 00(0), 2020, pp. 1–4

All these epidemics and their devastating consequences to the Indian population show the great vulnerability of these peoples to the introduction of new pathogens.[1]

The year 2020 brings a new disease, COVID-19, with high dissemination potential, which has mobilized health authorities worldwide. Since its emergence in China in December 2019, it has rapidly spread throughout the world, and, by May 11, 2020, it had affected 215 countries, with more than 4 million confirmed cases and more than 350,000 deaths as of June 1, 2020.[3] As in other countries, once it was introduced in Brazil, COVID-19 claimed many victims and raised many questions for its control, especially when dealing with the most susceptible groups, such as Indians. Based on these considerations, we discuss challenges in caring for the indigenous population in the context of the COVID-19 pandemic in Brazil.SARS-COV-2 AND COVID-19:

A NEW PANDEMIC IN BRAZIL Coronaviruses (CoVs) are the second leading cause of the common cold, behind rhinoviruses.[3,4] The CoVs mostly cause mild respiratory infections. However, the emergence of three new species of CoVs that infect humans has altered this reality, with serious outbreaks of SARS-CoV, Middle East respiratory syndrome, and now COVID-19, caused by SARSCoV-2. The newly discovered SARS-CoV-2 is capable of causing severe respiratory symptoms, with an important lethality rate, although most infections are mild to moderate. Infection with this pathogen first appeared in December 2019 in Wuhan, Hubei Province, China. On January 30, 2020, the outbreak was declared a public health emergency of international importance by the WHO, and, on March 11, COVID-19 was characterized by the WHO as a pandemic.[3,5] In Brazil, the first case of COVID-19 was confirmed on February 26, 2020, but retrospective analyses have suggested that the first cases occurred in January. Considering the growing number of suspect cases and the country's continental dimension, population density, disparities between rural and urban areas, and great socioeconomic inequality, the current scenario points to a multitude of vulnerabilities for this pandemic. Therefore, there is a need for broad and effective measures to contain the advance of COVID-19 throughout the country.[6,7]

HEALTH OF INDIGENOUS PEOPLE IN BRAZIL

The Special Secretariat of Indigenous Health (SESAI) of the Ministry of Health, created in 2010, reports the existence of 416 distinct indigenous ethnic groups currently in Brazil.[6] According to the National Indian Foundation (FUNAI), the latest census conducted by the Brazilian Institute of Geography and Statistics shows an indigenous population of 817,963 distributed throughout the country.[2] Although Indians are present in all states of the federation, the Northern Region has the largest number, with the largest concentration in the state of Amazonas.[2]

In Brazil, the assistance given to this population is the responsibility of FUNAI. Created in 1967, FUNAI is the official body of the Brazilian state related to the indigenous people, and its mission is to protect and promote the rights of indigenous peoples in the country. In the area of health, SESAI is responsible for coordinating and executing the National Policy for the Health Care of Indigenous Peoples (PNASPI), with the mission of ensuring that indigenous health care is integral, resolute, and humanized. Access to health services for members of the indigenous population, as well as for any Brazilian citizen, is guaranteed, with one of the largest and most complex public health systems in the world.[6] Healthcare coverage includes [3, 4,] Special Indigenous Health Districts, strategically divided by territorial criteria, based on the geographical occupation of indigenous communities:

1,199 basic indigenous health units and 67 indigenous health support houses.[2] Although advances in indigenous health care in the country are renowned, there are still numerous challenges in working with this population. Whether at the organizational, cultural, or geographical level, there is still much to be done. Even if the current PNASPI contemplates differentiated attention to indigenous populations based on sociocultural diversity and the epidemiological and logistical particularities of these peoples, with the guarantee of completeness of assistance, one can observe that care is still focused on palliative and emergency practices.[9-11]

In addition, despite the growing financial resources made available to implement care, the actions have presented few results in health indicators, reflecting the historical inequalities that mark these peoples in relation to the other inhabitants of Brazil, especially when dealing with the scarcity of demographic and epidemiological data. Another important point concerns social participation, which reflects users' dissatisfaction with the discontinuity of care, the lack of inputs, equipment limitations, the shortage and high turnover of professionals, and deficits in intercultural dialogues that promote consideration of the traditional knowledge of these peoples. There is still a difficulty of access to health services, both at the level of primary care in the villages and of specialized actions and services requiring medium and high complexity. Thus, these ethnic minorities remain at high risk in the fight against all diseases.[9-11]

SARS-COV-2 AND COVID-19: A DANGER TO BRAZILIAN INDIGENOUS PEOPLE

The COVID-19 pandemic brings great concern to the indigenous population of Brazil. This is nothing new, as infectious and parasitic diseases are among those most responsible for deaths among Indians, especially when compared with the rest of the national population.[1] Outbreaks of respiratory diseases such as H1N1 influenza, in 2009, reinforce the fragility of this portion of the population and suggest that Indians are more susceptible to diseases of the respiratory tract.[1] Therefore, it should be observed that typical cultural behaviours, such as the sharing of gourds and other household utensils, as well as community housing and diverse hygiene practices justify the fear that COVID-19 may spread widely in these communities, causing another stage of decimation.

In addition to the cultural and behavioural aspects of the indigenous people capable of promoting the dissemination of SARS-CoV-2, there is great fear for the socioeconomic relations of communities with non-natives. Commercial activities in the cities to supply the tribes, without the proper recommended prevention measures, and the proximity of the villages to cities where the virus already circulates, can expedite the dissemination of COVID-19 in indigenous lands and tribes. Furthermore, even with social isolation in different regions of the country, missionary actions, the constant invasions of indigenous lands, nonstop hunting, and exploitation activities by logging companies and mines—especially illegal ones—have not ceased in the country. These and other obstacles that have made it difficult to contain the COVID-19 pandemic increase the burden on governments—and especially on FUNAI—for measures to protect native communities.[6]

On April 11, 2020, SESAI reported the death of two indigenous people by COVID-19 in Manaus: a 44-year-old Kokama indigenous woman hospitalized since February 28 for autoimmune haemolytic anaemia and a 78-year-old Ticuna indigenous woman hospitalized for cardiovascular treatment. On May 15, 340 confirmed cases, 159 suspected cases, and 21 deaths from COVID-19 were reported in indigenous peoples.

The data show a frightening progression of cases, with great concentration in the northern region, especially in the Upper Solimões River (145 cases and 10 deaths), Manaus (38 cases and one death), and Yanomami territory (19 cases and one death).[8]

In this context, government actions have been directed to expand the capacity to attend to COVID-19 cases and avoid the collapse of the health network, which is imminent. Especially in the capital city of Manaus, the number of people in need of hospitalization is increasing daily, and the health system is already operating at the limits of its capacity. As damage containment measures, by May 11, three multidisciplinary teams of the Brazilian National Health System had already been sent to the capital to reinforce care. There was also availability of an online platform that allows physicians to discuss management of each patient in the intensive care unit with other health professionals. Also ongoing are the expansion of hospital beds; hiring of private beds; increases in the transfer of financial resources; sending of supplies, respirators, molecular tests, and individual protection equipment; construction of a campaign hospital with a capacity of 200 beds; convening of health professionals enrolled in the strategic action O Brasil Conta Comigo ("Brazil depends on me"); and intensification of recommendations to the population for the adoption of preventive measures.[8]

Despite these actions, rapid progression to chaos is feared among indigenous people, and this possibility becomes even more worrying, given the high prevalence of risk factors for COVID-19 in this population, such as obesity, hypertension, and diabetes mellitus.[12-14]

This may lead to worse prognosis and increased need for hospitalization and advanced life support, as observed in China and Italy.[15,16] Added to these factors are the social vulnerability of indigenous peoples in the face of disrespect for the social distancing of thousands of miners, lumbermen, and land invaders who continue to exploit indigenous territory illegally; the lack of a protective policy for indigenous peoples by the federal government[17]; the lack of structure and limited access to health care, especially high complexity care; a communal lifestyle; lack of an adequate drinking water supply system, poor hygiene conditions, and difficult access to soap and alcohol gel; and exposure in urban centres during searches for emergency financial aid offered by the federal government.[18,19]

The disaster chronicle can be properly understood when considering the consequences of the H1N1 pandemic in 2009 in Brazil. On that occasion, 34,506 cases of influenza and 1,567 deaths were recorded among indigenous peoples.[20] Among the most affected groups were children younger than 5 years, patients with respiratory and metabolic comorbidities, pregnant women, and indigenous people. In Brazil, the epidemiological behaviour of H1N1 assumed a seasonal pattern, with the highest number of cases in the South and Southeast regions, where the climate is more temperate.[21] Although these are the two Brazilian regions with the smallest indigenous population, during the course of H1N1, Indians in these regions were subjected to notoriously higher risks for severe infection, with higher rates of hospitalization and lethality, than the nonindigenous population.[20-22] Therefore, similar to what occurred with the H1N1 pandemic in 2009, the current prospects for COVID-19 in the indigenous population are of more serious consequence than other segments of the Brazilian population.

Statistically, Indians were 4.5 times more affected than others by severe acute respiratory disease during the 2009 pandemic.[23]Thus, if the strategies to contain the advance of COVID-19 for indigenous peoples are not successful, then it is possible that we will experience another historical tragedy,[24] especially when considering the propagation speed of the virus, and limitations of the Brazilian health system, with a significant overload of patients and scarce resources.

CONCLUSION

Indigenous peoples are highly vulnerable to the advancement of SARS-CoV-2 infection. If there is not an immediate implementation of a serious care policy for the Brazilian indigenous people, there will be a real possibility of a new wave of decimation of this population, as thousands of deaths caused by other epidemics throughout history have shown. It is imperative that every effort be made to contain the advance of COVID-19 among Brazilian Indians, otherwise the genocide prophetically announced by the brilliant artist Sebastião Salgado[25] will come to pass. Authors' addresses: Graziela Almeida Cupertino, School of Medicine, Faculdade Dinamica do Vale do Piranga, Ponte Nova, Brazil, E-mail:ˆ gacupertino@gmail.com. Marli do Carmo Cupertino and Rodrigo Siqueira-Batista, School of Medicine, Faculdade Dinamica do Vale doˆ Piranga, PonteNova, Brazil, and Department of Medicine and Nursing, Federal University of Viçosa, Viçosa, Brazil, E-mails: marli.cupertino. vet@gmail.com and rsiqueirabatista@yahoo.com.br. Andr´eia Patrı´cia Gomes and Luciene Muniz Braga, Department of Medicine and Nursing, Federal University of Viçosa, Viçosa, Brazil, E-mails: andreiapgomes@ gmail.com and luciene.muniz@ufv.br.

REFERENCES

1. Ministry of Health Brazil, 2016. Health Disease and Attention in Indigenous Territories. Available at: http://bvsms.saude.gov.br/ bvs/publicacoes/saude_doenca_atencao_territorios_indigenas. pdf. Accessed May 04, 2020.

2. FUNAI, 2020. Indians in Brazil: Who They Are. Available at: http:// www.funai.gov.br/. Accessed April 20, 2020.

3. World Health Organization, 2020. Coronavirus Disease (COVID19) Outbreak Situation. Available at: https://www.who.int/ emergencies/diseases/novel-coronavirus-2019. Acessed May 11, 2020.

4. Falsey, A.R., Walsh, E.E., Hayden, F.G. (2002).Rhinovirus and coronavirus infection-associated hospitalizations among older adults. J Infect Dis 185: 1338–1341.

5. Zou L et al., 2020. SARS-CoV-2 viral load in upper respiratoryspecimens of infected patients. N Engl J Med 382: 1177–1179. 6. Ministry of HealthBrazil, 2020. Coronavirus Panel - COVID-19. Available at: https://covid.saude.gov.br/. Accessed May 15, 2020.

7. Cupertino, M.C., Cupertino, G.A., Gomes, A.P., Mayers, N.A.J., SiqueiraBatista, R. (2020). COVID-19 in Brazil: epidemiological update and perspectives. Asian Pac J Trop Med 13: 193–196.

8. SESAI - Special Secretariat for Indigenous Health. Ministry of Health, 2020. Coronavirus Disease (COVID-19) in Indigenous Populations - SESAI Epidemiological Bulletin. Available at: http://www.saudeindigena.net.br/coronavirus/mapaEp.php. Accessed May 15, 2020.

9. Gomes, S.C., Esperidião MA, (2017). Access of indigenous users to health services in Cuiab´a, Mato Grosso, Brazil. Cadernos de Sa´ude P´ublica 33: 1–20.

10. Mendes, A.M., Leite, M.S., Langdon, EJ, Grisotti M, (2018). The challenge of primary care in indigenous health in Brazil. Rev Panam Salud Publica 42: e184.

11. Badanta-Romero, B., Moreno-Moreno, B., Soto-Dı´az V, BarrientosTrigo S, (2020). Nursing care for the community health approach in the indigenous population of the Peruvian Amazon. Clin Nurs S1130–8621: 30519–30524.

12. Oliveira, G.F, Oliveira, T.R.R., Rodrigues, F.F., Correa, L.F., Ikejiri, A.T.,ˆ Casulari, L.A., (2011). Prevalence of diabetes mellitus and decreased glucose tolerance in the indigenous people of Jaguapiru Village, Brazil. Rev Panam Salud Publica 29: 315–321.

13. Freitas, G.A., Souza, M.C.C., Lima, R.C., (2016). Prevalence of diabetesmellitus and associated factors in indigenous women in the municipality of Dourados, Mato Grosso do Sul, Brazil. Cad Sa ́ude P ́ublica 32: e00023915.

14. Chagas, C.A., Castro, T.G., Leite, M.S., Viana, M.A.C.B.M, Beinner, M.A, Pimenta, A.M. ((2020). Estimated prevalence and factors associated with hypertension in indigenous Krenak adults in the state of Minas Gerais, Brazil. Cad Sa ́ude P ́ublica 36: e00206818.

15. WU Z; McGoogan J, (2020). Characteristics of and important lessons from the coronavirus disease 2019 (COVID-19). Outbreak in China: summary of a report of 72314 cases from the Chinese Centre for Disease Control and Prevention. JAMA 323: 1239–1242.

16. Cecconi, M et al., (2020). Baseline characteristics and outcomes of1591 patients infected with SARS-CoV-2 admitted to ICUs of the lombardy region, Italy. JAMA 323: 1574–1581.

17. Oliveira, R.N.C, Rosa LCS, 2014. Indigenous health in times ofbarbarity: public policy, scenarios and perspectives. RevPoli ́ticas P ́ublicas 18: 481–495.

18. Basta PC, (2020). COVID-19 Moves Towards Indigenous Lands. Report ENSP. Available at: https://www.arca.fiocruz.br/handle/ icict/40837. Accesse April 20, 2020.

19. Korap, A., (2020). Sanitation and COVID-19: Challenges and Strategies for Indigenous Communities. Ana Paula Evangelista. Interviewed:RosanaLima. Rio de Janeiro,Brazil: OswaldoCruz Foundation. Escola Polit ́ecnica de Sa ́ude Joaquim Venancio.ˆ Podcast.

20. Baker, M., Kelly, H., Wilson, N., (2009). Pandemic H1N1 influenza lessons from the southern hemisphere. Euro Surveill 14: 19370.

21. Schuck-Paim C, Viboud C, Simonsen L, Miller MA, Moura FEA,Fernandes RM, Carvalho ML, Alonso WJ, 2012. Were equatorial regions less affected by the 2009 influenza pandemic? The Brazilian experience. PLoS One 7: e41918.

22. GogginL,S., Carcione.D., Mak,D.B.,Dowse, G.K.,Giele, C.M., Smith, D.W.,Effler, P.V., (2011). Chronic disease and hospitalisation for pandemic (H1N1) 2009 influenza in Indigenous and nonIndigenous Western Australians. Commun Dis Intell Q Rep 35: 172–176.

23. La Ruche, G., Tarantola, A., Barboza, P., Vaillant, L., Gueguen, J. ,Gastellu-Etchegorry, M (2009). Epidemic Intelligence Team at InVS,
    2009. The 2009 pandemic H1N1 influenza and indigenous populations of the Americas and the Pacific. Euro Surveill 14: 19366.

24. Left, D., 2020. Indian Day: COVID-19 Is a New Threat to Exterminate the Lives of Indians. Editorial, April 19, 2020. Edition of the day. Available at: http://www.esquerdadiario.com.br/Dia-do-indio-COVID-19-e-nova-ameca-de-exterminio-a-vida-dos-indigenas. Accessed May 02, 2020.

25. The Guardian, 2020. 'We Are on the Eve of a Genocide': Brazil Urged to Save Amazon Tribes from COVID-19. Available at: https://www.theguardian.com/world/2020/may/03/eve-ofgenocide-brazil-urged-save-amazon-tribes-COVID-19-sebastiaosalgado. Accessed May 20, 2020.

3. Brazil's Indigenous Peoples Face A Triple Threat From COVID-19, The Dismantling Of Socio-Environmental Policies, And International Inaction

[762]Grace Iara Souza[763]

(LSE Latin America and Caribbean Centre).

With the Brazilian state failing to protect them from coronavirus, indigenous groups have been forced to find ways to monitor and care for their own communities while also putting up serious resistance to destructive government policies. But these peoples already face increased risks because of longstanding discrimination, inequality, and the recent intensification of efforts to dismantle environmental protections. For the sake of indigenous groups and the environment that they do so much to protect, now is the time for decision-makers in the UK and Europe to implement stronger environmental and human rights regulations instead of continuing to farm out the problem for someone else to deal with,

Even before the arrival of COVID-19, the native peoples of Brazil were in a perilous situation, not least because of high-level attempts to use racism[764] to legitimise the dismantling of socio-environmental protections. But the pandemic has only intensified this persecution, and despite the impressive efforts of these guardians[765] of global biodiversity to adapt[766] their strategies of resistance, they cannot be expected to fight the climate crisis and coronavirus alone.

On the contrary, the connections[767] between COVID-19, deforestation, and global perceptions of nature should be central to the thinking of policymakers and investors[768] the world over.

This moment when states and societies begin to chart their post-pandemic journey towards recovery represents a chance to move away from the "business as usual" that led to the current environmental-health crisis[769] and to make sure that climate commitments are treated as more than words alone.

COVID-19, The State, And Indigenous Groups In Brazil

Sadly, Brazil has gone in the opposite direction, with the Bolsonaro government trying to control the information shared with the public in order to avoid dealing with the consequences of coronavirus, particularly when it comes to the fate of indigenous peoples. This has meant that

---

[762]

[763] The authors wish to acknowledge Bruce Albert, author with Davi Kopenawa of "The Falling Sky", and Fiona Watson, of Survival International, for their contribution.

[764] https://movimentorevista.com.br/2020/05/odiar-o-termo-povos-indigenas-e-apagar-a-cultura-e-historia-de-nossos-povos/

[765] https://www.sciencedirect.com/science/article/pii/S0959378020301424

[766] http://apib.info/2020/05/01/indigenas-realizam-edicao-historica-do-acampamento-terra-livre/

[767] https://www.weforum.org/agenda/2020/04/covid-19-nature-deforestation-recovery/

[768] https://www.unpri.org/

[769] https://www.theguardian.com/environment/2020/may/26/world-health-leaders-urge-green-recovery-from-coronavirus-crisis

indigenous movements themselves have had to take responsibility for documenting[770] cases in their own communities and highlighting failings in official reporting. By early July, Brazil had seen over 64,000 deaths from COVID-19[771] at the national level.

According to the Articulation of Indigenous Peoples in Brazil[772] (APIB), as of 4 July 2020 there had been 426 recorded deaths amongst indigenous peoples and 11,385 confirmed cases across a total of 124 indigenous groups. In contrast, the Special Secretariat for Indigenous Health[773] (SESAI) had recorded 171 deaths and 7,598 confirmed cases. In the Amazonian region alone, the Coordination of the Indigenous Organisations of the Brazilian Amazon[774] (COIAB) recorded 225 deaths on top of the 146 declared by SESAI. Aside from under-reporting cases of COVID-19 amongst indigenous peoples in its so-called Special Indigenous Sanitary Districts, the federal government has failed to assist those living in communities not legally classified as indigenous lands as well as those living in urban centres.

This effectively discriminates against indigenous peoples outside of titled lands as if their physical location made them somehow less indigenous, which is consistent with a wider tendency to define indigeneity in the process of denying indigenous rights to self-determination[775] and differentiated health care[776]. This approach also overlooks the fact that the federal government has made little progress in the demarcation of indigenous territories, increasing the vulnerability even of the largest indigenous group in the country, the Guarani. Many Guarani people live on campsites near motorways or on small plots of land whose boundaries are increasingly infringed by urban expansion. Some groups, such as the Guarani Kaiowa, have precarious access to water,[777] while several other groups have precious little space to produce food, leading them to depend on the sale of handicrafts to pay for supplies.

Neither has the government put in place preventative protocols nor a plan to treat indigenous peoples who have the infection. A lack of adequate testing has directly contributed to infection of indigenous groups by health-workers[778], as has happened with the Yanomami, Kokama, and Kanamari peoples. Nor has any adaptation of the "coronavoucher" emergency basic income[779] been introduced to address the particular conditions of river-dwelling communities[780], indigenous peoples, and descendants of Afro-Brazilian runaways (*quilombolas*)[781]. Instead, they are forced to travel from villages to urban centres to receive this subsistence payment of $600 Brazilian reals (roughly £90) even though the process can significantly increase the chance of infection. Rather than attempting to protect indigenous and Afro-descendant peoples, which would be consistent with the Brazilian state's historic debt to these groups, many members of the Bolsonaro administration have expressed racism[782] and an associated desire to eliminate indigenous groups

---

[770] http://quarentenaindigena.info/
[771] https://www.nytimes.com/interactive/2020/world/americas/brazil-coronavirus-cases.html#cases
[772] http://quarentenaindigena.info/casos-indigenas/
[773] http://www.saudeindigena.net.br/coronavirus/mapaEp.php
[774] https://coiab.org.br/
[775] https://www.mpil.de/files/pdf3/mpunyb_06_godinho_12.pdf
[776] https://www.scielo.br/scielo.php?script=sci_arttext&pid=S0100-55022020000200401&lng=en&nrm=iso
[777] https://news.trust.org/item/20200421152440-mcbrq
[778] https://www.nationalgeographic.co.uk/science-and-technology/2020/06/disaster-looms-for-indigenous-amazon-tribes-as-covid-19-cases
[779] mailto:https://www.opendemocracy.net/en/democraciaabierta/covid-19-brazil-implements-basic-income-policy-following-massive-civil-society-campaign/
[780] http://casaninjaamazonia.org/2020/06/12/600-familias-de-resex-na-amazonia-ameacadas-pelo-coronavirus-e-abandonadas-pelo-governo/
[781] https://news.mongabay.com/2020/05/coronavirus-puts-brazils-quilombos-at-risk-will-assistance-come/
[782] https://www.bbc.co.uk/news/world-latin-america-51501111

through assimilation[783] and homogenisation[784] of the Brazilian population. This denial of the richness and cultural diversity of Brazilian society disregards the lives of almost 900,000 indigenous people, with over 300 culturally specific ethnic indigenous groups[785] living in areas both rural (64%) and urban (36%). Bolsonaro's specific pledge not to demarcate "one single centimetre of indigenous territory[786]" also runs contrary to the government's constitutional obligation to do so. Of course, using social isolation as a means of preventing the spread of infectious diseases is anything but new for indigenous peoples.

The elders in particular have an ancestor memory[787] of previous pandemics that decimated many of their peoples, especially those brought by the European invasion[788] and the land grabbers, loggers, ranchers and miners that arrived during the dictatorship[789]. It is no coincidence that some indigenous groups have remained in voluntary isolation[790] right up to the present day. However, despite their expectation of finding safety deep in the rainforest, isolated indigenous groups like those in the Javari Valley [791]have increasingly found their culture and health security threatened. First, there is the threat from radical American evangelical missionary groups[792] such as Ethnos 360 that have received open government support[793] in their attempts to access the area. Then there is the presence of thousands of illegal gold miners[794], with roughly 20,000

in the territories of the Yanomami and Ye'kwana peoples, which could see them become one of the indigenous communities worst affected by COVID-19[795] on a global level. The wilful jeopardising of indigenous peoples' lives is particularly grave when you consider that the death of each elder represents the "burning of a library[796]". Whereas a neoliberal logic values those capable of paying taxes and contributing to society financially, the cosmological wisdom that indigenous elders carry is invaluable. These elders ensure the survival of the language, history, and traditions of their ancestors, preserving the cultural and socio-environmental richness of entire peoples. Every premature death represents an unimaginable loss not only for particular families and communities but also for the collective memory of the whole indigenous movement.[797]

---

[783] https://www.reuters.com/article/us-brazil-indigenous/brazils-indigenous-tribes-protest-bolsonaro-assimilation-plan-idUSKCN1S22B5
[784] https://www.gazetadopovo.com.br/wiseup-news/bolsonaro-raised-the-issue-do-natives-own-too-much-land-in-brazil/
[785] http://funai.gov.br/arquivos/conteudo/ascom/2013/img/12-Dez/pdf-brasil-ind.pdf
[786] https://www.nytimes.com/2020/04/19/world/americas/bolsonaro-brazil-amazon-indigenous.html
[787] https://amazoniareal.com.br/lembrancas-do-passado-e-o-medo-do-presente-nos-indigenas-diante-da-pandemia/
[788] https://www.survivalinternational.org/tribes/brazilian
[789] http://comissaodaverdade.al.sp.gov.br/relatorio/tomo-i/parte-ii-cap2.html
[790] https://unpo.org/article/21899
[791] https://www.theguardian.com/world/2020/apr/17/brazil-judge-bans-missionaries-coronavirus-amazon-indigenous-reserve
[792] https://news.mongabay.com/2020/03/bringing-christ-and-coronavirus-evangelicals-to-contact-amazon-indigenous/
[793] https://www.theguardian.com/global-development/2020/mar/23/the-isolated-tribes-at-risk-of-illness-from-amazon-missionaries
[794] http://www.digitaljournal.com/news/world/brazil-s-yanomamis-say-endangered-by-miners-spreading-coronavirus/article/572603#ixzz6OJT7gybg
[795] https://acervo.socioambiental.org/acervo/publicacoes-isa/o-impacto-da-pandemia-na-terra-indigena-yanomami-foragarimpoforacovid
[796] https://news.mongabay.com/2020/06/every-time-an-elder-dies-a-library-is-burnt-amazon-covid-19-toll-grows/
[797] https://www.bbc.co.uk/news/world-latin-america-53087933?fbclid=IwAR3qcAEHLGCQwm2VAXyYdllveKz6cYguOlIYYFKQDvRMB3u8fUlcdlqNKog

The Dual Health And Environmental Crisis

Scientists[798] all around the world have been quick to highlight the link between the current COVID-19 health crisis and the wider environmental one. They have emphasised the damaging effects[799] of practices linked to large monocultures such as poaching, logging, and deforestation[800] in terms of irrigation, respiratory problems, and destruction of wider ecosystems. Just a week before the World Health Organization declared COVID-19 a public health pandemic in March, climate scientists warned that the Amazon could become a net source of carbon dioxide as soon as the next decade[801], whereas the Brazilian National Institute of Space Research (INPE) has recently confirmed[802] that Amazon deforestation is rapidly increasing.

Despite already having to deal with the lethal effects of COVID-19, indigenous movements continue to energetically resist government retrenchment of socio-environmental law and policy. Even in the face of attempts to strip them of their constitutional rights[803], indigenous peoples and their allies have fought back[804] against attempts to scale back environmental monitoring and regularise "land-grabbers[805]" and invaders[806] in Mato Grosso, for example. With the Amazon fire[807]s of summer 2019 still fresh in the memory, and following the remarkable visit of indigenous leaders to twelve European countries[808]

in late 2019, there is growing awareness and pressure on these issues from environmental movements around the world. Greta Thunberg's Fridays for Future[809] movement, Extinction Rebellion[810], many campaigning NGOs (such as Greenpeace, Reporter Brasil [811], WWF,[812] Global Witness [813], Global Canopy [814], and Fern [815]), companies[816], investors [817], and even some EU governments[818] have recently threatened to boycott Brazil if the government fails to curb deforestation and protect indigenous rights.

[798] https://www.theguardian.com/world/2020/apr/27/halt-destruction-nature-worse-pandemics-top-scientists
[799] https://ipbes.net/covid19stimulus
[800] https://www.npr.org/2020/06/22/875961137/the-worrisome-link-between-deforestation-and-disease?t=1592831786828&t=1593015958492
[801] https://www.theguardian.com/environment/2020/mar/04/tropical-forests-losing-their-ability-to-absorb-carbon-study-finds
[802] https://www.documentcloud.org/documents/6937202-Aragao-Et-Al-Desmatamento-Fogo-E-COVID-19-Na.html
[803] https://www.uol.com.br/ecoa/ultimas-noticias/2020/06/02/o-que-e-o-marco-temporal-e-como-ele-impacta-indigenas-brasileiros.htm
[804] https://news.mongabay.com/2020/06/brazilian-government-taken-to-court-for-assault-on-environment-climate/
[805] https://news.mongabay.com/2020/05/brazils-land-grabbers-law-threatens-amazonia-commentary/
[806] http://amazonia.org.br/2020/06/projeto-do-governo-de-mt-amplia-vulnerabilidade-das-terras-indigenas-em-meio-a-pandemia/
[807] https://www.bbc.co.uk/news/world-latin-america-49971563
[808] http://apib.info/2019/10/09/indigenous-leaders-travel-to-europe-to-report-violations-in-brazil/
[809] https://www.theguardian.com/environment/2019/sep/27/climate-crisis-6-million-people-join-latest-wave-of-worldwide-protests
[810] https://rebellion.earth/2019/10/14/extinction-rebellion-target-institutions-funding-ecological-destruction-in-city-of-london/
[811] https://www.thebureauinvestigates.com/projects/food-and-farming-industry
[812] https://www.independent.co.uk/news/uk/home-news/british-food-consumption-wildlife-deforestation-wwf-a9342611.html
[813] https://www.ft.com/content/73f237dc-73f8-4092-ac0b-009e98681c95
[814] http://resources.trase.earth/documents/issuebriefs/TraseIssueBrief4_EN.pdf
[815] https://www.climatechangenews.com/2020/07/01/eu-must-not-sacrifice-amazon-rainforest-altar-trade-brazil/
[816] https://www.ft.com/content/ca84017c-94c5-48ca-80c6-2ac31ea20cd9
[817] https://www.theguardian.com/environment/2020/jun/23/trillion-dollar-investors-warn-brazil-over-dismantling-of-environmental-policies
[818] https://www.theguardian.com/environment/2020/jun/23/trillion-dollar-investors-warn-brazil-over-dismantling-of-environmental-policies

International reluctance to make serious changes

As much as these threats to sever commercial relations[819] with Brazil might delay damaging policies like the land reform bill[820] or trigger promises to use the armed forces[821] to fight deforestation, it remains to be seen how seriously those in power will be in tackling the climate emergency post-coronavirus. In the past, big words [822] have often failed to result in big actions.

Making threats about commercial relations while diverting business elsewhere[823] seems to offer an easy way out for governments, investors, and companies. When it comes to real changes like strengthening accountability[824] in supply chains[825], establishing tougher financial regulations, or even simply complying with existing commitments.

Evidence[826] shows that companies are still lagging[827] on their voluntary commitments to the 2020 deforestation goals for the consumer goods sector as well as on the 2030 United Nations Sustainable Development Goals (SDGs). Particularly important here is SDG12 on sustainable production and consumption, which includes a host of targets to encourage more responsible use of resources and better management of supply chains. Clearly, Bolsonaro's government and Minister of the Environment Ricardo Salles are to blame for "running the cattle herd[828]" through the Amazon, which threatens the health and human security of indigenous peoples and rainforest dwellers in Brazil.

Behind closed doors the international community is also responsible for financing[829] environmental destruction and human rights[830] violations in the Amazon and the Brazilian savanna. British and EU banks[831] and investors[832] are linked to the cattle industry[833], and the UK government has even been feeding its military personal[834] with beef sourced from illegal lands in Brazil. Soya[835] used to feed chicken[836] in the UK continues to contribute to deforestation, while mining giant Anglo-American has expressed its interest in mining on indigenous lands. Even the British Environmental Agency Active Pension Fund[837], amongst other pension funds such as TIAA[838], has financed farmlands linked to deforestation and displacement of local communities.

---

[819] https://climatenewsnetwork.net/uk-food-giants-mull-brazil-boycott-to-protect-forests/
[820] https://www.ft.com/content/ca84017c-94c5-48ca-80c6-2ac31ea20cd9
[821] https://www.ft.com/content/9dda2eaa-2ef1-45c3-bc6f-c19c88ece527
[822] https://www.ceres.org/news-centre/press-releases/investors-call-corporate-action-deforestation-signaling-support-amazonhttps://news.mongabay.com/2020/07/covid-19-lockdown-precipitates-deforestation-across-asia-and-south-america/
[823] https://news.mongabay.com/2020/07/covid-19-lockdown-precipitates-deforestation-across-asia-and-south-america/
[824] https://theecologist.org/2020/jun/08/due-diligence-overseas-agribusiness?utm_source=hootsuite&utm_medium=linkedin_
[825] https://engagethechain.org/investor-guide-deforestation-and-climate-change
[826] https://forest500.org/publications/forest-500-annual-report-2019-companies-getting-it-wrong-deforestation
[827] https://www.businessgreen.com/news/3083828/consumer-goods-sectors-2020-deforestation-goal-impossible-cdp-warns
[828] https://news.mongabay.com/2020/05/brazil-minister-advises-using-covid-19-to-distract-from-amazon-deregulation/
[829] https://www.ft.com/content/73f237dc-73f8-4092-ac0b-009e98681c95
[830] https://en.mercopress.com/2020/07/04/outbreaks-of-coronavirus-at-brazilian-pork-and-chicken-slaughter-plants
[831] https://www.theguardian.com/environment/2020/jun/04/revealed-uk-banks-and-investors-2bn-backing-of-meat-firms-linked-to-amazon-deforestation
[832] https://www.globalwitness.org/en/press-releases/open-letter-global-investors-and-financial-service-providers/
[833] https://www.theguardian.com/environment/2020/jun/04/revealed-uk-banks-and-investors-2bn-backing-of-meat-firms-linked-to-amazon-deforestation
[834] https://news.mongabay.com/2020/04/uk-military-beef-supplier-buys-from-sanctioned-brazilian-farmers-investigation-shows/
[835] https://www.globalcanopy.org/press-centre/five-most-powerful-soy-traders-must-do-more-address-land-conversion-brazilian-cerrado
[836] https://www.independent.co.uk/news/uk/home-news/chicken-forests-greenpeace-supermarket-fast-food-wildlife-trees-climate-deforestation-a9292576.html
[837] https://medium.com/@foe_us/harvard-and-tiaas-farmland-grab-in-brazil-goes-up-in-smoke-52dbfe57debf
[838] https://chainreactionresearch.com/wp-content/uploads/2020/01/Radar-company-report-2.pdf

These kinds of investments are increasing illegal deforestation, exacerbating the climate emergency, exploiting the current government's dismantling of socio-environmental policies, and further contributing to the genocide[839] of Brazil's indigenous peoples. The question that remains unanswered is whether these processes will continue unabated in the post-pandemic world, with a supposed "green recovery[840]" obscuring continued exporting of deforestation[841] and human rights violations. The signs coming from Europe via the EU-Mercosur free-trade agreement are not especially encouraging, as the indigenous leader Kretã Kaingang of APIB has pointed out[842]: The EU needs to know what they want. How long will our continent continue being economically colonised by Europe? How long will our blood and territories be taken by Europe?

The EU needs to think of how its capital continues enslaving Latin America and African countries. We, the indigenous peoples, know what we want: our territories demarcated, our environment protected, the planet alive through our biodiversity. The EU needs to decide what they want. Decision-makers the world over face this critical health and environmental crisis with the clock ticking on global warming of 1.5 oC[843] and the sixth mass extinction of wildlife[844]. What is needed now is not only a global coalition[845] to protect indigenous peoples' health in Brazil but also the real delivery of climate emergency commitments[846] already promised to British and European voters. To avoid indigenous genocide and secure the lands of rainforest peoples, governments and the financial sector must implement stronger environmental and human rights regulations that at last prevent issues of deforestation and environmental injustice from simply being farmed out to become someone else's problem.

---

[839] https://reporterbrasil.org.br/2020/06/dos-frigorificos-as-plantacoes-de-cana-como-o-agronegocio-expos-indigenas-a-covid-19/?utm_campaign=shareaholic&fbclid=IwAR13meuYg3II7kFALQctNYC7XzZEvNNklUXVQOFCBy66KrMSAJWZccI55iY
[840] https://www.theguardian.com/environment/2020/jun/15/leading-uk-charities-urge-pm-seek-green-recovery-covid-19
[841] https://news.mongabay.com/2012/11/exporting-deforestation-china-is-the-kingpin-of-illegal-logging/
[842] https://www.youtube.com/watch?v=EkatIn4NHio&feature=youtu.be
[843] hhttps://www.theguardian.com/environment/2020/jun/01/sixth-mass-extinction-of-wildlife-accelerating-scientists-warnhttps://www.ipcc.ch/sr15/
[844] https://www.theguardian.com/environment/2020/jun/01/sixth-mass-extinction-of-wildlife-accelerating-scientists-warnhttps://amazonialatitude.com/2020/06/16/indigenous-people-from-the-amazon-only-a-global-coalition-will-save-them/
[845] https://amazonialatitude.com/2020/06/16/indigenous-people-from-the-amazon-only-a-global-coalition-will-save-them/
[846] https://www.bbc.co.uk/news/uk-politics-48126677

4. Indigenous And Afro-Brazilian Lands Are Under Greater Threat In Brazil During COVID-19

Elielson Pereira da Silva

Doutorando, Desenvolvimento Socioambiental,
Federal University of Pará

Diana Cordoba

Assistant Professor, Global Development Studies, Queen's University, Ontario

The far right-wing government of Jair Bolsonaro in Brazil has used the COVID-19 pandemic as a smokescreen to undo environmental regulations and undermine the territorial rights of Indigenous Peoples and traditional Afro-Brazilian communities in the Amazon. The strategy of the Bolsonaro's government and its allies in congress is very clear: to take 9.8 million hectares from Indigenous and traditional territories in the Amazon to seize more land for agribusiness. These actions pose an existential threat to Indigenous Peoples and others living in communities in the Amazon, as the new policies would effectively disintegrate their territories and lead to more deforestation in the coming years.

Turning Crime Into Legal Activities

During the COVID-19 pandemic, Bolsonaro's government has ushered in a rapid process of dismantling of policies that protect Indigenous and traditional communities. There are 305 Indigenous groups in Brazil and 35 per cent of the territories they claim have not been recognized by the government[847].On April 22, the National Indian Foundation (FUNAI), the Brazilian government agency that oversees policies relating to Indigenous peoples, introduced new guidelines[848] that would encourage land-grabbing of undemarcated Indigenous lands. On May 12, the so-called "ruralist bench," a group of wealthy landholders with an important presence in congress, failed to approve a measure (MP910)[849] that would have legalized the occupation of Indigenous lands by land-grabbers, usually for the purpose of deforestation, agribusiness or mining. This temporary victory, the result of public pressure[850], was overshadowed by the presentation of another proposed bill, with the same intentions, on May 14.

---

[847] http://www.funai.gov.br/index.php/indios-no-brasil/terras-indigenas
[848] http://www.in.gov.br/web/dou/-/instrucao-normativa-n-9-de-16-de-abril-de-2020-253343033
[849] https://www.camara.leg.br/proposicoesWeb/fichadetramitacao?idProposicao=2233488
[850] https://www.congressonacional.leg.br/materias/medidas-provisorias/-/mpv/140116

FUNAI and the secretary of land affairs are controlled by two representatives from the ruralist bench. They have openly opposed[851] agrarian reform and the demarcation of Indigenous lands. They also have acknowledged their intentions to undo environmental and Indigenous protections, and are aligned with Bolsonaro who said, "I will not demarcate an extra square centimetre of Indigenous land. Period[852]."Environment Minister Ricardo Salles reiterated this position in April[853], when he advised Bolsonaro and his cabinet to take advantage of the media's attention on COVID-19. He argued COVID-19 was an opportunity to "run the cattle herd" through the Amazon, and change "all the rules and simplifying standards" in all the ministries to facilitate agribusiness and mining projects.

Quilombola Afro-Brazilian Territories At Risk

These measures will also have devastating impacts on the 3,658 territories that are home to Quilombola, descendants of escaped slaves. Only 180[854] of them have been fully titled. The plight of the Quilombola under Bolsonaro's government has received little press. Land conflicts that involved some form of violence, caused by alleged landowners and/or land-grabbers, peaked in 2019. According to data from the Pastoral Land Commission[855], 13,687 Quilombola families were involved in land conflicts and the lives of 15 leaders were threatened in that year alone. This was the highest number of land conflicts recorded by the commission since 1985.

Our research[856] shows how the Quilombola community of Nova Betel in the municipality of Tomé-Açu, in the Amazonian state of Pará — as well as many Quilombola territories that are not yet demarcated and fully recognized by the Brazilian state — could disappear under Bolsonaro's government. Nova Betel contains 1,850 hectares of land, certified in 2016 by Fundação Cultural Palmares (FCP) — the first (and easiest) step on the long path to collective land rights. Despite this, deforestation and land-grabbing have accelerated in Nova Betel since 2007.

For example, Biopalma da Amazônia S.A, owned by Vale, one of the world's largest mining companies, has planted palm oil trees in 75 per cent of Nova Betel's territory[857].nOther projects also threaten to take land from the Quilombola community. A pipeline, power transmission line[858] and even a government-proposed railway[859] cut through their territory. Each of these initiatives pushes the Quilombola members towards selling their lands.Our interviews in May with Quilombola leaders in Nova Betel revealed how employees of the Transmission Company of Energy of Pará S.A (ETEP)[860] pressured eight families to allow a power line to cross through their territory. ETEP offered each family about US$580 as financial compensation, but they refused. Not only did ETEP violate the Quilombola right to self-determination and prior consultation as

[851] https://www.reuters.com/article/us-brazil-politics-indigenous/brazils-bolsonaro-hands-indigenous-land-decisions-back-to-farm-sector-idUSKCN1TK37O

[852] https://www.reuters.com/article/us-brazil-election-landrights-deforestat/indigenous-land-culture-at-stake-in-brazil-election-experts-idUSKCN1N0241

[853] https://www.youtube.com/watch?v=nfgv7DLdCqA

[854] http://cpisp.org.br/direitosquilombolas/observatorio-terras-quilombolas/?terra_nome=&situacao=0&ano_de=1995&ano_ate=2020&orgao_exp=0

[855] https://www.cptnacional.org.br/component/jdownloads/send/41-conflitos-no-campo-brasil-publicacao/14195-conflitos-no-campo-brasil-2019-web?Itemid=0

[856] http://novacartografiasocial.com.br/tag/quilombolas/

[857] https://eventpilotadmin.com/web/page.php?page=Session&project=LASA20&id=312419c

[858] http://www2.aneel.gov.br/aplicacoes/siget/arq.cfm?arquivo=35490

[859] https://agenciapara.com.br/noticia/16323/

[860] http://www.tbe.com.br/conteudo_pti.asp?idioma=0&conta=45&tipo=66233

enshrined in the International Labour Organization's Indigenous and Tribal Peoples Convention[861], but it also breached the health protocols introduced by the community during the pandemic, putting at risk the health of isolated and vulnerable Quilombola families.

Quilombola Lives Matter

The racist discourse of the Bolsonaro government[862] together with the COVID-19 pandemic wreaks havoc on Quilombola communities in the Amazon. According to the COVID-19 Observatory in Quilombos[863], a joint initiative of the National Organization for the Coordination of Black Rural Quilombola Communities (CONAQ) and the Socio-Environmental Institute, an independent non-profit civil society organization, the mortality rate among Quilombola is 25.1 per cent, the highest among all social groups within Brazil. In the states of Pará and Amapá, Quilombola account for 54.9 per cent of COVID-19-verified deaths. The inequality in the fight against COVID-19 caused by historic dynamics of institutional racism will have a devastating impact on Quilombola people if the disease maintains this rate of spread and lethality. Taking inspiration from the Black Lives Matter movement, CONAQ launched on May 12 the campaign #Vidas Quilombolas Importam (Quilombola Lives Matter) to condemn the racism against Afro-Brazilians. Bolsonaro's government, however, has refused to take urgent measures to safeguard the lives of Quilombola during COVID-19 and to provide protection to their land rights.

---

[861] https://www.ilo.org/dyn/normlex/en/f?p=NORMLEXPUB:12100:0::NO::P12100_ILO_CODE:C169
[862] https://grist.org/article/4-indigenous-leaders-on-what-bolsonaro-means-for-brazil/
[863] https://quilombosemcovid19.org/

CHAPTER 27

THE ECONOMIC FUTURE ISN'T BRIGHT

1.The Impact of Coronavirus in Brazil: Uneven Prospects Across Industries

Angelica Salado
Elton Morimitsu
Guilherme Machado
Marcel Motta
Marília Borges
Pedro Alves
Ricardo Sfeir
Rodrigo Mattos

As the coronavirus (COVID-19) incidence advances in Brazil, economic fallout and major impacts are expected in different consumer goods and services industries. This comes not long after industries were showing signs of recovery following the country's economic crisis in 2014-2018. Euromonitor International forecasts another year of negative real GDP growth for Brazil in 2020. While we foresee some categories benefiting from spikes in short-term demand, most industries foresee major negative impacts on sales in 2020. This is especially true in services industries, where consumption occasions that did not take place due to the lockdown cannot be made up in future consumption events. Regardless of the industry, however, important common denominators should drive consumer behaviour in Brazil over the next few months:

•Bottlenecks in production chains and distribution: Reduced workforces may create or worsen pre-quarantine scenarios;
•Sales concentration in some industries in Q1 and Q2 2020 may not be sustained throughout the whole year: The level of product inventories is unprecedented for Brazilian industry, and manufacturers were not prepared to manage unexpected production;
•Reframing of consumption occasions: While there are new occasions boosting demand for products like streaming and video games, others, like restaurants, hotels and entertainment, are being harmed by lost opportunities;
•Resistance test for retailing: Omnichannel structures have become more important than ever and will consistently be tested in a scenario where non-essential stores must remain closed;
•First things first: Prioritisation of essential items may offset the timid signs of recovery many industries were trying to accomplish after the economic crisis in 2014-2018 – the result of unsustainable government expenditures, political instability and economic model failure.

Unemployment And Confidence Levels Are The
Key Indicators of Brazilian Market Resilience

According to Euromonitor International's Macro Model, the impact of COVID-19 on our baseline forecast for Brazilian real GDP will lead to a decline of 1.0% in 2020, while the impact of a COVID-19 Deep Recession would lead to a similar downturn to that seen during the crisis of 2014-2018.
If a COVID-19 Crisis scenario consolidates, however, unemployment rates and real GDP growth will be significantly worse than in 2016 (the worst year of the crisis), leading the Brazilian market to generally collapse. The Latin American outlook will be subject to further downgrade revisions if COVID-19 outbreaks worsen.

Beverages: Prioritisation of Essential Items

As the COVID-19 outbreak intensifies in Brazil, consumers are returning to "crisis mode", copying many habits acquired during the economic crisis of 2014-2018. This means prioritisation of essential items, especially due to concerns about unemployment.
Bottled water and coffee are set to see the greatest rises in demand in the short term, especially through larger pack sizes, as these are considered essential items for most Brazilians, who are looking for the most affordable unit prices. In the case of bottled water, bulk sales are expected to offset volume declines seen in the last couple of years, while intermediary packs (5-8 litres) should continue to grow in volume terms. Spirits, however, might struggle. On-trade establishments will suffer the biggest impact due to mandatory lockdowns in major cities, which are set to be followed by others in the coming weeks. Such a scenario might have a negative impact on ever-rising volumes of gin and recovery of vodka, previously boosted due to the popularity of Gin & Tonic and Moscow Mule cocktails respectively. Additionally, the US dollar exchange rate has reached BRL5.0, compared to a previous rate of BRL4.49 before the first case was confirmed on 26 February 2020, with a significant impact on prices of imported drinks, mainly spirits and wine.

Packaged Food: Sales Concentration on
Non-Perishable Items In Q1 And Q2 2020

Packaged food will undoubtedly benefit in the short term, as consumers are staying at home and replacing "eating out" occasions with homemade food. The most important items have been staples (rice, pasta and sauces/condiments), shelf-stable vegetables (the first items that supermarkets set purchase limits on), frozen ready meals and snacks. In general, products with longer shelf life are preferred during the quarantine, while chilled products such as yoghurts and ice cream are not considered cost beneficial at this point. Such a positive scenario in the short term, however, does not necessarily mean peaks in year-based sales in the second half of the year due to leftovers of longer shelf-life products. Other challenges are distribution logistics affected by a reduced workforce, raw materials shortage (especially those which are harvest dependent) and bottlenecks in packaging supply, as with glass manufacturers, for instance.

Technology And Connectivity:
Digital Services Rise At The Expense Of Technology-Based Products

With quarantine stipulated in most states in the country, digitalisation and online commerce and services have been greatly favoured by the "stay-at-home policy", with both e-commerce, delivery and streaming platforms seeing a surge in demand. It will also strengthen online adoption and mitigate concerns surrounding digital consumption in the long term, which are still quite common in Brazil. On the other hand, technology-based products – like smartphones, wearables and other small consumer appliances – have felt the COVID-19 blow, with the first quarter forecasting retraction within the industry. This is because of reduced production and distribution efficiency (due to a reduced logistics workforce), fewer import products making their way from China, postponement of product launches and devaluation of the Brazilian currency, increasing manufacturing and import costs. However, there are outliers to this scenario, such as computer peripherals (as more people adopt home office standards), food preparation appliances and video games.

Home Care And Hygiene:
Intensification Of Home Care And Focus On Basic Hygiene Products

As replication of other countries' scenarios, toilet paper has become one of the main demanded products in the weeks of quarantine in Brazil, resulting in disruptions of supply and availability in many grocery stores. While the unforeseen spike in the short term should not reflect a peak in year-based volume sales for the category, such strong demand in Q1 should contribute to concentrated production and distribution efforts for this category. As many consumers already stocked significant volumes of toilet paper, positive performance should be followed by a sales drop as the situation stabilises. In the week after the first COVID-19 case in Brazil in February 2020, general home cleaning products already presented significant volume sales rises, in anticipation of the quarantine period. Concerns with home cleaning and personal hygiene are high, benefitting sales of dishwashing items (as more people cook and eat at home), bleach and surface care. However, for these categories, a year-based volume sales increase is expected as consumers are developing the habit of cleaning their households more frequently.

Fashion: One Of The Brazilian Sectors Most Impacted By Lockdown

If the slow-paced growth of fashion categories was a concern related to the weak macroeconomic indicators in Brazil over the last couple of years, the pandemic scenario represents a big shock. Apparel, footwear, personal accessories and eyewear have been completely deprioritised at a time when most families are focused on stockpiling food and hygiene items. As fashion categories' operations are strongly concentrated in physical channels, and the main retailers are closing all their stores for an undetermined period, expectations rely on the quarantine duration to foresee when and how the industry can minimise impacts. In the first semester, Mothers' Day sales (celebrated in May) are expected to be severely harmed. In the best-case scenario, a shorter return to fashion categories' pre-COVID-19 sales level in 2-3 months would bring possibilities for recovery in Q2. Retailers are already engaged in negotiating sector agreements with the federal government to reduce costs (taxes and rental fees) to soften the losses.

Beauty and personal care:
distinct scenarios based on the essential nature of products

COVID-19's impact on the beauty and personal care industry will mostly present two distinct scenarios. In the personal care space, sales should not present a negative performance. In fact, sales of categories such as bath and shower are expected to grow in the short term, with many consumers looking for items such as bar and liquid soaps. According to Euromonitor International's price tracking system, Via Pricing, sales of liquid soap presented over a 20% weekly price increase between February and March 2020, showing the effects of high demand for items considered essential to prevent contamination.

Bath and Shower Items: Weekly Price Variations During COVID-19 Scenario

As for beauty-related items, a different scenario is expected. With several consumers staying at home, categories like colour cosmetics and fragrances are expected to perform poorly, as these are usually related to "going out". Due to lost "going out" occasions during the quarantine, sales of these products should not see a year-based recovery. Together, these two categories represent almost one-third of total beauty and personal care value sales in Brazil, potentially contributing to negative overall sales for the industry in 2020.

Consumer Health: Consumers Look For Immune System-Boosting Solutions

Consumer health is one of the few industries to have been boosted by the outbreak. Consumers rushed to drugstores aiming to purchase all sorts of products that claim to boost immune systems and potentially target COVID-19 symptoms. Items such as Vitamin C, multivitamins and even natural products such as propolis were hardly seen in many outlets from the beginning of March onwards. Since confirmation of the first case in February, prices have soared in the country. Vitamin C, for instance, posted a growth rate of almost 200% on a weekly basis, from February to March 2020, according to Euromonitor International's Via Pricing system. However, with the heated demand, there might be a lack of important raw materials to sustain production and supply in the medium term, potentially offsetting short-term positive results throughout 2020.

Immunity-System Boosting:
Weekly Pricing Variations During COVID-19 Scenarios

Unlike goods, which consumers can buy after the crisis, services such as travel and tourism and consumer foodservice will not benefit from the recovery of pent-up demand. The consumer foodservice industry expects the government to announce a package of emergency measures, capable of bearing a monthly benefit to restaurant workers for the next three months, to prevent mass layoffs. Although delivery activities are still allowed, even in cities where a quarantine has been established, the delivery market in Brazil is composed mainly of independent players that rely on delivery as a complementary operation, making it insufficient to compensate for the loss of revenues associated with the closure of dining areas. Therefore, although players are looking for diversification into delivery options, most of them do not have delivery operations that are robust enough to rely only on delivery activities .Retailing, in turn, is seeing heated activity for most grocery channels, as well as for drugstores and pharmacies. However, nearly all other store-based channels are expected to face months of sales at record lows. Players which demonstrate greater robustness in their operations in digital channels, both in terms of user experience and logistics operations, will be able to mitigate part of the impact of the lockdown. E-commerce represented 8% of total Brazilian retailing value sales in 2019, with this ratio expected to increase in 2020 as the crisis boosts demand for this channel. Digital payments are expected to benefit from this movement as well. Lastly, the travel and tourism industry see a much less encouraging outlook. With about 80% of lodging players closed and all parks and tourist attractions have had operations suspended, the industry expects the government to help pay employees' salaries within the next few months. According to trade association estimates, tourism in Brazil could lose around USD6.2 billion without the support of government aid. Euromonitor International's Travel Industry Forecast Model expects that the baseline scenario for inbound arrivals to Brazil will decrease by 50% in 2020, while the deep recession scenario presents a 54% decrease for the category in the same year.

2. The Impact Of COVID-19 On Franchising In Emerging Markets: An Example From Brazil

Vanessa Pilla Galetti BretasIlan Alon

ABSTRACT

The outbreak of COVID-19, the disease caused by the SARS-CoV-2 virus, has had significant economic, political, and social consequences worldwide. The franchising sector, consisting mostly of retail and service businesses, is an example of an industry that has been deeply affected. The experiences of franchising stakeholders in Brazil highlight the strengths of the franchising model in such situations. This study is based on primary data from webinars with food service, education, retail, and business-to-business service companies in Brazil, coupled with reports from commercial and franchising entities, reveals how the COVID-19 outbreak has affected the franchising sector. It illustrates the measures that were taken, the negotiations that take place between suppliers and landlords, the adaptation of business models, the effects on franchisor-franchisee relationships, and the impact the pandemic has had on relationships with customers. The strategies adopted by Brazilian franchisors and franchisees suggest lessons for other franchising companies in similar situations, such as those in developing and emerging economies.

INTRODUCTION

The COVID-19 pandemic is one of the greatest challenges the modern world has faced. The disease, caused by the severe acute respiratory syndrome coronavirus 2 (SARS-CoV-2), can be traced back to December 2019, when the first case was reported in Wuhan, China. In March 2020, the World Health Organization declared a pandemic, meaning that the disease was spreading worldwide.

In order to slow down the infections and "flatten the curve" of the epidemic, that is reduce the rate of transmission, several countries have suspended business activities, and adopted social distancing to reduce person-to-person contact. Governments are struggling to simultaneously save lives and mitigate the economic impact of the virus (Anderson, Heesterbeek, Klinkenberg, & Hollingsworth, 2020; Rodriguez-Morales et al., 2020; Surico & Galeotti, 2020). Numerous uncertainties surround the disease. Many of the characteristics of COVID-19, such as the duration of the infectious period, symptomatology, and the possibility of asymptomatic transmission, are either speculative or unknown. The development of a vaccine or possible treatment is a long-term project, which might take years to accomplish. Thus, social distancing measures such as isolation, the banning of mass gatherings, and the closing of schools and stores are, at present, the most effective ways to reduce the rate of transmission, avoid the collapse of healthcare systems, and minimize the number of deaths (Anderson et al., 2020).

COVID-19 In Emerging Economies

COVID-19 has had a damaging effect on the economy of countries around the world, but perhaps more particularly so in emerging economies. Although emerging economies are heterogeneous, they do share some common characteristics, such as weaker institutional and legal settings, lower levels of economic development, and higher levels of financial and social risk (Hevia & Neumeyer, 2020; Surico & Galeotti, 2020). These challenging economic and institutional conditions limit the range of their responses to the COVID-19 outbreak. Governments have fewer alternatives with which to confront the pandemic, guarantee health care, offer adequate social protection, and deal with the economic consequences of a pandemic (Buchanan, Anwar, & Tran, 2013; CuervoCazurra, 2012; Ramamurti, 2012; Stiglitz, 2020).

Besides the devastating impact of the pandemic on the weak health infrastructure in these countries, the need for prolonged social distancing and other mitigation policies have led to an economic slump, which in turn has had adverse effects on levels of unemployment.

Moreover, most emerging economies are dependent on exports; they are also affected by the contraction of international trade, the fall of commodity prices, currency devaluations, and disruptions to the global supply chain. A report from the United Nations Conference on Trade and Development (UNCTAD, 2020) projects that, due to the pandemic, developing countries (excluding China) will lose USD 800 billion in export revenue in 2020.Furthermore, these countries have other constraints that make it harder for them to take the necessary measures. Many jobs are informal and consist of the type of work that cannot be done from home. Most have poor housing and sanitary conditions, where people live in close proximity, making social distancing difficult or impossible.

Their economies are characterized by high levels of social inequality, which contributes to the risk of further disruption. Control measures that require the suspension of business activities and social isolation have very different consequences in a developed economy, where the workforce might expect access to free healthcare and income protection, than in an economy where people have to choose between starvation or going to work and risking their health. Throughout the world, COVID-19 has presented governments with a choice between preserving lives and the capacity of the health care system to deal with the pandemic, and the financing of policies to mitigate the costs of social distancing and shuttering businesses. However, it is important to recognize that the implementation of such measures is significantly more challenging for an emerging economy (Hevia & Neumeyer, 2020; Lemos, Almeida-Filho, & Firmo, 2020; Stiglitz, 2020).

Effects on The Franchising Sector

Franchising as a commercial and social model has several economic and social effects, such as job creation, economic modernization, and the development of entrepreneurship (Alon, 2004; Naatu & Alon, 2019). The direct impacts on income, employment, and the achievement of social goals are most noticeable in emerging and developing markets (Alon, Welsh, & Falbe, 2010; Elango, 2019; Naatu & Alon, 2019). According to the World Franchise Council's 2017 survey on the economic impact of franchising worldwide, India, Taiwan, and Brazil ranks among the top five countries worldwide in the number of franchise brands (Exhibit 1).

South Africa is the country with the second highest share of the country's overall GDP generated by the franchising sector, 15.3%. Brazil ranks fifth in terms of job creation by the franchising sector, employing almost1.2 million people in 2017 (ABF, 2020; FASA, 2020a).

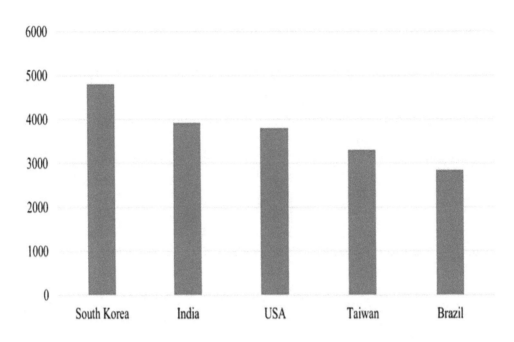

EXHIBIT 1 Top five countries by number of franchise brands [Color figure can be viewed at wileyonlinelibrary.com]

Due to the size of their population, per capita income, urbanization rates, and income distribution, emerging markets offer the largest markets for international franchisors. Emerging economies have used global franchising as a tool for economic and entrepreneurial development, job creation, and global integration (Alon, 2004, 2006; Alon & Lattemann, 2016; Alon, Toncar, & McKee, 2000; Baena, 2012; Welsh & Alon, 2001).

The negative effects of the pandemic on the economies of developing and emerging countries are worrying. One of the first consequences of the crisis has been the withdrawal of investment from countries considered to be at greatest risk. Countries that depend on exports of commodities or manufacturing goods, such as China, Mexico, and Brazil, are suffering from a drop in demand. Furthermore, tourism, which is an essential source of revenue for many developing and emerging countries, is paralyzed (Fariza, 2020; Stiglitz, 2020). The effects of the COVID-19 outbreak on other services and retail industries are also severe. Construction, food service, fashion, and retail are some of the sectors most affected by the pandemic. The franchising sector is also strongly impacted, with consequences for the business activities and integrity of the franchise system. The crisis also creates additional challenges to the dynamic between franchisors and franchisees.

Although mostly related to services and retail, franchising covers a broad spectrum of business activities, and is affected by the crisis to different degrees (Abell, 2020; Sebrae, 2020; Surico & Galeotti, 2020; Teixeira, 2020).

A study (Teixeira, 2020) by FIAF, the Ibero-American Franchising Federation, which represents the franchise associations of Portugal, Mexico, Guatemala, Costa Rica, Panama, Colombia, Venezuela, Ecuador, Peru, Brazil, Uruguay, Paraguay, and Argentina, showed that retail franchisors are the most affected by the coronavirus crisis, followed by food service franchises (Exhibit 2).

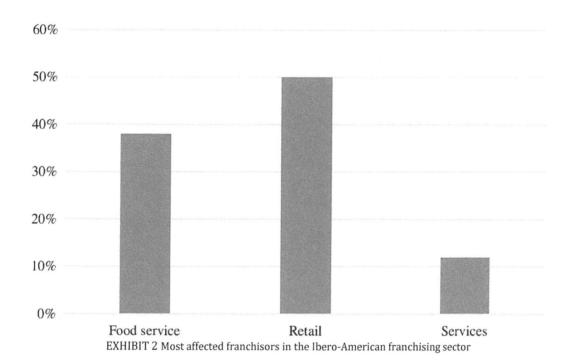

EXHIBIT 2 Most affected franchisors in the Ibero-American franchising sector

In this context, the impact of COVID-19 on the BRICS nations—Brazil, Russia, India, China, and South Africa—are of concern because they account for a large share of the global GDP and population. The social distancing measures are severely impacting the franchising, retail, and services sectors in these countries. In South Africa, since the implementation of the COVID-19 emergency policies, approximately 94% of the franchising industry has not been operating. The lockdown measures included food deliveries. The Franchising Association of South Africa made a public statement asking for the takeout and fast food sectors to be included as essential services (FASA, 2020b).

The joint report from the China Chain Store & Franchise Association and Deloitte China (Deloitte, 2020a) shows that retail businesses are facing several operational and financial challenges in the country. Among the companies surveyed, 90% said that the pandemic had impacted the number of customers, especially stores and food service chains operating in shopping centres. The Retailers' Association of India (2020) surveyed retail companies to understand the impact of COVID-19 on their businesses. More than 95% of non-food retailers have had their stores closed. Food retailers expect to earn only 56% of last year's revenues. The country is facing a massive decline in restaurant and food service businesses. Deliveries have become the primary source of income for these companies (Deloitte, 2020b). In Russia, all retail stores are closed, except for food stores and stores providing essential goods. Restaurants are open only for takeaways (Dentons, 2020).

The Impact of COVID-19 In Brazil

In Brazil, the first confirmed case of COVID-19 was a 61 year-old man, who had been traveling in Lombardy, Italy, and arrived in Sao Paulo on February 21, 2020. The Brazilian Ministry of Health confirmed the case on February 26, 2020. On March 13, the state health departments across the country announced recommendations to limit the spread of the disease. The government recognized community transmission across the country on March 20 (Croda et al., 2020; Rodriguez-Morales et al., 2020). To try to reduce the number of cases and flatten the pandemic curve, the Brazilian health authorities reacted by implementing measures such as isolation, quarantine, and temporary restrictions on entering and leaving the country. Despite this, the country still faces some major challenges when trying to alleviate the worst effects of the pandemic (Croda et al., 2020; Surico & Galeotti, 2020).

At the end of February, when the first case of COVID-19 was confirmed, the projections for the growth of Brazil's GDP in 2020 were around 2%, already signaing a weak expansion (Banco Central do Brasil, 2020).The coronavirus outbreak generated a supply and demand crisis, and will have a strong negative impact on the Brazilian GDP, resulting in unemployment and income losses.

More than 40% of Brazil's workforce is employed in the informal sector (IBGE, 2020). Consequently, the effects of prolonged quarantine are devastating (Surico & Galeotti, 2020).Moreover, like other emerging economies, Brazil is characterized by sizeable social inequality.

It is a country the size of some continents, with an estimated population of 209 million in 2018; it also has the most populous city in South America, S~ao Paulo, with a population of more than 21 million people in the greater metropolitan area. The wealthiest part of the country, around the capital Brasília, has a GDP per person equivalent to Italy, while the most impoverished region, the States of Maranh~ao and Piauí, have a GDP per capita comparable to Jordan (Economist, 2014; Rodriguez Morales et al., 2020).A large part of the population lives in deplorable conditions in the cities' outskirts or "favelas," where, in addition to poor healthcare and sanitation, overcrowding is such that it is almost impossible to implement social distancing.

According to a study developed by the Trata Brasil Institute, 16.38% of the Brazilian population does not have access to a clean water supply, and only 46% of the volume of sewage generated in the country is treated. Since hygiene is one of the most important measures against the spread of the disease, these conditions impose severe limitations on the ability of many people to take preventive actions (Instituto Trata Brasil, 2020; Macedo, Ornellas, & do Bomfim, 2020).As in some other emerging economies, such as Africa, South Asia, and Latin America, the capacity of the Brazilian health care system to deal with a pandemic is severely limited. The Brazilian population consists mainly of young adults with a high incidence of diseases such as diabetes, hypertension, obesity, HIV, and tuberculosis. The country has a universal health care system; however, in terms of the availability of intensive care units, equipment, and diagnostic tests, the outbreak of COVID-19 has placed additional pressure on an already vulnerable system (Croda et al., 2020; Surico & Galeotti, 2020). In response to these challenges, the Brazilian government has adopted some measures to mitigate the impact of the crisis on the economy. The main provisions include direct and indirect tax measures, employment related measures, and an economic stimulus (KPMG Global, 2020).

- **Tax Measures**

The indirect and direct tax measures include payment deferrals and rate reductions. The economic stimulus package announced on March 26 includes funds to replace the extension or suspension of the payment of taxes, a Guarantee Fund (FGTS), and a reduction in contributions.

- **Employment-Related Measures**

Several provisional measures were enacted to adapt labour regulations during the pandemic, and to provide aid to employers, employees, informal workers, and autonomous social services. These measures include the possibility of working remotely, provision for individual and collective vacations, and compensation for working unusual hours. Other provisions include the payment of job and income preservation benefits, permitting a proportional reduction of working hours and wages, and the temporary suspension of employment contracts. Emergency aid to informal workers and a reduction to the rate of contributions by autonomous social services were also granted.

- **Economic stimulus measures**

Among the measures to stimulate the economy are credit lines and loans for micro, small, and medium-sized companies, a simplification of the requirements to obtain credit, flexibility in the rules for obtaining loans, a moratorium on debt repayments, and credit lines for small and medium-sized companies to pay salaries. A list of all of the measures adopted so far appears in "Brazil's policy responses to COVID-19" published by the Secretariat for International Economic Affairs (Ministério da Economia, 2020).

The Response of Brazil's Franchising Stakeholders

In 2019, the Brazilian franchising sector's revenue was USD 46.3 billion, with 2,918 franchisors operating 160,958 establishments in the country. Brazilian franchisors were responsible for 1.36 million direct jobs in the country (Brazilian Franchising Association [ABF], 2019).
A recession in this sector has a significant negative impact on the Brazilian economy in terms of employment and revenue losses. The ABF, which represents the industry's stakeholders and has contributed to their best practices since 1987, took several measures to minimize the impact of this crisis on the franchising system.
It is developing advocacy initiatives with the federal and state-level governments, and with banks and other associations. Another effort centres on webinars and online roundtable discussions with franchisors, franchisees, and other relevant players.
Three webinars and five roundtable discussions were conducted online from April 7 to April 27; the participants included 17 franchisors, 7 franchisees, and 5 consultants. The discussions focused the strategies being adopted by companies and gaining insights for the future. The franchisors and franchisees that participated represented the food service, education, retail, and business-to-business service sectors. In the following sections, we review the main ideas discussed regarding

five topics: initial measures adopted, negotiations with suppliers and landlords, business model adaptations, the franchisor–franchisee relationship, and the relationship with customers. Some direct quotations of the participants' opinions are provided to illustrate certain points.

The First Measures Were Emergency Care

Both franchisors and franchisees had to close the doors of their stores at the end of March. In general, the first measures they took were revising their budgets and dealing with their employees. A primary concern was to find ways to preserve their cash flow, by reducing costs, and by maintaining at least part of their revenue through alternative channels. The franchise chains started by reducing or eliminating all nonessential expenses such as consulting services, communication services, store repairs, and maintenance. Several companies decided to terminate temporary and work-experience contracts, while permanent employees were encouraged to take their vacation days or to work remotely. After the isolation measures were introduced, the franchising firms began a temporary suspension of employment contracts and a reduction in work hours and wages.

Both franchisors and franchisees regarded layoffs as a last resort. At the same time, franchisors and franchisees started to apply for credit lines to finance salaries. As part of the Brazilian government's economic stimulus measures, private banks, serving as intermediaries between the public banks and enterprises, started offering credit. However, several companies reported difficulty in accessing these credit lines due to differences between the public and private sector banks about how to manage the process. The ABF began negotiating with the banks to release working capital lines for franchisees. There is a general perception that these were initial strategies that needed to be revised continuously. One franchisee stated, "We are living in the moment. After 30 days, we must revisit some decisions that we made. There is great uncertainty regarding our decisions since the paths are not very clear."

Relations With All Of The Players Are Becoming Increasingly Close

Negotiations with suppliers and commercial property landlords are essential to guarantee financial breathing room for franchisors and franchisees. These negotiations are complicated because all of the parties involved are trying to reduce expenses and maintain at least part of their income.

The suppliers of franchise chains are also strongly affected by the crisis. The shopping malls depend on rents and fees. Some of the street stores' landlords are individuals or family owners for whom rent is their primary income. A franchisee of a food service chain commented, "Many are family properties, many people who depend on that income, that rent." In this context, the risk that negotiations will end in a lose–lose situation is high. Thus, despite specificities of each negotiation process, because every stakeholder is facing an extraordinary situation, a shared vision has emerged among franchising companies of the importance of flexibility. Another franchisee stated, "We are looking for a negotiation with all our partners, service providers, and suppliers where the two parties lose less." Being part of a franchise is an advantage in the negotiations because of the benefits of scale; it is better to negotiate as part of a network than to negotiate individually. Several shopping malls are allowing food operations to open for a delivery-only service and offering to delay, discount, or cancel the payment of rent for March and April. Other suppliers are negotiating the postponement or a temporary suspension of payments.

However, according to the franchisees, most of the suppliers and landlords have not put forward any alternatives for the long term. Franchising companies are concerned about how to renegotiate their contracts and manage the return to business after COVID-19. The franchisee of a cosmetic company noted, "We are looking forward to more transparent negotiations when the moment for activities return. The criteria that are in our contracts now will not enable our recovery."

The ABF asked Abrasce, the association representing the shopping malls, for measures to cover the immediate future. Some of the suggested measures include the payment of proportional rent until the end of 2020, exemption from the advertising fund, proportional deductions from the condominium, discounts related to opening hours, and the elimination of transfer fees for 2020.

It Was Necessary, But Now It Is Inevitable

Franchisors and franchisees have begun implementing adaptations to their business models to lessen the effects of the crisis. Many developments that were seen as necessary in the medium or long term are considered inevitable now. The most significant change is the speed with which franchisors and franchisees have embraced technology. The crisis has intensified already-existing trends related to consumer behaviour, organizational structure, and the supply chain, and have affected every part of the businesses. Processes and technologies that were previously seen as experimental, such as digitalization, online purchasing, mobile technology, and omnichannel marketing, are now being more widely implemented due to the challenges posed by the pandemic. In the food service sector, some restaurants are offering delivery for the first time and the delivery model is seen as one that is likely to continue. Other chains that had been working with delivery before are now increasing their investment in this model.

A franchisee of a food service chain said, "We are specializing in delivery using a lot of [different types of] technology." Retail franchise companies are also investing in delivery, using marketplaces as a sales channel, or developing their own delivery structure. Another model being discussed by firms in the food sector is the "dark kitchen" model, where meals are prepared to order and exclusively for delivery. According to a franchisee of a food company that sells açaí "We have a plan to open a dark kitchen that operates only on delivery. The occupancy cost decreases, with reduced operation hours." However, some companies believe that the revenue from delivery sales will begin to diminish as ordering food is a nonessential expense for a significant part of the Brazilian population, especially with the expected growth of unemployment.

In the education sector, which includes second-language schools, academic tutoring, and training institutes, franchise chains are rapidly developing online classes. Most schools will offer payment renegotiation, or the possibility of postponing courses, to students who do not feel comfortable having online courses. Franchisors consider online courses to be a temporary measure, claiming that students prefer face-to-face interaction. For example, the franchisor of a second-language school said "Our intention, as soon as possible, is to return to traditional classes. We believe that face-to-face courses will rarely be replaced." However, the move toward an online environment is a source of concern for some franchisees. The online platform becomes a direct channel between the franchisor and the final consumer, which could impact on the role of the franchisee after the crisis. In sectors such as retail, companies are also adopting digital tools, and e-commerce sales are increasing. In 2019, 61% of the franchisors operating in Brazil used ecommerce as a sales channel. This figure will undoubtedly rise in 2020.

A strategy adopted by some franchising companies is "future sales": customers buy products with discounts now and take them later when the stores reopen. In addition, both franchisors and franchisees have started using tools such as WhatsApp and Instagram for sales, and are developing virtual catalogues and adapting their distribution, delivery, and payment routines. According to a franchisee of a beauty company, "WhatsApp is a tool for selling that is very efficient, very agile."

Building bridges between franchisors and franchisees

The structure of the franchise model facilitates the exchange of information and ideas which can help to reduce the negative impact of the crisis. The collaboration between franchisors and franchisees allows them to react more quickly and make decisions with greater certainty.

The franchisor offers financial and managerial support to the franchisees. On the other hand, the franchisees help the franchisors identify threats and opportunities for the network. The words of the president of the ABF highlight how the franchising system in Brazil is dealing with the crisis: "Franchisors and franchisees are working together, being flexible and adapting rules, models, concepts." In general, franchisors are renegotiating or suspending the payment of royalties and fees. Several franchise chains have created crisis committees that include franchisees and members of different areas of the franchisor to exchange ideas and discuss measures. The crisis committees accelerate processes. In addition, franchisors are investing in communication with the franchisees. They share information about their business and other topics, such as health, personal care, negotiation, and legal advice, through webinars, live discussions, and podcasts. For instance, a franchising group that includes accessories and fashion brands implemented a three-phase process with the franchisees. The first phase consisted of postponing or renegotiating the payments of royalties and fees. The next step was the analysis of the franchisees' financial situation and the need for working capital. And the last one consisted of individual guidance for each franchisee.

A second-language school devised a plan to offer online classes in 3 weeks. During the development of the strategy, the franchisor discovered that one franchisee already offered online courses. In this way, the network was able to shorten the path by learning from what the franchisee had done and replicating it with other franchisees. So far, the franchisees' overall perception of the franchisors' actions regarding the pandemic is positive. "There is a very healthy exchange between franchisor and franchisee to redesign the business."

They asserted that most of the franchisors had opened communication channels, were negotiating measures, and were trying to understand the franchisees' needs. Franchisors are helping in the negotiations with suppliers and landlords. Some of them are giving franchisees legal advice and commercial support.

The Customer's Behaviour Will Change; Our Behaviour Will Change

Franchising firms believe that during the crisis and the recovery period, customers will be primarily concerned with basic necessities. A second-language school franchisee asserted: "We have a considerable challenge because customers will prioritize [goods and services] that will meet their basic needs." Consumer confidence is eroding. Due to large numbers of informal workers without an income, the suspension of employment contracts, and an unemployment rate that will continue to rise, a substantial part of the Brazilian population is cutting out all nonessential expenses.

According to Instituto Brasileiro de Economia (FGV-IBRE, 2020), 80% of Brazilian consumers are only buying essential goods, such as food and health care products; consequently, franchise chains in sectors that offer goods or services that are considered superfluous are facing enormous difficulties. Most franchisors and franchisees are intensifying communication with their customers, trying to get closer, and to maintain their relationship. The franchisor of an accessories brand decided not to focus on sales at this moment, understanding that their customers have other priorities, "Our communications are concentrated on embracing our customers, to say that we are together right now."

Franchisors in the education sector are also investing in maintaining communication with the students, offering special payment plans to keep enrolments. Franchise chains in business-to business industries are adjusting their marketing campaigns, to target those clients who are in sectors where there is still a demand. Currently, changes in the amount of face-to-face interaction mean that businesses have shifted toward online shopping and delivery, investments in omnichannel marketing, and the digitalization of sales.

However, in the longer term, other aspects related to the interaction with customers are expected to emerge. For example, companies will need to encourage stores to accept digital payments, guarantee hygiene measures, rethink the provision of food, and experiment with new ideas for clothing outlets. A retail franchisor that sells glazed roasted nuts is revising several of its processes for the recovery period: "We will have to change our tasting process, the product display, and the packaging assembly. Our idea is to show customers everything we do, so the customer will be sure that the product is made in a safe way, and that he or she is not taking any risks."

Another unanswered question about the consequences of the pandemic is how this crisis will affect consumer behaviour in the long term. As a result of the health crisis, will companies have to deal with a more environmentally conscious consumer; one that is more concerned with sustainability and social issues? Will pre-existing trends such as a reduction in consumption, the change from ownership to rental services, and the repurposing of items be intensified? Stakeholders in the franchising sector believe that consumer behaviour or will inevitably change, and that companies will have to change too. The comments by the head of the ABF digital transformation committee highlight this perception, "The crisis is making people think about what they are consuming, and why they are consuming it."

EXHIBIT 3:Best practices from Brazil

Create a multidisciplinary crisis committee

Evaluate the budget, preserve cash flow where possible, and cut nonessential expenses

Understand the emergency aid packages available

Connect with relevant commercial and sectorial associations

Contact suppliers and landlords to renegotiate contracts to reduce losses

Modify existing business models to maintain revenue

Invest in and build upon franchisor–franchisee relationship

Invest in communication and transparency with employees

Adapt and improve of communication with clients

The situation can change quickly; it is necessary to regularly reassess strategies

Best Practices And The Implications For Franchising Companies

The experiences of the Brazilian franchising stakeholders, from food services, education, retail, and business-to-business services, offer a number of lessons to other companies facing the same challenges in similar contexts. A synthesis of their best practices appears in Exhibit 3.

- Several franchisors created multidisciplinary crisis committees, which included a number of different franchisees, to discuss alternatives, establish necessary measures, and create strategies. Having these committees accelerated the speed with which decisions could be taken.
- A thorough evaluation of the company's budget is crucial. The main concern for franchisors and franchisees, from all business areas, was to preserve their cash flow by reducing expenses and maintaining at least part of their revenue. Non-essential and temporary contracts were reviewed or cancelled. Employee-related measures such as salary reductions and the suspension of employment contracts were widely adopted.
- Franchising firms also had to make use of government emergency aid, such as credit lines to pay employees' salaries and cover fixed costs. To achieve this, franchisors and franchisees needed to understand what aid packages were available and how to apply for them.
- Commercial and sectorial associations play an important role in communicating the needs of companies to government and other public entities. They can also help in the negotiation with other players, such as banks and other associations.
- Companies need to negotiate with suppliers and landlords to prevent avoidable losses, by both parties, by reducing fees, offering discounts on rent, and postponing payments.
- To adapt to and exploit changing circumstances, franchising companies need to modify their existing business model, for example, by embracing technology, operating dark kitchens, or offering future sales.

- Franchisors need to help franchisees find appropriate financial responses to the crisis. The opening of new communication channels, such as webinars, podcasts, and multi-stakeholder online "round-table" meetings, are one way to achieve this; flexibility in the payment of fees will also help to reduce the immediate pressure on franchisees.
- Communication and transparency with employees is essential. Franchisors and franchisees need to help employees adapt to new modes of working by providing information about what is happening to the business, and about health and welfare.
- Franchisors and franchisees should adapt and intensify their communication with customers by, for example, the use of online tools.
- Much remains unknown about the characteristics of COVID-19, and new scenarios emerge daily; it is therefore essential that business strategies are reviewed periodically to take account of changes in circumstances.

To summarize, each business sector has its own particular characteristics, will suffer different effects from the crisis, and will need to take its own distinctive actions in response. However, looking at the experience of Brazil, three broad strategies stand out. The first is the acceleration of digital transformation. Franchisors and franchisees, from all business sectors, have increased the speed with which they have adopted technology to run their business. Trends that were viewed as experimental before the crisis, such as online sales, omnichannel marketing, and mobile technology, have now become essential components for a businesses' continued operation.

Second, collaboration and communication has become more widespread, and relationships have become more horizontal than vertical. Teamwork between franchisor and franchisees has become a central theme for the franchising sector. One example of this is the creation of crisis committees by franchise chains to consider alternatives to the challenges created by the COVID-19 outbreak.

A similar trend can be seen inside companies, with the relationships between managers and employees becoming more horizontal too. The third strategy concerns flexibility. The situation created by the pandemic requires stakeholders to be more proactive and adaptable. In addition to the need to adapt business models, flexibility is essential in consultations between franchisors and franchisees, negotiations with suppliers and landlords, and in dialog with employees and customers. These three strategies embracing technology, collaboration, and flexibility are vital for companies trying to keep up with the current changes in the business environment, and for dealing with whatever may come in the future. It remains unclear how long the crisis will last, and what its eventual impact will be; however, as we have seen, stakeholders in Brazil have been able to use the strengths of the franchising model to respond to the challenges. We believe their experiences will be of value to other franchising companies in similar situations.

ACKNOWLEDGMENTS

This work was supported in part by the Coordenaç~ao de Aperfeiçoamento de Pessoal de Nível Superior - Brasil (CAPES) - Finance Code 001.

REFERENCES

Abell, M. (2020). How franchisors should deal with the impact of COVID-19. Retrieved from http://www.twobirds.com/en/news/ articles/2020/global/how-franchisors-should-deal-with-the-impactof-COVID-19

ABF. (2020). Números do franchising mostrando o desempenho do setor. Retrieved from https://www.abf.com.br/numeros-dofranchising/

Alon, I. (2004). Global franchising and development in emerging and transitioning markets. Journal of Macromarketing, 24(2), 156–167.

Alon, I. (2006). Executive insight: Evaluating the market size for service franchising in emerging markets. International Journal of Emerging Markets, 1(1), 9–20.

Alon, I., & Lattemann, C. (2016). Tchibo goes global: Implementing a hybrid franchising strategy at Germany's leading coffee retailer. Global Business and Organizational Excellence, 35(2), 18–30.

Alon, I., Toncar, M., & McKee, D. (2000). Evaluating foreign-market environments for international franchising expansion. Foreign Trade Review, 35(1), 1–11.

Alon, I., Welsh, D. H. B., & Falbe, C. M. (2010). Franchising in emerging markets. In I. Alon (Ed.), Franchising globally: Innovation, learning and imitation (pp. 11–35). Basingstoke, UK: Palgrave Macmillan.

Anderson, R. M., Heesterbeek, H., Klinkenberg, D.,&Hollingsworth, T. D. (2020). How will country-based mitigation measures influence the course of the COVID-19 epidemic? The Lancet, 395(10228), 931–934.

Baena, V. (2012). Market conditions driving international franchising in emerging markets. International Journal of Emerging Markets, 7(1), 49–71.

Banco Central do Brasil. (2020, February 28). Focus—Relatório de mercado. Retrieved from https://www.bcb.gov.br/publicacoes/ focus/28022020

Buchanan, F. R., Anwar, S. T., & Tran, T. X. (2013). Spotlight on an emerging market: Assessing the footwear and apparel industries in Vietnam. Global Business and Organizational Excellence, 32(2), 38–51.

Croda, J., de Oliveira, W. K., Frutuoso, R. L., Mandetta, L. H., Baiada-Silva, D. C., Brito-Sousa, J. D., ... Lacerda, M. V. G. (2020). COVID-19 in Brazil: Advantages of a socialized unified health system and preparation to contain cases. Revista Da Sociedade Brasileira de Medicina Tropical, 53, e20200167. https://doi.org/ 10.1590/0037-8682-0167-2020

Cuervo-Cazurra, A. (2012). Extending theory by analyzing developing country multinational companies: Solving the goldilocks debate. Global Strategy Journal, 2(3), 153–167.

Deloitte. (2020a). COVID-19's impact on China's consumer products & retail industries. Retrieved from https://www2.deloitte.com/ global/en/pages/about-deloitte/articles/COVID-19/COVID-19-impacton-china-consumer-products-retail-industries.html

Deloitte. (2020b). Impact of COVID-19 on India's economic growth. Retrieved from https://www2.deloitte.com/in/en/pages/ consumer-business/articles/impact-of-COVID-19-on-consumerbusiness-in-india.html

Dentons. (2020). Retail: Country-by-country summary of the impact of COVID-19. Retrieved, from https://www.dentons.com/en/ insights/alerts/2020/march/30/COVID-19-retail-country-by-countrysummary

Economist (2014, June 12). Comparing Brazil's states: Welcome to Italordan. Retrieved from https://www.economist.com/theamericas/2014/06/12/welcome-to-italordan Elango, B. (2019). A bibliometric analysis of franchising research (1988–2017). The Journal of Entrepreneurship, 28(2), 223–249.

Fariza, I. (2020, May 4). Crise nos emergentes, o ângulo cego da pandemia do coronavírus. Retrieved from https://brasil.elpais.com/ economia/2020-05-04/crise-nos-emergentes-o-angulo-cego-da-crisedo-coronavirus.html

FASA. (2020a, February 12). Franchising's massive contribution to global economic output. Retrieved from https://www.fasa.co.za/ franchisings-massive-contribution-to-global-economic-output/

FASA. (2020b, April 18). Franchise sector appeals to government for urgent intervention. Retrieved from https://www.fasa.co.za/ franchise-sector-appeals-to-government-for-urgent-intervention/

FGV-IBRE. (2020, April 7). Webinar discute impactos do coronavírus no comportamento dos preços e na confiança de empresários e consumidores. Retrieved from https://portal.fgv.br/noticias/ webinar-discute-impactos-coronavirus-comportamento-precos-econfianca-empresarios-e

Hevia, C., & Neumeyer, P. A. (2020, April 21). A perfect storm: COVID-19 in emerging economies. Retrieved from https://voxeu. org/article/perfect-storm-COVID-19-emerging-economies

IBGE. (2020, February 14). Desemprego cai em 16 estados em 2019, mas 20 têm informalidade recorde. Retrieved from https:// agenciadenoticias.ibge.gov.br/agencia-noticias/2012-agenciade-noticias/noticias/26913-desemprego-cai-em-16-estados-em-2019-mas-20-tem-informalidade-recorde

Instituto Trata Brasil. (2020). Ranking do saneamento 2020. Retrieved from http://www.tratabrasil.org.br/blog/2020/03/12/ instituto-trata-brasil-lanca-mais-um-ranking-do-saneamentobasico/

KPMG Global. (2020, April 21). Brazil: Government and institution measures in response to COVID-19. Retrieved from https:// home.kpmg/xx/en/home/insights/2020/04/brazil-governmentand-institution-measures-in-response-to-covid.html

Lemos, P., Almeida-Filho, N., & Firmo, J. (2020). COVID-19, desastre do sistema de saúde no presente e tragédia da economia em um futuro bem próximo. Brazilian Journal of Implantology and Health Sciences, 2(4), 39–50.

Macedo, Y. M., Ornellas, J. L., & do Bomfim, H. F. (2020). COVID – 19 no Brasil: O que se espera para populaç~ao subalternizada? Revista Encantar - Educaç~ao. Cultura e Sociedade, 2, 01–10.

Ministério da Economia. (2020, April 14). Brazil's policy responses to COVID-19. Retrieved from https://www.gov.br/economia/ptbr/centrais-de-conteudo/publicacoes/publicacoes-em-outrosidiomas/COVID-19/brazil2019s-policy-responses-to-COVID-19/view

Naatu, F., & Alon, I. (2019). Social franchising: A bibliometric and theoretical review. Journal of Promotion Management, 25(5), 738–764.

Ramamurti, R. (2012). What is really different about emerging market multinationals? Global Strategy Journal, 2(1), 41–47.

Retailers Association of India. (2020). Impact of COVID-19 on Indian retail. Retrieved from https://rai.net.in/insightsrepository.php

Rodriguez-Morales, A. J., Gallego, V., Escalera-Antezana, J. P.,

Méndez, C. A., Zambrano, L. I., Franco-Paredes, C., ... Cimerman, S. (2020). COVID-19 in Latin America: The implications of the first confirmed case in Brazil. Travel Medicine and Infectious Disease, 101613 [published online ahead of print], https://doi.org/10.1016/j.tmaid.2020.101613

Sebrae. (2020). Veja quais setores serao mais afetados pela crise~ . Retrieved from https://m.sebrae.com.br/sites/PortalSebrae/ artigos/veja-quais-setores-serao-mais-afetados-pela-crise,c7c3f1b 0a59f0710VgnVCM1000004c00210aRCRD

Stiglitz, J. E. (2020, April 6). Internationalizing the crisis. Retrieved from https://www.project-syndicate.org/commentary/covid19impact-on-developing-emerging-economies-by-joseph-e-stiglitz-2020-04

Surico, P., & Galeotti, A. (2020, March). The economics of a pandemic: The case of COVID-19. Presented at the International Council for Small Business, London Business School. Retrieved from https://icsb.org/theeconomicsofapandemic/

Teixeira, R. (2020, March 24). FIAF: Efectos del COVID-19 sobre la industria de franquicias en Ibero-América. Retrieved from https://www.abf.com.br/fiaf-efectos-del-COVID-19-sobre-la-industriade-franquicias-en-ibero-america/

UNCTAD. (2020). The COVID-19 shock to developing countries: Towards a "whatever it takes" programme for the two-thirds of the world's population being left behind. Retrieved from https:// unctad.org/en/PublicationsLibrary/gds_tdr2019_covid2_en.pdf

Welsh, D. H. B., & Alon, I. (2001). International franchising in emerging markets: Central and Eastern Europe and Latin America. Chicago, IL: CCH Incorporated.

3. Economic Impact of COVID-19 On Tourism In Brazil

Luiz Carlos S. Ribeiro
Professor Adjunto do Departamento de Economia da Universidade Federal de Sergipe,
Coordenador do Laboratório de Economia Aplicada e Desenvolvimento Regional e Pesquisador de Produtividade em Pesquisa do CNPq. E-mail: ribeiro.luiz84@gmail.com.

Gervásio F. Santos
Professor Associado do Departamento de Economia da Universidade Federal da Bahia (UFBA);
Grupo de Pesquisa em Economia Espacial/UFBA e Grupo de Economia Aplicada. E-mail: gervasios@ufba.br.

Rodrigo B. Cerqueira
Mestre em Economia pela UFBA e Pesquisador da Superintendência de Estudos Econômicos e Sociais da Bahia
/SEI-BA. E-mail: rbcerqueira@gmail.com.

Kênia B. Souza
Professora Adjunta do Departamento de Economia da Universidade Federal do Paraná,
Pesquisadora do Núcleo de Estudos em Desenvolvimento Urbano e Regional e Pesquisadora de Produtividade em Pesquisa do CNPq.
E-mail: keniadesouza@gmail.com.

ABSTRACT

This research note aims to estimate the economic impact of pandemic COVID-19 on the tourism sector in Brazil. Tourist activities were the first to be strongly affected by the pandemic, and these impacts are expected to be the most prolonged among economic activities. In developing economies like Brazil, tourism services are supplied by a mix of formal and informal activities and workers that help to sustain important economic and social indicators. In this research, the method of partial hypothetical extraction, underling the input-output modelling, was used to simulate the economic impacts of two scenarios affecting the tourist activities and workers in this sector. First, we simulate the withdrawal of informal tourism workers, in a partial lockdown scenario, combined with the contraction in touristic demand. Second, we maintain the restrictions of the first scenario and simulate how government social and compensatory policies could offset the economic effects of tourist activities. The results show a potential decline of 31% in Gros Domestic Product (GDP) of tourist activities derived from the withdrawal of informal workers and touristic demand contraction. In addition, the government compensatory policy could mitigate these negative effects reducing it to 17%. Lodging services would be the most affected tourist activity.

INTRODUCTION

The World Health Organization (WHO) classified COVID-19 as a pandemic in March 2020 after which lockdown measures began to be taken. Such measures have allowed the functioning only of essential sectors to decrease the speed of virus transmission in the country. Brazil had more than half million confirmed cases by the beginning of June 2020, one of the highest number of cases of COVID19 in the world. Tourist activities were one of the first to be immediately impacted, and given the intrinsic features of this sector, it will also suffer greatly and longer due to people's uncertainty to travel in the post-pandemic period and as such its economic recovery will be slow and gradual. The intensity of the economic impacts will depend on the length of interruption of activities, on the implementation of economic policies to support the sector, and compensatory policies for individual workers.

At the international level, the impact on the sector is expected to be heterogeneous among countries due to the relative economic importance of the sector. According to the World Travel and Tourism Council (WTTC, 2019), tourism accounted for 8.1% of Brazilian GDP in 2018.Regarding the potential impact of pandemic COVID-19, it is necessary to highlight the high rate of informality in the sector, which was about 30% in 2015 and 51.4% in 2018. Informal workers are more vulnerable and immediately affected by the intensity of lockdown measures (ILO, 2020).While formal workers' losses are mitigated by social protection measures, informal workers have no access to them. Additionally, from the demand side, people reduce their movements and reorganize their budgets to prioritize more immediate subsistence goods and services because of reduced income in the economy. Consequently, the supply and demand for tourism-related services are reduced almost simultaneously.

Thus, two important questions can be posed: (i) *what would the economic cost caused by the COVID-19 partial lockdown measures be? (ii) how do compensatory policies of income transference mitigate these effects?*

Federal government rules and the varying intensities of the pandemic in regional and local economies make the simulations of lockdown policies difficult to model for the whole country at the sectoral level. Sectors and regions are unevenly affected by the spread of the virus. In addition, according to the Brazilian Constitution, the lockdown policies should be defined by local governments, at the municipal level[864]. However, tourism and informal activities and workers are among the most homogeneously affected groups in the pandemic throughout the country.

METHOD AND DATASET

To answer the research questions, the simulation method is based on the partial extraction approach for input-output systems, developed by Haddad *et al.* (2020), to evaluate the impacts of the COVID19 pandemic. Haddad *et al.* (2000) introduce imbalances in the supply and demand input-output system by internalizing lockdown policies. First, the labour supply (and respective payments) is constrained for different age risk groups of workers during the pandemic, as well as for informal workers. Second, the system is rebalanced, by a new set of constraints in the final demand vectors, based on the constrained income and supply of goods and services. A new equilibrium is generated in a constrained economy, which also results a new Leontief Inverse Matrix. Moreover, we use the advances proposed by Santos *et al.* (2020)[2] and we incorporate the following methodological improvements.

---

[864] Brazil has 5,570 municipalities. [2] See supplementary material.

Following Haddad *et al.* (2020), the demand effect is calculated based on foregone wages. To improve this measure, we disaggregate sectorial labour pay and consumption by income levels.

For each household $h = 1, \ldots, 10$, the percentage change in consumption is weighed such that:

$$F_{ch} = \sum F_n w_{nh} \, n$$

Where F_{ch} is the share of non-restricted consumption by household h, F_n is the share of non-restricted demand by sector and w_{nh} represents labour pay from sector n to household h. Therefore, each F_{ch} is used to calibrate the reduction in consumption by household h, assuming that the consumption drop is equivalent to the income change by household. By doing so, it is possible to adjust consumption considering the diversity of household income and consumption profiles and to better fit the compensatory policy effects. Additionally, this work introduces a new vector of demand constraints relative to the share of tourism expenditure in household consumption and exports. This new constraint aims to measure the specific impacts of the lockdown on tourist activities restricting the demand side.

2.1 Dataset

The economic model is parameterized using the most recent and official input-output matrix for Brazil, base year 2015, with 67 economic sectors (IBGE, 2018). The absence of a tourism satellite account in the matrix led to the use of the classification and data from IPEA (2015) to identify the tourist activities and measure its rate of informality. According to the IPEA, the total informality rate in the Brazilian tourist activities was 30% in 2015. As can be seen, there also are heterogeneities among these activities[865], ranging from 3% in the Air transportation to 48% in Culture[866]land recreation. To measure the demand values, the surveys of domestic (FIPE, 2012) and international tourism demand (MTUR, 2016) were used. Domestic tourism expenditure accounted for R$ 66.5 billion in 2011, updated to R$ 87.6 billion at 2015 values. International tourism expenditure accounted for R$ 18.9 billion in 2015. The employment share of tourist activities was used to breakdown the expenditure by sector, as in Ribeiro *et al.* (2017).The labour incomes were disaggregated according to data from the Continuous National Household Sample Survey (PNADC), while household consumption was broken down into different income deciles using from data of Household Budget Survey (POF) from the Brazilian Institute of Geography and Statistics (IBGE) for 2019 and 2008-2009, respectively. This is essential to map the income of informal workers by income deciles, as well as to identify eligible households to receive emergency assistance from the government. According to InLoco, the social distancing index in Brazil in April 2020[4] was on average 47%, well below the 70% recommended by WHO. In order to measure the economic impact of COVID-19 on tourist activities we define two scenarios:

---

[865] In December 2018, most recent data, the informality rate was 51.4%.
[866] https://www.ipea.gov.br/extrator/arquivos/160204_caracterizacao_br_re.pdf

Scenario 1: withdrawal of 47% of informal workers and the contraction of domestic and international tourist demand.

Scenario 2: taking into account the main compensatory policy of the Brazilian government, in addition to the same restrictions imposed in scenario 1.

3. RESULTS AND DISCUSSION

The compensation policy for informal workers was implemented by the Brazilian federal government for a period of three months. The results are therefore presented in a cumulative manner by quarter. Figure 1 presents the impact on GDP of the Brazilian tourist activities for the scenarios 1 and 2. Tourist activities represented 6.45% of the Brazilian GDP in 2015. The tourism GDP would accumulate a decrease in the quarter of R$ 35.3 billion in scenario 1 and R$ 20.1 billion in scenario 2. The most impacted activities in absolute values would be those with the largest share in the sector: road transport and food services.

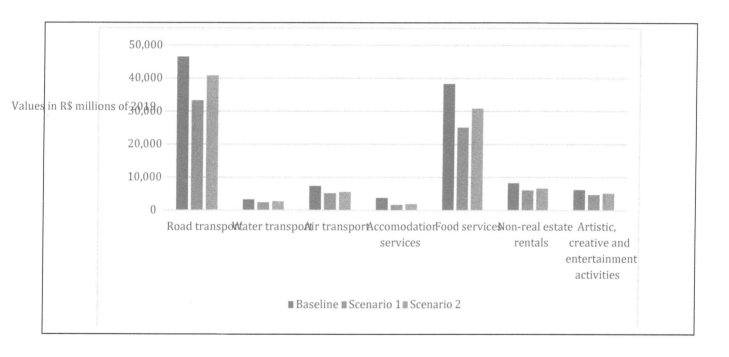

Figure 1: Economic impact of COVID-19 on tourist activities' GDP in Brazil .

Figure 2 shows the importance of the compensatory policy in mitigating the effects of the COVID19 pandemic on tourist activities in Brazil. In general, the compensatory policy (scenario 2) would mitigate the pandemic's effects on all tourist activities. The 31% drop in tourism GDP in Brazil in the scenario 1 would be mitigated to 17.7% with the compensatory policy. The most impacted activity in relative terms would be accommodation services with a 55.2% reduction in GDP in scenario 1 to 50.9% in scenario 2.

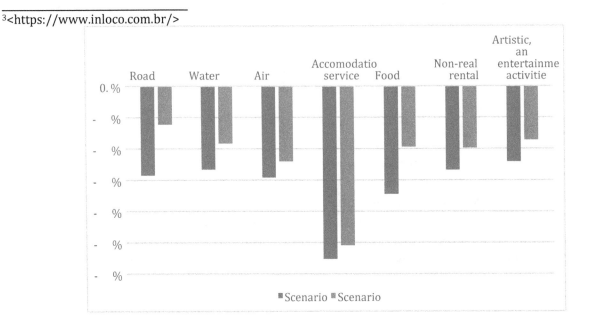

Figure 2: Relative economic impact of COVID-19 on tourist activities in Brazil (%) Authors' own.

The activities in which the compensatory policy would have the greatest mitigation effect would be road transport and accommodation services. The latter was the activity with the second highest rate of informality, 40% (see Table 1), among the tourist activities.

4. POLICY IMPLICATIONS

On the supply side, our results point out the importance of government assistance in order to mitigate the impact of the pandemic on the tourism sector in Brazil (Fig 2). On the demand side and following Yang *et al.* (2020), a tourism consumption subsidy could be created in a post-crisis scenario. A tourism consumption voucher for residents, for instance, was effective in the recovery of the Chinese tourism sector after the global financial crisis (Yan & Zhang, 2012).

REFERENCES

FIPE. (2012). Caracterização e dimensionamento do turismo doméstico no Brasil – 2010/2011. Relatório Executivo Produto 6.

Haddad, E. A., Perobelli, F. S., Araújo, I. F. (2020). Input-output analysis of COVID-19: Methodology for assessing the impacts of lockdown Measures. Discussion Paper NEREUS 01-2020, São Paulo.

IBGE. Instituto Brasileiro de Geografia e Estatística. (2018). Matriz de insumo-produto: Brasil: 2015. Rio de Janeiro: IBGE.

International Labor Organization (2020). COVID-19 crisis and the informal economy: Immediate responses and policy challenges. ILO policy brief. Retrieved from https://www.ilo.org/global/topics/employment-promotion/informal-economy/publications/lang-en/index.htm

IPEA. Instituto de Pesquisa Econômica Aplicada. (2015). Relatório com as estimativas da caracterização da ocupação formal e informal do turismo, com base nos dados da RAIS e da PNAD 2013, para o Brasil e regiões. Retrieved from http://www.ipea.gov.br/extrator/arquivos/160204_caracterizacao_br_re.pdf.

MTUR. Ministério do Turismo. Anuário Estatístico de Turismo 2016 - Ano Base 2015, 2016.

Ribeiro, L. C. S., Silva, E. O. V., Andrade, J. R. L. & Souza, K. B. (2017). Tourism and regional development in the Brazilian Northeast. *Tourism Economics*, 23(3): 717–727.

Santos, G. F., Ribeiro, L. C. S. & Cerqueira, R. (2020). Modelagem de impactos econômicos da pandemia COVID-19: aplicação para o estado da Bahia. (Preprint), 23p. Retrieved from: < https://www.researchgate.net/publication/341078147_Modelagem_de_impactos_economicos_da_p andemia_COVID-19_aplicacao_para_o_estado_da_Bahia>.

World Health Organization (2020). Coronavirus disease (COVID-2019) situation reports. Retrieved from https://www.who.int/emergencies/diseases/novel-coronavirus-2019/situation-reports/

World Travel and Tourism Council - WTTC. (2019). Travel and tourism economic impact 2019. Retrieved from https://wttc.org/Research/Economic-Impact.

Yan, Q. & Zhang, H. Q. (2012). Evaluation of the economic effectiveness of public tourism coupons in China in 2009 – A corrected DEA approach. *Asia Pacific Journal of Tourism Research*, 17(5), 534–550.

Yang, Y., Zhang, H. & Chenc, X. (2020). Coronavirus pandemic and tourism: Dynamic stochastic general equilibrium modeling of infectious disease outbreak. *Annals of Tourism Research*, 102913, http://dx.doi.org/10.1016/j.annals.2020.10291

4.Entrepreneurship And Small Business In The Context Of Post Covid-19:
Is There Light At The End Of The Tunnel?[867]

[868]Vânia Maria Jorge Nassif
[869]Eduardo Armando
[870]Jefferson Lopes La Falce

We want to contribute with entrepreneurs and public policy agents, in the face of the current chaos and offer reflections, recommendations and subsidies, anchored in scientific articles. However, we are still not sure of what is ahead and are optimistic and believe we will have a different future. Our previous editorial (v. 9, n. 2, 2020) questioned whether entrepreneurs and small businesses were prepared for contextual adversities, providing a reflection in light of the COVID-19 pandemic (Nassif, Corrêa, & Rossetto, 2020). This issue remains on the agenda in this issue, not as a past, but as a present and, in a way, looking ahead to the future.

The crisis is ongoing, as of this writing, especially in Brazil, which makes it difficult to locate references on how to act, in such a difficult time.

We have already experienced other crises, such as that of 2008-2009, which brought learning and new paths, aimed at a better future, in addition to suggestions to managers of small companies and to public policy agents. In the fight against Coronavirus, a large part of the research, performed in developed countries, such as, Germany and the United Kingdom, and in emerging countries, such as China (whose classification coincides with that of Brazil), the confrontation actions present substantial differences. Small businesses, despite their important contribution to job creation, are more susceptible to declining demand.

However, although the effects of the recession are severe, the evidence points to the fact that entrepreneurs have a quick recovery capacity (Cowling, Liu, Ledger, & Zhang, 2015). In addition, the idea that periods of imbalance create opportunities for entrepreneurs is not new (Cowling et al., 2015; Parker, Congregado, & Golpe, 2012; Schumpeter, 1942); however, for this to occur, it is necessary to seek a minimum of preparation, such as the domain of technology, to keep business,

---

[867] **Doi:** https://doi.org/10.14211/regepe.v9i3.1940 **Translator: Eliane Herrero Lopes**

[868] Associação Nacional de Estudos em Empreendedorismo e Gestão de Pequenas Empresas – ANEGEPE, São Paulo, (Brasil). Universidade Nove de Julho – UNINOVE, São Paulo. E-mail: vania.nassif@gmail.com Orcid id: https://orcid.org/0000-0003-3601-2831

[869] Instituto de Tecnologia y de Estudios Superiores de Monterrey – ITESM, Monterrey: Pequenas Empresas e Estratégia Empreendedora, (Mexico). E-mail: earmando@terra.com.br

[870] Universidade FUMEC, Minas Gerais, (Brasil). E-mail: jefferson.la.falce@gmail.com

partnerships and cooperation active. As a result, we ask whether entrepreneurs, small business owners and public policy agents are really prepared for the demands arising from this crisis.

The article by Rocha, Olave and Ordonez (2020), entitled "Innovation Strategies: An Analysis in Information Technology Startups", works not only on the idea of innovation, but on the quality of start ups and relationships. For the authors, among the most prominent practices are cooperation and organizational partnerships, which may follow an informal implementation, as the parties involved provide knowledge and skills to address any deficiencies.

This can be understood as an opportunity to strengthen relationships with customers and other organizations. This is possibly one of the paths to be followed by entrepreneurs who in difficult times, fight for the survival of their businesses. Neeley (2020) raises important aspects regarding remote work, which is to be considered as a model prevalent in current and future times. Among 15 questions, we selected those pertinent to our reflections in this editorial: Are companies able to make this sudden transition? How to prepare yourself psychologically when remote work is not part of your experiences? How will these changes affect productivity?

If the policies of social detachment continue for a while, how to measure the gains and, eventually, how to reinvent or revise the work? We wanted to address if these questions are present in the routine of entrepreneurs, small business managers and public policy agents.

When analyzing this social and economic paralysis, in a broad perspective, related to public policies of regional development, we find evidence in the literature that entrepreneurship is fundamental to promote diversification and capacity building in more resilient economies. It is also suggested to replace regional development agencies with partnerships, which mediate between the public and the private, to involve and coordinate other stakeholders (Williams & Vorley, 2014). In this context, this issue brings three articles that contribute to reflect on aspects of the COVID-19 post-crisis scenario. The first one, by Bendor, Lenzi and Souza (2020), presents factors for the formation of entrepreneurs, presenting instruments and guidelines for this, in addition to discussing the role of the state in social and economic development.

Although the entrepreneur is a social agent capable of developing the local / regional economy, he will not be able to solve all the problems of the same locality. To complement these discussions, the second article, by Mineiro, Dornelas, Arantes and Cougo (2020) highlights the importance of social entrepreneurship, indicating that in times of crisis and aggravated social problems, it becomes fundamental to search for alternatives and solutions that reduce the impact of the moment. This study shows a contrast between the discursive practices of social entrepreneurship compared to the managerial and instrumental discourse of the administration. The third article, by Barakat, Parente & Sarturi (2020), assumes that a fair share of the entrepreneurial businesses are housed in families; therefore, it's important to prioritize stakeholders, identifying similarities and differences between family and non-family companies.

In addition, the authors discuss that organizations should logically manage family and business, reflecting on values, goals and needs. Furthermore, in times of crisis, it is essential to have a long-term orientation, concerned with the reputation of the family and the company; that takes care of the non-financial objectives, seeking to preserve the socio-emotional investment of both institutions. Williams and Vorley (2014) bring another pertinent aspect to the discussions in this editorial: the importance of government support for the creation of companies with high growth potential, flexibility and adaptability for survival. These are aspects considered more relevant than the number of metrics created for startups.

This is because in crisis, small companies lose the ability not only to grow, but to keep going. Cowling et al. (2015) warn that only small companies with access to financial resources are able to achieve their goals and achieve a significant growth factor, as observed in countries that have incorporated these actions into their policies. In this sense, government support for angel investors is crucial, in the form of tax incentives, stimulating not only those who work, but increasing the amount invested (Mason & Harrison, 2015). When comparing entrepreneurial experiences in Brazil and the United States, particularly in South Florida, Rocha and Andreassi (2020) produce interesting information regarding the cultural and financial aspects of entrepreneurship in these two countries. For the authors, the perception of entrepreneurial activity proved to be better in the USA than in Brazil, with the entrepreneur considered as someone who invests and creates jobs in the country and this view is shared by public bodies. In contrast, in Brazil, laws, bureaucracy and the labour system contribute to the low articulation between the various agents of the Brazilian entrepreneurial ecosystem, formed by: government, companies, startups, universities, among others.

Reiterating the idea that this editorial presents a perspective of articulating discussions to overcome the crisis, looking at post COVID-19, another aspect addressed is support for research and development (R&D), especially in the sphere of countercyclical innovation policies, which can promote, in the post-crisis, a stabilizing effect on the economy, helping the survival and growth of small companies (Huda & Hussinger, 2015). Government investment in innovation, specifically in the form of support for technology parks and incubators, can help commercialize innovations. In companies, the incorporation of innovation in the organizational strategy, including in periods of crisis, contributes to improving the competitive position and financial performance in the post-crisis (MadridGuijarro, García-Pérez-de-Lema, & Van Auken, 2013).

In the current scenario, models that help project management become great allies for small and medium-sized enterprises (SMEs). Souza, Maccari, Mazieri and Santos (2020) present one of these models that, among the proposals for the development of skills in project management and for business management, highlights aspects relevant to the discussion promoted by this editorial, such as de-bureaucracy, flexibility, focus on people and management by non-specialists. This reinforces the premise that such models must be simplified, with low cost of implementation, to allow SMEs to anticipate problems.

Other surveys, referring to the 2008-2009 crisis, concluded that the chance of survival is greater when small companies develop and manage to sustain competitive advantages. This is something easy to say and complex to do, but it is a start. In addition, marketing innovations contribute to this process, regardless of the generic strategy pursued, the differentiation or the cost advantage. The training for innovation in marketing has been improved, since the small companies analyzed were oriented towards competition and cross-functional adjustments (Naidoo, 2010). The analysis of contemporary marketing practices was the object of investigation by Cittadin, Sarquis, Coelho and Pizzinatto (2020), in a multi-case study, entitled "Contemporary Marketing Practices: the Case of Small Garment Manufacturing Companies", in which the authors identified interaction, network and digital marketing practices, which indicated the presence of entrepreneurial and market orientations in these organizations. At the end of this edition, Menegon, Cernev, Ferreira and Balian (2020) present a teaching case, "Low-Income Female Entrepreneurship: When Business is Privacy", which discusses the management challenges faced by entrepreneurs at the beginning of its operations.

Furthermore, it also considers different retail business models, inviting students to discuss and reflect on the ability to solve management problems, of medium and high complexity, with regard to an enterprise with scalable growth potential. In addition, they make provocations about e-commerce strategies, logistical solutions, facing Chinese competition, supply and sales channels, favourable to the current scenario. Even without a light at the end of the tunnel, we hope that not only our country, but the world as a whole, will learn great lessons, including: how to greatly value interpersonal relationships and understanding the need to establish solid and effective partnerships with thrift and focus. Respect for others can provide social, financial, learning and survival balance, and, moreover, the experiences of social isolation can turn into opportunities and solidity for entrepreneurial businesses. In times of uncertainty, emotional balance and resilience are configured as coping strategies and foster reflection, both necessary for the prospect of a better future, as human beings.

REFERENCES

Cowling, M., Liu, W., Ledger, A., & Zhang, N. (2015). What really happens to small and mediumsized enterprises in a global economic recession? UK evidence on sales and job dynamics *International Small Business Journal, 33*(5), 488-513.

Huda, M., & Hussinger, K. (2015). The impact of R&D subsidies during the crisis. *Research Policy 44*(10), 1844-1855.

Madrid-Guijarro, A., García-Pérez-de-Lema, D., & Van Auken, H. (2013). An Investigation of Spanish SME Innovation during Different Economic Conditions. *Journal of Small Business Management, 51*(4), 578-601.

Mason, C. M., & Harrison, R. T. (2015). Business angel investment activity in the financial crisis: UK evidence and policy implications. *Environment and Planning C: Government and Policy, 33*(1), 43-60.

Naidoo, V. (2010). Firm survival through a crisis: The influence of market orientation, marketing innovation and business strategy. *Industrial Marketing Management, 39*(8), 1311-1320.

Nassif, V. M. J., Corrêa, V. S., & Rossetto, D. E. (2020). Estão os empreendedores e as pequenas empresas preparados para as adversidades contextuais? Uma reflexão à luz da pandemia do Covid-19. *Revista de Empreendedorismo e Gestão de Pequenas Empresas, 9*(2), 1-12.

Neeley, T. (2020). 15 Questions about remote work, answered. *Harvard Business Review*. Recuperado de https://hbr.org/2020/03/15-questions-about-remote-work-answered

Parker, S., Congregado, E., & Golpe, A. (2012). Is entrepreneurship a leading or lagging indicator of the business cycle? Evidence from UK self-employment data. *International Small Business Journal,30*(7), 736-753.

Schumpeter, J. (1942). *Capitalism, Socialism and Democracy.* New York: Harper & Row.

Souza, R. M., Santos, T. A., Maccari, E. A., & Mazieri, M. R. (2020). Proposição de um modelo de gerenciamento de projetos para pequenas e médias empresas (PME). *Revista de Empreendedorismo e Gestão de Pequenas Empresas, 10*(3), página.

Williams, N., & Vorley, T. (2014). Economic resilience and entrepreneurship: lessons from the Sheffield City Region. *Entrepreneurship & Regional Development, 26*(3-4), 257-281.

5. How To Reactivate The Economy Of Brazil After The New Coronavirus Pandemic

Fernando Alcoforado*

Brazil is a country that has its economic system in a terminal stage due to the vertiginous wave of mass unemployment and the general bankruptcy of companies aggravated by the government's restrictive measures of economic activity to face the spread of the new Coronavirus that is taking Brazil to the economic depression unprecedented in the history of the country. The main internal problem in Brazil today is the stagnation of the economy with its consequences related to the closure of industries and commercial activities and services and, above all, to the mass unemployment of millions of workers that got even worse with the spread of the new Coronavirus. The crisis of the new Coronavirus shows that Brazil is threatened with having collapsed its health system and unable to produce inputs for the manufacture of drugs, respirators and even masks to protect health professionals and the population.

Today, as in much of the world, many governments lament the lack of a national development project that makes the country self-sufficient because they have left the free market to make decisions such as closing factories in the country and taking them to places where the margins of profits would be higher, as is the case of China, India and Southeast Asian countries. This stance was dictated by the vision that started to prevail in Brazil and in the world after 1990, which was that of globalization and the opening of markets according to the neoliberal ideology. It is evident the misunderstanding of the governments of Brazil from 1990 to the present moment of adopting the economic policy of not producing locally, transferring it to places where the profit margins would be higher, a fact that was a determining factor in the decision not to invest in the production of materials and medical equipment in the country, transferring it to countries with lower production costs, such as China.

The result is being catastrophic because there is a lack of supplies for the manufacture of drugs, respirators and even masks to protect health professionals and the population. In Brazil, the situation is deplorable because industry, science and national technology have been scrapped since 1990 with the adoption by the various governments of neoliberal policies that have contributed to increasing technological and industrial dependence in relation to the outside.

Due to the misunderstandings practiced by the different governments of Brazil since 1990, the country's Gross Domestic Product (GDP) will suffer a steep drop due to the huge reduction in household consumption (C) and private investments (I) resulting from the new Coronavirus and, also, export earnings (X) resulting from the drop in international trade due to the new Coronavirus. It is worth noting that the Gross Domestic Product (GDP) is calculated based on the sum of all its components: GDP = C + I + G + X - M. In this formula, C corresponds to household expenditure on consumer goods (consumption private sector), I corresponds to the expenditure of companies in investment, either in capital goods, or in stocks of raw materials and products, G corresponds to the expenditure of the State (federal, state and municipal governments) in consumer goods (public consumption), X corresponds to export revenue and M to import expenditure.

Based on this formula, it can be said that the resumption of GDP growth after the new Coronavirus pandemic can only be achieved with the expansion of private consumption (C), the increase in investment in productive activity (I), the increase in spending 2 government (G), the increase in export revenue (X) and the reduction in spending on imports (M). Therefore, in order to increase household consumption (C), it is necessary to increase the wage mass of the population, whether by generating jobs and also by distributing basic income to vulnerable and unemployed populations and to adopt a credit policy that encourages consumer to buy. To raise the level of private sector investments (I), it is necessary for the government to reduce the tax burden and implement a policy of tax incentives and attractive interest for businessmen. Economic growth can also be achieved by raising the level of exports and reducing imports with the policy of substituting imported goods aimed at expanding economic activities. However, in order to reactivate the economy after the new Coronavirus pandemic, the State must act as if it were a locomotive capable of leveraging consumption in general and private investment. In this sense, the State must increase the State's expenditure (G) with the realization of massive investments in economic infrastructure (energy, transport and communications) and social infrastructure (education, health, housing and basic sanitation). The State must act as an inducer of the resumption of economic growth in Brazil. To promote the reactivation of the Brazilian economy, the Brazilian government should draw up an economic plan that contributes to the resumption of Brazil's development that presents to the population and the productive sectors a perspective of overcoming the current crisis and resumption of economic growth. The development plan should guide and coordinate companies in the country that, organized in networks, and helped with trade, technology and credit policies can successfully compete in the national and world economy.

The Brazilian government should consider as a number one priority to reactivate the economy with the immediate execution of a broad program of public infrastructure works (energy, transportation, housing, basic sanitation, etc.) with the participation of the private sector to combat the current situation of mass unemployment raising the levels of employment and income of families and companies to, consequently, promote the expansion of the consumption of families and companies resulting, respectively, from the increase in the salary mass of families and the income of companies with investments in public works to make Brazil grow economically again. In addition to the public works program, the Brazilian government should develop a broad export program, especially in agribusiness and the mineral sector, the drastic reduction in bank interest rates to encourage household consumption and investment by companies, the reduction of the burden taxation, the freezing of high salaries in the public sector and the cut of perks and public administration organs.

Therefore, there is an urgent need to make the Brazilian State take the reins of the national economy, abandoning the failed neoliberal economic model to reactivate the Brazilian economy and full employment, putting an end to the economic depression that will occur during the spread of the new Coronavirus. The entire set of measures to reactivate the Brazilian economy after the economic depression resulting from the fight against the new Coronavirus must be complemented with measures to combat unemployment and extreme poverty to avoid the social debacle. Given this perspective, what would be the solution to alleviate unemployment and poverty in the current situation?

The solution would consist of the adoption by the federal government, state governments and municipal governments of public policies aimed at the development of the social and solidarity economy to alleviate unemployment and the implementation of basic income or universal minimum income to alleviate the population's poverty. Without the adoption of these measures, Brazil will inevitably be driven to political and social upheaval. Regarding the Social and Solidarity Economy, it is important to note that it is a different way of generating work and income, in several sectors, be it in the productive activity, in 3 community banks, in credit cooperatives, in family farming cooperatives, in the question of trade fair, in exchange clubs, etc. The Social and Solidarity Economy is an important alternative for the inclusion of workers in the labour market, giving them a new opportunity, through self-management. Based on the Social and Solidarity Economy, there is the possibility of recovering bankrupt companies, and to continue them, with a new mode of production, in which profit maximization is no longer the main objective, giving rise to maximizing the quantity and the quality of work. The Social and Solidarity Economy is a possible alternative to generate employment for workers who are mostly excluded from the formal labour market and consumption. In France, for example66, it accounts for 10% of GDP and is responsible for 12.7% of that country's employment. The Social and Solidarity Economy emerged in various parts of the world with practices of economic and social relations that are promoting the survival and improving the quality of life of millions of people. In turn, the basic income policy or universal minimum income for the population is one of the solutions to alleviate poverty.

The cash transfer program, Bolsa Família, is an example of the application of the basic income policy. Among the reasons for this idea to become reality, lies in the fact that distributing money reduces crime, improves the health of the population and allows everyone to invest in themselves. The adoption of the basic income policy or universal minimum income for the poor population is one of the solutions to alleviate poverty, since it would allow the poor to start having money to meet their basic needs in terms of food, health, housing, etc. By having a basic income, the poor population will be able to supply their basic needs by increasing consumption that contributes to the reactivation of the economy.

From the above, actions aimed at reactivating the economy must be complemented with actions aimed at combating unemployment and extreme poverty that have worsened in Brazil with the fight against the new Coronavirus. These actions should be taken forward when there is the eradication of the new Coronavirus from Brazil.

As long as the virus is present in the country, the Brazilian government must act to minimize the drop in consumption by the population and companies by maintaining essential economic activities by adopting measures to benefit the unemployed and the poor so as not to starve to death and also for the benefit of micro, small and medium-sized companies in order not to succumb to the crisis that is already happening at an insufficient level. Measures for the benefit of the unemployed and the poor include transferring government income to families and suspending payment of taxes for a specified period and granting low interest loans to companies with the counterpart of not firing employees during isolation Social. This set of measures, which has been adopted in several countries of the world, must be maintained as long as the social distancing of the population persists so as not to aggravate their social conditions, especially of the most vulnerable populations, and the economic conditions of micro, small and medium-sized companies.

To cope with the drop in tax collection by the government at all levels resulting from the reduction of economic activities, the Brazilian government must allocate resources in the volume necessary for state and city governments to face the problems with the health system and, also, the social problems concerning the most vulnerable populations while the social isolation of the population endures. To finance all the actions necessary to reactivate the Brazilian economy and to fight unemployment and extreme poverty, the Brazilian government could adopt two strategies; 1) suspend for 5 years the payment of the internal public debt that corresponds to 48% of the federal government budget or renegotiate with its creditors in order to 4 extend its payment so that the government will have the necessary resources for investments aimed at reviving the economy and combating unemployment and extreme poverty; and, 2) use the international reserves of US$ 362.5 billion existing in February 2020. Without the adoption of this set of actions, Brazil will not resume its growth and will inevitably be driven to economic ruin. With Bolsonaro and his ministerial team in power and, above all, Paulo Guedes in charge of the Brazilian economy, Paulo Guedes, who did not present before and after the pandemic any economic development plan for Brazil, the country will be taken to bankruptcy economic and political and social breakdown. The ministerial meeting on March 22 shown on television demonstrated that Brazil is governed by a band of irresponsible, ill-educated and incompetent people who act uncoordinated thanks to the incompetence of the President of the Republic. Government un coordination does not only happen in the health area with its disastrous performance in the fight against the new Coronavirus, but also in the whole government. In addition, at the ministerial meeting, the attempt by some ministers to elaborate the program they called pro Brazil, which would represent an inductive action by the federal government to reactivate the Brazilian economy, was torpedoed by Paulo Guedes at the meeting which, driven by neoliberal thinking, does not admit that the government takes a proactive attitude in promoting national development.

Index

THINK DOCTOR PUBLICATIONS

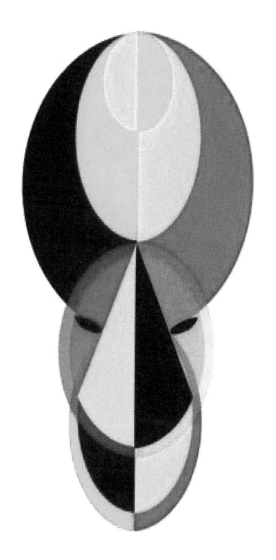

WWW.THINKDOCTORPUBLICATIONS.COM/KEEPBOOKSFREE

FEATURED BOOKS

Rice and Peas For The Soul 1: A collection of 150 Motivational, Inspirational and Moral Stories To make You Think, Reflect and Wonder

Rice and Peas for the Soul 2

Rice and Peas For The Soul 3: A Collection of 80 Motivational, Inspirational Stories That Empower, Enthuse and Engage

Rice and Peas For The Soul 4: A Collection of More Than 45 Motivational, Inspiration and Moving Stories, Which Aim to Stimulate, Stir and Confound.

Happy To Be Me: A Collection of 50 Poems Reflecting Love Hope and Faith: Volume 1

Happy To Be Me II: A Collection of 50 Poems Reflecting Love Hope and Faith (Poetry For The Soul Book 2)

Incidents in the Life of a Slave Girl

Behind The Scenes

Fifty Years In Chains: "Includes Interviews With Thirty Former Slaves

Hearts and Minds: A Resource Book Of 60 Learning Activities To Affirm Diversity and Promote Equality: Volume 1

Hearts and Minds (Vol. 2): A Resource Book of 30 Learning Activities To Affirm Diversity and Promote Equality.

Hearts and Minds (Vol. 3): 50 Diversity and Equality Case Studies (Volume 3)

Changing Hearts and Minds: More Than 90 Training Activities Which Promote Diversity and Equality (Volume 4)

How To Turn Your I Can't Into I Believe I Can: 30 Excellent Strategies That Will Enable You To Achieve Your True Potential

Fruit of the Soul 1: A Collection of 30 Stories Which Proves That God's Words Are Not Wasted But Richly RewardedFruit of the Soul 2: A Collection of 50 Stories of Humility, Compassion and Kindness

The WILLY LYNCH LETTER

How To Make African-Americ an Slaves For A 1000 Years

(Ed.) Delroy Constantine-Simms

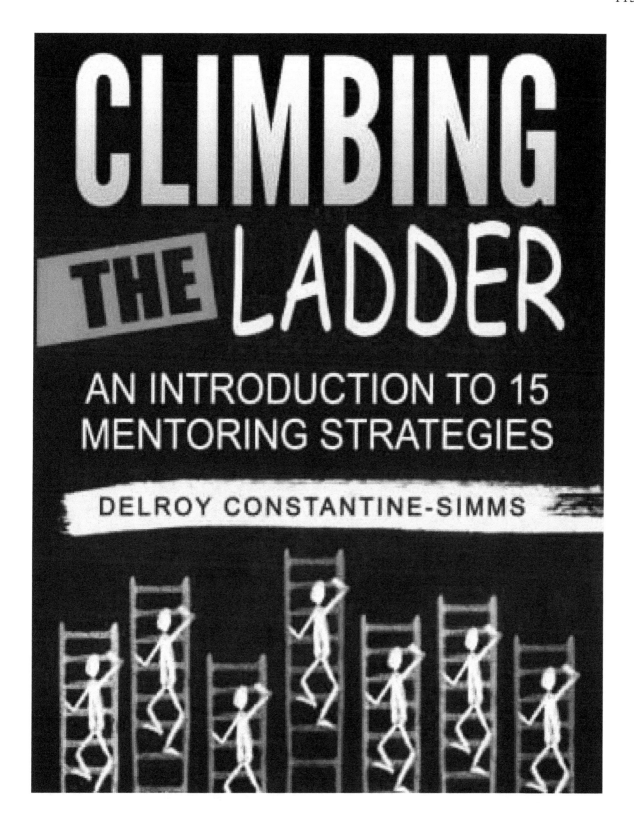

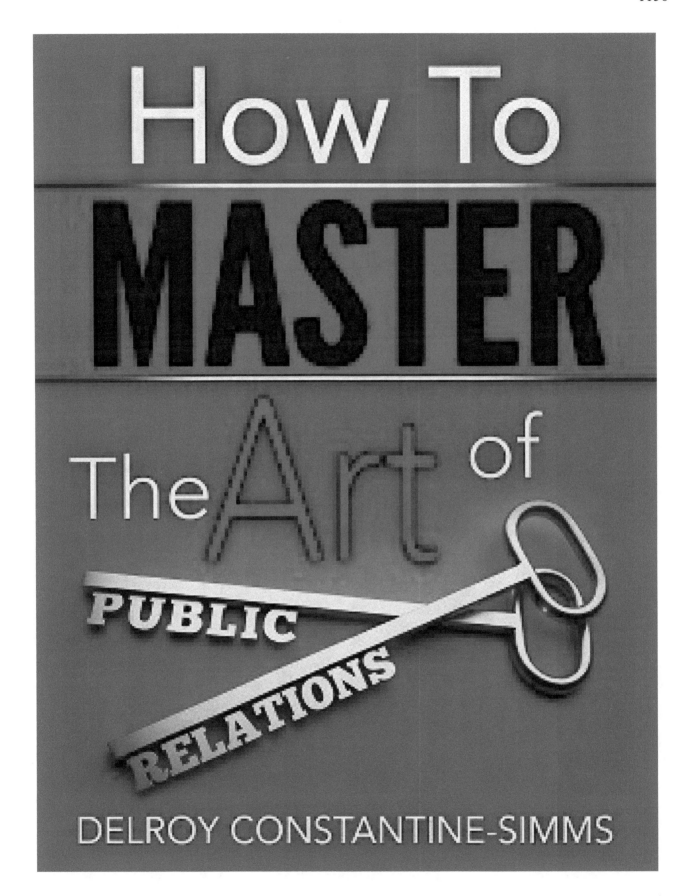

A SAMPLE

CASE STUDY FOR
STUDENT
COUNSELLING

Psychologists and Therapists

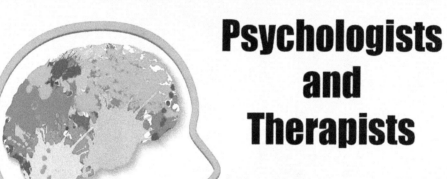

Delroy Constantine-Simms

TAKE A KNEE

A COLLECTION OF ESSAYS INFLUENCED BY
THE POLITICAL AWAKENING OF COLIN KAEPERNICK

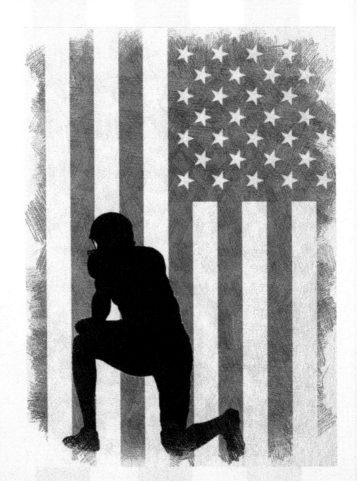

DELROY CONSTANTINE-SIMMS

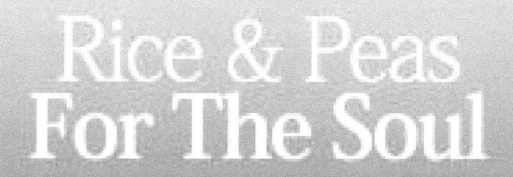

Rice & Peas
For The Soul

A Collection of more than 150 Motivational,
Inspirational and Moral Stories To Make You Think,
Reflect and Wonder

Edited by
D. Constantine-Simms

For *Think Doctor Publications*

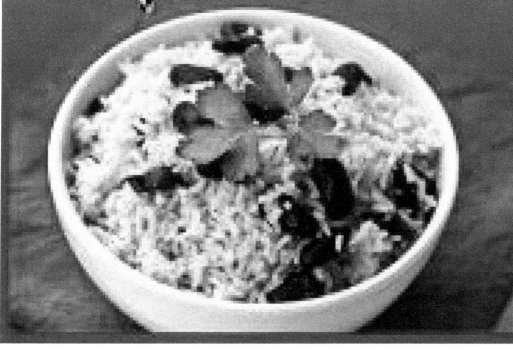

CPSIA information can be obtained
at www.ICGtesting.com
Printed in the USA
LVHW060402241020
669244LV00048BA/22